193.99

The GALE ENCYCLOPEDIA of CANCER

A GUIDE TO CANCER AND ITS TREATMENTS

FOURTH EDITION

The GALE ENCYCLOPEDIA of CANCER

A GUIDE TO CANCER AND ITS TREATMENTS

FOURTH EDITION

VOLUME

2

F–O

KRISTIN FUST, EDITOR

GALE
CENGAGE Learning·

Farmington Hills, Mich • San Francisco • New York • Waterville, Maine
Meriden, Conn • Mason, Ohio • Chicago

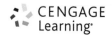
CENGAGE
Learning·

© 2015 Gale, Cengage Learning
WCN: 01-100-101

Gale Encyclopedia of Cancer: A Guide to Cancer and Its Treatments, Fourth Edition

Project Editor: Kristin Fust

Acquisitions Editor: Christine Slovey

New Product Manager: Douglas Dentino

Editorial Support Services: Andrea Lopeman

Indexing Services: Andriot Indexing, LLC

Rights Acquisition and Management:
Moriam Aigoro

Composition: Evi Abou-El-Seoud

Manufacturing: Wendy Blurton

Imaging: John Watkins

Product Design: Pam Galbreath, Kris Julien

Vice President & Publisher, New Products &
GVRL: Patricia Coryell

For product information and technology assistance, contact us at
Gale Customer Support, 1-800-877-4253.
For permission to use material from this text or product,
submit all requests online at **www.cengage.com/permissions.**
Further permissions questions can be emailed to
permissionrequest@cengage.com

While every effort has been made to ensure the reliability of the information presented in this publication, Gale, a part of Cengage Learning, does not guarantee the accuracy of the data contained herein. Gale accepts no payment for listing; and inclusion in the publication of any organization, agency, institution, publication, service, or individual does not imply endorsement of the editors or publisher. Errors brought to the attention of the publisher and verified to the satisfaction of the publisher will be corrected in future editions.

LIBRARY OF CONGRESS CATALOGING-IN-PUBLICATION DATA

The Gale encyclopedia of cancer : a guide to cancer and its treatments. --
Fourth edition / Kristin Fust, editor.
    p. ; cm.
  Encyclopedia of cancer
  Includes bibliographical references and index.
    ISBN 978-1-4103-1740-7 (hardback : set) -- ISBN 978-1-4103-1741-4 (vol. 1) --
ISBN 978-1-4103-1742-1 (vol. 2) -- ISBN 978-1-4103-1743-8 (vol. 3) -- ISBN 978-
1-4103-1744-5 (e-book)
  I. Fust, Kristin, editor.   II. Title: Encyclopedia of cancer. [DNLM:
1. Neoplasms--Encyclopedias--English.   2. Medical Oncology--Encyclopedias--
English. QZ 13]
  RC262
  616.99'4003--dc23
                                    2014047836

Gale
27500 Drake Rd.
Farmington Hills, MI, 48331-3535

ISBN-13: 978-1-4103-1740-7 (set)
ISBN-13: 978-1-4103-1741-4 (vol. 1)
ISBN-13: 978-1-4103-1742-1 (vol. 2)
ISBN-13: 978-1-4103-1743-8 (vol. 3)

This title is also available as an e-book.
ISBN-13: 978-1-4103-1744-5
Contact your Gale, a part of Cengage Learning sales representative for ordering information.

Printed in China
1 2 3 4 5 6 7 19 18 17 16 15

ADVISORY BOARD

A number of experts in the medical community provided invaluable assistance in the formulation of this encyclopedia. Our advisory board performed myriad duties, from defining the scope of coverage to reviewing individual entries for accuracy and accessibility. The editor would like to express her appreciation to them.

CONTENTS

PLEASE READ—IMPORTANT INFORMATION

The *Gale Encyclopedia of Cancer: A Guide to Cancer and Its Treatments* is a health reference product designed to inform and educate readers about a wide variety of cancers; other diseases and conditions related to cancers; diagnostic tests and procedures; nutrition and dietary practices beneficial to cancer patients; and various cancer treatments, including drugs. Cengage Learning believes the product to be comprehensive, but not necessarily definitive. It is intended to supplement, not replace, consultation with a physician or other healthcare practitioner. While Cengage Learning has made substantial efforts to provide information that is accurate, comprehensive, and up to date, Cengage Learning makes no representations or warranties of any kind, including without limitation, warranties of merchantability or fitness for a particular purpose, nor does it guarantee the accuracy, comprehensiveness, or timeliness of the information contained in this product. Readers should be aware that the universe of medical knowledge is constantly growing and changing, and that differences of opinion exist among authorities. Readers are also advised to seek professional diagnosis and treatment for any medical condition, and to discuss information obtained from this book with their healthcare provider.

FOREWORD

Unfortunately, man must suffer disease. Some diseases are totally reversible and can be effectively treated. Moreover, some diseases with proper treatment have been virtually annihilated, such as polio, rheumatic fever, smallpox, and, to some extent, tuberculosis. Other diseases seem to target one organ, such as the heart, and there has been great progress in either fixing defects, adding blood flow, or giving medications to strengthen the diseased pump. Cancer, however, continues to frustrate even the cleverest of doctors or the most fastidious of health-conscious individuals. Why?

By its very nature, cancer is a survivor. It has only one purpose: to proliferate. After all, that is the definition of cancer: unregulated growth of cells that fail to heed the message to stop growing. Normal cells go through a cycle of division, aging, and then selection for death. Cancer cells are able to circumvent this normal cycle and escape recognition to be eliminated.

There are many mechanisms that can contribute to this unregulated cell growth. One of these mechanisms is inheritance. Some individuals can be programmed for cancer due to inherited disorders in their genetic makeup. In its simplest terms, a person can inherit a faulty gene or a missing gene whose role is to eliminate damaged cells or to prevent imperfect cells from growing. Without this natural braking system, the damaged cells can divide and lead to more damaged cells with the same abnormal genetic makeup as the parent cells. Given enough time, and our inability to detect them, these groups of cells can grow to a size that will cause discomfort or other symptoms.

Inherited genetics are obviously not the only source of abnormalities in cells. Humans do not live in a sterile world devoid of environmental attacks or pathogens. Humans must work, and working environments can be dangerous. Danger can come in the form of radiation, chemicals, or fibers to which we may be chronically exposed with or without our knowledge. Moreover, humans must eat, and if our food is contaminated with these environmental hazards, or if we prepare our food in a way that may change the chemical nature of the food to hazardous molecules, then chronic exposure to these toxins could damage cells. Finally, humans are social. They have found certain habits that are pleasing because they are relaxing or help release inhibitions. Such habits, including smoking and alcohol consumption, can have a myriad of influences on the genetic makeup of cells.

Why the emphasis on genes in the new century? Because they are potentially the reason as well as the answer for cancer. Genes regulate our micro- and macrosopic events by eventually coding for proteins that control our structure and function. If environmental events cause errors in those genes that control growth, then imperfect cells can start to take root. For the majority of cases, a whole cascade of genetic events must occur before a cell is able to outlive its normal predecessors. This cascade of events could take years to occur, in a silent, undetected manner until the telltale signs and symptoms of advanced cancer are seen, including pain, lack of appetite, cough, loss of blood, or the detection of a lump. How did these cells get to this state where they are now dictating the everyday physical, psychological, and economic events for the person afflicted?

At this time, the sequence of genetic catastrophes is much too complex to comprehend or summarize, because it is only in the past decade that we have even been able to map what genes we have and where they are located in our chromosomes. We have learned, however, that cancer cells are equipped with a series of self-protection mechanisms. Some of the altered genes are actually able to express themselves more than in the normal situation. These genes could then code for more growth factors for the transforming cell, or they could make proteins that could keep our own immune system from eliminating these interlopers. Finally, these cells are chameleons: if we treat them with drugs to try to kill them, they can "change their colors" by mutation, and then be resistant to the drugs that may have harmed them before.

Then what do we do for treatment? Humans have always had a fascination with grooming, and grooming involves removal—dirt, hair, waste. The ultimate removal involves cutting away the spoiled or imperfect portion. An abnormal growth? Remove it by surgery . . . make sure the edges are clean. Unfortunately, the painful reality of cancer surgery is that it is most effective when performed in the early stages of the disease. "Early stages of the disease" implies that there is no spread, or, hopefully, before there are symptoms. In the majority of cases, however, surgery cannot eradicate all the disease because the cancer is not only at the primary site of the lump, but also has spread to other organs. Cancer is not just a process of growth, but also a metastasizing process that allows for invasion and spread. The growing cells need nourishment so they secrete proteins that allow for the growth of blood vessels (angiogenesis); once the blood vessels are established from other blood vessels, the tumor cells can make proteins that will dissolve the imprisoning matrix surrounding them. Once this matrix is dissolved, it is only a matter of time before the cancer cells will migrate to other places, making the use of surgery fruitless.

Since cancer cells have a propensity to spread to other organs, therapies must be geared to treat the whole body and not just the site of origin. The problem with these chemotherapies is that they are not selective and wreak havoc on tissues that are not affected by the cancer. These therapies are not natural to the human host, and result in nausea, loss of appetite, fatigue, and a depletion in the cells that protect us from infection and those that carry oxygen. Doctors who prescribe such medications must walk a fine line between helping the patient (causing a "response" in the cancer by making it smaller) or causing "toxicity," which, due to effects on normal organs, causes the patient problems. Although these drugs are far from perfect, we are fortunate to have them because when they work, their results can be remarkable.

But that's the problem—"when they work." We cannot predict who is going to benefit from our therapies, and doctors must inform the patient and his/her family about countless studies that have been done to validate the use of these potentially beneficial/potentially harmful agents. Patients must suffer the frustration that oncologists have because each individual afflicted with cancer is different, and each cancer is different. This makes it virtually impossible to personalize an individual's treatment expectations and life expectancy. Cancer, after all, is a very impersonal disease, with little regard to sex, race, age, or any other "human" characteristics.

Cancer treatment is in search of "smart" options. Like modern-day instruments of war, successful cancer treatment necessitates the construction of therapies that can do three basic tasks: search out the enemy, recognize the enemy, and kill the enemy without causing "friendly fire." The successful therapies of the future will involve the use of "living components," "manufactured components," or a combination of both. Living components, white blood cells, will be educated to recognize where the cancer is, and help our own immune system fight the foreign cells. These lymphocytes can be educated to recognize signals on the cancer cell that make them unique. Therapies in the future will be able to manufacture molecules with these signature, unique signals that are linked to other molecules specifically for killing the cells. Only the cancer cells are eliminated in this way, hopefully sparing the individual from toxicity.

Why use these unique signals as delivery mechanisms? If they are unique and are important for growth of the cancer cell, why not target them directly? This describes the ambitious mission of gene therapy, whose goal is to supplement a deficient, necessary genetic pool or diminish the number of abnormally expressed genes fortifying the cancer cells. If a protein is not being made that slows the growth of cells, gene therapy would theoretically supply the gene for this protein to replenish it and cause the cells to slow down. If the cells can make their own growth factors that sustain them selectively over normal cells, then the goal is to block the production of this growth factor. There is no doubt that gene therapy is the wave of the future, and it is under intense investigation and scrutiny. The problem, however, is that there is no way to tell when this future promise will be fulfilled.

No book can fully describe the medical, psychological, social, and economic burden of cancer, and if this is your first confrontation with the enemy, you may find yourself overwhelmed with its magnitude. Books are only part of the solution. Newly enlisted participants in this war must seek proper counsel from educated physicians who will inform the family and the patient of the risks and benefits of a treatment course in a way that can be understood. Advocacy groups of dedicated volunteers, many of whom are cancer survivors, can guide and advise. The most important component, however, is an intensely personal one. The afflicted individual must realize that he/she is responsible for charting the course of his/her disease, and this requires the above described knowledge as well as great personal intuition. Cancer comes as a series of shocks: the symptoms, the diagnosis, and the treatment. These shocks can be followed by cautious optimism or profound disappointment. Each one of these shocks either reinforces or chips away at one's resolve, and how an individual reacts to these issues is as unique as the cancer that is being dealt with.

While cancer is still life-threatening, strides have been made in the fight against the disease. Thirty years ago, a young adult diagnosed with testicular cancer had few options for treatment that could result in cure. Now, chemotherapy for good-risk stage II and III testicular cancer can result in a complete response of the tumor in 98% of the cases and a durable response in 92%. Sixty years ago, there were no regimens that could cause a complete remission for a child diagnosed with leukemia, but now, using combination chemotherapy, complete remissions are possible in 96% of these cases. Progress has been made, but more progress is needed. The first real triumph in cancer care will be when cancer is no longer thought of as a life-ending disease, but as a chronic disease whose symptoms can be managed. Anyone who has been touched by cancer or who has been involved in the fight against it lives in hope that that day will arrive.

Helen A. Pass, MD, FACS
Director, Breast Care Center
William Beaumont Hospital
Royal Oak, MI

INTRODUCTION

The *Gale Encyclopedia of Cancer: A Guide to Cancer and Its Treatments* is a unique and invaluable source of information for anyone touched by cancer. This collection of more than 600 entries provides in-depth coverage of specific cancer types, diagnostic procedures, treatments, cancer side effects, and cancer drugs. In addition, entries have been included to facilitate understanding of related concepts, such as cancer biology, carcinogenesis, and cancer genetics, as well as cancer issues such as clinical trials, home health care, fertility issues, and cancer prevention. This easy-to-read encyclopedia defines medical concepts and terminology in language that general readers can understand while still providing thorough coverage.

SCOPE

Entries follow a standardized format to help users find information quickly. Rubrics include the following headings (as applicable):

Cancer types

- Definition
- Description
- Demographics
- Causes and symptoms
- Diagnosis
- Treatment team
- Clincial staging
- Treatment
- Prognosis
- Coping with cancer treatment
- Clinical trials
- Prevention
- Special concerns
- Resources

Drugs, herbs, and supplements

- Definition
- Description
- Recommended dosage
- Precautions
- Side effects
- Interactions
- Resources

Tests, treatments, and other procedures

- Definition
- Purpose
- Description
- Benefits
- Precautions
- Preparation
- Aftercare
- Risks
- Results
- Alternatives
- Health care team roles
- Research and general acceptance
- Caregiver concerns
- Training and certification

INCLUSION CRITERIA

A preliminary list of cancers and related topics was compiled from a wide variety of sources, including professional medical guides and textbooks as well as consumer guides and encyclopedias. The advisory board, made up of medical doctors and oncology pharmacists, evaluated the topics and made suggestions for inclusion. Final selection of topics to include was made by the advisory board in conjunction with the editor.

ABOUT THE CONTRIBUTORS

The essays were compiled by experienced medical writers, including physicians, pharmacists, nurses, and other healthcare professionals. Medical advisors reviewed the completed essays to ensure that they are appropriate, up to date, and accurate.

HOW TO USE THIS BOOK

The *Gale Encyclopedia of Cancer* has been designed with ready reference in mind.

- Straight **alphabetical arrangement** of topics allows users to locate information quickly.

- **Bold-faced terms** within entries indicate that full-length articles exist for those topics.

- **Cross-references** placed throughout the encyclopedia direct readers from alternate names and related topics to their intended entries.

- A list of **key terms** is provided in most entries to define unfamiliar or complicated terms or concepts.

- A **glossary**, located at the end of volume 3, contains a list of all key terms, arranged alphabetically.

- **Questions to Ask Your Doctor** sidebars are provided when appropriate to help facilitate patient discussions with physicians and other healthcare providers.

- **See also** suggestions at the end of some entries point readers toward similar or related topics.

- **Resources** sections at the end of entries direct readers to additional sources of information on a topic.

- Valuable **contact information** for organizations and support groups is included with most entries. All of the contact information is compiled in an appendix in the back of volume 3, arranged alphabetically.

- A comprehensive **general index** guides readers to all topics mentioned in the text.

- **Author and advisor bylines** provide information on who updated and reviewed the entries, including their credentials. Advisor bylines are new to this edition and are not yet present in every article, but the absence of an advisor byline does not mean that the entry was never reviewed.

A note about **drug entries**: Drug entries are listed in alphabetical order by common **generic names**. However, because many oncology drugs have more than one common generic name, and because the brand name may be used interchangeably with a generic name, drug entries may be located in three ways: The reader may find the intended entry under the generic drug name in alphabetical order; may be directed to the entry from an alternate name cross-reference; or may use the **index** to look up a **brand name**, which will direct the reader to the appropriate entry.

GRAPHICS

The *Gale Encyclopedia of Cancer* is enhanced by 275 color photographs, illustrations, and tables.

ALPHABETICAL LIST OF ENTRIES

A

Abarelix
Accelerated partial breast irradiation
Acoustic neuroma
Acute erythroblastic leukemia
Acute lymphocytic leukemia
Acute myelocytic leukemia
Adenocarcinoma
Adenoma
Adjuvant chemotherapy
Ado-trastuzumab emtansine
Adrenal fatigue
Adrenal tumors
Adrenocortical carcinoma
Adult cancer pain
Advance directives
Afatinib
AIDS-related cancers
Alcohol consumption and cancer
Aldesleukin
Alemtuzumab
Allopurinol
Alopecia
Altretamine
Amantadine
Amenorrhea
American Joint Committee on Cancer
Amifostine
Aminoglutethimide
Amitriptyline
Amputation
Amsacrine
Anagrelide
Anal cancer
Anemia

Angiogenesis
Angiogenesis inhibitors
Angiography
Anorexia
Anoscopy
Antiandrogens
Antibiotics
Anticancer drugs
Antidiarrheal agents
Antiemetics
Antiestrogens
Antifungal therapy
Antimicrobials
Antineoplastic agents
Antioxidants
Antiviral therapy
Aromatase inhibitors
Arsenic trioxide
Ascites
Asparaginase
Astrocytoma
Axillary dissection
Azacitidine
Azathioprine

B

Bacillus Calmette-Guérin
Barium enema
Barrett's esophagus
Basal cell carcinoma
BCR-ABL inhibitors
Bendamustine hydrochloride
Benzene
Benzodiazepines

Bevacizumab
Bexarotene
Bile duct cancer
Biological response modifiers
Biopsy
Bisphosphonates
Bladder cancer
Bleomycin
Body image/self image
Bone marrow aspiration and biopsy
Bone marrow transplantation
Bone pain
Bone survey
Bortezomib
Bowen disease
Brain and central nervous system tumors
BRCA1 and *BRCA2*
Breast cancer
Breast reconstruction
Breast self-exam
Breast ultrasound
Bronchoalveolar lung cancer
Bronchoscopy
Burkitt lymphoma
Buserelin
Busulfan

C

Calcitonin
Cancer
Cancer biology
Cancer cluster
Cancer diet

Fibrosarcoma
Filgrastim
Flow cytometry
Floxuridine
Fludarabine
Fluorouracil
Fluoxymesterone
Folic acid

G

Gabapentin
Gallbladder cancer
Gallium nitrate
Gallium scan
Gastrectomy
Gastroduodenostomy
Gastrointestinal cancers
Gastrointestinal complications
Gefitinib
Gemcitabine
Gemtuzumab
Gene therapy
Genetic testing
Germ cell tumors
Gestational trophoblastic tumors
Giant cell tumors
Global cancer incidence and
    mortality
Glossectomy
Glutamine
Goserelin acetate
Graft-versus-host disease
Gynecologic cancers

H

Hairy cell leukemia
Hand-foot syndrome
Head and neck cancers
Health insurance
Hemolytic anemia
Hemoptysis
Heparin
Hepatic arterial infusion
Herpes simplex
Herpes zoster
Histamine 2 antagonists

Hodgkin lymphoma
Home health services
Horner syndrome
Hospice care
Human growth factors
Human papillomavirus
Hydroxyurea
Hypercalcemia
Hypercoagulation disorders
Hyperthermia
Hypocalcemia

I

Ibritumomab
Idarubicin
Ifosfamide
Imaging studies
Imatinib mesylate
Immune globulin
Immune response
Immunoelectrophoresis
Immunohistochemistry
Immunotherapy
Incontinence, cancer-related
Infection and sepsis
Intensity-modulated radiation
    therapy
Interferons
Interleukin 2
Intrathecal chemotherapy
Intravenous urography
Investigational drugs
Irinotecan
Itching

K

Kaposi sarcoma
Ki67
Kidney cancer

L

Lambert-Eaton myasthenic
    syndrome
Laparoscopy
Lapatinib

Laryngeal cancer
Laryngeal nerve palsy
Laryngectomy
Laryngoscopy
Late effects of cancer treatment
Laxatives
Leiomyosarcoma
Leucovorin
Leukemias, acute
Leukemias, chronic
Leukoencephalopathy
Leukotriene inhibitors
Leuprolide acetate
Levamisole
Li-Fraumeni syndrome
Limb salvage
Lip cancer
Liver biopsy
Liver cancer
Lobectomy
Lomustine
Lorazepam
Low molecular weight heparins
Lumbar puncture
Lumpectomy
Lung biopsy
Lung cancer, non-small cell
Lung cancer, small cell
Lymph node biopsy
Lymph node dissection
Lymphangiography
Lymphocyte immune globulin
Lymphoma

M

Magnetic resonance imaging
Male breast cancer
Malignant fibrous histiocytoma
MALT lymphoma
Mammography
Mantle cell lymphoma
Mastectomy
Matrix metalloproteinase inhibitors
Mechlorethamine
Meclizine
Mediastinal tumors
Mediastinoscopy

Medroxyprogesterone acetate
Medulloblastoma
Megestrol acetate
Melanoma
Melphalan
Memory change
Meningioma
Meperidine
Mercaptopurine
Merkel cell carcinoma
Mesna
Mesothelioma
Metastasis
Methotrexate
Methylphenidate
Metoclopramide
Micronutrients and cancer prevention
Mistletoe
Mitomycin-C
Mitotane
Mitoxantrone
Modified radical mastectomy
Mohs surgery
Monoclonal antibodies
Mucositis
Multiple endocrine neoplasia
Multiple myeloma
Myasthenia gravis
Mycophenolate mofetil
Mycosis fungoides
Myelodysplastic syndromes
Myelofibrosis
Myeloma
Myeloproliferative diseases
Myelosuppression

N

Nasal cancer
Nasopharyngeal cancer
National Cancer Institute
National Comprehensive Cancer
    Network
Nausea and vomiting
Nephrectomy
Nephrostomy
Neuroblastoma
Neuroendocrine tumors

Neuropathy
Neurotoxicity
Neutropenia
Night sweats
Nilotinib
Non-Hodgkin lymphoma
Nonsteroidal anti-inflammatory
    drugs
Nuclear medicine scans
Nutritional support

O

Obesity and cancer risk
Obinutuzumab
Occupational exposures and cancer
Ofatumumab
Oligodendroglioma
Omega-3 fatty acids
Ommaya reservoir
Oncologic emergencies
Oophorectomy
Opioids
Oprelvekin
Oral cancers
Orchiectomy
Oropharyngeal cancer
Osteosarcoma
Ovarian cancer
Ovarian epithelial cancer

P

Paget disease of the breast
Pain management
Pancreatectomy
Pancreatic cancer
Pancreatic cancer, endocrine
Pancreatic cancer, exocrine
Panitumumab
Pap test
Paracentesis
Paranasal sinus cancer
Paraneoplastic syndromes
Parathyroid cancer
PC-SPES
Pegaspargase
Pemetrexed

Penile cancer
Pentostatin
Percutaneous transhepatic
    cholangiography
Pericardial effusion
Pericardiocentesis
Peritoneovenous shunt
Pesticides
Peutz-Jeghers syndrome
Pharyngectomy
Phenytoin
Pheochromocytoma
Pheresis
Photodynamic therapy
Physical therapy
Pilocarpine
Pineoblastoma
Pituitary tumors
Plerixafor
Pleural biopsy
Pleural effusion
Pleurodesis
Plicamycin
Ploidy analysis
Pneumonectomy
Pneumonia
Polyomavirus hominis type 1 (BK
    virus) infection
Pomalidomide
Porfimer sodium
Positron emission tomography
Pregnancy and cancer
Primary site
Procarbazine
Prostate cancer
Prostatectomy
Protein electrophoresis
Proteomics
Psycho-oncology

Q

Quadrantectomy

R

Radiation dermatitis
Radiation therapy

CONTRIBUTORS

Margaret Alic, PhD
Science Writer
Eastsound, WA

Lisa Andres, MS, CGC
*Certified Genetic Counselor and
    Medical Writer*
San Jose, CA

Racquel Baert, MSc
Medical Writer
Winnipeg, Canada

Julia R. Barrett
Science Writer
Madison, WI

Nancy J. Beaulieu, RPh, BCOP
Oncology Pharmacist
New Haven, CT

Linda K. Bennington, CNS, MSN
Clinical Nurse Specialist
Department of Nursing
Old Dominion University
Norfolk, VA

Kenneth J. Berniker, MD
Attending Physician
Emergency Department
Kaiser Permanente Medical Center
Vallejo, CA

Olga Bessmertny, PharmD
Clinical Pharmacy Manager
Pediatric Hematology/Oncology/
    Bone Marrow Transplant
Children's Hospital of New York
Columbia Presbyterian Medical
    Center
New York, NY

Patricia L. Bounds, PhD
Science Writer
Zürich, Switzerland

Cheryl Branche, MD
Retired General Practitioner
Jackson, MS

Tamara Brown, RN
Medical Writer
Boston, MA

Diane M. Calabrese
*Medical Sciences and Technology
    Writer*
Silver Spring, MD

**Rosalyn Carson-DeWitt, BSN,
    MD**
Medical Writer
Durham, NC

Lata Cherath, PhD
Science Writer
Franklin Park, NY

Lisa Christenson, PhD
Science Writer
Hamden, CT

Rhonda Cloos, RN
Medical Writer
Austin, TX

David Cramer, MD
Medical Writer
Chicago, IL

L. Lee Culvert, PhD
Medical Writer
Portland, ME

Tish Davidson, AM
Medical Writer
Fremont, CA

Dominic DeBellis, PhD
Medical Writer and Editor
Mahopac, NY

Tiffani A. DeMarco, MS
Genetic Counselor
Cancer Control
Georgetown University
Washington, DC

Lori DeMilto
Medical Writer
Sicklerville, NY

Stefanie B. N. Dugan, MS
Genetic Counselor
Milwaukee, WI

Janis O. Flores
Medical Writer
Sebastopol, CA

Paula Ford-Martin
Medical Writer
Chaplin, MN

Rebecca J. Frey, PhD
*Research and Administrative
    Associate*
East Rock Institute
New Haven, CT

Jason Fryer
Medical Writer
Lubbock, TX

Jill Granger, MS
Senior Research Associate
University of Michigan
Ann Arbor, MI

David E. Greenberg, MD
Medicine Resident
Baylor College of Medicine
Houston, TX

Maureen Haggerty
Medical Writer
Ambler, PA

Kevin Hwang, MD
Medical Writer
Morristown, NJ

Michelle L. Johnson, MS, JD
*Patent Attorney and Medical
    Writer*
Portland, OR

Paul A. Johnson, EdM
Medical Writer
San Diego, CA

Cindy L. A. Jones, PhD
Biomedical Writer
Sagescript Communications
Lakewood, CO

Crystal H. Kaczkowski, MSc
Medical Writer
Montreal, Canada

David S. Kaminstein, MD
Medical Writer
Westchester, PA

Beth Kapes
Medical Writer
Bay Village, OH

Janet M. Kearney
Writer
Gainesville, FL

Bob Kirsch
Medical Writer
Ossining, NY

Melissa Knopper
Medical Writer
Chicago, IL

Monique Laberge, PhD
Research Associate
Department of Biochemistry and
    Biophysics
University of Pennsylvania
Philadelphia, PA

Jill S. Lasker
Medical Writer
Midlothian, VA

G. Victor Leipzig, PhD
Biological Consultant
Huntington Beach, CA

Lorraine Lica, PhD
Medical Writer
San Diego, CA

John T. Lohr, PhD
Utah State University
Logan, UT

Warren Maltzman, PhD
Consultant, Molecular Pathology
Demarest, NJ

Richard A. McCartney MD
*Fellow, American College of
    Surgeons*
Diplomat, American Board of Surgery
Richland, WA

Sally C. McFarlane-Parrott
Medical Writer
Mason, MI

Monica McGee, MS
Science Writer
Wilmington, NC

Alison McTavish, MSc
Medical Writer and Editor
Montreal, Quebec

Molly Metzler, RN, BSN
*Registered Nurse and Medical
    Writer*
Seaford, DE

Beverly G. Miller, MT (ASCP)
Technical Writer
Charlotte, NC

Mark A. Mitchell, MD
Medical Writer
Seattle, WA

Laura J. Ninger
Medical Writer
Weehawken, NJ

Nancy J. Nordenson
Medical Writer
Minneapolis, MN

Melinda G. Oberleitner
Associate Dean and Professor
College of Nursing and Allied
    Health Professions
University of Louisiana at Lafayette
Lafayette, LA

Teresa G. Odle
Medical Writer
Albuquerque, NM

Lee Ann Paradise
Science Writer
Lubbock, TX

J. Ricker Polsdorfer, MD
Medical Writer
Phoenix, AZ

Elizabeth J. Pulcini, MS
Medical Writer
Phoenix, AZ

Kulbir Rangi, DO
Medical Doctor and Writer
New York, NY

**Esther Csapo Rastegari, EdM,
    RN, BSN**
Registered Nurse and Medical Writer
Holbrook, MA

Toni Rizzo
Medical Writer
Salt Lake City, UT

Martha Floberg Robbins
Medical Writer
Evanston, IL

Richard Robinson
Medical Writer
Tucson, AZ

Edward R. Rosick, DO, MPH, MS
*University Physician and Clinical
    Assistant Professor*
Student Health Services
Pennsylvania State University
University Park, PA

Nancy Ross-Flanigan
Science Writer
Belleville, MI

Belinda Rowland, PhD
Medical Writer
Voorheesville, NY

Andrea Ruskin, MD
Whittingham Cancer Center
Norwalk, CT

Laura Ruth, PhD
*Medical, Science, and Technology
    Writer*
Los Angeles, CA

Kausalya Santhanam, PhD
Technical Writer
Branford, CT

Marc Scanio
Doctoral Candidate in Chemistry
Stanford University
Stanford, CA

Joan Schonbeck, RN
Medical Writer
Massachusetts Department of
  Mental Health
Marlborough, MA

**Kristen Mahoney Shannon, MS,
CGC**
Genetic Counselor
Center for Cancer Risk
  Analysis
Massachusetts General Hospital
Boston, MA

Judith Sims, MS
Science Writer
Logan, UT

Genevieve Slomski, PhD
Medical Writer
New Britain, CT

**Anna Rovid Spickler, DVM,
PhD**
Medical Writer
Salisbury, MD

Laura L. Stein, MS
Certified Genetic Counselor
Familial Cancer Program-
  Department of Hematology/
  Oncology
Dartmouth Hitchcock Medical
  Center
Lebanon, NH

Phyllis M. Stein, BS, CCRP
Affiliate Coordinator
Grand Rapids Clinical Oncology
  Program
Grand Rapids, MI

Kurt Sternlof
Science Writer
New Rochelle, NY

Deanna M. Swartout-Corbeil, RN
Medical Writer
Thompsons Station, TN

Jane M. Taylor-Jones, MS
Research Associate
Donald W. Reynolds Department of
  Geriatrics
University of Arkansas for Medical
  Sciences
Little Rock, AR

Carol Turkington
Medical Writer
Lancaster, PA

Samuel Uretsky, PharmD
Medical Writer
Wantagh, NY

Marianne Vahey, MD
Clinical Instructor
Medicine
Yale University School of
  Medicine
New Haven, CT

Malini Vashishtha, PhD
Medical Writer
Irvine, CA

Ellen S. Weber, MSN
Medical Writer
Fort Wayne, IN

Ken R. Wells
Writer
Laguna Hills, CA

Barbara Wexler, MPH
Medical Writer
Chatsworth, CA

Wendy Wippel, MSc
*Medical Writer and Adjunct
  Professor of Biology*
Northwest Community College
Hernando, MS

Debra Wood, RN
Medical Writer
Orlando, FL

Kathleen D. Wright, RN
Medical Writer
Delmar, DE

Jon Zonderman
Medical Writer
Orange, CA

Michael V. Zuck, PhD
Writer
Boulder, CO

ILLUSTRATIONS OF BODY SYSTEMS

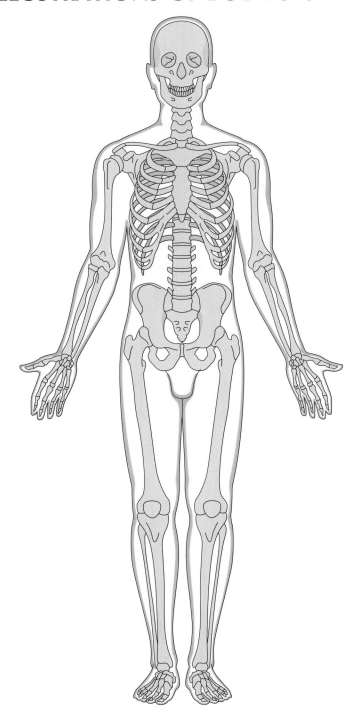

HUMAN SKELETON and SKIN. Some cancers that affect the skeleton are: Osteosarcoma; Ewing sarcoma; Fibrosarcoma (can also be found in soft tissues like muscle, fat, connective tissues, etc.). Some cancers that affect tissue near bones: Chondrosarcoma (affects joints near bones); Rhabdomyosarcoma (formed from cells of muscles attached to bones); Malignant fibrous histiocytoma (common in soft tissues, rare in bones). SKIN CANCERS: Basal cell carcinoma; Melanoma; Merkel cell carcinoma; Squamous cell carcinoma of the skin; and Trichilemmal carcinoma. Precancerous skin condition: Bowen disease. Lymphomas that affect the skin: Mycosis fungoides; Sézary syndrome. *(Illustration by Argosy Publishing. © Cengage Learning®.)*

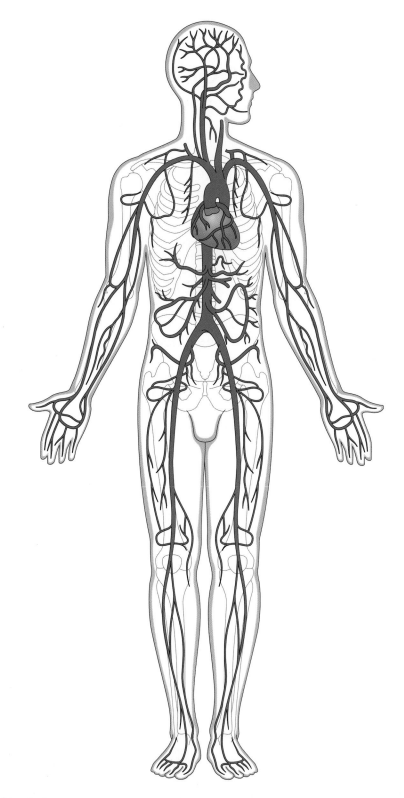

HUMAN CIRCULATORY SYSTEM. Some cancers of the blood cells are: Acute erythroblastic leukemia; Acute lymphocytic leukemia; Acute myelocytic leukemia; Chronic lymphocytic leukemia; Chronic myelocytic leukemia; Hairy cell leukemia; and Multiple myeloma. One condition associated with various cancers that affects blood is called Myelofibrosis. *(Illustration by Argosy Publishing. © Cengage Learning®.)*

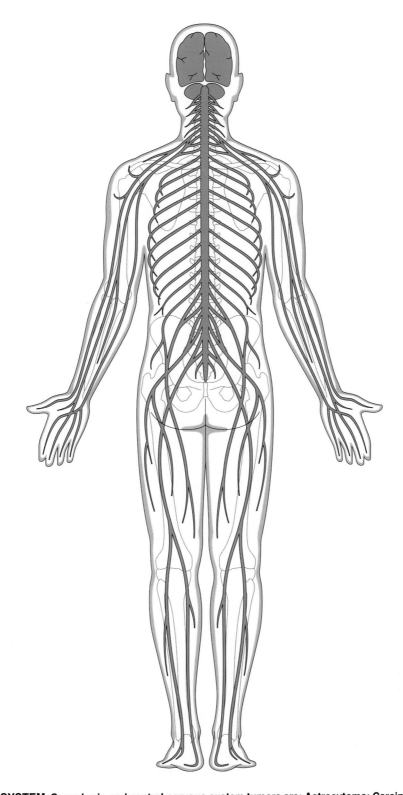

HUMAN NERVOUS SYSTEM. Some brain and central nervous system tumors are: Astrocytoma; Carcinomatous meningitis; Central nervous system carcinoma; Central nervous system lymphoma; Chordoma; Choroid plexus tumors; Craniopharyngioma; Ependymoma; Medulloblastoma; Meningioma; Oligodendroglioma; and Spinal axis tumors. One kind of noncancerous growth in the brain: Acoustic neuroma. *(Illustration by Argosy Publishing. © Cengage Learning®.)*

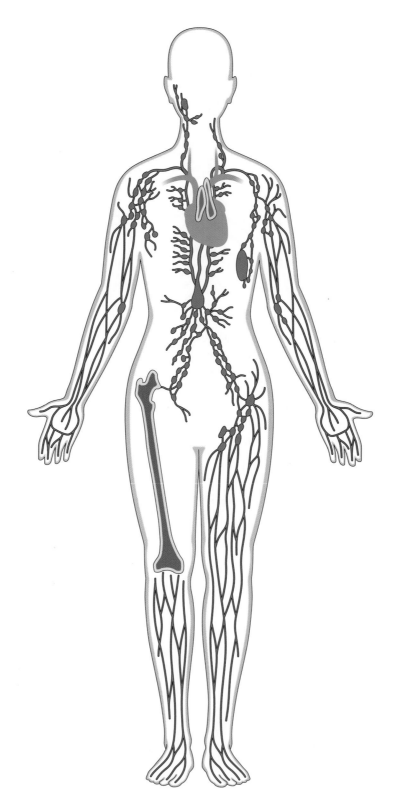

HUMAN LYMPHATIC SYSTEM. The lymphatic system and lymph nodes are shown here in pale green, the thymus in deep blue, and one of the bones rich in bone marrow (the femur) is shown here in purple. Some cancers of the lymphatic system are: Burkitt lymphoma; Cutaneous T-cell lymphoma; Hodgkin lymphoma; MALT lymphoma; Mantle cell lymphoma; Sézary syndrome; and Waldenström macroglobulinemia. *(Illustration by Argosy Publishing. © Cengage Learning®.)*

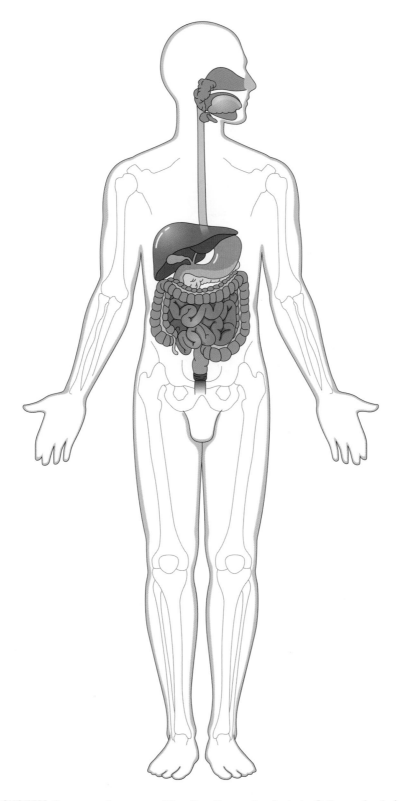

HUMAN DIGESTIVE SYSTEM. Organs and cancers of the digestive system include: Salivary glands (shown in turquoise): Salivary gland tumors. Esophagus (shown in bright yellow): Esophageal cancer. Liver (shown in bright red): Bile duct cancer; Liver cancer. Stomach (pale gray-blue): Stomach cancer. Gallbladder (bright orange against the red liver): Gallbladder cancer. Colon (green): Colon cancer. Small intestine (purple): Small intestine cancer; can have malignant tumors associated with Zollinger-Ellison syndrome. Rectum (shown in pink, continuing the colon): Rectal cancer. Anus (dark blue): Anal cancer.
(Illustration by Argosy Publishing. © Cengage Learning®.)

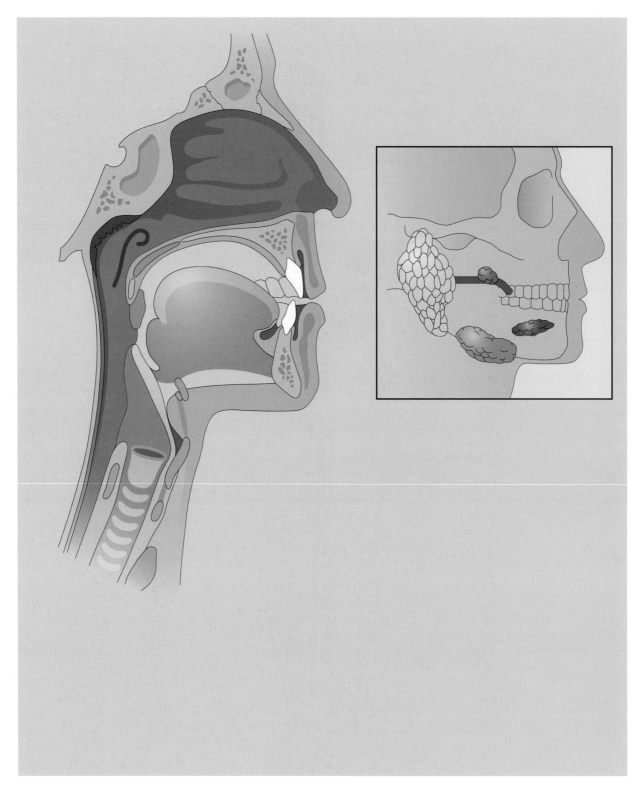

HEAD AND NECK. The pharynx, the passage that leads from the nostrils down through the neck, is shown in orange. This passage is broken into several divisions. The area behind the nose is the nasopharynx. The area behind the mouth is the oropharynx. The oropharynx leads into the laryngopharynx, which opens into the esophagus (still in orange) and the larynx (shown in the large image in medium blue). The cancers that affect these regions include: Nasopharyngeal cancer; Oropharyngeal cancer; Esophageal cancer; and Laryngeal cancer. Oral cancers can affect the lips, gums, and tongue (pink). Referring to the inset picture of the salivary glands, salivary gland tumors can affect the parotid glands (shown in yellow), the submandibular glands (turquoise), and the sublingual glands (purple). *(Illustration by Argosy Publishing. © Cengage Learning®.)*

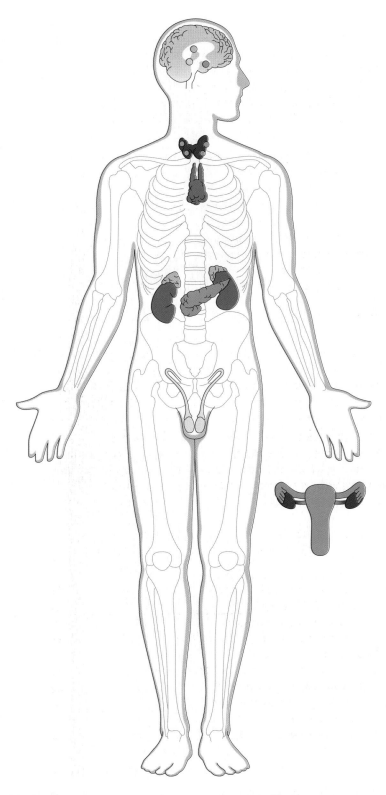

HUMAN ENDOCRINE SYSTEM. The glands and cancers of the endocrine system include (in the brain): the pituitary gland shown in blue (pituitary tumors), the hypothalamus in pale green, and the pineal gland in bright yellow. Throughout the rest of the body: Thyroid (shown in dark blue): Thyroid cancer. Parathyroid glands, adjacent to the thyroid: Parathyroid cancer. Thymus (green): Thymic cancer; Thymoma. Pancreas (turquoise): Pancreatic cancer; Zollinger-Ellison syndrome tumors can also be found in the pancreas. Adrenal glands (shown in apricot, above the kidneys): Neuroblastoma; Pheochromocytoma. Testes (in males, shown in yellow): Testicular cancer. Ovaries (in females, shown in dark blue in inset image): Ovarian cancer. *(Illustration by Argosy Publishing. © Cengage Learning®.)*

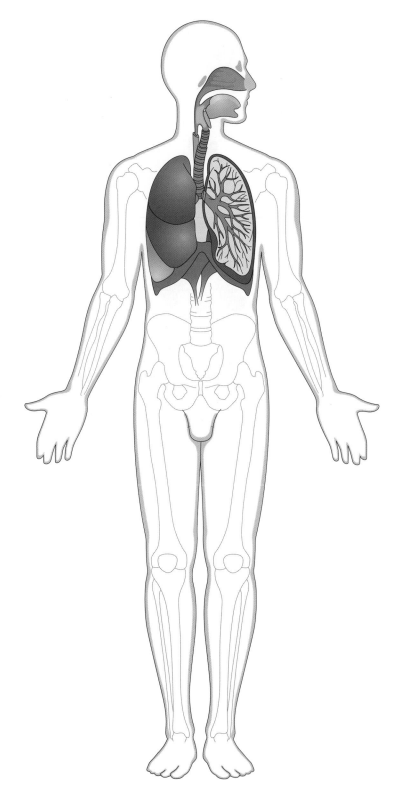

HUMAN RESPIRATORY SYSTEM. Air is breathed in through the nose or mouth, enters the pharynx (shown in orange), and passes through the larynx (shown as the green tube with a ridged texture; the smooth green tube is the esophagus, which is posterior to the larynx but is involved in digestion instead of breathing). The air then passes into the trachea (purple), which divides into two tubes called bronchi. One bronchus passes into each lung and continues to branch within the lung. These branches are called bronchioles, and each bronchiole leads to a tiny cluster of air sacs called alveoli. This is where the air and gases breathed in get diffused to the blood. The lungs (deep blue) are spongy and can be affected by Lung cancer, both the non-small cell and small-cell types. *(Illustration by Argosy Publishing. © Cengage Learning®.)*

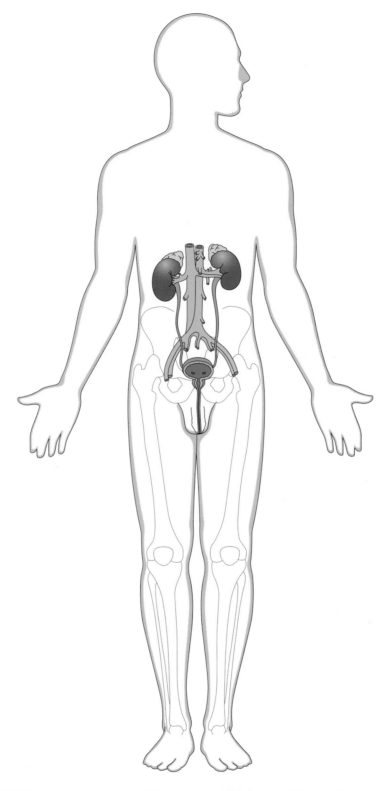

HUMAN URINARY SYSTEM. Organs and cancers of the urinary system include: Kidneys (shown in purple): Kidney cancer; Renal pelvis tumors; Wilms tumor. Ureters are shown in green. Bladder (blue-green): Bladder cancer. The kidneys, bladder, or ureters can be affected by Transitional cell carcinoma. *(Illustration by Argosy Publishing. © Cengage Learning®.)*

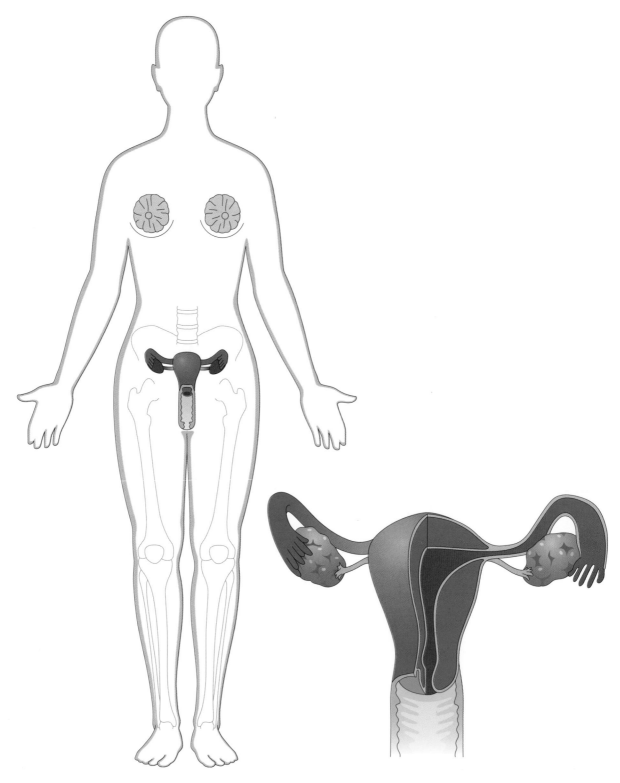

FEMALE REPRODUCTIVE SYSTEM. Organs and cancers of the female reproductive system include: Uterus, shown in red with the uterine or Fallopian tubes: Endometrial cancer. Ovaries (blue): Ovarian cancer. Vagina (shown in pink with a yellow interior or lining): Vaginal cancer. Breasts: Breast cancer; Paget disease of the breast. Shown in detailed inset only (in turquoise), Cervix: Cervical cancer. *(Illustration by Argosy Publishing. © Cengage Learning®.)*

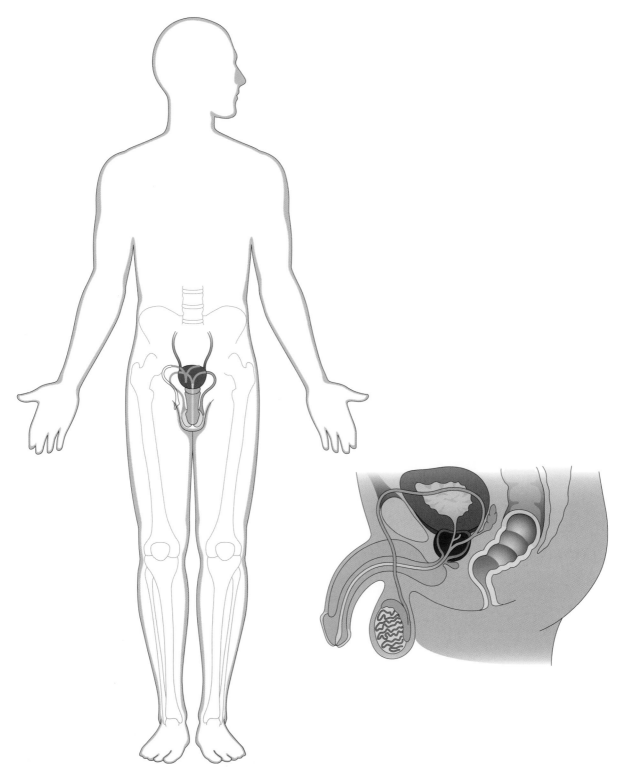

MALE REPRODCTIVE SYSTEM. Organs, glands, and cancers of the male reproductive system include: Penis (shown in pink): Penile cancer. Testes (shown in yellow): Testicular cancer. Prostate gland (shown in full-body illustration in a peach/apricot color, and in the inset as the dark blue gland between the bladder and the penis): Prostate cancer. *(Illustration by Argosy Publishing. © Cengage Learning®.)*

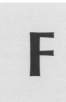

Famciclovir *see* **Antiviral therapy**

Familial cancer syndromes

Definition

Familial **cancer** syndromes—also called family or familial cancer susceptibility syndromes or hereditary cancer syndromes—are inherited genetic mutations that increase the risk for specific types of cancers.

Demographics

Familial cancer syndromes are rare in the general population, but they account for 5%–10% of all cancers. Colorectal cancer is the third most common cancer and second most lethal cancer in the United States, and 11% of colon cancers and 18% of rectal cancers occur in people under age 50; of these, about 20% are caused by familial cancer syndromes.

Description

More than 50 different familial cancer syndromes have been identified. Although genetic mutations play a role in the development of all cancers, most cancer-promoting mutations occur during a person's lifetime and are neither inherited nor passed on to offspring. Genetic mutations responsible for familial cancer syndromes are inherited from a parent and can be passed on to offspring. In addition to increasing the risk for specific cancers, these syndromes may cause other medical problems, such as non-cancerous (benign) tumors.

Major types

Hereditary breast and ovarian cancers were among the first recognized familial cancer syndromes. Breast and/or ovarian cancers sometimes occur in multiple women in one family, often at younger-than-expected ages, and sometimes separate breast cancers develop in each breast. These observations led to the discovery of the BRCA1 and BRCA2 genes. Certain mutations in either gene—especially in BRCA1—result in a very high risk for breast and/or **ovarian cancer**. They also increase the risk of fallopian tube, primary peritoneal, pancreatic, prostate, and male breast cancers, as well as certain others. **Pancreatic cancer** and male breast and prostate cancers are more common in people with BRCA2 mutations. In the United States, BRCA mutations are more common in people of Ashkenazi Jewish background.

Lynch syndrome or hereditary nonpolyposis colorectal cancer (HNPCC) is the most common familial cancer syndrome that increases the risk of colorectal cancer, usually before age 50. Lynch syndrome is also associated with endometrial (uterine lining), ovarian, renal pelvic, pancreatic, small intestinal, liver and biliary tract, stomach, brain, ureter, and breast cancers. Lynch syndrome can be caused by mutations in various genes, including MSH2, MLH1, MSH6, PMS2, or EPCAM. Most of these genes are involved in DNA repair, which is

Suppressor genes that, when deleted, predispose families to cancers

Gene	Consequence of gene loss
Rb	Retinoblastoma and osteosarcoma
TP53	Li-Fraumeni syndrome
Wt1	Wilms' tumor
VHL	von Hippel-Lindau syndrome; renal cell carcinoma
NF1	von Recklinghausen's disease; neurofibromatosis type 1; schwannoma and glioma
NF2	Neurofibromatosis type 2; acoustic neuroma and meningiomas
APC	Familial adenomatous polyposis; colorectal tumors
MMR	Hereditary nonpolyposis-colorectal cancer

Table listing different types of suppressor genes and the cancers that may occur if a gene is deleted. *(Table by GGS Creative Resources. © Cengage Learning®.)*

one of the body's defense mechanisms against cell mutations and other abnormalities.

Li-Fraumeni syndrome is a rare condition associated with many different cancers, including breast and ovarian cancers, soft-tissue **sarcoma**, **osteosarcoma** (bone cancer), leukemia, **brain tumors**, **adrenocortical carcinoma**, and others. The cancers seen in Li-Fraumeni syndrome most often develop during childhood, although breast cancers occur in young adults. Patients can develop more than one cancer and appear to be at higher risk of cancer from **radiation therapy**. Li-Fraumeni syndrome is most often caused by mutations in the TP53 gene that encodes a tumor suppressor protein called p53, which normally halts the growth of abnormal cells. Li-Fraumeni syndrome can also be caused by mutations in the CHEK2 gene.

Other common familial cancer syndromes for which **genetic testing** is available include:

- Cowden Syndrome, caused by mutations in the PTEN gene and associated with breast, thyroid, endometrial, and other cancers
- familial adenomatous polyposis caused by mutations in the APC gene and associated with colorectal cancer, multiple nonmalignant colon polyps, and both benign and cancerous tumors in the small intestine, brain, stomach, bone, skin, and other tissues
- retinoblastoma, caused by mutations in the RB1 gene and associated with cancer of the retina, pineal gland cancer, osteosarcoma, melanoma, and soft-tissue sarcoma
- Wermer syndrome or multiple endocrine neoplasia type 1, caused by mutations in the MEN1 gene and associated with pancreatic endocrine tumors and (usually benign) parathyroid and pituitary gland tumors
- Sipple syndrome or multiple endocrine neoplasia type 2, caused by mutations in the RET gene and associated with medullary thyroid cancer and pheochromocytoma (generally benign adrenal gland tumors), as well as overactive parathyroid glands and benign parathyroid gland tumors
- von Hippel-Lindau syndrome, caused by mutations in the VHL gene and associated with kidney cancer and multiple benign tumors

Other familial cancer syndromes include:

- Peutz-Jeghers syndrome, associated with colorectal, breast, and ovarian cancers
- Wilms tumor
- Gorlin-Goltz syndrome or basal cell nevus syndrome
- Bloom syndrome, a skin cancer
- Fanconi anemia, associated with skin cancer

- familial hyperparathyroidism, associated with endocrine and neuroendocrine neuroplasias
- familial medullary thyroid cancer
- hereditary melanoma
- hereditary paraganglioma
- familial juvenile polyposis, associated with colorectal cancer
- MYH-associated polyposis, associated with colorectal cancer
- hereditary prostate cancer
- hereditary renal cell cancer, associated with uterine leiomyomas
- xeroderma pigmentosum, associated with skin cancer
- attenuated familial adenomatous polyposis, associated with colorectal cancer

Risk factors

Different familial cancer syndromes carry different risks for developing cancer and associated symptoms. In general, someone who inherits a gene for a familial cancer syndrome has a higher risk of developing associated cancers than the general population; however, this does not mean that the individual will necessarily develop cancer. Furthermore, multiple cancers in one family are not usually indicative of a familial cancer syndrome—they are most often due to chance or to exposure to a common carcinogen such as cigarette smoking. Common cancers—such as prostate cancers in brothers in their 80s—are unlikely to be familial cancer syndromes.

Risk factors for a familial cancer syndrome include:

- many cases of an uncommon or rare cancer, such as kidney cancer, within a family
- an unusual number of cancers diagnosed in a single family
- even one case of a very rare cancer, such as cancer of the adrenal cortex
- two or more close relatives on the same side of the family (parent and child or siblings) with the same type of cancer
- cancer diagnosed at an earlier-than-usual age, such as colon cancer under age 30
- multiple primary cancers (not recurrences) in an individual, such as breast and ovarian cancers
- primary cancers in a pair of organs (bilateral), such as both eyes, both breasts, or both kidneys
- multiple tumors in an organ, such as the breast, arising from a single primary tumor
- childhood cancers such as sarcomas in siblings
- male breast cancer

- a cluster of cancers associated with a known familial cancer syndrome, such as breast and ovarian cancers

- tumors with rare cell types

- cancer in an individual with birth defects or cancers associated with birth defects

- cancers associated with other genetic traits

Causes and symptoms

Familial cancer syndromes are caused by mutations in individual genes or damage to one or more sections of specific chromosomes. The symptoms depend on the affected organ(s) or systems, the inheritance pattern, the number of genes involved, the specific mutations within a gene, and other factors.

Inheritance patterns

The majority of familial cancer syndromes show autosomal dominant inheritance and are caused by gene mutations that are known as highly penetrant. This means that the mutated gene inherited from one parent overrides the effects of the normal gene inherited from the other parent. It also means that each child of the individual with the mutated gene has a 50% chance of inheriting the abnormal gene. Autosomal means that the gene is not carried on the X or Y sex chromosomes and so affects males and females equally.

Some familial cancer syndromes have autosomal recessive inheritance. This means that the normal gene overrides the effects of the mutant gene, and the syndrome occurs only in people who have inherited two mutated copies of the same gene, one from each parent. If each parent has a single copy of the same mutated gene, the parents themselves will not be affected by the syndrome, but each of their children has a 25% chance of inheriting both mutated genes and may develop the associated cancer syndrome.

Diagnosis

An accurate family medical history is important for diagnosing a familial cancer syndrome. The family history should include types of cancer and ages at diagnosis for children, siblings, parents, aunts, uncles, grandparents, nieces, nephews, and cousins on both sides of the family. Birth defects, unusual skin conditions, benign tumors, and results of screening tests—such as colonoscopies to detect colon polyps—should also be noted. An online tool from the U.S. Surgeon General— "My Family Health Portrait"—can assist in creating a family health history. It is available at https://familyhis tory.hhs.gov/FHH/html/index.html.

QUESTIONS TO ASK YOUR DOCTOR

- Could I be at risk for a familial cancer syndrome?
- Should I be tested for possible mutations related to a familial cancer?
- What information will genetic testing provide?
- Can you recommend a hospital or clinic that provides genetic testing and counseling?

Many hospitals have familial cancer clinics that may include geneticists, genetic counselors, oncologists, and social workers. They assist individuals and families by providing risk assessment, support, screening and prevention recommendations, and possible genetic testing options.

Tests

Genetic testing is available for many familial cancer syndromes; however for others, the responsible genes have not yet been identified. When genetic testing is available, it can determine whether someone from a cancer syndrome family carries the gene mutation. A genetic counselor, physician, or other healthcare professional trained in genetics can assist individuals and families in understanding test results.

There are particular issues surrounding genetic testing for each familial cancer syndrome, such as:

- the risk, benefits, and limitations of genetic testing

- insurance coverage

- the age when testing should be performed

- how the results will affect medical management

- how the results will affect other family members

- the potential effects of rapid progress in identifying genes and developing genetic testing for familial cancer syndromes

Since inherited mutations that cause familial cancer syndromes affect all cells in the body, genetic testing can usually be performed on blood samples. Close relatives of an individual diagnosed with a familial cancer syndrome should be examined for signs of the syndrome. Sometimes the patient is the first in the family to be affected by the syndrome. Parents and siblings may not be affected, but the patient can pass the mutated gene on to offspring. Depending on the syndrome, genetics professionals can determine who in the family is at risk. For example, women with a strong family history of breast and/or ovarian cancers can undergo genetic counseling to estimate the risk that they carry a BRCA mutation. Based on this estimate, they may choose to undergo genetic testing.

Genetic testing is available for gene mutations that cause HNPCC. Physicians or genetic counselors can determine whether cases of nonpolyposis colorectal cancer are likely to be familial using the Amsterdam criteria and the revised Bethesda guidelines. People with colorectal or endometrial cancers can also have their tumor tissues tested for characteristics called microsatellite instability that are associated with Lynch syndrome.

Prevention

Since the completion of the Human Genome Project in mid-2002, there have been rapid advances in the identification of genes responsible for familial cancer syndromes, leading to new genetic screens and eventually to improved preventive and therapeutic interventions. The U.S. National Library of Medicine's Genetics Home Reference Website at http://ghr.nlm.nih.gov has extensive information about familial cancer syndromes, including the genes responsible, inheritance patterns, and information about genetic testing and counseling.

When genetic tests indicate that family members carry gene mutations that put them at risk for familial cancer syndromes, preventive measures may include:

- lifestyle changes, including diet, exercise, and other factors
- preventive drugs
- monitoring and screenings to detect cancers at the earliest—and most curable—stage
- clinical trials
- education on risk reduction and monitoring
- psychological counseling
- further genetic testing

Genetic testing that reveals gene mutations responsible for some familial cancer syndromes, such as familial **breast cancer** or HNPCC, indicates that close relatives (parents, siblings, and children) may have a 50% risk of also carrying the gene mutation. Women at risk for familial breast cancer because of BRCA gene mutations can undergo frequent screenings by **mammography** or **magnetic resonance imaging** (MRI) beginning at a young age. Some women choose prophylactic **mastectomy** and/or **oophorectomy** (ovary removal). Patients who carry a gene mutation that causes HNPCC can be screened for colorectal cancer beginning in their early 20s or take other steps that may help prevent cancer development. Women with HNPCC gene mutations can also undergo regular screening for **endometrial cancer**. Some at-risk individuals choose

KEY TERMS

Autosomal dominant—A gene located on a chromosome other than the X or Y sex chromosomes and whose expression is dominant over that of a second copy of the same gene.

Autosomal recessive—A gene located on a chromosome other than the X or Y sex chromosomes and carrying a trait that is not expressed unless the second copy of the same gene inherited from the other parent is also recessive or mutated.

BRCA1 and BRCA2—Breast cancer susceptibility genes; specific inherited mutations in these genes greatly increase the risk of breast and ovarian cancer.

Hereditary nonpolyposis colorectal cancer; HNPCC—Lynch syndrome; the most common familial cancer syndrome that increases the risk of colorectal cancer, especially at a younger age; caused by inherited mutations in any of several genes, most of which are involved in DNA repair.

Li-Fraumeni syndrome—A rare familial cancer syndrome characterized by high risk for early onset breast cancer and soft-tissue sarcomas.

Magnetic resonance imaging (MRI)—A diagnostic technique that provides cross-sectional images of structures such as the breasts using a magnetic imaging device.

Mammography—X-ray screening to detect breast cancer.

Mastectomy—Surgical removal of part or all of the breast and possibly associated lymph nodes and muscle.

Mutation—An inherited or spontaneous change in the DNA sequence of a gene.

Polyps—Projecting tissue masses that can occur with colorectal cancers.

Tumor suppressor—A protein such as p53 that helps prevent cancer; mutations that cause familial cancer syndromes are often in genes encoding tumor suppressors.

to have regular cancer screenings or take other precautions to lower their risk, even if they decide not to have genetic testing.

Prenatal genetic counseling may be very important for prospective parents who have a familial cancer syndrome or who may carry a mutated gene that puts their offspring at risk. Preimplantation genetic diagnosis can help couples undergoing in vitro fertilization techniques to avoid having a child with a familial cancer syndrome.

Resources

BOOKS

Nosé, Vania, Joel K. Greenson, and Gladell P. Paner. *Familial Cancer Syndromes.* Philadelphia: Lippincott Williams & Wilkins, 2013.

Schneider, Katherine A. *Counseling About Cancer: Strategies for Genetic Counseling.* 3rd ed. Hoboken, NJ: Wiley-Blackwell, 2012.

PERIODICALS

Ahnen, Dennis J., et al. "The Increasing Incidence of Young-Onset Colorectal Cancer: A Call to Action." *Mayo Clinic Proceedings* 89, no. 2 (February 2014): 216–24.

Beattie, Mary S., et al. "Genetic Counseling, Cancer Screening, Breast Cancer Characteristics, and General Health among a Diverse Population of BRCA Genetic Testers." *Journal of Health Care for the Poor and Underserved* 24, no. 3 (August 2013): 1150–66.

Rich, Thereasa A., et al. "Comparison of Attitudes Regarding Preimplantation Genetic Diagnosis Among Patients with Hereditary Cancer Syndromes." *Familial Cancer* 13, no. 2 (2014): 291–9.

Shipman, Hannah Elizabeth, et al. "On the Limits of Genetic Responsibility: Communication and Consent for Tumour Testing for Lynch Syndrome." *Communication & Medicine* 10, no. 3 (2013): 225–35.

Walcott, Farzana L., et al. "The Affordable Care Act and Genetic Testing for Inheritable Cancer Syndromes: Impact on High-Risk Underserved Minorities." *Journal of Health Care for the Poor and Underserved* suppl. 25, no. 1 (February 2014): 36–62.

WEBSITES

"Cancer Genetics Overview (PDQ)." National Cancer Institute. July 21, 2014. http://www.cancer.gov/cancertopics/pdq/genetics/overview/healthprofessional (accessed August 10, 2014).

"Family Cancer Syndromes." American Cancer Society. June 25, 2014. http://www.cancer.org/cancer/cancercauses/geneticsandcancer/heredity-and-cancer (accessed August 10, 2014).

"Genetic Testing for Hereditary Cancer Syndromes." National Cancer Institute. April 11, 2013. http://www.cancer.gov/cancertopics/factsheet/Risk/genetic-testing (accessed August 10, 2014).

Lindor, Noralane M., et al. *Concise Handbook of Familial Cancer Susceptibility Syndromes.* 2nd ed. *Journal of the National Cancer Institute Monographs* no. 38 (2008). http://jncimono.oxfordjournals.org/content/2008/38/3.full.pdf+html (accessed August 10, 2014).

ORGANIZATIONS

American Cancer Society, 250 Williams Street NW, Atlanta, GA 30303, (800) 227-2345, http://www.cancer.org.

National Cancer Institute, 6116 Executive Boulevard, Suite 300, Bethesda, MD 20892-8322, (800) 4-CANCER (422-6237), http://www.cancer.gov.

Office of Rare Diseases Research, National Center for Advancing Translational Sciences, 6701 Democracy Boulevard, Suite 1001, MSC 4874, Bethesda, MD 20892, (301) 402-4336, Fax: (301) 480-9655, (888) 205-2311, ordr@nih.gov, http://rarediseases.info.nih.gov.

University of Chicago Medicine, Comer Children's Hospital, 5721 South Maryland Avenue, Chicago, IL 60637, (773) 702-1000, (888) 824-0200, https://www.uchicagokidshospital.org.

Laura L. Stein, M.S., C.G.C.
Teresa G. Odle
REVISED BY REBECCA J. FREY, PhD
Margaret Alic, PhD

▌Family and caregiver issues

Definition

Family and caregiver issues affect the family members and friends who are not trained health care professionals but nonetheless care for a **cancer** patient at home during inpatient treatment and near the end of life. These persons are sometimes referred to as "informal caregivers" to distinguish them from the medical or social service professionals also entrusted with care for cancer patients. The issues caregivers confront include not only care of the cancer patient (decision making, communicating with the health care team, providing hands-on care for the patient, advocating for the patient, and providing companionship and social support) but also self-care and the resolution of family conflicts that might arise during cancer treatment.

Demographics

The **National Cancer Institute** (NCI) notes that about 1.6 million persons in the United States are expected to be diagnosed with cancer in 2014. Most of these persons will receive care from one or more caregivers, usually family members, neighbors, or friends. The Family Caregiver Alliance (FCA) estimates that caregivers (for all patients suffering from chronic illnesses including cancer) number about 45 million Americans over the age of 18, and that their unpaid caregiving services are worth about $310 billion each year—more than the combined annual costs of home health care and nursing home care.

KEY TERMS

Caregiver burden—The high level of emotional and physical stress experienced by a person who is caring for someone (most often a family member) with a long-term serious illness.

Distress—A condition marked by emotional, social, spiritual, or physical pain or suffering that may affect caregivers as well as cancer patients.

Hospice—A program that provides specialized medical and spiritual care for patients at the end of life. Hospice care may be delivered in the patient's home, in hospitals, or in separate facilities.

Palliative care—Care intended to relieve the symptoms of a disease rather than cure the disease.

Respite care—Temporary care provided to a patient so that the regular caregiver(s) can be relieved for a short time. Respite care may be given in the patient's home, in a nursing home, or in an adult day care facility.

Role strain—The experience of someone who is filling a specific role (here, the role of caregiver) that is frustrated by excessive obligations or multiple demands on time, energy, or availability.

Supportive care—The prevention or management of the adverse effects of cancer and cancer treatment.

Although there is considerable variation in educational level, occupation, age, race, and other demographic features of caregivers, the statistically average caregiver is female, between the ages of 46 and 55, employed full-time, and either married or related to the cancer patient. Two-thirds of all caregivers in the United States are women, and 35% of all caregivers are in poor health themselves.

Description

Caring for cancer patients has become more difficult in recent years. Hospital stays are shorter and technological advances make it possible to provide more in-home care. Patients are also living longer. This means heavier demands are placed on caregivers for longer periods of time than was the case in the 1980s. Family structure and the workplace have changed too, which adds to the difficulty in caring for cancer patients. Cancer patients are not necessarily part of a nuclear family; the number of single adults and childless adults has increased markedly since the 1960s. According to the Bureau of the Census, as of 2011, there were 102 million Americans over the age of 18; fifty-five million households were headed by unmarried men and women. Thirty-three million Americans lived alone in 2011—up from 17% in 1970. Most caregivers are either employed full time or seeking full-time work, complicating their responsibilities as caregivers.

Decision making and administrative tasks

Caregivers may be unprepared for the number of decisions that the patient's care requires or the variety of tasks involved in running the household and coordinating the patient's care (sometimes called case management). Hospital and medical bills must be paid; insurance claims need to be filed. Sometimes decisions need to be reached about which family member will become the primary caregiver.

Large extended families can often divide the caregiving tasks among several members, or one family member will become the primary caregiver while others assume responsibility for communication with the health care team or social support for the patient. This division of responsibilities can be complicated by distance if some family members live far away from the patient. Sometimes the patient must travel to a specialized cancer center in a distant city. The NCI suggests periodic family meetings to resolve disagreements and frustrations and deal with painful emotions. The NCI also suggests that one member assume the role of family spokesperson.

Instrumental tasks

Instrumental caregiving tasks include driving and accompanying the patient to doctors' appointments; shopping and running personal errands; laundry; cooking, cleaning, child and pet care; home and automobile maintenance; and other chores entailed in running a household.

Commonly, adult caregivers must manage these tasks while continuing full-time employment. While some large companies grant paid or unpaid leave for care of a seriously ill cancer patient, people who own small businesses or work as independent contractors or consultants face loss of income if they must take time off. In some cases, the cancer patient may continue to work part-time during treatment. It is important that individual family members consult with employers to protect their job security and their own **health insurance**.

Hands-on care

Although some families can afford professional home health care, most home caregivers are family members. Medications must be stored and administered; careful records of all medications administered and their side effects must be kept, and the patient's symptoms must be documented. Caregivers may also be required to lift or carry, feed, bathe, groom, dress, and toilet the patient. In some cases, the caregiver will operate oxygen tanks, assistive devices, or other medical equipment in the home.

Care of patients in the later stages of treatment may include management of side effects of therapy, including nausea, vomiting, loss of appetite and other nutritional problems, chronic pain, and sleep disorders. In addition to identifying new or intensified symptoms, the caregiver must also report to the patient's health care team. In the best-case scenario, the patient is compliant with the caregiver's home health care, but sometimes patients disagree or refuse to comply with the treatment team's recommendations. In these high-risk situations, the treatment team may need to intervene to resolve the conflict.

Communication and navigating the health care system

The NCI suggests that one family member take on the responsibility of communicating with the health care providers and the rest of the family about the course of treatment, the patient's progress, and other relevant information. In this way, the possibility of duplicated messages, misunderstandings, and family conflicts are minimized.

Navigating the health care system is a process that begins for everyone when the patient is diagnosed with cancer. Most caregivers are not health care professionals. Therefore, they must learn medical terms and concepts while also struggling to absorb all the financial, emotional, and social consequences of the patient's disease. Family caregivers often take it upon themselves to research the patient's cancer and its treatment; various treatment options; and the location of specialized cancer centers.

Social support

Providing social support for the patient also adds to the strain of caring for a sick family member. Although some patients are able to work or continue limited outside activities, others become dependent solely on caregivers for companionship and household tasks, as well as hands-on care. When the patient is in pain or depressed, this can be particularly stressful and a burden that increases over time. In addition to serving as the patient's primary source of social support, many caregivers become gradually isolated from their own friends and former activities.

Respite care is care that provides relief for the caregiver from 24/7 responsibility for home care of the patient. Respite care may be provided by a companion who comes to the home, temporary placement in a nursing home, or adult day care for the patient.

End-of-life care

According to the NCI, care for a patient at the end-of-life stage is the most difficult and stressful time for caregivers. Stress-related illnesses increase. Anxiety and **depression** are highest in caregivers of patients with lung, blood, or **head and neck cancers**. Caregivers as well as patients have benefited from the recent development of hospice and palliative care as a medical specialty, as many hospital-based palliative care programs provide much-needed emotional support to both patients and caregivers.

Caregivers and self-care

Stress associated with caregiving has been well documented since the 1990s. According to the FCA, between 40% and 70% of caregivers eventually develop symptoms of depression; many have coexisting anxiety disorders and are at increased risk of alcohol or **substance abuse**. About 22% of caregivers report that they are physically exhausted and 10% report short-term memory loss, difficulty concentrating at work, or while driving. As a result of high stress levels, caregivers are at twice the risk (45% versus 22%) as non-caregivers for chronic disorders, such as heart attack, arthritis, diabetes, and cancer. The NCI reports that the risk of dying from stress-related illness within five years is 63% higher for caregivers than non-caregivers.

Caregivers often need reminders to attend to their own health care and emotional needs. American Cancer Society has published a caregiver distress checklist, available on the website listed below. The purpose of the checklist is to help caregivers with self-assessment and provide suggestions about how to ask for help. Caregivers with high scores on the distress checklist are encouraged to consult a mental health professional and seek assistance with the caregiving responsibilities.

Special concerns

Some caregivers and cancer patients have special needs.

Cultural differences

The NCI points to cultural differences that sometimes complicate caregiving. In some Asian cultures, for example, discussion about symptoms is considered bad luck, which makes it difficult to discuss the condition honestly with the patient. Pride or cultural tradition also prevents some families from seeking help from outside agencies. According to the NCI, African American and Hispanic caregivers are more likely to give up employment than place their patients in nursing homes, and they suffer from higher levels of distress and caregiver burden than Caucasian caregivers.

Single caregivers

Changes in family structure have resulted in increased isolation for some cancer patients and their caregivers. Single caregivers may have few resources outside the home. Sometimes friendship networks, neighbors, or church and synagogue groups are available to help with care or errands.

Abusive or dysfunctional families

Health care teams are alert to the need to evaluate troubled families when treating a patient's cancer. The strain of patient's diagnosis and treatment can reopen old family conflicts and trigger new ones. An assessment instrument known as the Cancer Communication Assessment Tool for Patients and Families (CCAT-PF) was published in 2008, and can be used by the patient's health care team to evaluate the family's situation. A high score on the CCAT-PF, indicates the likelihood of conflict, less ability to communicate, and low levels of family cohesion. High scores also suggest the likelihood of depression and reduced quality of life.

The ACS notes that dysfunction sometimes results in abuse; the patient may be the target of the abuse or the abuser. When abuse is present in any form, caregivers should consult the health care team for help.

Resources

Fortunately, resources for caregivers of cancer patients have increased in the last few years. In addition to local support groups and community social service agencies, the ACS and the NCI offer brochures, checklists, dictionaries of cancer terms, and other materials online that can be downloaded free of charge. Many materials are intended especially for caregivers. In addition to the cancer organizations, such organizations as the Family Caregiver Alliance (FCA) and the Caregiver Action Network (CAN; formerly the National Family Caregivers Association, offer plentiful online materials to help caregivers identify community resources and cope with the stresses related to caregiving. Although the FCA and CAN were originally founded to help caregivers for patients with Alzheimer's disease, lupus, Parkinson's disease, multiple sclerosis, traumatic brain injuries, and other chronic conditions, the

---

QUESTIONS TO ASK YOUR DOCTOR

- Can you recommend a local support group for caregivers of cancer patients?
- Caring for the cancer patient in my family has caused a number of heated arguments and disagreements about which member should be responsible for what aspect of care. Where can we go for help in resolving our conflicts?
- I can't afford to quit my job in order to take care of a parent with terminal cancer. What financial resources might be available?
- My own health is starting to suffer because I feel guilty about taking time for myself or eating properly. What resources are available for respite care?
- How can I explain my spouse's diagnosis and treatment to young children?
- The cancer patient in my family is becoming increasingly angry as well as depressed and refuses to cooperate with the recommended treatments. Can we ask his health care team to intervene?

---

information is also valuable for caregivers of cancer patients. One particularly useful resource is the Plugged-In Caregiving website, a joint project of CAN and Philips Lifeline, which offers information about high-tech devices and services that can simplify and streamline caregiving tasks.

A psychoeducational program called COPE (Creativity, Optimism, Planning, and Expert) provides caregivers with problem-solving strategies to improve their effectiveness as caregivers. The COPE program provides handouts for caregivers to use at home and education sessions to guide them through the complexities of cancer treatment plans. Other COPE sessions provide instruction in medication and symptom management. The COPE program was first introduced in 1996; it has been shown to reduce levels of stress in caregivers and improve their quality of life.

Resources

BOOKS

Bucher, Julia A., Peter S. Houts, and Terri Ades, eds. *American Cancer Society Complete Guide to Family Caregiving: The Essential Guide to Cancer Caregiving at Home*, 2nd ed. Atlanta, GA: American Cancer Society/Health Promotions, 2011.

Maxwell, Tracy. *Single, with Cancer: A Solo Survivor's Guide to Life, Love, Health, and Happiness.* New York: Demos Health, 2014.

Talley, Ronda C., Ruth McCorkle, and Walter F. Baile, eds. *Cancer Caregiving in the United States: Research, Practice, Policy.* New York: Springer, 2012.

PERIODICALS

Angelo, J., and R. Egan. "Family Caregivers Voice Their Needs: A Photovoice Study." *Palliative and Supportive Care,* May 20, 2014: 1–12 [E-publication ahead of print].

Bevans, M.F., and E.M. Sternberg. "Caregiving Burden, Stress, and Health Effects Among Family Caregivers of Adult Cancer Patients." *Journal of the American Medical Association* 307 (January 25, 2012): 398–403.

Girgis, A., et al. "Physical, Psychosocial, Relationship, and Economic Burden of Caring for People with Cancer: A Review." *Journal of Oncology Practice* 9 (July 2013): 197–202.

Kim, Y., et al. "Prevalence and Predictors of Depressive Symptoms among Cancer Caregivers 5 Years after the Relative's Cancer Diagnosis." *Journal of Consulting and Clinical Psychology* 82 (February 2014): 1–8.

Laudenslager, M.L. "'Anatomy of an Illness': Control from a Caregiver's Perspective." *Brain, Behavior, and Immunity* 36 (February 2014): 1–8.

Longacre, M.L., E.A. Ross, and C.Y. Fang. "Caregiving Choice and Emotional Stress Among Cancer Caregivers." *Western Journal of Nursing Research* 36 (November 11, 2013): 806–824.

McMullen, C.K., et al. "Caregivers as Healthcare Managers: Health Management Activities, Needs, and Caregiving Relationships for Colorectal Cancer Survivors with Ostomies." *Supportive Care in Cancer* 22 (September 2014): 2401–2408.

Meyers, F.J., et al. "Effects of a Problem-solving Intervention (COPE) on Quality of Life for Patients with Advanced Cancer on Clinical Trials and Their Caregivers: Simultaneous Care Educational Intervention (SCEI): Linking Palliation and Clinical Trials." *Journal of Palliative Medicine* 13 (April 2011): 465–473.

Pagano, E., et al. "The Economic Burden of Caregiving on Families of Children and Adolescents with Cancer: A Population-based Assessment." *Pediatric Blood and Cancer* 61 (June 2014): 1088–1093.

Tang, S.T., et al. "Trajectories of Caregiver Depressive Symptoms While Providing End-of-life Care." *Psycho-oncology* 22 (December 2013): 2702–2710.

WEBSITES

American Cancer Society (ACS). "Being a Caregiver." http://www.cancer.org/acs/groups/content/@editorial/documents/document/acspc-031602.pdf (accessed August 1, 2014).

American Cancer Society (ACS). "Caregiver Distress Checklist." http://www.cancer.org/treatment/treatmentsandside effects/emotionalsideeffects/copingchecklistforpatients andcaregivers/distress-checklist-for-caregivers (accessed August 3, 2014).

American Cancer Society (ACS). "Caregivers." http://www.cancer.org/treatment/caregivers/index (accessed August 1, 2014).

Caregiver Action Network (CAN). "Toolbox." http://www.caregiveraction.org/resources/toolbox (accessed August 2, 2014).

Family Caregiver Alliance (FCA). "Fact Sheet: Caregiver Health." https://www.caregiver.org/caregiver-health (accessed August 1, 2014).

Family Caregiver Alliance (FCA). "Women and Caregiving: Facts and Figures." https://www.caregiver.org/women-and-caregiving-facts-and-figures (accessed August 1, 2014).

National Cancer Institute (NCI). "Family Caregivers and Cancer: Roles and Challenges (PDQ)." http://www.cancer.gov/cancertopics/pdq/supportivecare/caregivers/health professional/page1/AllPages (accessed August 2, 2014).

Plugged-In Caregiving. "Technology for Family Caregivers." http://nfca.typepad.com/pluggedin_caregiving (accessed August 2, 2014).

ORGANIZATIONS

American Cancer Society (ACS), 250 Williams Street NW, Atlanta, GA 30303, (800) 227-2345, http://www.cancer.org/aboutus/howwehelpyou/app/contact-us.aspx, http://www.cancer.org/index.

Caregiver Action Network (CAN)[formerly the National Family Caregivers Association], 2000 M Street NW, Suite 400, Washington, DC 20036, (202) 772-5050, info@caregiveraction.org, http://www.caregiveraction.org.

Family Caregiver Alliance (FCA), 785 Market Street, Suite 750, San Francisco, CA 94103, (800) 445-8106, https://www.caregiver.org/contact, https://www.caregiver.org.

National Cancer Institute (NCI), BG 9609 MSC 9760, 9609 Medical Center Drive, Bethesda, MD 20892-9760, (800) 4-CANCER (422-6237), http://www.cancer.gov/global/contact/email-us, http://www.cancer.gov.

National Hospice and Palliative Care Organization (NHPCO), 1731 King Street, Alexandria, VA 22314, (703) 837-1500, Fax: (703) 837-1233, http://www.nhpco.org.

Rebecca J. Frey, PhD.

Famotidine *see* **Histamine 2 antagonists**

Fanconi anemia

Definition

Fanconi **anemia** is an inherited form of aplastic anemia characterized by an abnormally low number of cellular components in the blood due to failing bone marrow.

Description

Fanconi anemia (FA) is a rare genetic disease caused by mutations or alterations in one of seven different genes. The disease is an autosomal recessive condition, meaning that the genes are not located on the sex chromosomes and a mutated gene copy must be inherited from both parents in order for a person to be affected. Test results of cells from FA patients suggest that the genetic defects of FA reduce the cell's ability to repair damaged deoxyribonucleic acid (DNA), the primary chemical component of chromosomes. Five of the seven genes associated with FA have been isolated.

Demographics

With only approximately 1,000 cases documented in the literature, FA is a rare disease with varied frequency in different ethnic groups. It is particularly prevalent in the Ashkenazi Jewish population, where carriers are 1 in 89 persons, compared to an overall carrier frequency of 1 in 100 to 600. A carrier is a person unaffected by the disease who has one mutated and one normal gene in their genome. Both parents must be carriers in order to produce a child with FA.

Causes and symptoms

FA is caused by inheriting two abnormal copies of one of seven different genes, all thought to be involved in DNA repair. About 67% of children with FA are born with some sort of congenital defect. The problems seen include:

- short stature
- abnormalities of the thumb or arm

- other skeletal abnormalities such as of the hip or ribs
- kidney malformations
- skin discoloration
- small eyes or head
- mental retardation
- low birth weight and failure to thrive
- abnormalities of the digestive system
- heart defects

The defining characteristic of FA is progressive pancytopenia, a gradual reduction of the cellular components of the blood. A reduction in red blood cells is typically noted first, then white blood cells, and finally, platelets. Complete bone marrow failure in FA patients is usually seen between the ages of three and twelve, with a median of seven.

Later in life, FA patients have delayed sexual maturity and an increased probability of developing **cancer**. For FA patients surviving into adulthood, 50% develop leukemia (a malignancy of the white blood cells) and/or myelodysplastic syndrome (MDS, a pre-leukemic state). Persons with FA also have an elevated chance of developing squamous cell cancers (originating in the outer layer of the skin), particularly gynecological cancers (for females); head, neck and throat cancers; **gastrointestinal cancers**; and liver cancers.

Diagnosis

Diagnosis can be made upon the appearance of the characteristic congenital defects, but is more common upon development of aplastic anemia (when the bone marrow fails to produce normal numbers of blood cells). Definitive diagnosis involves a showing of an unusual level of chromosome breakage when cells are exposed to DNA damaging agents. Additionally, with five of the seven genes associated with FA isolated, genetic engineering techniques can often be used to determine exactly what gene mutation is responsible for the disease. An estimated 90% of FA patients have mutations within the FANCA, FANCC and FANCG genes, all of which have been isolated.

Treatment team

FA is usually treated by pediatricians, hematologists, and, if a bone marrow transplant (BMT) is performed, a specialized teams of physicians, nurses, and medical assistants who are experienced in BMT.

Treatment

BMT and androgen therapy are two long-term non-experimental treatments for FA. BMT involves the suppression of the patient's own marrow and replacement with stem cells of the donor. The effectiveness of BMT is highly dependent on the existence of a donor that is closely matched to the patient. For sibling match (full match) transplants, the two-year survival rate is about 80%, compared to about 37% for less than a full match. The difference is due the prevalence of graft versus host disease (GVHD), where the recipient's body rejects the donor cells. The use of T-cell (a type of immune cell) depletion before transplantation and the drug **fludarabine** have significantly reduced the occurrence of GVHD. BMT does not alter the tendency of FA patients to develop other malignancies later in life.

Androgen therapy involves the administration of male hormones to stimulate the production of blood cells. Most FA patients respond for at least some time to this therapy; however, the cell increase lasts a few years at most and the hormones have serious side effects, including masculinization of female patients and liver disease.

Clinical trials

Growth factor therapy and **gene therapy** are two treatments being tested in **clinical trials**. Two growth factors—granulocyte/macrophage colony stimulating factor (GM-CSF) and granulocyte colony stimulating factor (G-CSF)—were shown to increase blood cell production. Patients with low neutrophil counts particularly benefit from this treatment.

A clinical trial for gene therapy of FA patients is ongoing. The normal copy of the mutated gene is introduced into the patient's own bone marrow stem cells using a viral vector. When the virus infects the stem cells, the normal FANC gene is integrated into the stem cell's DNA. This therapy will—theoretically—correct the defect in the stem cells and prevent their premature death, curing the aplastic anemia seen in FA patients. As with BMT, however, this gene therapy will not reduce the development of other cancers in FA patients.

Prevention

The only known method of prevention of this disease is prenatal diagnosis and termination of pregnancies for affected embryos. Preimplantation genetic diagnosis, where one or two cells are tested from *in vitro* fertilized embryos, is also available. This method avoids the need for abortion, but carries more risk.

Special concerns

Because FA can be present without any outward symptoms, it is essential that any potential sibling donor for BMT be carefully tested for the disease using white blood cell exposure to DNA damaging agents or direct examination of their FANC gene copies before the transplant.

See also Bone marrow transplantation; Genetic testing.

Resources

PERIODICALS

Schneider, M., et al. "Fanconi Anaemia: Genetics, Molecular Biology, and Cancer: Implications for Clinical Management in Children and Adults." *Clinical Genetics* (October 2014): e-pub ahead of print. http://dx.doi.org/10.1111/cge.12517 (accessed November 3, 2014).

WEBSITES

National Heart, Lung, and Blood Institute. "What Is Fanconi Anemia?" http://www.nhlbi.nih.gov/health/health-topics/topics/fanconi (accessed November 3, 2014).

ORGANIZATIONS

Fanconi Anemia Research Fund, Inc., 1801 Willamette St., Ste. 200, Eugene, OR 97401, (541) 687-4658, 888-FANCONI (326-2664), info@fanconi.org, http://www.fanconi.org.

Michelle Johnson, M.S., J.D.

Fareston *see* **Toremifene**

Fatigue

Definition

Fatigue in the general population is a nonspecific symptom of tiredness or exhaustion. It is considered a subjective symptom in that it is reported by the patient rather than demonstrated by test results or laboratory findings. It is important to distinguish between normal or healthy fatigue, which is relieved by rest and sleep; and cancer-related fatigue, which can last for a long period of time, interferes with the patient's daily life, and is not relieved by rest or sleep. The term *chronic fatigue* is not useful in the context of **cancer** because it is easily confused with chronic fatigue syndrome, which is a condition unrelated to cancer. Health care professionals prefer to use the term *cancer fatigue* or *cancer-related fatigue* (CRF) when discussing the lack of energy and other symptoms of fatigue associated with cancer.

Description

Cancer-related fatigue (CRF) is a feeling of physical and psychological exhaustion or loss of strength. According to the American Cancer Society, CRF affects between 70% and 100% of cancer patients during their course of treatment. The duration of fatigue for a patient with cancer is generally one to two times the length of time between diagnosis and completion of treatment, so it is common for fatigue to persist beyond a patient's treatment regimen—although there are significant individual differences. Cancer-related fatigue or CRF also has emotional and cognitive dimensions, with 15% to 25% of cancer patients meeting the diagnostic criteria for **depression**. In regard to cognitive disturbances, many patients have memory lapses or difficulty paying attention as a side effect of **chemotherapy** or **radiation therapy**. This type of mental fatigue is sometimes called "chemo brain."

Causes

Many people experience fatigue as a side effect of cancer treatment. It is the single most common side effect in patients treated with chemotherapy, radiation therapy, or **biological response modifiers** (BRMs). Scientists believe fatigue also occurs because the body devotes so much of its energy to fighting the cancer that little remains for daily life. Often the feelings of CRF are more intense immediately following a chemotherapy treatment but gradually ease over time as strength returns. The pattern of CRF with radiation therapy is different, with patients typically reporting an increase in fatigue that reaches its peak about halfway through the course of therapy and remains until radiation therapy is completed.

In the course of chemotherapy, **anticancer drugs** kill both cancer cells and healthy cells, including red blood cells. This treatment can lead to **anemia**, or low red blood cell counts, which causes fatigue. Chemotherapy agents also attack white blood cells, weakening the immune system. Chemotherapy-induced anemia is the only medical cause of CRF that has been demonstrated through research as of 2014. Other physical causes that have been proposed include increased inflammatory activity affecting the immune system and changes in

the regulation of cortisol by the hypothalamic-pituitary-adrenal (HPA) axis.

Pain, poor nutrition resulting from nausea and loss of appetite, depression, sleep disorders, lack of exercise, hormonal changes, dehydration, infections, and the stress of the diagnosis and treatment also result in fatigue. Some cancer patients develop increased fatigue as the result of coexisting disorders, such as diabetes, arthritis, high blood pressure, asthma, or heart disease. Side effects of medication also contribute to CRF. These medications include antidepressants, **antiemetics**, pain relievers, steroids, antihistamines, beta blockers, antiseizure drugs, and sleeping medications.

Although a number of research studies on CRF in patients undergoing active treatment for cancer have been conducted in recent years, fatigue in cancer survivors (post-treatment fatigue) is poorly understood. While some survivors return to their pre-treatment levels of energy and activity, others suffer for months or years with ongoing fatigue that resembles the symptoms of chronic fatigue syndrome. Patients who received bone marrow transplants appear to be at particularly high risk for post-treatment fatigue, with 56% of transplant recipients in one study reporting chronic fatigue as long as 18 years after treatment. More research is necessary to better understand the mechanisms of fatigue in cancer survivors, since survivors often manage their own care and the late effects of treatment on their own.

Treatment

Before treating CRF, the patient's doctor may administer one or more quality-of-life instruments in order to measure the level of the patient's fatigue and identify its major contributing factors. Common assessment tools include the Brief Fatigue Inventory, the Piper Fatigue Scale, the Schwartz Cancer Fatigue Scale, and the Fatigue Symptom Inventory.

If blood tests indicate that the patient is anemic, or has a low red blood cell count, physicians may prescribe iron supplements or drugs such as erythropoietin to stimulate blood cell growth. In some cases, blood transfusions are necessary.

Many cancer patients find that they must pace themselves, alternating periods of activity with small naps and scheduling essential activities for the times of day when their energy level is highest. Earlier bed times seems to help. Patients with depression may find antidepressants or such psychostimulant medications as pemoline (Cylert), modafinil (Provigil), or **methylphenidate** (Concerta) helpful. Cognitive behavioral therapy (CBT) is a psychoeducational intervention that has been found helpful in relieving CRF associated with insomnia, fear of cancer recurrence, or dysfunctional beliefs about fatigue. If physical pain is the primary contributing factor to CRF, increased doses of pain medication may be prescribed.

Research indicates that physical exercise improves cancer-related fatigue. Walking, t'ai chi, yoga, or using an exercise bicycle are good choices. For those with severe weakness, even a few minutes of gentle stretching in bed can make a difference. A physical therapist can design an exercise program tailored to the individual patient's level of strength, flexibility, and endurance.

Eating nutritious food is another way to get an energy boost to better fight cancer. The patient's diet should include a variety of fruits and vegetables, whole grains and plenty of protein, as long as **nausea and vomiting** are not a problem. High-calorie liquid meals can help offset severe **weight loss** for those who cannot tolerate solid foods. Drinking plenty of water also helps prevent **diarrhea** and dehydration, which add to fatigue.

Patient education is an important aspect of treating CRF in cancer patients. Patients benefit from guidance in adjusting and adapting to their condition; some may need to confront the possibility that their fatigue may be a chronic, or ongoing. Cancer patients and their family members benefit from information about techniques of self-care and symptom management before CRF occurs. The effectiveness of specific interventions to manage fatigue should be monitored and evaluated on a regular basis so that they can be modified or changed if necessary.

When to call the doctor

It is normal for cancer patients to feel some fatigue as a result of the changes in their body caused by cancer treatments as well as by the cancer itself. Patients should, however, call their doctor at once if they notice any of the following symptoms, as they are not a normal part of CRF:

• shortness of breath or painful breathing

• dizziness

• severe mental confusion or disorientation

• inability to get out of bed that lasts 24 hours or longer

• loss of balance

• worsening of signs and symptoms associated with the cancer

Alternative and complementary therapies

Complementary and alternative (CAM) therapies are an increasingly popular part of supportive care for cancer patients with CRF. Movement therapies like yoga and t'ai chi have proven effective in reducing stress, thereby increasing energy and improving relaxation and sleep.

Marijuana has been used to help ease nausea in cancer patients. Since a loss of appetite can cause weakness and fatigue, marijuana may help indirectly. As of 2014, however, only some states permit the use of marijuana for medical reasons. Physicians will be aware of these regulations.

Treatment with American ginseng (*Panax quinquefolius*) was found to be helpful in relieving CRF in one Phase II trial conducted in 2013. The patients in the experimental group received capsules containing 2000 mg of ground ginseng root in a capsule form while those in the control group received a placebo. At the end of 8 weeks, the patients receiving the ginseng had significantly lower levels of fatigue with no side effects.

Such other complementary therapies as massage, aromatherapy, meditation, or prayer, help people with cancer relax, relieve muscle tension, and ultimately reduce fatigue. Patients may also benefit from such pleasurable activities as music therapy or art therapy. In addition, a growing number of cancer centers employ therapy animals for patients to hug, cuddle, or play with. Pet therapy has been shown to reduce the patients' blood pressure as well as provide companionship and comfort.

See also Complementary cancer therapies.

Resources

BOOKS

Matzo, Marianne, and Deborah Witt Sherman, eds. *Palliative Care Nursing: Quality Care to the End of Life*. 4th ed. New York: Springer, 2014.

Nathan, Neil, M.D. *Healing Is Possible: New Hope for Chronic Fatigue, Fibromyalgia, Persistent Pain, and Other Chronic Illnesses*. Laguna Beach, CA: Basic Health Publications, 2013.

Noggle, Chad A., and Raymond S. Dean, eds. *The Neuropsychology of Cancer and Oncology*. New York: Springer, 2013.

Preedy, Victor R., ed. *Diet and Nutrition in Palliative Care*. Boca Raton, FL: CRC Press, 2011.

PERIODICALS

Barton, D.L., et al. "Wisconsin Ginseng (*Panax quinquefolius*) to Improve Cancer-related Fatigue: A Randomized, Double-blind Trial, N07C2." *Journal of the National Cancer Institute* 105 (August 21, 2013): 1230–1236.

Bower, J.E. "Cancer-related Fatigue—Mechanisms, Risk Factors, and Treatments." *Nature Reviews. Clinical Oncology*, August 12, 2014. [E-publication ahead of print].

Foster, C., et al. "Cancer Survivors' Self-efficacy to Self-manage in the Year Following Primary Treatment." *Journal of Cancer Survivorship*, July 16, 2014 [E-publication ahead of print].

Garland, S.N., et al. "Sleeping Well with Cancer: A Systematic Review of Cognitive Behavioral Therapy for Insomnia in Cancer Patients." *Neuropsychiatric Disease and Treatment* 10 (June 18, 2014): 1113–1124.

Hoffman, A.J., et al. "Home-based Exercise: Promising Rehabilitation for Symptom Relief, Improved Functional Status and Quality of Life for Post-surgical Lung Cancer Patients." *Journal of Thoracic Disease* 6 (June 2014): 632–640.

Krigel, S., et al. "'Cancer Changes Everything!' Exploring the Lived Experiences of Women with Metastatic Breast Cancer." *International Journal of Palliative Nursing* 20 (July 2014): 334–342.

Reeve, B.B., et al. "The Piper Fatigue Scale-12 (PFS-12): Psychometric Findings and Item Reduction in a Cohort of Breast Cancer Survivors." *Breast Cancer Research and Treatment* 136 (November 2012): 9–20.

Stubbs, C.E., and M. Valero. "Complementary Strategies for the Management of Radiation Therapy Side Effects." *Journal of the Advanced Practitioner in Oncology* 4 (July 2013): 219–231.

Wright, F., et al. "Associations between Multiple Chronic Conditions and Cancer-related Fatigue: An Integrative Review." *Oncology Nursing Forum* 41 (July 1, 2014): 399–410.

WEBSITES

American Cancer Society (ACS). "Fatigue in People with Cancer." http://www.cancer.org/acs/groups/cid/documents/webcontent/002842-pdf.pdf (accessed August 18, 2014).

Cancer.Net. "Fatigue." http://www.cancer.net/navigating-cancer-care/side-effects/fatigue (accessed August 19, 2014).

Mayo Clinic. "Cancer Fatigue: Why It Occurs and How to Cope." http://www.mayoclinic.org/diseases-conditions/cancer/in-depth/cancer-fatigue/ART-20047709 (accessed August 19, 2014).

National Cancer Institute (NCI). "Fatigue (PDQ)." http://www.cancer.gov/cancertopics/pdq/supportivecare/fatigue/HealthProfessional/page1/AllPages (accessed August 18, 2014).

Seidman Cancer Center. "Pet Therapy." http://www.uhhospitals.org/seidman/services/supportive-oncology/our-services/integrative-oncology-services/pet-therapy (accessed August 20, 2014).

ORGANIZATIONS

American Cancer Society (ACS), 250 Williams Street NW, Atlanta, GA 30303, (800) 227-2345, http://www.cancer.org/aboutus/howwehelpyou/app/contact-us.aspx, http://www.cancer.org/index.

American Society of Clinical Oncology (ASCO), 2318 Mill Road, Suite 800, Alexandria, VA 22314, (571) 483-1300, (888) 651-3038, Fax: (571) 366-9537, contactus@cancer.net, http://www.asco.org.

National Cancer Institute (NCI), BG 9609 MSC 9760, 9609 Medical Center Drive, Bethesda, MD 20892-9760, (800) 4-CANCER (422-6237), http://www.cancer.gov/global/contact/email-us, http://www.cancer.gov.

Food and Drug Administration (FDA), 10903 New Hampshire Avenue, Silver Spring, MD 20993, (888) INFO-FDA (463-6332), http://www.fda.gov/AboutFDA/ContactFDA/default.htm, http://www.fda.gov/default.htm.

Melissa Knopper, M.S.

REVISED BY REBECCA J. FREY, PHD.

Fecal occult blood test

Definition

The fecal occult blood test (FOBT) is performed as part of the routine physical examination during the examination of the rectum. It is used to detect microscopic blood in the stool and is a screening tool for colorectal **cancer**.

Purpose

FOBT uses chemical indicators on stool samples to detect the presence of blood not otherwise visible—the word "occult" in the test's name means that the blood is hidden from view. Blood originating from or passing through the gastrointestinal tract can signal many conditions requiring further diagnostic procedures and, possibly, medical treatment. These conditions may be benign or malignant and some of them include:

• colon, rectal, and gastric (stomach) cancers

• ulcers

• hemorrhoids

• polyps

• inflammatory bowel disease

• irritations or lesions of the gastrointestinal tract caused by medications, such as nonsteroidal anti-inflammatory drugs, also called NSAIDs

• irritations or lesions of the gastrointestinal tract caused by stomach acid disorders, such as reflux esophagitis

The FOBT is used routinely—in conjunction with a rectal examination performed by a physician—to screen for colorectal cancer, particularly after age 50. The ordering of this test should not be taken as an indication that cancer is suspected. The FOBT must be combined with regular screening endoscopy, such as a **sigmoidoscopy**, to detect cancers at an early stage.

Precautions

Certain foods and medicines can influence the test results. Some fruits contain chemicals that prevent the guaiac, the chemical in which the test paper is soaked, from reacting with the blood. Aspirin and some NSAIDs irritate the stomach, resulting in bleeding, and should be avoided prior to the examination. Red meat and many vegetables and fruits containing vitamin C also should be avoided for a specified period of time prior to the test. All of these factors could result in a false-positive result.

QUESTIONS TO ASK YOUR DOCTOR

• What kinds of foods should I avoid prior to the FOBT?

• How much stool should I collect for the stool samples?

• What is the next step if my test is positive?

Description

Feces for the stool samples is obtained either by the physician at the rectal examination or by the patient at home, using a small spatula or a collection device. In most cases, the collection of stool samples can easily be done at home, using a kit supplied by the physician. The standard kit contains a specially prepared card on which a small sample of stool will be spread, using a stick provided in the kit. The sample is placed in a special envelope and either mailed or brought in for analysis. When the physician applies hydrogen peroxide to the back of the sample, the paper will turn blue if an abnormal amount of blood is present.

Types of fecal occult blood tests

Hemoccult is the most commonly used fecal occult blood test. The Hemoccult test takes less than five minutes to perform and may be performed in the physician's office or in the laboratory. The Hemoccult blood test can detect bleeding from the colon as low as 0.5 mg per day.

Tests that use anti-hemoglobin antibodies—or immunochemical tests—to detect blood in the stool are also used. Immunochemical tests can detect up to 0.7 mg of hemoglobin in the stool and do not require dietary restrictions. Immunochemical tests

• are not accurate for screening for stomach cancer

• are more sensitive than Hemoccult tests in detecting colorectal cancer

• are more expensive than Hemoccult tests

Hemoquant, another fecal occult blood test, is used to detect as much as 500 mg/g of blood in the stool. Like the Hemoccult, the Hemoquant test is affected by red meat. It is not affected by chemicals in vegetables.

Fecal blood may also be measured by the amount of chromium in the red blood cells in the feces. The stool is collected for three to ten days. The test is used in cases where the exact amount of blood loss is required. It is the only test that can exclude blood loss from the gastrointestinal area with accuracy.

Medicare coverage began on January 1, 2004, for a newer fecal occult blood test based on immunoassay. This technique does not rely on guiaic, so it is not influenced by diet or medications used prior to the test. The immunoassay test also requires fewer specimen collections. At a conference of gastroenterologists—physicians who specialize in diseases of the stomach and related digestive systems—a company announced a new fecal occult blood test that was based on DNA and appeared more sensitive than traditional tests. Widespread use of these new tests remains to be seen; the traditional guiaic test has been in place for about 30 years.

Preparation

For 72 hours prior to collecting samples, patients should avoid red meats, NSAIDs (including aspirin), antacids, steroids, iron supplements, and vitamin C, including citrus fruits and other foods containing large amounts of vitamin C. Foods like uncooked broccoli, uncooked turnips, cauliflower, uncooked cantaloupe, uncooked radish, horseradish, and parsnips should be avoided and not eaten during the 72 hours prior to the examination. Fish, chicken, pork, fruits (other than melons) and many cooked vegetables are permitted in the diet.

Results

Many factors can result in false-positive and false-negative findings.

Positive results

It is important to note that a true-positive finding only signifies the presence of blood—it is not an indication of cancer. The **National Cancer Institute** states that, in its experience, less than 10% of all positive results were caused by cancer. The FOBT is positive in 1%–5% of the unscreened population and 2%–10% of those are found to have cancer. The physician will want to follow up on a positive result with further tests, as indicated by other factors in the patient's history or condition.

Negative results

Alternatively, a negative result—meaning no blood was detected—does not guarantee the absence of **colon** cancer, which may bleed only occasionally or not at all. Only 50% of colon cancers are FOBT-positive.

Conclusions

Screening using the FOBT has been demonstrated to reduce colorectal cancer. However, because only half of colorectal cancers are FOBT-positive, FOBT must be combined with regular screening endoscopy to increase the detection of pre-malignant colorectal polyps and cancers.

Resources

WEBSITES

Mayo Clinic staff. "Fecal Occult Blood Test." http://www.mayoclinic.org/tests-procedures/fecal-occult-blood-test/basics/definition/prc-20014429 (accessed December 4, 2014).

ORGANIZATIONS

American Association for Clinical Chemistry, 1850 K St. NW, Ste. 625, Washington, DC 20006, (800) 892-1400, Fax: (202) 887-5093, custserv@aacc.org, http://www.aacc.org.

American Cancer Society, 250 Williams St. NW, Atlanta, GA 30303, (800) 227-2345, http://www.cancer.org.

National Cancer Institute, 9609 Medical Center Dr., BG 9609 MSC 9760, Bethesda, MD 20892-9760, (800) 4-CANCER (422-6237), http://www.cancer.gov.

Jill S. Lasker
Cheryl Branche, MD

Fentanyl *see* **Opioids**

Fentanyl transdermal *see* **Opioids**

Fertility issues

Overview

Any procedure or medication that interferes with the functioning of the testes or ovaries affects fertility. The choices made before **cancer** treatment begins can determine whether the patient will remain fertile after treatment. Prior to deciding on a treatment plan, it is important for the patient to discuss the issue of fertility with the treatment team so that all options, with their associated risks, can be considered.

Conventional cancer treatments and their effects on fertility

Cancer is usually treated with surgery, **chemotherapy**, and/or radiation, with the type and stage of the cancer dictating the treatment regimen recommended. While some physicians may routinely take into consideration alternatives to spare a patient's fertility, others may not, feeling that to differ from the treatment norm may compromise the patient's best chances for survival. Patients for whom fertility preservation is important, or for whom fertility-sparing measures could compromise treatment outcome, must discuss this issue fully with their treatment team.

Surgery

Surgery for cancer usually involves removal of the cancerous area, with some sampling of the adjacent area and lymph nodes to check for **metastasis**. If surgery must involve the removal of both of the testes or ovaries, the man will not be able to provide his own sperm, and the woman her own egg, towards the development of a biological child; however, a couple may be able to use donated sperm or egg when attempting a future pregnancy. Fertility-sparing surgery may be an option for some individuals, depending on the type and stage of their cancer. For example, a woman with **ovarian cancer** contained to one ovary may be able to have just that one removed. The same is true for a man with **testicular cancer** contained to one testicle. In the case of testicular cancer, removal of retroperitoneal lymph nodes during surgery may damage the nerves affecting ejaculation. Men may wish to discuss nerve-sparing surgery and their concerns for fertility with their surgeon prior to surgery.

Chemotherapy

Chemotherapy affects the whole body, but certain drugs are less harmful to the reproductive tract than others. The drugs used in chemotherapy are highly toxic, in order to kill any cancer cell. However, they are not very selective, meaning that in addition to cancerous cells, normal cells are killed as well. It may take a few years after chemotherapy has finished to understand its temporary or permanent effect on fertility. It is generally recommended that women wait about two years after chemotherapy before attempting to become pregnant to avoid the risk of a pregnancy that may end in miscarriage or a fetal malformation. Men who have had chemotherapy can have their sperm analyzed after treatment has finished to check sperm counts and motility.

There is a concern that individuals may delay treatment in order to undergo various fertility-preserving measures, such as sperm banking or egg retrieval and cryopreservation, and that this delay could result in a poorer treatment outcome. Some women undergo attempts at egg retrieval and embryo cryopreservation after an initial dose of chemotherapy. Some treatment centers offer the option of doing the chemotherapy in

---

Chemotherapy drugs associated with fertility issues

- Busulfan (Myleran, Busulfex)
- Carmustine (BCNU, BiCNU)
- Chlorambucil (Leukeran)
- Cisplatin (Platinol, CDDP)
- Cyclophosphamide (Cytoxan, Neosar, CTX)
- Cytarabine (Ara-C, Cytosar-U)
- Ifosfamide (Ifex, Isophosphamide)
- Lomustine (CCNU, CeeNU)
- Mechlorethamine (Mustine)
- Melphalan (L-Phenylalanine Mustard, L-PAM, Alkeran, L-Sarcolysin)
- Nitrosoureas (streptozocin)
- Procarbazine (Matulane)
- Vinblastine (Velban, Velbe, Velsa)

SOURCE: National Cancer Institute, "Sexuality and Reproductive Issues (PDQ®): Fertility Issues," http://www.cancer.gov/cancertopics/pdq/supportivecare/sexuality/HealthProfessional/page6.

Table listing chemotherapy drugs associated with fertility issues. (Table by Lumina Datamatics Ltd. © 2015 Cengage Learning®.)

stages. The first stage of chemotherapy uses medications that are considered less toxic. Then the more intensive treatment follows after the harvesting of egg or sperm. However, it is still not yet clear what kind of damage may have been endured by tissue harvested right after some chemotherapy.

Radiation

Radiation is known to damage the highly sensitive sperm and eggs. Just as chemotherapy attacks healthy cells, so does radiation; however, radiation technology is able to focus very tightly on the cancerous area, which decreases risk to healthy tissue. When radiation for cancer does not involve the pelvic area, it may be possible to successfully shield the reproductive organs to preserve fertility. If the area needing irradiation is the pelvis, the reproductive organs are at great risk of damage.

When radiation is done to the pelvic area, women often experience a pause in menstruation, along with other symptoms of menopause. There may also be vaginal dryness, **itching**, and burning. Radiation may affect sexual desire as well. Men may experience a decrease in sperm count and motility, and difficulty in having or maintaining an erection. These changes may be temporary or permanent, and it may take up to a few years to determine if the effects were temporary or permanent. Sperm banking or cryopreservation of eggs may allow the individual reproductive success in the future.

Since radiation can be harmful to the fetus, pregnancy during **radiation therapy** is contraindicated, and because the full effect of the radiation on fertility

QUESTIONS TO ASK YOUR DOCTOR

- What is the type and stage of my cancer?
- What treatment options do I have that would retain my fertility?
- Is my survival compromised if I choose fertility-sparing treatment?
- Would the health of future child/children be compromised if I undergo this treatment?
- Can you provide me with research studies of others who had this treatment and went on to have children?
- How long should I wait after treatment before attempting a pregnancy?
- If treatment is successful, what can I expect in terms of survival and quality of life?
- If treatment is unsuccessful, what can I expect in terms of survival and quality of life?
- What is the type and stage of my child's cancer?
- Does the treatment of this cancer have a risk of developing another cancer later on?
- How will this treatment affect my child's development during puberty?
- What effect will this treatment have on my child's future fertility?

cannot be predicted, individuals should use contraception during sexual relations while receiving radiation therapy.

Bone marrow transplant

A bone marrow transplant (BMT) may be part of the suggested treatment regimen. If so, patients need to understand its potential impact on future fertility. While the actual BMT does not jeopardize fertility, chemotherapy or radiation done prior to the BMT in preparation for the body's receiving of the new marrow can damage fertility. This pretreatment can destroy cells in the reproductive organs, rendering the individual infertile. While each case is unique, patients may wish to discuss the impact of their treatment on their reproductive future, and consider sperm banking or egg cryopreservation.

Alternative and complementary therapies

Individuals undergoing cancer treatment may turn to alternative therapies for a number of reasons.

Techniques such as meditation, therapeutic touch, yoga, t'ai chi, and guided imagery can be very helpful in reducing stress and its effects on the body. Acupuncture has been shown through research studies to be effective in reducing the **nausea and vomiting** associated with chemotherapy. A study reported in the March 1999 issue of the medical journal *Fertility and Sterility* investigated several herbal remedies and their effect on sperm and ova. While this study was involved in animal research, the finding that high concentrations of St. John's wort—an herbal supplement used for mild to moderate **depression**—Echinacea, and ginkgo biloba damaged reproductive cells raised concern for its effect on humans. In particular, St. John's wort was found to be mutagenic to sperm cells.

Children's cancers and future fertility

In the case of children, chemotherapy and radiation for childhood cancer can cause permanent damage to the ovaries or testes. In boys who have become sexually mature, sperm banking may provide future reproductive options. Options such as sperm aspiration, and cryopreservation of female ova are still considered experimental in children. While they may be effective, researchers are concerned that parents and their children may be unrealistic in their hopes for future fertility, and that the reintroduction of the harvested tissue may return latent cancer cells into the body. While research may bring new options, obtaining true informed consent involving children and their parents is an issue of moral and practical concern.

Special concerns

Some cancers, such as testicular cancer, affect primarily young men. Most men diagnosed with testicular cancer are between the ages of 15 and 40. Sperm banking is highly recommended for these men. The method intracytoplasmic sperm injection uses just one sperm to fertilize one egg by injecting the sperm directly into the egg. This can result in a fertilized egg for insemination, even when the sperm has decreased motility. It has a success rate of 30%.

Fertility issues and the development of cancer

Fertility issues can also play a role in the development of cancer. For example, women having their first child after 30 are at slightly higher risk of developing ovarian cancer than those having their first child before age 30. The number of ovulatory cycles a woman experiences also appears to affect her risk for ovarian cancer. A longer reproductive period—meaning early menarche and late menopause—appears to raise the risk. Conversely, having children, since there is no ovulation during pregnancy; breastfeeding, because of some suppression of ovulation during breastfeeding; and the use of oral contraceptives for at least five years decreases the risk of developing ovarian cancer.

Women who used the infertility medication clomiphene citrate without becoming pregnant were found in some studies to have a greater risk of developing a low malignancy potential ovarian cancer. In a November 1999 issue of the medical journal *Lancet*, researchers reported that women whose infertility remained unexplained were found to have more ovarian and uterine cancers, irrespective of whether or not they had been treated for the infertility. Also, more breast cancers were detected in the first year after treatment for infertility terminated than was expected. The lead author of the study speculated that these cancer diagnoses may be due to closer medical supervision that resulted in early detection. In some cases it was believed that the infertility was a symptom of the undiagnosed cancer.

Resources

PERIODICALS

Munch, Joe. "Addressing Fertility Issues in Cancer Patients." *OncoLog* 59, no. 1 (2014). http://www2.mdanderson.org/depts/oncolog/articles/14/1-jan/1-14-1.html (accessed December 4, 2014).

WEBSITES

Breastcancer.org. "Fertility Issues." http://www.breastcancer.org/treatment/side_effects/fertility_issues (accessed December 4, 2014).

National Cancer Institute. "Fertility Issues." http://www.cancer.gov/cancertopics/pdq/supportivecare/sexuality/Patient/page5 (accessed December 4, 2014).

ORGANIZATIONS

American Cancer Society, 250 Williams St. NW, Atlanta GA 30303, (800) 227-2345, http://www.cancer.org.

Esther Csapo Rastegari, R.N., B.S.N., Ed.M.

Fever

Definition

Fever is a condition in which the body's temperature rises above its normal thermoregulatory set point, usually by about 1.8°F to 3.6°F (1°C to 2°C). It is also known as pyrexia. Fever is sometimes categorized as a form of **hyperthermia**—any elevation of body temperature above normal—but it is distinguished from hyperthermia

caused by exposure to heat from the environment. The latter condition represents a failure of thermoregulation; that is, the body absorbs or produces more heat than it can dissipate. Fever, on the other hand, represents the immune system's response to an internal threat, usually a disease organism. The role of fever in the body's response to disease was first understood and described by a German physician named Carl Wunderlich (1815–1877) in a report published in 1868.

Demographics

Fever is an extremely common condition worldwide. Almost all children have at least one febrile illness during childhood, and many adults have low-grade fevers with such widespread illnesses as the common cold. According to one estimate, as many as 11% of adults who travel abroad return home with a febrile illness, usually an upper respiratory infection or community-acquired **pneumonia**.

Description

A healthy person's body temperature fluctuates between 97 °F (36.1 °C) and 100 °F (37.8 °C), with the average being 98.6 °F (37 °C). The body maintains stability within this range by balancing the heat produced by the metabolism with the heat lost to the environment. Body temperature in humans also varies according to the time of day as well as from individual to individual. Early morning body temperature may be as low as 97°F, and as high as 99.3°F in the afternoon hours, yet still be considered normal.

It is also important to note that normal human body temperature varies somewhat in different locations in the body. Depending on where a thermometer is inserted, fever can be defined as:

• Rectal: a temperature above 100°F (37.8°C).

• Oral: a temperature above 99.5°F (37.5°C).

• Armpit: a temperature at or above 99°F (37.2°C).

• Ear: a temperature at or above 99°F (37.2°C).

The set point or "thermostat" that controls this process is located in the hypothalamus, a small structure located deep within the brain just above the brain stem. The nervous system constantly relays information about the body's temperature to the thermostat, which in turn activates different physical responses designed to cool or warm the body, depending on the circumstances. These responses include: decreasing or increasing the flow of blood from the body's core, where it is warmed, to the surface, where it is cooled; slowing down or speeding up the rate at which the body turns food into energy (metabolic rate); inducing shivering, which generates heat through muscle contraction; and inducing sweating, which cools the body through evaporation.

A fever occurs when the thermostat resets at a higher temperature, primarily in response to an infection. To reach the higher temperature, the body moves blood to the warmer interior, increases the metabolic rate, and induces shivering. The chills that often accompany a fever are caused by the movement of blood to the body's core, leaving the surface and extremities cold. Once the higher temperature is achieved, the shivering and chills stop. When the infection has been overcome or such drugs as aspirin or acetaminophen (Tylenol) have been taken, the thermostat resets to normal and the body's cooling mechanisms switch on: the blood moves to the surface and sweating occurs.

Fever is an important component of the **immune response**, though its role is not completely understood. Physicians believe that an elevated body temperature has several effects. The immune system chemicals that react with the fever-inducing agent and trigger the resetting of the thermostat also increase the production of cells that fight off the invading bacteria or viruses. Higher temperatures also inhibit the growth of some bacteria, while at the same time speeding up the chemical reactions that help the body's cells repair themselves. In addition, the increased heart rate that may accompany the changes in blood circulation also speeds the arrival of white blood cells to the sites of infection.

How long a fever lasts and how high it may go depends on several factors, including its cause, the age of the patient, and his or her overall health. Most fevers caused by infections are acute, appearing suddenly and then resolving as the immune system defeats the infectious agent. An infectious fever may also rise and fall throughout the day, reaching its peak in the late afternoon or early evening. A low-grade fever that lasts for several weeks is associated with such autoimmune diseases as lupus or rheumatoid arthritis, or with some cancers, particularly leukemia and **lymphoma**.

It is important to note that the degree of a fever in an adolescent or adult does not necessarily reflect the seriousness of the underlying cause. It is possible for relatively minor illnesses to produce high fevers and for serious conditions to produce relatively low fevers.

Risk factors

Risk factors for fever include:

- Living or working in close contact with others with febrile illnesses, particularly small children.

- Having a weakened immune system.

- Frequent travel abroad, particularly to countries with poor sanitation, high rates of malaria, and high rates of other febrile illnesses.

- Being treated for cancer.

- Being hospitalized for any illness or injury. Many people contract pneumonia or other febrile illnesses during a hospital stay.

- Having an autoimmune disorder.

- Having Parkinson's disease or other severe neurological disorder.

Causes and symptoms

Causes

Fevers in the general population are primarily caused by viral or bacterial infections, such as pneumonia or influenza. Other conditions can also induce a fever, including allergic reactions; autoimmune diseases; trauma, such as breaking a bone; **cancer**; excessive exposure to the sun; intense exercise; hormonal imbalances; certain drugs; and damage to the hypothalamus. When an infection occurs, fever-inducing agents called pyrogens are released, either by the body's immune system or by the invading cells themselves, that trigger the resetting of the thermostat. In other circumstances, the immune system may overreact (allergic reactions) or become damaged (autoimmune diseases), causing the uncontrolled release of pyrogens. A stroke or tumor can damage the hypothalamus, causing the body's thermostat to malfunction. Malignant hyperthermia is a rare inherited condition in which a person develops a very high fever when given certain anesthetics or muscle relaxants in preparation for surgery.

Fever associated with cancer can generally be categorized into four major causal groups: infection, tumors, allergic reactions to a drug, or allergic reaction to blood components in transfusion therapies. For cancer patients, fever should be considered a result of infection until an alternative cause is diagnosed. When a fever develops in a cancer patient, the individual must be thoroughly examined to determine the cause. A comprehensive physical examination should be administered by the physician and blood drawn for laboratory analysis.

Symptoms

The most common symptoms of fever in addition to a high temperature include:

- sweating
- shivering

- headache
- muscle cramps or aches
- loss of appetite
- thirst/dehydration
- general feeling of tiredness and weakness

Symptoms that may appear with high fevers (103°F to 106°F; 39.4°C to 41.1°C):

- mental confusion
- hallucinations
- irritability
- seizures or convulsions

SYMPTOMS REQUIRING EMERGENCY TREATMENT. A fever requires emergency treatment under the following circumstances:

- newborn (three months or younger) with a fever over 100.5 °F (38 °C)
- infant or child with a fever over 103 °F (39.4 °C)
- fever accompanied by severe headache, neck stiffness, mental confusion, or severe swelling of the throat
- hyperpyrexia: fever at or over 105°F (41°C) in anyone
- the fever has lasted three days or longer
- unusual skin rash
- inability to swallow or take liquids by mouth
- unusual sensitivity to bright light
- persistent vomiting
- difficulty breathing or chest pain
- abdominal pain or pain when urinating

A very high fever in a small child can trigger seizures (febrile seizures) and therefore should be treated immediately. A fever accompanied by the above symptoms can indicate the presence of a serious infection, such as meningitis, and should be brought to the immediate attention of a physician.

FEVER IN CHILDREN. Children's temperatures are generally higher than those of adults and fluctuate more widely. They may vary depending on the time of day, the child's emotional state or level of physical activity, the amount of clothing worn, or the surrounding room temperature. In general, temperatures under 100°F (37.7°C) are considered subfebrile (i.e., not indicating fever). Rectal temperatures of up to 100.4°F (38°C) may be considered normal.

A child's temperature can be taken in several ways. Rectal temperatures are about one-half a degree higher than oral ones. A rectal reading is considered more accurate than an oral one, which may be affected by previously eaten hot or cold foods or by a child's

breathing. Underarm temperatures are considered reliable for young infants, and electronic thermometers can measure temperature through the ear. Although fever is generally a cause for concern among parents, high fevers are not necessarily a sign of serious illness. A mild cold may produce a fever as high as 105°F (40.5°C), while the fever accompanying pneumonia may only be 100°F (37.7°C). The temperatures of newborn infants are particularly unreliable because the baby's temperature control mechanism is not yet adequately developed.

Diagnosis

A fever is usually diagnosed using a thermometer. A variety of different thermometers are available, including traditional glass and mercury ones used for oral or rectal temperature readings and more sophisticated electronic ones that can be inserted in the ear to quickly register the body's temperature. For adults and older children, temperature readings are usually taken orally. Younger children who cannot or will not hold a thermometer in their mouths can have their temperature taken by placing an oral thermometer under their armpit. Infants generally have their temperature taken rectally using a rectal thermometer.

Examination

The cause of fever in adults or adolescents is generally diagnosed during an office visit by a careful patient history including recent travel, a history of autoimmune disorders, recent immunizations, or exposure to persons with contagious illnesses, and taking the patient's vital signs—temperature, pulse, breathing rate, and blood pressure. The doctor will examine the inside of the patient's mouth and throat for signs of an infectious illness, and may swab the patient's throat to obtain a sample for culture.

In terms of office visits for children, most experts agree that a doctor should be notified immediately when fever appears in an infant under the age of eight weeks. Children at this age are susceptible to serious, even life-threatening, infections that can come on suddenly and need immediate attention. For children up to the age of three years, a doctor should be notified of any fever over 103°F (39.4°C). In older children, a fever of 105°F (40.5°C) or over requires prompt medical attention, as does any fever that lasts longer than four or five days. Medical attention should also be sought for any fever accompanied by unusual irritability or sleepiness, listlessness, pain, a stiff neck, difficulty breathing, reduced urination, or any other symptoms that arouse suspicion.

Tests

Blood tests can aid in identifying an infectious agent by detecting the presence of antibodies against it or providing samples for growth of the organism in a culture. Blood tests can also provide the doctor with white blood cell counts. A urine sample may be collected for testing if the patient's fever is related to a urinary tract infection. A stool sample may be taken if the doctor suspects intestinal parasites or gastrointestinal bleeding. Ultrasound tests, **magnetic resonance imaging** (MRI) tests, or **computed tomography** (CT) scans may be ordered if the doctor cannot readily determine the cause of a fever.

Treatment

Traditional

Most cases of fever are treated with medications of one type or another, at least initially.

Drugs

Physicians agree that the most effective treatment for a fever is to address its underlying cause, such as through the administration of **antibiotics**. Antibiotics are usually given to treat fevers related to ear infections, urinary tract infections, and other illnesses caused by bacteria. Because a fever helps the immune system fight infection, it usually should be allowed to run its course.

Drugs to lower fever (antipyretics) can be given if a patient (particularly a child) is uncomfortable. These include aspirin, acetaminophen (Tylenol), and ibuprofen (Advil). Bathing a patient in cool water can also help alleviate a high fever.

DRUGS IN CHILDREN. Although fevers in children are generally not dangerous, they are treated because they cause discomfort and can prevent children from getting the sleep and nourishment they need in order to get well. Aspirin was the medication most commonly used to lower fevers until 1980, when researchers found that the use of aspirin to treat children's fevers caused by influenza and chicken pox was associated with Reye's syndrome, a dangerous condition that causes liver impairment and brain damage and can result in coma and eventual death. Since then, acetaminophen (sold under such brand names as Tylenol) has become the most widely recommended drug for treating fever in children. Acetaminophen, which is available in liquid form, tablets, and capsules for oral use, and as suppositories, is effective in treating fever but does not share aspirin's inflammation-reducing properties.

Ibuprofen (Advil, Motrin, etc.) is an effective fever reducer that is also an anti-inflammatory agent; however, it has been known to produce allergic and gastrointestinal side effects. Studies have shown that ibuprofen can be more effective than acetaminophen in reducing fever in children, but it does have more potential side effects. This fact has led some physicians to recommend alternating the two drugs for the best effect. Parents can give the drugs every four to six hours over three days; this dosage pattern has been shown to be more effective in lowering fever in infants and children than using either drug alone. Doctors caution, however, that parents may become confused when alternating the medicines and accidentally miss a dose or give the child an extra dose.

Children's fever can also be reduced one or two degrees by sponging the child with room-temperature water (about 70°F [21°C]) while he or she sits in a tub filled with water up to waist level.

FEVER IN CANCER PATIENTS. Once a diagnosis has been made and treatment initiated, it is important to address problems created by the fever itself. It may be necessary to increase fluids and nutritional supplements. Because fever places increased demands on the body, this can be critical in restoring normal health for patients who may already be nutritionally compromised. Fever in a patient with **neutropenia** (low white blood cell count) represents the potential for a critical, life-threatening situation, and treatment should begin as quickly as the patient can reach the emergency room.

Physicians do not fully understand how tumors can cause fever, but certain correlations are well documented. Fever spikes may indicate that a tumor has grown or spread to other areas of the body, or that the tumor has produced some type of blockage. The fever associated with a tumor tends to be cyclic, and subsides with tumor treatment and recurs when the tumor returns or increases in size. In the case of drug-associated fever, the fever is an allergic-type reaction to a particular medication or combination of medications. Similarly, an immune response to donor blood cells is the typical cause of fever associated with blood components.

Each of the major causes for fever associated with cancer has recommended conventional treatment procedures. For infection-related fever, broad-spectrum antibiotics, given orally, rectally, or intravenously, are the principle method of control. Some antibiotics may be started before a definitive diagnosis is made to retard additional complications caused by the infection. Treatment typically is administered for five to seven days as long as the fever and infection show a positive response.

Fever from a tumor is best treated by treating the tumor itself. Supplemental treatment for the fever may include the use of **nonsteroidal anti-inflammatory drugs** (NSAIDs) and acetaminophen. Aspirin should only be used in patients with no risk of bleeding problems. The allergic responses manifesting in drug- or blood-associated fever may be treated by various methods: antihistamines and acetaminophen may be administered prior to drug therapy or blood **transfusion therapy**; discontinuing the present drug and choosing alternate medication may be required; blood may require irradiation or removal of white blood cells from the donor blood.

Alternative

There are several different types of alternative approaches to fever:

- Herbal remedies: Western herbalists commonly recommend teas or tinctures made from catnip, yarrow, feverfew, sage, wormwood, and chamomile. These herbs and preparations made from them are sometimes referred to as febrifuges, from two Latin words that mean "to drive away fever."

- Homeopathy: Homeopathic practitioners usually recommend *Aconite* or *Belladonna* for fevers that come on suddenly; *Pulsatilla* for patients with symptoms of a cold or ear infection related to the fever; *Ferrum phos.* for fever accompanied by a severe cough; and *Nux vomica* for fevers associated with gastrointestinal symptoms, heavy drinking, or the use of recreational drugs.

- Naturopathy: Naturopaths generally regard fever as one of the body's self-regulatory mechanisms. They usually prescribe treatment of the underlying cause of the fever along with self-care at home and extra vitamin or mineral supplements to support the body's immune system, rather than drugs or medications intended to suppress the fever.

- Traditional Chinese medicine (TCM): Practitioners of TCM distinguish between fever caused by disease organisms, fever related to menstruation in women, and fever caused by disorders of the blood or the internal organs (including cancer). There are a number of different herbal remedies prescribed according to the type of condition and its severity. Unlike Western herbal formulations, which tend to be based on a single herb, traditional Chinese medicines typically contain five or more ingredients. In addition to a traditional medicine, the practitioner of TCM will also usually recommend acupuncture, changes in the patient's diet, and in some cases a form of massage known as *tui na*.

- Ayurveda: Practitioners of Ayurveda, the traditional medical system of India, typically regard fever as caused by external infections, disorders of the internal organs, or an imbalance in the three energetic principles within humans known as doshas. To treat fever, an Ayurvedic practitioner may recommend herbal remedies (cumin seeds, coriander, turmeric, or ginger), abstention from sexual activity as well as heavy meals or exercise, and mild sweating. Sweating in Ayurvedic practice is done by covering the patient with a light blanket for 10–20 minutes and giving him or her a hot beverage to drink made from a mixture of raisins and ginger.

- Native American: traditional Native American healers typically boiled fever wort, dogwood, or willow tree bark in water and gave the resulting liquid to the patient to drink. Willow was most commonly used by tribes living in the southern or western parts of North America, while dogwood was used in the Northeast.

Some cancer patients are investigating and adhering to the use of alternative treatments and complementary therapies. These choices may include holistic healing and therapy utilizing biofeedback, relaxation therapy, prayer and meditation, and imagery techniques. Still other complementary therapies include pet therapy, humor therapy, art therapy, and journaling. Patients maintain that these alternative and complementary therapies add a sense of control to their life during a period when they have little control over anything. No conclusive data exists on the effectiveness of the therapies used alone; however, in conjunction with conventional methods of fever management, they do not appear to hinder mainstream therapy and may provide the patient increased goodwill and a positive outlook.

Prognosis

Most fevers caused by infection end as soon as the immune system rids the body of the pathogen and do not produce any lasting effects. The prognosis for fevers associated with such chronic conditions as autoimmune disease depends upon the overall outcome of the disorder. Hyperpyrexia caused by sepsis or other severe infections has a guarded prognosis.

Prevention

The most effective way to prevent fever is to avoid exposure to infectious diseases, follow proper techniques for food storage and preparation, maintain good personal hygiene, and wash the hands frequently.

Resources

BOOKS

Goroll, Allan H., and Albert G. Mulley Jr., eds. *Primary Care Medicine: Office Evaluation and Management of the Adult Patient.* 6th ed. Philadelphia : Wolters Kluwer Health/ Lippincott Williams and Wilkins, 2009.

Landau, Elaine. *Fever.* New York: Marshall Cavendish Benchmark, 2010.

Porter, Robert S., ed. *The Merck Manual of Patient Symptoms: A Concise, Practical Guide to Etiology, Evaluation, and Treatment.* Whitehouse Station, NJ: Merck Laboratories, 2008.

PERIODICALS

Barone, J.E. "Fever: Fact and Fiction." *Journal of Trauma* 67 (August 2009): 406–9.

Fumagalli, R., et al. "Which Drugs for the Control of Fever in Critical Patients?" *Current Drug Targets* 10 (September 2009): 881–86.

Laupland, K.B. "Fever in the Critically Ill Medical Patient." *Critical Care Medicine* 37 (July 2009): S273–S278.

WEBSITES

American Cancer Society. "Signs and Symptoms of Cancer." http://www.cancer.org/cancer/cancerbasics/signs-and-symptoms-of-cancer (accessed November 4, 2014).

Mayo Clinic. "Fever." http://www.mayoclinic.org/diseases-conditions/fever/basics/definition/con-20019229 (accessed November 4, 2014).

ORGANIZATIONS

American Academy of Pediatrics, 141 Northwest Point Blvd., Elk Grove Village, IL 60007-1098, (847) 434-4000, (800) 433-9016, Fax: (847) 434-8000, http://www.aap.org.

American Cancer Society, 250 Williams St. NW, Atlanta, GA 30303, (800) 227-2345, http://www.cancer.org.

Centers for Disease Control and Prevention (CDC), 1600 Clifton Rd., Atlanta, GA 30333, (800) CDC-INFO (232-4636), http://www.cdc.gov.

National Cancer Institute, 9609 Medical Center Dr., BG 9609 MSC 9760, Bethesda, MD 20892-9760, (800) 4-CANCER (422-6237), http://www.cancer.gov.

National Center for Complementary and Alternative Medicine, 9000 Rockville Pike, Bethesda, MD 20892, (888) 644-6226, TTY: (866) 464-3615, http://nccam.nih.gov.

World Health Organization (WHO), Avenue Appia 20, 1211 Geneva 27, Switzerland, 41 22 791 21 11, info@who.int, http://www.who.int/en.

Rebecca J. Frey, PhD.

Fibrocystic breast disease *see* **Fibrocystic condition of the breast**

Fibrocystic condition of the breast

Definition

Fibrocystic condition of the breast is a term that may refer to a variety of symptoms including breast swelling, lumpiness, tenderness, and pain. It is not a specific diagnosis because a wide range of vaguely defined benign breast conditions can be labeled as fibrocystic condition. It is not a **cancer**, and the majority of types of fibrocystic conditions do not increase the risk of **breast cancer**.

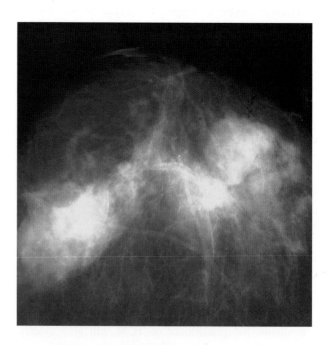

A mammogram of a female breast indicating multiple cysts (shown in white). *(CMSP/Custom Medical Stock Photo)*

KEY TERMS

Advanced breast biopsy instrument (ABBI)—A rotating circular knife and thin heated electrical wire used to remove a large cylinder of abnormal breast tissue.

Lobule—A small lobe or subdivision of a lobe (often on a gland) that may be seen on the surface of the gland as a bump or bulge.

Lymph nodes—Rounded, encapsulated bodies consisting of an accumulation of lymphatic tissue.

Mammotome—Also known as a vacuum-assisted biopsy; a method for performing breast biopsies using suction to draw tissue into an opening in the side of a cylinder inserted into the breast tissue. A rotating knife then cuts tissue samples from the rest of the breast.

Stereotactic biopsy—A biopsy performed by precisely locating areas of abnormal growth through the use of delicate instruments.

Description

Defining normal or typical breast tissue is difficult, because the tissues of the female breast change over time. The normal breast contains milk glands, with their accompanying ducts, or pipelines, for transporting milk. These complex structures can change in size and increase or decrease in number as needed. Fibrous connective tissue, fatty tissue, nerves, blood and lymph vessels, and lymph nodes, with their different shapes and textures, are found among the ever-changing milk glands. Thus, a woman's breasts might not be uniform in texture, and feelings of "lumpiness" may change over time. Breast tissue can also change in response to hormone levels, aging, weight fluctuation, and injury. Further, several different types of tissue occur in breasts, and each of these tissue types may respond differently to changes in body chemistry.

Fibrocystic breast condition is sometimes called fibrocystic disease, although it is not a single, specific diagnosis. Variations or changes in the way the breast feels or looks on x-ray may cause the condition to be called "fibrocystic change." Other names used to refer to this condition include mammary dysplasia, mastopathy, chronic cystic mastitis, indurative mastopathy, physiologic nodularity and, most commonly, fibrocystic breasts.

Demographics

Estimates vary, but 40%–90% of all women have some evidence of a fibrocystic condition, change, or disease. It is most common among women between the ages of 30 and 50, but it may be seen in older or younger women.

Causes and symptoms

The fibrocystic condition refers to the tenderness, enlargement, and/or changing degree of lumpiness that many women encounter just before or during their menstrual periods. At this time, female hormones are preparing the breasts for pregnancy by stimulating the milk-producing cells and storing fluid. Each breast can contain as much as three to six teaspoons of excess fluid. Swelling with increased sensitivity or pain can result. If pregnancy does not occur, the body reabsorbs the fluid, and the engorgement and discomfort are relieved.

Symptoms of fibrocystic breast condition range from mild discomfort in some women to extreme pain in others. The severity of discomfort may vary from month to month in the same woman. Although sometimes distressing, this experience is the body's normal response to routine hormonal changes.

This cycle of breast sensitivity, pain, and/or enlargement can also result from medications. Some hormone replacement therapies (estrogen and progesterone) used for postmenopausal women can produce these effects. Other medications, primarily but not exclusively those involving hormones, can also provoke these symptoms.

Breast pain unrelated to hormone shifts is called noncyclic pain. "Trigger-zone breast pain" is a term that may also be used to describe this area-specific pain. This type of pain may be continuous or it may be felt intermittently. Trauma (such as a blow to the chest area), a prior breast **biopsy**, or sensitivity to certain medications may also underlie this type of pain. Fibrocystic condition of the breast may be cited as the cause of otherwise unexplained breast pain.

Lumps, apart from those clearly associated with hormone cycles, can also be placed under the heading of fibrocystic condition. These lumps stand out from enlarged general breast tissue. Although noncancerous lumps may occur, the obvious concern with such lumps is cancer.

Types of noncancerous breast lumps include:

- Adenosis is a condition characterized by the enlargement of breast lobules, which contain a greater number of glands than usual. If groups of lobules are found near each other, the affected area may be large enough to be felt.
- Cysts are fluid-filled sacs in the breast. They may develop as ducts that become clogged with old cells in

the process of normal emptying and filling. Cysts usually feel soft and round or oval. A cyst deep within the breast can feel hard, however, as it pushes up against firmer breast tissue. A woman with a cyst may experience pain, especially if it increases in size before her menstrual cycle, as is often the case. Women between the age of 30 and 50 are most likely to develop cysts.

- Epithelial hyperplasia is a condition characterized by the overgrowth of cells lining either the ducts or the lobules; it is also called proliferative breast disease.

- Fibroadenomas are tumors that form in the tissues outside the milk ducts. The cause of fibroadenomas is unknown. They generally feel smooth and firm, with a somewhat rubber-like texture. Typically a fibroadenoma is not attached to surrounding tissue and moves slightly when touched. They are most commonly found in adolescents and women in their early 20s but can occur at any age.

- Fibrosis refers to a situation where one area of breast tissue persistently feels thicker or more prominent than the rest of the breast. This feeling may be caused by old hardened scar tissue and/or dead fat tissue as a result of surgery or trauma. Often the origin of this type of breast tissue is unknown.

- Miscellaneous other benign (noncancerous) breast problems may be classified as a fibrocystic condition. These problems include disorders that may lead to breast inflammation (mastitis), infection, and/or nipple discharge.

Atypical ductal hyperplasia

Atypical ductal hyperplasia (ADH) is a condition in which the cells lining the milk ducts of the breast are growing abnormally. This condition may appear as spots of calcium (calcifications) on a mammogram. A biopsy removed from the breast would confirm the diagnosis. Atypical ductal hyperplasia is not a cancer, and in most women, this condition causes no problems. For some women, however, especially women with family histories of breast cancer, the risk of developing breast cancer is increased by ADH. For women with ADH and a family history of breast cancer, more frequent mammograms and closer monitoring may be required.

Diagnosis

Breast cancer is the most common concern of women who feel a breast lump or experience an abnormal breast symptom. Any newly discovered breast lump or other abnormality should be brought to the attention of a physician. He or she will obtain a history and conduct a thorough physical examination of the area.

Depending on the findings of the physical examination, the patient may be referred for tests. These may include:

- A mammogram is an x-ray examination of the breasts. The two major types of abnormalities doctors look for are masses and calcifications; these may be either benign or malignant (cancerous). The size, shape, and edges of these masses help doctors determine whether cancer is present. Sometimes, however, this test can be difficult to interpret due to dense breast tissue.

- If a suspicious lump is detected during mammography, an ultrasound—the use of high-frequency sound waves to outline the shape of various organs and tissues in the body—is useful, although not definitive, in distinguishing benign from cancerous growths.

- A ductogram (also called a galactogram) is a test that is sometimes useful in evaluating nipple discharge. A very fine tube is threaded into the opening of the duct onto the nipple. A small amount of dye is injected, outlining the shape of the duct on an x-ray to indicate whether there is a mass in the duct.

- If a lump cannot be proven benign by mammography and ultrasound, a breast biopsy may be considered. Usually a tissue sample is removed through a needle (fine-needle aspiration biopsy, or FNAB) to obtain a sample of the lump. The sample is examined under the microscope by a pathologist, and a detailed diagnosis regarding the type of benign lesion or cancer is established. In some cases, however, FNAB may not provide a clear diagnosis, and another type of biopsy such as a surgical biopsy, core-needle biopsy, or other stereotactic biopsy method—such as the Mammotome or Advanced Breast Biopsy Instrument—may be required.

Breast conditions such as inflammation or infection are usually recognized on the basis of suspicious history, breastfeeding, or such characteristic symptoms as pain, redness, and swelling. A reduction in symptoms in response to treatment often confirms the diagnosis.

Treatment

Once a specific disorder is identified, treatment can be prescribed. There are a number of treatment options for women with a lump that has been diagnosed as benign. If it is not causing a great deal of pain, the growth may be left in the breast. Some women, however, choose to have a lump like a fibroadenoma surgically removed, especially if it is large. Another option to relieve the discomfort of a painful benign lump is to have the cyst aspirated or drained. If there is any uncertainty regarding diagnosis, the fluid may be sent to the lab for analysis.

Over-the-counter pain medication such as acetaminophen (Tylenol) or ibuprofen (Advil) may be recommended. In some cases, treatment with prescription drugs such as hormones or hormone blockers may prove successful. Oral contraceptives may also be prescribed.

Infections are often treated with warm compresses and **antibiotics**. Lactating women are encouraged to continue breastfeeding because it promotes drainage and healing. A serious infection, however, can progress to form an abscess that may require surgical drainage.

Warm soaks or ice packs may provide comfort. A well-fitted support bra can minimize physical movement and do much to relieve breast discomfort. Breast massage may promote removal of excess fluid from tissues and alleviate symptoms. Massaging the breast with oil can help reduce and dissipate fibroadenomas as well as keep women aware of changes in their breast tissue.

Alternative

Although there are no scientific data to support this claim, many women have reported relief of symptoms when they reduced or eliminated their intake of caffeine. Decreasing salt intake before and during the period when breasts are most sensitive may also ease swelling and discomfort. Low-fat diets and elimination of dairy products also appear to decrease soreness for some women. It can take several months to realize the effects of these various treatments.

Some studies of alternative or complementary treatments, although controversial, have indicated that **vitamins** A, B complex and E, and mineral supplements may reduce the risk of developing fibrocystic condition of the breast. Evening primrose oil (*Oenothera biennis*), flaxseed oil, and fish oils have been reported to be effective in relieving cyclic breast pain for some women. Women should consult with their physician before attempting any form of alternative treatment.

Prognosis

Most benign breast conditions carry no increased risk of development of breast cancer; the exception is unusually dense breast tissue, which is an independent risk factor for breast cancer. A small percentage of biopsies, however, uncover overgrowth of tissue in a particular pattern in some women; this pattern indicates a 15%–20% increased risk of breast cancer over the next 20 years. Strict attention to early detection measures such as annual mammograms is especially important for these women.

Prevention

There is no proven method of preventing the various manifestations of fibrocystic condition from occurring.

QUESTIONS TO ASK YOUR DOCTOR

- How common is this condition?
- Can fibrocystic condition of the breast lead to cancer?
- How can I tell the difference between cysts and cancer when I perform my breast self-exam?
- Can I do anything to prevent this condition?
- What are my treatment options?
- Will I have this condition for the rest of my life?

Some alternative health care practitioners believe that eliminating foods high in methyl xanthines (primarily coffee and chocolate) can decrease or reverse fibrocystic breast changes, but this has not been proven.

See also Breast self-examination.

Resources

BOOKS

Heywang-Köbrunner, Sylvia H. *Diagnostic Breast Imaging: Mammography, Sonography, Magnetic Resonance Imaging, and Interventional Procedures.* 3rd ed. New York: Thieme, 2014.

Ikeda, Debra M. *Breast Imaging.* 2nd ed. Philadelphia: Elsevier/Mosby, 2011.

Love, Susan M., with Karen Lindsey. *Dr. Susan Love's Breast Book.* 5th ed. Cambridge, MA: Da Capo Press, 2010.

PERIODICALS

Athanasiou, A., et al. "Complex Cystic Breast Masses in Ultrasound Examination." *Diagnostic and Interventional Imaging* 95 (February 2014): 169–79.

Cho, S. H., and S. H. Park. "Mimickers of Breast Malignancy on Breast Sonography." *Journal of Ultrasound in Medicine* 32 (November 2013): 2029–36.

O'Brien, S., and G. C. Cowdley. "Benign Breast Diseases and Body Mass Index: Is There a Correlation?" *American Surgeon* 80 (May 2014): 461–65.

Tice, J. A., et al. "Benign Breast Disease, Mammographic Breast Density, and the Risk of Breast Cancer." *Journal of the National Cancer Institute* 105 (July 17, 2013): 1043–49.

WEBSITES

A.D.A.M. Medical Encyclopedia. "Fibrocystic Breast Disease." MedlinePlus. http://www.nlm.nih.gov/medlineplus/ency/article/000912.htm (accessed October 15, 2014).

Diagnostic Imaging Centers. "Breast Health: Fibrocystic Breasts." YouTube video, 3:49. June 20, 2013. https://www.youtube.com/watch?v=ioFutYhS19w (accessed October 15, 2014).

Mayo Clinic staff. "Fibrocystic Breasts." Mayo Clinic. http://www.mayoclinic.org/diseases-conditions/fibrocystic-breasts/basics/definition/CON-20034681 (accessed October 15, 2014).

MedicineNet. "Fibrocystic Breast Condition/Fibrocystic Changes." http://www.medicinenet.com/fibrocystic_breast_condition/article.htm (accessed August 24, 2014).

ORGANIZATIONS

American Congress of Obstetricians and Gynecologists (ACOG), P.O. Box 70620, Washington, DC 20024-9998, (202) 638-5577, (800) 673-8444, resources@acog.org, http://www.acog.org.

Foundation for Women's Cancer, 230 W. Monroe, Suite 2528, Chicago, IL 60606-4902, (312) 578-1439, (800) 444-4441, Fax: (312) 578-9769, info@foundationforwomenscancer.org, http://www.foundationforwomenscancer.org.

Susan G. Komen, 5005 LBJ Freeway, Suite 250, Dallas, TX 75244, (877) 465-6636, http://ww5.komen.org/Contact.aspx, http://ww5.komen.org.

Ellen S. Weber, M.S.N.
Genevieve Slomski, PhD.
REVISED BY REBECCA J. FREY, PhD.

Fibrosarcoma

Definition

A fibrosarcoma is a malignant tumor that arises from fibroblasts (cells that produce connective tissue). This is a type of **sarcoma** that is predominantly found in the area around bones or in soft tissue.

Demographics

In general, fibrosarcomas are an uncommon type of **cancer** in humans; they are relatively more common in dogs and cats. Soft-tissue fibrosarcomas are extremely rare in people, with approximately 500 new cases reported in the United States each year. Sarcomas of the bone are also rare and represent about 0.2 percent of all new cancer cases each year.

Fibrosarcomas typically develop in people between the ages of 25–79. The peak age of occurrence is the fourth decade of life. Generally, fibrosarcomas develop equally in men and women, though they are rare in children. They occur with equal frequency in all races and ethnic groups.

Infantile fibrosarcoma, also known as congenital fibrosarcoma or juvenile fibrosarcoma, is unique. Under microscopic examination, it is similar to fibrosarcomas seen in adults. However, infantile fibrosarcomas have a

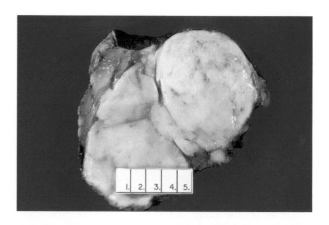

Excised specimen of a skin tumor known as a **fibrosarcoma, sliced open (white).** (DR. WALKER/Science Source)

more positive prognosis with a post-treatment, five-year survival rate of 83% to 94%.

Description

Fibrosarcomas develop from fibroblasts, cells that produce such connective tissues as collagen. Fibrosarcoma tumors are consequently rich in collagen fibers. The immature proliferating fibroblasts take on an interlacing or herringbone pattern.

Fibrosarcomas can form from fibroblasts in such soft tissue as muscles, connective tissues, blood vessels, joints, and fat. Soft-tissue fibrosarcoma normally occurs in fibrous tissue of the body's trunk and the extremities (arms and legs). About 43% of fibrosarcomas are found on the arms and legs.

Fibrosarcomas can also occur in bones. While a bone is made up of such inorganic substances as calcium phosphate, it also has an organic element made up of 95% collagen, similar to the collagen found in the skin. Fibrosarcomas of the bone usually occur in the long bones in the bone marrow cavity where collagen is formed. The bones that predominantly yield fibrosarcomas are those in the legs, arms, pelvis, and hip.

The two most common forms of bone cancer are **osteosarcoma** and **Ewing sarcoma**. Among the less common are **chondrosarcoma**, fibrosarcoma, and **malignant fibrous histiocytoma**, all of which arise from spindle cell neoplasms.

Risk factors

Risk factors for fibrosarcoma include:

- Genetic factors.
- Exposure to radiation therapy for an area of bone or soft tissue.

- Age. Fibrosarcomas are most common in adults between 35 and 45.
- Paget disease and other preexisting diseases of the bone.
- Having metallic implants for joint fixation or reconstruction.

Causes and symptoms

The exact cause(s) of fibrosarcomas is still unknown, but many sarcomas are associated with genetic mutations, particularly **chromosome rearrangements**. Fibrosarcomas of the bone are sometimes connected with underlying benign bone tumors. Both fibrosarcomas of soft tissue and of the bone can develop as a result of exposure to radiation. This may represent a side effect from previous **radiation therapy** for unrelated primary cancer treatment. Individuals with such other bone diseases as Paget's disease and osteomyelitis are at a higher risk for developing fibrosarcomas.

There are many symptoms associated with the onset of fibrosarcomas. The following is a list of the main symptoms that may be present:

- pain (more common in fibrosarcomas of bone; soft-tissue fibrosarcomas are typically painless)
- swelling
- a firm lump just under the skin or on a bone
- broken bone
- loss of normal range of motion
- limping or other difficulties in walking or using the arms or legs normally
- neurologic symptoms
- gastrointestinal bleeding (seen in soft tissue abdominal fibrosarcomas)
- urinary frequency (seen in pelvic fibrosarcomas)
- urinary obstruction (seen in pelvic fibrosarcomas)

Diagnosis

In order to diagnose fibrosarcoma, a doctor will take the patient's medical history and will conduct a thorough physical exam. Blood tests will be performed to rule out other conditions and to identify cancer markers.

The most revealing initial exam is an x-ray. It can show the location, size, and shape of the tumor. If a malignant tumor is present, the x-ray will expose a soft tissue mass with ill-defined edges. This procedure takes less than an hour and can be performed in the doctor's office.

Once there is evidence of a tumor, one or more of several other procedures may be performed, including

computed tomography (CT) scans, **magnetic resonance imaging** (MRI), angiograms, and biopsies.

Treatment

Treatment team

The patient's primary care physician may perform the initial diagnostic tests; however, in order to comprehensively diagnose and treat fibrosarcomas, the primary care physician will refer the patient to an oncologist (cancer specialist). Radiologists, pathologists, and orthopedic surgeons will also be involved to read x-rays, examine tissue samples, and, if needed, remove the tumor.

Other individuals might be involved with the treatment of fibrosarcoma, including nurses, dieticians, and physical or vocational therapists.

Staging

After the physician makes the diagnosis, it is important to determine the stage of the cancer. Staging will help reveal how far the cancer has progressed and how much tissue has been affected.

The **American Joint Committee on Cancer** developed the most widely used staging system for fibrosarcomas. The foremost categories of this system include grade (G), size of the tumor (T), lymph node involvement (N), and presence of metastases (M). Low grade and high grade are designated G1 and G3, respectively. The size of the tumor can be less than 5 centimeters (2 inches), designated as T1, or greater than 5 centimeters, designated as T2. If the lymph nodes are involved, N1 is designated, while no lymph involvement is designated N0. Finally, there may be a presence of distant metastases (M1), or no metastases (M0). The following is a list of stages and their indications:

- Stage IA: (G1, T1, N0, M0)
- Stage IB: (G1, T2, N0, M0)
- Stage IIA: (G2, T1, N0, M0)
- Stage IIB: (G2, T2, N0, M0)
- Stage IIIA: (G3, T1, N0, M0)
- Stage IIIB: (G3, T2, N0, M0)
- Stage IVA: (Any G, any T, N1, M0)
- Stage IVB: (Any G, any T, N1, M1)

Tumors with lower stage numbers, such as IA and IB, contain cells that look very similar to normal cells, while tumors with higher stage designations are composed of cells that appear very different from normal cells. In higher staged tumors, the cells appear undifferentiated.

Traditional

Physicians can employ several courses of treatment to remove fibrosarcomas. The most effective treatment is surgical removal; this is used as a primary treatment for all stages of fibrosarcoma. When performing the surgery, the surgeon will remove the tumor and some healthy soft tissue or bone around it to ensure that the tumor does not recur near the original site.

Prior to surgery, large tumors (greater than 5 centimeters, or 2 inches) may be treated with **chemotherapy** or radiation in order to shrink them, thus rendering the surgical procedure more effective. Chemotherapy is particularly effective in shrinking fibrosarcomas in children.

Even individuals with low-grade fibrosarcoma who have undergone surgery experience a 60% risk of local recurrence. To combat recurrence, **adjuvant chemotherapy** (the use of one or more cancer-killing drugs) and radiation therapy (the use of high-energy rays), such as irradiation and brachytherapy, are also used to complement surgery. Employing chemotherapy or radiation therapy individually without surgery is much less effective.

After therapy, low-stage fibrosarcomas (stages IA and IB) have greater five-year survival rates than high stages (Stages IVA and IVB). Because high-grade tumors are more aggressive and more highly metastatic than lower grade tumors, patients with high-grade tumors have a lower survival rate. Not only is the grade of the tumor (the estimate of its aggressiveness) important in determining prognosis, the age of the patient is also crucial. Generally, fibrosarcomas that occur in childhood and infancy have a lower mortality rate than those that occur in adults. Additionally, patients with fibrosarcomas that occur in the extremities have a better survival rate than those with fibrosarcomas in the visceral region.

Metastases appear later in the development of fibrosarcomas. The lungs are the primary sites of **metastasis** for fibrosarcomas that develop in the extremities. Once metastasis to the lungs has occurred, the chances of survival are significantly decreased.

Patients treated for fibrosarcomas are monitored for at least five years after treatment.

Alternative

Many individuals choose to supplement traditional therapy with complementary methods. Often, these methods improve the patient's tolerance of side effects and symptoms, as well as enrich their quality of life. The American Cancer Society recommends that patients talk to their doctor to ensure that the methods they choose are safely supplementing their traditional therapy. Some **complementary cancer therapies** include the following:

- yoga
- meditation
- religious practices and prayer
- music therapy
- art therapy
- pet therapy
- massage therapy
- aromatherapy

Coping with cancer treatment

Chemotherapy often results in several side effects, depending on the drug used and the patient's individual tolerance. Patients may have to deal with nausea, vomiting, loss of appetite (**anorexia**), and hair loss (**alopecia**). Many times, chemotherapy as well as radiation therapy are better handled if patients are eating well. Nurses and dieticians can aid patients in choosing healthful foods to incorporate into their diet.

If the fibrosarcoma necessitated a limb **amputation**, then patients will need to learn how to cope with a prosthetic device. Both physical and vocational therapists can effectively help patients adjust and learn how to use the prosthetic device to perform their daily activities.

Clinical trials

Fibrosarcomas are rare, but advances are being made in both diagnostic and curative procedures. Although surgery is the most effective treatment, both pre- and post-operative adjuvant therapies are being researched to complement surgery—specifically, chemotherapy and radiation therapy. There were two active **clinical trials** for fibrosarcoma treatment in progress as of late 2014. Drugs being studied included pazopanib (Votrient) and **bevacizumab** (Avastin).

Patients should consult with their physicians or contact the American Cancer Society or **National Cancer Institute** to learn what procedures are currently being investigated in clinical trials. In some cases, insurance companies will not cover procedures that are part of clinical trials. Patients should talk with their doctor and insurance company to determine which procedures are covered.

Prognosis

The prognosis of a fibrosarcoma depends on its location, stage, and whether it has metastasized.

QUESTIONS TO ASK YOUR DOCTOR

- What diagnostic procedures are best for the location and type of tumor suspected?
- What treatments are best for the location and type of tumor suspected?
- What kinds of side effects will this course of treatment cause?
- Are there support services available?
- What treatments are currently in clinical trials?
- What treatments will my health care insurance cover?
- What alternative treatments are safe?

Prevention

The prevention of cancer can be assisted by avoiding such known chemical **carcinogens** as alpha-naphthylamine, carbon tetrachloride, and **benzene**. Another way to avoid developing cancer is to minimize exposure to penetrating radiation such as x-rays and radioactive elements. Medical x-rays revolutionized the field of medicine and are used to detect and treat many diseases. In most cases, the benefits of medical x-rays outweigh the risks.

Special concerns

Treatment, especially surgical amputation, can take a physical and psychological toll on cancer patients and their families. To deal with the psychological impact, there are many different support groups and psychotherapists that can help. Some therapists will consider amputation a posttraumatic stress disorder, and treat it accordingly. To deal with their condition, relying on faith practices can also be beneficial for cancer patients. Patients should discuss all options with their physician to determine what is available.

For patients whose fibrosarcoma affected their face or head, Look Good...Feel Better is a free public service program approved by the American Cancer Society. It helps patients with any kind of cancer cope with changes in their looks related to cancer treatment. It began in 1987 when a doctor asked the president of the Personal Care Products Council to help a patient who was so depressed by her appearance during chemotherapy that she refused to leave her hospital room. The president sent a makeup artist to visit the patient, who was so delighted with her makeover that she began to respond better to her cancer treatment. Look Good...Feel Better has expanded to include programs for teens, men, and Spanish-speaking patients; groups are

available in all 50 states, the District of Columbia, and Puerto Rico. The main website is http://www.lookgoodfeelbetter.org/.

Once the cancer has been treated, patients should make sure to schedule follow-up appointments with their physicians. Physicians will want to monitor the patient for side effects or possible recurrence that may develop years after treatment.

Resources

BOOKS

Hasegawa, Sota, ed. *Soft Tissue Cancers: Etiology, Pathogenesis and Interventions*. New York: Nova Science Publishers, 2008.

PERIODICALS

Collini, P., et al. "Sarcomas with Spindle Cell Morphology." *Seminars in Oncology* 36 (August 2009): 324–37.

Russell, H., et al. "Infantile Fibrosarcoma: Clinical and Histologic Responses to Cytotoxic Chemotherapy." *Pediatric Blood and Cancer* 53 (July 2009): 23–27.

Stein-Wexler, R. "MR Imaging of Soft Tissue Masses in Children." *Magnetic Resonance Imaging Clinics of North America* 17 (August 2009): 489–507.

WEBSITES

Boston Children's Hospital. "Fibrosarcoma." http://www.childrenshospital.org/health-topics/conditions/fibrosarcoma (accessed November 4, 2014).

National Cancer Institute (NCI). "Childhood Soft Tissue Sarcoma Treatment (PDQ®)." http://www.cancer.gov/cancertopics/pdq/treatment/child-soft-tissue-sarcoma/Patient (accessed November 4, 2014).

ORGANIZATIONS

American Academy of Orthopaedic Surgeons, 6300 N. River Rd., Rosemont, IL 60018, (847) 823-7186, Fax: (847) 823-8125, orthoinfo@aaos.org, http://www.aaos.org.

American Cancer Society, 250 Williams St. NW, Atlanta, GA 30303, (800) 227-2345, http://www.cancer.org.

National Cancer Institute, 9609 Medical Center Dr., BG 9609 MSC 9760, Bethesda, MD 20892-9760, (800) 4-CANCER (422-6237), http://www.cancer.gov.

Sally C. McFarlane-Parrott
REVISED BY REBECCA J. FREY, PhD.

Filgrastim

Definition

Filgrastim is a medicine used to increase the white blood cell count in the body, which will help prevent infection. Filgrastim is known by the brand name Neupogen.

Purpose

Filgrastim is a drug approved by the U.S. Food and Drug Administration (FDA) to increase white blood cell counts. If a patient has a lower than normal white blood cell count it is referred to as **neutropenia**.

Filgrastim can be used to treat neutropenia caused by cancer chemotherapy treatment. In these patients the filgrastim increases the recovery of white blood cells after **chemotherapy**. Filgrastim can also be used to treat patients who have a neutropenia not related to chemotherapy. In both cases, the filgrastim decreases the risk of **fever** and infection.

Filgrastim is not usually used in leukemia patients; however, in patients with the disease known as acute myelocytic leukemia, it is approved for use after chemotherapy. Filgrastim can increase the recovery of the white blood cell count thereby decreasing the length of time a patient may have a fever associated with a low white count.

Filgrastim can also be used after **bone marrow transplantation**. Once the new healthy bone marrow has been given back to a patient, filgrastim can be administered to help increase the white blood cell count and decrease the risk of fever and infection.

Filgrastim can be used for patients who will receive a peripheral blood stem cell transplant. Patients will receive the filgrastim before the transplant. The filgrastim in these patients causes young, non-developed blood cells, known as stem or progenitor cells, to move from the bone marrow to the blood where they will then be removed from a patient by the process of apheresis. These blood cells are stored until after the patient receives large doses of chemotherapy that destroy the bone marrow and the **cancer**. The patient then receives these stored cells back by an intravenous infusion. The stored cells repopulate the bone marrow and develop into the many types of functioning blood cells.

Description

Filgrastim has been available to cancer patients since the 1990s and is highly effective at decreasing neutropenia. Filgrastim may be referred to as G-CSF, granulocyte colony stimulating factor. This compound is manufactured by recombinant DNA methods using E. coli as the host organism. Chemotherapy destroys white blood cells temporarily. These white blood cells will grow again, but during the time that the levels are low, patients are at an increased risk of developing fevers and infection. Filgrastim acts to stimulate the bone marrow to make more white blood cells, which can either prevent the white count from dropping below normal or decrease the time that the level is low. By effectively avoiding fevers

and infections, patients are able to receive their next doses of chemotherapy without delay.

Recommended dosage

Filgrastim is a clear colorless liquid that is dosed on body weight in kilograms. It is kept refrigerated until ready to use, and it is administered to patients as a subcutaneous injection (directly underneath the skin). It is usually administered in the back of the arms, upper legs, or stomach area. Filgrastim can also be given to patients as a short intravenous infusion into a vein over 15 to 30 minutes.

Chemotherapy-caused neutropenia

The starting dose for patients who have just finished chemotherapy is 5 micrograms per kilogram of body weight per day. This is given as a subcutaneous injection under the skin daily for up to 14 consecutive days, and sometimes longer. The doctor will inform the patient when it is time to stop the filgrastim.

Bone marrow transplants

The recommended dose is 10 micrograms per kilogram per day. This can be administered as a 4- to 24-hour infusion intravenously, or as a 24-hour subcutaneous infusion.

Peripheral blood stem cell transplant

The recommended dose is 10 micrograms per kilogram per day. This can be given either as an under the skin injection, intravenously, or as a continuous infusion over 24 hours. This dosing should begin four days before the first apheresis collection process and continue until the last day of collection.

Other neutropenia

The dose recommendation is variable based on the reason for neutropenia. The range of filgrastim doses has been from 5 micrograms per kilogram per day up to 100 microgram per kilogram per day. Doctors may increase the filgrastim dose based on how the white blood cell count responds to the treatment. Other factors that play a role in filgrastim dosing include how low the white blood cell count is and the length of time the white blood cell count remains low.

Precautions

Filgrastim should not be received by a patient in the 24-hour time frame before or after receiving chemotherapy or reinfusion of bone marrow or stem cells.

Blood counts will be monitored while on the drug filgrastim. This allows the doctor to determine if the drug is working and when to stop the drug.

It is not recommended to give filgrastim to patients who have certain types of leukemias.

Patients with a known previous allergic reaction to filgrastim or to any other substance derived from the bacteria *E. coli* should not take filgrastim.

Patients who may be pregnant, or trying to become pregnant, should tell their doctor before receiving filgrastim.

Side effects

The most common side effect from filgrastim is **bone pain**. The filgrastim causes the bone marrow to produce more white blood cells, and as a result, patients may experience pain in their bones. Tylenol, an over-the-counter pain reliever, can usually control mild to moderate pain that occurs with standard dosed filgrastim. Larger doses of filgrastim, like those given for bone marrow transplant patients, can cause severe bone pain that may need a prescription pain reliever to ease the pain.

Another common side effect due to filgrastim administration is pain or burning at the site of the injection. This can be decreased by bringing the filgrastim to room temperature before administering the injection, icing the area of injection to numb it before receiving the injection, and moving the site of the injection with each dose.

Patients who have received filgrastim after cancer chemotherapy have reported fever, **nausea and vomiting**, muscle pain, **diarrhea**, hair loss (**alopecia**), mouth sores, **fatigue**, shortness of breath, weakness, headache, cough, rash, constipation, and pain. These side effects may be due to the chemotherapy administration.

Interactions

Filgrastim should not be given at the same time as chemotherapy or **radiation therapy**. Dosing should begin at least 24 hours after the last dose of treatment.

Patients on the drug lithium should tell their doctor before starting filgrastim therapy.

Filgrastim use for delayed **myelosuppression** has not been studied after the use of the chemotherapy agents **mitomycin-C**, and nitrosoureas, or after the drug **fluorouracil**.

Resources

BOOKS

Wilkes, Gail M., and Margaret Barton-Burke. *2013 Oncology Nursing Drug Handbook*. Burlington, MA: Jones & Bartlett Learning, 2013.

WEBSITES

AHFS Consumer Medication Information. "Filgrastim Injection." American Society of Health-System Pharmacists. Available from: http://www.nlm.nih.gov/medlineplus/druginfo/meds/a692033.html (accessed November 4, 2014).

American Cancer Society. "Filgrastim." http://www.cancer.org/treatment/treatmentsandsideeffects/guidetocancerdrugs/filgrastim (accessed November 4, 2014).

Nancy J. Beaulieu, RPh., BCOP

Firmagon *see* **Degarelix**

5-Azacitidine *see* **Azacitidine**

5-Fluorouracil *see* **Fluorouracil**

Flow cytometry

Definition

Flow cytometry is a method of sorting and measuring types of cells by fluorescent labeling of markers on their surfaces. It is sometimes referred to as fluorescent-activated cell sorting (FACS) analysis or flow cytometric immunophenotyping.

Purpose

Flow cytometric analysis is most often used clinically to:

- analyze blood or bone-marrow cells to determine whether a high white blood cell count is due to a blood cancer
- classify the type of lymphocytes (immune-system white blood cells) to distinguish lymphomas from infections or non-cancerous diseases of the lymph nodes
- diagnose acute and chronic leukemias, lymphoid cancers (including non-Hodgkin lymphoma), and myelodysplastic and myeloproliferative syndromes (cancers in which bone marrow overproduces white blood cells), and to distinguish them from immunodeficiency disorders
- determine the type of leukemia, lymphoma, or myeloma cells present in bone marrow, lymph nodes, or blood samples to help with treatment plans and prognosis
- analyze characteristics of a leukemia to help determine its aggressiveness
- detect rare cell types and residual levels of disease
- identify disease relapses following treatment
- analyze certain solid (non-blood), benign (non-cancerous), and malignant (cancerous) tumors

Precautions

Drugs that suppress the immune system (such as steroids) will affect the number of white blood cells in the patient's sample.

Description

Flow cytometry is performed on a blood or **biopsy** sample. For leukemia, analysis is performed on a blood sample from which the red blood cells have been removed. For **lymphoma**, the sample may be collected by fine-needle aspiration biopsy, and the tissue sample is separated into single cells. The blood or biopsy cells are mixed with different antibodies that can bind to markers (antigens) on the surfaces of the cells. Different types of cells have characteristic antigens, so a particular cell type

KEY TERMS

Aneuploid—An abnormal number of chromosomes or amount of DNA in a cell.

Antibody—A protein produced by immune-system white blood cells that binds to a specific antigen.

Antigen—A protein or other molecule, often located on the cell surface, that binds specific antibodies.

Biopsy—A procedure for removing potentially cancerous tissue for examination by a pathologist.

Cytometer—An instrument that measures cells.

Fluorescence—Light absorbed at one wavelength and emitted at another so that it glows.

Fluorescent-activated cell sorting (FACS)—Flow cytometry or immunophenotyping.

Leukemia—An acute or chronic blood cancer that is classified according to the type of white blood cell that is overproduced.

Lymphoma—Cancer of lymphatic tissue.

Myeloma—Cancer of the bone marrow.

can be identified by the antibodies that bind to it. The antibodies are labeled so that they will emit fluorescent light (glow) as they pass through the laser beam in the cytometer. The cytometer measures the number of live cells and the numbers and percentages of each cell type in the sample, according to the specific tumor antigens or biomarkers on their surfaces. It also measures the sizes of the cells and their shapes and provides some information about the interiors of the cells. The information is analyzed by a computer and used to determine the

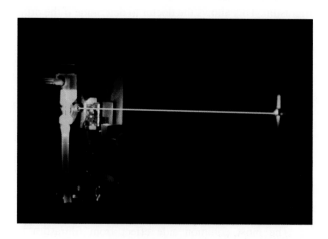

Laser used in flow cytometry. (*©CMSP/Custom Medical Stock Photo – All rights reserved.*)

specific type of leukemia—such as myelogenous or lymphocytic—or other **cancer** type. This helps determine the most appropriate treatment. Solid tumor samples can be analyzed with a laser-scanning cytometer attached to a microscope.

Flow cytometry is also used to measure the DNA content of cells to determine how fast the cells are growing and dividing (proliferating) and whether the amount of DNA in the cells is normal (diploid) or abnormal (aneuploid). Rather than using antibodies that detect cell-surface antigens, the cells are treated with dyes that react with DNA.

Preparation

Flow cytometry performed on a blood sample requires a blood draw. A biopsy of a solid tumor or a bone-marrow aspiration is a more complicated procedure for which the patient must be appropriately prepared.

Aftercare and risks

The only aftercare and risks associated with flow cytometry are those associated with the sample collection procedure.

Results

A pathology report may include flow cytometry results indicating several different cell types with a variety of antigens on their surfaces. A normal result will indicate no increase in the number of any particular type of immune cell. The pathologist will report the presence and percentages of several different types of cells, but no one type will be present in increased numbers. This indicates that the sample is less likely to contain leukemia or lymphoma cells.

Abnormal results

Abnormal results are an unusually large number of one particular cell type with identical antigens on the cell surface. The types of markers present on the cell provide further information about the type of leukemia or lymphoma and can suggest a prognosis. For example, leukemic cells that have markers that are normally found on less mature cell types may suggest a poorer prognosis, and more aggressive therapy might be recommended. DNA content that indicates rapidly proliferating cells can suggest a more aggressive cancer. Aneuploid cells tend to indicate more aggressive cancers that spread faster and are harder to treat.

See also Tumor grading.

QUESTIONS TO ASK YOUR DOCTOR

- What information will flow cytometry provide?
- Is this the best way to determine if I have cancer and what type of cancer?
- What type of sample will be tested?
- Are there any special preparations for this test or risks or possible complications?
- Is it possible that the test may give unclear or inaccurate results?

Resources

BOOKS

Bartek, Jiri, and André Lieber. "Analysis of EMT by Flow Cytometry and Immunohistochemistry." In *Ovarian Cancer: Methods and Protocols*, Anastasia Malek and Oleg Tchernitsa, eds. New York: Humana, 2013.

WEBSITES

"Immunophenotyping." Lab Tests Online. http://labtestsonline.org/understanding/analytes/immunophenotyping/tab/glance (accessed September 30, 2014).

"Testing Biopsy and Cytology Specimens for Cancer." American Cancer Society. http://www.cancer.org/acs/groups/cid/documents/webcontent/003185-pdf.pdf (accessed September 30, 2014).

ORGANIZATIONS

American Cancer Society, 250 Williams Street NW, Atlanta, GA 30303, (800) 227-2345, http://www.cancer.org.

Leukemia & Lymphoma Society, 1311 Mamaroneck Avenue, Suite 310, White Plains, NY 10605, (914) 949-5213, Fax: (914) 949-6691, (800) 955-4572, infocenter@lls.org, http://www.lls.org.

National Cancer Institute, 6116 Executive Boulevard, Suite 300, Bethesda, MD 20892-8322, (800) 4-CANCER (422-6237), http://www.cancer.gov.

Racquel Baert, MS
REVISED BY MARGARET ALIC, PhD.

Floxuridine

Definition

Floxuridine is an anti-cancer drug that is injected directly into the artery that carries blood to the liver or the abdominal cavity. The brand names of floxuridine are Fluorodeoxyuridine, FUDR, and Floxuridine For

KEY TERMS

Catheter—Tube used to inject medicine into the body.

Hepatic intra-arterial infusion—Injection of medicine into the artery to the liver.

Intraperitoneal—Within the abdominal cavity.

Metastasis—Spread of cancer from its point of origin to other parts of the body.

Injection USP. The generic name product may be available in the United States.

Purpose

Floxuridine is used to treat **gastrointestinal cancers** that have metastasized, or spread, to the liver. These cancers include **rectal cancer** and Stage IV **colon cancer**. Floxuridine also has been used to treat cancerous gastrointestinal tumors; however the response rate is poor and usually the drug is used only to relieve symptoms.

Description

Floxuridine is approved by the United States Food and Drug Administration.

Floxuridine is a type of medicine called an antimetabolite because it interferes with the metabolism and growth of cells. Floxuridine prevents the production of DNA in cells. The cells cannot reproduce and eventually they die.

Floxuridine sometimes is used in conjunction with the drugs **fluorouracil (5-FU)**, **cisplatin**, and/or **leucovorin**. Leucovorin increases the activity of floxuridine. In general, floxuridine is more effective than other chemotherapies against liver metastases, but its use does not improve overall survival rates. Ongoing studies are comparing floxuridine with other chemotherapies. The drug may be used in conjunction with surgery. Its use in conjunction with **radiation therapy** is being evaluated.

Recommended dosage

Floxuridine is injected directly into the liver. This is called hepatic intra-arterial infusion, or **hepatic arterial infusion**. A special pump delivers the drug through an implanted infusion port or catheter into an artery that goes to the liver. Injection of floxuridine into a vein is being evaluated. Floxuridine also may be injected into the abdominal cavity (intraperitoneal therapy). The dosage of floxuridine depends on a number of factors including body weight, type of **cancer**, and any other medicines that are being used.

Precautions

Floxuridine may lower the number of white blood cells and therefore reduce the body's ability to fight infection. Immunizations (vaccinations) should be avoided during or after treatment with floxuridine because of the risk of infection. It also is important to avoid contact with individuals who have recently taken an oral polio vaccine. Treatment with floxuridine may cause chicken pox or shingles (**Herpes zoster**) to become very severe and spread to other parts of the body.

Kidney or liver diseases may increase the effects of floxuridine, since the drug may be removed from the body at a slower rate. Floxuridine also may put an individual at an increased risk for hepatitis.

Floxuridine can cause birth defects in animals; therefore, this drug should not be taken by pregnant women or by either the man or the woman at the time of conception. Women usually are advised against breast-feeding while receiving this drug.

Side effects

Since floxuridine may affect the growth of normal cells as well as cancer cells, side effects may occur during or after drug treatment. Some effects may occur months or even years after the drug is administered. Floxuridine increases the risk of later developing certain types of cancer, such as leukemia.

The more common side effects of floxuridine include:

• diarrhea

• loss of appetite (anorexia)

• sores in the mouth or on the lips

• stomach pain or cramps

• numbness or tingling in the hands and feet

Less common side effects of floxuridine include:

• nausea and vomiting

• black, tar-like stools

• heartburn

• redness or scaling of the hands or feet

• sore, swollen tongue

• skin rash or itching

• temporary thinning of hair (alopecia)

• bleeding at the site of the catheter

• infection from the catheter

• closing off of the catheter

Other, rare side effects of floxuridine include:

- blood in urine or stools
- hiccups
- hoarseness or coughing
- fever or chills
- sore throat
- difficulty swallowing
- blurred vision
- lower back or side pain
- painful or difficult urination
- small red skin spots
- difficulty walking
- bleeding or bruising
- yellow eyes or skin
- seizures
- depression

In addition to lowering the white blood cell count, increasing the risk of infection, floxuridine may reduce the level of blood platelets that are necessary for normal blood clotting. This can increase the risk of bleeding. The drug also may lead to abnormalities in liver function. Intraperitoneal floxuridine therapy has been associated with the development of fibrous masses in the abdomen.

Interactions

Previous treatment with radiation or other anti-cancer drugs can increase the effects of floxuridine on the blood.

Drugs that may interact with floxuridine include:

- amphotericin B (Fungizone)
- antithyroid drugs that are used to treat an overactive thyroid
- azathioprine (Imuran)
- chloramphenicol (Chloromycetin)
- colchicine
- flucytosine (Ancobon)
- ganciclovir (Cytovene)
- interferon (Intron A, Roferon-A)
- plicamycin (Mithracin)
- zidovudine (AZT, Retrovir)

Resources

BOOKS

Wilkes, Gail M., and Margaret Barton-Burke. *2013 Oncology Nursing Drug Handbook*. Burlington, MA: Jones & Bartlett Learning, 2013.

WEBSITES

AHFS Consumer Medication Information. "Floxuridine." American Society of Health-System Pharmacists. Available from: http://www.nlm.nih.gov/medlineplus/druginfo/meds/a682006.html (accessed November 4, 2014).
American Cancer Society. "Floxuridine." http://www.cancer.org/treatment/treatmentsandsideeffects/guidetocancer-drugs/floxuridine (accessed November 4, 2014).

Margaret Alic, PhD.

Fluconazole *see* **Antifungal therapy**
Fludara *see* **Fludarabine**

Fludarabine

Definition

Fludarabine is a **chemotherapy** medicine used to treat certain types of **cancer** by destroying cancerous cells. It is known as the brand name Fludara. Fludarabine may also be referred to as Fludarabine phosphate, 2-fluoroadenine aribinoside 5-phosphate, and FAMP.

Purpose

Fludarabine is approved by the U.S. Food and Drug Administration (FDA) to treat refractory **chronic lymphocytic leukemia** (CLL). Patients must have a disease that did not respond to other treatment or a disease that became worse during other treatment. Fludarabine has also been used to treat **Hodgkin lymphoma**, **non-Hodgkin lymphoma**, **cutaneous T-cell lymphoma**, macroglobulinemic **lymphoma**, **mycosis fungoides**, and **hairy cell leukemia**.

Description

Fludarabine has been available for use since the early 1990s, and is a member of the group of chemotherapy drugs known as antimetabolites. Antimetabolites interfere with the genetic material (DNA) inside the cancer cells and prevent them from further dividing and growing more cancer cells.

Recommended dosage

Fludarabine is a clear solution that is administered through a vein.

A fludarabine dose can be determined using a mathematical calculation that measures a person's body surface area (BSA). This number is dependent upon a patient's height and weight. The larger the person, the

KEY TERMS

Anemia—A red blood cell count that is lower than normal.

Chemotherapy—Specific drugs used to treat cancer.

Deoxynucleic acid (DNA)—Genetic material inside of cells that carries the information to make proteins that are necessary to run the cells and keep the body functioning smoothly.

Electrolytes—Elements normally found in the body (sodium, potassium, calcium, magnesium, phosphorus, chloride, and acetate) that are important to maintain the many cellular functions and growth.

Food and Drug Administration (FDA)—The government agency that oversees public safety in relation to drugs and medical devices, and gives the approval to pharmaceutical companies for commercial marketing of their products.

Gout—A disease caused by the build up of uric acid in the joints causing swelling and pain.

Intravenous—To enter the body through a vein.

Neutropenia—A white blood cell count that is lower than normal.

Refractory—Cancer that no longer responds to treatment.

greater the body surface area. BSA is measured in the units known as square meter (m^2). The body surface area is calculated and then multiplied by the drug dosage in milligrams per square meter (mg/m^2). This calculates the actual dose a patient is to receive.

The approved dose for chronic lymphocytic leukemia is 25 milligrams per square meter per day for 5 days in a row. The fludarabine is given intravenously into a vein over a 30-minute to 2-hour time period. This 5-day cycle is repeated every 4 weeks.

The dose of fludarabine may need to be decreased in patients who have kidney problems.

Precautions

Blood counts will be monitored regularly while on fludarabine therapy. During a certain time period after receiving fludarabine, there is an increased risk of getting infections. Caution should be taken to avoid unnecessary exposure to crowds and people with infections.

Patients with a known previous allergic reaction to chemotherapy drugs should tell their doctor.

Patients who may be pregnant or are trying to become pregnant should tell their doctor before receiving fludarabine. Chemotherapy can cause men and women to be sterile, or unable to have children. It is unknown if fludarabine has this effect on humans.

Patients should check with their doctors before receiving live virus vaccines while on chemotherapy.

Side effects

The most common side effect expected from taking fludarabine is low blood counts (**myelosuppression**). When the white blood cell count is lower than normal (**neutropenia**), patients are at an increased risk of developing a **fever** and infections. Patients may need to be treated with **antibiotics** at this point. The platelet blood count can also be decreased due to fludarabine administration, but generally returns to normal within 2 weeks after the end of the infusion. Platelets are blood cells that cause clots to form to stop bleeding. When the platelet count is low, patients are at an increased risk for bruising and bleeding. Fludarabine causes low red blood cell counts (**anemia**). Low red counts make people feel tired and dizzy.

Fludarabine can cause the development of autoimmune **hemolytic anemia**, which occurs when the body begins to destroy its own red blood cells. It is an uncommon side effect, but very serious when it occurs.

Common side effects from fludarabine include **nausea and vomiting**. If nausea and vomiting are a problem, patients can be given **antiemetics** before receiving fludarabine. This medication helps prevent or decrease these side effects. Other common side effects include fever, chills, joint pain, fluid gain, **fatigue**, sleepiness, pain, muscle ache, weakness, and infection. Other less common side effects include loss of appetite (**anorexia**), **diarrhea**, abnormal touch sensation, cough, **pneumonia**, and shortness of breath.

Damage to the nerves and nervous system tissues can occur with fludarabine. Side effects due to this nerve damage include sleepiness, confusion, weakness, fatigue, irritability, numbness or tingling in the hands and feet, visual changes, and difficulty walking.

Infrequent side effects of fludarabine are skin rashes, pain, **itching**, fever, lung problems, insomnia, headache, muscle and joint aches, swelling, and decreased blood pressure.

Rare side effects of fludarabine include mouth sores, constipation and abdominal cramping, bleeding from the bladder, hair loss, hearing problems, and liver and kidney problems.

Fludarabine can cause the rapid breakdown of cancer cells. Patients who have large numbers of cancer cells in their bloodstream can develop a problem known as **tumor lysis syndrome**. The symptoms of this syndrome include pain in the lower back and blood in the urine. A patient can develop high or low levels of electrolytes and high levels of uric acid, which can lead to gout and kidney damage. The drug **allopurinol** may be given to patients prior to fludarabine treatment to prevent this from occurring. Drinking an increased amount of liquids also may help prevent the kidney damage.

All side effects a patient experiences should be reported to the doctor.

Interactions

Fludarabine should not be used in combination with the drug **pentostatin**. The combination causes severe lung damage.

Resources

BOOKS

Wilkes, Gail M., and Margaret Barton-Burke. *2013 Oncology Nursing Drug Handbook*. Burlington, MA: Jones & Bartlett Learning, 2013.

WEBSITES

American Cancer Society. "Fludarabine." http://www.cancer. org/treatment/treatmentsandsideeffects/guidetocancer-drugs/fludarabine (accessed November 4, 2014).

The Scott Hamilton CARES Initiative. "Fludarabine." Chemo-care.com. http://chemocare.com/chemotherapy/drug-info/fludarabine.aspx (accessed November 3, 2014).

Nancy J. Beaulieu, R.Ph., B.C.O.P.

Fluorodeoxyuridine *see* **Floxuridine**

▌Fluorouracil

Definition

Fluorouracil is a medication that kills **cancer** cells. It is also known as 5-FU or 5-fluourouracil, and as the brand name Adrucil.

Purpose

5-FU may be used in combination with other **chemotherapy** agents to treat cancers of the breast, stomach, colon, rectum, and pancreas.

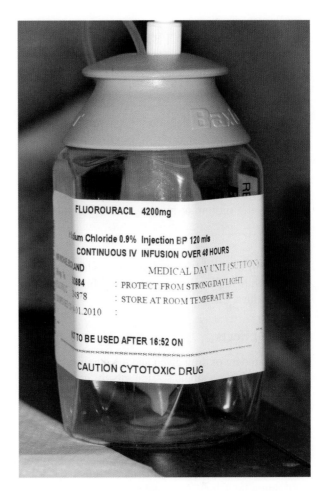

Bottle containing fluorouracil. (*Dr. P. Marazzi/Science Source*)

Description

5-FU is a cytotoxic drug. 5-FU kills cells by interfering with the activities of DNA and RNA, which are molecules in the cells important in expressing genetic material.

Recommended dosage

Most frequently, 5-FU is given as an injection into the vein (intravenous injection or IV). Many different doses and regimens are used depending on the cancer diagnosis, and patients should discuss with their physician the dose based on the individual protocol used. A sample dose is 500 to 1,000 mg per square meter of body surface area given as a 24-hour infusion for four to five days every three weeks. A dose of 425 mg per square meter of body surface area per day for five days given along with the drug **leucovorin** is also common.

Precautions

Patients with allergic reaction to 5-FU should not be administered this drug. It is also inadvisable for pregnant

KEY TERMS

Cytotoxic drug—A medicine that kills (cancer) cells.

DNA—A molecule found in all living cells that contains tiny bits of genetic information.

Infusion therapy—Administration of a medication as a liquid through an intravenous (IV) device.

RNA—A molecule found in all living cells that plays a role in transmitting information from the DNA to the protein-forming system of the cell.

women. 5-FU should be administered with caution to patients with impaired liver or kidney function, or in patients with a history of heart problems.

Side effects

The amount of drug given and the duration of which it is given during a single session greatly influences the side effects seen. For example, when given as a 24-hour continuous infusion, the most common side effects are **diarrhea** and mouth ulcers. If 5-FU is given as a bolus infusion (a high quantity of the drug all at once), the most common side effect is bone marrow suppression; this results in a decrease of the white blood cells responsible for fighting infections, the platelets responsible for blood clotting, and the red blood cells responsible for providing oxygen to the cells of the body.

The severity of the side effects is increased when 5-FU is given with the drug leucovorin. Vomiting, diarrhea, nausea, and loss of appetite (**anorexia**) may occur regardless of how 5-FU is administered. The diarrhea side effect may be severe in some patients, and it is important for them to alert their doctor immediately so that appropriate medications for the diarrhea can be prescribed.

5-FU may cause rashes, increased sensitivity to sunlight, changes in skin color, changes to the fingernails, and redness and swelling in the palms of the hands and soles of the feet. Patients who have had heart disease before starting therapy with 5-FU may have problems with blood flow to the heart. Rarely, 5-FU may cause an allergic reaction, dry eyes, sleepiness, confusion, headache, changes in walking gait, involuntary rapid movement of the eyes, and difficulty speaking. When 5-FU is applied directly on the skin, there are usually no side effects except for those to the skin itself. These may include burning sensations, pain, and darkening of the skin color.

Some authorities recommend discontinuation of 5-FU therapy as soon as mild side effects are observed as a way of reducing the extent of injury to the digestive tract. Administration may then be restarted at a lower dose after the side effects have stopped.

Interactions

People taking fluorouracil should consult their doctor before taking any other prescription drug, over-the-counter drug, or herbal remedy.

Resources

BOOKS

Chu, Edward, and Vincent T. DeVita Jr. *Physicians' Cancer Chemotherapy Drug Manual 2014*. Burlington, MA: Jones & Bartlett Learning, 2014.

Wilkes, Gail M., and Margaret Barton-Burke. *2013 Oncology Nursing Drug Handbook*. Burlington, MA: Jones & Bartlett Learning, 2013.

WEBSITES

American Cancer Society. "Fluorouracil (5-FU)." http://www.cancer.org/treatment/treatmentsandsideeffects/guidetocancerdrugs/fluorouracil (accessed November 4, 2014).

Cancer Research UK. "Fluorouracil." http://www.cancerresearchuk.org/about-cancer/cancers-in-general/treatment/cancer-drugs/fluorouracil (accessed November 3, 2014).

ORGANIZATIONS

American Cancer Society, 250 Williams St. NW, Atlanta, GA 30303, (800) 227-2345, http://www.cancer.org.

Bob Kirsch

Fluoxymesterone

Definition

Fluoxymesterone is a synthetic male hormone used to treat women with hormone-dependent **breast cancer**, and may also be used as a **testosterone** replacement for men. Fluoxymesterone is sold as Halotestin, Android-F, and Ora-Testryl.

Purpose

Fluoxymesterone is used to manage metastatic breast **cancer** in menopausal women who have hormone receptor–positive tumors. It may also be used as a supplement to **chemotherapy** for metastatic breast cancer, or as a hormone replacement for men. Additionally, it is sometimes used to treat **anemia**.

KEY TERMS

Androgen—A male hormone.

Hypercalcemia—High levels of calcium in the blood.

Description

Fluoxymesterone is a synthetic androgen, or male hormone, similar in action to testosterone. Fluoxymesterone works by attaching itself to androgen receptors; this causes it to interact with the parts of the cell involved in the making of proteins. It may cause an increase in the synthesis of some proteins or a decrease in the synthesis of others. These proteins have a variety of effects, including blocking the growth of some types of breast cancer cells, stimulating cells that cause male sexual characteristics, and stimulating the production of red blood cells.

When used as a breast cancer treatment, this drug blocks the growth of tumor cells that are dependent on female hormones to grow. It can only be used on female breast cancer patients who have reached menopause one to five years earlier, or as a result of surgery. It may be used in addition to other chemotherapeutic drugs, such as **tamoxifen** or **cyclophosphamide**, **doxorubicin**, and **fluorouracil**.

Fluoxymesterone may be used to treat men; it replaces male hormones that are not being released in the body as a result of tumors, radiation, or surgery affecting the pituitary or hypothalamus.

Recommended dosage

The recommended dosage will depend on the age, sex, and diagnosis of the patient, as well as the response to treatment and occurrence of side effects. Treatment is usually with a full therapeutic dose initially, then adjusted to the individual needs of the patient.

Women being treated for breast cancer usually take 10–40 mg per day orally, divided into several doses. Up to three months may be required for a response to treatment.

Androgen replacement therapy for men is usually started at 5–20 mg per day, taken orally in divided doses.

If a dose is missed, it should be taken as soon as it is remembered, unless it is more than two hours late. If it is more than two hours late, the patient should skip that dose and continue to follow the normal dosing schedule.

Precautions

Fluoxymesterone may be taken with food if it causes stomach upset. Patients taking this medication should ensure that they see their physician regularly during treatment and receive appropriate laboratory tests. Liver function should be monitored and cholesterol and red blood cell levels may need to be examined during treatment. Female breast cancer patients should have their serum and urine calcium levels checked. Prepubescent males will require x-rays to determine the rate of their bone maturation. Diabetics should be aware that this medication may affect blood sugar levels.

Fluoxymesterone should not be taken by pregnant women as it will affect the sexual development of the fetus. The hormone may also pass into the milk of nursing mothers, affecting sexual development of the infant. Fluoxymesterone should not be taken by people with liver, kidney, heart or blood vessel disease, prostate problems, or sensitivity to the dye tartrazine. Patients with migraines or epilepsy should discuss these conditions with their physician before using the drug. Senior male patients using fluoxymesterone have an increased risk of prostate enlargement.

Patients should consult their physician before discontinuing the drug.

Side effects

Patients who use fluoxymesterone have an increased risk of developing liver disease, and should report symptoms such as yellowing of the eyes and skin to their physicians immediately. Women being treated for breast cancer and patients who are immobilized may develop **hypercalcemia**. Other side effects that may occur include the following:

• fluid retention

• nausea and vomiting

• diarrhea

• anxiety

• depression

• changes in sex drive

• dizziness

• suppression of blood clotting factors II, V, VII, and X

• headache

• itching

• reduction in number of white blood cells

• increase in number of red blood cells

Women who take this medication may also experience menstrual irregularities, acne, enlarged clitoris, and masculine characteristics such as deepening of the voice, increased hair growth, and male pattern baldness. Some of these changes may go away if the medication is stopped, while others may remain.

Men taking fluoxymesterone may experience breast growth, erections of excessive frequency and duration, impotence, decreased ejaculatory volume, and bladder irritation.

Interactions

A large number of medications may cause interactions with fluoxymesterone, including acetaminophen, anabolic steroids, anticoagulants, antidiabetic agents, and many others. Patients should notify their physicians of any medications they are taking before using fluoxymesterone.

Resources

BOOKS

Wilkes, Gail M., and Margaret Barton-Burke. *2013 Oncology Nursing Drug Handbook*. Burlington, MA: Jones & Bartlett Learning, 2013.

WEBSITES

AHFS Consumer Medication Information. "Fluoxymesterone." American Society of Health-System Pharmacists. Available from: http://www.nlm.nih.gov/medlineplus/druginfo/meds/a682690.html (accessed November 4, 2014).

The Scott Hamilton CARES Initiative. "Fluoxymesterone." Chemocare.com. http://chemocare.com/chemotherapy/drug-info/fluoxymesterone.aspx (accessed November 4, 2014).

ORGANIZATIONS

U.S. Food and Drug Administration, 10903 New Hampshire Ave., Silver Spring, MD 20993, (888) INFO-FDA (463-6332), http://www.fda.gov.

Racquel Baert, M.Sc.

Flutamide *see* **Antiandrogens**

Folex *see* **Methotrexate**

Folic acid

Definition

Folic acid is a water-soluble B vitamin essential in the human diet. It is an important cofactor in the synthesis of DNA and RNA of dividing cells, particularly during pregnancy and infancy when there is an increase in cell division and growth.

Purpose

Folic acid is important to the field of oncology in two ways. First, prior to neoplasm formation, folic acid is important in the synthesis of DNA and RNA and the repair of damaged DNA. Second, after a tumor develops, a form of folic acid is used to counter the side effects of **methotrexate** and 5-fluorouracil (also called **fluorouracil** or 5-FU).

Description

Prior to tumor formation

Since folic acid is a cofactor in DNA replication and biosynthesis of purines and also in DNA repair, there is an increasing amount of research (epidemiological, clinical, and experimental) that suggests a folic acid deficiency might be a factor that predisposes the formation of tumors in normal epithelial tissue. There is an inverse relationship associated with low folate diets and an increase in DNA breakage and mutation that is unable to be effectively repaired. The preventative influence of dietary folic acid on the formation of **colon cancer** is currently under heavy research. Although a correlation is observed, it has not yet been proven to show cause and effect. However, there is enough evidence to encourage consuming minimal daily dietary requirements of folic acid to potentially reduce the risk. When choosing supplements, other names for folic acid that may be encountered are folate and folacin.

After tumors form

Once a neoplasm forms, folic acid levels need to be decreased. In neoplasms, DNA replication and cell division are both occurring in an uncontrolled manner. Folate, which assists in this process, needs to be inhibited, causing an interruption in DNA synthesis and slowing the growth of the tumor. Chemotherapeutic agents called antimetabolites, or folic acid antagonists, such as methotrexate and 5-fluorouracil (5-FU), inhibit the enzymatic pathways for biosynthesis of nucleic acids by substituting for folic acid and sabotaging the reaction. Unfortunately, drugs that inhibit the biosynthesis of **cancer** cells also inhibit the biosynthesis of normal cells, resulting in extremely toxic side effects. To counter the side effects, a drug called **leucovorin** (a form of folate also known as Wellcovorin, Citrovorum, and folinic acid) opposes the toxic effects of methotrexate on normal tissue. Leucovorin also increases the anticancer effect of 5-FU.

Recommended dosage

Non-cancer individuals supplementing their diet with folic acid may reduce the risk of cancer. Supplemental folic acid can be purchased over the counter and is also fortified in breakfast cereals and whole grain products produced in the United States. The recommended intake for adults is 400 micrograms (mcg) each day. While the risk of upper limit toxicity is low, adult men and women should not exceed the advised upper limit of 1,000 mcg per day. It is especially important that individuals diagnosed with cancer seek the advice of medical professionals before commencing or continuing supplemental folic acid use because it may interact with **chemotherapy**.

Cancer patients treated with methotrexate may be given leucovorin as a "rescue" treatment approximately 24 hours later to counteract the toxic side effects on normal tissues of the gastrointestinal system and bone marrow. Leucovorin is only available by prescription. It is a systemic drug available in oral form (tablets) or via injections. The dosage varies from person to person and is based on body size.

Precautions

Patients should inform their physician of the following conditions before they begin to take leucovorin:

- Pregnancy or breast-feeding.
- Pernicious anemia.
- Allergies to leucovorin or any other drugs.

- Vitamin B_{12} deficiency. Folic acid may mask hematologic signs of B_{12} deficiency while neurologic damage progresses.

Side effects

Folic acid in general and specifically leucovorin are usually well-tolerated; however, there are some uncommon side effects that include skin rashes, **itching**, vomiting, nausea, **diarrhea**, and difficulty breathing. Although extremely rare, seizures have occurred in some patients taking leucovorin. Since leucovorin is taken with chemotherapeutic drugs, some side effects may be due to drug interaction.

Interactions

Supplemental folic acid can interact with anticonvulsant medications such as dilantin, **phenytoin**, and primidone. It also complicates the effects of metformin (used in individuals with type 2 diabetes), sulfasalazine (used in individuals with Crohn's disease), and triamterene (a diuretic).

Leucovorin enhances the effects of 5-FU and antagonizes the effects of methotrexate. It additionally interacts with barbiturate medications that may be taken by people with sleep disorders.

Resources

PERIODICALS

Durda, K., et al. "Folic Acid and Breast Cancer Risk." *Hereditary Cancer in Clinical Practice* 10, suppl. 4 (2012): A7. http://dx.doi.org/10.1186/1897-4287-10-S4-A7 (accessed November 4, 2014).

WEBSITES

American Cancer Society. "Folic Acid." http://www.cancer.org/treatment/treatmentsandsideeffects/complementaryandalternativemedicine/herbsvitaminsandminerals/folic-acid (accessed November 4, 2014).

Sally C. McFarlane-Parrott

Fortical *see* **Calcitonin**
Foscarnet *see* **Antiviral therapy**

G

Gabapentin

Definition

Gabapentin is an antiseizure or anticonvulsant medication that is used to help manage epilepsy and to treat certain types of nerve pain as well as some other conditions.

Purpose

The U.S. Food and Drug Administration (FDA) first approved gabapentin in 1993 as an antiepileptic to help prevent and manage partial seizures, with or without generalization, in combination with other antiseizure drugs in adults and children over age 12. Partial seizures are caused by brief abnormal electrical activity in localized areas of the brain. They usually do not result in loss of consciousness, but may cause rhythmic contractions in one area of the body or abnormal numbness or tingling sensations. When gabapentin is used along with other drug therapies for managing epileptic partial seizures, improvements are usually observed within 12 weeks. A liquid formulation and its use in children aged three to 12 was approved by the FDA in 2000.

The FDA has also approved gabapentin for the treatment of nerve pain that sometimes accompanies herpes infections (post-herpetic neuralgia from shingles). Gabapentin is used off-label (without specific FDA approval) to treat severe chronic nerve pain due to nerve damage, diabetic **neuropathy**, multiple sclerosis, **cancer**, and trigeminal neuralgia. It is also used as an acute treatment for bipolar mood disorder (manic-depressive disorder), to treat tremors associated with multiple sclerosis, and to prevent migraine headaches. Gabapentin is sometimes prescribed off-label for other mood disorders and for post-menopausal hot flashes.

Gabapentin has begun to replace tricyclic antidepressants (TCAs)—such as **amitriptyline**, nortriptyline, and desipramine—as a first-line treatment for neuropathic pain. Although both gabapentin and TCAs take from one to three weeks to provide pain relief, gabapentin appears to be the safer drug, especially in the elderly and those taking multiple medications. However, gabapentin is more expensive than TCAs.

Description

Gabapentin is structurally similar to gamma-aminobutyric acid (GABA), a neurotransmitter in the central nervous system (brain and spinal cord) that decreases the firing of neurons and prevents excitatory electrical impulses from spreading to neighboring cells. Although this could theoretically lead to a decrease in seizure activity, gabapentin does not interact with GABA receptors and its exact mechanism of action for controlling seizures and reducing pain is not known. However, gabapentin does appear to alter the activity of nerve cells.

Gabapentin is available as 100, 300, and 400 milligram (mg) capsules; as 600 and 800 mg tablets; and as a 250 mg per 5 mL liquid solution.

U.S. brand names

- Gabarone
- Neurontin

Canadian brand names

- Apo-Gabapentin
- Neurontin
- Novo-Gabapentin
- Nu-Gabapentin
- PMS-Gabapentin

International brand names

- Gabapentin
- Neurontin

Recommended dosage

For seizure control in those over age 12, the initial gabapentin dose may be 300 mg three times daily. This may be gradually increased as necessary, usually to no more than a total of 1,800 mg daily in three doses. However, some patients may need even higher doses to control their seizures. Doses up to 3,600 mg per day have been well-tolerated in research studies. For children ages three to 12, the dosage is based on body weight, initially 10–15 mg per kilogram (kg; 2.2 lb.) per day in three equal doses, increased as necessary until an effective dosage is reached, typically 25–40 mg per kg per day. For children under the age of three, use and dosage of gabapentin is determined by the physician.

To treat neuropathic pain, gabapentin is usually gradually increased from an initial dose of 300 mg on the first day, two 300 mg doses on the second day, and three 300 mg on the third day, up to a maximum daily dose of 1,800 mg. Research studies have found effective doses to range from 300 to 3,600 mg per day. The optimal dosage appears to be 1,200–2,400 mg per day in three doses.

The optimal dosage for treatment of bipolar disorder is not well-established. Doses up to 4,800 mg per day have been used.

To minimize side effects the first dose should be taken at bedtime and doses should be taken at even intervals. If a dose is missed, it should be taken as soon as remembered. However, double dosing can be hazardous and should be avoided. Capsules should not be chewed or crushed.

Precautions

- Gabapentin should be taken only as prescribed.
- Gabapentin should not be used alone for the treatment of seizures unless the patient cannot tolerate other anticonvulsant drugs.
- Patients should avoid driving, operating dangerous machinery, or participating in hazardous activities until they learn how gabapentin affects their alertness, reaction time, and judgment.
- Gabapentin should not be discontinued suddenly, since this can increase the risk of seizures; rather, the dosage should be gradually decreased over at least one week.
- Gabapentin has caused the development of tumors in experimental animals, although it is not known whether this occurs in humans.
- In 2008, the FDA issued a warning that gabapentin and other antiepileptic drugs posed an increased risk for suicidal thoughts and behaviors.

Pediatric

Gabapentin should be used with caution in children under 12 years-of-age, due to the lack of safety and efficacy studies in this population.

Pregnant or breastfeeding

Gabapentin has caused fetal abnormalities in mice, rats, and rabbits. Although it has not been studied in pregnant women, it should only be used by women who are pregnant or may become pregnant if its potential benefits outweigh the risks. Breastfeeding mothers should discuss the risks and benefits of gabapentin with their physicians.

Other conditions and allergies

Gabapentin should be used with caution in patients with severe kidney disease and the dosage should be reduced.

Side effects

Gabapentin is usually well-tolerated. The most common side effects are nervous system symptoms including:

- drowsiness
- dizziness
- fatigue
- trembling or shaking
- unsteadiness
- clumsiness
- uncontrollable back-and-forth eye movements or eye rolling
- double or blurred vision
- swelling of the hands, feet, or legs
- muscle weakness or pain

These side effects appear to be dose-related and usually disappear after the first several weeks.

Less common side effects that may occur when first taking gabapentin include:

- dry mouth and eyes
- runny nose
- frequent urination
- indigestion
- nausea and/or vomiting
- constipation or diarrhea
- low blood pressure
- back pain
- decreased sexual drive

- ringing in the ears
- slurred speech
- difficulty concentrating
- insomnia
- weight gain
- twitching

Other less common side effects of gabapentin include:

- irritability
- mood changes
- memory loss
- impotence
- depression
- changes in thinking

Rare side effects of gabapentin include:

- pain in the lower back or side
- difficulty urinating
- fever and/or chills
- cough
- hoarseness

A patient experiencing any of the following should contact their physician or pharmacist immediately:

- mental or mood changes
- tingling or numbness in the hands or feet
- swelling of ankles
- vision problems
- fever or unusual bleeding

Signs of gabapentin overdose may include:

- double vision
- slurred speech
- drowsiness
- diarrhea

Pediatric

Gabapentin can cause behavioral and emotional disorders in children, including hostility and hyperactivity. Children under age 12 who experience the following more common side effects should see a doctor immediately:

- aggressive behavior
- irritability
- anxiety
- difficulty concentrating or paying attention
- crying
- depression

QUESTIONS TO ASK YOUR DOCTOR

- How should I take this medication?
- What side effects might I experience?
- When should I call my doctor about side effects?
- Can I drink alcohol while taking this medication?
- Can I stop taking this medication on my own?

- mood swings
- increased emotionality
- hyperactivity
- suspiciousness or distrust

Geriatric

Elderly patients may be more sensitive to the side effects of gabapentin.

Interactions

Among the advantages of gabapentin are that it is not broken down in the body and unlike many other drugs that are used to treat epilepsy, it has few interactions with other drugs. In particular, gabapentin does not interfere with other commonly used anticonvulsants such as **phenytoin**, **carbamazepine**, valproic acid, and phenobarbital. However antacids such as Mylanta and Maalox can interfere with the absorption of gabapentin, lowering its level in the blood, and should be taken at least two hours after taking gabapentin to avoid compromising its effectiveness.

Alcohol should be limited or avoided while taking gabapentin since it can intensify drowsiness and dizziness caused by the drug. Foods do not appear to affect the absorption of gabapentin.

The following herbs should be avoided when taking gabapentin:

- evening primrose
- valerian
- St. John's wort
- kava kava
- gotu kola

Resources

BOOKS

Corey, E. J., et al. *Molecules and Medicine.* Hoboken, NJ: John Wiley & Sons, 2007.

Hales, Robert E., et al. *What Your Patients Need To Know About Psychiatric Medications.* Washington, DC: American Psychiatric Publishing, 2007.

Schatzberg, Alan F., and Charles B. Nemeroff. *Essentials of Clinical Psychopharmacology.* 2nd ed. Washington, DC: American Psychiatric Publishing, 2006.

PERIODICALS

Kirkey, Sharon. "Off-Label Drug Use Can Have Painful Consequences; Many Drugs Are Used to Treat Illnesses They Were Not Intended For." *Vancouver Sun* (January 2, 2009): B3.

Steinman, Michael A., et al. "Narrative Review: The Promotion of Gabapentin: An Analysis of Internal Industry Documents." *Annals of Internal Medicine* 145, no. 4 (August 15, 2006): 284–293.

WEBSITES

American Society of Health-System Pharmacists. "Gabapentin." MedlinePlus. http://www.nlm.nih.gov/medlineplus/druginfo/meds/a694007.html (accessed November 4, 2014).

U.S. Food and Drug Administration. "Suicidal Behavior and Ideation and Antiepileptic Drugs." http://www.fda.gov/Drugs/DrugSafety/PostmarketDrugSafetyInformationforPatientsandProviders/UCM100190 (accessed November 4, 2014).

ORGANIZATIONS

American Chronic Pain Association, PO Box 850, Rocklin, CA 95677, (800) 533-3231, Fax: (916) 632-3208, ACPA@pacbell.net, http://www.theacpa.org.

American Pain Foundation, 201 North Charles Street, Suite 710, Baltimore, MD 21201-4111, (888) 615-PAIN (7246), info@painfoundation.org, http://www.painfoundation.org.

U.S. Food and Drug Administration, 10903 New Hampshire Ave., Silver Spring, MD 20993, (888) INFO-FDA (463-6332), http://www.fda.gov.

Rosalyn Carson-DeWitt, MD.
Emily Jane Willingham, PhD.
REVISED BY MARGARET ALIC, PHD.

Galactogram *see* **Ductogram**

Gallbladder cancer

Definition

Cancer of the gallbladder is cancer of the pear-shaped organ that lies on the undersurface of the liver. The basic function of the gallbladder is to store bile, a fluid produced by the liver that is essential in the proper digestion of fats. The gallbladder in adult humans is about 3.1–4 inches long (7.9–10.2 centimeters) and 1.6 inches (4 centimeters) in diameter when it is completely filled.

Description

The human gallbladder serves primarily as a storage vessel for bile, a yellowish-brown or dark green fluid that aids in the digestion of fats in the small intestine. The gallbladder is not, however, essential to life and can be surgically removed when needed to treat recurrent gallstones or other disorders. Bile from the liver is funneled into the gallbladder by way of the cystic duct. Between meals, the gallbladder stores a large amount of bile. To do this, it must absorb much of the water and electrolytes from the bile. In fact, the inner surface of the gallbladder is the most absorptive surface in the body. After a meal, the gallbladder's muscular walls contract to deliver the bile back through the cystic duct and eventually into the small intestine, where the bile can help digest fatty foods.

Demographics

Gallbladder cancer is relatively uncommon compared to other cancers. About 10,650 new cases of gallbladder cancer will be diagnosed in the United States in 2014, making it the sixth most common gastrointestinal cancer; about 3,630 of these patients will die during the year. It is two to six times more common in females than males, and most patients are elderly. The average age of patients with gallbladder cancer in the United States and Canada is 72, and the risk increases with age. Southwest American Indians have a particularly high incidence—six times that of the general American population. Other high-risk populations include American Hispanics and people from Southeast Asia. Caucasians and African Americans have lower rates of gallbladder cancer than other ethnic groups in the United States.

Worldwide, there is considerable variation in the incidence of gallbladder cancer. Areas with the highest rates include India, Korea, Japan, the Czech Republic, Slovakia, Spain, Colombia, Chile, Peru, Bolivia, and Ecuador. The high incidence rates reported in Peru and Chile are thought to reflect their large Hispanic populations with Indian heritage. The United Kingdom, Norway, and Denmark have the lowest rates of gallbladder cancer.

Causes and symptoms

Although the basic cause of gallbladder cancer is not well understood as of 2014, chronic inflammation plays an important role. Gallstones are the most significant risk factor for the development of gallbladder cancer. Roughly 75 to 90 percent of patients with gallbladder cancer also have gallstones. Larger gallstones are

KEY TERMS

Adenocarcinoma—A type of cancerous tumor that develops in the gland-like cells of epithelial tissue, which is the tissue that lines the inner and exterior surfaces of body organs.

Cholangiography—Radiographic examination of the bile ducts after injection with a special dye. It is used to determine whether the bile ducts are enlarged, narrowed, or blocked.

Cholecystectomy—The medical term for surgical removal of the gallbladder.

Cholecystitis—Inflammation of the gallbladder, usually due to infection.

Computed tomography—A radiology test by which images of cross-sectional planes of the body are obtained.

Congenital—Present at birth.

Jaundice—Yellowish staining of the skin and eyes due to excess bilirubin in the bloodstream.

Metastasis (plural, metastases)—The spread of tumor cells from one part of the body to another through blood vessels or lymphatic vessels.

Pancreatitis—Inflammation of the pancreas.

Porcelain gallbladder—A condition in which calcium is deposited in the walls of the gallbladder, causing the organ to become whitish or bluish-white in appearance and brittle. It is a risk factor for gallbladder cancer.

Resection—The surgical removal of a portion of an organ or body part.

Stent—Slender hollow catheter or rod placed within a vessel or duct to provide support or maintain patency.

Tumor marker—A type of protein found in blood, urine, or body tissues that can be measured and used to detect the presence of cancer.

Ultrasound—A radiology test utilizing high-frequency sound waves.

associated with a higher chance of developing gallbladder cancer. Chronic inflammation of the gallbladder from infection or parasitic infestation also increases the risk of gallbladder cancer.

Other risk factors include:

- Family history of gallbladder cancer.
- Obesity.
- History of heavy smoking.
- Congenital abnormalities in the structure of the gallbladder.
- Porcelain gallbladder. This is a condition in which calcium is deposited in the gallbladder wall, causing the organ to become bluish-white in appearance and brittle.
- In women, a high number of pregnancies.
- In men, Korean ethnicity.

Unfortunately, sometimes cancer of the gallbladder does not produce symptoms until late in the disease; this is one reason for the high mortality rate of this type of cancer. When symptoms are evident, the most common is pain in the upper right portion of the abdomen, underneath the right rib cage. Patients with gallbladder cancer may also report symptoms such as nausea, vomiting, weakness, jaundice, skin **itching**, **fever**, chills, poor appetite, black or tarry stools, and **weight loss**. In some cases, the patient's gallbladder may become so enlarged that the physician can feel it during an examination of the abdomen.

Diagnosis

Diagnosis of gallbladder cancer is difficult because it mimics other more common conditions such as gallstones, cholecystitis, and pancreatitis. The imaging tests that are utilized to evaluate these other conditions, however, can also detect gallbladder cancer. For example, ultrasound is a quick, noninvasive imaging test that reliably diagnoses gallstones and cholecystitis. It can also detect the presence of gallbladder cancer, as well as show how far the cancer has spread. If cancer is suspected, a **computed tomography** scan is useful in confirming the presence of an abnormal mass and further demonstrating the size and extent of the tumor. The wide variation in appearance of gallbladder tumors on CT scans, however, complicates the use of this imaging modality as a diagnostic tool; some gallbladder cancers appear as a general thickening of the wall of the organ rather than a well-defined mass. Cholangiography, usually performed to evaluate a patient with jaundice, can also detect gallbladder cancer.

There are no specific laboratory tests for gallbladder cancer as of 2014, although researchers are testing two **tumor markers**, CA242 and CA199, as possible screening tools. Other tumor markers that are presently used are carcinoembryonic antigen (CEA) and CA 19-9, although these are not specific for gallbladder cancer. Blood tests are sometimes useful because tumors in the gallbladder can obstruct the normal flow of bile from the liver to the small intestine. Bilirubin, a component of bile, builds up within the liver and is absorbed into the bloodstream in excess amounts. Bilirubin can be detected in a blood test, but it can also manifest clinically as jaundice. Elevated bilirubin levels and clinical jaundice can also occur with such other conditions as gallstones.

On occasion, gallbladder cancer is diagnosed incidentally. About 1% of all patients who have their gallbladder removed for symptomatic gallstones are found to have gallbladder cancer. The cancer is found either by the surgeon or by the pathologist who inspects the gallbladder with a microscope.

Treatment team

The main member of the treatment team is the surgeon, since surgical removal of the cancer is the only measure that offers a significant chance of cure. Because gallbladder cancer is a relatively uncommon cancer, patients diagnosed with it should consider seeking treatment at a major cancer center with surgeons who are experienced in performing surgery for gallbladder cancer.

Sometimes the cancer is so advanced that surgery would be of no benefit, though the patient might suffer from jaundice or blockage of the stomach. In this case, the gastroenterologist or interventional radiologist may be able to provide nonsurgical alternatives to address these complications. In limited scenarios, the oncologist or radiation therapist may treat the patient with **chemotherapy** or **radiation therapy**.

Other members of the treatment team include the anesthesiologist, nurses, and hospital pharmacists. A physical therapist and dietitian may be part of the treatment team during recovery, as appropriate exercise is beneficial to patients, and removal of the gallbladder may require changes in the patient's diet.

Clinical staging

About 90% of gallbladder cancers are adenocarcinomas, which means that they are a type of cancer that begins in the gland-like cells that line the interiors of such organs as the gallbladder. The remaining 10% are sarcomas or squamous cell carcinomas. The prognosis of gallbladder cancer that has progressed beyond stage 0 is poor. At the time of diagnosis, about 40% of gallbladder cancers have perforated the gallbladder wall, and another 30% have metastasized to distant organs.

Staging of gallbladder cancer is determined by how far the cancer has spread. The effectiveness of treatment declines as the stage progresses. Most gallbladder cancers begin in the innermost wall of the organ and grow through the various layers of tissue toward the outside of the gallbladder. Stage 0 gallbladder cancer is very small and confined to the inner wall of the gallbladder. Approximately 20% of cancers are at this stage at the time of diagnosis; the 5-year survival rate is 80%. Stage I cancer has grown into the intermediate walls of the organ; its 5-year survival rate is 50%. Stage II cancer has penetrated the full thickness of the wall, but has not spread to nearby lymph nodes or invaded adjacent organs; its 5-year survival rate is 28%. Stage III cancer has spread to nearby lymph nodes or has invaded the liver, stomach, colon, small intestine, or large intestine; its 5-year survival rate is 7%–8%. Stage IV disease has invaded very deeply into two or more adjacent organs, has grown into the main blood vessels leading into the liver, or has spread to distant lymph nodes or organs by way of **metastasis**; its 5-year survival rate is 2%–4%. The median survival for patients with stage IV gallbladder cancer is only 2–5 months.

Treatment

Early stage I cancers involving only the innermost layer of the gallbladder wall can be cured by simple removal of the gallbladder; this procedure is called a cholecystectomy. Cancers at this stage are sometimes found incidentally when the gallbladder is removed in the treatment of gallstones or cholecystitis. Late stage I cancers, which involve the outer muscular layers of the gallbladder wall, are generally treated in the same way as stage II or III cancers. Removal of the gallbladder is not sufficient for these stages. The surgeon also removes nearby lymph nodes, as well as a portion of the adjacent liver; this is called an extended or radical cholecystectomy. Patients with early stage IV disease may benefit from radical surgery, but the issue is controversial. One reason why radical surgery for patients with advanced gallbladder cancer is a subject of debate is the relative rarity of the cancer; it is difficult for clinicians to gather a large enough patient sample to obtain statistically significant results. Late stage IV cancer has spread too extensively to allow complete resection. Surgery is not an option for these patients.

Other therapies

When long-term survival is not likely, the focus of therapy shifts to improving quality of life. Jaundice and blockage of the stomach are two problems faced by patients with advanced cancer of the gallbladder. These can be treated with surgery, or alternatively, by special interventional techniques employed by the gastroenterologist or radiologist. A stent can be placed across the bile ducts in order to re-establish the flow of bile and relieve jaundice. A small feeding tube can be placed in the small intestine to allow feeding when the stomach is blocked. Pain may be treated with conventional pain medicines or a celiac ganglion nerve block. Another palliative treatment that is sometimes used to relieve pain in

QUESTIONS TO ASK YOUR DOCTOR

- What stage of cancer do I have?
- How will my cancer be treated?
- What side effects can I expect as a result of my treatment?
- Will I need to make changes to my diet?
- What is my prognosis?

gallbladder cancer is alcohol injections to deaden the nerves that carry pain sensations from the gallbladder and digestive tract to the brain.

Current chemotherapy or radiation therapy cannot cure gallbladder cancer, but these modalities may offer some benefit in certain patients. For cancer that is too advanced for surgical cure, treatment with such chemotherapeutic agents as 5-fluorouracil, **gemcitabine**, **cisplatin**, or **capecitabine** may lengthen survival for a few months. The limited benefit of chemotherapy must be weighed carefully against its side effects. Radiation therapy is sometimes used after attempted surgical resection of the cancer to extend survival for a few months or relieve jaundice. The most common form of radiation therapy used to treat gallbladder cancer is external beam radiation therapy. Radiation therapy may be used as a palliative treatment to relieve pain in patients with advanced gallbladder cancer.

Complementary and alternative (CAM) treatments cannot cure gallbladder cancer, but may be helpful in relieving the emotional and spiritual distress of patients with this type of cancer. Acupuncture is reported to relieve nausea associated with chemotherapy, and essential oils used in aromatherapy (particularly lavender and Roman chamomile) are calming and relaxing for some patients. Prayer, meditation, journaling or expressive writing, and guided imagery are helpful for others.

Coping with cancer treatment

After cancer treatment, many patients find that good nutrition and a strong support system (which may include a support group) improve their quality of life. Treatment team members, social workers, or hospital chaplains can often recommend local resources that can be of assistance to the patient. Many larger cancer centers have staff members specifically assigned to assist patients and their family members with finding nearby housing during the patient's treatment, dealing with financial questions, and coping with the stress of the patient's illness and the side effects of radiation or chemotherapy.

Clinical trials

More **clinical trials** are needed to define the role of chemotherapy and radiation therapy after attempted surgical resection of stage II and III cancer. Of the 182 clinical trials of therapies for gallbladder cancer registered with the National Institutes of Health as of mid-2014, most are investigations of different combinations of chemotherapy drugs, or of chemotherapy combined with radiation therapy. There are no trials presently underway of radical cholecystectomy as a treatment, or of CAM therapies for gallbladder cancer.

Prevention

Preventive surgery is recommended for patients with porcelain gallbladder even when it is asymptomatic, because of the high risk of it progressing into cancer. Some surgeons also recommend a preventive cholecystectomy in patients over the age of 50 with large polyps in the gallbladder.

Special concerns

After the removal of the gallbladder, patients may experience a temporary change in bowel habits. The bowel movements may be more frequent or more liquid than before surgery. This situation usually resolves within about six months. In some cases, a change in diet may help, and patients may wish to consult a registered dietitian for advice about a nutritious and easily digested diet.

Patients with metastatic gallbladder cancer should be referred for **hospice care** as soon as possible after diagnosis because their typical length of survival is six months or less.

Resources

BOOKS

Abeloff, Martin D., et al. *Clinical Oncology*. 4th ed. New York: Churchill Livingstone/Elsevier, 2008.

Herman, Joseph M., Timothy M. Pawlik, and Charles L. Thomas, Jr., eds. *Biliary Tract and Gallbladder Cancer*, 2nd ed. New York: Springer, 2014.

Sabiston, David C., et al. *Sabiston Textbook of Surgery: The Biological Basis of Modern Surgical Practice*, 19th ed. Philadelphia: Saunders/Elsevier, 2012.

Spiliotis, John D., and Konstantinos Tepetes, eds. *Cancer Surgery in the Elderly*. New York: Nova Science Publishers, 2011.

Thomas, Charles R., Jr., and Clifton David Fuller, eds. *Biliary Tract and Gallbladder Cancer: Diagnosis and Therapy*. New York: Demos Medical, 2009.

PERIODICALS

Andrén-Sandberg, A., and Y. Deng. "Aspects on Gallbladder Cancer in 2014." *Current Opinion in Gastroenterology* 30 (May 2014): 326–331.

Hundal, R., and E. A. Shaffer. "Gallbladder Cancer: Epidemiology and Outcome." *Clinical Epidemiology* 6 (March 7, 3014): 99–109.

Mitchell, C. H., et al. "Features Suggestive of Gallbladder Malignancy: Analysis of T1, T2, and T3 Tumors on Cross-sectional Imaging." *Journal of Computer-assisted Tomography* 38 (March-April 2014): 235–241.

Wang, Y. F., et al. "Combined Detection Tumor Markers for Diagnosis and Prognosis of Gallbladder Cancer." *World Journal of Gastroenterology* 20 (April 14, 2014): 4085–4092.

Wernberg, J. A., and D. D. Lucarelli. "Gallbladder Cancer." *Surgical Clinics of North America* 94 (April 2014): 343–360.

WEBSITES

American Cancer Society (ACS). "Gallbladder Cancer." http://www.cancer.org/acs/groups/cid/documents/webcontent/003101-pdf.pdf (accessed August 8, 2014).

Denshaw-Burke, Mary. "Gallbladder Cancer." Medscape Reference. http://emedicine.medscape.com/article/278641-overview (accessed August 8, 2014).

Mayo Clinic. "Gallbladder Cancer." http://www.mayoclinic.org/diseases-conditions/gallbladder-cancer/basics/definition/con-20023909 (accessed August 8, 2014).

National Cancer Institute (NCI). "Gallbladder Cancer." http://www.cancer.gov/cancertopics/types/gallbladder (accessed August 8, 2014).

ORGANIZATIONS

American Cancer Society (ACS), 250 Williams Street NW, Atlanta, GA 30303, (800) 227-2345, http://www.cancer.org/aboutus/howwehelpyou/app/contact-us.aspx, http://www.cancer.org/index.

American College of Gastroenterology (ACG), 6400 Goldsboro Road, Suite 200, Bethesda, MD 20817, (301) 263-9000, info@acg.gi.org, http://gi.org/.

National Cancer Institute (NCI), BG 9609 MSC 9760, 9609 Medical Center Drive, Bethesda, MD 20892-9760, (800) 4-CANCER (422-6237), http://www.cancer.gov/global/contact/email-us, http://www.cancer.gov.

Office of Cancer Complementary and Alternative Medicine (OCCAM), 9609 Medical Center Dr., Room 5-W-136, Rockville, MD 20850, (240) 276-6595, Fax: (240) 276-7888, ncioccam1-r@mail.nih.gov, http://cam.cancer.gov.

Kevin O. Hwang, MD.
REVISED BY REBECCA J. FREY, PhD.

Gallium nitrate

Definition

Gallium nitrate is a drug that is used to treat **hypercalcemia**, or too much calcium in the blood. This condition may occur when individuals develop **cancer** that spreads to or affects the bones, such as **multiple**

myeloma. Gallium nitrate is also known by the common brand name Ganite.

Purpose

The purpose of gallium nitrate is to reduce the level of calcium in a patient's blood. It is a liquid medication that is injected into a person's vein.

Description

Hypercalcemia is a serious condition that can be fatal, so it is very important that it is effectively treated. Hypercalcemia is a common complication of cancer, affecting approximately 10%–20% of all cancer patients. The condition can affect many systems of the body and has various signs and symptoms.

Symptoms of hypercalcemia include frequent urination, thirst, dizziness, constipation, nausea, and vomiting. Sometimes, these symptoms may be thought to be associated with the cancer, and therefore the hypercalcemia itself may go undiagnosed. Another symptom is disruptions in cardiac rhythm; if severe, this complication can lead to seizure, cardiac arrest, coma, or death.

Hypercalcemia should first be treated with fluids, but fluid treatment alone is usually not effective to treat this condition. Therefore, some physicians may recommend that their patients take gallium nitrate to establish a normal balance of calcium in the blood.

Recommended dosage

The recommended dosage of gallium nitrate differs depending on the patient and should be determined by a physician. For adults and teenagers, the dosage of this medication is based on body weight/size and must be calculated by a doctor. The medication is injected into a patient's vein at a slow pace for 24 hours over a period of five days. If a patient's calcium level is still too high, this process can be repeated in two to four weeks. For younger children, up to the age of 12, there are no specific studies to determine the effects of gallium nitrate. Therefore, use and dosage of this medication must be determined by the treating physician.

While undergoing treatment with gallium nitrate, patients' calcium levels should be checked at regular intervals. Even if a patient's condition has improved, he or she may still need to undergo regular examinations to make sure that the hypercalcemia does not redevelop.

Precautions

Patients should let their physicians know if they are allergic to any foods, preservatives or dyes. In addition, patients with certain medical problems, specifically kidney disease, should make sure that the prescribing physician is aware of this, as use of gallium nitrate can exacerbate this condition. Adequate hydration may minimize toxic effects on the kidney.

Use of gallium nitrate has not been studied in pregnant animals or humans. It is not recommended for women who are pregnant or breast-feeding, as it may cause negative side effects.

Side effects

Individuals who are considering taking gallium nitrate should discuss its use in detail with their physician. This includes talking about the potential benefits versus any potential side effects. Some individuals may experience all, some, or none of these side effects, and side effects may lessen as a person's body adjusts to the medication. It is important to be aware of all potential side effects, as some of them may require medical interventions.

More common side effects include:

- blood in the urine
- pain in the bones
- change in urination frequency
- feeling thirsty
- loss of appetite (anorexia)
- weakness of muscles
- feeling nauseous
- diarrhea
- metallic taste in the mouth
- nausea and vomiting
- decrease of phosphate levels in the blood

Less common side effects include:

- cramps in the abdomen
- a feeling of confusion
- muscle spasms

Rare side effects include:

- excessive fatigue or weakness

Interactions

Patients should tell their physician if they are taking any other medications on a regular basis, especially the ones listed below, as they could cause a negative interaction if taken with gallium nitrate:

- certain medications taken for infections
- cisplatin
- medications for pain that contain acetaminophen or aspirin
- cyclosporine
- deferoxamine
- some medications for treatment of arthritis
- lithium
- methotrexate
- penicillamine
- gentamicin
- amphotericin B
- nephrotoxic agents

Resources

WEBSITES

American Cancer Society. "Gallium Nitrate." http://www. cancer.org/treatment/treatmentsandsideeffects/guidetocancerdrugs/gallium-nitrate (accessed September 26, 2014).

Tiffani A. DeMarco, MS

Gallium scan

Definition

A gallium scan of the body is a nuclear medicine test that is conducted using a camera that detects gallium, a form of radionuclide, or radioactive chemical substance.

Purpose

Most gallium scans are ordered to detect cancerous tumors, infections, or areas of inflammation in the body. Gallium is known to accumulate in inflamed, infected, or cancerous tissues. The scans are used to determine whether a patient with an unexplained **fever** has an infection and the site of the infection, if present. Gallium scans also may be used to evaluate **cancer** following **chemotherapy** or **radiation therapy**.

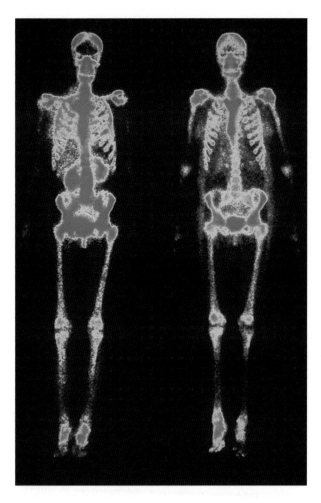

Nuclear medicine scan of the skeleton. A radioisotope, like gallium, is used to produce this image. This scan reveals that lung cancer has spread to ribs and there is osteomyelitis in ankle. *(Scott Camazine/Science Source)*

Precautions

Children and women who are pregnant or breast-feeding are only given gallium scans if the potential diagnostic benefits will outweigh the risks.

Description

The patient will usually be asked to come to the testing facility 24–48 hours before the procedure to receive the injection of gallium. Sometimes, the injection will be given only four to six hours before the study or as long as 72 hours before the procedure. The time frame is based on the area or organs of the body being studied.

For the study itself, the patient lies very still for approximately 30–60 minutes. A camera is moved across the patient's body to detect and capture images of concentrations of the gallium. The camera picks up signals from any accumulated areas of the radionuclide.

In most cases, the patient is lying down throughout the procedure. Back (posterior) and front (anterior) views will usually be taken, and sometimes a side (lateral) view is used. The camera may occasionally touch the patient's skin, but will not cause any discomfort. A clicking noise may be heard throughout the procedure; this is only the sound of the scanner registering radiation.

Preparation

The intravenous injection of gallium is done in a separate appointment prior to the procedure. Generally, no special dietary requirements are necessary. Sometimes the physician will ask that the patient have light or clear meals within a day or less of the procedure. Many patients will be given **laxatives** or an enema prior to the scan to eliminate any residual gallium from the bowels.

Aftercare

There is generally no aftercare required following a gallium scan. Women who are breastfeeding who have a scan will be cautioned against breastfeeding for four weeks following the exam.

Risks

There is a minimal risk of exposure to radiation from the gallium injection, but the exposure from one gallium scan is generally less than exposure from x-rays.

Results

A radiologist trained in nuclear medicine or a nuclear medicine specialist will interpret the exam results and compare them to other diagnostic tests. It is normal for gallium to accumulate in the liver, spleen, bones, breast tissue, and large bowel.

Abnormal results

An abnormal concentration of gallium in areas other than those where it normally concentrates may indicate the presence of disease. Concentrations may be due to inflammation, infection, or the presence of tumor tissue. Often, additional tests are required to determine if the tumors are malignant (cancerous) or benign.

Even though gallium normally concentrates in organs such as the liver or spleen, abnormally high concentrations will suggest certain diseases and conditions. For example, **Hodgkin lymphoma** or **non-Hodgkin lymphoma** may be diagnosed or staged if there is abnormal gallium activity in the lymph nodes. After a patient receives cancer treatment, such as radiation therapy or chemotherapy, a gallium scan may help to find new or recurring tumors or to record regression of a treated tumor. Physicians can narrow causes of liver problems by noting abnormal gallium activity in the liver. Gallium scans also may be used to diagnose lung diseases or a disease called sarcoidosis, in the chest.

Resources

WEBSITES

MedlinePlus. "Gallium Scan." http://www.nlm.nih.gov/medline plus/ency/article/003450.htm (accessed December 4, 2014).

ORGANIZATIONS

American Cancer Society, 250 Williams St. NW, Atlanta, GA 30303, (800) 227-2345, http://www.cancer.org.

American College of Nuclear Medicine, 1850 Samuel Morse Dr., Reston, VA 20190-5316, (703) 326-1190, Fax: (703) 708-9015, http://www.acnmonline.org.

American Liver Foundation, 39 Broadway, Ste. 2700, New York, NY 10006, (212) 668-1000, (800) GO-LIVER (465-4837), Fax: (212) 483-8179, http://www.liverfoundation.org.

Society of Nuclear Medicine and Molecular Imaging, 1850 Samuel Morse Dr., Reston, VA 20190, (703) 708-9000, Fax: (703) 708-9015, http://www.snmmi.org.

Teresa G. Odle

Ganciclovir *see* **Antiviral therapy**

Ganite *see* **Gallium nitrate**

Gardasil *see* **Cancer vaccines; Human papillomavirus**

Gastrectomy

Definition

Gastrectomy is the surgical removal of all or part of the stomach.

Purpose

Gastrectomy is performed most often to treat the following conditions:

- stomach (gastric) cancer
- bleeding gastric ulcer
- perforation of the stomach wall
- noncancerous tumors

Demographics

According to the World Health Organization (WHO), **stomach cancer** is the second leading cause of **cancer** deaths in the world, accounting for about 8.8% of all deaths from cancer—lung cancer accounts for 17.8% of cancer deaths. Although stomach cancer is a worldwide problem, the incidence rates vary considerably in different countries. In the 2000s, the highest death rates from stomach cancer were found in Japan, South America (especially Chile), and parts of the former Soviet Union. In the United States, the American Cancer Society expected about 22,220 new cases of stomach cancer to be diagnosed in 2014, with 10,990 deaths attributed to the disease. Since gastrectomy is most often done to treat stomach cancer, gastrectomy rates should mirror stomach cancer rates.

Description

Gastrectomy for cancer

Surgery is the only curative treatment for gastric (stomach) cancer. If the cancer is diagnosed early and limited to one part of the stomach, the tumor and only part of the stomach may be removed (partial or subtotal gastrectomy). More often, the entire stomach is removed (total gastrectomy) along with the surrounding lymph nodes. When the entire stomach is removed, the esophagus is attached directly to the small intestine.

A gastrectomy is performed under general anesthesia. Once the patient is anesthetized, a urinary catheter is usually inserted to monitor urine output. A thin

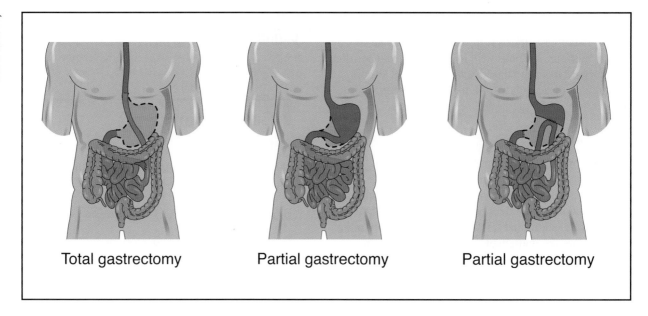

Total gastrectomy   Partial gastrectomy   Partial gastrectomy

Illustration showing total gastrectomy (removal of the stomach) and two types of partial gastrectomy. *(Illustration by Electronic Illustrators Group. © Cengage Learning®.)*

nasogastric tube is inserted into the nose, through the esophagus, and into the stomach. The abdomen is cleansed with an antiseptic solution. The surgeon makes a large incision from just below the breastbone down to the navel. The surgeon then removes all or part of the stomach and attaches either the remaining piece of stomach or the esophagus to the small intestine.

Gastrectomy for gastric cancer is almost always done using the traditional open surgery technique, which requires a wide incision to open the abdomen. Some surgeons use a laparoscopic technique that requires only a small incision. The laparoscope is connected to a tiny video camera that relays a picture of the abdomen to a monitor to guide the surgeon who then operates through this incision.

The potential benefits of laparoscopic surgery include less postoperative pain, decreased hospitalization, and earlier return to normal activities. The use of laparoscopic gastrectomy is limited—only patients with early-stage gastric cancers or those whose surgery is intended only as palliative treatment (pain and symptomatic relief rather than cure) are considered for this minimally invasive technique.

Gastrectomy for ulcers

Gastrectomy is also used occasionally in the treatment of severe peptic ulcer disease or its complications. While the vast majority of peptic ulcers (gastric ulcers in the stomach or duodenal ulcers in the duodenum) are managed with medication, partial gastrectomy is sometimes required for peptic ulcer patients who have complications. These include patients who do not respond satisfactorily to medical therapy, those who develop a bleeding or perforated ulcer, and those who develop pyloric obstruction (a blockage to the exit from the stomach). The surgical procedure for severe ulcer disease is also called an antrectomy. An antrectomy is a limited form of gastrectomy in which the antrum, or lower portion of the stomach that produces digestive juices, is removed.

Preparation

Before undergoing gastrectomy, patients require a variety of tests such as **x-rays**, **computed tomography** (CT) scans, **ultrasonography**, or endoscopic biopsies (microscopic examination of tissue) to confirm the diagnosis and localize the tumor or ulcer. **Laparoscopy** and tissue **biopsy** may be used to diagnose a malignancy or to determine the extent of a tumor that is already diagnosed. When a tumor is strongly suspected, laparoscopy is often performed immediately before the surgery to remove the tumor. This avoids the need to anesthetize the patient twice, and sometimes avoids the need for surgery completely if the tumor found through laparoscopy is deemed inoperable.

Aftercare

After gastrectomy surgery, patients are taken to the recovery unit and vital signs are closely monitored by the nursing staff until the anesthesia wears off. Patients

KEY TERMS

Adenocarcinoma—A form of cancer that involves cells from the lining of the walls of many different organs of the body.

Antrectomy—A surgical procedure for ulcer disease in which the antrum, a portion of the stomach, is removed.

Biopsy—Surgical removal of a small piece of tissue so that it can be examined under the microscope for malignancy (cancer).

Laparoscopy—The examination of the inside of the abdomen through a lighted tube (endoscope) inserted through a small incision, sometimes accompanied by surgery.

Lymphoma—Malignant tumor of lymphoblasts derived from B lymphocytes, a type of white blood cell.

commonly feel pain from the incision. Pain medication is prescribed to provide relief and is usually delivered intravenously (IV, directly into a vein). Upon waking from anesthesia, patients have an intravenous line, a urinary catheter, and a nasogastric tube in place. They cannot eat or drink immediately following surgery. In some cases, oxygen is delivered through a mask that fits over the mouth and nose. The nasogastric tube is attached to intermittent suction to keep what remains of the stomach empty.

If the whole stomach has been removed, the tube goes directly to the small intestine and remains in place until bowel function returns. This can take two to three days and is monitored by listening with a stethoscope for bowel sounds. When bowel sounds return, the patient can drink clear liquids. If the liquids are tolerated, the nasogastric tube is removed and the diet is gradually changed from liquids to soft foods, and then to more solid foods. Dietary adjustments may be necessary, as certain foods may now be difficult to digest. Overall, gastrectomy surgery usually requires a stay of 7–10 days in the hospital and recuperation time of at least several weeks.

Risks

Surgery for peptic ulcer is effective, but it may result in a variety of postoperative complications. Following gastrectomy surgery, as many as 30% of patients have significant symptoms. An operation called highly selective vagotomy, in which a nerve that stimulates the stomach is cut, is now preferred for ulcer management, as it is safer than gastrectomy.

After a gastrectomy, several abnormalities may develop that produce symptoms related to food intake. They happen largely because the stomach, which serves as a food reservoir, has been reduced in its capacity by the surgery. Other surgical procedures that often accompany gastrectomy for ulcer disease can also contribute to later symptoms. These other surgical procedures include vagotomy, which lessens acid production and slows stomach emptying, and pyloroplasty, which enlarges the opening between the stomach and small intestine to facilitate emptying of the stomach.

Some patients experience light-headedness, heart palpitations (racing heart), sweating, nausea, and vomiting after a meal. These may be symptoms of dumping syndrome, as food is rapidly moved into the small intestine from the remaining stomach or directly from the esophagus. Dumping syndrome is treated by adjusting the diet and pattern of eating—for example, eating smaller, more frequent meals, and limiting liquids.

Patients who have abdominal bloating and pain after eating, followed frequently by **nausea and vomiting**, may have afferent loop syndrome, a serious condition that must be corrected surgically. Patients who have early satiety (feeling of fullness after eating), abdominal discomfort, and vomiting may have bile reflux gastritis (also called bilious vomiting), which is also surgically correctable. Many patients experience **weight loss** after gastrectomy.

Reactive hyperglycemia is a condition that results when blood sugar levels become too high after a meal, stimulating the release of insulin, occurring about two hours after eating. Should this occur after gastrectomy, changing to a high-protein diet and smaller meals is advised.

Ulcers recur in a small percentage of patients after partial gastrectomy for peptic ulcer. Recurrence is usually within the first few years after surgery. Further surgery is usually necessary.

Vitamin and mineral supplementation is necessary after gastrectomy to correct certain deficiencies, especially vitamin B_{12}, iron, and folate. Vitamin D and calcium are also needed to prevent and treat the bone problems that often occur. These include softening and bending of the bones, which can produce pain and osteoporosis, which is a loss of bone mass. According to one study, the risk for spinal fracture after gastrectomy may be as high as 50%.

Results

Overall, survival after gastrectomy for gastric cancer varies greatly by the stage of disease at the time of

QUESTIONS TO ASK YOUR
DOCTOR

- What happens on the day of surgery?
- What type of anesthesia will be used?
- How long will it take to recover from the surgery?
- When can I expect to return to work and/or resume normal activities?
- What are the risks associated with a gastrectomy?
- How many gastrectomies do you perform in a year?
- What is the rate of postsurgical complications among your patients?
- Will there be a scar?

surgery. For early gastric cancer, the five-year survival rate is as high as 77%. For late-stage disease, the five-year survival rate is only 3%. The five-year survival rate for cancers in the lower stomach is better than for those found in the upper stomach, and the survival rate for gastric **lymphoma** is better than for gastric adenocarcinomas.

Most studies have shown that patients can have an acceptable quality of life after gastrectomy for a potentially curable gastric cancer. Many patients maintain a healthy appetite and eat a normal diet. Others lose weight and do not enjoy meals as much as before gastrectomy. Some studies show that patients who have total gastrectomies have more disease-related or treatment-related symptoms after surgery and poorer physical function than patients who have subtotal gastrectomies. There does not appear to be much difference, however, in emotional status or social activity level between patients who have undergone total versus subtotal gastrectomies.

Morbidity and mortality rates

Depending on the extent of surgery, the risk for postoperative death after gastrectomy for gastric cancer has been reported as 1%–3%, and the risk of non-fatal complications as 9%–18%.

Health care team roles

A gastrectomy is performed by a board-certified surgeon trained in gastroenterology, the branch of medicine that deals with the diseases of the digestive tract. An anesthesiologist is responsible for administering anesthesia. The operation is always performed in a hospital setting.

Resources

BOOKS

Beers, Mark H., Robert S. Porter, and Thomas V. Jones, eds. "Disorders of the Stomach and Duodenum." In *The Merck Manual*, 18th ed. Whitehouse Station, NJ: Merck, 2007.

Feldman, M., et al. *Sleisenger & Fordtran's Gastrointestinal and Liver Disease*. 9th ed. Philadelphia: Saunders/Elsevier, 2010.

PERIODICALS

Choi, Yoon Young. "Laparoscopic Gastrectomy for Advanced Gastric Cancer: Are the Long-Term Results Comparable with Conventional Open Gastrectomy? A Systematic Review and Meta-Analysis." *Journal of Surgical Oncology* (September 24, 2013): e-pub ahead of print. http://dx.doi.org/10.1002/jso.23438 (accessed October 3, 2014).

WEBSITES

A.D.A.M. Medical Encyclopedia. "Gastrectomy." MedlinePlus. http://www.nlm.nih.gov/medlineplus/ency/article/002945. htm (accessed October 3, 2014).

American Cancer Society. "Surgery for Stomach Cancer." http://www.cancer.org/cancer/stomachcancer/detailedguide/ stomach-cancer-treating-types-of-surgery (accessed October 3, 2014).

Cleveland Clinic. "Post-Gastrectomy Syndrome Overview." http://www.cancer.org/cancer/stomachcancer/detailed-guide/stomach-cancer-treating-types-of-surgery (accessed October 3, 2014).

NHS (UK National Health Service). "Gastrectomy." http:// www.nhs.uk/Conditions/Gastrectomy/Pages/Introduction. aspx (accessed October 3, 2014).

ORGANIZATIONS

American Cancer Society, 250 Williams St. NW, Atlanta, GA 30303, (800) 227-2345, http://www.cancer.org.

American College of Gastroenterology, 6400 Goldsboro Rd., Ste. 200, Bethesda, MD 20817, (301) 263-9000, info@acg.gi.org, http://gi.org.

American Gastroenterological Association, 4930 Del Ray Ave., Bethesda, MD 20814, (301) 654-2055 Fax: (301) 654-5920, member@gastro.org, http://www. gastro.org.

Caroline A. Helwick
Monique Laberge, PhD.
REVISED BY TISH DAVIDSON, AM

Gastric cancer *see* **Stomach cancer**

Gastrinoma *see* **Zollinger-Ellinger syndrome**

Gastroduodenostomy

Definition

A gastroduodenostomy is a surgical reconstruction procedure by which a new connection between the stomach and the first portion of the small intestine (duodenum) is created.

Purpose

A gastroduodenostomy is a gastrointestinal reconstruction technique. It may be performed in cases of **stomach cancer**, a malfunctioning pyloric valve, gastric obstruction, and peptic ulcers.

As a gastrointestinal reconstruction technique, it is usually performed after a total or partial **gastrectomy** (stomach removal) procedure. The procedure is also referred to as a Billroth I procedure. For benign (noncancerous) diseases, a gastroduodenostomy is the preferred type of reconstruction because of the restoration of normal gastrointestinal physiology. Several studies have confirmed the advantages of this procedure, because it preserves the duodenal passage. Compared to a gastrojejunostomy (Billroth II) procedure—meaning the surgical connection of the stomach to the jejunum—gastroduodenostomies have been shown to result in less modification of pancreatic and biliary functions, as well as decreased incidence of ulceration and inflammation of the stomach (gastritis). However, gastroduodenostomies performed after gastrectomies for **cancer** have been the subject of controversy. Although there seems to be a definite advantage of performing gastroduodenostomies over gastrojejunostomies, surgeons have become reluctant to perform gastroduodenostomies because of possible obstruction at the site of the surgical connection due to tumor recurrence.

As for gastroduodenostomies specifically performed for the surgical treatment of malignant gastric tumors, they follow the general principles of oncological surgery, aiming for at least 0.8 in. (2 cm) of margins around the tumor. Because gastric adenocarcinomas tend to metastasize quickly and are locally invasive, it is rare to find good surgical candidates. Gastric tumors of such patients are thus only occasionally excised via a gastroduodenostomy procedure.

Gastric ulcers are often treated with a distal gastrectomy followed by gastroduodenostomy or gastrojejunostomy, which are the preferred procedures because they remove both the ulcer (mostly on the lesser curvature) and the diseased antrum.

Demographics

Stomach cancer was the most common form of cancer in the world in the 1970s and early 1980s. The incidence rates show substantial variations worldwide. Rates are currently highest in Japan and eastern Asia, but other areas of the world have high incidence rates, including eastern European countries and parts

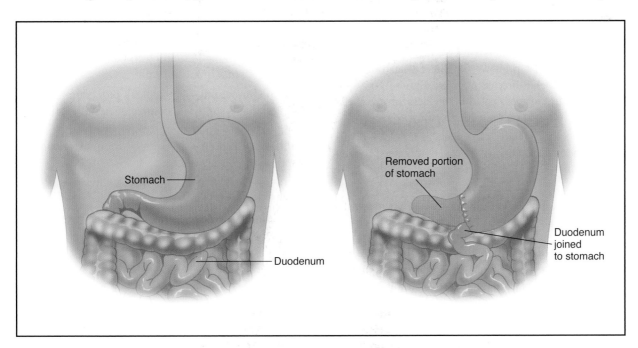

Illustration showing gastroduodenostomy, a surgical procedure that removes a portion of the stomach and reconnects the stomach to the upper portion of the small intestine (duodenum) *(Illustration by Electronic Illustrators Group. © Cengage Learning®.)*

of Latin America. Incidence rates are generally lower in western European countries and the United States. Stomach cancer incidence and mortality rates have been declining for several decades in most areas of the world.

Description

After removing a piece of the stomach, the surgeon reattaches the remainder to the rest of the bowel. The Billroth I gastroduodenostomy specifically joins the upper stomach back to the duodenum.

Typically, the procedure requires ligation (tying) of the right gastric veins and arteries as well as of the blood supply to the duodenum (pancreaticoduodenal vein and artery). The lumen of the duodenum and stomach is occluded at the proposed site of resection (removal). After resection of the diseased tissues, the stomach is closed in two layers, starting at the level of the lesser curvature, leaving an opening close to the diameter of the duodenum. The gastroduodenostomy is performed in a similar fashion as small intestinal end-to-end anastomosis, meaning an opening created between two normally separate spaces or organs. Alternatively, the Billroth I procedure may be performed with stapling equipment (ligation and thoracoabdominal staplers).

Diagnosis

If a gastroduodenostomy is performed for gastric cancer, diagnosis is usually established using the following tests:

- Endoscopy and barium x-rays. The advantage of endoscopy is that it allows for direct visualization of abnormalities and directed biopsies. Barium x-rays do not facilitate biopsies, but they are less invasive and may give information regarding motility.

- Computed tomography (CT) scan. A CT scan of the chest, abdomen, and pelvis is usually obtained to help assess tumor extent, nodal involvement, and metastatic disease.

- Endoscopic ultrasound (EUS). EUS complements information gained by CT. Specifically, the depth of tumor invasion, including invasion of nearby organs, can be assessed more accurately by EUS than by CT.

- Laparoscopy. This technique allows examination of the inside of the abdomen through a lighted tube.

The diagnosis of gastric ulcer is usually made based on a characteristic clinical history. Routine laboratory tests such as a complete blood cell count and iron studies can help detect **anemia**, which is indicative of the condition. By performing high-precision endoscopy and

KEY TERMS

Adenocarcinoma—The most common form of gastric cancer.

Anastomosis—An opening created by surgical, traumatic, or pathological means between two normally separate spaces or organs.

Antrum—The lower part of the stomach that lies between the pylorus and the body of the stomach. It is also called the gastric antrum or antrum pyloricum.

Barium swallow—An upper gastrointestinal series (barium swallow) is an x-ray test used to define the anatomy of the upper digestive tract; the test involves filling the esophagus, stomach, and small intestines with a white liquid material (barium).

Computed tomography (CT) scan—An imaging technique that creates a series of pictures of areas inside the body, taken from different angles. The pictures are created by a computer linked to an x-ray machine.

Duodenum—The first part of the small intestine that connects the stomach above and the jejunum below.

Endoscopy—The visual inspection of any cavity of the body by means of an endoscope.

Gastrectomy—A surgical procedure in which all or a portion of the stomach is removed.

Gastroduodenostomy—A surgical procedure in which the doctor creates a new connection between the stomach and the duodenum.

Gastrointestinal—Pertaining to or communicating with the stomach and intestine.

Gastrojejunostomy—A surgical procedure where the stomach is surgically connected to the jejunum.

Laparoscopy—The examination of the inside of the abdomen through a lighted tube, sometimes accompanied by surgery.

Lumen—The cavity or channel within a tube or tubular organ.

Small intestine—The small intestine consists of three sections: duodenum, jejunum, and ileum. All are involved in the absorption of nutrients.

by obtaining multiple mucosal **biopsy** specimens, the diagnosis of gastric ulcer can be confirmed. Additionally, upper gastrointestinal tract radiography tests are usually performed.

Preparation

Preparation for the surgery includes nasogastric decompression prior to the administration of anesthesia, intravenous or intramuscular administration of **antibiotics**, insertion of intravenous lines for administration of electrolytes, and a supply of compatible blood. Suction provided by placement of a nasogastric tube is necessary if there is any evidence of obstruction. Thorough medical evaluation, including hematological studies, may indicate the need for preoperative transfusions. All patients should be prepared with systemic antibiotics, and there may be some advantage in washing out the abdominal cavity with tetracycline prior to surgery.

Aftercare

After surgery, the patient is brought to the recovery room where vital signs are monitored. Intravenous fluid and electrolyte therapy is continued until oral intake resumes. Small meals of a highly digestible diet are offered every 6 hours, starting 24 hours after surgery. After a few days, a more normal diet is gradually introduced. Medical treatment of associated gastritis may continue in the immediate postoperative period.

Risks

A gastroduodenostomy has many of the same risks associated with any other major abdominal operation performed under general anesthesia, such as wound problems, difficulty swallowing, infections, nausea, and blood clotting.

More specific risks associated with gastroduodenostomy include:

- duodenogastric reflux, which results in persistent vomiting
- dumping syndrome, which occurs after a meal and is characterized by sweating, abdominal pain, vomiting, light-headedness, and diarrhea
- low blood sugar levels (hypoglycemia) after a meal
- alkaline reflux gastritis, which is marked by abdominal pain, vomiting of bile, diminished appetite, and iron-deficiency anemia
- malabsorption of necessary nutrients, especially iron, in patients who have had all or part of the stomach removed

Results

Results of a gastroduodenostomy are considered normal when the continuity of the gastrointestinal tract is reestablished.

Morbidity and mortality rates

For gastric obstruction, a gastroduodenostomy is considered the most radical procedure. It is recommended in the most severe cases and has been shown to provide good results in relieving gastric obstruction in most patients. Overall, good to excellent gastroduodenostomy results are reported in 85% of cases of gastric obstruction. In cases of cancer, a median survival time of 72 days has been reported after gastroduodenostomy following the removal of gastric **carcinoma**, although a few patients had extended survival times of three to four years.

Alternatives

In the case of ulcer treatment, the need for a gastroduodenostomy procedure has diminished greatly over the past 20–30 years due to the discovery of two new classes of drugs and the presence of the responsible germ (*Helicobacter pylori*) in the stomach. The drugs are the H_2 blockers such as cimetidine and ranitidine and the proton pump inhibitors such as omeprazole; these effectively stop acid production. *H. pylori* can be eliminated from most patients with combination therapy that includes antibiotics and bismuth.

If an individual requires gastrointestinal reconstruction, there is no alternative to a gastroduodenostomy.

Health care team roles

Gastroduodenostomy is performed by a surgeon trained in gastroenterology, the branch of medicine that deals with the diseases of the digestive tract. An anesthesiologist is responsible for administering anesthesia, and the operation is performed in a hospital setting.

Resources

BOOKS

Benirschke, R., et al. *Embracing Life: Great Comebacks from Ostomy Surgery*. Rancho Santa Fe, CA: Rolf Benirschke Enterprises, 2009.

Schumpelick, Volker. *Atlas of General Surgery*. New York: Thieme, 2009.

PERIODICALS

Huddy, Jeremy R., Karim Jamal, and Yuen Soon. "Single Port Billroth I Gastrectomy." *Journal of Minimal Access Surgery* 9, no. 2 (2013): 87–90. http://dx.doi.org/10.4103/0972-9941.110971 (accessed October 3, 2014).

Kim, Dae Hoon, et al. "Circular Stapler Size and Risk of Anastomotic Complications in Gastroduodenostomy for Gastric Cancer." *World Journal of Surgery* 36, no. 8 (2012): 1796–99. http://dx.doi.org/10.1007/s00268-012-1584-2 (accessed October 3, 2014).

Xiong, Jun-Jie, et al. "Roux-en-Y versus Billroth I Reconstruction after Distal Gastrectomy for Gastric Cancer: A Meta-Analysis." *World Journal of Gastroenterology* 19, no. 7 (2013): 1124–34. http://dx.doi.org/10.3748/wjg.v19.i7.1124 (accessed October 3, 2014).

WEBSITES

American Cancer Society. "Stomach Cancer." http://www.cancer.org/cancer/stomachcancer/index (accessed October 3, 2014).

ORGANIZATIONS

American College of Gastroenterology, 6400 Goldsboro Rd., Ste. 200, Bethesda, MD 20817, (301) 263-9000, info@acg.gi.org, http://gi.org.

American Gastroenterological Association, 4930 Del Ray Ave., Bethesda, MD 20814, (301) 654-2055, Fax: (301) 654–5920, member@gastro.org, http://www.gastro.org.

Society of American Gastrointestinal Endoscopic Surgeons (SAGES), 11300 West Olympic Blvd., Ste. 600, Los Angeles, CA 90064, (310) 437-0544, Fax: (310) 437-0585, webmaster@sages.org, http://www.sages.org.

United Ostomy Associations of America, Inc. (UOAA), PO Box 512, Northfield, MN 55057-0512, (800) 826-0826, info@ostomy.org, http://www.ostomy.org.

Monique Laberge, PhD.

Gastrointestinal cancers

Definition

Gastrointestinal (GI) cancers include cancers of the esophagus, stomach, small intestine, colon, rectum, and anus as well as cancers of the liver, pancreas, gallbladder, and biliary system.

Description

The GI tract, or digestive tract, processes all the food a person consumes. It starts from the oral cavity (mouth) and proceeds to the esophagus, stomach, small intestine, large intestine (colon and rectum), and anus. As it travels through the tract, food is digested, nutrients and water are extracted, and waste is eliminated from the body in the form of stool and urine. **Cancer** can affect any of the gastrointestinal organs. The **National Cancer Institute** estimates that 25% of all cancers are gastrointestinal, with the majority of these occurring in the colon and rectum (colorectal cancers). Other sites most commonly affected by GI cancers are the pancreas, stomach, liver, and esophagus.

Types of cancers

Esophageal cancer

The esophagus is a muscular, hollow tube that carries food from the oropharynx (area behind the mouth and soft palate) to the stomach. It consists of several layers. **Esophageal cancer** usually develops in the inner layer cells and grows outward. There are two major types of esophageal cancer. The first occurs in the cells found in the lining of the esophagus (squamous cells) and is called squamous cell **carcinoma**. It can develop anywhere along the entire length of the esophagus and represents approximately half of all reported esophageal cancers. The second type of cancer known to occur in the esophagus is **adenocarcinoma**, which is cancer of the glandular cells that line the inside of organs. Adenocarcinoma occurs near the stomach entrance and may be associated with a condition known as **Barrett's esophagus**. This is a disorder in which the lining of the esophagus undergoes cellular changes as a result of chronic irritation and inflammation resulting from a backwash of acidic stomach gastric juices. Esophageal adenocarcinomas cannot develop unless squamous cells have been transformed by the acid reflux of the stomach juices. The American Cancer Society (ACS) predicted the occurrence of approximately 18,170 new cases of esophageal cancer in 2014 that will result in some 15,450 deaths in the United States.

Stomach cancer

Stomach cancer is also called gastric cancer. The stomach is located in the upper abdomen under the ribs. It is the most expandable organ of the digestive system. Food reaches the stomach from the esophagus and is broken down by gastric juices secreted by the stomach. After leaving the stomach, partially broken down food passes into the small intestine and afterwards

Gastrointestinal cancers

Cancer	Types
Esophageal cancer	Squamous cell carcinoma
	Adenocarcinoma
Stomach cancer	Adenocarcinoma
Liver cancer	Angiosarcoma
	Hepatoblastoma
	Cholangiocarcinoma
	Hepatocellular carcinoma (hepatoma)
Gallbladder cancer	Adenocarcinoma
	Squamous cell carcinoma
	Carcinosarcoma
	Small cell (oat cell) carcinoma
Pancreatic cancer	Adenocarcinoma
	Insulinoma
	Gastrinoma
	Glucagonoma
	Vipoma
	Somatostinoma
	Acinar cell carcinoma
	Cystic tumors
	Papillary tumors
	Pancreatoblastoma
Colorectal cancer	Adenocarcinoma
	Carcinoid tumors
	Gastrointestinal stromal tumors
	Lymphomas
Anal cancer	Squamous cell carcinoma
	Basal cell carcinoma
	Melanoma
	Adenocarcinoma

Table listing different types of gastrointestinal cancers.
(Table by GGS Creative Resources. © Cengage Learning®.)

into the colon (first part of the large intestine). In cancer of the stomach, cancerous cells are found in the tissues of the stomach and the cancer can develop anywhere in the organ. It may grow along the stomach wall into other organs such as the esophagus or small intestine or go through the stomach wall and invade the nearby lymph nodes or organs such as the liver, pancreas, and colon. It may also metastasize (spread) to more distant organs, such as the lungs, the lymph nodes, and the ovaries.

The major type of stomach cancer is adenocarcinoma (90% of all stomach cancers). The American Cancer Society predicted that approximately 22,220 new cases of stomach cancer would be diagnosed in the United States in 2014, with about 10,990 deaths occurring in the same year. The number of cases, as well as the death rate, has declined significantly over the past several decades. A cure is possible if the cancer is found before spreading to other organs. Unfortunately, the early symptoms are not very noticeable, and by the time stomach cancer is diagnosed, it has in many cases already metastasized.

Liver cancer

The liver is one of the largest organs in the body. In normal adults, it weighs about three pounds and is located in the upper right side of the abdomen, under the right lung and rib cage. It plays a major role in digestion, in the transformation of food into energy and in filtering and storing blood. It is also responsible for processing nutrients and drugs, producing bile, controlling the level of glucose (sugar) in the blood, detoxifying blood, and regulating blood clotting. When cancer of the liver occurs, cancerous cells are found in the tissues of the liver. Primary **liver cancer** is cancer that starts in the liver. As such, it is different from cancer that starts somewhere else and spreads to the liver. Liver cancer is an uncommon form of GI cancer in the United States with only about 33,190 new cases predicted to be diagnosed in 2014 and 23,000 deaths occurring in the same year.

Primary cancers of the liver and of the bile ducts are far more common in Africa and Asia than in the United States, where they only represent 1.5% of all cancer cases. Worldwide, about 700,000 new cases of liver cancer are diagnosed each year. The highest occurrence rate is in Vietnamese men, most likely as a result of the high incidence of viral hepatitis infections in Vietnam. Asian American groups also have higher liver cancer incidence rates than the Caucasian population. Liver cancer mortality rates calculated for populations for which statistics are available are highest in China.

There are four main types of liver cancer: angiosarcoma, a rare type of cancer that starts in the blood vessels of the liver; hepatoblastoma, another rare type of liver cancer occurring chiefly in young children; cholangiocarcinoma, which starts in the bile ducts and accounts for approximately 13% of liver cancers; and finally, hepatocellular carcinoma, also known as hepatoma. The most common liver cancer is hepatocellular carcinoma, which accounts for approximately 84% of liver cancers. As is the case with stomach cancer, liver cancer is hard to diagnose early because there are seldom any clear-cut symptoms.

Some diseases have been identified as liable to increase a person's risk of liver cancer. They include: hepatitis B, hepatitis C, and cirrhosis of the liver. Exposure to certain chemicals such as aflatoxins (a substance made by a fungus in tropical regions and that can infect wheat, peanuts, soybeans, corn, and rice), vinyl chloride, thorium dioxide, anabolic steroids, and arsenic. Some types of birth control pills have been found to cause noncancerous tumors in the liver (known as hepatic adenomas), but a causative link between oral contraceptive use and liver cancer has not been found.

Abdomen—A part of the body that lies between the thorax and the pelvis. It contains a cavity (abdominal cavity) which holds organs such as the pancreas, stomach, intestines, liver, and gallbladder. It is enclosed by the abdominal muscles and the vertebral column (backbone).

Bile—A greenish-yellow fluid produced by the liver and stored in the gallbladder.

Bile ducts—Passages external to the liver for the transport of bile.

Digestion—The conversion of food in the stomach and in the intestines into substances capable of being absorbed by the blood.

Digestive system—Organs and paths responsible for processing food in the body. These are the mouth, esophagus, stomach, liver, gallbladder, pancreas, small intestine, colon, and rectum.

Gastric juice—An acidic secretion of the stomach that breaks down the proteins contained in ingested food, prior to digestion.

Gland—An organ that produces and releases substances for use in the body, such as fluids or hormones.

Lymph nodes—Small, bean-shaped organs surrounded by a capsule of connective tissue. Also called lymph glands. Lymph nodes are spread out along lymphatic vessels and store special cells (lymphocytes), which filter the lymphatic fluid (lymph).

Lymphatic system—The tissues and organs that produce, store, and carry white blood cells that fight infection. It includes the bone marrow, spleen, thymus, and lymph nodes as well as a network of thin vessels (lymphatic vessels) that carry lymph and white blood cells into all the tissues of the body.

Metastasis—The transfer of cancer from one location or organ to another one not directly related to it.

Ovary—One of two small oval-shaped organs located on either side of the uterus. They are female reproductive glands in which the ova (eggs) are formed.

Small intestine—The part of the digestive tract located between the stomach and the large intestine.

Squamous cells—Flat, thin cells, such as those found on the outer layer of the skin.

Stage—The extent to which a cancer has spread from its original site to other parts of the body. A Stage 1 cancer is less advanced than a Stage 4 cancer.

Gallbladder cancer

The gallbladder is a pear-shaped organ located just under the liver in the upper abdomen. Its role in digestion is to store and release the bile produced by the liver into the stomach to help break down fat. In **gallbladder cancer**, the cancer cells develop in the tissues of the gallbladder. Several types of cancer can occur, such as adenocarcinoma, squamous cell carcinoma, carcinosarcoma, and small cell (oat cell) carcinoma, all of them uncommon. The American Cancer Society predicted that about 6,000 new cases of gallbladder cancer would be diagnosed in 2014 in the United States. Women are affected twice as often as men. Most diagnosed individuals are elderly.

Pancreatic cancer

The pancreas is a tongue-shaped glandular organ lying below and behind the stomach. It consists of two areas, the exocrine and endocrine regions. The endocrine pancreas secretes the hormones insulin and glucagon, which regulate blood sugar. The exocrine pancreas secretes pancreatic juice into the small intestine. The juice contains enzymes that break down fats and proteins so that the body can use them. In **pancreatic cancer**, the cancer can develop either in the cells that secrete the pancreatic juice (**exocrine pancreatic cancer**) or in the cells that release the hormones (**endocrine pancreatic cancer**). Exocrine pancreatic cancer is much more common than endocrine. Several types can develop, the majority being various types of carcinomas. The American Cancer Society predicted that, in 2014, about 46,240 people in the United States would be diagnosed with pancreatic cancer and the same year, pancreatic cancer would cause 39,590 deaths. Pancreatic cancer was estimated to be the third leading cause of cancer death in 2014. Because the pancreas is located deep inside the body, it cannot be felt during a routine physical exam, and no tests are presently available to allow early detection.

Colorectal cancers

The colon, the first part of the large intestine, extends from the end of the small intestine to the rectum.

The colon has four major divisions. The first is called the ascending colon; it starts where the small intestine attaches and extends upward on the right side of the abdomen. The second part is the transverse colon and it extends across the body to the left side where it joins the third section, called the descending colon, which continues downward on the left side. The fourth part of the colon is the sigmoid colon, which joins the rectum. The rectum joins the anus, where stool passes out of the body.

Each of the divisions of the colon and rectum has several layers of tissue. Colorectal cancers usually start in the innermost layer and can grow through some or all of the other layers. Colorectal cancers are common, and occur more frequently in people over the age of 50. The American Cancer Society estimated that in 2014 in the United States, about 96,830 new cases of **colon cancer** would be diagnosed along with 40,000 new cases of **rectal cancer**. Combined, these cancers are expected to cause 50,310 deaths in 2014. The number of new colorectal cancer cases and reported deaths has declined in recent years due to improved screening and diagnostic methods. Colorectal cancers are highly treatable when detected early through screening, but the symptoms are often not obvious in early stages.

Over 95% of colorectal cancers are adenocarcinomas. Other, less common types of colorectal cancers are: carcinoid tumors, which develop from the hormone-producing cells of the intestine, gastrointestinal stromal tumors, which start in the connective tissue and muscle layers located in the wall of the colon and rectum, and lymphomas, which are cancers of the immune system cells that usually occur in the lymph nodes but may also start in the colon.

Anal cancer

The anus has several types of tissues. Each type of tissue also contains several types of cells and cancer can develop in each of these kinds of tissues. The American Cancer Society estimated that approximately 7,210 new cases of **anal cancer** would be diagnosed in the United States in 2014 and that about 950 Americans would die as a result of anal cancers in that year. Anal cancer accounts for about 2% of the cancers of the digestive system. The cancer is rare in individuals under age 35. The average age at diagnosis is in individuals over 50 years old. Approximately half of all anal cancers are squamous cell carcinomas. This type of cancer is found in the surface cells that line the anus and most of the anal canal. Another 15% of anal cancers consist of adeno-carcinomas and usually start in glands found in the anus area. The remaining anal cancers are accounted for by basal cell carcinomas and malignant melanomas. People who have the **human papillomavirus** (HPV) infection have a greater chance of developing anal cancer as well as men who practice anal sex. How treatable the cancer is depends partly on where it starts.

See also Bile duct cancer; Carcinoid tumors, gastrointestinal; Human papillomavirus; Laryngeal cancer; Liver cancer, primary; Melanoma; Pancreatic cancer, endocrine; Pancreatic cancer, exocrine; Small intestine cancer; Upper gastrointestinal endoscopy.

Resources

BOOKS

Jankowski, Janusz and Ernest Hawk, eds. *Handbook of Gastrointestinal Cancer*. Wiley-Blackwell, 2012.

WEBSITES

American College of Gastroenterology. "Gastrointestinal Cancers." http://patients.gi.org/topics/gastrointestinal-cancers/ (accessed January 29, 2015).

ORGANIZATIONS

American Cancer Society, 1599 Clifton Rd., NE, Atlanta, GA 30329, (404) 320-3333, (800) ACS-2345 (227-2345), http://www.cancer.org.

National Cancer Institute, BG 9609 MSC 9760, 9609 Medical Center Drive, Bethesda, MD 20892-9760, (800) 4-CANCER (422-6237); TTY: (800) 332-8615, http://www.cancer.gov.

National Digestive Diseases Information Clearinghouse (NDDIC), 2 Information Way, Bethesda, MD 20892-3570, (800) 891-5389, TTY: (866) 569-1162, Fax: (703) 738-4929, info@niddk.nih.gov, http://digestive.niddk.nih.gov.

Society of American Gastrointestinal and Endoscopic Surgeons, 11300 West Olympic Boulevard, Suite 600, Los Angeles, CA 90064, (310) 437-0544, Fax: (310) 437-0585, webmaster@sages.org, http://www.sages.org.

Monique Laberge, PhD.
REVISED BY TISH DAVIDSON, AM

Gastrointestinal carcinoid tumors *see* Carcinoid tumors, gastrointestinal

Gastrointestinal complications

Description

Constipation, fecal impaction, bowel obstruction, and **diarrhea** are common gastrointestinal complications faced by **cancer** patients due to either their cancer or the treatment of it. The seriousness of these complications varies from mildly uncomfortable to life threatening.

Constipation is the slow and infrequent passage of small, dry bowel movements through the large intestine. Unpleasant and sometimes painful, constipation often causes people to strain while trying to have a bowel movement. Constipation itself is generally not life threatening; however, fecal impaction can be.

Fecal impaction is the collection of hard, dry stool in the colon or rectum that can't be excreted. Patients with fecal impaction may or may not experience the typical gastrointestinal symptoms usually associated with constipation, such as cramping and pressure. For example, if the impaction is pressing on a nerve, there may be back pain. If the impaction is pressing on the urethra or bladder, there may be an increase or decrease in urination. There may be nausea and abdominal pain, stool that leaks out when the patient coughs, and explosive diarrhea, which is the result of stool moving around the impaction. When movement of the diaphragm is restricted due to abdominal distention (swelling of the abdomen), the patient may not be getting enough oxygen. Breathing, heart, and circulation problems may develop, such as dizziness, hypotension (low blood pressure), hypoxia (a lack of oxygen to the brain), and angina. If left untreated, fecal impaction can cause death.

Bowel obstruction, as defined by the **National Cancer Institute**, is "a partial or complete blockage of the small or large intestine by a process other than fecal impaction." Classified by type, cause, and location, bowel obstructions can be caused by tumors inside or outside of the bowel, as well as the development of scar tissue after surgery. Patients with colostomies have an increased risk of becoming constipated. Therefore, they need to be especially proactive and report any signs of constipation to their physicians in order to avoid developing bowel obstruction.

Diarrhea is loose, watery stool, which results in abdominal cramps and frequent trips to the bathroom. For cancer patients, diarrhea tends to be especially bothersome. It can affect their eating patterns, as well as cause them to become dehydrated and lose weight. Although it can usually be managed, it sometimes leads to life threatening problems.

Causes

Constipation and fecal impaction

Constipation can have many causes. It can be a symptom of cancer or the result of a growing tumor. It can be linked to certain cancer treatments as well. Sometimes the medications given to cancer patients, such as **opioids** for pain, diuretics, or **chemotherapy** drugs, can cause constipation. Medications prescribed for anxiety and **depression**, not to mention the depression

itself, can be the culprits, too. Patients may find it difficult or painful to move and may put off going to the bathroom. Physical illness, exacerbated by depression, can also alter eating habits, resulting in dietary changes that aren't healthy, such as drinking too little water or not eating enough. In addition, certain muscle and nerve damage, such as **spinal cord compression** from a tumor, can lead to a loss of muscle tone in the bowel, making it difficult for a patient to complete a bowel movement. Environmental factors can worsen constipation. For example, patients who are in unfamiliar surroundings, or need assistance getting to the bathroom, or use a bedpan may have difficulty relaxing and this may affect their ability to defecate. Treating cancer patients with dignity and allowing them as much privacy as possible can be very helpful in these situations.

The National Cancer Institute has identified five major factors that can lead to fecal impaction:

- opioid pain medications
- inactivity over a long period of time
- changes in diet
- mental illness
- long-term use of laxatives

Oddly enough, using **laxatives** over a long period of time actually contributes to the development of constipation and fecal impaction, because the higher doses necessary to do the job "make the colon less able to signal the need to have a bowel movement," according to the National Cancer Institute. It may be difficult for cancer patients to avoid repeated bouts of constipation during their cancer treatment, especially if they are taking opioids for pain. However, patients should talk with their physicians about the specific preventative measures that would be the most suitable for them. Every effort should be made to avoid fecal impaction.

Bowel obstruction

According to the National Cancer Institute, "a bowel obstruction may be caused by a narrowing of the intestine from inflammation or damage of the bowel, tumors, scar tissue, hernias, twisting of the bowel, or pressure on the bowel from outside the intestinal tract." Most bowel obstructions, usually due to scar tissue and hernias, occur in the small intestine. Tumors, volvulus (twisting of the bowel), or diverticulitis account for most of the bowel obstructions in the large intestine. Cancers of the colon, stomach, and ovary are the ones that most frequently cause bowel obstructions. When lung and breast cancers spread to the abdomen, they too can cause bowel obstructions. Abdominal surgery or abdominal radiation may put patients at a greater risk of developing a bowel obstruction.

Diarrhea

Most often when cancer patients have diarrhea, the cause is related to their cancer therapy (i.e., chemotherapy drugs, especially fluoropyrimidines or **irinotecan**, **radiation therapy**, or surgery). Intestinal surgery, for example, can cause diarrhea by negatively affecting the way the bowel functions. Chemotherapy drugs, which can alter the way food is broken down and absorbed in the small intestine, can cause indigestion and diarrhea. According to Tuchmann and Engelkind, the stress and anxiety associated with cancer diagnosis and treatment can also cause diarrhea. Unfortunately, antibiotic therapy to treat infection, as the National Cancer Institute points out, "can cause inflammation of the lining of the bowel, resulting in diarrhea that often does not respond to treatment." In other cases, the cause can be directly tied to the patient's diet or use of laxatives. Severe diarrhea may result from concurrent chemotherapy and radiation therapy.

Treatment

Constipation and fecal impaction

A physician can diagnose the causes of constipation by performing a physical examination and reviewing a patient's medical history. The patient's stool can be tested for the presence of blood, which is done by asking the patient to provide a sample. In some cases, the physician might suspect that constipation has progressed to fecal impaction. In that case, an examination might include **x-rays** of the abdomen or chest, blood tests, and an electrocardiogram, which is a painless test that shows the activity of the heart. Another way to check for fecal impaction is to perform a rectal examination, which involves the physician inserting a lubricated, gloved finger into the rectum. If there is an impaction, there may be some discomfort; however, in general, the worst part of this examination is the embarrassment some people might feel.

A **colonoscopy** might be scheduled to see if cancer is present or to simply rule it out. A colonoscopy takes about thirty minutes to complete and is performed in a clinic or hospital setting. It is relatively painless, because patients are given a sedative and/or pain medicine. By inserting a flexible lighted tube into the patient's anus, the physician is able to see the entire large intestine all the way to the lower end of the small intestine.

Treatments options for patients with constipation may include a combination of preventative measures. Patients will probably be advised to keep track of their bowel movements in a journal. If they are too ill to do so, their caregivers may be asked to perform the task on their behalf. When the patient is trying to defecate, caregivers should be careful to respect their privacy, allowing them enough time and space to encourage success. Some patients find it helpful to run water in the sink or tub; the sound relaxes them and creates a sound barrier. If it is not contraindicated, patients may be advised to add fiber to their diets. Patients may be referred to nutritionists who are familiar with addressing the needs of cancer patients and can create individualized meal plans based on a patient's medical profile.

Adequate fluid intake is critical for patients prone to developing constipation, as well as fecal impaction. Patients may be asked to reduce their use of laxatives. In addition, patients should seek the approval of their physicians before they take any over-the-counter medications. According to the National Cancer Institute, "impactions are usually treated by moistening and softening the stool with an enema." A physician needs to be consulted before an enema is given, because too many enemas can damage the bowel. Nonstimulating bowel softeners may be needed. In some cases, it may be necessary for the fecal material to be manually removed by a physician, although it is understandable that many patients may dislike the thought of it.

Bowel obstruction

To make a diagnosis of bowel obstruction, the physician will need to perform a physical exam to determine if the patient has abdominal pain, gas, or stool in the bowel. The physician will most likely want to draw blood in order to check for infection and body chemistry imbalances. If an obstruction is diagnosed, a **barium enema** may need to be performed to ascertain its location.

Bowel obstruction can be classified into two categories: acute (short term) and chronic (long term). Patients with acute bowel obstruction must be monitored carefully. If their condition cannot be stabilized, it may necessary to insert a lubricated nasogastric tube through the patient's nose and esophagus until it reaches the stomach. Many patients find this procedure initially unpleasant, which is understandable. It is a brief procedure, but it causes many patients to gag and sometimes vomit. Some patients may respond better to a tube inserted in their rectum to relieve the pressure. The purpose of inserting the tube is to reduce the patient's swelling, gas, and excess fluid; however, surgery may be unavoidable, if the obstruction worsens and completely blocks the bowel. The insertion of a stent may be required in patients with advanced cancer, if the obstruction cannot be removed through surgical means.

A chronically ill patient may need to have a gastrostomy tube (or feeding tube) inserted through the wall of the abdomen into the stomach. This is done to help the patient eat and to alleviate painful symptoms. A gastroenterologist performs the procedure while the patient is under general anesthesia; therefore, it is completely painless. The tube may need to be temporary or permanent, depending on the patient's condition.

Diarrhea

Many factors can play a part in causing diarrhea, making its treatment challenging. Because severe diarrhea can be very upsetting and even life threatening, physicians will try to establish the cause of the problem as quickly as possible. Patients can expect to be asked a series of questions and to be physically examined. Their vital signs, such as blood pressure and pulse, will be taken and compared to previous readings. The patient may need to provide a stool sample so that it can be tested for the presence of blood or bacteria.

Dietary changes are likely to be suggested. The patient may be given a list of foods to avoid and a list of foods that are acceptable in small quantities. Patients with severe diarrhea may need to monitored closely by their caretakers or admitted to the hospital where intravenous fluids will be administered.

Alternative and complementary therapies

RELAXATION THERAPY. Some patients find that relaxation therapy helps them cope with the anxiety associated with cancer treatments and their side effects. A well-established psychogenic modality, relaxation therapy has been said to help cancer patients alleviate pain. When patients are in pain, they tend to tense up. This increases the pain, which causes even more stress. Learning relaxation techniques can help reverse this negative cycle. For example, some patients have found that by utilizing progressive muscle relaxation techniques, they are better able to handle physical and emotional pain, such as constipation and anxiety.

COMFORT MEASURES. Utilizing comfort measures to help patients heal is grounded in the belief that a patient should be seen as a whole person, not just someone with a disease and symptoms. Those who practice Eastern medicine have traditionally embraced this holistic approach, which considers the patient's mind, body, and spirit. Indeed, many Eastern philosophies have begun to greatly influence Western society. Some physicians have begun to change their personal philosophies to incorporate holistic concepts in their therapeutic handling of pain. For example, some cancer patients suffer not only from physical pain, but they also feel anxious and show signs of depression. In an article published by the *New England Journal of Medicine*, Dr. Campion promotes comfort measures as a way to help alleviate depression, recognizing that a person's state of mind affects his or her physical health. Comfort measures that embrace dignity, such as showing the patient kindness and respect, go a long way to promote healing. Patients with diarrhea, for example, can benefit from comfort measures that include a bedside commode, frequently changed sheets, and adjustable beds.

ACUPUNCTURE. Over 10,000 acupuncture and Oriental medicine practitioners currently practice in the United States. In a 1997 consensus statement issued by the National Institutes of Health, acupuncture was recognized as being an effective treatment for pain and nausea. It has also been used successfully to treat bowel obstructions. Developed by the Chinese as far back as 3000 B.C., acupuncture is thought to correct an imbalance of energy flow in the body. The technique involves inserting fine, sterile needles into a person's energy points, sometimes referred to as meridians. Some people fear acupuncture because they think the procedure will be painful, but in actuality it is not painful and tends to relax many people. Some people even fall asleep during the procedure.

Not everyone agrees on how acupuncture works, but research has shown that acupuncture increases the body's electromagnetic flow, which could cause the release of endorphins, the body's natural painkillers. Acupuncture is performed in a clinical setting. Patients interested in receiving acupuncture treatments should talk with their doctors to obtain suitable referrals to reputable, well-trained medical practitioners.

Resources

BOOKS

Jacobson, E. *Progressive Relaxation.* Chicago, IL: Chicago University Press, 1938.

Tuchmann L., Engelking, C. Cancer-related diarrhea. In *Oncology Nursing Secrets, edited by R. A. Gates and R. M. Fink.* Philadelphia, PA: Hanley and Belfus, 2001, pp. 310–322.

PERIODICALS

Campion, E. W. "Why unconventional medicine?" *New England Journal of Medicine* 328 (1993): 282–283.

Ripamonti, C., De Conno, F., Ventafridda, V., et al. "Management of bowel obstruction in advanced and terminal cancer patients." *Annals of Oncology* 4 (1993): 15–21.

WEBSITES

National Cancer Institute. "Gastrointestinal Complications (PDQ®)." http://www.cancer.gov/cancertopics/pdq/

supportivecare/gastrointestinalcomplications/Patient
(accessed December 3, 2014).

National Institutes of Health. "Acupuncture. National Institutes
of Health Consensus Development Conference Statement."
http://consensus.nih.gov/1997/1997Acupuncture107html.
htm (accessed December 3, 2014).

Lee Ann Paradise

Gazyva *see* **Obinutuzumab**

G-CSF *see* **Filgrastim**

Gefitinib

Definition

Gefitinib, which is sold under the brand name Iressa, is an anticancer drug used to inhibit the growth of lung **cancer** cells and reduce the size of a cancerous tumor.

Purpose

Gefitinib is used as a single agent for the treatment of advanced **non-small cell lung cancer** that has advanced or failed to respond to other kinds of treatment. It is not suitable for use as an initial treatment, but it may help to shrink tumors by as much as 10% when used as a third-line therapy in patients with advanced non-small lung cancer.

Description

In May 2003, gefitinib was approved for use in the United States under the U.S. Food and Drug Administration's (FDA) accelerated approval program. Generally speaking, before the FDA approves a drug for use, a great deal of data regarding the safety, efficacy, and quality of the drug is usually compiled. In fact, it is typical for the FDA to review thousands of pages of data about a medicine under consideration for approval. One of the reasons for this is the FDA's extremely strict approval process. FDA approval means that the regulators have decided that the new drug's potential benefits outweigh its risks. When a drug is approved under the accelerated program it is done so because, as Mark B. McClellan, MD and FDA Commissioner states, the "FDA believes it is critical for patients to have many safe and effective treatment options available to them in their battles against disease."

Gefitinib was approved by the FDA, as all drugs approved under the accelerated program, with the condition that further studies would be conducted to measure the drug's clinical benefit. According to the manufacturer, once these studies were conducted, gefitinib was found to benefit only about 10% of patients. It continues to be available, but only through a special distribution program and only for patients who have had previous success with gefitinib.

Recommended dosage

Gefitinib is available in 250 mg tablets. Dosage levels may vary, depending on the needs of the patient; however, patients generally take one 250 mg tablet a day. The tablets should not be crushed or broken and the patient should be certain to drink plenty of fluids throughout the day.

Precautions

Women who are pregnant or may become pregnant should not use gefitinib. Patients receiving gefitinib should not breast-feed their babies during the treatment cycle and for a substantial time after the treatment.

This drug has been associated with high toxicity. In rare cases, using gefitinib resulted in severe side effects, including inflammation of the lungs (interstitial **pneumonia**) and difficulty breathing. Patients should report any side effects, whether they seem severe or not, to their physician.

Side effects

The most common side effects of gefitinib include:

- skin rash
- acne
- dry skin

More severe side effects include:

- loss of appetite
- nausea and vomiting
- diarrhea
- eye problems
- swelling

Interactions

Gefitinib increases the effect of metoprolol and may increase the risk of bleeding in patients taking the anticoagulant drug **warfarin**. The following drugs may decrease gefitinib's effectiveness:

- carbamazepine (Tegretol)
- cimetidine (Tagamet)
- dexamethasone (Decadron)

KEY TERMS

Non-small cell lung cancer (NSCLC)—The most common type of lung cancer; includes squamous cell carcinoma, adenocarcinoma, and large cell carcinoma.

U.S. Food and Drug Administration—A government agency that oversees public safety in relation to drugs and medical devices.

• phenobarbital (Luminal)

• phenytoin (Dilantin)

• rifampin (Rifadin)

• ranitidine (Zantac)

• sodium bicarbonate

Several drugs can cause levels of gefitinib to build up in the body to toxic levels. These include:

• antiretroviral drugs (used to treat human immunodeficiency syndrome [HIV])

• certain antibiotics (including ketolide, macrolide, and antifungal antibiotics)

• nefazodone (Serzone)

Resources

BOOKS

Hodgson, B. B., Kizior, R. J., Foley, M., et al. *Mosby's 2005 Drug Consultant for Nurses.* St. Louis, MO: Mosby, 2005.

Koda-Kimbl, M. A., Young, L. Y., Kradjan, W. A., Guglielmo, B. J., editors. *Applied Therapeutics: The Clinical Use of Drugs.* 10th ed. Baltimore, MD: Lippincott Williams & Wilkins, 2005.

PERIODICALS

Giorgianni, S. J., editor. "Enhancing pharmaceutical safety." *The Pfizer Journal* 8 (2004): 4–13.

WEBSITES

Public Citizen. "Cancer Drug Iressa Should Not Be Approved, Public Citizen Tells FDA." http://www.citizen.org/pressroom/pressroomredirect.cfm?ID=1417 (accessed December 3, 2014).

U.S. Food and Drug Administration. "About FDA Product Approval." http://www.fda.gov/NewsEvents/Products Approvals/ucm106288.htm (accessed December 3, 2014).

U.S. Food and Drug Administration. "Information for Healthcare Professionals: Gefitinib (marketed as Iressa)." http://www.fda.gov/Drugs/DrugSafety/PostmarketDrugSafety InformationforPatientsandProviders/DrugSafetyInformation forHeathcareProfessionals/ucm085197.htm (accessed December 3, 2014).

ORGANIZATIONS

U.S. Food and Drug Administration, 10903 New Hampshire Ave., Silver Spring, MD 20993, (888) INFO-FDA (463–6332), http://www.fda.gov.

Lee Ann Paradise

Gemcitabine

Definition

Gemcitabine is a drug that is used to treat advanced stages of pancreatic, lung, and other cancers. Its brand name is Gemzar.

Purpose

Gemcitabine is used to treat **pancreatic cancer**, particularly when it has metastasized, or spread to other parts of the body (Stage IVB). In combination with the drug **cisplatin**, gemcitabine is the first-line treatment for inoperable, metastasized **non-small cell lung cancer**. Sometimes it is used to treat cancers of the bladder or breast, or epithelial **ovarian cancer**.

Description

Gemcitabine is a type of medicine called a pyrimidine antimetabolite because it interferes with the metabolism and growth of cells. It does this by replacing the pyrimidine deoxycytidine in DNA, thereby preventing the DNA from being manufactured or repaired. As a result, cells cannot reproduce and eventually die.

Gemcitabine was approved by the U.S. Food and Drug Administration (FDA) to treat pancreatic **cancer** in 1998 and non-small cell lung cancer in 2002. Gemzar may relieve pain and other symptoms of advanced pancreatic cancer and increase survival time by several weeks to two months. Clinical studies of pancreatic cancer are comparing the effectiveness of combination treatments using gemcitabine with **fluorouracil** (5-FU), cisplatin, **streptozocin**, or **radiation therapy**. Gemcitabine has activity against metastatic **bladder cancer** and recurrent ovarian cancer, and further **clinical trials** are underway. Gemcitabine is being evaluated for its effectiveness in the treatment of uterine, stomach, laryngeal and hypopharyngeal, and colon and rectal cancers.

KEY TERMS

Deoxycytidine—Component of DNA, the genetic material of a cell, that is similar in structure to gemcitabine.

Metastasis—Spread of cancer from its point of origin to other parts of the body.

Platelet—Blood component that aids in clotting.

Pyrimidine—Class of molecules that includes gemcitabine and deoxycytidine.

Vasculitis—Inflammation of a blood or lymph vessel.

Recommended dosage

Gemcitabine is administered by injection over a period of 30 minutes. The dosage and number of administrations depend on a variety of factors, including the type of cancer, body size, the patient's sex, and other concurrent treatments.

Precautions

Gemcitabine may temporarily reduce the number of white blood cells, particularly during the first 10–14 days after administration. A low white blood cell count reduces the body's ability to fight infection. Thus, it is very important to avoid exposure to infections and to receive prompt medical treatment. Immunizations (vaccinations) should be avoided during or after treatment with gemcitabine. It also is important to avoid contact with individuals who have recently taken an oral polio vaccine. Treatment with gemcitabine may cause chicken pox or shingles (**herpes zoster**) to become very severe and spread to other parts of the body.

Gemcitabine also may lower the blood platelet count. Platelets are necessary for normal blood clotting. The risk of bleeding may be reduced by using caution when cleaning teeth, avoiding dental work, and avoiding cuts, bruises, or other injuries.

Gemcitabine can cause birth defects and fetal death in animals. Therefore, this drug should not be taken by pregnant women or by either the man or woman at the time of conception. Women usually are advised against breastfeeding while taking this drug.

Side effects

Gemcitabine affects normal cells as well as cancer cells, resulting in various side effects. The most common side effects are related to reduction in red and white blood cells and blood platelets. These side effects may include symptoms of infection or unusual bleeding or bruising. Older patients are more likely to suffer from low blood cell counts after treatment.

Flu-like symptoms are common following the first treatment with gemcitabine. Other common side effects of gemcitabine may include:

- nausea
- vomiting
- chills and fever
- constipation
- diarrhea
- loss of appetite (anorexia)
- headache
- muscle pain
- weakness or fatigue
- shortness of breath
- blood in urine or stools
- skin rash
- swelling of the hands, feet, legs, or face
- insomnia

Less common side effects of gemcitabine may include:

- cough or hoarseness
- lower back or side pain
- painful or difficult urination
- chest, arm, or back pain
- difficulty with speech
- fast or irregular heartbeat
- high blood pressure
- pain or redness at the site of injection
- numbness or tingling in hands or feet
- sores or white spots on lips and in mouth
- hair loss (alopecia)
- itching

Some of these side effects may occur or continue after treatment with gemcitabine has ended. **Itching**, hives, swelling, or a skin rash, particularly if accompanied by breathing problems, may indicate an allergic reaction to gemcitabine. Some researchers have coined the term gemcitabine-induced severe pulmonary toxicity, or GISPT, to describe an inflammatory reaction in the lungs following treatment with gemcitabine. The incidence of GISPT is estimated to range between 0.5% and 5% of patients receiving the drug.

Additional side effects of gemcitabine may be symptoms associated with liver or kidney malfunction. Furthermore, kidney or liver disease may cause gemcitabine to be removed from the body at a slower rate, thus increasing the effects of the drug.

Another potentially fatal side effect of gemcitabine is vasculitis, or inflammation of blood or lymph vessels. A group of physicians in Iowa reported on two cases of women who died of necrotizing enterocolitis resulting from vasculitis associated with gemcitabine treatment for ovarian cancer. A case of vasculitis in a male patient treated with gemcitabine for bladder cancer was reported in Turkey.

Interactions

Previous treatment with radiation or other anti-cancer drugs can increase the risk of very low blood counts with gemcitabine. Serious problems may develop in areas previously treated with radiation.

Drugs that may interact with gemcitabine, or that may increase the risk of infections while being treated with gemcitabine, include live vaccines and **warfarin**. Because some other medications have a tendency to interact with gemcitabine, patients should alert their doctor to any drugs they are taking.

It is also important not to take any medicines containing aspirin during treatment with gemcitabine, since aspirin can increase the chances of excessive bleeding.

Resources

BOOKS

Beers, Mark H., MD, and Robert Berkow, MD, editors. "Pancreatic Tumors." Section 3, Chapter 34 In The Merck Manual of Diagnosis and Therapy Whitehouse Station, NJ: Merck Research Laboratories, 2007.

Karch, A. M. *Lippincott's Nursing Drug Guide*. Springhouse, PA: Lippincott Williams & Wilkins, 2003.

PERIODICALS

Barlesi, F., P. Villani, C. Doddoli, et al. "Gemcitabine-Induced Severe Pulmonary Toxicity." *Fundamental and Clinical Pharmacology* 18 (February 2004): 85–91.

Birlik, M., S. Akar, E. Tuzel, et al. "Gemcitabine-Induced Vasculitis in Advanced Transitional Cell Carcinoma of the Bladder." *Journal of Cancer Research and Clinical Oncology* 130 (February 2004): 122–125.

Geisler, J. P., D. F. Schraith, K. J. Manahan, and J. I. Sorosky. "Gemcitabine Associated Vasculitis Leading to Necrotizing Enterocolitis and Death in Women Undergoing Primary Treatment for Epithelial Ovarian/Peritoneal Cancer." *Gynecologic Oncology* 92 (February 2004): 705–707.

Li, D., K. Xie, R. Wolff, and J. L. Abbruzzese. "Pancreatic Cancer." *Lancet* 363 (March 27, 2004): 1049–1057.

ORGANIZATIONS

ASHP (formerly the American Society of Health-System Pharmacists), 7272 Wisconsin Ave., Bethesda, MD 20814, (301) 664-8700, (866) 279-0681, custserv@ashp.org, http://www.ashp.org.

U.S. Food and Drug Administration, 10903 New Hampshire Ave., Silver Spring, MD 20993, (888) INFO-FDA (463-6332), http://www.fda.gov.

Margaret Alic, PhD.
Rebecca J. Frey, PhD.

Gemtuzumab

Definition

Gemtuzumab ozogamicin was a humanized monoclonal antibody used to treat patients with acute myeloid leukemia (AML). It was marketed in the United States under the brand name Mylotarg but was discontinued by the manufacturer in 2010.

Purpose

Gemtuzumab is a monoclonal antibody used to treat AML that is characterized by expression of the CD33 protein on the cancerous cells, called leukemic blasts. The CD33 protein is found on the surface of the leukemic blasts of about 80% of patients with AML. After the gemtuzumab antibody was produced in the laboratory, a chemical reaction was used to link it to an antitumor drug called calicheamicin. About half of the antibody acquired the antitumor drug.

When the antibody-calicheamicin molecule bound to the cancerous cells, both the antibody and the drug were taken into the cell. There, the drug bound to the cell's genetic material (deoxyribose nucleic acid or DNA), inducing breaks in the molecule and killing it. This method is known as antibody-targeted **chemotherapy**.

Gemtuzumab was also used to induce remission (remove cancerous cells) in AML patients to prepare them for **stem cell transplantation**. It was indicated for refractory AML (AML that does not readily yield to treatment). The use of antibody-targeted chemotherapy has been shown to have fewer side effects than traditional chemotherapy courses and does improve the disease-free survival time after transplantation.

KEY TERMS

Antibody—A protective protein made by the immune system in response to an antigen, also called an immunoglobulin.

Blasts—A type of immature cell that lacks some of the outward characteristics of the mature cell.

Calicheamicin—An antitumor drug that binds to DNA within the tumor cells, causing breaks in the strands and killing the cell.

Monoclonal—Genetically engineered antibodies specific for one antigen.

Description

Gemtuzumab was approved by the U.S. Food and Drug Administration (FDA) in 2000 as a method of treating relapsed AML in older patients (over 60 years of age) that were not candidates for other cytotoxic chemotherapy. It was withdrawn by the manufacturer in 2010 due to lack of effectiveness and an increased number of deaths in patients taking Mylotarg.

See also Monoclonal antibodies.

Resources

WEBSITES

National Cancer Institute. "Gemtuzumab Ozogamicin." http://www.cancer.gov/cancertopics/druginfo/gemtuzumabozo-gamicin (accessed September 26, 2014).

U.S. Food and Drug Administration. "Mylotarg (gemtuzumab ozogamicin): Market Withdrawal." http://www.fda.gov/Safety/MedWatch/SafetyInformation/SafetyAlertsforHumanMedicalProducts/ucm216458.htm (accessed September 26, 2014).

Michelle Johnson, M.S., J.D.

Gemzar *see* **Gemcitabine**

Gene therapy

Definition

Gene therapy is the insertion of genetic material (DNA or RNA) into cells of the body to prevent or treat disease. Although gene therapy is still experimental, **cancer** is the most common disease being treated with gene therapy in **clinical trials**.

Purpose

Gene therapy has the potential to efficiently and specifically target cancer cells without harming healthy cells. The primary purposes of cancer gene therapy are:

• eliminating cancer cells

• blocking tumor vascularization—blood vessel formation or angiogenesis—to prevent tumor growth

• boosting immune system responses to target and destroy cancer cells

As of 2014, approximately two-thirds of gene therapy clinical trials being conducted at the **National Cancer Institute** (NCI), academic medical centers, and biotechnology companies were testing cancer treatments. These included phase 3 trials for head and neck cancer and metastatic **melanoma** treatments and prostate and **pancreatic cancer** gene vaccines, as well as phase 1 and 2 trials of various technologies for treating brain, liver, colon, breast, kidney, and other cancers.

Description

Cancer results from damage (changes or mutations) to oncogenes or tumor suppressor genes. In their normal states, oncogenes are involved in controlling cell growth, and tumor suppressors prevent cells from turning cancerous. Damage to these genes results in uncontrolled cell growth. A mutated gene can be inherited, as with the BRCA **breast cancer** genes, or damaged by environmental toxins, such as smoking, or by various assaults that accumulate with age. It usually takes mutations in multiple genes to change a cell into one that is cancerous. Different types of cancer may share some mutations, but even the same type of cancer may have different mutations in different individuals. For this reason, multiple strategies for cancer gene therapy are being pursued. These include:

• introducing therapeutic genetic material into cancer cells

• reprogramming cancer cells to self-destruct

• replacing cancer-causing genes with normal genes

• silencing or suppressing cancer gene expression

• directly killing cancer cells

• boosting or reprogramming the immune system to fight the cancer

The introduction or alteration of genetic material in cells is sometimes called oligonucleotide therapy. In vivo therapy uses a vector to introduce the genetic material (oligonucleotides) into cells within the patient's body. Ex vivo therapy removes cells from the patient, genetically alters them and grows them in the laboratory, and then transfers (infuses) them back into the patient.

Addition of genetic material

Gene therapy strategies often involve the introduction of genes or oligonucleotides into cells.

• Genes or oligonucleotides (specific strands of RNA or DNA) can be introduced into cancer cells to alter their metabolic state and increase their susceptibility to chemotherapy, radiation therapy, or other treatments.

• Genes can be inserted into cancer cells to prevent them from developing new blood vessels to nurture their growth.

• Genes can be inserted into healthy blood-forming stem cells to increase their resistance to the toxic effects of cancer treatments, such as high-dose chemotherapy.

• Genes for producing immune-system-stimulating proteins called cytokines are introduced into cells to boost the immune system's ability to recognize and destroy cancer.

Gene replacement and reprogramming

Gene-replacement therapies substitute a normal gene for a mutated gene that is causing cancer. For example, the tumor-suppressor gene that encodes the p53 protein—which normally causes damaged cells to undergo programmed cell death (apoptosis)—is mutated in about half of all cancers, enabling the cancer cells to survive and multiply. As of 2014, clinical trials involved the insertion of a normal p53 gene into these cancer cells to promote apoptosis, with the goals of inhibiting cancer growth, promoting cancer regression, or making the cells more sensitive to **chemotherapy** and/or radiation.

Gene silencing

Gene silencing is the blockage or suppression of the expression (activity) of a mutated gene, such as an oncogene, whose activity or overexpression is promoting tumor growth, **angiogenesis**, cancer **metastasis**, or resistance to chemotherapy. For example, the oncogenes encoding the proteins c-myc or epidermal growth factor receptor (EGFR) are amplified or "upregulated" in some cancers, and reducing their expression can inhibit tumor growth. Suppressing genes that promote angiogenesis can also inhibit tumor growth. Gene silencing may be accomplished with genes or with oligonucleotides that are complementary to a messenger RNA (mRNA). The oligonucleotides pair with the target mRNA and cause it to be degraded or prevent its translation into a cancer-promoting protein.

Eliminating cancer cells

Several gene therapies are designed to directly destroy cancer cells. Oncolytic viruses are genetically engineered viruses that infect and kill cancer cells but do not harm healthy cells. These viruses can reach cells deep inside tumors. There are many different kinds of oncolytic viruses. Some engineered viruses have mutations that enable them to selectively grow in tumor cells and burst out (oncolysis), releasing millions more viruses to invade and kill other tumor cells while avoiding normal cells. Other oncolytic viruses deliver genes that encode toxic proteins to tumor cells, including proteins that induce apoptosis. Typically, these proteins are produced under the control of a DNA regulatory sequence—called a promoter—that functions in cancer cells but not in normal cells. Another method, known as the "bystander effect," introduces into the body genetically modified cells that release factors that kill tumor cells in their vicinity.

Viruses can also selectively deliver "suicide genes" to cancer cells. These genes encode enzymes that convert a prodrug into a cancer-killing drug. The enzyme remains inactive until the prodrug is administered to the patient. Since the prodrug is converted into a toxic drug only in cells infected with the suicide gene, drug concentrations are only high in cancer cells, thereby reducing toxic side effects elsewhere in the body. Examples of prodrugs and their activating enzymes include:

• ganciclovir activated by thymidine kinase from a herpes simplex virus

• fludarabine phosphate activated by purine nucleoside phosphorylase from the bacterium *Escherichia coli*

• 5-fluorocytosine activated by cytosine deaminase

• cyclophosphamide activated by cytochrome p450

• tirapazamine activated by cytochrome p450 reductase

• CMDA activated by carboxypeptidase

Immunological approaches

Immunological approaches are often ex vivo gene therapies using cell transfer techniques.

• Cells that have been genetically modified to express tumor antigens can be used as vaccines to stimulate the immune system to destroy cancer cells carrying the antigens.

• Genes for factors such as cytokines can be introduced into healthy immune-system cells to enhance the immune response. In combination with the introduction of immune cells that express tumor antigens, the response can be targeted at cancer cells.

• Immune cells called cytotoxic T cells can be isolated from a patient's blood and modified with a gene for a receptor that recognizes an antigen specific to the patient's cancer. The T cell receptors bind to the antigen on tumor cells and destroy them. This method is under

KEY TERMS

Angiogenesis—Blood vessel formation.

Antibodies—Immune-system proteins that recognize specific antigens, such as proteins on tumor cells.

Antigen—A protein or other molecule that evokes a specific immune response.

Apoptosis—Programmed self-destruction of a cell when DNA damage is detected.

Chimeric antigen receptor (CAR) cells—Immune cells that are genetically modified with receptors that bind a specific cancer-cell antigen; the binding activates the immune cell to destroy the cancer cell.

c-myc—An oncogene that is a master regular of cell- cycle progression, apoptosis, and cellular transformation.

Cytokines—Proteins that regulate immune responses and mediate intercellular communication.

Epidermal growth factor receptor (EGFR)—A protein on the cell surface that can initiate growth and proliferation.

Ex vivo—Combined gene and cell-transfer therapy, in which cells are removed from the patient's blood, genetically modified, and returned to the patient.

In vivo—Gene therapy in which a vector is used to introduce genetic material into cells within the body.

Oligonucleotide—A relatively short single-stranded nucleic acid chain, either RNA or DNA.

Oncogene—A gene that has the potential, if mutated, to transform a cell into cancer; proto-oncogenes promote normal cell growth and division.

Oncolytic virus—A viral vector that can destroy cancer cells by infecting them and either bursting the cell directly or carrying a gene that destroys the cell.

p53—A tumor suppressor gene that, when mutated, is associated with a high risk for certain cancers.

Prodrug—An inactive drug that is enzymatically converted to its active form within a target cell.

Suicide gene—A gene that produces an enzyme that converts a prodrug to its active toxic form that kills the cell.

T cells—Immune-system cells that originate in the thymus gland; killer or cytotoxic T cells can destroy cancer cells.

Tumor suppressor genes—Genes that encode proteins such as p53 that inhibit cell division and replication; tumor suppressor genes are damaged or inactive in many types of cancer.

Vector—A carrier, such as a virus, that can transfer genetic material into cells in the body.

study for the treatment of metastatic melanoma, other solid tumors, and blood cancers.

- Chimeric antigen receptor (CAR) cells are immune cells with an added gene that both recognizes cancer cells and activates the immune cell when it binds to the cancer cell.

- Immune system cells can be infected with antibodies that bind to cancer cells. In 2013, scientists announced the remission of four leukemia cases treated with this method.

Gene vectors

Efficiently delivering therapeutic genes or oligonucleotides into cancer cells has been a major roadblock to the development of cancer gene therapies. Genetic material cannot usually be directly inserted into cells in the body—it must be transferred by a carrier or vector. Fatty particles called liposomes, or nanoparticles, are sometimes used. More often, the vector is a virus. Oncolytic viruses are engineered both to increase their ability to recognize and infect cancer cells and to inactivate genes that would enable them to reproduce in healthy cells or cause disease. Viral vectors used in gene therapy include:

- adenovirus

- adeno-associated virus

- herpes simplex virus

- lentiviruses such as the human immunodeficiency virus (HIV)

In addition to ex vivo cell-transfer techniques, certain cells, such as neuroprecursor and mesenchymal cells, are attracted to tumor cells, in part because of factors released by the cancer cells. These can be used as delivery cells to carry latent oncolytic viruses or therapeutic genes to the vicinity of the cancer.

Precautions

Failed or fatal clinical trials have, at times, threatened the future of gene therapy. Although certain gene therapies are available in a few countries, as of 2014, gene therapy was available in the United States only as part of a clinical trial.

Preparation

As of 2014, there were 64 active NCI-sponsored gene therapy trials listed at: http://www.cancer.gov/clinicaltrials/search/results?protocolsearchid=11898166&vers=1.

Risks

A major risk of gene therapy is partial or total ineffectiveness. The vector may not reach the cancer cells or the genetic material may not be expressed or may be expressed for too brief a time period. There may be an insufficient response to immunological gene therapies, or the cancer cells may become resistant to the therapy. It is possible that disease symptoms will worsen or be prolonged or that adverse effects of the therapy will further complicate the cancer. With the vectors in clinical trials as of 2014, there was no way to "turn off" gene expression that was producing undesirable effects. Retroviral and lentiviral gene-therapy vectors carry the risk that the genetic material will be inserted into the patient's DNA in a manner that causes "insertional mutagenesis" and produces a secondary cancer—for example, by insertion next to an oncogene or tumor suppressor gene. Other risks include:

- side effects such as flu-like symptoms

- gene introduction into healthy cells, including reproductive cells

- overexpression of an introduced gene such that it harms healthy tissues

- toxicity from high doses of some viral vectors, particularly in patients with compromised immune systems

- transmission of the viral vector to other people or its escape into the environment

Research and general acceptance

Clinical trials of cancer gene therapies have met with both modest success and failures.

- Many patients with blood and bone marrow cancers, including acute and chronic lymphocytic leukemias, have remained in remission for up to three years following ex vivo gene therapies using their own T cells modified with genes to target and destroy cancer cells. This method holds promise for treatment of acute lymphoblastic leukemia and could be approved as early as 2016; however, it is very expensive, since the therapy is individualized for each patient, and it can cause temporary severe flu-like symptoms and other side effects.

- In 2013, the biotech company Amgen announced a successful advanced clinical trial for metastatic melanoma, using a herpes virus engineered to infect cancer cells. After replicating (reproducing) inside the cells and producing a protein that causes an immune response, the viruses burst the cancer cell and attract immune cells to the tumor site. The cancer disappeared completely in 11% of late-stage melanoma patients, and tumors shrank by at least 50% in another 15% of patients. Some tumors that were not injected with the virus also disappeared, indicating that the viruses might spread through the body.

- In 2012, a phase 2 trial for advanced cancer pain proved no more effective than a placebo, in part, due to a profound placebo effect on pain reduction. This novel gene therapy used a modified herpes simplex virus that selectively targets nerve cells to deliver a gene for enkephalin, an endogenous painkiller, to the dorsal root ganglion. There were only minor adverse reactions, and the researchers speculated that the dose may have been too low or the cancers were too far advanced.

- Gene therapy for glioblastoma multiforme, a highly invasive and invariably fatal brain tumor, proved ineffective in phase 3 clinical trials.

As of 2014, there was renewed optimism over the future of gene therapies. Hospitals and companies were constructing manufacturing plants to produce viral-based gene-therapy products on a commercial scale. Fred Hutchinson Cancer Research Center, Seattle Children's Hospital, and Memorial Sloan-Kettering Cancer Center announced a partnership in a new company that will use patient's T cells to make CAR cells that target a protein called CD19 on the surface of some leukemia and other blood cancer cells and destroy the cells. Trials in patients with advanced leukemia and **non-Hodgkin lymphoma** were very promising. Similar early-stage trials were being launched for some prostate, lung, breast, and pancreatic cancers.

Resources

BOOKS

Abeloff, M. D., et al. *Clinical Oncology.* 5th ed. New York: Churchill Livingstone, 2014.

Gerdemann, Ulrike, Martin Pule, and Malcolm K. Brenner. "Gene Therapy: Methods and Applications." In *Childhood Leukemias,* edited by Ching-Hon Pui. 3rd ed. New York: Cambridge University, 2012.

Goldman, L., and D. Ausiello, eds. *Cecil Textbook of Internal Medicine.* 24th ed. Philadelphia: Saunders, 2012.

Krimsky, Sheldon, and Jeremy Gruber. *Biotechnology in Our Lives: What Modern Genetics Can Tell You About Assisted Reproduction, Human Behavior, Personalized Medicine, and Much More.* New York: Skyhorse, 2013.

López-Camarillo, César, and Laurence A. Marchat. *MicroRNAs in Cancer.* Boca Raton, FL: CRC/Taylor & Francis, 2013.

McPherson, R. A., et al. *Henry's Clinical Diagnosis and Management By Laboratory Methods.* 22nd ed. Philadelphia: Saunders, 2011.

Niederhuber, J. E., et al. *Clinical Oncology.* 5th ed. Philadelphia: Elsevier, 2014.

Piquet, Pascale, and Philippe Poindron. *Genetically Modified Organisms and Genetic Engineering in Research and Therapy.* New York: Karger, 2012.

PERIODICALS

"Ingenious; Gene Therapy." *Economist* 410, no. 8873 (February 8, 2014): 75–6.

Kwiatkowska, Aneta, et al. "Strategies in Gene Therapy for Glioblastoma." *Cancers* 5, no. 4 (2013): 1271–1305.

Tobias, Alex, et al. "The Art of Gene Therapy for Glioma: A Review of the Challenging Road to the Bedside." *Journal of Neurology, Neurosurgery, and Psychiatry* 84, no. 2 (2013): 213–22.

Young, Susan. "The Slow and Steady Revival of Gene Therapy." *Technology Review* 116, no. 6 (November/December 2013): 15–16.

WEBSITES

"Biological Therapies for Cancer." National Cancer Institute. June 12, 2013. http://www.cancer.gov/cancertopics/factsheet/Therapy/biological (accessed September 7, 2014).

"Cancer Gene Therapy and Cell Therapy." American Society of Gene & Cell Therapy. http://www.asgct.org/general-public/educational-resources/gene-therapy-and-cell-therapy-for-diseases/cancer-gene-and-cell-therapy (accessed September 8, 2014).

"Cell & Gene Therapy FAQ." Alliance for Cancer Gene Therapy. 2014. http://www.acgtfoundation.org/cell-and-gene-therapy/faq (accessed September 8, 2014).

"FAQS." American Society of Gene & Cell Therapy. http://www.asgct.org/general-public/educational-resources/faqs (accessed September 8, 2014).

"Gene Therapy and Children." KidsHealth. April 2014. http://kidshealth.org/parent/system/medical/gene_therapy.html# (accessed September 8, 2014).

"Gene Therapy Shows Promise Against Leukemia, Other Blood Cancers." HealthDay. *U.S. News & World Report.* December 9, 2013. http://health.usnews.com/health-news/news/articles/2013/12/09/gene-therapy-shows-promise-against-leukemia-other-blood-cancers (accessed September 8, 2014).

Mayo Clinic Staff. "Gene Therapy." Mayo Clinic. http://www.mayoclinic.org/tests-procedures/gene-therapy/basics/definition/prc-20014778 (accessed September 8, 2014).

ORGANIZATIONS

Alliance for Cancer Gene Therapy, 96 Cummings Point Road, Stamford, CT 06902, (203) 358-8000, http://www.acgtfoundation.org.

American Society of Gene & Cell Therapy, 555 East Wells Street, Suite 1100, Milwaukee, WI 53202, (414) 278-1341, Fax: (414) 276-3349, info@asgct.org, http://www.asgct.org.

National Cancer Institute, 6116 Executive Boulevard, Suite 300, Bethesda, MD 20892-8322, (800) 4-CANCER (422-6237), http://www.cancer.gov.

Margaret Alic, PhD.

Genetic testing

Definition

Genetic testing is a process that involves the examination of an individuals' genetic material for the presence of a change that might explain the development of a disease or disorder. Genetic testing may also help patients understand that they are at increased risk of developing a disease such as **cancer** in the future, even though they presently have no symptoms.

Description

Genetic testing usually involves taking a sample of a person's blood or saliva. The changes in the genetic material that can be detected by this testing vary in size. Sometimes parts or even entire chromosomes may be altered or missing completely. Other times, a mutation is present on a gene that causes it to malfunction. One type of mutation is known as a hereditary mutation. Hereditary mutations may also be called germline mutations since they are found in all the cells of a person's body, including the reproductive or germ cells, the sperm for a male and the egg for a female. This is why hereditary mutations can

KEY TERMS

Autosomal dominant—A non-sex-linked gene copy whose expression predominates over the other copy of the same gene, inherited from the other parent.

Cancer—The process by which cells grow out of control and subsequently invade nearby cells and tissue.

Cancer susceptibility gene—The type of genes involved in cancer. If a mutation is identified in this type of gene it does not diagnose the cancer, but reveals that an individual is at increased risk (is susceptible) of developing a new or recurring (developing again) cancer in the future.

Chromosome—Structures found in the center of a human cell on which genes are located.

Colonoscopy—A screening test performed with a tube called a colonoscope that allows a doctor to view a patient's entire colon and rectum.

DNA repair genes—A type of gene that usually corrects the common mistakes the body makes in the process of the DNA copying itself. If these genes are mutated and the mistakes are not corrected, those mistakes may accumulate and result in cancer.

Epigenetics—The study of heritable changes in genes caused by functional changes in the genome that do not involve alterations in the DNA sequence itself. Certain chemical reactions can cause a gene to "turn on" or "turn off" without any changes in the underlying DNA sequence. Epigenetics is the study of these changes.

Genes—Packages of DNA that control the growth, development and normal function of the body.

Genetic counselor—A specially trained health care provider who helps individuals understand whether a disease (such as cancer) runs in their family and their risk of inheriting this disease. Genetic counselors also discuss the benefits, risks and limitations of genetic testing with patients.

Germline mutation—A mutation that affects the germ cells (sperm or eggs) of an organism that reproduces by sexual reproduction. This type of mutation is inherited but is responsible for only a minority of cancers.

Hepatoblastoma—A cancerous tumor of the liver. Individuals with FAP are at increased risk for developing this type of tumor at a young age.

Mammogram—A screening test that uses X-rays to look at a woman's breasts for any abnormalities, such as cancer.

Mutation—An alteration in the number or order of the DNA sequence of a gene.

Oncogenes—Genes that typically promote cell growth. If mutated, they may promote cancer development.

Pedigree—A family tree. Often used by a genetic counselor to determine whether a disease may be passed from a parent to a child.

Penetrance—The likelihood that a person will develop a disease (such as cancer), if they have a mutation in a gene that increases their risk of developing that disorder.

Polyp—A growth that may develop in the colon. These growths may be benign or cancerous.

Prophylactic surgery—The preventive removal of an organ or tissue before a disease such as cancer develops.

Sequencing—A method of performing genetic testing in which the chemical order of a patient's DNA is compared to that of normal DNA.

Sigmoidoscopy—A screening test performed with a flexible scope called a sigmoidoscope that allows a doctor to view a limited portion of a patient's colon or rectum for the presence of polyps.

Tumor suppressor genes—Genes that typically prevent cells from growing out of control and forming tumors that may be cancerous.

be inherited, or passed from a parent to a child. Genetic testing involves looking for the presence or absence of these of mutations in genes.

Genes and cancer

Cancer is defined as one cell that grows out of control and subsequently invades nearby cells and tissue. There are several steps involved in the process that causes a normal cell to become malignant (cancerous). It is believed that different genes play a role in this specialized process. Oncogenes typically promote or encourage cell growth. If they are overexpressed or mutated, however, they may cause cancer to develop. Tumor suppressor genes when working properly prevent cells from growing

QUESTIONS TO ASK YOUR DOCTOR

- What is the likelihood that the cancer in my family is due to a mutation in a cancer susceptibility gene?

- If the cancer in my family is hereditary, what is the chance that I carry a mutation in a cancer susceptibility gene?

- What are the benefits, limitations, and risks of undergoing genetic testing?

- What is the cost of genetic testing and how long will it take to obtain results?

- If I undergo genetic testing, will my insurance company pay for testing? If so, will I want to share my results with them?

- What does a positive test result mean for me?

- What does a negative test result mean for me?

- If I test positive for a mutation in a cancer susceptibility gene, what are the best options available for screening and prevention? What research studies may I be eligible to participate in?

- What legislation is in effect to protect me against discrimination by my insurer or employer?

too quickly or out of control. They are often compared to brakes in a car. If these genes cannot perform their function because of the presence of a mutation, cells may grow out of control and become cancerous. Finally, cancer is sometimes caused by faulty DNA repair genes. These genes function to correct the common mistakes that are made by the body as the DNA copies itself, a normally occurring process. If these genes do not correct mistakes, however, the mistakes may accumulate and lead to cancer.

It is important to remember that while all cancer is genetic, or caused by changes in genes, just a small number of cancers is hereditary, or passed from parent to child. In fact, only about 5%–10% of cancer falls into this category. Therefore, the majority of cancer cases are not hereditary but sporadic. Most cancer is the result of mutations from environmental exposures or lifestyle choices. It is usually difficult to determine the exact cause of cancer that is not known to be the result of an altered gene.

Identifying individuals and families at risk of hereditary cancer

Although scientists have identified genetic tests for common cancers, such as breast and **colon cancer**,

genetic testing is not an option offered to all people with cancer, or even to those who may have a history cancer in the family. Since most cancer is not hereditary, genetic testing is not helpful for the majority of cancer patients. In order to determine who will benefit from genetic testing for cancer, health care providers need information about an individual's personal and family history of cancer.

Someone considering genetic testing for cancer usually meets with a genetic counselor, a specially trained health care provider. The genetic counselor asks about the personal and family history of cancer and creates a detailed family tree, also known as a pedigree. The family tree is then examined to determine the existence of certain "clues" that the cancer may be hereditary.

Some of those clues are listed below; **breast cancer** is used as the example:

- Multiple relatives in more than one generation with the same type of cancer, or related cancers. For example, a grandmother, mother, and daughter with breast cancer. Or, relatives with both breast and ovarian cancer; or a male relative with cancer of the male breast.

- Cancer occurring in the family at younger ages than is typically observed in the general population. For example, breast cancer usually occurs in women as they get older, most commonly in their 60s to 70s. In families with an alteration in a gene, the risk of developing breast cancer is increased; however, the disease may occur in women at much younger ages.

- Cancer that occurs in paired organs. For example, breast cancer that occurs in both of a woman's breasts, also known as bilateral breast cancer.

- Development of more than one type of related cancer in the same person within a family. For example, female relatives with both breast and ovarian cancer diagnosed at young ages.

- Specific ethnic background. Mutations in certain cancer susceptibility genes may be more likely to occur in individuals of specific ethnic backgrounds. For this reason, it is important that a complete family tree includes the country of family origin.

If a genetic counselor or other health care provider observes one or more of the above features in an individual's family tree, the option of genetic testing with the patient may be explored. Cancer genetic testing is offered only to patients if options exist to screen for the specific cancer and detect it early, or if screening has the potential to prevent the cancer from occurring.

Process of genetic testing

Genetic testing for genes that increase the risk of cancer is unique among medical tests. Genes involved in cancer are called cancer susceptibility genes. A mutation in one of these genes indicates an increased risk of developing cancer in the future, not the presence of cancer. Genetic testing in someone who has had cancer in the past may determine an increased risk of developing cancer again; however, the risk of developing a future cancer can not be determined with 100% accuracy. Penetrance is the term that describes the likelihood that a person will develop cancer if they carry an altered gene. Penetrance may differ even among relatives in the same family for reasons are not well understood. For example, a mother with a mutation in a cancer susceptibility gene may never develop cancer, but may pass this mutation on to her daughter, who is then diagnosed with cancer at a young age.

In a family in which an inherited mutation has not been previously identified, it is best to begin genetic testing by obtaining a blood sample from a person in the family who was diagnosed with cancer at a young age. DNA is extracted from this blood sample and examined for the presence of a mutation. One method of examining DNA is sequencing, in which the chemical sequence of a patient's DNA is compared to DNA that is known to be normal. Scientists search for differences, including missing or extra pieces of DNA in the patient's gene.

Testing can be very expensive; as of 2014, typical laboratory fees for genetic testing related to cancer range from $400 to $1100 for patients without **health insurance**. In general, it costs less to test for a genetic variant known to run in a family than to order a comprehensive test to predict a person's future likelihood of developing cancer. In addition, it may take several weeks or months to obtain results. Also, insurance companies are sometimes reluctant to cover the cost of genetic testing. Some families participate in research studies that offer genetic counseling and testing at a lower cost or free of charge.

Since 2007, direct-to-consumer or DTC genetic testing has emerged. This involves companies that offer genetic testing kits online or through consumer networks. According to a journal article published in 2013, the cost of these kits ranges from less than $100 to slightly more than $1000. The U.S. Food and Drug Administration (FDA) and the Centers for Disease Control and Prevention (CDC) have expressed serious reservations about the quality of these tests; some lack scientific validity; others yield results that are meaningful only when interpreted by a medical professional or trained genetic counselor. People who are considering a DTC genetic test should first consult a health professional and check the privacy policy of the online or network marketer to determine the security of their genetic information. The Federal Trade Commission (FTC) maintains a web page (listed below) with detailed information about and advice regarding DTC genetic testing.

Categories of results

A positive result indicates the presence of a genetic mutation that is known to be associated with an increased risk for developing cancer. Once this type of mutation has been identified in an individual, it is possible to test this person's relatives, such as children, for the presence or absence of that particular mutation. This testing is completed in brief period of time and provides results that are clearly positive or negative for a particular mutation.

A true negative result is defined as a family member who tests negative for a mutation in a cancer susceptibility gene that was previously identified in a family member. In other words, that individual did not inherit the mutation in the gene responsible for the cancer in a family member. Someone who receives a true negative result has the same risk of cancer as anyone in the general population. Since the individual tests negative for the mutation, the mutation will not be passed on to that individual's children. The term *true negative* distinguishes this test result from a negative or indeterminate result, described below.

If the first person tested within a family is found not to have an alteration in a cancer susceptibility gene, this result is negative; however, this result is also indeterminate. *Indeterminate* is used because a negative test result cannot completely rule out the possibility of hereditary cancer in a family. The interpretation of this result is complex. A negative result could mean that the method used to detect mutations may not be sensitive enough to identify all mutations in the gene; or the mutation may be located in a part of the gene that is difficult to analyze. It is also possible that the mutation is located in a cancer susceptibility gene that has not yet been identified or is very rare. Finally, a negative result could indicate that the mutation exists in a single cancer susceptibility gene, meaning that there is not an increased risk of future cancer.

Sometimes mutations are identified in cancer genes but scientists do not know how to interpret the results. They do not know whether these types of mutations affect the functioning of the gene and thereby increase a person's risk of cancer, or whether they are normal changes in the DNA that account only for slight variations. When this type of mutation identification occurs, the genetic counselor may work with the laboratory to determine whether future research might help interpret the patient's test result.

In general, a genetic counselor will help a patient to understand the meaning of his or her genetic test result, whether positive, negative, or indeterminate.

Benefits and limitations of genetic testing for cancer susceptibility genes

There are potential benefits for patients who undergo genetic testing, but limitations and risks exist too. A genetic counselor will discuss these issues in detail with a patient. Before undergoing genetic testing, a patient signs a consent form. This is a written agreement indicating that the patient understands the benefits and risks of genetic testing and has decided independently to undergo testing. The informed consent process is an aspect of genetic counseling and testing. With the exception of familial adenomatous polyposis (FAP), a disorder in which polyps and subsequently colon cancer occur in children or adolescents, the cancers associated with carrying an altered breast or colon cancer susceptibility gene do not typically occur at young ages. Therefore, genetic testing for mutations in these genes is usually offered to men and women 18 years of age or older, legally capable of providing informed consent.

Benefits of participation in genetic testing for alterations in cancer susceptibility genes:

- Results of genetic testing may provide additional information about the increased risk of developing cancer in the future. It may also provide relief from anxiety once someone learns that he or she does not carry an altered gene.
- Once discovery of an altered cancer susceptibility gene alerts an individual that he or she is at increased risk of developing cancer, that person may choose to be screened for this cancer at a younger age and more frequently. These results may also aid decisions about prophylactic surgery.
- Testing may provide information about cancer risks for children, brothers and sisters, and other relatives.
- Genetic testing may benefit knowledge about the origins of a family history of cancer. This information may lighten the emotional burden associated with the diagnosis of cancer.

Limitations and risks of participating in genetic testing for cancer susceptibility genes:

- Sometimes the results of genetic testing are difficult to interpret. Even a positive test result is not a guarantee that someone will develop cancer.

- In the process of genetic testing, people learn information about themselves or their family members that may have not been known before. Genetic testing sometimes reveals a previously unknown adoption or new information about the identity of an individual's biological parent. Strained family relationships sometimes result.
- Information about the presence of a cancer susceptibility gene sometimes causes emotions such as sadness, anger, or anxiety. Psychological counseling may be helpful when feelings are very intense.
- Genetic testing sometimes results in risk of discrimination by health or life insurers or employers. The completion of the Human Genome Project, which has mapped all the genes in the human body, has increased the number of available genetic tests. Two major laws at the federal level address the issue of privacy as well as discrimination. The Health Information Portability and Accountability Act of 1996 (HIPAA) requires health care providers and others with access to personal health information (PHI) to protect the privacy of this information. It also limits the conditions under which PHI can be shared or released and grants individuals some power over the release of PHI to other persons or entities. In May 2008, Congress passed the Genetic Information Nondiscrimination Act (GINA), which prohibits insurers from charging higher premiums or denying coverage to healthy persons on the basis of a genetic predisposition to developing a disease at some point in the future. GINA also prohibits employers from basing hiring and promotion decisions on genetic information. The statute does not, however, cover members of the Armed Forces. Detailed information about GINA's provisions may be found at the National Human Genome Research Institute (NHGRI) link listed below.
- Recent findings regarding cancer susceptibility genes increase the complications associated with genetic testing. For example, genes other than the well-known BRCA genes associated with breast cancer are now known to affect risk of breast cancer. Some genes interact with one another as well as with the BRCA genes, which adds to the complexity of identifying persons at risk of hereditary breast cancer. Another layer of complications is added by the epigenetic factors that influence gene behavior. Epigenetics is the study of chemical reactions that can turn genes "on" or "off" without altering the sequence of the nucleotides (subunits) in DNA or RNA. These epigenetic changes are heritable, however, in the same way as alterations in the DNA sequence. Some epigenetic factors are environmental in nature, but others are as yet not fully understood. In sum, it is highly unlikely that any

method of genetic testing will allow perfect predictions about the likelihood of developing breast cancer or any other form of cancer.

Genes and cancer types

Genes have been discovered that are associated with or responsible for several types of cancer, including **chronic myelocytic leukemia**, Burkitt **lymphoma**, **retinoblastoma**, **Wilms tumor**, **prostate cancer**, **stomach cancer**, and breast and colon cancers. As of 2014, about 100 hereditary cancer syndromes have been identified; however, genetic testing is available for fewer than half of these conditions. The remainder of this entry will focus on genetic testing for two of the most common cancers, breast and colon cancer.

Breast cancer genetic testing

Breast and ovarian cancer statistics

All women are at some risk of developing breast and **ovarian cancer** during their lifetime. While breast cancer is a common cancer among women in the United States, ovarian cancer is not. Most women are diagnosed with breast or ovarian cancer after the age of 50, and the great majority of cases are not hereditary. Of the 5%–10% of breast and ovarian cancer that is family related, most result from mutations in two genes, the BReast CAncer–1 gene (**BRCA1**) and the BReast CAncer–2 gene (**BRCA2**). The *BRCA1* gene is located on chromosome 17 and was discovered in 1994. The *BRCA2* gene is on chromosome 13 and was discovered in 1995.

BRCA1 and BRCA2 genes

The **BRCA1 and BRCA2** genes are tumor suppressor genes and are inherited in an autosomal dominant fashion. This means that children of a parent with a mutation in one of the breast cancer genes have a 50% chance of inheriting this mutation. These mutations can be passed from either mother or father, and can be inherited by both males and females. The mutations may be detected by performing genetic testing on a patient's blood or saliva sample.

Mutations in these genes are more common in Jewish people of Ashkenazi (Eastern or Central European) descent. While these mutations are more common in this population, they are also identified in other ethnic groups.

Cancer risks

Females who inherit a mutation in the *BRCA1* or the *BRCA2* gene are at increased risk of developing breast and/or ovarian cancer during their lifetimes. The lifetime risk of breast cancer in this group may be as high as 85%, as compared to about 13% in the general population. The lifetime risk of developing ovarian cancer may be as high as 60%, compared to 1.5% in the general population. Males who inherit a mutation in one of these genes are also at increased risk of developing certain cancers, including prostate, colon, and breast cancer.

Men and women who inherit an alteration in the *BRCA2* gene are also at increased risk of developing such rare cancers as pancreatic and stomach cancer. However, the risks for these cancers are lower than those for breast, ovarian, and prostate cancer.

Screening and prevention options

It is recommended that individuals who are at increased risk of developing breast cancer undergo increased surveillance, which means undergoing medical screening at an earlier age and more frequently than they would if they did not have an altered gene. For example, it is recommended that women with an altered *BRCA1* or *BRCA2* gene undergo mammograms at a younger age than is recommended for the general population. It is also recommended that these women see their doctors more often for breast exams and perform breast self-exams regularly. Because women who have a mutation in *BRCA1* or *BRCA2* are also at increased risk for developing ovarian cancer, they may also elect to be screened closely for this cancer. Screening includes a CA-125 test, which detects tumor marker protein in a woman's blood. Women may also undergo pelvic ultrasounds to examine the size and shape of the ovaries to determine the presence of cancer. Since ovarian cancer is difficult to detect, screening methods do not always find the cancer at a stage early enough for successful treatment.

Men with an altered *BRCA1* or *BRCA2* gene may also choose earlier and more frequent screening for cancers they are at risk for developing. Prostate screening consists of a test called prostate-specific antigen (PSA) that measures protein levels in a man's blood. Men may also undergo an examination by a physician. There are no standard screening recommendations for males who are at increased risk of breast cancer. It is recommended that they learn to conduct breast self-exams and consult their doctors about changes in breast tissue.

Some women at increased risk of developing breast or ovarian cancer may decide to have prophylactic or preventive surgery. This approach entails removal of healthy breasts or ovaries before cancer develops; however, even the best surgeon is unable to remove completely all of the breast or ovarian tissue. Therefore, even preventive breast or ovary removal does not completely eliminate all risk of cancer, though the risk is believed to be small.

Finally, some healthy women who are at increased risk of developing breast or ovarian cancer may decide to take certain medications that have been shown to reduce risk. Some of these medications have been studied only in the general population; further research is underway to assess the effectiveness these medications for women known to have an inherited risk of developing cancer.

Colon cancer genetic testing

Colon cancer statistics

Males and females in the general population have a 6% risk for developing colon cancer over their lifetime; the average age at diagnosis 60 to 70. Similar to breast and ovarian cancer, most colon cancer is not hereditary. Some colon cancer does run in families, however, and may be due to a mutation in a colon cancer susceptibility gene. Three of the more common hereditary colon cancer syndromes are described below.

Familial adenomatous polyposis (FAP)

FAP is a syndrome in which individuals develop numerous polyps (growths) in their colon or rectum. This disorder is sometimes called familial polyposis or Gardner's syndrome. Males or females with FAP often have hundreds of precancerous polyps when they are teenagers or young adults.

FAP is due to a mutation in a gene called *APC*. Mutations in this gene are dominantly inherited. In about 80% of families, genetic testing performed on a blood sample finds the alteration in the *APC* gene that causes this disorder. It is believed that two-thirds of people with FAP have inherited a mutated gene from a parent. The remaining one-third of individuals with FAP are believed to be new (sporadic) mutations, meaning that the alteration in the *APC* gene was not inherited from a parent. Individuals with sporadic mutations, however, can pass the mutation to their children.

Cancer risks

Since individuals with FAP develop multiple polyps in their colons, the risk that these polyps will develop into colon cancer if not removed is high. Individuals with FAP may also develop precancerous polyps in other organs, such as stomach or small intestine. Young people with FAP may also be at increased risk of developing a tumor in the liver (hepatoblastoma), as well as the thyroid gland or pancreas. Males or females with FAP may manifest the disease in other ways. For example, they may have cysts or bumps on their skin or on the bones of their legs or arms, or freckle-like spots in their eyes.

APC I1307K mutation

In 1997, scientists identified another mutation of the *APC* gene known as I1307K. This mutation is found only in individuals of Ashkenazi Jewish descent. It is estimated that about 6% of Jewish individuals have this particular mutation. The I1307K mutation itself does not cause an increased risk of colon cancer, but rather makes the *APC* gene more likely to undergo other genetic changes that increase risk of developing colon cancer. Genetic testing can be performed on a blood sample to determine whether an individual carries the I1307K mutation. A person with this mutation has a 50% chance of passing it on to his or her children.

Cancer risks

Individuals who carry the I1307K mutation have an 18%–30% risk of developing colon cancer during their lifetime. Research is ongoing to determine whether individuals with this mutation may also be at risk of developing other cancers, such as breast cancer.

Hereditary nonpolyposis colorectal cancer (HNPCC)

HNPCC, also known as Lynch syndrome, is a condition in which individuals are at increased risk of developing colon cancer even with few or no polyps present in the colon. It is believed that mutations in one of five cancer susceptibility genes are associated with most cases of HNPCC. These genes are known as *MSH2*, *PMS1*, *MSH6* (all on chromosome 2), *TGFBR2* (chromosome 3), *MLH1* (chromosome 1), and *PMS2* (chromosome 7). It is possible that other genes may be found that are also associated with HNPCC. Mutations in these genes are dominantly inherited and may be detected through genetic testing performed on a blood sample.

Cancer risks

Individuals with an altered HNPCC gene are at higher risk of colon cancer, often at a younger age (less than 50) than people in the general population. Those with an HNPCC mutation are at increased risk of developing other types of cancer, including stomach, urinary tract, bile duct, uterine and ovarian cancer. It is recommended that men and women are screened closely for these cancers.

Screening and prevention options

All individuals who are at increased risk of developing colon cancer should undergo screening for this cancer. Screening for colon cancer consists of two main tests. The first test is called a **sigmoidoscopy**. It is performed by inserting a flexible tube, called a sigmoidoscope into the anus to examine the rectum and lower colon. The doctor can use the scope to visualize polyps but cannot remove these growths with this test. The second test, a **colonoscopy** is similar to a sigmoidoscopy but allows a doctor to see the entire colon. The colonoscope, which the doctor uses to see the polyp enables the doctor to remove the polyp at the same time. Patients are sedated during this test. Patients considered at increased risk of developing colon cancer are encouraged to undergo this screening at younger ages and more frequently than individuals in the general population. Individuals with FAP are encouraged to have undergo sigmoidoscopy beginning at age 11.

Finally, men and women with a mutation in a colon cancer susceptibility gene may take certain medications that have been approved for use in individuals with an increased risk of developing colon cancer.

The only way to prevent colon cancer from developing is to remove the colon entirely. If a person with FAP, HNPCC, or the I1307K mutation develops colon cancer, he or she may elect to have the colon removed. Individuals who are especially anxious about the possibility of developing colon cancer may elect to have the colon removed before cancer develops. There are several different procedures for removing the colon that allow a person to function normally. Women with an HNPCC mutation may also consider prophylactic removal of their ovaries and uterus.

See also Cancer genetics; Familial cancer syndromes.

Resources

BOOKS

Ahuja, Nita, and Brenda S. Nettles. *Johns Hopkins Patients' Guide to Colon and Rectal Cancer*. Burlington, MA: Jones and Bartlett Learning, 2014.

Cummings, Michael R. *Human Heredity: Principles and Issues*, 10th ed. Belmont, CA: Brooks/Cole, Cengage Learning, 2014.

Hesse-Biber, Sharlene. *Waiting for Cancer to Come: Women's Experiences with Genetic Testing and Medical Decision Making for Breast and Ovarian Cancer*. Ann Arbor: University of Michigan Press, 2014.

Klitzman, Robert L. *Am I My Genes?: Confronting Fate and Family Secrets in the Age of Genetic Testing*. New York: Oxford University Press, 2012.

Matloff, Ellen T., ed. *Cancer Principles and Practice of Oncology: Handbook of Clinical Cancer Genetics*. Philadelphia: Wolters Kluwer Health/Lippincott Williams and Wilkins, 2013.

Mozersky, Jessica. *Risky Genes: Genetics, Breast Cancer, and Jewish Identity*. New York: Routledge, 2013.

PERIODICALS

Arnold, A.G., et al. "Assessment of Individuals with *BRCA1* and *BRCA2* Large Rearrangements in High-risk Breast and Ovarian Cancer Families." *Breast Cancer Research and Treatment* 145 (June 2014): 625–634.

Edwards, K.T., and C.J. Huang. "Bridging the Consumer-Medical Divide: How to Regulate Direct-to-Consumer Genetic Testing." *Hastings Center Report* 44 (May-June 2014): 17–19.

Feldman, E.A. "The Genetic Information Nondiscrimination Act (GINA): Public Policy and Medical Practice in the Age of Personalized Medicine." *Journal of General Internal Medicine* 27 (June 2012): 743–746.

Friebel, T.M., S.M. Domchek, and T.R. Rebbeck. "Modifiers of Cancer Risk in *BRCA1* and *BRCA2* Mutation Carriers: Systematic Review and Meta-analysis." *Journal of the National Cancer Institute* 106 (June 2014): dju091.

Giardiello, F.M., et al. "Guidelines on Genetic Evaluation and Management of Lynch Syndrome: A Consensus Statement by the US Multi-Society Task Force on Colorectal Cancer." *Diseases of the Colon and Rectum* 57 (August 2014): 1025–1048.

Kean, S. "The 'Other' Breast Cancer Genes." *Science* 343 (March 28, 2014): 1457–1459.

McCarthy, A.M., and K. Armstrong. "The Role of Testing for *BRCA1* and *BRCA2* Mutations in Cancer Prevention." *JAMA Internal Medicine* 174 (July 1, 2014): 1023–1024.

Su, P. "Direct-to-Consumer Genetic Testing: A Comprehensive View." *Yale Journal of Biology and Medicine* 86 (September 2013): 359–365.

Turgeon, D.K., and M.T. Ruffin 4th. "Screening Strategies for Colorectal Cancer in Asymptomatic Adults." *Primary Care* 41 (June 2014): 331–353.

Yee, J., et al. "ACR Appropriateness Criteria Colorectal Cancer Screening." *Journal of the American College of Radiology* 11 (June 2014): 543–551.

WEBSITES

American Cancer Society (ACS). "Genetic Testing for Cancer: What You Need to Know." http://www.cancer.org/acs/groups/cid/documents/webcontent/002548-pdf.pdf (accessed July 15, 2014).

American Cancer Society (ACS). "Heredity and Cancer." http://www.cancer.org/cancer/cancercauses/geneticsandcancer/heredity-and-cancer (accessed July 15, 2014).

Federal Trade Commission (FTC). "Direct-to-Consumer Genetic Tests." http://www.consumer.ftc.gov/articles/0166-direct-consumer-genetic-tests (accessed July 15, 2014).

National Cancer Institute (NCI). "Fact Sheet: *BRCA1* and *BRCA2*: Cancer Risk and Genetic Testing." http://www.cancer.gov/cancertopics/factsheet/Risk/BRCA (accessed July 12, 2014).

National Cancer Institute (NCI). "Fact Sheet: Genetic Testing for Hereditary Cancer Syndromes."

http://www.cancer.gov/cancertopics/factsheet/Risk/genetic-testing (accessed July 15, 2014).

National Human Genome Research Institute (NHGRI). "Genetic Discrimination." http://www.genome.gov/10002077 (accessed July 15, 2014).

National Human Genome Research Institute (NHGRI). "Learning about Breast Cancer." http://www.genome.gov/10000507 (accessed July 12, 2014).

National Society of Genetic Counselors (NSGC) and the Genetic Alliance. "Making Sense of Your Genes: A Guide to Genetic Counseling." http://www.geneticalliance.org/sites/default/files/publicationsarchive/guidetogcfinal.pdf (accessed July 14, 2014).

ORGANIZATIONS

American Cancer Society (ACS), 250 Williams Street NW, Atlanta, GA 30303, (800) 227-2345, http://www.cancer.org/aboutus/howwehelpyou/app/contact-us.aspx, http://www.cancer.org/index.

American College of Medical Genetics (ACMG), 7220 Wisconsin Avenue, Suite 300, Bethesda, MD 20814, (301) 718-9603, Fax: (301) 718-9604, acmg@acmg.net, https://www.acmg.net.

National Cancer Institute (NCI), BG 9609 MSC 9760, 9609 Medical Center Drive, Bethesda, MD 20892-9760, (800) 4-CANCER (422-6237), http://www.cancer.gov/global/contact/email-us, http://www.cancer.gov.

National Human Genome Research Institute (NHGRI), Building 31, Room 4B09, 31 Center Drive, MSC 2152, 9000 Rockville Pike, Bethesda, MD 20892-2152, (301) 402-0911, Fax: (301) 402-2218, http://www.genome.gov/10005049, http://www.genome.gov.

National Society of Genetic Counselors (NSGC), 330 N. Wabash Avenue, Suite 2000, Chicago, IL 60611, (312) 321-6834, Fax: (312) 673-6972, nsgc@nsgc.org, http://www.nsgc.org.

Tiffani A. DeMarco, M.S.
REVISED BY REBECCA J. FREY, PhD.

Genetics of cancer *see* **Cancer genetics**

Gentamicin *see* **Antibiotics**

Germ cell tumors

Definition

Germ cell tumors are a diverse group of tumors that originate in the developing embryo or fetus from cells that would normally become the cells of the gonads—testes (including sperm) in males and ovaries (including eggs [ova]) in females. Germ cell tumors can occur in many parts of the body and can be either benign (non-cancerous) or malignant (cancerous).

Demographics

Germ cell tumors are rare; their incidence has declined since the early 2000s. The incidence of germ cell tumors in the United States and worldwide is about 2.4 children in one million per year. The peak occurrences of germ cell tumors appear in infancy and adolescence. They account for about 4% of all cancers in children and adolescents under age 20. Germ cell tumors outside of the brain account for about 16% of all cancers in teenagers aged 15–19. The most common type of germ cell tumors are benign and malignant teratomas in the region of the tailbone during the first few years of life. These are about four times more common in girls than in boys. The second peak incidence reflects testicular cancers in teenage and young adult males. Other relatively common childhood germ cell tumors are abdominal, vaginal, and testicular tumors in infants, **brain tumors** in children, and ovarian tumors in young adolescent girls. Adult germ cell tumors usually occur in the testes or ovaries.

Description

Germ cells are the specialized cells in an embryo or fetus that develop into the testes and ovaries. Although most ovarian and testicular tumors are germ cell tumors, most germ cell ovarian tumors are benign. Less than 2% of ovarian cancers are germ cell tumors. In contrast more than 90% of testicular cancers are germ cell tumors.

During embryonic development, germ cells can move along the midline to other parts of the body, including the brain, where they may eventually form tumors. These are called **extragonadal germ cell tumors** because they are outside of the gonads (testes and ovaries). More than 60% of germ cell tumors in children are extragonadal. Germ cell tumors that occur outside of the brain are called **extracranial germ cell tumors**. In addition to the gonads and brain, germ cell tumors can occur in other parts of the body's midline:

• other reproductive organs such as the cervix, uterus, vagina, or prostate
• middle of the chest
• center back wall of the abdominal cavity
• center of the pelvis
• oral or nasal cavities
• lips

Germ cell tumors are usually discovered either during the first few years of life or shortly after puberty when they grow in response to increasing hormone levels. Extragonadal, extracranial germ cell tumors in early childhood usually originate in the sacrum and coccyx at the lower end of the spinal cord. Extragonadal,

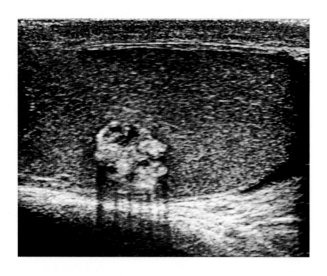

An ultrasound scan revealing a germ cell tumor (shown in purple) in a male testicle. *(Du Cane Medical Imaging Ltd./ Science Source)*

extracranial germ cell tumors in teenagers and young adults often originate in the chest. Some germ cell tumors are almost always malignant and others are almost always benign, depending on where in the body they occur.

There are two major types of germ cell tumors: germinomas, which contain only immature germ cells, and embryonic germ cell tumors, which contain both germ cells and some cells that have begun to develop into other tissues, as they normally would in a fetus. Germinomas—also called dysgerminoma if located in the ovaries and seminoma if located in the testes—are malignant tumors. Most embryonic germ cell tumors are a mixture of tissue types:

- Teratomas contain each of the three layers of the developing embryo—the endoderm (inner layer), mesoderm (middle layer), and ectoderm (outer layer). Mature teratomas are usually benign and immature teratomas are usually cancerous

- Endodermal sinus or yolk sac tumors, also called infantile embryonal carcinomas or orchidoblastomas, consist of cells that resemble the yolk sac of an early embryo and are usually malignant, often aggressively so.

- Embryonal carcinomas look like the tissue of very early embryos and are usually malignant and mixed with other types of germ cell tumors.

- Choriocarcinomas are very rare but often malignant tumors that arise from the chorion layer of the placenta during pregnancy and can spread to the mother and infant. They also occasionally develop in the ovaries or testes of young children.

- Gonadoblastomas and polyembryomas are rare types of embryonic germ cell tumors.

In general any type of germ cell tumor can develop at any germ cell tumor site; however some germ cell tumor types are much more common at particular locations:

- About 40% of all germ cell tumors are teratomas in the area of the tailbone and are typically diagnosed in the first month or two of life.

- Teratomas are also the most common type of ovarian germ cell tumor.

- Germinomas and endodermal sinus tumors are most common in the ovaries. Endodermal sinus tumors are also common in the testes.

- Embryonal carcinomas are most common in the testes, usually mixed with endodermal sinus tumors or choriocarcinomas.

Diagnosis, treatment, and prognosis for germ cell tumors depend on the major cell type in the tumor and the most malignant type of cell in the tumor. Malignant germ cell tumors can spread or metastasize to other parts of the body, most often to the lungs, liver, lymph nodes, and central nervous system. Rarely, they metastasize to the bone, bone marrow, and other organs.

Risk factors

The known risk factors for germ cell tumors include a number of inherited conditions, especially malformations of the central nervous system and genitourinary tract. Some types of germ cell tumors tend to run in families. Conditions involving extra or missing sex chromosomes (such as Klinefelter syndrome) can result in abnormal or incomplete reproductive system development, increasing the risk of germ cell tumors. Boys with cryptorchidism—failure of the testes to descend into the scrotal sac—are at increased risk for testicular germ cell tumors.

Causes and symptoms

The causes of germ cell tumors are not well understood. Since germ cell tumors usually consist of several different types of **cancer** cells, there are probably multiple causes. Increases in hormone levels at puberty are thought to play a role in the development of ovarian and testicular tumors in adolescents. Some germ cell tumors have a high frequency of certain genetic sequences or abnormal chromosome numbers that may lead to cancer. Testicular germ cell tumors can have structural abnormalities involving chromosome 12, which may play a role in tumor development.

Symptoms of germ cell tumors vary greatly depending on the size and location of the tumor. The most common symptom of germ cell tumors is a mass somewhere along the midline of the body, possibly accompanied by abdominal pain or bloating. Other possible symptoms include:

• constipation, incontinence, and leg weakness if the tumor is located in the sacrum and is compressing structures
• abnormally shaped or irregularly sized testes
• early entry into puberty
• vaginal bleeding
• late onset of menstruation
• menstrual problems
• excessive hair growth
• shortness of breath or other breathing problems
• diabetes
• hormonal abnormalities
• stunted growth
• headaches or vision problems

Diagnosis

Examination

Most germ cell tumors are initially identified by a lump in the testicles in boys or somewhere else along the midline of the body. Childhood teratomas of the tailbone are often visible from the outside. A doctor will perform a complete medical history and physical examination.

Tests

There are two **tumor markers** that are suggestive of germ cell tumors. Tumor markers are proteins that are produced by tumor cells and often found at elevated levels in the blood. Teratomas and endodermal sinus tumors produce high levels of alpha-fetoprotein (AFP). Germ cell tumors containing embryonal **carcinoma** or choriocarcinoma are associated with elevated levels of beta-human chorionic gonadotropin (beta-HCG). These markers are also used to monitor the effectiveness of surgery or other therapies and to monitor patients for a recurrence of the tumor.

Other blood tests may include:

• complete blood count (CBC)
• blood chemistries
• liver and kidney function
• cytogenetic analysis to look for changes in chromosomes
• immunohistochemistry to identify subtypes of tumors

Procedures

Procedures to identify germ cell tumors often include a **biopsy** of an identified lump. A small piece of tissue is removed and cut into thin sections. A specialist examines these sections under a microscope for the presence of abnormal cells. The degree to which the biopsied tissue differs from healthy tissue is an indication of the probable severity of the disease. Biopsy results are used to grade tumors and provide a prognosis.

Imaging procedures for the diagnosis and staging of germ cell tumors include x-rays, **computed tomography** (CT) scans, **magnetic resonance imaging** (MRI), ultrasound, bone scans, and **positron emission tomography** (PET) scans. X-rays can reveal calcium deposits in normally soft tissues. CT scans and ultrasound can provide details about the tumor, such as its site of origin, whether it is solid or cystic, and whether its borders are well-defined. Tumors with well-defined borders are more likely to be removed completely with surgery.

Staging

Grading and staging of malignant tumors determine treatment and prognosis. Tumor grades are based on the tissue types present in the tumor. Staging indicates the spread of the cancer. Separate staging systems exist for childhood and adult ovarian and testicular cancers, which are treated by pediatric and adult oncologists, respectively.

Pediatric testicular cancers are typically staged as follows:

• Stage I tumors are limited to the testes. Postoperative tumor marker levels are within the normal range.
• Stage II tumors have spread to the abdominal lymph nodes and tumor markers are elevated.
• Stage III tumors have greater involvement of the abdominal lymph nodes.
• Stage IV tumors have spread to other organs such as the lungs.

Adult testicular cancers are commonly staged according to a simplified TNM system:

• Stage T, with several sub-levels, is a localized tumor.
• Stage N is a cancer that has spread to local lymph nodes.
• Stage M is a cancer that has spread to distant lymph nodes and organs.

Treatment

Traditional

The treatment and prognosis of germ cell tumors depend on the types of tissues in the tumor, the tumor's location, and the stage of the cancer. The age of the patient, overall health and medical history, prognosis, and the issue of future childbearing also affect treatment choice. Most germ cell tumors require surgical removal of the tumor. More advanced cancers are treated with additional radiation or **chemotherapy**. Sometimes it is possible to completely remove all cancerous tissue with surgery. In other cases **debulking surgery** is performed to reduce the size of the tumor before it is treated with chemotherapy or radiation. Sometimes a **second-look surgery** is performed after **radiation therapy** or chemotherapy to confirm that cancerous tissues have been eradicated.

Germinomas are especially sensitive to radiation and this may be the primary treatment for these types of tumors. However, germinomas in the brain are the only type of childhood germ cell tumors that are routinely treated with radiation.

Drugs

Chemotherapy is administered with pills taken by mouth, by injection, or intravenously (IV). Chemotherapy kills cancerous cells, including those that have moved from the initial site. In more advanced stages of disease, chemotherapy is sometimes the primary treatment. It usually involves a platinum-based drug such as **cisplatin** in combination with one or two other anticancer medications. A combination of drugs reduces the risk of serious side effects from high doses of a single drug, since each drug includes different side effects. Drug combinations also decrease the risk of the cancer developing resistance to a particular drug. Various combinations of drugs are used to treat different types of tumors.

Clinical trials for germ cell cancer treatment are underway to evaluate a therapy called "peripheral stem cell rescue," in which the patient's red blood cells are removed before high-dose chemotherapy and replaced once the chemotherapy is complete. This decreases the side effects of the medications and improves the patient's chances of successful treatment. **Bone marrow transplantation** also allows the administration of higher-dose chemotherapy. Other clinical trials for germ cell cancer treatments are evaluating different combinations of chemotherapy drugs and new types of drug treatments.

Some of the more common side effects of chemotherapy include:

• hair loss (alopecia)

• fatigue and weakness

• nausea and vomiting

• bedwetting

Hair loss can be especially difficult for teenage patients. Other sources of hair damage—such as curling, blow-drying, or chemical treatments—should be avoided to slow the rate of hair loss. Children should be presented options for coping with hair loss and their choices should be supported. They may choose to remain bald or to wear hats or scarves. Schools may need to be persuaded to allow a child to wear a head covering. If a young patient chooses to wear a wig, a sample of pretreatment hair can be used to match color and texture. It is important to assure the child that the hair loss is temporary and a sign that the medication is working. Children should be prepared for the possibility that their hair may grow back a different color or texture.

Drugs may be prescribed to combat **nausea and vomiting** from chemotherapy. Desensitization, hypnosis, guided imagery, and relaxation techniques can also help treat nausea and vomiting. Video games are often an effective means of distracting children who are undergoing treatment.

Bedwetting can be especially distressing for older children. The child should be assured that this is insignificant and temporary. Extra linens and towels should be kept by the bed in case of an accident. Limiting fluids for a few hours before bedtime or waking the child in the night can help prevent bedwetting.

Alternative and complementary therapies

Common complementary therapies in the treatment of germ cell tumors involve reducing anxiety and increasing feelings of well-being. They may include:

• aromatherapy

• art therapy

• massage

• meditation

• music therapy

• prayer

• t'ai chi

• yoga

• other forms of exercise

There are numerous alternative therapies for cancer:

• Vitamins A, C, and E and selenium are believed to act as antioxidants.

• Vitamin E, melatonin, aloe vera, and beta-1,3-glucan may stimulate the immune system.

• Some practitioners believe that substances such as garlic and ginger shrink tumors. Any supplements should be discussed with the attending physician.

- Is the germ cell tumor benign or malignant?
- What are the treatment options?
- What treatments do you recommend?
- What are the side effects of treatment?
- Are there clinical trials that might be appropriate?
- What is the prognosis?
- Are there any complementary therapies that you would recommend?

Home remedies

Home treatment of children with germ cell tumors includes:

- a well-balanced diet
- small frequent meals with light nourishing food such as soup to combat nausea and vomiting
- plenty of rest
- avoidance of stress
- allowing the child to pursue normal activities to the extent possible, including participation in activities that are most important to the child and availability of backup activities or alternative mobility (such as a stroller or wheelchair) if the child becomes too fatigued

Prognosis

The prognosis for germ cell tumors depends on the type of tumor, its size and location, and whether a cancerous tumor has metastasized. The overall prognosis for germ cell tumors has improved dramatically in recent decades. About 90% of patients diagnosed with localized tumors are cured and the cure rate for metastasized germ cell cancers is approaching 80%:

- Childhood teratomas of the tailbone are usually diagnosed and treated very early and have a very favorable prognosis.
- Mature teratomas of the ovaries—by far the most common type of ovarian tumor—are almost always benign, unless mixed with other more malignant germ cell tumor types.
- Malignant germ cell ovarian tumors are usually diagnosed at a late stage and have the worst prognosis of all germ cell tumors.
- Embryonal carcinomas and choriocarcinomas are particularly malignant. Without treatment, the average survival time is only a few months.

Since most germ cell tumor patients are children or young adults, future fertility is a major concern. Radiation, in particular, destroys fertility and therefore is not usually used to treat children except in cases of brain germinomas. The surgical removal of reproductive organs to treat germ cell tumors can have major psychological consequences and cause altered feelings of sexuality.

Prevention

There are no methods for preventing germ cell tumors. Patients who have been successfully treated for germ cell cancers require frequent follow-ups to check for recurrences. Boys or young men who have had **testicular cancer** can improve their chances of detecting a recurrence at an early stage by performing regular self-examinations.

Health care team roles

The treatment team for a germ cell cancer patient typically involves the referring physician (often a pediatrician or gynecologist), an oncologist, a pathologist, and nurses. Radiation therapy involves a radiation oncologist, radiation therapist, radiation nurse, radiation physicist, and a dosimetrist. Treatment may also include a psychologist, nutritionist, social worker, and chaplain.

Resources

BOOKS
Bope, E. T. *Conn's Current Therapy*. Philadelphia: Saunders Elsevier, 2014.

Ferri, Fred, ed. *Ferri's Clinical Advisor 2015*. Philadelphia: Mosby Elsevier, 2015.

Goldman, L., and D. Ausiello, eds. *Cecil Textbook of Internal Medicine*. 24th ed. Philadelphia: Saunders, 2012.

Lentz, S. G., et al. *Comprehensive Gynecology*. 6th ed. Philadelphia: Elsevier, 2013.

Niederhuber, J. E., et al. *Clinical Oncology*. 5th ed. Philadelphia: Elsevier, 2014.

Rakel, R. *Textbook of Family Medicine 2011*. 8th ed. Philadelphia: Saunders Elsevier, 2011.

PERIODICALS
Feldman, Darren R., and Robert J. Motzer. "Good-Risk-Advanced Germ Cell Tumors: Historical Perspectives and Current Standards of Care." *World Journal of Urology* 27, no. 4 (August 2009): 463-470.

Schrader, Mark, et al. "Germ Cell Tumors of the Gonads: A Selective Review Emphasizing Problems in Drug Resistance and Current Therapy Options." *Oncology* 76, no. 2 (February 2009): 77-84.

Westermann, Dirk H., and Urs E. Studer. "High-Risk Clinical Stage I Nonseminomatous Germ Cell Tumors: The Case for Chemotherapy." *World Journal of Urology* 27, no. 4 (August 2009): 455-461.

WEBSITES

"Childhood Extracranial Germ Cell Tumors Treatment." National Cancer Institute. http://www.cancer.gov/cancer-topics/pdq/treatment/extracranial-germ-cell/patient/ (accessed December 3, 2014).

"Extragonadal Germ Cell Tumors Treatment." National Cancer Institute. http://www.cancer.gov/cancertopics/pdq/treatment/extragonadal-germ-cell/patient/ (accessed December 3, 2014).

"Germ Cell Tumors." Lucile Packard Children's Hospital. http://www.lpch.org/DiseaseHealthInfo/HealthLibrary/oncology/gct.html (accessed December 3, 2014).

"General Information About Childhood Extracranial Germ Cell Tumors." National Cancer Institute. http://www.cancer.gov/cancertopics/pdq/treatment/extracranial-germ-cell/HealthProfessional (accessed September 25, 2014).

"Germ Cell Tumors—Childhood." Cancer.Net. http://www.cancer.net/patient/Cancer+Types/Germ+Cell+Tumor+Childhood?sectionTitle=Overview (accessed December 3, 2014).

"Ovarian Germ Cell Tumors Treatment." National Cancer Institute. http://www.cancer.gov/cancertopics/pdq/treatment/ovarian-germ-cell/patient/ (accessed December 3, 2014).

"Testicular Cancer." MedlinePlus. http://www.nlm.nih.gov/medlineplus/ency/article/001288.htm (accessed December 3, 2014).

ORGANIZATIONS

American Cancer Society, 250 Williams St. NW, Atlanta, GA 30303, (800) 227-2345, http://www.cancer.org.

National Cancer Institute, 9609 Medical Center Dr., BG 9609 MSC 9760, Bethesda, MD 20892-9760, (800) 4-CANCER (422-6237), http://www.cancer.gov.

National Children's Cancer Society (NCCS), 500 N. Broadway, Ste. 800, St. Louis, MO 63102, (314) 241-1600, http://www.thenccs.org.

Wendy Wippel, MS
Margaret Alic, PhD.
REVISED BY TERESA G. ODLE

Gestational trophoblastic tumors

Definition

A gestational trophoblastic tumor (GTT)—also called gestational trophoblastic disease (GTD) or gestational trophoblastic neoplasm (GTN)—is a rare **cancer** that develops in the trophoblastic cells that help attach the embryo to the uterus and form the placenta.

Demographics

GTTs account for less than 1% of all **gynecologic cancers**. GTTs are significantly more common in some African and Asian countries than in Europe and North America. In the United States and Europe:

- Hydatidiform moles—the most common type of GTT—occur in about one out of every 1,000 pregnancies.
- About 15% of hydatidiform moles become invasive moles.
- Choriocarcinoma, a malignant form of GTT, occurs in 4% of women who have had a hydatidiform mole that was surgically removed or treated with radiation therapy.
- The overall incidence of choriocarcinoma is about one in 40,000 pregnancies.

GTTs occur only in women of childbearing age, almost always following a failed pregnancy. They are most common in women who:

- are under age 20
- are over age 40
- have had a previous GTT
- have had difficulty becoming pregnant or have had prior miscarriage
- have type A or AB blood
- have taken birth control pills
- have a family history of GTT
- are of lower socioeconomic status

Description

GTTs are highly curable malignancies that originate inside the uterus in cells called trophoblasts that make up one layer of the placenta. The most common types of GTTs are hydatidiform moles, also called molar pregnancies, and choriocarcinomas. A placental-site trophoblastic tumor is an extremely rare type of GTT that originates at the site where the placenta was attached to the wall of the uterus.

A hydatidiform mole can form when a sperm and egg cell unite but a fetus does not develop. If all of the tissue is not expelled, the cells that form the placenta can continue to grow until they look something like a cluster of grapes. Hydatidiform moles are classified as partial or complete. A hydatidiform mole does not spread beyond the uterus, but it can develop into an invasive mole in the uterine muscle or into a choriocarcinoma. Between 2% and 4% of hydatidiform moles progress to choriocarcinomas.

A choriocarcinoma is a malignancy of the trophoblastic cells. It usually originates in a hydatidiform mole; however, it can also develop in tissue that remains in the uterus following normal pregnancy and delivery, miscarriage, abortion, or an ectopic pregnancy. A choriocarcinoma is an aggressive, invasive tumor characterized by rapid growth and heavy bleeding. It can spread (metastasize) to any part of the body. **Metastasis** begins at an early stage of the disease and usually involves the lungs, vagina, pelvis, brain, and/or liver. Less frequently a choriocarcinoma spreads to the kidneys, spleen, and/or gastrointestinal tract.

Risk factors

Although the exact cause of GTTs is unknown, the risk of a GTT is higher than normal if a woman's blood group is A and her partner's is O. A woman's risk of a second GTT is twice that of a first GTT, although the risk is still very low.

Causes and symptoms

A partial hydatidiform mole can develop when two sperm fertilize a normal egg cell. Although fetal development may be initiated, the extra genetic material from the second sperm results in early miscarriage.

A complete hydatidiform mole most often develops when one or two sperm fertilize an empty egg cell that has no internal genetic material. Since all of the genetic material is from the father's sperm, no fetal tissue forms.

Choriocarcinomas develop from tissue that remains behind following pregnancy:

- About 50% develop after molar pregnancies.
- About 25% develop following a miscarriage, abortion, or tubal pregnancy (an ectopic pregnancy in a fallopian tube).
- The remaining 25% of choriocarcinomas develop after normal pregnancy and birth.

Although molar pregnancy is almost always diagnosed during the first trimester, it is often difficult to distinguish it from the early stages of a normal pregnancy. The most common symptoms of a hydatidiform mole are vaginal bleeding and severe morning sickness. Other symptoms may include:

- an unusually large uterus for the pregnancy stage
- a uterus that is enlarged on only one side
- absence of a fetal heartbeat
- absence of a visible fetus on a sonogram
- absence of fetal movement at the appropriate stage of pregnancy
- passage of clots with the color and consistency of prune juice or of finger-like structures (villi) containing fetal blood cells
- toxemia
- ovarian cysts
- hyperthyroidism
- iron-deficiency anemia from recurrent bleeding

Choriocarcinomas most often occur following a molar pregnancy. Persistent vaginal bleeding after giving birth can be a symptom of a choriocarcinoma. Irregular, abnormal bleeding can indicate that the choriocarcinoma has invaded the vagina. Other symptoms include lesions that can be seen on a chest x-ray but do not cause shortness of breath or other symptoms. Symptoms of lung metastasis include severe shortness of breath (respiratory insufficiency) and coughing up blood. The central nervous system (CNS) is rarely affected by choriocarcinoma unless the disease has spread to one or both lungs. Metastasis to the brain may cause headaches, seizures, and stroke-like symptoms.

Diagnosis

Examination

An internal pelvic examination is performed to detect lumps or abnormalities in the size or shape of the uterus.

Tests

Blood and urine tests measure levels of beta-human chorionic gonadotropin (beta-HCG). This hormone—which is normally produced by the placenta during pregnancy and is the basis for pregnancy tests—is abnormally elevated in the blood and urine of women with a GTT. The presence of beta-HCG in the blood of a woman who is not pregnant is indicative of a GTT. Beta-HCG is a sensitive marker for the presence of a GTT before, during, and after treatment.

Procedures

Imaging studies such as chest x-rays, **computed tomography** (CT) scans, **magnetic resonance imaging** (MRI), ultrasound, and **positron emission tomography** (PET) scans may be used to locate tumors.

Staging

Cancer centers commonly use the following system to describe the stage or extent of a GTT:

- Hydatidiform mole: Cancer is found only in the space inside the uterus.
- Invasive mole or choriocarcinoma destruens: Cancer is in the muscle of the uterus.
- Placental-site gestational trophoblastic tumor: Cancer is found in the muscle of the uterus and at the site where the placenta was attached.
- Nonmetastatic: Cancer is derived from cells remaining after treatment of a hydatidiform mole or following an abortion or delivery of a baby. Cancer has not spread beyond the uterus.

- Metastatic, good prognosis: Cancer cells have grown inside the uterus from tissue remaining after treatment of a hydatidiform mole or following an abortion or delivery and have invaded tissues outside of the uterus, but have not spread to the liver or brain; blood levels of beta-HCG are low; less than four months have passed since the last pregnancy; the patient has not received previous chemotherapy.

- Metastatic, poor prognosis: Cancer cells have invaded tissues outside of the uterus, including the liver or brain; blood levels of beta-HCG are high; more than four months have passed since the last pregnancy; previous chemotherapy has not eradicated the disease; or the tumor developed after the completion of a normal pregnancy.

- Recurrent: The cancer came back after treatment, in the uterus or elsewhere in the body.

Treatment

Traditional

The choice of treatment for a GTT is determined by the following factors:

- the woman's age and general health

- tumor type

- stage of the disease

- areas of the body where the cancer has spread

- blood levels of beta-HCG

- length of time between conception and initiation of treatment

- prior pregnancy-related problems and their treatments

- whether the woman plans to become pregnant in the future

A GTT is usually treated with surgery to remove the tumor. If the woman does not wish to become pregnant in the future, a hysterectomy may be performed to remove the uterus. If she does wants to become pregnant in the future, a **dilatation and curettage** (D&C) with suction evacuation is performed. This is used only for molar pregnancies. It involves:

- stretching the cervix—the opening of the uterus

- using a small vacuum-like device to remove material from inside the uterus

- gently scraping the walls of the uterus to remove any remaining material.

Radiation therapy is sometimes used to treat a GTT that has spread to other parts of the body. The radiation is either from a machine outside of the body (external beam) or from radiation-producing pellets (radioisotopes)

inserted into the area of the body where cancer cells have been found.

In the case of a recurrent GTT that has spread to the liver, radiation does not improve survival and may make **chemotherapy** less effective. The prognosis is even worse if both the liver and brain are affected.

Following diagnosis and treatment of a GTT, blood tests are performed weekly, pelvic exams every other week, and chest x-rays every four to six weeks until the blood level of beta-HCG has returned to normal. Once beta-HCG levels have normalized, monthly blood tests are continued for the next year and medical monitoring, including blood tests, with decreasing frequency for the next three years. Women who have been treated for a GTT should wait at least a year before becoming pregnant and should see a doctor as soon as they think they may be pregnant.

Drugs

Following D&C or hysterectomy for a hydatidiform mole, the blood levels of beta-HCG are carefully monitored. Chemotherapy is initiated if:

- Beta-HCG levels continue to rise for two weeks or remain constant for three weeks.

- Beta-HCG levels become elevated after having fallen to normal values.

- Analysis of tissue removed during surgery indicates the presence of invasive disease (choriocarcinoma).

- Heavy, unexplained bleeding occurs.

Chemotherapy may be in oral pill form or administered intravenously to kill any cancer cells remaining after surgery. Chemotherapy is started as early in the course of the disease as possible and administered every 14–21 days until beta-HCG blood levels drop to normal:

- Nonmetastatic disease, the most common form of choriocarcinoma, is usually treated with single-agent chemotherapy.

- Metastatic disease with good prognosis may be treated with chemotherapy alone, hysterectomy followed by chemotherapy, or chemotherapy followed by hysterectomy. Patients are carefully monitored because 40%–50% of the cancers will become resistant to the first chemotherapy drug used.

- Metastatic disease with poor prognosis is usually treated with combination chemotherapy.

Metastatic GTT may be further classified as low-risk, medium-risk, or high-risk. High-risk patients are treated with combination chemotherapy regardless of the stage of their disease. Factors used to determine risk include:

- age
- prior pregnancy experiences
- time elapsed between conception and initiation of treatment
- blood beta-HGC levels
- the size of the largest tumor
- the locations of metastasized cancer
- previous chemotherapy

A woman who develops one or more new GTTs after chemotherapy is considered high risk with a poor prognosis and is treated with aggressive chemotherapy, as well as possible surgery. If recurrent disease has spread to the central nervous system, whole brain radiation and systemic chemotherapy are administered simultaneously.

Research into GTT treatment is addressing the following questions:

- How effective are certain chemotherapy drugs for treating a GTT that has not responded to other therapies or that has recurred after treatment?
- At what dosages do specific chemotherapy drugs become toxic?
- How does the frequency of chemotherapy treatments affect a patient's prognosis?
- What is the relationship between the start of chemotherapy and an immediate drop in a woman's beta-HCG levels?

Prognosis

A GTT is one of the most curable cancers of the female reproductive system. This is because GTT cells respond well to chemotherapy and beta-HCG blood tests are a reliable means of determining whether cancer cells are still present and whether therapy should continue. Although it can be life-threatening, with early specialized treatment a GTT is highly curable even when it has spread far beyond the uterus:

- A hydatidiform mole is 100% curable by surgery. Partial hydatidiform moles are usually completely removed by the initial surgery. With about 20% of complete hydatidiform moles, some persistent molar material remains after surgery, usually as an invasive mole and rarely as choriocarcinoma, both of which require further treatment.
- Placental-site GTTs do not generally spread to other parts of the body; however they do not respond well to chemotherapy and can be fatal.
- Nonmetastatic GTT has a cure rate of almost 100%.
- About 80% of patients with widely metastasized disease are cured by prompt, aggressive chemotherapy, sometimes combined with surgery and radiation.

About 70% of patients with high-risk disease go into remission:

- Combination chemotherapy is effective in 74% of patients who have not responded to other forms of treatment and in 76% of those who have not been treated previously with chemotherapy.
- The survival rate for patients treated with combination chemotherapy is 84%.
- When recurrent GTT has spread to the central nervous system, simultaneous whole-brain radiation and systemic chemotherapy result in sustained remission in 50%–60% of cases.

About 85% of GTT recurrences are within 18 months of remission and almost all are within 36 months of remission. A GTT recurs in about:

- 2.5% of women treated for nonmetastatic disease
- 3.7% of women treated for metastatic disease, good prognosis
- 13% of women treated for metastatic disease, poor prognosis

Prevention

There are no known preventions for a GTT, other than never becoming pregnant. Women who have had previous molar pregnancies should speak to their doctors about future risks.

Health care team roles

A GTT is typically treated by a team of gynecologists, gynecologic oncologists, medical oncologists, and surgeons. Women with poor prognoses should be treated at a specialized trophoblastic disease center by a physician experienced in caring for high-risk GTT patients.

Resources

BOOKS

Bellenir, Karen. *Cancer Sourcebook.* 5th ed. Detroit: Omnigraphics, 2007.

Johnson, Tara, and Meredith Celene Schwartz. *Gestational Trophoblastic Neophasia: A Guide for Women Dealing with Tumors of the Placenta, such as Choriocarcinoma, Molar Pregnancy and Other Forms of GTN.* Victoria, BC: Trafford, 2007.

Sutton, Amy L. *Cancer Sourcebook for Women.* 3rd ed. Detroit: Omnigraphics, 2006.

PERIODICALS

El-Helw, L. M., and B. W. Hancock. "Treatment of Metastatic Gestational Trophoblastic Neoplasia." *Lancet Oncology* 8 (2007): 715-724.

Shih, I. M. "Gestational Trophoblastic Neoplasia—Pathogenesis and Potential Therapeutic Targets." *Lancet Oncology* 8 (2007): 642-650.

WEBSITES

American Cancer Society. "What is Gestational Trophoblastic Disease?" http://www.cancer.org/cancer/gestational trophoblasticdisease/detailedguide/gestational-trophoblastic-disease-what-is-g-t-d? (accessed November 4, 2014).

National Cancer Institute. "Gestational Trophoblastic Disease." http://www.cancer.gov/cancertopics/types/gestational trophoblastic (accessed November 4, 2014).

ORGANIZATIONS

American Cancer Society, 250 Williams St. NW, Atlanta, GA 30303, (800) 227-2345, http://www.cancer.org.

American College of Obstetricians and Gynecologists, PO Box 96920, Washington, DC 20090-6920, (202) 638-5577, resources@acog.org, http://www.acog.org.

National Cancer Institute, 9609 Medical Center Dr., BG 9609 MSC 9760, Bethesda, MD 20892-9760, (800) 4-CANCER (422-6237), http://www.cancer.gov.

Maureen Haggerty
Margaret Alic, PhD.

Giant cell tumors

Definition

Giant cell tumor generally refers to a bone tumor and is typically found in the end of arm and leg bones.

Description

Giant cell tumor of the bone is also referred to as an osteoclastoma as it contains a large number of giant

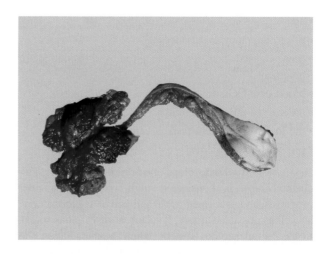

An excised giant cell tumor. *(CMSP/Custom Medical Stock Photography)*

cells resembling a type of bone cells called osteoclasts. Half of all giant cell tumors occurs in the knee, at the lower end of femur (thigh bone) or upper tibia (one of the bones of the lower leg). The tumor is usually located eccentrically and often causes expansion of the bone end. The tumor destroys the bony structure and thus could lead to fractures, even in the absence of stress. Other giant cell tumors can occur in virtually any other bone, including the sacrum, pelvis, and small bones of hands and feet. The growth of this tumor is variable and unpredictable. It is considered to be benign, but can recur following surgical removal. It can also have pulmonary metastases that are mostly curable. Some of the giant cell tumors may change into malignant sarcomas, especially when they recur after high-dose radiation treatment.

Giant cell tumor of tendon sheath

Giant cell tumor of tendon sheath is also referred to a localized nodular tenosynovitis. It usually occurs as a single, painless mass that grows slowly. It is mainly found in the wrist and fingers. These are benign growths that can be easily excised (surgically removed). This type is not discussed further in this entry.

Demographics

Giant cell tumor of bone is mostly seen in adults between the ages of 20 and 40 years. It is slightly more common among women than men and is seen in Asians more than other ethnic groups. It is very uncommon in children.

Causes and symptoms

The cause of giant cell tumors of bone is unknown.

The following symptoms may be seen in patients with giant cell tumors:

- Pain: As this tumors mainly occurs in the joints, arthritic pain is usually the first symptom.
- Swelling: Giant cell tumor causes enlargement of the bone and, as it grows, the patient may find a swelling at the site of the tumor.
- Fracture: Giant cell tumors destroy the surrounding bone and, unlike other bone cancers, fractures are common as the tumor grows. Initially the patient may have a sore or painful joint and the fracture could make it suddenly, severely painful.

Diagnosis

Typically the patient with giant cell tumor will go to the doctor because of pain. The doctor will perform routine physical tests and test the affected area for tenderness, swelling, warmth, redness, and mobility. An x-ray of the affected area will be obtained. Certain other imaging tests could be done, including **magnetic resonance imaging** (MRI) and **computed tomography** (CT scan) to see extent of growth. CT scan of the chest will also be done to test for **metastasis** to the lungs. An isotope scan may be also done to test for extent of damage. These techniques are noninvasive and can be performed within a day. A surgical **biopsy** is always done either before or during surgical removal of the tumor. The biopsy determines whether the tumor is malignant and identifies the stage of the tumor. This may done under either local or general anesthesia, depending upon the location of the tumor and the condition and age of the patient.

Treatment team

The treatment team will consist primarily of radiation oncologist, orthopedic oncologist, and oncology nurse. Following surgical removal of the tumor, recovery may be aided by physical therapists.

Clinical staging

Most giant cell tumors are initially classified as benign (grade 0). The tumor may progress in three stages. Stage 1, or latent stage, consists of a very slow growing tumor. It is well demarcated and there is little destruction of the outer surface of the bone. Stage 2, or the active stage, is the most commonly found stage. In this stage the tumor grows more steadily and the cortex (or outer layer of the bone) is lost. Stage 3 is the aggressive stage and accounts for about 20% of all giant cell tumors. In this

---

KEY TERMS

Computed tomography—Commonly known as CT or CAT scan. It uses a rotating beam of x-ray to get internal images of the body from different angles. During this test a harmless dye may be injected to increase contrast between normal and abnormal tissues.

Curettage—Surgical method in which a tumor is scraped away from the healthy tissue.

Magnetic resonance imaging—Also referred to as MRI. A procedure using a powerful magnetic field and radio waves to produce images of internal organs. MRI images can be used to look at soft tissues like muscle and fat.

Sarcoma—Uncommon, malignant tumors that begin in bones, or soft tissues such as muscle or fat.

---

stage the tumor grows rapidly and extends beyond the bone into the soft tissue. This stage is also associated more frequently with fractures.

Treatment

Treatment of giant cell tumors is mainly surgical. Most stage 1 and 2 and some stage 3 tumors are treated by aggressive curettage, and the bone may be treated chemically and filled with cement. In some stage 2 and most stage 3 lesions the affected section of the bone may have to be removed (en bloc resection). In very rare cases the tumor may be so expanded that **amputation** may be necessary. Radiation is used to treat giant cell tumors in a location difficult to treat surgically. **Chemotherapy** has not been shown to be effective against giant cell tumors.

Alternative and complementary therapies

There are no alternative or complementary therapies available for giant cell tumors.

Coping with cancer treatment

As the treatment for giant cell tumors is mainly surgical, **physical therapy** with strengthening exercises to restore range of motion is extremely important. If amputation is required, resulting psychological effects will also have to be addressed, especially as this disease occurs in adults who are physically and sexually active.

Prognosis

Prognosis following resection is excellent, with less than 5% chance of recurrence. When the tumor is removed by curettage followed by aggressive chemical treatment, there is a 5%–10% chance of local recurrence. When the tumors recur locally it is usually within three years of surgical removal and the patient needs to be monitored closely during this time. A small percentage of giant cell tumors can metastasize to the lungs. The metastases can be removed surgically and most can be cured.

When a rare case of malignant **sarcoma** develops from a giant cell tumor, it is treated aggressively by surgery. In these cases, prognosis is poor and long-term survival rate is as low as 20%–30%.

Clinical trials

In 2014, there were two ongoing **clinical trials** for treatment of giant cell tumors. More information is available from the **National Cancer Institute** website at: http://www.cancer.gov/clinicaltrials/search.

Prevention

As the cause of giant cell tumors is not known, there is no known method for prevention. When adults in the age group of 20 to 40 years notice pain and swelling in the joints, prompt radiological evaluation could identify giant cell tumors in early stages and lead to a complete cure.

Special concerns

Whenever a giant cell tumor is suspected, a chest CT scan should also be performed to check for metastasis to the lungs. During pregnancy the tumor can grow more rapidly, in which case it may be better to wait to perform surgery until the baby can be safely delivered by induction. If a patient with giant cell tumor suffers a fracture at the affected area, it may be best to wait until the fracture is healed before performing the surgery.

Resources

BOOKS

Campanacci, Mario. *Bone and soft tissue tumors.* New York: Springer-Verlag Wien Publishing, 1999.

PERIODICALS

Blackley, H. R., et al. "Treatment of giant cell tumors with curettage and bone grafting." *Journal of Bone and Joint Surgery* American, 81, no. 6 (1999): 811-20.

ORGANIZATIONS

American Academy of Orthopaedic Surgeons, 6300 N. River Rd., Rosemont, IL 60018, (847) 823-7186, Fax: (847) 823-8125, orthoinfo@aaos.org, http://www.aaos.org.

Malini Vashishtha, PhD.

Gilotrif *see* **Afatinib**

Gleevec *see* **Imatinib mesylate**

Gliadel Wafers *see* **Carmustine**

Gliomas *see* **Astrocytoma; Brain and central nervous system tumors**

Global cancer incidence and mortality

Definition

Cancer is a leading cause of death worldwide, with an estimated 14.1 million new cancer cases and 8.2 million deaths in 2012. Many countries, regions, and international organizations maintain registries of cancer incidence and mortality. These registries track the number of newly diagnosed cancer cases and cancer deaths in a given population.

Description

Cancer incidence is the number of new cases diagnosed over a given period in a specified population, determined from information routinely collected by cancer registries. Incidence can be expressed as the absolute number of cases diagnosed each year or as the cancer rate per 100,000 people per year. Mortality is the number of cancer deaths occurring in a given period in a specified population. It can be expressed as an absolute number of deaths per year or as a rate per 100,000 people per year. Mortality data are maintained by national statistical

Countries with the highest cancer rates

Country	Rate per 100,000 people
Denmark	338.1
France (metropolitan)	324.6
Australia	323.0
Belgium	321.1
Norway	318.3
United States of America	318.0
Ireland	307.9
Korea, Republic of	307.8
Netherlands	304.8
New Caledonia	297.9

SOURCE: World Cancer Research Fund International, "Data for Cancer Frequency by Country." Available online at: http://www .wcrf.org/int/cancer-facts-figures/data-cancer-frequency-country.

Table listing the ten countries with the highest cancer rates. *(Table by Lumina Datamatics Ltd. © 2015 Cengage Learning®.)*

offices. Measurements of "cancer burden" are based on both incidence and mortality rates and also on the total number of new cases and deaths in a given year, which indicates needs for medical care and social services.

Surveillance

The primary databases for global cancer incidence and mortality are compiled and managed by the Section of Cancer Surveillance (CSU) of the International Agency for Research on Cancer (IARC) of the World Health Organization (WHO). There are three major CSU databases.

- GLOBOCAN estimates the worldwide incidence, mortality, and prevalence for 28 types of cancer.
- Cancer Incidence for Five Continents (CI5) includes detailed statistics on cancer incidence from regional and national cancer registries that collect high-quality data. The CI5 covers approximately 11% of the global population.
- The WHO database features selected cancer mortality statistics over time for selected countries, along with trends and future predictions.

The CSU also maintains collaborative databases, including the:

- Automated Childhood Cancer Information System (ACCIS) of cancer incidence and survival in children, collected from European cancer registries
- International Incidence of Childhood Cancer (IICC) from regional and national cancer registries worldwide
- European Cancer Observatory (ECO) of cancer data from Europe
- NORDCAN—cancer incidence, mortality, prevalence, and survival for 40 cancers over time from Nordic countries, along with predictions

- SurvCan—cancer survival data from cancer registries in low- and middle-income regions of the world

GLOBOCAN data

GLOBOCAN is the most comprehensive and reliable source for data on global cancer incidence and mortality. It estimates national incidence, mortality, and prevalence for major cancers in 184 countries; however, since data collection is continuously improving, estimates may not be comparable over time. Furthermore, data collection varies significantly among countries. GLOBOCAN provides scores that indicate rough assessments of the quality of data from different countries. There are no data for cancer incidence and mortality in many developing countries. In these cases, estimates are made using frequency data or rates from neighboring countries. GLOBOCAN rates its incidence data as:

- high-quality national or regional data with coverage of more than 50%
- high-quality regional data with coverage of 10%–50%
- high-quality regional data with coverage below 19%
- national data (rates)
- regional data (rates)
- frequency data
- no data

Cancer mortality data are available for all industrialized countries and for some developing countries, covering approximately one-third of the global population. The quality of mortality data depends on the accuracy of underlying causes of death. The data are highly accurate for developed countries and of low accuracy for developing countries. GLOBOCAN rates its mortality data as:

- high-quality complete vital registration
- medium-quality complete vital registration
- low-quality complete vital registration
- incomplete or sample vital registration
- sources other than vital registration, such as cancer registries or verbal autopsy surveys
- no data

GLOBOCAN data are available by gender, country, WHO regions (Africa, the Americas, South-East Asia, Europe, the Eastern Mediterranean, and the Western Pacific), and the 24 IARC member countries. Data are also available by more and less developed regions and by the human development index (HDI). Economic development is categorized as low, lower-middle, upper-middle, and high income, based on 2008 gross national income per capita. Cancer rates for more economically developed regions are estimated as the population-weighted average of all of Europe, North America, Australia/New Zealand, and Japan. The rates for less-developed regions are estimated as the population-weighted average of all of Africa, all of Asia except Japan, the Caribbean, Central and South America, Melanesia, Micronesia, and Polynesia. The HDI is based on a population's life expectancy at birth, educational attainment (a combination of the adult literacy rate and enrollment rates in primary through tertiary education), and income (based on the gross domestic product per capita adjusted for purchasing-power parity in U.S. dollars). Countries are grouped into four HDI categories by the United Nations Development Programme as very high, high, medium, and low.

GLOBOCAN data are available for the most common cancers:

- breast
- cervical/uterine
- colorectal
- liver
- lung
- esophageal
- prostate
- stomach

Cancer statistics

Cancer incidence and mortality rates are usually standardized for age. This is because different populations vary in their age composition—some countries, especially in the developing world, have very young populations; other countries, such as Japan, have a high proportion of elderly people. Since the risk of various cancers increases significantly with age, populations with higher proportions of younger people would be expected to have lower cancer incidence or rates than populations with higher proportions of older people. Age standardization allows cancer incidence and mortality to be compared among different populations. Age standardization applies the age-specific cancer rates in a given population to a standard based on a common age distribution in a population. This yields the hypothetical cancer incidence and mortality rates that would be observed if the population had an age distribution equal to that of the standard population; however, data from different sources do not necessarily use the same standard age composition. IARC and some other data sources standardize to a 1960 world standard population. Incidence and mortality data in the United States and several European countries are standardized to the 2000 U.S. and European standard populations, respectively.

Top ten most common cancers worldwide

Type of cancer	Percentage of all cancer diagnoses*
Lung cancer	13.0%
Breast cancer	11.9%
Colorectal cancer	9.7%
Prostate cancer	7.9%
Stomach cancer	6.8%
Liver cancer	5.6%
Cervical cancer	3.7%
Esophageal cancer	3.2%
Bladder cancer	3.1%
Non-Hodgkin lymphoma	2.7%

*Does not include non-melanoma skin cancer.

SOURCE: World Cancer Research Fund International, "Worldwide Data." Available online at: http://www.wcrf.org/int/cancer-facts-figures/worldwide-data.

Table listing the most common cancers throughout the world. *(Table by Lumina Datamatics Ltd. © 2015 Cengage Learning®.)*

In addition to incidence and mortality, cancer databases often include prevalence and survival. GLOBOCAN makes available one-, three-, and five-year cancer prevalence data for ages 15 and over. Survival rates are the proportion of people alive at a specific time—usually five years—following cancer diagnosis. The observed survival rate is the proportion of cancer patients living after five years of follow-up, without regard to deaths from causes other than cancer. The relative survival rate is the proportion of people alive five years after diagnosis compared to the population of the same age and sex without cancer, which takes into account deaths from other causes. Cancer survival data are available for North American and European countries and some developing countries. Survival rates vary tremendously among countries and regions, due to different rates of specific types of cancer and differences in the availability of screening, diagnosis, and effective timely treatments, as well as large variability in cancer registration and follow-up.

Incidence

There were an estimated 7.4 million new cancer cases in males and 6.7 million in females in 2012 in a global population of 7.1 billion (3.6 billion males and 3.5 billion females). The age-standardized rate for new cancer cases was 182 per 100,000 people—205 per 100,000 males and 165 per 100,000 females. This yields an overall 18.5% risk of cancer diagnosis before age 75—a 21% risk for males and a 16% risk for females. Thus, the overall age-standardized cancer incidence rate in 2012 was almost 25% higher for men than for women. Incidence rates for cancer in males varied nearly five-fold among different regions, from a low of 79 per 100,000 in Western Africa to 365 per 100,000 in Australia/New Zealand, with **prostate cancer** accounting for much of the higher rates. Female incidence rates varied nearly three-fold, from 103 per 100,000 in South-Central Asia to 295 per 100,000 in North America.

Absolute 2012 global incidences for all cancers except **non-melanoma skin cancer** were as follows:

- United States: 1.6 million—825,000 in men and 779,000 in women
- China: 3.1 million—1.8 million in men and 1.2 million in women
- India: 1 million—477,000 in men and 537,000 in women
- European Union: 2.7 million—1.4 million in men and 1.2 million in women
- WHO Africa Region: 645,000—265,000 in men and 381,000 in women
- WHO Americas Region: 2.9 million—1.5 million in men and 1.4 million in women
- WHO South-East Asia Region: 1.7 million—816,000 in men and 908,000 in women
- WHO Europe Region: 3.7 million—2 million men and 1.8 million women
- WHO Eastern Mediterranean Region: 555,000—263,000 in men and 293,000 in women
- WHO Western Pacific Region: 4.5 million—2.6 million in men and 1.9 million in women
- more-developed regions: 6.1 million—3.2 million in men and 2.8 million in women
- less-developed regions: 8.0 million—4.2 million in men and 3.8 million in women

Lung, female breast, colorectal, and stomach cancers accounted for more than 40% of all newly diagnosed cancers. Lung cancer was the most common cancer in men, accounting for 16.7% of all new male cases. **Breast cancer** was by far the most commonly diagnosed cancer in women, accounting for 25.2% of all new female cancers. Lung and breast cancers were the overall first and second most frequently diagnosed cancers, respectively. Prostate cancer was the second most common cancer in males. Colorectal cancer was the second most common cancer in females and the third most common overall. Lung cancer was the third most common in females, and colorectal cancer was the third most common in males. Prostate cancer, which only affects males, was the overall fourth most commonly diagnosed cancer worldwide. Cervical/uterine cancers were the fourth most common in females, and **stomach cancer**

was the fourth most common in males. Stomach cancer was the fifth most common overall and in females. **Liver cancer** was the fifth most common in males.

Mortality

There were 4.7 million male cancer deaths and 3.5 million female deaths globally in 2012. The age-standardized rate was 102 deaths per 100,000 population—126 per 100,000 for males and 83 per 100,000 for females. Overall, there was a 10.4% risk of dying from cancer before age 75—12.7% for males and 8.4% for females. More than half of all cancer mortality was due to lung, stomach, liver, colorectal, and female breast cancers. Tobacco consumption is estimated to be a causal factor in 21% of all cancer deaths worldwide.

There was less regional variation in cancer mortality than in incidence. Mortality rates were 15% higher for men and 8% higher for women in more-developed regions compared with less-developed regions. Mortality rates for men were highest in Central and Eastern Europe, at 173 per 100,000, and lowest in Western Africa, at 69 per 100,000. The highest mortality rates for women varied from 119 per 100,000 in Melanesia and 111 per 100,000 in Eastern Africa to lows of 72 per 100,000 in Central America and 65 in South-Central Asia.

QUESTIONS TO ASK YOUR DOCTOR

- What is the cancer incidence and mortality for my population?
- What are the most common cancers in my population?
- What is my risk of developing cancer before age 75?
- What is the incidence and mortality for my type of cancer?
- What is the survival rate for my type of cancer?

The absolute number of global deaths from all cancers except non-melanoma **skin cancer** in 2012 were as follows:

- United States: 617,000—324,000 men and 293,000 women
- China: 2.2 million—1.4 million men and 776,000 women
- India: 683,000—357,000 men and 326,000 women
- European Union: 1.3 million—715,000 men and 560,000 women
- WHO Africa Region: 456,000—205,000 men and 250,000 women
- WHO Americas Region: 1.3 million—677,000 men and 618,000 women
- WHO South-East Asia Region: 1.2 million—616,000 men and 555,000 women
- WHO Europe Region: 1.9 million—1.1 million men and 852,000 women
- WHO Eastern Mediterranean Region: 367,000—191,000 men and 176,000 women
- WHO Western Pacific Region: 3 million—1.9 million men and 1.1 million women
- more-developed regions: 2.9 million—1.6 million men and 1.3 million women
- less-developed regions: 5.3 million—3.1 million men and 2.3 million women

Trends

About 44% of cancer cases and 53% of cancer deaths occur in countries with a low or medium HDI. If recent trends for major cancers continue globally, 23.6 million new cancer cases can be expected annually by 2030. This is an increase of 68% over 2012—a 66% increase in low- to medium-HDI countries and a 56% increase in high- to very-high-HDI countries.

Projections of cancer incidence in 2030 are based on expected demographic changes, as well as on assumptions about trends in the rates of six cancers, based on the changing annual age-adjusted incidence determined from 101 cancer registries from 1988 to 2002. These assumptions include:

- worldwide annual decreases of 2.5% for stomach cancer and 2% for cervical cancer
- 1% annual decreases in lung cancer in men in high- and very-high-HDI regions
- worldwide annual increases of 1% for colorectal cancer, 2% for female breast cancer, and 3% for prostate cancer
- 1% annual increases in lung cancer in women in high- and very-high-HDI regions

As low-HDI countries become more developed through rapid economic and social changes, they tend to become "westernized," and cancer incidence trends move toward patterns seen in countries with a high HDI. As a result, incidence rates for cervical/uterine cancers tend to decline, and incidence rates for female breast cancer and prostate and colorectal cancers tend to increase. Cancers associated with infection, such as **cervical cancer**, tend to decline; however, increases in cancers associated with reproductive, hormonal, and dietary risk factors outweigh declines. Thus, cancer incidence is rising rapidly in developing economies, including China, India, and Russia. Furthermore, cancer mortality rates are twice as high in these countries as in the United States and the United Kingdom. WHO projects that by 2032, more than 60% of new cancers and 70% of cancer deaths will occur in Central and South America, Africa, and Asia.

Resources

BOOKS

Miller, Kenneth D., and Miklos Simon. *Global Perspectives on Cancer: Incidence, Care, and Experience.* Santa Barbara, CA: Praeger, 2015.

Stewart, Bernard W., and Christopher P. Wild, editors. *World Cancer Report 2014.* Lyon, France: International Agency for Research on Cancer, 2014.

PERIODICALS

Bender, Eric. "Global Warning." *Nature suppl. Outlook: Cancer* 509, no. 7502 (May 29, 2014): S64–5.

Shi, Yuankai, and Frank B. Hu. "The Global Implications of Diabetes and Cancer." *Lancet* 383, no. 9933 (June 7, 2014): 1947–8.

WEBSITES

"Global Cancer Facts & Figures." 2nd ed. American Cancer Society. 2011. http://www.cancer.org/acs/groups/content/@epidemiologysurveilance/documents/document/acspc-027766.pdf (accessed September 12, 2014).

"GlOBOCAN 2012: Estimated Cancer Incidence, Mortality and Prevalence Worldwide in 2012." International Agency for Research on Cancer. http://globocan.iarc.fr/Default.aspx (accessed September 12, 2014).

"World Cancer Factsheet." Cancer Research UK. January 2014. http://publications.cancerresearchuk.org/downloads/product/CS_REPORT_WORLD.pdf (accessed September 12, 2014).

ORGANIZATIONS

American Cancer Society, 250 Williams Street NW, Atlanta, GA 30303, (800) 227-2345, http://www.cancer.org.

International Agency for Research on Cancer, 150 Cours Albert Thomas, Lyon, FranceCEDEX 0869372, 33 (0)4 72 73 84 85, Fax: 33 (0)4 72 73 85 75, http://www.iarc.fr.

Margaret Alic, PhD.

Glossectomy

Definition

A glossectomy is the surgical removal of all or part of the tongue.

Purpose

A glossectomy is performed to treat **cancer** of the tongue. Removal of the tongue is indicated if the patient has a cancer that does not respond to other forms of treatment. In most cases, however, only part of the tongue is removed (partial glossectomy). Cancer of the tongue is considered very dangerous due to the fact that it can easily spread to nearby lymph glands. Most cancer specialists recommend surgical removal of the cancerous tissue.

Demographics

According to the American Cancer Society, 36,000 people in the United States were diagnosed with oral cavity or **oropharyngeal cancer** in 2013. Oral and pharyngeal cancers are more common in men than women. Rates of new cases have been fairly stable for several years, but there has been a recent increase in the number of **oral cancers** associated with **human papillomavirus** (HPV).

The most important risk factors for cancer of the tongue are alcohol consumption and smoking. The risk is significantly higher in patients who use both alcohol and tobacco than in those who consume only one.

Description

Glossectomies are always performed under general anesthesia. A partial glossectomy is a relatively simple operation. If the "hole" left by the excision of the cancer is small, it is commonly repaired by sewing up the tongue

KEY TERMS

Biopsy—A diagnostic procedure that involves obtaining a tissue specimen for microscopic analysis to establish a precise diagnosis.

Fistula (plural, fistulae)—An abnormal passage that develops either between two organs inside the body or between an organ and the surface of the body. Fistula formation is one of the possible complications of a glossectomy.

Flap—A piece of tissue for grafting that has kept its own blood supply.

Lymph—The almost colorless fluid that bathes body tissues. Lymph is found in the lymphatic vessels and carries lymphocytes that have entered the lymph glands from the blood.

Lymph gland—A small bean-shaped organ consisting of a loose meshwork of tissue in which large numbers of white blood cells are embedded.

Lymphatic system—The tissues and organs (including the bone marrow, spleen, thymus and lymph nodes) that produce and store cells that fight infection, together with the network of vessels that carry lymph throughout the body.

Oncology—The branch of medicine that deals with the diagnosis and treatment of cancer.

immediately or by using a small graft of skin. If the glossectomy is more extensive, care is taken to repair the tongue so as to maintain its mobility. A common approach is to use a piece of skin taken from the wrist together with the blood vessels that supply it. This type of graft is called a radial forearm free flap. The flap is inserted into the hole in the tongue. This procedure requires a highly skilled surgeon who is able to connect very small arteries. Complete removal of the tongue, called a total glossectomy, is rarely performed.

Diagnosis

If an area of abnormal tissue has been found in the mouth, either by the patient or by a dentist or doctor, a **biopsy** is the only way to confirm a diagnosis of cancer. A pathologist, who is a physician who specializes in the study of disease, examines the tissue sample under a microscope to check for cancer cells.

Preparation

If the biopsy indicates that cancer is present, a comprehensive physical examination of the patient's head and neck is performed prior to surgery. The patient will meet with the treatment team before admission to the hospital so that they can answer questions and explain the treatment plan.

Aftercare

Patients usually remain in the hospital for seven to ten days after glossectomy. They often require oxygen during the first 24–48 hours after the operation. Oxygen is administered through a face mask or through two small tubes placed in the nostrils. The patient is given fluids through a tube that goes from the nose to the stomach until he or she can tolerate taking food by mouth. Radiation treatment is often scheduled after the surgery to destroy any remaining cancer cells. As patients regain the ability to eat and swallow, they also begin speech therapy.

Risks

Risks associated with glossectomy include:

- Bleeding from the tongue. This is an early complication of surgery; it can result in severe swelling leading to blockage of the airway.

- Poor speech and difficulty swallowing. This complication depends on how much of the tongue is removed.

- Fistula formation. Incomplete healing may result in the formation of a passage between the skin and the mouth cavity within the first two weeks following a glossectomy. This complication often occurs after feeding has resumed. Patients who have had radiotherapy are at greater risk of developing a fistula.

- Flap failure. This complication is often due to problems with the flap's blood supply.

Results

A successful glossectomy results in complete removal of the cancer, improved ability to swallow food, and restored speech. The quality of the patient's speech is usually very good if at least one-third of the tongue remains and an experienced surgeon has performed the repair.

Total glossectomy results in severe disability because the "new tongue" (a prosthesis) is incapable of movement. This lack of mobility creates enormous difficulty in eating and talking.

Morbidity and mortality rates

Even in the case of a successful glossectomy, the long-term outcome depends on the stage of the cancer and the involvement of lymph glands in the neck. Five-year survival data reveal overall survival rates of less than 60%, although the patients who do survive often endure major functional, cosmetic, and psychological burdens as a result of their difficulties in speaking and eating.

Alternatives

An alternative to glossectomy is the insertion of radioactive wires into the cancerous tissue. This is an effective treatment but requires specialized surgical skills and facilities.

Health care team roles

A glossectomy is performed in a hospital by a treatment team specializing in head and neck oncology surgery. The treatment team usually includes an ear, nose, and throat (ENT) surgeon; an oral-maxillofacial (OMF) surgeon; a plastic surgeon; a clinical oncologist; a nurse; a speech therapist; and a dietitian.

Resources

BOOKS

Harrison, Louis B., Roy B. Sessions, and Merrill S. Kies. *Head and Neck Cancer: A Multidisciplinary Approach.* 4th ed. Philadelphia: Lippincott Williams & Wilkins, 2014.

PERIODICALS

Acher, Audrey, et al. "Speech Production after Glossectomy: Methodological Aspects." *Clinical Linguistics & Phonetics* (July 9, 2013): e-pub ahead of print. http://dx.doi.org/10.3109/02699206.2013.802015 (accessed October 3, 2014).

Joo, Young-Hoon, et al. "Functional Outcome after Partial Glossectomy with Reconstruction Using Radial Forearm Free Flap." *Auris Nasus Larynx* 40, no. 3 (2013): 303–7. http://dx.doi.org/10.1016/j.anl.2012.07.012 (accessed October 3, 2014).

Navach, Valeria, et al. "Total Glossectomy with Preservation of the Larynx: Oncological and Functional Results." *British Journal of Oral and Maxillofacial Surgery* 51, no. 3 (2013): 217–23. http://dx.doi.org/10.1016/j.bjoms. 2012.07.009 (accessed October 3, 2014).

Rihani, Jordan, et al. "Flap Selection and Functional Outcomes in Total Glossectomy with Laryngeal Preservation." *Otolaryngology—Head and Neck Surgery* (July 24, 2013): e-pub ahead of print. http://dx.doi.org/10.1177/0194599813498063 (accessed October 3, 2014).

WEBSITES

American Cancer Society. "What are the Key Statistics about Oral Cavity and Oropharyngeal Cancers?" http://www.cancer.org/cancer/oralcavityandoropharyngealcancer/detailedguide/oral-cavity-and-oropharyngeal-cancer-key-statistics (accessed October 3, 2014).

Cohen, Robert B. "Cancerous Mouth Growths." *The Merck Manual Home Health Handbook for Patients and Caregivers* (online). http://www.merckmanuals.com/home/mouth_and_dental_disorders/mouth_growths/cancerous_mouth_growths.html (accessed October 3, 2014).

Griffin Kellicker, Patricia. "Glossectomy." NYU Langone Medical Center. http://www.med.nyu.edu/content?ChunkIID=446187 (accessed October 3, 2014).

ORGANIZATIONS

American Academy of Otolaryngology—Head and Neck Surgery, 1650 Diagonal Rd., Alexandria, VA 22314-2857, (703) 836-4444, http://www.entnet.org.

American Cancer Society, 250 Williams St. NW, Atlanta, GA 30303, (800) 227-2345, http://www.cancer.org.

Oral Cancer Foundation, 3419 Via Lido, #205, Newport Beach, CA 92663, (949) 646-8000, info@oralcancerfoundation.org, http://oralcancerfoundation.org.

Monique Laberge, PhD.

Glutamine

Definition

Glutamine is an amino acid that is used as a nutritional supplement in the treatment of a variety of diseases, including **cancer**.

Purpose

Glutamine is the most abundant free amino acid in the human body. In addition to its role as a component of protein, it serves a variety of functions in the body. It is a non-essential amino acid because it is made by body cells. In addition, most dietary protein contains ample amounts of glutamine and healthy people usually obtain all the additional glutamine that they need in their diet.

Cancer and other diseases and injuries induce a state of physiologic stress that is characterized by glutamine deficiency. This deficiency is aggravated by **chemotherapy** and **radiation therapy** used to treat cancer. Therefore, glutamine is sometimes described as a conditionally essential amino acid that needs to be supplemented when the body is stressed.

Cancer-related glutamine deficiency can reduce the tolerance of normal tissues to cancer treatment, necessitating reduced doses and possibly diminishing the effects of treatment. Glutamine supplementation may help protect normal tissues from chemotherapy and radiation while sensitizing tumor cells to these agents.

Glutamine has been increasingly considered an important component of both oral and parenteral (intravenous) nutrition (PN) therapy during high-dose chemotherapy and radiation treatment. It also is used as a nutritional supplement for bone marrow transplant (BMT) patients, particularly those with leukemia or **lymphoma** whose bone marrow has been destroyed with high-dose chemotherapy.

Glutamine supplementation appears to do the following:

- improve nitrogen retention
- decrease the incidence of infection
- decrease the length of hospitalization, saving thousands of dollars

Glutamine supplementation also appears to reduce the incidence of gastrointestinal, nervous system, and heart complications arising from cancer therapy. Oral glutamine may reduce **diarrhea** and the duration and severity of other gastrointestinal side effects of chemotherapy. In particular it appears to help prevent the intestinal toxicity of the cancer drug **fluorouracil**. Glutamine may reduce the incidence and severity of **mucositis**, a common, painful inflammation of the membranes of the oral cavity that can result from chemotherapy. Rinsing with a glutamine-containing mouthwash can help reduce mouth sores from radiation and chemotherapy treatments. Glutamine also appears to reduce the need for antifungal agents during chemotherapy.

Description

Glutamine (Gln) or L-glutamine is available by prescription as a powder called NutreStore. It is taken as an oral suspension for treating short bowel syndrome. It also is available in nutritional formulas and as an individual nutritional supplement. As an intravenous

KEY TERMS

Arginine—An essential amino acid derived from dietary protein; sometimes used in combination with glutamine to boost the immune system.

Beta-hydroxy-beta-methylbutyrate, HMB—A nutritional supplement used to buildup muscles and to treat muscle-wasting caused by disease.

Bone marrow transplant, BMT—The destruction of bone marrow by high-dose chemotherapy or radiation and its replacement with healthy bone marrow taken from the patient prior to chemotherapy or from a donor.

Cachexia—Severe malnutrition, weakness, and muscle-wasting caused by disease.

Gluconeogenesis—The formation of glucose from non-carbohydrates such as protein or fat.

Glutaminase—The enzyme that breaks down glutamine; high glutaminase activity may be correlated with the proliferation of cancer cells.

Glutathione (GSH)—A three-amino-acid tripeptide that reduces harmful oxygen radicals and activates some proteins, including natural killer cells.

Hepatic veno-occlusive disease—Liver failure caused by chemotherapy that may benefit from glutamine supplementation.

Lymphocyte—A white blood cell of the immune system, making up 25%–33% of all adult white blood cells.

Mucositis—A common, painful inflammation of the membranes of the mouth caused by chemotherapy.

Natural killer cell—A type of lymphocyte that kills cancer cells and certain microorganisms.

Parenteral nutrition (PN)—Intravenous feeding.

Short bowel syndrome—A condition that occurs after a large segment of the small intestine has been removed; it is treated with glutamine.

Tryptophan—An essential amino acid that is sometimes used in combination with glutamine supplementation.

supplement it may be supplied in the form of alanyl-glutamine dipeptide or glycyl-glutamine dipeptide.

Metabolic effects

There is much speculation about why glutamine appears to be a beneficial adjunct for cancer treatment.

Glutamine is required for numerous metabolic processes, including the following:

• Regulation of cell growth and function.

• Synthesis of proteins and nucleic acids (DNA and RNA).

• Movement of nitrogen in the body. Glutamine is the body's primary means of transferring ammonia in a nontoxic form.

• Gluconeogenesis—the formation of glucose from protein and fat.

• Maintenance of acid-base equilibrium in the body.

• As a major fuel for intestinal mucosal cells.

• Improved kidney cell function.

Tumors cause major disruptions in nitrogen and glutamine metabolism. The high rate of protein synthesis in rapidly growing tumors requires a continuous supply of amino acids. Tumors are referred to as nitrogen traps because they actively compete with normal tissues for nitrogen-containing compounds such as glutamine. Tumors also are referred to as glutamine traps because glutamine moves from normal tissues to tumors. Some evidence suggests that glutamine supplementation may diminish tumor growth, in part by improving overall protein metabolism.

Cancer cells generally move glutamine across their cell membranes at a faster rate than normal cells. Glutaminase—the enzyme that breaks down glutamine—has increased activity in cancerous cells, and there is evidence that glutaminase activity correlates with the proliferation of malignant cells.

Immunological effects

Glutamine and arginine may be referred to as immunonutrients because of their important roles in the functioning of the immune system that protects the body from foreign entities, including cancer cells. Glutamine helps to regulate the immune system and is a major fuel for lymphocytes (a type of white blood cell) and other immune system cells. In cancer patients undergoing chemotherapy and total body irradiation, glutamine has been shown to boost the immune system by increasing the levels of circulating lymphocytes and other cells of the immune system.

In patients undergoing chemotherapy with radioactive drugs for advanced **esophageal cancer**, oral glutamine supplementation helped to protect immune system function by causing lymphocytes to divide and multiply. Glutamine supplementation also reduced the permeability of the gastrointestinal tract in these patients.

Antioxidative effects

Glutamine appears to be the rate-limiting factor for the production of liver and intestinal glutathione (GSH), a chemical that protects cells against the damaging effects of oxidation. As cancer cells deplete the glutamine in normal cells, the levels of GSH drop. It has been suggested that PN without added glutamine may itself decrease GSH levels and increase oxidative damage. By increasing GSH levels, oral glutamine supplementation also may increase the selectivity of **anticancer drugs** by protecting normal cells from oxidative damage caused by the drugs. Glutamine supplementation also appears to protect normal cells from radiation-induced oxidative damage. Since GSH depletion reduces the activity of natural killer cells (immune system cells that destroy cancer cells) glutamine supplementation may increase GSH levels and restore natural-killer-cell activity. Some evidence suggests that this may diminish tumor growth.

Effectiveness

Glutamine supplementation during cancer therapy and bone marrow or **stem cell transplantation** remains under investigation. Although some studies have demonstrated specific benefits in at least some types of cancer, numerous animal and human studies have shown no clear benefit or any effect on tumor response, or on the side effects of chemotherapy. However, one study suggested that glutamine supplementation could increase the likelihood of long-term survival in patients with cancers of the blood.

Other studies have found that glutamine supplementation in cancer patients receiving high-dose chemotherapy and BMT decreases the incidence and/or severity of the following:

• chemotherapy-associated mucositis

• diarrhea associated with irinotecan, a drug used to treat colon and rectal cancers

• nervous system damage caused by the anticancer drug paclitaxel

• cardiac toxicity caused by the drug anthracycline

Combination supplements

Cancer-related cachexia (severe malnutrition, weakness, and muscle-wasting) is caused by the increased breakdown of proteins and reduced protein synthesis in patients with advanced cancer. One study demonstrated that supplementation with specific nutrients, including a combination of glutamine, beta-hydroxy-beta-methylbutyrate (HMB), and arginine, could reverse these processes. Patients with stage IV cancer who received this combination gained significant fat-free body mass in four weeks and continuing over a period of 24 weeks, as compared to control patients who lost body mass.

Case studies have reported that the administration of glutamine orally and intravenously, in combination with oral vitamin E, decreases the signs and symptoms of hepatic veno-occlusive disease. This is an often-fatal type of liver failure that occurs in patients treated with high-dose chemotherapy in preparation for BMT.

Recommended dosage

Glutamine supplementation generally is started three to five days before chemotherapy. The glutamine dosage used to treat short bowel syndrome is 5 g, six times per day for up to 16 weeks. It is taken with food, every two to three hours while awake. Nutritional guidelines for cancer patients generally recommend 2–4 g of glutamine per day to protect against radiation-induced **enteritis** (intestinal inflammation).

Dosages used in clinical studies of glutamine supplementation in cancer patients vary:

• 18–30 g per day, orally

• 10 g three times per day, orally

• 0.57 g per kg (2.2 lb.) of body weight per day

• 50 g per day of dipeptide glycyl-glutamine, intravenously

• 0.4 g per kg (2.2 lb.) of body weight per day of dipeptide glycyl-glutamine, intravenously

• 14 g of glutamine per day in combination with arginine and HMB for up to 24 weeks

Precautions

Glutamine, taken orally or by injection, appears to be safe; however, precautions include the following:

• Excess amino acids may be excreted in the urine without being absorbed by the body.

• Excess amino acids can harm the kidneys.

• Glutamine, like any drug, can potentially cause an allergic reaction.

• It is not known whether glutamine supplementation is safe during pregnancy or while breastfeeding.

• Elderly patients may be more sensitive to glutamine supplementation, requiring lower doses.

• Glutamine can worsen liver disease.

Since glutamine is essential for the growth of both healthy and cancerous cells, it is theoretically possible that glutamine could fuel tumor cells, leading to more rapid growth. However, there is no evidence to suggest this, nor is there evidence that glutamine supplementation adversely affects treatment or clinical outcomes.

Side effects

Glutamine supplementation in cancer patients does not appear to cause side effects or adversely affect quality of life.

Interactions

Glutamine supplementation is not known to negatively interact with other medications.

Resources

WEBSITES

A.D.A.M. Medical Encyclopedia. "Glutamine." University of Maryland Medical Center. http://umm.edu/health/medical/altmed/supplement/glutamine (accessed November 4, 2014).

Memorial Sloan Kettering Cancer Center. "Glutamine." http://www.mskcc.org/cancer-care/herb/glutamine (accessed November 4, 2014).

ORGANIZATIONS

Office of Cancer Complementary and Alternative Medicine (OCCAM), 9609 Medical Center Dr., Rockville, MD 20850, (240) 276-6595, ncioccam1-r@mail.nih.gov, http://cam.cancer.gov.

Margaret Alic, PhD.

GM-CSF *see* **Sargramostim**

Gonadal dysfunction *see* **Fertility issues**

Goserelin acetate

Definition

Goserelin acetate is a synthetic (man-made) hormone that acts similarly to the naturally occurring gonadotropin-releasing hormone (GnRH). It is available in the United States under the tradename Zoladex.

Purpose

Goserelin acetate is used primarily to counter the symptoms of late-stage **prostate cancer** in men or is offered as an alternative to treat prostate **cancer** when surgery to remove the testes or estrogen therapy is not an option or is unacceptable for the patient. Goserelin is also given as combination therapy with the drug flutamide to manage prostate cancer that is locally confined and not widespread. It is often used to ease the pain and discomfort of women suffering from endometriosis and to relieve symptoms in women with advanced **breast cancer**.

Description

Goserelin acetate is a man-made protein that mimics many of the actions of gonadotropin-releasing hormone (GnRH). In men, this results in decreased blood levels of the male hormone **testosterone**. In women, it decreases blood levels of the female hormone estrogen.

Recommended dosage

Goserelin acetate is given in the form of an implant containing 3.6 mg of the medication. This implant is placed just under the skin of the upper abdominal wall. The drug lasts for 28 days, after which a new implant has to be placed. Goserelin is also available in a dose of 10.8 mg, in which case the drugs lasts for three months.

Precautions

If a woman becomes pregnant while taking this drug, goserelin acetate may cause birth defects or the loss of the pregnancy. It is not known if goserelin is passed into breast milk; therefore, it is not recommended to breast feed while on this drug.

Goserelin acetate will also interfere with the chemical actions of birth control pills. For this reason, sexually active women who do not wish to become pregnant should use some form of birth control other than birth control pills during treatment with goserelin acetate and for at least 12 weeks after the completion of treatment.

Goserelin acetate will cause sterility in men, at least for the duration of the treatment.

Side effects

In patients of both sexes, common side effects of goserelin acetate include:

• sweating accompanied by feelings of warmth (hot flashes)
• a decrease in sex drive
• depression or other mood changes
• headache
• tumor flare, which is exhibited as bone pain (this is due to a temporary initial increase in testosterone/estrogen before its production is finally decreased)

Other common side effects in men include:

• impotence (erectile dysfunction)
• sterility
• breast enlargement

Other common side effects in women include:

• light, irregular, vaginal bleeding
• no menstrual period

- vaginal dryness and/or itching

- emotional instability

- depression

- change in breast size

- an increase in facial or body hair

- deepening of the voice

Less common side effects, in patients of either sex, include:

- nausea and vomiting

- insomnia

- weight gain

- swollen feet or lower legs

- acne or other skin rashes

- abdominal pain

- increased appetite

A doctor should be consulted immediately if the patient experiences any of the above symptoms.

Interactions

There are no known interactions of goserelin acetate with any food or beverage.

Patients taking goserelin acetate should consult their physician before taking any other prescription, over-the-counter, or herbal medication. Patients taking any other hormone or steroid-based medications should not take goserelin acetate without first consulting their physician.

See also Endometrial cancer; Ovarian cancer.

Paul A. Johnson, Ed.M.

Graft-versus-host disease

Definition

Cancer patients sometimes receive stem cells, which are immature blood cells, from a donor as part of their cancer treatment. Sometimes the patient's immune system—the body's natural defense against infection and disease—attacks the new stem cells, causing graft-versus-host disease (GVHD).

Description

Patients with certain types or stages of cancer can be treated with stem cell transplants with high-dose **chemotherapy**. Also called a bone marrow transplant, the treatment replaces a patient's stem cells as a way to treat and even cure cancer. Stem cells are the immature cells that form blood cells. They are produced in the bone marrow, which is the spongy tissue inside the larger bones in the body.

One step in **stem cell transplantation** is to destroy a patient's existing cells with high doses of chemotherapy, and sometimes using **radiation therapy**. Some patients who have stem cell transplants are able to use their own stem cells, which are removed before the therapy begins, frozen, and stored. Once the chemotherapy and radiation therapy are complete, the patient's stem cells are returned to the body. This type of stem cell transplant is called an autologous transplant.

Many patients cannot have an autologous transplant, partly because there is a danger of removing and reinfusing cancerous stem cells. A more popular type of transplant is an allogeneic transplant, in which cells come from a donor. Doctors carefully match the bone marrow or stem cell donor to the patient, and the donor is often a relative. If no matched relative is available, they seek a matched donor from a national registry. The transplanted cells are known as the graft, and the patient's immune system is the host for the new cells.

Although doctors attempt to match donor and patient, sometimes immune cells from the donor, or graft, attack the patient's healthy cells along with the cancer cells. A patient with graft-versus-host-disease can become quite ill.

The tissues most affected by bone marrow GVHD are the skin, the liver, and the intestines. One of these forms of tissue is affected in nearly half of the patients who receive bone marrow transplants.

Bone marrow GVHD comes in both an acute and a chronic form. The acute form usually appears within weeks of the transplant, while the chronic form appears within three months or several years. The acute disease produces a skin rash, liver abnormalities, and **diarrhea** that can be bloody. The skin rash is primarily a patchy thickening of the skin. Chronic disease can produce a similar skin rash, a tightening or an inflammation of the skin, lesions in the mouth, drying of the eyes and mouth, hair loss (**alopecia**), liver damage, lung damage, and indigestion. The symptoms are similar to an autoimmune disease called scleroderma.

Both forms of GVHD increase risk of infections in patients, either because of the immune system reaction or because of treatment with cortisone-like drugs and medications called immunosuppressives that inhibit the **immune response**. Patients can die from liver failure, infection, or other severe disturbances of their immune system.

Causes

Cells from a donor who has an active immune system may be transplanted along with the bone marrow and stem cells into the host who has a suppressed immune system. These transplanted cells attack the host's body, causing GVHD. Substances made in the body called cytokines are thought to play a role in the development of this reaction. Cytokines are protein substances made by cells that affect other cells. Several proteins may play a role in immune system acceptance of new cells.

Even if the donor and recipient are well matched, GVHD can still occur. There are many different components involved in generating immune reactions, and all people (except identical twins) are different. Testing can often find donors who match all the major components, but there are many minor ones that can be different. Making a close match between a donor and recipient depends upon the urgency of the need for a transplant and the chance that a suitable donor will be found.

Treatment

Both the acute and chronic forms of the disease are treated with cortisone-like drugs, immunosuppressive agents, or with **antibiotics** and immune chemicals from donated blood (gamma globulin). **Cyclosporine** and prednisone are two immunosuppressive drugs that are often used, and **methotrexate** can make them work better. Another way to prevent GVHD is to rid donor bone marrow of the immune cells (T cells) that would attack the recipient's body before transplantation.

New directions in research may help to solve the problem of GVHD. In 2013, a clinical trial at the University of Michigan and Washington University in St. Louis showed that a new drug called **vorinostat** worked at fighting cancer and inflammation. The drug could help fight GVHD. A potential source for new stem cells is the umbilical cord. Cord blood cells do not provoke such strong immune reactions and can be useful for re-establishing cell populations. Another potential treatment would use genetically engineered cells to correct genetic defects in stem cells within the marrow.

Alternative and complementary therapies

Alternative and complementary therapies range from herbal remedies, vitamin supplements, and special diets to spiritual practices, acupuncture, massage, and similar treatments. When these therapies are used in addition to conventional medicine, they are called complementary therapies. When they are used instead of conventional medicine, they are called alternative therapies.

Complementary or alternative therapies are widely used by people suffering with illness. Good nutrition and activities, such as yoga, meditation, and massage, that reduce stress and promote a positive view of life have no unwanted side effects and appear to be beneficial. Alternative and experimental treatments are often not covered by insurance.

Special concerns

If GVHD is suspected as a complication to a cancer treatment, a skin punch **biopsy** can be performed to confirm this diagnosis. This is a relatively minor procedure in which the skin is anesthetized in a local area and a small piece is removed for testing in the laboratory.

Infection with one particular virus, called cytomegalovirus (CMV), is such a common complication of GVHD that some experts recommend treating it in advance, using ganciclovir or valacyclovir.

Bone marrow transplant patients who do not have a graft-versus-host reaction gradually return to normal immune function in a year. A graft-versus-host reaction may prolong the diminished immune capacity indefinitely, requiring supplemental treatment with immunoglobulins (gamma globulin). The grafted cells develop a tolerance to the recipient's body after 6–12 months, and the medications can be gradually withdrawn.

Prognosis

Doctors base a patient's prognosis, or outlook, on a grade they assign to the graft-versus-host disease. These grades predict how well the patient will respond to treatment. Patients whose disease continues to worsen after beginning treatment tend to fare worse than those whose disease improves with medication. Research from the University of North Carolina in 2012 showed that B cells, which produce certain proteins called antibodies, are much more active in patients who have graft-versus-host disease. This might offer clues to targeting new therapies that can better prevent and treat the disease.

Prevention

As research into genetics improves, cancer centers and bone marrow registries can better match donors and patients at more precise levels. Doctors can give patients immunosuppressive medications and immunoglobulins immediately after transplantation to prevent immune reactions that cause GVHD.

See also Bone marrow transplantation; Transfusion therapy.

Resources

BOOKS

Anderson, William L. *Immunology.* Madison, CT: Fence Creek Publishing, 1999.

Janeway, Charles A., et al. *Immunobiology:The Immune System in Health and Disease.* New York, NY: Current Biology Publications; London, England: Elsevier Science London/Garland Publishing, 1999.

Roitt, Ivan, and Arthur Rabson. *Really Essential Medical Immunology.* Malden, MA: Blackwell Science, 2000.

WEBSITES

"About Stem Cell Transplantation." Memorial Sloan Kettering Cancer Center. http://www.mskcc.org/cancer-care/blood-marrow-stem-cell-transplantation/about-stem-cell-transplantation (accessed September 30, 2014).

"B Cell Survival Holds Key to Chronic Graft Vs. Host Disease." University of North Carolina School of Medicine. http://news.unchealthcare.org/news/2012/august/b-cell-survival-holds-key-to-chronic-graft-vs.-host-disease (accessed September 30, 2014).

"Graft-Vs.-Host Disease: An Overview in Bone Marrow Transplant." Cleveland Clinic. http://my.clevelandclinic.org/services/bone_marrow_transplantation/hic_graft_vs_host_disease_an_overview_in_bone_marrow_transplant.aspx (accessed September 30, 2014).

"GVHD (Graft-Vs.-Host Disease): A Guide for Patients and Families After Stem Cell Transplant." National Institutes of Health. http://www.cc.nih.gov/ccc/patient_education/pepubs/gvh.pdf (accessed September 30, 2014).

"New Drug Cuts Risk of Deadly Transplant Side Effect in Half." University of Michigan Health System. http://www.uofmhealth.org/news/archive/201312/new-drug-cuts-risk-deadly-transplant-side-effect-half (accessed September 30, 2014).

"Stem Cell Transplant." American Cancer Society. http://www.cancer.org/acs/groups/cid/documents/webcontent/003215-pdf.pdf (accessed September 30, 2014).

J. Ricker Polsdorfer, MD
Jill Granger, MS
REVISED BY TERESA G. ODLE

Granisetron *see* **Antiemetics**

GVHD *see* **Graft-versus-host disease**

Gynecologic cancers

Definition

Gynecologic cancers are malignant tumors within the female reproductive organs. Gynecologic cancers include cervical, endometrial (uterine), ovarian, vaginal, and vulvar cancers.

Demographics

In the United States the most commonly diagnosed **cancer** of the female reproductive organs is **endometrial cancer**, with approximately 52,630 new cases

Gynecologic cancers

Cancer type	Occurs in	Tumor types
Endometrial cancer	Uterus	Endometrioid tumors Clear-cell carcinomas Papillary serous Sarcomas Mixed tumors
Fallopian tube cancer	Fallopian tubes, but frequently spreads	Serous carcinomas Mucinous tumors Endometrioid tumors
Cervical cancer	Cervix	Squamous cell carcinomas Adenocarcinomas Clear-cell carcinoma Serous carcinoma Glassy-cell carcinoma
Ovarian cancer	Ovaries	Serous carcinomas Mucinous tumors Endometrioid tumors
Vaginal cancer	Vagina	Squamous cell carcinoma Adenocarcinoma Melanoma Sarcoma
Vulvar cancer	Vulva	Squamous cell carcinomas Melanoma Basal cell carcinoma Paget's disease Adenocarcinomas

Table listing different types of gynecologic cancers. *(Table by GGS Creative Resources. © Cengage Learning®.)*

KEY TERMS

Adenocarcinoma—A cancer that originates in glandular or mucus-producing cells.

Adjuvant therapy—Treatment involving radiation, chemotherapy (drug treatment), hormone therapy, biotherapeutics, or a combination of any of these given after the primary treatment in order to rid the body of residual microscopic cancer.

Biopsy—Removal of a small sample of tissue for examination under a microscope; used for the diagnosis and treatment of cervical cancer and precancerous conditions.

Brachytherapy—A form of radiation therapy in which small pellets of radioactive material are placed inside or near the area to be treated. It is also known as internal radiation therapy or sealed-source radiotherapy.

Cervix—The narrow lower end of the uterus forming the opening to the vagina.

Colposcopy—Diagnostic procedure using a hollow lighted tube (colposcope) to look inside the vagina, cervix, and uterus.

Conization—Cone biopsy; removal of a cone-shaped section of tissue from the cervix for diagnosis or treatment.

Endometrium—The inner mucous membrane that lines the uterus in humans and other mammals.

Estrogen—The primary female sex hormone, responsible for the buildup of endometrial tissue, the development of secondary sexual characteristics in women, and regulation of other aspects of the menstrual cycle.

Exenteration—Extensive surgery to remove the uterus, ovaries, pelvic lymph nodes, part or all of the vagina, and the bladder, rectum, and/or part of the colon.

Human papillomavirus (HPV)—Virus that causes abnormal cell growth (warts or papillomas); some types can cause cervical cancer.

Hysterectomy—Surgical removal of the uterus.

Laparoscopy—Laparoscopic pelvic lymph node dissection; insertion of a tube through a very small surgical incision to remove lymph nodes.

expected to be diagnosed in 2014. An American woman has one chance in 37 of developing endometrial cancer during her lifetime. About 50% of the new cases of endometrial cancer occur in women between the ages of 55 and 74 years. The average age at diagnosis is 60 years old. The incidence of this type of cancer is higher in Caucasians, but more African American women die from endometrial cancer than Caucasian women. Native Americans, Koreans, and Vietnamese have the lowest incidence. About 8,590 women are expected to die from endometrial cancer in the United States in 2014.

The estimated number of new cases of **ovarian cancer** (cancer of the ovaries) in the U.S. in 2014 is 21,980, with 14,270 deaths. In 2014, ovarian cancer was the ninth most common cancer among women in the United States. It accounted for about 2.8% of all new cancers in American women; however, because of poor early detection, ovarian cancer is the fifth most common cause of cancer death among women. About one in 71 American women will develop ovarian cancer during her lifetime, and one in 95 will die from it. Older women (over the age of 60) are most often diagnosed with this type of cancer. Incidence rates for ovarian cancers have been decreasing in recent years.

The American Cancer Society (ACS) estimates that 12,360 new cases of invasive **cervical cancer** will be diagnosed in the United States in 2014 and there will be 4,020 deaths from the disease. The death rate from cervical cancer has declined by almost 75% since the mid-1950s due to implementation of Pap (Papanicolaou) screening for cervical cancer detection. Most women are diagnosed with cervical cancer prior to the age of 50, but 20% of cases are diagnosed in women over the age of 65 years. Hispanic and African American women are considered high-risk groups for the development of cervical cancer. The actual occurrence of cervical cancer (as distinct from mortality) in the United States is highest among Hispanic women and lowest among Native American and Alaska Native women.

Cancers of the vulva and vagina account for 4% and 1% of all female reproductive tract cancers respectively. In 2014, the American Cancer Society estimates that 4,850 new cases of vulvar cancers and 3,170 new cases of vaginal cancers will be diagnosed. An American woman has 1 chance in 333 of developing **vulvar cancer** over the course of her lifetime. Approximately 1,030 women will die from vulvar cancer and about 880

Lichen sclerosus—A condition in which the skin of the vulva develops white patches and becomes thinner. It may be characterized by itching or have no symptoms. It is also known as kraurosis vulvae.

Lymph nodes—Small round glands, located throughout the body, that filter the lymphatic fluid; part of the body's immune defense.

Menarche—The medical term for a girl's first menstrual period.

Müllerian ducts—Paired ducts in the human embryo that give rise to the fallopian tubes, uterus, cervix, and the upper one-third of the vagina in females. The Müllerian ducts disappear in males.

Neoadjuvant therapy—The administration of chemotherapy or other treatment prior to surgery to shrink the tumor and improve the chances of successful treatment.

Pap (Papanicolaou) test—Pap smear; removal of cervical cells to screen for cancer. The test was invented by and named for a Greek physician, George Papanicolaou, who was an early pioneer in cancer detection.

Progestins—Synthetic hormones resembling progesterone used in the treatment of advanced endometrial cancer.

Salpingo-oophorectomy—Surgical removal of the fallopian tubes and the ovaries.

Squamous cells—Thin, flat cells found on the surfaces of the skin, the vagina and cervix, and the linings of various organs.

Targeted therapy—In cancer treatment, a type of drug therapy that blocks tumors by interfering with specific molecules that the cancer cells need for growth. Also called biologic therapy, targeted therapy is less harmful to normal cells than traditional chemotherapy.

Trachelectomy—A surgical procedure in which the cervix and upper portion of the vagina are removed but the uterus is left intact with an artificial purse-string opening. This procedure allows a woman to conceive after removal of a cancerous cervix.

Vulva—The outer part of the female genitals.

women will die from **vaginal cancer** in the United States in 2014. The average age of women with invasive cancer of the vulva is 70. About half of all cases of vaginal cancer occur in women over the age of 70.

Description

The female reproductive tract comprises the ovaries, fallopian tubes, uterus, cervix, vagina, and vulva. Together, these organs allow a woman to become pregnant, protect and nourish an unborn baby, and give birth. An understanding of each organ and its role in reproduction may help the patient to understand her particular gynecologic cancer. There are two ovaries, which are the internal organs dedicated to producing eggs. Released eggs are captured by the fallopian tubes, through which the egg (or fertilized egg) travels to the womb (uterus). The lining of the uterus (endometrium) responds to such female hormones as estrogen, and becomes thickened to allow for the implantation of a fertilized egg. The cervix is the opening of the uterus that opens (dilates) during labor to allow for passage of the baby. The vagina is a short tube between 3 and 4 inches

(7 and 10 cm) long that extends from the outer female genitalia (vulva) to the cervix.

Gynecologic cancers are defined not solely by the organ affected but also by the type of cancerous cells in the tumor. The type of cancer depends on the cell types that make up an organ. Adenocarcinomas are cancers that contain primarily cells originating from glands or ducts. Squamous cell carcinomas are tumors that arose from squamous cells, the main cell type found in skin. Sarcomas are cancers that originated from cells of basic connective tissue (mesenchymal cells). Sarcomas are comprised of cells that have become specialized (differentiated) and are named according to the predominant cell type. Endometrioid tumors are those that originate from the endometrium. Clear-cell **carcinoma** is a rare gynecologic tumor that contains cells from the Müllerian duct, which gives rise to the uterus, vagina, and fallopian tubes during development.

Because the reproductive organs are interconnected, the spread of cancer from one organ to another (direct extension) is not uncommon. Gynecologic cancer carries the name of the organ where the cancer originated (primary cancer site). For example, a tumor restricted to the vagina would be a "primary vaginal cancer," whereas one that has extended from the cervix to the vagina would be a "primary cervical cancer."

Risk factors

Risk factors for the different kinds of gynecologic cancer vary by type of cancer.

Risk factors related to the development of cervical cancer include:

- history of HPV infection
- history of smoking
- infection with human immunodeficiency virus (HIV)
- chlamydial infection
- diet low in fruits and vegetables
- long-term use of oral contraceptives
- history of multiple pregnancies
- women whose mothers used the drug diethylstilbestrol (DES) during pregnancy
- family history of cervical cancer

Risk factors related to the development of endometrial cancer include:

- use of estrogen replacement therapy
- history of early menarche (before age 12) and late menopause (after age 55)
- women who have never been pregnant
- obesity
- small risk (1 in 500) for women taking the drug tamoxifen
- history of polycystic ovary syndrome (PCOS)
- increasing age
- diet high in animal fat
- history of type 2 diabetes
- family history of endometrial cancer
- family history of hereditary nonpolyposis colon cancer (HNPCC)
- personal history of breast or ovarian cancer
- prior radiation therapy to the pelvic area of the body
- history of endometrial hyperplasia

Risk factors associated with the development of ovarian cancer include:

- increasing age
- obesity
- history of never being pregnant
- use of androgen drugs
- postmenopausal estrogen use
- family history of ovarian, breast or colorectal cancer
- personal history of breast cancer

Risk factors related to the development of vaginal cancer include:

- increasing age
- women whose mothers took DES in pregnancy have a small risk (1 in 1000)
- personal history of vaginal adenosis
- HPV infection
- HIV infection
- history of cervical cancer
- smoking and alcohol use

Risk factors related to the development of vulvar cancer include:

- increasing age
- HPV infection, especially in younger women
- smoking
- HIV infection
- presence of a precancerous condition called vulvar intraepithelial neoplasia (VIN), which is a precursor to squamous cell carcinoma of the vulva
- presence of a dermatologic condition of the vulva called lichen sclerosus
- history of cervical cancer
- personal or family history of melanoma

Types of cancers

Uterine cancer, also called endometrial cancer, is the most common gynecologic cancer. Endometrial cancer primarily affects postmenopausal women, however, 25% of cases are in premenopausal women. There are two types of endometrial cancer: estrogen-dependent and non-estrogen-dependent. Estrogen-dependent cancers are usually comprised of well-differentiated cells and are associated with a good outcome and a long survival time. Non-estrogen-dependent cancers are usually made up of poorly differentiated cells and are invasive and associated with a poor prognosis. Uterine tumors are most frequently endometrioid tumors, usually adenocarcinomas. Clear-cell carcinomas, papillary serous carcinomas, sarcomas, and mixed tumors also occur.

Ovarian cancer is the second most common cancer of the female reproductive organs. It accounts for 30% of all gynecologic cancers and 53% of the deaths in this group. The high death rate associated with ovarian cancer is due to the fact that most women are not diagnosed until the cancer has progressed to an advanced stage. The average age at diagnosis is 63 years. Serous carcinomas are the most common type of ovarian cancer. Other common types of ovarian cancer include mucinous tumors and endometrioid tumors.

Fallopian tube cancers, as primary cancers, are very rare. They frequently spread widely within the abdominal cavity. Although often diagnosed earlier than ovarian cancer, fallopian tube cancer produces similar symptoms and originates from similar cell types as ovarian cancer.

Cervical cancer is the third most common cancer of the female reproductive tract. Although cervical cancer can affect any adult woman, there are peaks of occurrence around the ages of 37 years and 62 years. Although cervical cancer used to be one of the most common causes of death among American women, in the past 50 years there has been a 75% decrease in mortality from cervical cancer. This decrease is primarily due to routine screening with Pap tests to identify precancerous and early-stage invasive cervical cancer. Between 60% and 80% of the cases of cervical cancer are squamous cell carcinomas, with the remainder being adenocarcinomas. Clear-cell carcinoma, serous carcinoma, and glassy-cell carcinoma are less common types of cervical cancers.

Cervical cancer is very strongly associated with the **human papillomavirus** (HPV). HPV infection accounts for approximately 90% of all cervical cancer cases. Two vaccines, introduced in 2006 and 2009 respectively, protect against the HPV strains that cause 70% of all cervical cancers. Gardasil, the older vaccine, is known to protect against HPV for at least five years while Cervarix is effective for at least seven years. However, it does not protect or treat women who are already infected with HPV. The vaccine is recommended for females ages 9 through 26 years prior to becoming sexually active.

Vulvar cancer is rare and accounts for 4% of the gynecologic cancers. It most often strikes women in their 60s and 70s. Squamous cell carcinoma is the most common type and **melanoma** is the second most common type of vulvar cancer. Other types of vulvar cancer include **basal cell carcinoma**, Paget's disease, and adenocarcinomas (arising from the Bartholin, Skene, and sweat glands). There is an association between vulvar cancer and human papillomavirus.

Vaginal cancer is also a rare type of cancer and accounts for just 1% of the gynecologic cancers. It most often strikes women in their sixties. Greater than 90% of the vaginal cancers are squamous cell carcinomas. **Adenocarcinoma**, melanoma, and **sarcoma** account for the remaining cases. There is an association between vaginal cancer and human papillomavirus; a study done in the United States reported in 2014 that 75% of a series of 60 cases of invasive vaginal cancer were

HPV-positive, and that many of these were in women below the age of 60.

Causes and symptoms

The exact cause of most cases of gynecologic cancers remain unknown at this time, although several risk factors that place women at higher risk for specific types of gynecologic cancers have been identified.

Symptoms associated with cervical cancer include abnormal vaginal bleeding, especially after sexual intercourse. Other symptoms include bleeding between periods or after menopause. Unusual vaginal discharge and pain after intercourse are also symptoms of cervical cancer.

Episodes of such unusual bleeding as bleeding between periods and after menopause are also symptoms of endometrial cancer, as is unusual vaginal discharge. Other symptoms, which may be indicative of advanced disease, include pain in the pelvic area and **weight loss**.

Symptoms of vaginal cancer are similar to the symptoms associated with other gynecologic cancers, including abnormal bleeding and vaginal discharge. Other symptoms include pain during intercourse, pain upon urination, constipation, and pain in the pelvic area.

Women with ovarian cancer may not experience any symptoms, or may experience only vague symptoms until the cancer spreads beyond the ovaries. Symptoms of ovarian cancer include bloating, pain in the abdomen or pelvis, and early satiety or the sensation of feeling full after eating very little. Other symptoms include back pain, pain during intercourse, constipation, and menstrual changes.

Symptoms associated with cancer of the vulva are somewhat different from that of the other gynecologic cancers. Symptoms associated with VIN include vulvar skin that is often lighter or thicker. There may also be lumps and/or bumps as well as other skin changes, including the appearance of cauliflower- or wart-like growths on the vulva. Other nondermatologic symptoms include persistent **itching**, pain, burning, bleeding, discharge, and/or painful urination.

Diagnosis

Examination

When a gynecologic cancer is suspected, a physical examination, often including an abdominal/pelvic examination will be conducted. The patient may be referred to a gynecologic oncologist for further examination and evaluation.

Tests

Blood tests that may be ordered include a complete blood count (CBC) with platelet count and blood chemistry profile with liver function tests. Other specialized blood tests such as testing for **tumor markers** may be done depending on the type of cancer. For example, CA-125 is considered a tumor marker for ovarian cancer. Levels of CA-125 may be elevated in some women with ovarian cancer.

Other tests may be done specific to a particular cancer, including cervical **cytology** tests (such as a **Pap test** or smear), to determine presence of cervical or uterine cancers. Evaluation of the gastrointestinal system may be clinically indicated as well.

Imaging tests that may be ordered include chest imaging, ultrasound, and/or computerized axial tomography (CT scans) of the abdomen and/or pelvis. **Positron emission tomography** scans (PET scans) may also be included in the workup for gynecologic cancers.

Procedures

Procedures that may be included in the work-up related to the diagnosis of gynecologic cancers include colposcopy (examination of the vagina and cervix with a lighted tube called a colposcope); endometrial **biopsy** of uterine tumors; cervical and cone biopsies (conization) for cervical cancer; and cystoscopy/proctoscopy if there is suspicion of bladder and/or bowel involvement of the tumor.

Treatment

Treatment of gynecologic cancers is dependent on several factors including: type of cancer, the extent of tumor involvement or stage of the cancer at time of diagnosis, and such patient characteristics as age and the presence of other concurrent medical conditions.

Modalities used in the treatment of an endometrial tumor considered to be operable include surgical removal of the uterus, cervix, fallopian tubes, and ovaries. Adjuvant treatment options that may be employed following surgery include vaginal brachytherapy with or without **radiation therapy** directed to the pelvis and may also include treatment with **chemotherapy**. Women who are less than 60 years old and who are diagnosed with minimal-sized tumors that have not invaded the lymph nodes may be observed prior to being offered further adjuvant treatment. Other treatment options for endometrial cancer include hormone treatment using progestins, hormones that slow the growth of endometrial cells; or **aromatase inhibitors**, drugs that lower estrogen levels in the body.

Primary treatment for ovarian cancer includes laparotomy with total abdominal hysterectomy and bilateral or unilateral salpingo-oophorectomy (performed in select patients to preserve fertility options). All suspicious and/or enlarged lymph nodes should be removed during surgery. Some patients may require surgical removal of the appendix, the spleen and/or parts of the bowel. Chemotherapy may be used prior to surgery to reduce the size of the tumor; this is called neoadjuvant therapy. Chemotherapy administered after surgery for ovarian cancer includes the drugs **cisplatin**, paclitaxel, **docetaxel** and **carboplatin**. Targeted therapy is a newer form of pharmacotherapy that treats cancers with drugs that target the changes in genes or proteins that cause cancer cells to grow and spread. As of 2014, targeted therapy is most often used to treat advanced or metastatic ovarian cancer. The drug most often used to treat ovarian cancer is **bevacizumab**, a drug that works by blocking the growth of new blood vessels that nourish the tumor. It can be given together with chemotherapy.

Treatment options for cervical cancer depend on tumor stage and include observation (for early Stage 1 tumors), hysterectomy, pelvic radiation/brachytherapy, and cisplatin-containing chemotherapy regimens. An option for some women who wish to become pregnant is an operation known as a trachelectomy. In a trachelectomy, the surgeon removes the cervix and the upper part of the vagina but not the uterus itself. The surgeon makes a purse-string closure to act as an artificial opening to the uterine cavity. About 70% of women who have had a trachelectomy are able to conceive afterward, but the baby must be delivered by cesarean section. A newer treatment modality for cervical cancer is targeted therapy, also called biologic therapy. The drugs used in targeted therapy work by affecting the changes in genes that cause cancer rather than killing the cells outright, as is the case in traditional chemotherapy. Targeted therapy drugs used to treat cervical cancer include pazopanib, which blocks the effect of growth factors on cancer cells; and bevacizumab, which prevents the formation of new blood vessels in cancerous tumors.

The preferred modality for the treatment of most vaginal cancers is radiation therapy. Radiation therapy for vaginal cancer can be delivered via external beam radiation, intracavitary brachytherapy, or by interstitial radiation. Surgery to treat this type of cancer is used only if the cancer is not cured by radiation. Surgery may be an option to remove small Stage 1 tumors. Chemotherapy has not proven to be an effective option in the treatment of vaginal cancers. However, chemotherapy may be used prior to surgery to shrink the tumor size and may be administered concurrently with radiation therapy to enhance the effects of the radiation. Laser surgery and such topical drugs as imiquimod and the chemotherapy drug 5-FU are used to treat cases of noninvasive vaginal cancer.

Surgical treatment options for vulvar cancer include laser surgery, surgical excision of the cancer and surrounding tissue margins, vulvectomy (removal of all or part of the vulva), and pelvic **exenteration**, a procedure that entails removal of the vulva, the pelvic lymph nodes, and possibly the lower colon, rectum, bladder, uterus, cervix, and vagina. Extent of the exenteration depends on the extent of cancer involvement. Radiation therapy may be given directed to lymph nodes in the groin and pelvis. Chemotherapy, utilizing drugs such as cisplatin, mitomycin, and 5-FU, has been used in the treatment of advanced vulvar cancer but with minimal positive results to date.

Prognosis

Prognosis related to the gynecologic cancers varies by cancer type and is determined by stage of diagnosis. Detection of the cancer in earlier stages is related to better overall survival. Pelvic exenteration has a five-year survival rate of 40% as of 2014. The overall five-year survival rate by specific gynecologic cancer type is as follows:

- cervical cancer – 71%
- endometrial cancer – 73%
- ovarian cancer – 46%
- vaginal cancer -50%

Prevention

The exact cause of most gynecologic cancers is not currently known. Certain risk factors have been identified that can place women at higher risk for the development of certain types of gynecologic cancers. When possible, steps should be taken to minimize the possibility for developing these cancers. Quitting smoking (or never starting), maintaining a normal body weight, and getting adequate physical exercise are helpful preventive lifestyle choices. Girls and young women between the ages of 9 and 26 years should be vaccinated with the cervical cancer vaccine. The American Cancer Society also recommends limiting the number of one's sexual partners and avoiding partners who have had a large number of sexual contacts. In addition, women should adhere to recommended annual screening guidelines and practices related to the early detection of specific gynecologic cancers as recommended by the American Cancer Society and other national organizations.

Resources

BOOKS

Elit, Laurie, ed. *Cervical Cancer: Screening Methods, Risk Factors and Treatment Options.* Hauppauge, NY: Nova Science Publishers, 2013.

Farghaly, Samir A., ed. *Advances in Diagnosis and Management of Ovarian Cancer.* New York: Springer, 2013.

Greggi, Stefano, ed. *Endometrial Cancer: Prevention, Diagnosis and Treatment.* Hauppauge, NY: Nova Science Publishers, 2013.

Karlan, Beth Y., Robert E. Bristow, and Andrew J. Li, eds. *Gynecologic Oncology: Clinical Practice and Surgical Atlas.* New York: McGraw-Hill, 2012.

Odunse, Kunle, and Tanja Pejovic, eds. *Gynecologic Cancers: A Multidisciplinary Approach to Diagnosis and Management.* New York: Demos Medical Publishing, 2013.

PERIODICALS

Aravantinos, G., and D. Pectasides. "Bevacizumab in Combination with Chemotherapy for the Treatment of Advanced Ovarian Cancer: A Systematic Review." *Journal of Ovarian Research* 7 (May 19, 2014): 57.

Banerjee, R., and M. Kamrava. "Brachytherapy in the Treatment of Cervical Cancer: A Review." *International Journal of Women's Health* 6 (May 28, 2014): 555–564.

Carlson, M.J., K.W. Thiel, and K.K. Leslie. "Past, Present, and Future of Hormonal Therapy in Recurrent Endometrial Cancer." *International Journal of Women's Health* 6 (May 2, 2014): 429–435.

Deppe, G., I. Mert, and I.S. Winer. "Management of Squamous Cell Vulvar Cancer: A Review." *Journal of Obstetrics and Gynaecology Research* 40 (May 2014): 1217–1225.

Frazer, I.H. "Development and Implementation of Papillomavirus Prophylactic Vaccines." *Journal of Immunology* 192 (May 1, 2014): 4007–4011.

Hodeib, M., R. Eskander, and R.F. Bristow. "New Paradigms in the Surgical and Adjuvant Treatment of Ovarian Cancer." *Minerva Ginecologica* 66 (April 2014): 179–192.

Marchetti, C., et al. "Targeted Drug Delivery Via Folate Receptors in Recurrent Ovarian Cancer: A Review." *Onco Targets and Therapy* 7 (July 10, 2014): 1223–1236.

Miccò, M., et al. "Role of Imaging in the Pretreatment Evaluation of Common Gynecological Cancers." *Women's Health (London, England)* 10 (May 2014): 299–321.

Sinno, A.K., et al. "Human Papillomavirus Genotype Prevalence in Invasive Vaginal Cancer from a Registry-based Population." *Obstetrics and Gynecology* 123 (April 2014): 817–821.

Tewari, K.S., et al. "Improved Survival with Bevacizumab in Advanced Cervical Cancer." *New England Journal of Medicine* 370 (February 20, 2014): 734–743.

van Gent, M.D., et al. "Nerve-sparing Radical Abdominal Trachelectomy Versus Nerve-sparing Radical Hysterectomy in Early-stage (FIGO IA2-IB) Cervical Cancer: A Comparative Study on Feasibility and Outcome." *International Journal of Gynecological Cancer* 24 (May 2014): 735–743.

Westin, S.N., et al. "Overall Survival after Pelvic Exenteration for Gynecologic Malignancy." *Gynecologic Oncology.* July 9, 2014 [E-publication ahead of print].

WEBSITES

American Cancer Society (ACS). "Cervical Cancer." http://www.cancer.org/acs/groups/cid/documents/webcontent/003094-pdf.pdf (accessed June 16, 2014).

American Cancer Society (ACS). "Endometrial (Uterine) Cancer." http://www.cancer.org/acs/groups/cid/documents/webcontent/003097-pdf.pdf (accessed June 22, 2014).

American Cancer Society (ACS). "Ovarian Cancer." http://www.cancer.org/acs/groups/cid/documents/webcontent/003130-pdf.pdf (accessed June 26, 2014).

American Cancer Society. "Vaginal Cancer." http://www.cancer.org/acs/groups/cid/documents/webcontent/003146-pdf.pdf (accessed July 17, 2014).

American Cancer Society (ACS). "Vulvar Cancer." http://www.cancer.org/acs/groups/cid/documents/webcontent/003147-pdf.pdf (accessed July 17, 2014).

American College of Obstetricians and Gynecologists (ACOG). "Frequently Asked Questions, FAQ 163: Cancer of the Cervix." http://www.acog.org/~/media/For%20Patients/faq163.pdf (accessed June 16, 2014).

Centers for Disease Control and Prevention (CDC). "Human Papillomavirus (HPV)." http://www.cdc.gov/hpv (accessed June 16, 2014).

National Cancer Institute (NCI). "What You Need to Know about Cancer of the Uterus." http://www.cancer.gov/cancertopics/wyntk/uterus/page1/AllPages (accessed June 22, 2014).

Ovarian Cancer National Alliance. "About Ovarian Cancer." http://www.ovariancancer.org/about (accessed June 26, 2014).

Society of Gynecologic Oncology (SGO). "Ovarian Cancer." https://www.sgo.org/ovarian-cancer (accessed June 26, 2014).

ORGANIZATIONS

American Cancer Society (ACS), 250 Williams Street NW, Atlanta, GA 30303, (800)-227-2345, http://www.cancer.org/aboutus/howwehelpyou/app/contact-us.aspx, http://www.cancer.org/index.

American Congress of Obstetricians and Gynecologists (ACOG), P.O. Box 70620, Washington, DC 20024-9998, (202) 638-5577, (800) 673-8444, resources@acog.org, http://www.acog.org.

American Society of Clinical Oncology (ASCO), 2318 Mill Road, Suite 800, Alexandria, VA 22314, (571) 483-1300, (888) 651-3038, contactus@cancernet http://www.asco.org.

Foundation for Women's Cancer, 230 W. Monroe, Suite 2528, Chicago, IL 60606-4902, (312) 578-1439, (800) 444-4441, Fax: (312) 578-9769, info@foundationforwomenscancer.org, http://www.foundationforwomenscancer.org.

National Cancer Institute (NCI), BG 9609 MSC 9760, 9609 Medical Center Drive, Bethesda, MD 20892-9760, (800) 4-CANCER (422-6237), http://www.cancer.gov/global/contact/email-us, http://www.cancer.gov.

Office of Cancer Complementary and Alternative Medicine (OCCAM), 9609 Medical Center Dr., Room 5-W-136, Rockville, MD 20850, (240)-276-6595, Fax: (240)-276-7888, ncioccam1-r@mail.nih.gov, http://cam.cancer.gov.

Ovarian Cancer National Alliance, 1101 14th Street NW, Suite 850, Washington, DC 20005, (202) 331-1332, (866) 399-6262, Fax: (202) 331-2292, http://www.ovariancancer.org.

Society of Gynecologic Oncology (SGO), 230 W. Monroe St., Suite 710, Chicago, IL 60606-4703, (312) 235-4060, Fax: (312) 235-4059, sgo@sgo.org, https://www.sgo.org.

Belinda Rowland, PhD.
Melinda Granger Oberleitner, R.N., D.N.S., A.P.R.N., C.N.S.
REVISED BY REBECCA J. FREY, PhD.

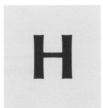

Hair loss *see* **Alopecia**

Hairy cell leukemia

Definition

Hairy cell leukemia is a disease in which a type of white blood cell called the lymphocyte, present in the blood and bone marrow, becomes malignant and proliferates. It is called hairy cell leukemia because the cells have tiny hair-like projections when viewed under the microscope.

Description

Hairy cell leukemia (HCL) is a rare **cancer**. It was first described in 1958 as *leukemic reticuloendotheliosis*, erroneously referring to a red blood cell because researchers were unsure of the cell of origin. It became more easily identifiable in the 1970s. There are approximately 600 new cases diagnosed every year in the United States, making up about 2% of the adult cases of leukemia each year.

HCL is found in cells located in the blood. There are three types of cells found in the blood: the red blood cells that carry oxygen to all the parts of the body; the white blood cells that are responsible for fighting infection and protecting the body from diseases; and the platelets that help in the clotting of blood. Hairy cell leukemia affects a type of white blood cell called the lymphocyte. Lymphocytes are made in the bone marrow, spleen, lymph nodes, and other organs. It specifically affects B-lymphocytes, which mature in the bone marrow. However, extremely rare variants of HCL have been discovered developing from T-lymphocytes, which mature in the thymus.

When hairy cell leukemia develops, the white blood cells become abnormal both in the way they appear (by acquiring hairy projections) and in the way they act (by proliferating without the normal control mechanisms). Further, the cells tend to accumulate in the spleen, causing it to become enlarged. The cells may also collect in the bone marrow and prevent it from producing normal blood cells. As a result, there may not be enough normal white blood cells in the blood to fight infection.

Demographics

The median age at which people develop HCL is 52 years. Though it occurs in all ages, HCL more commonly develops in the older population. Men are four times more likely to develop HCL than women. There have been reports of familial aggregation of disease, with higher occurrences in Ashkenazi Jewish men. A potential genetic link is undergoing further investigation.

Causes and symptoms

The cause of hairy cell leukemia is not specifically known. However, exposure to radiation is a known cause of leukemia in general. Familial involvement is another theory, suggesting that there is a genetic component associated with this disease.

HCL is a chronic (slowly progressing) disease, and the patients may not show any symptoms for many years. As the disease advances, the patients may suffer from one or more of the following symptoms:

- weakness
- fatigue
- recurrent infections
- fever
- anemia
- bruising
- pain or discomfort in the abdominal area
- weight loss (uncommon)
- night sweats (uncommon)

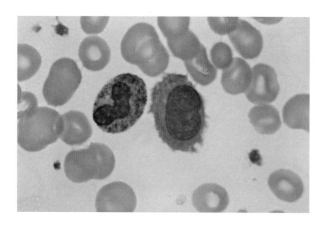

A magnified image of white blood cells with "hairy" projections. *(MICHAEL ABBEY/Science Source)*

Pain and discomfort are caused by an enlarged spleen, which results from the accumulation of the abnormal hairy cells in the spleen. Blood tests may show abnormal counts of all the different types of cells. This happens because the cancerous cells invade the bone marrow as well and prevent it from producing normal blood cells. Because of the low white cell count in the blood, the patient may have frequent infections. **Fever** often accompanies the infections. The patient is most susceptible to bacterial infections, but infections of any kind are the major cause of death. The low red cell count may cause **anemia**, **fatigue**, and weakness, and the low platelet count may cause the person to bruise and bleed easily.

Diagnosis

When a patient suffers from the above symptoms, the doctor will palpate (examine with fingers) the abdomen and may order scans to see if the spleen is enlarged (splenomegaly). An enlarged spleen is present in 80% of patients. An enlarged liver is less common, but can occur.

If the spleen is enlarged, the doctor may order several blood tests. In these tests, the total numbers of each of the different types of blood cells (CBC) are reported. Sixty to eighty percent of patients suffer from pancytopenia, which is a dramatic reduction in the number of red blood cells, white blood cells, and platelets circulating in the blood.

If the blood tests are abnormal, the doctor may order a **bone marrow aspiration and biopsy**. In order to establish a diagnosis, hairy cells must be present in the bone marrow.

Treatment team

If the patient is seeing a primary care provider, the provider may perform the initial diagnostic tests.

However, in order to diagnose and treat HCL comprehensively, the primary care provider will refer the patient to an oncologist (cancer specialist). Radiologists and pathologists will also be involved to read scans and examine tissue samples. Other specialists involved with the treatment of hairy cell leukemia will be nurses and dieticians who are available to explain side effects of treatment and offer suggestions on eating healthy meals that may help fight the side effects.

Clinical staging

When physicians perform blood tests, they will determine the level of hemoglobin (the oxygen-transporting molecule of red blood cells). Serum hemoglobin

816

QUESTIONS TO ASK YOUR DOCTOR

- How long will this course of treatment take?
- How long will the side effects last after treatment ends?
- What kinds of side effects will this course of treatment cause?
- Are there support services available?
- What treatments are currently in clinical trials?
- What treatments will my healthcare insurance cover?
- What alternative or complementary treatments are safe and effective?
- Why is this type of treatment being used?

levels and the size of the spleen, which can be measured on exam and by using an x-ray, are proposed criteria for determining the stage of HCL. The following are the three proposed stages and their criteria:

- Stage I: Hemoglobin greater than 12 g/dL (1 g = approximately 0.02 pint and 1 dL = approximately 0.33 ounce) and spleen less than or equal to 10 cm (3.9 inches).

- Stage II: Hemoglobin between 8.5 and 12 g/dL and spleen greater than 10 cm (3.9 inches).

- Stage III: Hemoglobin less than 8.5 g/dL and spleen greater than 10 cm (3.9 inches).

Since there is generally no accepted staging system, another method for evaluating the progression of HCL is to group patients into two categories: untreated HCL and progressive HCL, in which hairy cells are present after therapy has been administered.

Some people with hairy cell leukemia have very few or no symptoms at all, and it is reasonable to expect that 10% of patients may not need any treatment. However, if the patient is symptomatic and needs intervention, HCL is especially responsive to treatment.

Treatment

There are three main courses of treatment: **chemotherapy**, **splenectomy** (surgical removal of the spleen), and **immunotherapy**. Once a patient meets treatment criteria, purine analogues, particularly the drugs **pentostatin** and **cladribine**, are the first-line therapy. Pentostatin is administered at 5 mg/m^2 for two days every

other week until total remission is achieved. Patients may experience side effects such as fever, **nausea and vomiting**, photosensitivity, and keratoconjuctivitis. However, follow-up studies estimate a relapse-free survival rate at 76%. Cladribine (2-CdA) taken at 0.1 mg/kg/day for seven days also has an impressive response. Eighty-six percent of patients experience complete remission after treatment, while 16% experience partial remission. Fever is the principal side effect of 2-CdA.

Biological therapy (also called immunologic therapy or immunotherapy), where the body's own immune cells are used to fight cancer, is also being investigated in **clinical trials** for hairy cell leukemia. A substance called interferon that is produced by the white blood cells of the body was the first systemic treatment that showed consistent results in fighting HCL. The FDA approved interferon-alpha (INF-alpha) to fight HCL. The mechanism by which INF-alpha works is not clearly understood. However, it is known that interferon stimulates the body's natural killer cells that are suppressed during HCL. The standard dosage is 2 MU/m^2 three times a week for 12 months. Side effects include fever, myalgia, malaise, rashes, and gastrointestinal complaints.

If the spleen is enlarged, it may be removed in a surgical procedure known as splenectomy. This usually causes a remission of the disease. However, 50% of patients who undergo splenectomy require some type of systemic treatment such as chemotherapy or immunotherapy. Splenectomy is not the most widely used course of treatment as it was many years ago. Although the spleen is not an indispensable organ, it is responsible for helping the body fight infection. Therefore, other therapies are preferred in order to salvage the spleen and its functions.

Alternative and complementary therapies

Many individuals choose to supplement traditional therapy with complementary methods. Often, these methods improve the tolerance of side effects and symptoms as well as enrich the quality of life. The American Cancer Society recommends that patients talk to their doctors to ensure that the methods they are using are safely supplementing traditional therapy. Some complementary treatments include the following:

- yoga
- meditation
- religious practices and prayer
- music therapy
- art therapy

- massage therapy
- aromatherapy

Coping with cancer treatment

The treatment and the disease interfere with the patient's ability to produce red blood cells, white blood cells, and platelets, causing the patient to be vulnerable to anemia and life-threatening infection and bleeding. Transfusions can be given to patients in order to increase the number of red blood cells and platelets in the blood. In addition, colony-stimulating factors are being studied. These increase the number of the patient's own white blood cells.

Nausea and vomiting can result from chemotherapy and are often controlled by prescription drugs called **antiemetics**. Patients can also curb nausea and vomiting by eating slowly and avoiding large meals. Drinking water an hour before meals and staying away from foods that are sweet or fried is also helpful. Many times, chemotherapy is handled better if the patient is eating well. Nurses and dieticians can aid patients in choosing healthful foods to incorporate into their diet.

Patients can fight anemia and fatigue by getting plenty of rest and minimizing strenuous activities. A well-balanced diet can also counter anemia and fatigue.

Although physicians will do everything possible to keep a patient's blood count high, there are precautions that can be taken by patients in order to reduce their risk of infection. Patients should regularly wash their hands, especially before and after eating meals and after using the restroom. Patients should avoid individuals who are contagious with colds, the flu, or the chickenpox. It is also helpful if patients do not cut themselves or do anything to expose deeper layers of the skin where bacteria can contaminate and cause infection. Finally, patients should avoid large crowds.

Prognosis

Most patients have excellent prognosis and can expect to live ten years or longer. The disease may remain silent for years with treatment. Continual follow-up is necessary to monitor the patient for relapse and determine true cure rates.

Clinical trials

Clinical trials are being performed to improve the effectiveness of treatment and to minimize the side effects. Patients may choose to volunteer for a clinical trial if they do not respond to standard therapy or if they want to reduce side effects. Clinical trials for the treatment of HCL involving purine analogues were being researched in 2005. Clinical trials are being performed all over the United States, and patients should discuss options with their doctors or contact the Cancer Information Service at (800) 4-CANCER (800-422-6237).

In many cases, insurance companies will not cover procedures that are part of clinical trials. Patients should talk with their doctor and insurance company to determine which procedures are covered.

Prevention

Since the cause for the disease is unknown and there are no specific risk factors, there is no known prevention.

Special concerns

Cancer treatments and their side effects can take a physical and psychological toll on cancer patients and their families. To deal with the psychological impact, there are many different support groups and psychotherapists that can help. Psychiatrists can prescribe medication to help with **depression**. Support groups can encourage and strengthen the psyche by relating to one another through shared experiences and success stories. Relying on faith practices is also beneficial for cancer patients to deal with their condition. Patients should discuss all options with their physician to determine what is available to them.

See also Tumor staging.

Resources

BOOKS

Bast, Robert C. *Cancer Medicine*. Lewiston, NY: B.C. Decker Inc., 2000.

Haskell, Charles M. *Cancer Treatment*. 5th ed. Philadelphia: W.B. Saunders Company, 2001.

WEBSITES

National Cancer Institute. "Hairy Cell Leukemia Treatment (PDQ®)." http://www.cancer.gov/cancertopics/pdq/ treatment/hairy-cell-leukemia/Patient/page1 (accessed December 4, 2014).

ORGANIZATIONS

American Cancer Society, 250 Williams St. NW, Atlanta, GA 30303, (800) 227-2345, http://www.cancer.org.

Hairy Cell Leukemia Foundation, 790 Estate Drive, Suite 180, Deerfield, IL 60015, (224) 355-7201, info@ hairycellleukemia.org, http://www.hairycellleukemia.org.

Leukemia & Lymphoma Society, 1311 Mamaroneck Ave., Ste. 310, White Plains, NY 10605, (914) 949-5213, Fax: (914) 949-6691, infocenter@lls.org, http://www.lls.org.

National Cancer Institute, 9609 Medical Center Dr., BG 9609 MSC 9760, Bethesda, MD 20892-9760, (800) 4-CANCER (422-6237), http://www.cancer.gov.

Lata Cherath, PhD.
Sally C. McFarlane-Parrott

Haloperidol *see* **Antiemetics**

Halotestin *see* **Fluoxymesterone**

Hand-foot syndrome

Definition

Hand-foot syndrome (HFS), also called palmar-plantar erythrodysesthesia syndrome (PPES) or chemotherapy-induced acral erythema, is a relatively common side effect associated with high-dosage **chemotherapy** treatments involving **fluorouracil** (5-FU) and drugs belonging to the chemical class called anthracyclines. It was first reported in 1974.

Demographics

There are no reliable statistics about the frequency of hand-foot syndrome as a complication of **cancer** chemotherapy.

Description

Anthracyclines have been widely used since the 1960s as dose-limited chemotherapy drugs for a variety of cancers, particularly leukemia, metastatic **breast cancer**, **ovarian cancer**, and colorectal cancer. The most familiar anthracyclines are **capecitabine** (Xeloda), **daunorubicin** (Cerubidine), **doxorubicin** (Adriamycin), **idarubicin** (Idamycin), and **vinorelbine** (Navelbine). Each of these drugs is broken down into 5-FU by chemicals inside the cancer cells.

A dose-limited drug is a drug for which the maximum dose is determined by the reactions of an individual patient. Symptoms of HFS usually indicate that a patient is receiving too much 5-FU or a particular anthracycline. In such a case, the dosage of the drug that is causing HFS is usually decreased until these symptoms either disappear completely or become tolerable to the patient.

Risk factors

The primary risk factor for HFS is cancer therapy involving anthracycline medications. There are no indications that sex, race, or age affects a person's risk of developing HFS.

Causes and symptoms

Causes

The symptoms of HFS are believed to be caused by some of the chemicals that 5-FU is broken down into by the natural biochemical processes of the body. Since all anthracycline drugs chemically break down into 5-FU, these drugs will all eventually be broken down into the chemicals that can cause the symptoms of HFS. For reasons that are not clear, some patients seem more prone to developing symptoms of HFS than other patients.

The direct cause of HFS is leakage of the chemotherapy drug from tiny blood vessels called capillaries into the skin on the palms of the hands and soles of the feet. The amount of drug leakage from the capillaries is increased by friction or heat. The leakage results in redness, tenderness, and possibly peeling of the skin on the palms and soles. The rash often looks like sunburn.

Symptoms

The symptoms of HFS may begin anywhere from days to weeks after the beginning of chemotherapy. The primary symptom of HFS is a tingling sensation and/or numbness of the skin, particularly on the palms of the hands or the soles of the feet. Swelling and redness (erythema) often accompany this symptom. In severe cases, the skin may peel, develop ulcerations or blisters, and cause severe pain. In the most extreme cases, symptoms of HFS may make it difficult or impossible for the patient to grasp small objects, walk, or conduct other normal daily activities.

In a few cases, patients develop HFS on the knees and elbows as well as on the hands and feet.

Diagnosis

The diagnosis of HFS is based on a combination of the patient's history of chemotherapy and the appearance of the characteristic reddening and peeling of the skin on the extremities. It is important for cancer patients to consult their doctor as soon as they notice redness or tenderness on their palms or soles, before the skin starts to peel.

Treatment

Traditional

The symptoms of HFS are usually alleviated by lowering the dosage of the drug that the patient is receiving. In severe cases of HFS, it may be necessary to discontinue the use of the drug that is causing these symptoms. In some patients, but not all, the symptoms of HFS are reduced by treatment with such steroid-containing skin creams as hydrocortisone.

Other measures that help some patients are the application of cold in an ice pack or even a package of frozen food for 15–20 minutes at a time, or gently applying moisturizers like Lubriderm or Bag Balm to the palms and soles. It is important not to use pressure in applying moisturizers, however, as friction can worsen HFS.

Drugs

Some doctors recommend taking acetaminophen (Tylenol), an over-the-counter pain reliever, to ease the discomfort of HFS.

Alternative

Treatment of the hands and feet with an aloe vera-containing skin cream may help to alleviate some of the symptoms of HFS. Topical treatment of the skin with dimethyl sulfoxide (DMSO) has also been suggested as an alternative treatment.

Another alternative treatment that is sometimes recommended is vitamin therapy, specifically taking vitamin B_6.

Prognosis

HFS clears up in most cases when the medication dose is adjusted or the drug discontinued.

Prevention

Taking steps to reduce heat or friction on the hands and feet can help to prevent HFS:

- Avoid exposing the skin to hot water for long periods of time. Take short showers and baths, or bathe in lukewarm rather than hot water.
- Do not use rubber gloves when washing dishes as they trap heat against the skin.
- Avoid direct contact with detergents, bleach, ammonia, and other harsh household chemicals.
- Avoid jogging, power walking, jumping, tennis, softball, baseball, or aerobics as forms of exercise.
- Limit sun exposure.
- Make sure that shoes fit properly and do not put too much pressure on the feet.
- Wear loose, well-ventilated clothing.

QUESTIONS TO ASK YOUR DOCTOR

- Will my medication dose be adjusted?
- What would you recommend to stop the itching and peeling?
- What is your opinion of vitamin therapy for HFS?
- How many patients have you treated for HFS?

- Avoid using garden and household tools that force the hand against a hard surface, such as chopping knives, screwdrivers, and some power tools.

These preventive measures should be taken within a week of starting intravenous anthracycline drugs and should be followed all the time when taking oral anthracyclines.

Resources

BOOKS

Airley, Rachel. *Cancer Chemotherapy*. Hoboken, NJ: Wiley-Blackwell, 2009.

McKay, Judith, and Tamera Schacher. *The Chemotherapy Survival Guide: Everything You Need to Know to Get Through Treatment*. 3rd ed. Oakland, CA: New Harbinger Publications, 2009.

Spencer, Peter, and Walter Holt, eds. *Anticancer Drugs: Design, Delivery and Pharmacology*. Hauppauge, NY: Nova Science Publishers, 2009.

PERIODICALS

Cicek, D., et al. "Localized Palmar-Plantar Hyperplasia Associated with Use of Sorafenib." *Clinical Drug Investigation* 28 (December 2008): 803–07.

Eng, C. "Toxic Effects and Their Management: Daily Clinical Challenges in the Treatment of Colorectal Cancer." *Nature Reviews: Clinical Oncology* 6 (April 2009): 207–18.

Goutos, I., et al. "Hand-foot Syndrome—An Unusual Case of Plantar Pathology Presenting to a Burns Unit." *Journal of Burn Care and Research* 30 (May-June 2009): 529–32.

Sivaramamoorthy, C., et al. "Hand-foot Syndrome after Treatment with Docetaxel." *Medical Journal of Australia* 191 (July 6, 2009): 40.

OTHER

National Cancer Institute (NCI). *Managing Chemotherapy Side Effects: Skin and Nail Changes*. http://www.cancer.gov/cancertopics/coping/chemo-side-effects/skin-and-nail.pdf (accessed November 4, 2014).

WEBSITES

American Society of Clinical Oncology (ASCO). "Hand-Foot Syndrome or Palmar-Plantar Erythrodysesthesia." Cancer.

Net. http://www.cancer.net/navigating-cancer-care/side-effects/hand-foot-syndrome-or-palmar-plantar-erythrody-sesthesia (accessed November 4, 2014).

The Scott Hamilton CARES Initiative. "Hand-Foot Syndrome." Chemocare.com. http://chemocare.com/chemotherapy/side-effects/handfoot-syndrome.aspx (accessed November 4, 2014).

ORGANIZATIONS

American Cancer Society, 250 Williams St. NW, Atlanta, GA 30303, (800) 227-2345, http://www.cancer.org.

American Society of Clinical Oncology (ASCO), 2318 Mill Rd., Ste. 800, Alexandria, VA 22314, (571) 483-1300, (888) 651-3038, contactus@cancer.net, http://www.asco.org.

National Cancer Institute, 9609 Medical Center Dr., BG 9609 MSC 9760, Bethesda, MD 20892-9760, (800) 4-CANCER (422-6237), http://www.cancer.gov.

Paul A. Johnson, EdM
REVISED BY REBECCA J. FREY, PHD.

Head and neck cancers

Definition

The term head and neck cancers refers to a group of cancers found in the head and neck region, excluding tumors of the eyes and the thyroid gland, and tumors that originate in the brain.

Cancers of the head and neck

Cancer types	Cancer occurs in
Hypopharyngeal cancer	Lowest section of the pharynx (region behind mouth)
Laryngeal cancer	Larynx (front of neck, near Adam's apple)
Nasopharyngeal cancer	Behind nose
	Pharynx
Oral cancer	Lips
	Lining of lips and cheeks
	Front two-thirds of tongue
	Teeth
	Gums
	Under tongue
Oropharyngeal cancer	Back one-third of tongue
	Upper section of pharynx
	Area around tonsils
Parathyroid cancer	Parathyroid glands (found behind the thyroid gland)
Thyroid cancer	Thyroid gland (found at front of neck, below the Adam's apple)

Table listing cancers of the head and neck, by type and location of the cancer. (Table by GGS Creative Resources. © Cengage Learning®.)

Tumors classified as head and neck tumors are found in:

- The oral cavity (mouth). The lips, the tongue, the teeth, the gums, the lining inside the lips and cheeks, the floor of the mouth (under the tongue), the roof of the mouth, and the small area behind the wisdom teeth are all included in the oral cavity.
- The oropharynx, which includes the back one-third of the tongue, the back of the throat, and the tonsils.
- The nasopharynx, which includes the area behind the nose.
- The hypopharynx, the lower part of the throat.
- The larynx (voice box, located in front of the neck, in the region of the Adam's apple). In the larynx, the cancer can occur in any of the three regions: the glottis (location of the vocal cords); the supraglottis (the area above the glottis); and the subglottis (the area that connects the glottis to the windpipe).
- The paranasal sinuses, which include the ethmoid and maxillary sinuses.
- The salivary glands.

The most frequently occurring cancers of the head and neck area are **oral cancers** and laryngeal cancers. Almost half of all head and neck cancers occur in the oral cavity, and a third of the cancers are found in the larynx. By definition, the term "head and neck cancers" usually excludes tumors that occur in the brain.

Description

The tumors associated with head and neck cancers are found in several regions, including the lips, tongue, mouth, nasal passages, pharynx, larynx (voice box), and salivary gland. Many head and neck cancers interfere with the functions of eating and breathing. **Laryngeal cancer** affects speech. Because the loss of any of these functions is significant, early detection and appropriate treatment is of utmost importance.

Demographics

Roughly 3% of all cancers in the United States develop in the oral cavity, pharyngeal area, or in the larynx. The most common cancers of the head and neck area are oral cancers and laryngeal **cancer**. Half of all head and neck cancers occur in the oral cavity and pharynx and almost 20% originate in the larynx. With regard to the total number of head and neck cancers, the **National Cancer Institute** (NCI) estimates that between 52,000 and 55,000 men and women (40,220 men and 14,850 women) in this country are diagnosed with head and neck cancers each year and that 12,000 (8,600 men and 3,400 women) die from the disease. The American

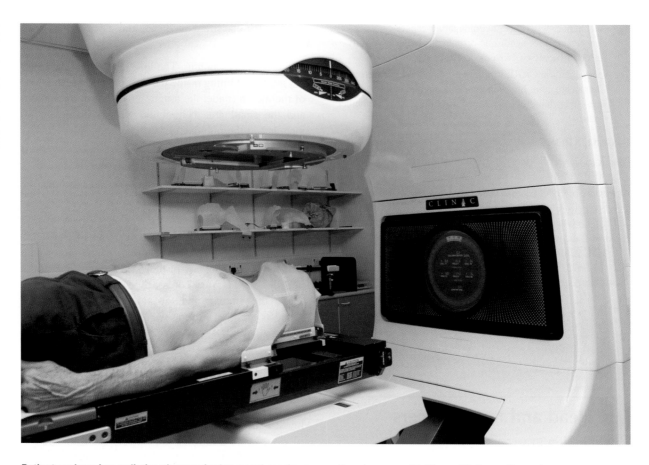

Patient undergoing radiation therapy for laryngeal carcinoma, or throat cancer. *(P. Marazzi/Science Source)*

Cancer Society estimated that about 37,000 new cases of oral cavity and pharyngeal cancers would be diagnosed in the United States in the year 2014 and that 7,300 people would die from them. The estimated number of cases worldwide is about 450,000.

The numbers of new cases and deaths from laryngeal and oral cancers, however, have been steadily decreasing in the last three decades. This decrease is attributed to the decrease in smoking. The demographics of oral cancer are changing, however, with nonsmokers below the age of 50 being the fastest-growing group among people recently diagnosed with oral cancer. It is thought that the spread of **human papillomavirus** (HPV) among younger people is a major factor in this demographic shift.

Risk factors

Tobacco is regarded as the single greatest risk factor contributing to the occurrence of oral and laryngeal cancer: 75%–80% of these patients are smokers. Heavy alcohol use has also been included as a risk factor. A combination of tobacco and alcohol use increases the risk

for oral cancer by 6 to 15 times more than for users of either substance alone. Exposure to asbestos also appears to increase the risk of developing laryngeal cancer. Infection with human papillomavirus (HPV)—particularly HPV16—is a recently recognized risk factor for oral cancer and is thought to be one of the leading causes of **oropharyngeal cancer**. Oral HPV infection is more common in men than in women. The risk of oral HPV infection is linked to such sexual behaviors as open mouth kissing and oral-genital contact (oral sex). The risk of HPV16 infection also increases with the number of a person's sexual partners.

For **lip cancer**, exposure to sunlight appears to be one of the risk factors. Geographical location and sex are also risk factors. While oral cancer is ranked as the sixth leading cancer among men in the United States, it is the fourth leading cancer in African American men. About 7% of oral cancers are thought to result from a genetic predisposition; two inherited syndromes linked to an increased risk of oral cancer are **Fanconi anemia** and dyskeratosis congenita. A family history of oral cancer is an additional risk factor for the disease.

Biopsy—Removal of a portion of tissue or cells for microscopic examination. Incisional biopsy is removal of only a sample tissue. Excisional biopsy is removal of an entire tumor or lesion. A sample of tissue or fluid removed with a needle is fine-needle biopsy.

Brachytherapy—A form of radiation therapy in which small pellets of radioactive material are placed inside or near the area to be treated. It is also known as internal radiation therapy or sealed-source radiotherapy.

Buccal—Pertaining to the mouth or cheeks. It is derived from the Latin word for cheek.

Erythroplakia—A flat red patch or lesion in the mouth.

Leukoplakia—A flat whitish-colored area of the oral mucosa that is not caused by thrush or any other specific disease.

Lymph node—Bean-shaped mass of lymphatic tissue surrounded by connective tissue. Lymph nodes contain lymphocytes, which are cells that help to maintain the immune system.

Oropharynx—A set of structures behind the oral cavity that lies between the upper portion of the pharynx and the lower portion of the throat. The oropharynx contains the tonsils, the base of the tongue, and the soft palate.

Otolaryngologist—A physician who diagnoses and treats disorders of the head and neck; sometimes called an ear, nose, and throat specialist or ENT.

Prosthesis—An artificial device used to replace a missing body part.

Prosthodontist—A dentist with specialized training in restoring dental function after surgery and making dental prostheses.

Resection—Surgical removal of a tumor.

Squamous cell—A flat, scale-like cell found in epithelial tissue. Squamous cells are polygon-shaped when viewed from above. Most head and neck cancers begin as squamous cell carcinomas.

Squamous cell carcinoma—A malignancy that arises from outer skin cells.

Targeted therapy—In cancer treatment, a type of drug therapy that blocks tumors by interfering with specific molecules that the cancer cells need for growth. Also called biologic therapy, targeted therapy is less harmful to normal cells than traditional chemotherapy.

Other factors that increase the risk of oral cancer include: poor oral hygiene; poor nutrition; gastroesophageal reflux disease (GERD); disorders of the immune system, including HIV infection; or taking medications following organ transplantation that weaken the immune system.

The risk of both oral cancer and laryngeal cancer seems to increase with age. Most of the cases occur in individuals over 40 years of age, and the average age at diagnosis is 60. While oral cancer is diagnosed in men twice as often as it is in women, laryngeal cancer is four times more common in men than in women. Both diseases are more common in African Americans than among Caucasians.

Causes and symptoms

The use of tobacco products and alcohol—and in particular, the combination of the two—play a major role in the development of cancers of the head and neck. Infection with HPV is linked to the development of oropharyngeal cancer.

There are many types of head and neck cancers. Signs and symptoms of the various types of cancer are often specific to the original location of the cancer:

• Oral cancers occur in the mouth, or oral cavity, which includes the lips, the lining inside the lips and cheeks (the buccal area), the front two-thirds of the tongue, the teeth, the gums, the floor of the mouth (under the tongue), the roof of the mouth, and the small area behind the wisdom teeth. Symptoms and signs include: a mouth sore that does not heal within two weeks; white or red patches on the oral mucosa (leukoplakia and erythroplakia); unusual bleeding from the teeth or gums; or a lump on the gums, mouth, or tongue.

• Lip cancers occur on the inside or outside surface of the lips. Signs of this cancer include a lump on the inside of the lip or a sore on the outside, which is usually a form of skin cancer.

• Oropharyngeal cancer is found on the back one-third of the tongue, the upper section of the pharynx, and the area around the tonsils. Symptoms include a lump in the back of the mouth or throat, ear pain, or difficulty swallowing.

• Nasopharyngeal cancer is found in the area behind the nose and the upper section of the pharynx, the area just behind the mouth. Symptoms include difficulty breathing or speaking, pain or ringing in ears, frequent headaches, or trouble hearing.

• Hypopharyngeal cancer is found only in the lower portion of the pharynx. Symptoms include a sore throat that does not subside, difficulty swallowing, a lump in the neck, or ear pain.

• Laryngeal cancer starts in the larynx, which is located in the front of the neck in the region of the Adam's apple. Symptoms include pain when swallowing, a sore throat that does not subside, a change in voice, or ear pain.

• Paranasal sinus cancer and nasal cancer develop in the small hollow spaces in the nose called the sinuses and in the nasal cavity, which is the passageway for air moving to the throat during breathing. Symptoms include frequent sinus infections, nosebleeds, a sore inside the nose that does not heal, or pain in the sinus area.

• Salivary gland tumors form in the salivary glands, which produce saliva to help prevent the mouth from drying out and to aid with digestion. They are located under the jaw, in front of the ears, underneath the tongue, and in other regions of the digestive tract. Symptoms include swelling under the chin or around the jawbone; facial numbness; inability to move the facial muscles; or persistent pain in the face, chin, or neck.

Diagnosis

Specific diagnostic tests that are used to detect cancers of the head and neck depend on the location of the cancer. The standard tests are:

Physical examination

The first step in diagnosis is a complete and thorough examination of the oral and nasal cavity, using mirrors and other visual aids. This examination may be performed by the patient's dentist or by an otolaryngologist, a doctor who specializes in disorders of the ear, nose, and throat. The tongue and the back of the throat are examined as well. Any suspicious-looking lumps or lesions are examined with fingers (palpation). In order to look inside the larynx, the doctor may sometimes perform a procedure known as **laryngoscopy**. In indirect laryngoscopy, the doctor looks down the throat with a small, long-handled mirror. Sometimes the doctor inserts a lighted tube (laryngoscope or a fiberoptic scope)

through the patient's nose or mouth. As the tube goes down the throat, the doctor can observe areas that cannot be seen by a simple mirror. This procedure is called a direct laryngoscopy. Sometimes patients may be given a mild sedative to help them relax, and a local anesthetic to ease any discomfort. An endoscopic examination under anesthesia may also be required as part of the workup for head and neck cancer.

Blood tests

The doctor may order blood or other immunological tests. In cases where oropharyngeal cancer is suspected, HPV testing is recommended.

Imaging tests

X-rays of the mouth, the sinuses, the skull, and the chest region may be required. **Computed tomography** scans (CT scans), a procedure in which a computer takes a series of x-ray pictures of areas inside the body, and/or **magnetic resonance imaging** (MRI) and **positron emission tomography** (PET scans) may be ordered. Patients with cancers of the nasopharynx may also undergo imaging tests with PET scans and/or CT scans to determine the presence of distant metastatic lesions. A positron emission tomography or PET scan involves the injection of a radioactive sugar into the patient's blood. Cancers take up sugar at a higher rate than normal tissue and therefore will emit higher levels of radioactivity that can be detected by the PET scanner. Some machines are designed to perform a CT scan and a PET scan at the same time. A bone scan may be done in patients with advanced cancer to determine whether the cancer has spread to the bones.

Dental, speech, and swallowing evaluations may also be conducted.

Biopsy

When a sore does not heal or a suspicious patch or lump is seen in the mouth, larynx, nasopharynx, or throat, a **biopsy** may be performed to rule out the possibility of cancer. The biopsy is the most definitive diagnostic tool for detecting the cancer. If cancerous cells are detected in the biopsied sample, the doctor may perform more extensive tests in order to find where the cancer may have spread.

Treatment team

The cancer care team for cancers of the head and neck typically involves a specialist surgeon, usually either an otolaryngologist or an oral surgeon; a dentist; a medical oncologist; and a radiation therapist. Because treatment of oral cancers often involves adjustments to the patient's diet, a dietitian will usually be consulted. If treatment of the cancer involves facial disfigurement, a plastic surgeon may perform follow-up surgery. If the patient requires **chemotherapy** and/or biologic agents, specially educated oncology nurses will administer the drugs.

Treatment

Most head and neck cancers are treated initially with surgery and/or **radiation therapy**. As of 2014, cancers of the oropharynx may be treated by resection using trans-oral robotic surgery or TORS. In the past, these cancers were difficult to treat with open surgery on the throat because of postoperative complications. TORS, however, allows the surgeon to remove cancerous tissue from the oropharynx through the mouth without having to open the throat.

Chemotherapy may be administered as primary systemic therapy or concurrently with radiation therapy. Chemotherapy drugs currently used in the treatment of head and neck cancers are **cisplatin, fluorouracil** (5-FU), **carboplatin, docetaxel**, paclitaxel, docetaxel, **methotrexate, ifosfamide, bleomycin**, and **gemcitabine**.

A newer form of radiotherapy that has proved beneficial to patients with head and neck cancer is **intensity-modulated radiation therapy**, or IMRT. IMRT allows the radiologist to deliver controlled doses of radiation to cancerous tissues, while leaving nearby normal tissues and organs unaffected. IMRT has proven especially useful in the treatment of oropharyngeal, paranasal sinus, and nasopharyngeal cancers by reducing radiation doses to adjacent non-cancerous tissues and structures. The use of IMRT to treat other head and neck cancers is evolving. 3D-conformal and 2D-conformal radiation therapy techniques may also be utilized. Another radiation technique that may be used is the Simultaneous Integrated Boost (SIB) technique, which integrates IMRT, target volume dosing, and fractionation of radiation therapy. Brachytherapy or internal radiation involves the surgical implant of metal rods or radioactive pellets that deliver radioactive materials to or near the cancer.

A newer form of pharmacotherapy is targeted therapy (sometimes called biologic therapy), which uses drugs that block the growth of cancer cells by targeting specific molecules that the cancer cells need for growth and reproduction. The targeted drug used most often to treat oral cancer is **cetuximab**, which may be combined with radiation therapy for earlier-stage cancers, or with cisplatin for advanced-stage oral cancers. Cetuximab works by targeting the epidermal growth factor receptor (EGFR), a protein on the surface of certain cells that helps them grow

QUESTIONS TO ASK YOUR DOCTOR

- What specific type of head and neck cancer do I have?
- What are the current treatment recommendations for this type of cancer?
- Will I require surgery? If so, how extensive will my surgery be?
- What types of treatment can I expect after surgery?
- How long will these treatments last?
- Will the surgery or any of my other treatments affect my ability to speak and/or swallow?

and divide. Cancers of the oral cavity usually have larger than normal amounts of EGFR, so they can be effectively treated with cetuximab. Other drugs that target EGFR, including **panitumumab**, are currently under investigation as treatments for oral cancer.

For many years, one of the most difficult aspects of treating head and neck cancer has been the necessity of **reconstructive surgery** and rehabilitation therapy following removal of the patient's lips, tongue, voice box, or other structures. In some cases, a prosthodontist may be able to make a prosthesis to replace the missing part of the oral cavity, lip, or nose. Recent advances in plastic and reconstructive surgery, however, have provided patients with better functioning as well as appearance, thus improving their quality of life as well as length of survival.

Prognosis

The survival rates for head and neck cancers vary from good to poor, depending on the specific cancer, stage of the cancer at diagnosis, and the overall physical condition of the patient. Five-year relative survival rates for laryngeal cancer range from 41%–83% for patients diagnosed in stage I to 20%–43% for patients diagnosed in stage IV. The average survival for patients diagnosed with laryngeal cancer has not improved significantly since the early 1970s. Five-year relative survival rates for patients diagnosed with oral/oropharyngeal cancers range from 57%–83% diagnosed in stage I to 27%–47% diagnosed in stage IV.

Prevention

Refraining from the use of all tobacco products (**cigarettes**, cigars, pipe tobacco, chewing tobacco), consuming alcohol in moderation, and practicing good oral hygiene are some of the measures that one can take to lower the risk of head and neck cancers. Better education of the public is important, as knowledge regarding the risk factors of head and neck cancers is limited. Only 25% of U.S. adults can detect early signs of abnormalities in the oral cavity, and only 13% understand the implications of regular alcohol consumption in developing oral cancer. **Cancer prevention** and control programs are growing rapidly with screening services for high-risk populations, health promotion, education, and intervention strategies. HPV vaccinations in both girls and boys should also help prevent against oropharyngeal cancers.

Because there is an association between excessive exposure to the sun and lip cancer, people who spend a lot of time outdoors in the sun should protect themselves from the sun's harmful rays. Regular physical examinations and oral examinations by the patient's doctor or dentist (or the patients themselves) can help detect oral cancer in its very early stages.

Because working with asbestos has been shown to increase one's risk of getting cancer of the larynx, asbestos workers should follow safety rules to avoid inhaling asbestos fibers. Also, malnutrition and vitamin deficiencies have been shown to have some association with an increased incidence of head and neck cancers. The American Cancer Society, therefore, recommends eating a healthy diet, consisting of at least five servings of fruits and vegetables every day, and six servings of food from other plant sources such as cereals, breads, grain products, rice, pasta, and beans. Reducing one's intake of high-fat food from animal sources is also advised.

Resources

BOOKS

Cummings, Louise, ed. *The Cambridge Handbook of Communication Disorders.* Cambridge, UK: Cambridge University Press, 2014.

Harrison, Louis B., et al., eds. *Head and Neck Cancer: A Multidisciplinary Approach.* 4th ed. Philadelphia, PA: Wolters Kluwer Health/Lippincott Williams and Wilkins, 2013.

Hinni, Michael L., and David G. Lott, eds. *Contemporary Transoral Surgery for Primary Head and Neck Cancer.* San Diego, CA: Plural Publishing, 2015.

Kesting, Marco. *Oral Cancer Surgery: A Visual Guide.* New York: Thieme, 2014.

Ward, Elizabeth C., and Corina J. van As-Brooks, eds. *Head and Neck Cancer: Treatment, Rehabilitation, and Outcomes,* 2nd ed. San Diego, CA: Plural Publishing, 2015.

Wolk, Burrell H. *A Patient's Guide to Skin Cancer: What You Need to Know: Your Essential Guide to the Prevention,* *Early Detection, and Treatment of Skin and Lip Cancer.* Phoenix, AZ: Skin and Cancer Center of Arizona Publishing, 2010.

PERIODICALS

Baumeister, P., et al. "Surgically Treated Oropharyngeal Cancer: Risk Factors and Tumor Characteristics." *Journal of Cancer Research and Clinical Oncology* 140 (June 2014): 1011–1019.

Brickman, D., and N. D. Gross. "Robotic Approaches to the Pharynx: Tonsil Cancer." *Otolaryngologic Clinics of North America* 47 (June 2014): 359–372.

Cohen, R. B. "Current Challenges and Clinical Investigations of Epidermal Growth Factor Receptor (EGFR)- and ErbB Family-targeted Agents in the Treatment of Head and Neck Squamous Cell Carcinoma (HNSCC)." *Cancer Treatment Reviews* 40 (May 2014): 567–577.

Deschler, D. G., et al. "The 'New' Head and Neck Cancer Patient—Young, Nonsmoker, Nondrinker, and HPV Positive: Evaluation." *Otolaryngology—Head and Neck Surgery* 151, no. 3 (2014): 375–80.

Fried, J. L. "Confronting Human Papilloma Virus/Oropharyngeal Cancer: A Model for Interprofessional Collaboration." *Journal of Evidence-based Dental Practice* 14 (June 2014): Suppl. 136–146.e1.

Hayes, D. N., et al. "An Exploratory Subgroup Analysis of Race and Gender in Squamous Cancer of the Head and Neck: Inferior Outcomes for African American Males in the LORHAN Database." *Oral Oncology* 50 (June 2014): 605–610.

Kelly, K., et al. "Oncologic, Functional and Surgical Outcomes of Primary Transoral Robotic Surgery for Early Squamous Cell Cancer of the Oropharynx: A Systematic Review." *Oral Oncology* 50, no. 8 (2014): 696–703.

Lubek, J. E., and R. A. Ord. "Lip Reconstruction." *Oral and Maxillofacial Surgery Clinics of North America* 25 (May 2013): 203–214.

Seiwert, T. Y., et al. "A Randomized, Phase 2 Study of Afatinib Versus Cetuximab in Metastatic or Recurrent Squamous Cell Carcinoma of the Head and Neck." *Annals of Oncology* 25, no. 9 (2014): 1813–20.

Selber, J. C., et al. "Transoral Robotic Reconstructive Surgery." *Seminars in Plastic Surgery* 28 (February 2014): 35–38.

Vainshtein, J. M., et al. "Refining Risk Stratification for Locoregional Failure after Chemoradiotherapy in Human Papillomavirus-associated Oropharyngeal Cancer." *Oral Oncology* 50 (May 2014): 513–519.

WEBSITES

American Cancer Society (ACS). "Nasal Cavity and Paranasal Sinus Cancers." http://www.cancer.org/acs/groups/cid/documents/webcontent/003123-pdf.pdf (accessed August 8, 2014).

American Cancer Society (ACS). "Oral Cavity and Oropharyngeal Cancer." http://www.cancer.org/acs/groups/cid/documents/webcontent/003128-pdf.pdf (accessed August 8, 2014).

American Dental Association (ADA). "Oral Cancer." http://www.ada.org/en/member-center/oral-health-topics/oral-cancer (accessed August 8, 2014).

Cancer.Net. "Head and Neck Cancer." http://www.cancer.net/cancer-types/head-and-neck-cancer (accessed August 8, 2014).

National Cancer Institute (NCI). "Fact Sheet: Head and Neck Cancers." http://www.cancer.gov/cancertopics/factsheet/Sites-Types/head-and-neck (accessed August 8, 2014).

National Cancer Institute (NCI). "Paranasal Sinus and Nasal Cavity Cancer Treatment (PDQ®)." http://www.cancer.gov/cancertopics/pdq/treatment/paranasalsinus/Health Professional/page1/AllPages (accessed August 8, 2014).

National Cancer Institute (NCI). "What You Need to Know About Oral Cancer." http://www.cancer.gov/cancertopics/wyntk/oral/WYNTK_oral.pdf (accessed August 8, 2014).

Oral Cancer Foundation (OCF). "Oral Cancer Facts." http://www.oralcancerfoundation.org/facts (accessed August 8, 2014).

Skin Cancer Foundation. "Lip Cancer: Not Uncommon, Often Overlooked." http://www.skincancer.org/skin-cancer-information/lip-cancer-not-uncommon (accessed August 8, 2014).

ORGANIZATIONS

American Academy of Facial Plastic and Reconstructive Surgery (AAFPRS), 310 South Henry Street, Alexandria, VA 22314, (703) 299-9291, Fax: (703) 299-8898, info@aafprs.org, http://www.aafprs.org.

American Academy of Otolaryngology—Head and Neck Surgery, 1650 Diagonal Road, Alexandria, VA 22314-2857, (703) 836-4444, http://entnet.org/content/contact_us, http://entnet.org.

American Cancer Society (ACS), 250 Williams Street NW, Atlanta, GA 30303, (800) 227-2345, http://www.cancer.org/aboutus/howwehelpyou/app/contact-us.aspx, http://www.cancer.org/index.

American Dental Association (ADA), 211 East Chicago Ave., Chicago, IL 60611-2678, (312) 440-2500, http://www.ada.org/en.

National Cancer Institute (NCI), BG 9609 MSC 9760, 9609 Medical Center Drive, Bethesda, MD 20892-9760, (800) 4-CANCER (422-6237), http://www.cancer.gov/global/contact/email-us, http://www.cancer.gov.

Oral Cancer Foundation, 3419 Via Lido #205, Newport Beach, CA 92663, (949) 723-4400, http://www.oralcancerfoundation.org/contact/index.html, http://www.oralcancerfoundation.org.

Support for People with Oral and Head and Neck Cancer (SPOHNC), PO Box 53, Locust Valley, NY 11560-0053, (800) 377-0928, Fax: (516) 671-8794, info@spohnc.org, http://www.spohnc.org.

Lata Cherath, PhD.
Melinda Granger Oberleitner, RN, DNS, APRN, CNS
REVISED BY REBECCA J. FREY, PhD.

Health insurance

Definition

Health insurance is insurance that pays for all or part of a person's healthcare bills. The types of health insurance are group health plans, individual plans, workers' compensation, and government health plans such as Medicare and Medicaid.

Health insurance can be further classified into fee-for-service (traditional insurance) and managed care. Both group and individual insurance plans can be either fee-for-service or managed care plans.

The following are types of managed care plans:

• Health Maintenance Organization (HMO)
• Preferred Provider Organization (PPO)

Purpose

The purpose of health insurance is to help people cover their healthcare costs. Healthcare costs include doctor visits, hospital stays, surgery, procedures, tests, home care, and other treatments and services.

Description

Health insurance is available to groups as well as individuals. Government plans, such as Medicare, are offered to people who meet certain criteria.

Group and individual plans can be further classified as either fee-for-service or managed care. **Cancer** patients may have specific concerns, such as the freedom to select specialists, that play a factor in choosing a healthcare plan. Fee-for-service plans traditionally offer greater freedom when choosing a healthcare professional. Managed care often limits a patient to healthcare professionals listed by the managed care insurance company.

Affordable Care Act

The Affordable Care Act (ACA) made several changes to health insurance. These include making insurers, which offer coverage through designated marketplaces, pay for certain prevention services such as some cancer screenings, and eliminating many clauses in coverage contracts for preexisting conditions that made it difficult for cancer survivors to retain or obtain health coverage. Though not without controversy, the law has guaranteed some rights for cancer patients, such as the right to appeal denial of payment for a service.

Group health plans

A group health plan offers healthcare coverage for employers, student organizations, professional associations, religious organizations, and other groups. Many employers offer group health plans to employees and their dependents as a benefit of working with that particular employer (medical benefits). The employer may pay for part or all of the insurance cost (premium).

When an employee leaves a job, he or she may be eligible for continued health insurance as a result of the Consolidated Omnibus Budget Reconciliation Act of 1986 (COBRA). This federal law protects employees and their families in certain situations by allowing them to keep their health insurance for a specified amount of time. The individual must, however, pay a premium to keep their insurance plan in effect. It is important to note that COBRA only applies under certain conditions, such as job loss, death, divorce, or other life events. The COBRA law usually applies to group health plans offered by companies with more than 20 employees. Some states have laws that require employers to offer continued healthcare coverage for people who do not qualify for COBRA. Each state's insurance board can provide additional information.

Individual plans

These type of healthcare plans are sold directly to individuals.

Fee-for-service

Fee-for-service is traditional health insurance in which the insurance company reimburses the doctor, hospital, or other healthcare provider for all or part of the fees charged. Fee-for-service plans may be offered to groups or individuals. This type of plan gives people the highest level of freedom to choose a doctor, hospital, or other healthcare provider. A person may be able to receive medical care anywhere in the United States and, often, in the world.

Under this type of insurance, a premium is paid and there is usually a yearly deductible, which means benefits do not begin until this deductible is met. After the person has paid the deductible (an amount specified by the terms of the insurance policy) the insurance company pays a portion of covered medical services. For example, the deductible may be $250, so the patient pays the first $250 of yearly covered medical expenses. After that, he or she may pay 20% of covered services while the insurance company pays 80%. The exact percentages and deductibles will vary with each policy. The person may have to fill out forms (claims) and send them to the insurance company to have their claims paid.

People who have cancer may be attracted to the freedom of choice that traditional fee-for-service plans

offer. However, they will most likely have higher out-of-pocket costs than they would in a managed care plan.

Managed care

Managed care plans are also sold to both groups and individuals. In these plans, a person's health care is managed by the insurance company. Approvals are needed for some services, including visits to specialist doctors, medical tests, or surgical procedures. In order for people to receive the highest level of coverage, they must obtain services from the doctors, hospitals, labs, imaging centers, and other providers affiliated with their managed care plan.

People with cancer who are considering a managed care plan should check with the plan regarding coverage for services outside of the plan's list of participating providers. For example, if a person wants to travel to a cancer center for treatment, he or she should find out what coverage will be available. In these plans, coverage is usually much less if a person receives treatment from doctors and hospitals not affiliated with the plan.

HEALTH MAINTENANCE ORGANIZATION (HMO). An HMO is a type of managed care called a prepaid plan. This type of coverage was designed initially to help keep people healthy by covering the cost of preventive care, such as medical checkups. The patient selects a primary care doctor, such as a family physician, from an HMO list. This doctor coordinates the patient's care and determines if referrals to specialist doctors are needed. People pay a premium, usually every month, and receive their healthcare services (doctor visits, hospital care, lab work, emergency services, etc.) when they pay a small fee called a copayment. The HMO has arrangements with caregivers and hospitals and the copayment only applies to those caregivers and facilities affiliated with the HMO. This type of coverage offers less freedom than fee-for-service, but out-of-pocket healthcare costs are generally lower and more predictable. A person's out-of-pocket costs will be much higher if he or she receives care outside of the HMO unless prior approval from the HMO is received.

PREFERRED PROVIDER ORGANIZATION (PPO). A PPO combines the benefits of fee-for-service with the features of an HMO. If patients use healthcare providers (doctors, hospitals, etc.) who are part of the PPO network, they will receive coverage for most of their bills after a deductible and perhaps a copayment are met. Some PPOs require people to choose a primary care physician who will coordinate care and arrange referrals to specialists when needed. Other PPOs allow patients to choose specialists on their own. A PPO may offer lower levels of coverage for care given by doctors and other professionals not affiliated with the PPO. In these cases the patient may have to fill out claim forms to receive coverage.

Government health plans

Medicare and Medicaid are two health plans offered by the U.S. government. They are available to individuals who meet certain age, income, or disability criteria. TRICARE Standard, formerly called CHAMPUS, is the health plan for U.S. military personnel.

MEDICARE. Medicare, created in 1965 under Title 18 of the Social Security Act, is available to people who meet certain age and disability criteria. Eligible people include:

- those who are age 65 years and older
- some younger individuals who have disabilities
- those who have end-stage renal disease (permanent kidney failure)

Medicare has several parts: Part A and Part B cover most medical services. Part A is hospital insurance and helps cover the costs of inpatient hospital stays, skilled nursing centers, **home health services**, and **hospice care**. Part B helps cover medical services such as doctors' bills; ambulances; outpatient therapy; and a host of other services, supplies, and equipment that Part A does not cover. Medicare Part C is also called Medicare Advantage, and is offered by private companies. A person covered under Part C receives all Medicare coverage from the private insurer as other Medicare beneficiaries receive under parts A and B, plus some additional services. Costs of the Advantage Plan vary. Medicare Part D is prescription drug coverage.

MEDICAID. Medicaid, created in 1965 under Title 19 of the Social Security Act, is designed for people receiving federal government aid such as Aid to Families with Dependent Children. This program covers hospitalization, doctors' visits, lab tests, and x-rays. Some other services may be partially covered.

TRICARE. Eligible military families may enroll in TRICARE Prime, which is an HMO; TRICARE Extra, which offers an expanded choice of providers; or TRICARE Standard, which is the new name for CHAMPUS.

Supplemental insurance

Supplemental insurance covers expenses that are not paid for by a person's health insurance. Cancer insurance is a specific form of supplemental insurance that covers expenses that are not normally covered by health insurance but are specifically related to cancer treatments.

Workers' compensation

Workers' compensation covers healthcare costs for an injury or illness related to a person's job. Medical conditions that are unrelated to work are not covered under this plan. In some cases an evaluation is done to determine whether or not the medical condition is truly related to a person's employment.

Special concerns

There are a variety of special concerns that people with cancer have regarding health insurance.

Waiting period

Insurance may not take effect immediately upon signing up for a policy. Sometimes a waiting period exists, during which time premiums are not paid and benefits are not available. Healthcare services received during this period are not covered.

Preexisting condition

A preexisting condition, such as cancer, has always been a concern when choosing insurance. If a person received medical advice or treatment for a medical problem within six months of enrolling in new insurance, this condition is called preexisting, and it could be excluded from the new coverage. Under the ACA, health insurers can no longer deny coverage to an adult or child because of a preexisting health condition such as cancer.

Experimental/investigational treatments

Experimental/investigational treatments are often a concern for people with cancer. These treatments may or may not be covered by a person's health insurance. Some states mandate coverage for investigational treatments. People should check with their insurance plans and state insurance boards to determine if coverage is available.

A clinical trial is a type of investigational treatment. Costs involved include patient care costs and research costs. Usual patient care costs that may be covered by insurance

QUESTIONS TO ASK YOUR DOCTOR

- What types of insurance do you accept?
- Does your office file claims for patients?
- Will your office get pre-authorization for procedures where it is required?
- Do you have a list of providers for my type of insurance in case a referral is necessary?
- If an experimental procedure is recommended, what costs will be involved?

are visits to the doctor, stays in the hospital, tests, and other procedures that occur whether a person is part of an experiment or is receiving traditional care. Extra patient care costs that may or may not be covered by insurance are the special tests required as part of the research study.

Health insurance plans have policies regarding coverage for **clinical trials**. People should determine their level of health insurance coverage for clinical trials, and they should learn about the costs associated with a particular study.

In 2000, Medicare began covering certain clinical trials. The trials must meet specific criteria in order to be covered. In eligible trials, federal law now prevents insurers from refusing to let patients take part in trials. There are certain limitations, but most plans must cover trials under the ACA.

Complementary therapies

Complementary cancer therapies are another coverage consideration. A cancer patient undergoing this type of therapy should check with his or her insurance policy regarding coverage.

Cancer screening coverage

The ACA requires all health plans sold in the new health insurance marketplaces to cover cancer screenings such as colorectal screenings and mammograms.

Healthcare regulations

The Health Insurance Portability and Accountability Act (HIPAA), passed by the U.S. Congress in 1996, offers people rights and protections regarding their healthcare plans. Because of HIPAA, there are limits on preexisting condition exclusions, people cannot be discriminated because of health factors, there are special enrollment requirements for people who lose other group

plans or have new dependents, small employers are guaranteed group health plan availability, and all group plans have guaranteed renewal if the employer wishes to renew. In summary these rights and protections include:

- Portability. This is the ability for a person to get new health insurance if a change is desired or needed.
- Availability. This refers to whether or not health insurance must be offered to a person and his or her dependents.
- Renewability. This refers to whether or not a person is able to renew his or her health plan.

The Women's Health and Cancer Rights Act of 1998 requires health insurance plans to cover **breast reconstruction** related to a **mastectomy** if the patient chooses to have reconstruction and if the health plan covered the mastectomy. The law became effective for different health plans on different dates, with the earliest date of effect being October 21, 1998.

Resources

PERIODICALS

Aizer, A. A., et al., "Cancer-Specific Outcomes Among Young Adults Without Health Insurance." *Journal of Clinical Oncology* 32, no. 19 (2014): 2025–30.

OTHER

American Cancer Society. "The Health Care Law: How It Can Help People with Cancer and Their Families." http://www.cancer.org/acs/groups/content/@editorial/documents/document/acspc-026864.pdf (accessed September 25, 2014).

WEBSITES

American Cancer Society. "Health Insurance and Financial Assistance for the Cancer Patient." http://www.cancer.org/treatment/findingandpayingfortreatment/managinginsuranceissues/healthinsuranceandfinancialassistanceforthecancerpatient/index (accessed September 25, 2014).

American Society of Clinical Oncology. "Health Insurance." Cancer.Net. http://www.cancer.net/navigating-cancer-care/financial-considerations/health-insurance (accessed September 25, 2014).

Centers for Medicare and Medicaid Services. "How Do Medicare Advantage Plans Work?" http://www.medicare.gov/sign-up-change-plans/medicare-health-plans/medicare-advantage-plans/how-medicare-advantage-plans-work.html (accessed September 25, 2014).

National Cancer Institute. "Insurance Coverage and Clinical Trials." http://www.cancer.gov/clinicaltrials/learning-about/payingfor/insurance-coverage (accessed September 25, 2014).

Rhonda Cloos, RN
REVISED BY TERESA G. ODLE

Hemolytic anemia

Definition

Hemolytic **anemia** is a form of red blood cell (RBC) deficiency in which the RBCs break down at a faster than normal rate either inside the blood vessels or elsewhere in the body. The term *hemolytic* comes from two Greek words that mean "blood" and "disintegration."

Red blood cells live on average about 120 days in the circulation and then die. They are replaced by new RBCs produced in the bone marrow. What happens in hemolytic anemia is that the bone marrow cannot produce enough RBCs quickly enough to keep pace with their early death. Premature destruction of the RBCs inside the blood vessels is called intravascular hemolytic anemia, while their destruction elsewhere in the body (usually in the spleen and liver) is called extravascular hemolytic anemia. Hemolytic anemia can also be classified according to whether it is inherited or whether it is acquired later in life as a complication of another disease or disorder.

Demographics

The overall incidence of hemolytic anemia is approximately 4 per 100,000 people in the United States and Canada. Hemolytic anemia accounts for about 5% of all cases of anemia.

Most types of hemolytic anemia are not sex-specific or specific to any race or ethnic group. The incidence of hemolytic anemia in other countries is thought to be close to the United States figures.

Description

Red blood cells (erythrocytes) transport oxygen and carbon dioxide in the bloodstream, maintain a normal acid-base balance, and determine how thick or thin the blood is. Hemolytic anemia refers to the premature increased destruction of erythrocytes. Hemolysis is the process in which these erythrocytes rupture with the release of hemoglobin into the plasma, and anemia is a reduced delivery of oxygen to the tissues. Some of the symptoms of hemolytic anemia include nosebleeds, bleeding gums, shortness of breath, **fatigue**, rapid heartbeat, pale skin color or yellow skin color (jaundice), chills, and dark-colored urine.

Risk factors

Risk factors for hemolytic anemia include:

- Race or ethnicity. A few types of inherited hemolytic anemia are more common in some racial or ethnic groups than in others. African Americans are at increased risk of sickle cell anemia, the Amish are at increased risk of pyruvate kinase deficiency, and people of Southeast Asian or Mediterranean ancestry are at increased risk of thalassemia.
- Sex. Men are at increased risk of G6PD deficiency while women over 40 are at increased risk of hemolytic anemia related to lupus and other autoimmune disorders.
- Having certain types of cancer, particularly non-Hodgkin lymphoma and chronic lymphocytic leukemia.
- Having certain viral infections, particularly Epstein-Barr virus (EBV), cytomegalovirus (CMV), and HIV infection.
- Having a form of bacterial pneumonia caused by *Mycoplasma pneumoniae*.
- Exposure to diseases caused by parasites, like malaria and babesiosis.
- Taking high doses of penicillin, methyldopa, ribavirin, or some other medications.
- Having artificial heart valves or extensive vascular surgery.
- Having liver disease.
- Working in an occupation that involves exposure to toxic chemicals or venomous snakes and insects.

Causes and symptoms

Causes

Erythrocyte (red blood cell) formation takes place in the red bone marrow in an adult and in the liver, spleen, and bone marrow of the fetus. Their formation requires an adequate supply of iron, cobalt, copper, amino acids, and certain **vitamins**. When the bone marrow loses its ability to compensate for the destruction of the erythrocytes by increasing their production, hemolytic anemia occurs. There are many types of hemolytic anemia, which are classified according to the location of this inability to produce red blood cells. If the problem lies within the red blood cell itself, it is referred to as an intrinsic factor, and if the problem is outside the red blood cell, it is referred to as an extrinsic factor.

Rh factor incompatibility refers to genetically deter-mined substances capable of producing an **immune response** (antigens). This can cause hemolytic anemia not only during pregnancy when the mother is Rh negative and the fetus is Rh positive, but in mismatched blood transfusions as well. There are a number of industrial poisons that produce hemolytic anemia. These include:

- antimalarial agents
- organic solvents (benzene)

- certain chemotherapies
- hypersensitivity to certain antibiotics
- metals (chromium, platinum salts, nickel, lead, copper)
- pyridium
- arsenic
- some herbs used in traditional Chinese medicines
- intravenous (IV) water (an IV that is not normal or half-normal saline)
- snake bites (if the venom contains hemolytic toxins)

These are all factors external to the red blood cell and thus are extrinsic in nature.

One important extrinsic factor in the cause of hemolytic anemia is in the course of widespread **cancer**, leukemia, **Hodgkin lymphoma**, acute alcoholism, and liver disease. Many of the **chemotherapy** agents (**cisplatin**, **carboplatin**, and nonplatinum drugs) utilized in treating various cancers have side effects that cause a suppression of bone marrow activity, which results in severe hemolytic anemia. In essence, an individual is not only anemic as a result of cancer, but this anemia is worsened by the treatment. Since nausea, vomiting, and lack of appetite are also side effects of chemotherapy, it is extremely difficult for the patient to overcome this type of anemia with diet and supplements. Eventually, severe hemolytic anemia is the end result.

Intrinsic factors would include disorders in the immune response and such genetically inherited disorders as glucose-6-phosphate dehydrogenase (G6PD) deficiency, an essential enzyme. People with this disorder do not display any symptoms until exposed to certain medications or stress. Aspirin and **nonsteroidal anti-inflammatory drugs** (NSAIDs) can precipitate this reaction. This disorder is more common among African American males, with approximately 10% to 14% of the population being affected. Other genetic disorders include sickle cell anemia, thalassemia, and spherocytosis. All of these produce structurally abnormal red blood cells to varying degrees.

Symptoms

The symptoms of hemolytic anemia depend on its severity and to some extent on its cause. People with only mild hemolytic anemia may not have any noticeable symptoms. The most common symptom of moderate to severe hemolytic anemia, however, is fatigue. It is a particularly troublesome symptom in cancer patients. Other symptoms of hemolytic anemia typically include shortness of breath; dizziness, especially when standing up; headache; cold, clammy hands or feet; pale skin, gums, and nail beds; and chest pain. Severe hemolytic anemia may produce jaundice or pain in the upper abdomen from an enlarged spleen. People with sickle cell anemia may also develop leg ulcers and severe pain in different parts of the body.

The low level of red blood cells in the patient's blood means that the heart must work harder to supply the body with oxygenated blood. This extra workload may lead to enlargement of the heart, heart murmurs, or abnormal heart rhythms.

Diagnosis

Hemolytic anemia is usually diagnosed by a combination of a careful patient history and the results of laboratory tests. The doctor will ask the patient about a family history of anemia as well as the patient's occupation; prescription and over-the-counter medications; and a history of liver disease, infections, or heart valve replacement or other procedures that can damage red blood cells. Hemolytic anemia can be diagnosed by family doctors, although in some cases the patient may be referred to a hematologist or infectious diseases specialist.

Examination

An office examination for hemolytic anemia will include listening to the patient's breathing and heartbeat for any irregularities, checking the skin and eyeballs for evidence of discoloration due to jaundice, feeling the patient's abdomen to see whether the spleen and liver are enlarged, and performing a rectal examination to check for occult (hidden) bleeding from the digestive tract.

Tests

There are several different types of blood tests that may be performed to diagnose the severity and cause of the patient's anemia:

- Complete blood count (CBC). This test measures the number of RBCs, white blood cells (WBCs), and platelets in the patient's blood. It also measures the hematocrit (proportion of blood volume occupied by red blood cells) and the amount of hemoglobin in the blood.
- Reticulocyte count. Reticulocytes are immature RBCs. Measuring the number of them in a blood sample tells whether the bone marrow is producing new RBCs at the correct rate.
- Peripheral smear. This test tells the doctor whether the red blood cells have normal or abnormal shapes.
- Coombs test. This test detects the presence of antibodies in the blood that may be destroying red blood cells. It can also be used to test blood prior to transfusions to prevent transfusion reactions.

• Tests for bilirubin (a breakdown product of hemoglobin) and liver function.

If blood tests do not help to diagnose the cause of the patient's hemolytic anemia, the doctor may order tests of the patient's bone marrow and kidney function, or have the patient tested for possible lead poisoning or vitamin deficiencies.

Treatment

Treatment of hemolytic anemia has three goals: stopping the premature destruction of red blood cells, raising the patient's RBC count to a healthy level, and treating the underlying condition. Inherited hemolytic anemias typically require lifelong treatment, while acquired hemolytic anemias often clear up once the cause is identified and treated.

Traditional

The treatment depends upon the cause and severity of the anemia. Medicines like **folic acid** and **corticosteroids** may be used to treat the anemia if it is not severe. Severe hemolytic anemia may be very quickly fatal and immediate hospitalization is required for transfusion of washed and packed red blood cells. Severe anemias can aggravate preexisting heart disease, lung disease, and cerebrovascular disease.

Frequently with cancer treatments, a patient may undergo numerous blood transfusions to make up for the severe anemia suffered as a result of chemotherapy. Researchers investigating ways to enhance the quality of life for chemotherapy patients have primarily looked at controlling pain and loss of appetite (**anorexia**). Recent studies, however, have examined the use of erythropoietin (also called epoetin alfa; a protein hormone that stimulates red blood cell production) in improving fatigue symptoms and enhancing overall quality of life. Once-weekly therapy with erythropoietin was found to increase hemoglobin levels, decrease transfusion requirements, and improve quality of life in patients with cancer and anemia undergoing chemotherapy. The downside of erythropoietin therapy is that it may stimulate some types of tumors and cause them to grow faster. The **National Cancer Institute** (NCI) recommends that cancer patients discuss the risks and benefits of this treatment with their doctor.

Alternative

Avoiding exposure to chemicals that precipitate the reaction; eating natural, whole grain foods; avoiding stress; and taking vitamin supplements can be helpful to patients with hemolytic anemia. With cancer patients, yoga and meditation provide a means of enhancing

---

QUESTIONS TO ASK YOUR DOCTOR

- What is causing the hemolytic anemia?
- How severe is it?
- If it is an inherited form, what are the risks of passing it on to children?
- What treatment do you recommend?
- What are the risks and benefits of the treatment?

---

relaxation, reducing stress, and incorporating visualization for healing. Those patients who attend and participate in support groups have an increased quality of life with better outcomes from mainstream treatments.

Prognosis

The prognosis of hemolytic anemia depends on its cause. Some inherited anemias like sickle cell anemia lead to shortened life spans, while some acquired anemias have an excellent prognosis. Few patients die as a direct result of hemolytic anemia; however, elderly people and those with heart disease are at increased risk of health crises brought about by increased strain on the heart caused by the anemia.

Prevention

Inherited types of hemolytic anemia cannot be prevented, with the exception of G6PD deficiency. People born with this deficiency can avoid fava beans, naphthalene (found in some brands of moth balls), and certain medications as advised by their doctor.

Acquired hemolytic anemia caused by a blood transfusion mismatch can be prevented by careful matching of blood donors and recipients. Hemolytic anemia caused by Rh-factor incompatibility can be prevented by prenatal care during pregnancy.

Resources

BOOKS
Bridges, Kenneth R., and Howard A. Pearson, eds. *Anemias and Other Red Cell Disorders.* New York: McGraw-Hill, 2007.

PERIODICALS
American Academy of Family Physicians. "Information from Your Family Doctor: Thalassemia." *American Family Physician* 80 (August 15, 2009): 371.

Elyassi, C. A., and M.H. Rowshan. "Perioperative Management of the Glucose-6-phosphate Dehydrogenase Deficient

Patient: A Review of Literature." *Anesthesia Progress* 56 (Fall 2009): 86–91.

Khurana, V., et al. "Microangiopathic Hemolytic Anemia Following Disseminated Intravascular Coagulation in Aluminum Phosphide Poisoning." *Indian Journal of Medical Sciences* 63 (June 2009): 257–59.

Kotwal, R.S., et al. "Central Retinal Vein Occlusion in an Army Ranger with Glucose-6-phosphate Dehydrogenase Deficiency." *Journal of Special Operations Medicine* 9 (Summer 2009): 59–63.

Lai, J. I., and W. S. Wang. "Acute Hemolysis After Receiving Oxaliplatin Treatment: A Case Report and Literature Review." *Pharmacy World and Science* 31 (October 2009): 538–41.

Shen, Y. "Autoimmune Hemolytic Anemia Associated with a Formulation of Traditional Chinese Medicines." *American Journal of Health-System Pharmacy* 66 (October 1, 2009): 1701–03.

WEBSITES

National Cancer Institute (NCI). "Fatigue (PDQ®)." http://www.cancer.gov/cancertopics/pdq/supportivecare/fatigue/patient/allpages (accessed November 4, 2014).

National Heart, Lung, and Blood Institute (NHLBI). "Hemolytic Anemia." http://www.nhlbi.nih.gov/health/health-topics/topics/ha (accessed November 4, 2014).

ORGANIZATIONS

American Cancer Society, 250 Williams St. NW, Atlanta, GA 30303, (800) 227-2345, http://www.cancer.org.

American Society of Hematology (ASH), 1900 M Street, NW, Washington, DC 20036, 202-776-0544, Fax: 202-776-0545, http://www.hematology.org.

National Cancer Institute, 9609 Medical Center Dr., BG 9609 MSC 9760, Bethesda, MD 20892-9760, (800) 4-CANCER (422-6237), http://www.cancer.gov.

National Heart, Lung, and Blood Institute, 31 Center Dr. MSC 2486, Bldg. 31, Rm. 5A52, Bethesda, MD 20892, (301) 592-8573, nhlbiinfo@nhlbi.nih.gov, http://www.nhlbi.nih.gov.

Linda K. Bennington, CNS, MSN
Rebecca J. Frey, PhD.

Hemoptysis

Definition

Hemoptysis is the coughing up of blood or bloody sputum from the respiratory tract. It is a symptom of a disease or disorder rather than a disease in its own right. The blood can come from the nose, mouth, throat, airway passages leading from the lungs, or the lungs themselves. Hemoptysis may be either self-limiting or recurrent. Massive hemoptysis is defined as 200–600 mL of blood coughed up within a period of 24 hours or less.

Description

Hemoptysis can range from small quantities of bloody sputum to life-threatening amounts of blood. The patient may or may not have chest pain. Massive hemoptysis is considered a medical emergency. Up to 75 percent of patients with massive hemoptysis die from asphyxiation (lack of oxygen) caused by too much blood in the airway.

Hemoptysis refers specifically to the spitting up of blood that comes from the respiratory tract. Often when persons spit up blood, they are not spitting up blood from the respiratory tract, but from somewhere else. When the blood comes from somewhere other than the respiratory tract, such as from a bloody nose or from the gastrointestinal tract, the symptom is called pseudohemoptysis. Vomiting blood from the gastrointestinal tract, which is called hematemesis, is one type of pseudohemoptysis. It is important to distinguish between true hemoptysis and pseudohemoptysis because they often involve very different parts of the body and the treatments are radically different. Hematemesis differs from hemoptysis in that the vomited blood is usually dark brown or black rather than pink or red, is usually mixed with food particles, and resembles coffee grounds rather than having a liquid or foamy appearance.

Risk factors

Risk factors for hemoptysis include:

• Smoking

• Occupational exposure to asbestos, nickel, or chromium

• Frequent travel to countries where parasitic and other infections are endemic

• HIV infection (This is a risk factor for Kaposi sarcoma of the lung and for such opportunistic infections as aspergillosis.)

• History of bronchitis or other lung disorders

Causes and symptoms

Hemoptysis can be caused by a range of disorders:

• Infections. These include pneumonia; tuberculosis; aspergillosis; and parasitic diseases, including ascariasis, amebiasis, and paragonimiasis. Infection is the most common single cause of hemoptysis in adults, accounting for 60%–70% of cases.

• Tumors that erode blood vessel walls. Cancers associated with hemoptysis include bronchial carcinoma, bronchial adenoma, respiratory tract hemangioma, and occasionally by metastatic cancer to the lungs. Primary lung cancers account for 23% of cases of hemoptysis in North America.

- Drug abuse. Cocaine can cause massive hemoptysis.
- Trauma. Chest injuries can cause bleeding into the lungs.
- Vascular disorders, including aneurysms, pulmonary embolism, and malformations of the blood vessels.
- Bronchitis. Its most common cause is long-term smoking.
- Foreign object(s) in the airway. This is a common cause of hemoptysis in children, second only to upper respiratory infections.
- Blood clotting disorders.
- Bleeding following such surgical procedures as bronchial biopsies and heart catheterization.
- Thoracic endometrial syndrome (TES). TES is a rare disorder marked by endometrial (uterine lining) tissue growing in the tissue covering the lungs or in the airway. A woman with TES will have catamenial hemoptysis, or hemoptysis related to her menstrual periods.

Diagnosis

The diagnosis of hemoptysis is complicated by the number of possible causes. For this reason, the doctor must take a thorough patient history, including the patient's occupation, recent travels, tobacco use, and a history of **cancer** or cancer treatment. It is important for the doctor to distinguish between blood from the lungs and blood coming from the nose, mouth, or digestive tract. Patients may aspirate, or breathe, blood from the nose or stomach into their lungs and cough it up. They may also swallow blood from the chest area and then vomit. The doctor will ask about stomach ulcers, repeated vomiting, liver disease, alcoholism, smoking, tuberculosis, mitral valve disease, or treatment with anticoagulant medications.

Examination

The doctor will examine the patient's nose, throat, mouth, and chest for bleeding from these areas and for signs of chest trauma. The most important consideration is to either identify or rule out bleeding from the upper airway. The doctor also listens to the patient's breathing and heartbeat for indications of heart abnormalities or lung disease. In some cases asking the patient whether they can identify the sensation of the bleeding may help the doctor pinpoint the location.

Tests

Laboratory tests for hemoptysis include blood tests to rule out clotting disorders, and to look for food particles or other evidence that the blood comes from the stomach. Sputum can be tested for fungi, bacteria, or parasites.

Procedures

Chest x-rays and **bronchoscopy** are the most important studies for evaluating hemoptysis. They are used to evaluate the cause, location, and extent of the bleeding. The bronchoscope is a long, flexible tube used to identify tumors or remove foreign objects.

Computed tomography scans (CT scans) are used to detect aneurysms and to confirm x-ray results. Ventilation-perfusion scanning is used to rule out pulmonary embolism. The doctor may also order an angiogram to rule out pulmonary embolism, or to locate a source of bleeding that could not be seen with the bronchoscope.

In spite of the number of different diagnostic tests, the cause of hemoptysis cannot be determined in 30%–40% of cases.

Treatment

Traditional

Massive hemoptysis is a life-threatening emergency that requires treatment in an intensive care unit. The patient will be intubated (the insertion of a tube to help breathing) to protect the airway, and to allow evaluation of the source of the bleeding. Patients with lung cancer, bleeding from an aneurysm (blood clot), or persistent traumatic bleeding require chest surgery.

The goal of treatment for patients with hemoptysis is to stop the bleeding as soon as possible while also treating the cancer or other underlying disorder that is causing the hemoptysis. When large amounts of blood have been lost, the patient may also require intravenous (IV) fluids and/or a blood transfusion.

Mild hemoptysis generally will stop spontaneously and no treatment is necessary, apart from reassurance of the patient that this condition will resolve on its own. Therefore, the general treatment for hemoptysis is to keep the patient calm and to ensure complete bed rest.

In the most severe cases of hemoptysis, surgery to remove the cancer that is causing the spitting up of blood may be necessary to relieve the symptoms of hemoptysis. Other treatment modalities include PDT (**photodynamic therapy**).

Foreign objects in the airway are removed with a bronchoscope.

If the cause of the bleeding cannot be determined, the patient is monitored for further developments.

Drugs

If the coughing that accompanies the hemoptysis is troublesome or aggravating the condition, cough suppressant medications may be recommended.

Patients with tuberculosis, aspergillosis, or bacterial **pneumonia** are given **antibiotics**.

Patients with pain associated with hemoptysis should not be given sedatives or opioid pain relievers (morphine, fentanyl, oxycodone, etc.) because these medications slow down respiration.

Alternative

Inhalation of the fumes of a tea made from the bark of the wild cherry (*Prunus virginiana*) tree has been an herbal remedy for many respiratory tract ailments, including tuberculosis and hemoptysis, among the Native Americans for centuries.

Hydrazine sulfate, a naturally occurring monoamine oxidase inhibitor (MAOI), has also been suggested as a treatment for hemoptysis.

Prognosis

The prognosis depends on the underlying cause. Patients with mild hemoptysis usually recover completely within six months of evaluation. In cases of massive hemoptysis, the mortality rate is about 15%. The rate of bleeding, however, is not a useful predictor of the patient's chances for recovery.

Prevention

Hemoptysis is a condition that is difficult to prevent because it has so many different possible causes. Avoiding or quitting smoking, however, is a preventive measure that can reduce a person's susceptibility to upper respiratory infections and lung cancer—two common causes of hemoptysis.

Resources

BOOKS

Fiebach, Nicholas H., et al, eds. *Principles of Ambulatory Medicine.* Philadelphia: Lippincott Williams and Wilkins, 2007.

Goroll, Allan H., and Albert G. Mulley Jr., eds. *Primary Care Medicine: Office Evaluation and Management of the Adult Patient,* 6th ed. Philadelphia: Wolters Kluwer Health/ Lippincott Williams and Wilkins, 2009.

Porter, Robert S., ed. *The Merck Manual of Patient Symptoms: A Concise, Practical Guide to Etiology, Evaluation, and Treatment.* Whitehouse Station, NJ: Merck Research Laboratories, 2008.

PERIODICALS

Gross, A.M., et al. "Management of Life-threatening Haemoptysis in an Area of High Tuberculosis Incidence." *International Journal of Tuberculosis and Lung Disease* 13 (July 2009): 875–80.

Izumi, N., et al. "Primary Pulmonary Meningioma Presenting with Hemoptysis on Exertion." *Annals of Thoracic Surgery* 88 (August 2009): 647–48.

Lane, M. A., et al. "Human Paragonimiasis in North America Following Ingestion of Raw Crayfish." *Clinical Infectious Diseases* 49 (September 15, 2009): 55–61.

Lau, E.M., et al. "Recombinant Activated Factor VII for Massive Hemoptysis in Patients with Cystic Fibrosis." *Chest* 136 (July 2009): 277–81.

Parker, C.M., et al. "Catamenial Hemoptysis and Pneumothorax in a Patient with Cystic Fibrosis." *Canadian Respiratory Journal* 14 (July-August 2007): 295–97.

Prasad, R., et al. "Lessons from Patients with Hemoptysis Attending a Chest Clinic in India." *Annals of Thoracic Medicine* 4 (January 2009): 10–12.

WEBSITES

A.D.A.M. Medical Encyclopedia. "Coughing Up Blood." MedlinePlus. http://www.nlm.nih.gov/medlineplus/ency/article/003073.htm (accessed November 4, 2014).

ORGANIZATIONS

American Cancer Society, 250 Williams St. NW, Atlanta, GA 30303, (800) 227-2345, http://www.cancer.org.

American College of Emergency Physicians, 1125 Executive Cir., Irving, TX 75038-2522, (972) 550-0911, (800) 798-1822, Fax: (972) 580-2816, membership@acep.org, http://www.acep.org.

American Lung Association, 55 W. Wacker Dr., Ste. 1150, Chicago, IL 60601, (800) LUNG-USA (586-4872), Fax: (202) 452-1805, http://www.lung.org.

Centers for Disease Control and Prevention (CDC), 1600 Clifton Rd., Atlanta, GA 30333, (800) CDC-INFO (232-4636), http://www.cdc.gov.

National Cancer Institute, 9609 Medical Center Dr., BG 9609 MSC 9760, Bethesda, MD 20892-9760, (800) 4-CANCER (422-6237), http://www.cancer.gov.

National Heart, Lung, and Blood Institute, 31 Center Dr. MSC 2486, Bldg. 31, Rm. 5A52, Bethesda, MD 20892, (301) 592-8573, nhlbiinfo@nhlbi.nih.gov, http://www.nhlbi.nih.gov.

Paul A. Johnson, EdM
Rebecca J. Frey, PhD.

Heparin

Definition

Heparin is a drug that helps prevent blood clots from forming and belongs to the family of drugs called anticoagulants (blood thinners), although it does not actually thin the blood. It is sold in the United States under the brand names of Calciparine, Liquaemin, Calciparine, Hepalean, and Heparin Leo, and Calcilean in Canada.

Purpose

Heparin is used to decrease the clotting ability of the blood and to help prevent harmful clots from forming in the blood vessels. Heparin will not dissolve blood clots that have already formed, but it may prevent the clots from becoming larger and causing more serious problems. Heparin possesses several antithrombotic mechanisms. It is often used as a treatment for certain blood vessel, heart, and lung conditions and is also used to prevent blood clotting during open-heart surgery, bypass surgery, and dialysis. Heparin is used in low doses to prevent the formation of blood clots in certain patients, especially those who must have certain types of surgery or who must remain in bed for a long time. It is also used for the long-term treatment of thromboembolic disease, a common side effect of **cancer**.

One of the most common hematological complications is disordered coagulation. Approximately 15% of all cancer patients are affected by thromboembolic disease, which is the second leading cause of death for cancer patients. However, thromboembolic disease may represent only one of many complications in end-stage patients. Thromboembolic disease includes superficial and deep venous thrombosis, pulmonary emboli, thrombosis of venous access devices, arterial thrombosis, and embolism. The cancer itself or cancer treatments may induce coagulation. For example, **chemotherapy** can increase the risk of thromboembolic disease. An

increased risk for arterial thrombosis has been observed with chemotherapy treatment.

Cancer and its treatment can affect all three causes of thromboembolic disease, including the alteration of blood flow, damage to endothelial cells (the cells in blood vessels), and enhancing procoagulants (causing the blood to clot). Cancer can affect blood flow by mechanically affecting blood vessels close to a tumor. In addition, tumors cause **angiogenesis**, which may create complexes of blood vessels that have a disordered appearance and flow (varying in magnitude and direction). Chemotherapy or tumors may directly damage endothelial cells. Procoagulants may be secreted into the blood stream by cancer cells or can be increased on the surface of cancer cells.

KEY TERMS

Angiogenesis—The formation of new blood vessels that occurs naturally under certain circumstances, for example, in the healing of a cut.

Anticoagulant—Anticoagulants are nonhabit-forming medications that prevent the formation of new blood clots and keep existing blood clots from growing larger.

Blood clot—A clump of blood that forms in or around a vessel as a result of coagulation. The formation of blood clots when the body has been cut is essential because without blood clots to cease the bleeding, a person would bleed to death from a relatively small wound.

Coagulation—The blood's natural tendency to clump and stick.

Embolism—An embolism occurs when a clump of material such as a broken-off piece of plaque, a blood clot, or air travels through the bloodstream and becomes lodged in a blood vessel.

Endothelial cells—The cells lining the inside of blood vessels.

Parenteral—Medications administered through intravenous, subcutaneous, or intramuscular injection.

Procoagulants—Inducing the blood to clot.

Thromboembolism—Another word for embolism (see embolism).

Thrombosis—The formation of a blood clot in an artery or vein that may be accompanied by inflammation. If untreated in arteries, thrombosis can lead to death of the nearby tissue.

Antithrombotic treatment, in the form of the low-molecular-weight heparin reviparin, has been shown for the first time to safely improve the outcomes of patients with an acute myocardial infarction. The new findings show that reviparin "clearly improves the outcomes of patients who undergo thrombolysis with streptokinase or urokinase, and it also appears to be a useful adjunct for patients treated with primary percutaneous coronary intervention (PCI)," said Dr. Anderson, associate chief of the division of cardiology at LDS Hospital in Salt Lake City. The study has some limitations.

Description

Heparin is the most common anticoagulant used and the generic name product may be available in the United States and Canada.

Mechanisms of action

Heparin increases the release of specific proteins, like tissue plasminogen activator and tissue factor pathway inhibitor (TFPI), into the blood in order to inhibit blood coagulation. It can also increase the activity of these proteins. Heparin augments the activity of anti-thrombin III, a natural compound that inhibits activated clotting factors from contributing to more coagulation. Furthermore, heparin has been found to inhibit substances that may contribute to angiogenesis, including vascular endothelial growth factor, tissue factor, and platelet-activating factor.

Whether anticoagulants like heparin may also improve cancer survival rates independent of their effect on thromboembolism has been investigated. In fact, experimental and clinical data have demonstrated that heparin is an effective compound in preventing metastases. Many investigators have shown that heparin inhibits tumor **metastasis** in experimental animals; a few **clinical trials** also suggest a positive effect in humans with cancer.

Recommended dosage

Heparin is available only with a doctor's prescription, in parenteral and injection (United States and Canada) dosage forms. A doctor will need to prescribe a specific dose for an individual based on the type of heparin, as well as the patient's medical condition and body weight.

Dosing schedule

Heparin should be taken under the doctor's direction and at the same time every day. If a dose is missed, take it as soon as possible. However, if a dose is missed until the following day, patients should not double-dose, but just take the usual daily dose. Double-dosing may cause bleeding.

Precautions

Some medications should not be combined. Over-the-counter medicines, **vitamins**, and herbal products may cause interactions when combined with heparin, so the patient should check with the doctor monitoring the heparin medication before taking any new medication, even when prescribed by another doctor.

Patients who are pregnant, breastfeeding, using an IUD for birth control, or who have given birth recently should consult their doctors. The doctor should also be notified if radiation treatments, surgery, or a fall or other injury has recently occurred.

The presence of other medical problems may affect the use of heparin. Patients should be sure to tell their doctors about any other medical problems, in particular:

• allergies or asthma (or history of)
• blood disease or bleeding problems
• colitis or stomach ulcer (or history of)
• diabetes mellitus
• high blood pressure (hypertension)
• kidney disease
• liver disease
• tuberculosis (active)

Side effects

The doctor should be contacted immediately if any of these side effects are present:

• wheezing or trouble breathing
• skin rash, itching, or hives
• red or "coffee ground" vomit
• unexplained nosebleeds
• swelling in the face, lips, or tongue
• blood in urine or stools
• black tarry stools

Interactions

Using any of the following medicines together with heparin may increase the risk of bleeding. Again, candidates for heparin should alert their physicians if they are taking any of these medications:

• aspirin
• persantine
• carbenicillin by injection (Geopen)
• cefamandole (Mandol)

- cefoperazone (Cefobid)
- cefotetan (Cefotan)
- dipyridamole (Persantine)
- divalproex (Depakote)
- medicine for inflammation or pain (Motrin, Aleve), except narcotics
- medicine for overactive thyroid
- pentoxifylline (Trental)
- plicamycin (Mithracin)
- probenecid (Benemid)
- sulfinpyrazone (Anturane)
- ticarcillin (Ticar)
- valproic acid (Depakene)
- medicines via intramuscular injection

See also Low molecular weight heparin; Warfarin.

Crystal Heather Kaczkowski, MSc

Hepatic arterial infusion

Definition

Hepatic arterial infusion (HAI) therapy delivers chemotherapeutic agents directly to the liver through a catheter placed in the hepatic artery. The hepatic artery is the main route of blood supply to liver tumors. HAI is also known as regional **chemotherapy**.

Purpose

Approximately 106,000 patients are diagnosed with **colon cancer** in the United States each year. The **cancer** spreads to the liver in about 70% of those patients. For patients with colorectal liver metastases, tumor progression within the liver is typically the primary cause of death.

Systemic chemotherapy using various agents has some efficacy, but the side effects can have a profound negative impact on the patient's quality of life during treatment. HAI therapy may be an effective option because it delivers chemotherapy medication directly to the site of the tumor, making it appropriate as an alternative or adjuvant treatment to systemic chemotherapy. When metastases is limited to the liver, HAI with **floxuridine** (FUDR) or radioactive microspheres through an implantable pump under the skin or an external pump worn on the belt may be a better option than systemic chemotherapy.

KEY TERMS

Adjuvant treatment—A treatment that is added to increase effectiveness of the first treatment.

Cancer—A term for diseases in which abnormal cells divide without control. Cancer cells can invade nearby tissues and can spread through the bloodstream and lymphatic system to other parts of the body.

Catheter—A flexible tube used to administer or withdraw fluids. During a course of chemotherapy, an indwelling catheter can be placed in a vein to administer intravenous fluids and chemotherapy. Catheters can stay in place for several weeks or months with proper care.

Chemotherapy—A cancer treatment using medicines.

Hepatic—Refers to the liver.

Implant—A device inserted into the body to either treat cancer or to replace or substitute for a lost part or ability.

Metastases—The spread of cancer to other body parts.

Tumor—An abnormal mass of tissue that serves no purpose. Tumors may be either benign (noncancerous) or malignant (cancerous).

HAI may extend life expectancy and reduce the chance that more liver tumors will develop.

Precautions

- Strict aseptic techniques should be used to prevent infection during all procedures.

- Pump flow rate will vary depending on factors such as body temperature, altitude, arterial pressure at the catheter tip, and solution viscosity.

- Patients should not attempt to resterilize the pump.

- The manufacturer's instructions should be followed regarding drug preparation, dosage, and administration.

- FUDR should be used with added caution in patients with impaired liver or kidney function.

Systemic therapy should be considered for patients with disease known to extend beyond the area capable of being infused.

Description

HAI enhances cancer therapy by increasing drug delivery directly to the site of the tumor (the liver) while minimizing systemic drug exposure and side effects. Development of fully implanted infusion systems have allowed for long-term delivery of hepatic regional chemotherapy.

Benefits of HAI therapy include:

• yields higher tumor response rates and delays cancer progression
• trend toward increased survival rates
• enhances quality of life
• reduced systemic side effects

Preparation

Patient selection criteria

Successful results depend on careful patient selection. Candidates for HAI therapy should:

• have primary liver cancer or liver metastases from primary colorectal cancer
• show an absence of tumors outside the liver
• have demonstrated portal vein patency
• be a suitable surgical candidate
• show no evidence of infection
• be willing to participate in frequent pump refill appointments

Studies have demonstrated that patients with metastatic colorectal cancer who had liver disease only, had less than 70% of their liver involved with metastases, and had a good performance status responded best to HAI. When metastases are also located outside of the liver, HAI does not offer an advantage over systemic chemotherapy.

Aftercare

During the course of treatment, pump pocket infections occur rarely. At the first sign of infection at the pump pocket, systemic **antibiotics** need to be started. The pump needs to be moved to a new location in a newly created pocket if the infection does not resolve itself. The old pocket should be opened and drained.

Risks

The major problems with HAI are not surgical. They include gastritis, duodenitis, and biliary sclerosis.

Drug toxicity and medication side effects may occur. The most commonly reported side effects for FUDR are **nausea and vomiting**, **diarrhea**, and intestinal inflammation.

Other possible complications include:

• Arterial thromboses.
• Catheter dislodgement.
• The catheter may erode through the wall of the duodenum when the pump has been in place for more than a year.
• Overdose or underdose of medication if certain conditions affect the rate at which the pump delivers medication, i.e., pump damage due to strenuous activity, high heat, or a change in air pressure.
• Disruption in therapy if the pump is damaged by improper handling or filling.

Results

Morbidity or mortality occurring as a result of this procedure should be close to zero. Appropriate selection of patients and new combinations of chemotherapy should provide at least a 70% response rate from HAI for the treatment of hepatic metastases from colorectal primary tumors. This response rate is at least twice that of current systemic chemotherapies.

When used in conjunction with traditional chemotherapy, HAI therapy has been shown to extend life expectancy and reduce recurrence of liver tumors after two years for certain patients.

Abnormal results

Complications that can occur with surgery include:

• infection
• fluid build up around the implant site
• skin erosion over the site of the implant
• incision breakdown
• drugs may be delivered to organs other than the liver

Resources

WEBSITES

University of Southern California Center for Pancreatic and Biliary Diseases. "Hepatic Artery Infusion Chemotherapy (HAI)." http://www.surgery.usc.edu/divisions/tumor/pancreasdiseases/web%20pages/laparoscopic%20liver%20surgery/HAI.html (accessed December 4, 2014).

Crystal Heather Kaczkowski, MS

Hepatocellular carcinoma *see* Liver cancer
Herceptin *see* Trastuzumab

Herpes simplex

Definition

Herpes simplex is a virus that causes blister-like open sores, usually on the mouth or genitals of the infected person.

Demographics

There are two distinct types: herpes simplex virus type 1 (HSV-1) and herpes simplex virus type 2 (HSV-2). Both types of HSV are common worldwide. HSV-1 is transmitted from person to person by close contact, such as kissing. In the United States, by age 30, half of all individuals of high socioeconomic status are infected with HSV-1, and 80% of all individuals of low socioeconomic status carry the virus, although many of those infected do not show symptoms.

HSV-2 is transmitted through sexual contact, thus its distribution is related to the age at which sexual activity begins and the extent of sexual activity within a population. Infection is more common in women than men, and in the United States infection is more common among blacks than whites. As many as 90% of people infected with HSV-2 are unaware that they carry the virus because they have either no symptoms or very mild symptoms. The number of people infected with HSV-2 has been increasing worldwide since the mid-1990s.

Description

HSV-1 usually is associated with infections of the lips, mouth, and face. HSV-1 sores are referred to as oral herpes, cold sores, or **fever** blisters. HSV-2, or genital herpes, is a sexually transmitted disease (STD) and usually is associated with genital ulcers or sores. The first symptoms often occur within 2–20 days after contact with an infected person, although individuals may be infected with HSV-1 and/or HSV-2 and not develop any symptoms or the development of symptoms may be delayed.

Risk factors

Risk factors for HSV-2 infection include having many sexual partners and having unprotected sex. HSV-2 can also be transmitted by oral sex and cause sores on the lips. **Cancer** patients, especially those who are undergoing **chemotherapy** or radiation treatments, are at greater risk of primary (first) and secondary (recurrent) herpes infections, as are individuals with HIV/AIDS or other conditions in which the immune system is weakened.

Causes and symptoms

HSV virus causes sores on mucous membranes, most often in the mouth and in the genital region. Once HSV enters the body it spreads to nearby mucosal areas through nerve cells. Typically, 50%–80% of people with oral herpes experience a prodrome (symptoms of oncoming disease) of pain, burning, **itching**, or tingling at the site where blisters will form. This prodrome stage may last anywhere from a few hours to one to two days. The herpes infection prodrome occurs in both the primary infection and recurrent infections.

Symptoms of the primary infection usually are more severe than those of recurrent infections. The primary infection can cause symptoms similar to those experienced in other viral infections, including lack of energy, headache, fever, and swollen lymph nodes in the neck. The first sign of infection is formation of fluid-filled blisters that may last up to two weeks. However, the pain in the area may last much longer.

Once an individual becomes infected with HSV, the virus remains in the body for the life of that individual. During periods of latency there are no symptoms. At times the infected person may shed the virus, even in the absence of visible symptoms, and infect others. Individuals infected with the virus can have recurrent infections or flare-ups; however, recurrent infections usually have milder and shorter symptoms. Nevertheless, cancer patients and others with compromised immune systems can have severe recurrences and serious complications.

Women who develop their first (primary) HSV-2 infection during pregnancy are at greater risk of delivering babies with birth defects. An active genital herpes sore at the time of birth can cause extremely serious results, including blindness, birth defects, and even death. Cesarean section may be advisable for mothers with active herpes sores at the time of delivery.

Diagnosis

Often, herpes infection is diagnosed from symptoms and by visually examining the sores.

Tests

Testing for neonatal herpes infections may include special smears and/or viral cultures, blood antibody levels, and polymerase chain reaction (PCR) testing of spinal fluid. Cultures are usually obtained from skin vesicles, eyes, mouth, rectum, urine, stool, and blood. For older children and adults, if there is a question as to the cause of a sore, a tissue sample or culture can be taken to determine what type of virus or other microorganism is responsible. For herpes, it is preferable

Herpes simplex

to have this test done within the first 48 hours after symptoms first show up for a more accurate result.

Treatment

Drugs

There is no cure for HSV infection, although antiviral drugs have some effect in lessening the symptoms, decreasing the length of herpes outbreaks, and preventing complications in immunocompromised individuals. There is evidence that some of these drugs, also may prevent future outbreaks. For the best results, drug treatment should begin during the prodrome stage before blisters are visible. Depending upon the length of the outbreak, drug treatment could continue up to ten days.

Acyclovir (Zovirax) is often the drug of choice for herpes infection and can be given intravenously or taken by mouth. It can be applied directly to sores as an ointment but is not very useful in this form. A liquid form for children is also available. Acyclovir is effective in treating both the primary infection and recurrent outbreaks. When taken by mouth to prevent an outbreak, acyclovir reduces the frequency of herpes outbreaks. Other antiviral drugs used to treat HSV infection include penciclovir (Denavir), valacyclovir (Valtrex), and famciclovir (Famvir).

Alternative and complementary therapies

A number of steps may relieve the symptoms of herpes infections. It is important to keep the blisters or sores clean and dry with an agent such as cornstarch. One should avoid touching the sores, and wash hands frequently. Local application of ice may relieve the pain. Over-the-counter medication for fever, pain, and inflammation, such as aspirin, acetaminophen, or ibuprofen, may help. Children should never be given aspirin because of the possible development of Reye's syndrome.

Sexual intercourse should be avoided during both the active stage and the prodrome stages. During an outbreak of cold sores, salty foods, citrus foods (oranges etc.), and other foods that irritate the sores should be avoided. Over-the-counter lip products that contain the chemical "phenol" (such as Blistex Medicated Lip Ointment) and numbing ointments (such as Anbesol) help to relieve the pain of cold sores. A bandage may be placed over the sores to protect them and prevent spreading the virus to other sites on the lips or face.

A diet rich in the amino acid lysine may help prevent recurrences of cold sores. Foods that contain high levels of lysine include most vegetables, legumes, fish, turkey,

QUESTIONS TO ASK YOUR DOCTOR

- How do I know which type of HSV I have?
- How will HSV infection affect my sex life?
- What can I do to help prevent spreading HSV-1 to family members?
- What are the possible serious complications of this infection, and when should I call the doctor?

and chicken. Oral lysine supplements in the amount of 1000 mg per day may help sores heal faster. There is a belief that foods with high lysine-to-arginine ratio will help prevent outbreaks of herpes simplex. That has not been proven, and it is important to include foods that have a low lysine-to-arginine ratio also, such as nuts, onion, garlic, and green vegetables. It is also suggested that the amount of arginine in the diet be limited as there is a belief that arginine is needed for herpes virus growth. This amino acid is found in peanuts, beer, chocolate, gelatin, and raisins.

Prognosis

Infection is permanent. Although symptom-free periods are common, during these times individuals may still shed the virus into their saliva and genital secretions and infect others. Life-threatening neurological complications may occur in individuals who are immunocompromised, and HSV-2 infection during pregnancy and delivery can cause birth defects or serious harm to the infant.

Prevention

It is almost impossible to prevent HSV-1 infection. Limiting the number of sexual partners reduces the likelihood of becoming infected with HSV-2. Using a condom may help discourage infection, but does not fully protect against spread of the virus.

Resources

BOOKS

Ebel, Charles and Anna Wald. *Managing Herpes: Living and Loving with HSV.* Research Triangle Park, NC: American Social Health Association, 2007.

Warren, Terri. *The Good News About the Bad News: Herpes: Everything You Need to Know.* Oakland, CA: New Harbinger Publications, 2009.

WEBSITES

"Genital Herpes." U.S. Centers for Disease Control and Prevention. http://www.cdc.gov/std/Herpes (accessed November 4, 2014).

"Herpes Simplex." MedlinePlus. http://www.nlm.nih.gov/medlineplus/herpessimplex.html. (accessed November 4, 2014).

ORGANIZATIONS

American Social Health Association, PO Box 13827, Research Triangle Park, NC 27709, (919) 361-8400, (800) 227-8922, Fax: (919) 361-8425, http://www.ashastd.org.

National Institute of Allergy and Infectious Diseases Office of Communications and Government Relations, 6610 Rockledge Drive, MSC 6612, Bethesda, MD 20892-6612, (301) 496-5717, (866) 284-4107, TDD: (800) 877-8339 (for hearing impaired), Fax: (301) 402-3573, http://www3.niaid.nih.gov.

Belinda M. Rowland, PhD.

REVISED BY TISH DAVIDSON, AM

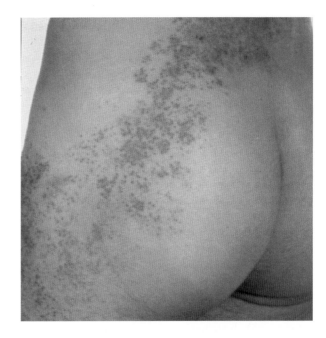

Shingles, or herpes zoster, on patient's buttocks and thigh. *(Wellcome Image Library/Custom Medical Stock Photography)*

Herpes zoster

Description

Herpes zoster, also called shingles, and referred to as "zosteer," gets its name from both the Latin and French words for belt or girdle and refers to belt-like skin eruptions that may occur on the trunk of the body. The virus that causes chickenpox, the varicella zoster virus (VSV), can become dormant in nerve cells after an episode of chickenpox and later reemerge as shingles. Any individual who has had chickenpox can develop shingles. People of all ages, even children, can be affected, but the incidence increases with age. There are many other conditions that can predispose people to developing shingles, including newborn infants, bone marrow and other transplant recipients, and individuals with immune systems weakened by diseases like HIV or **cancer**, or drugs, such as those used in **chemotherapy**.

Shingles erupts along the course of the affected nerve, producing lesions anywhere on the body, and may cause severe nerve pain. The most common areas to be affected are the face and trunk, which correspond to the areas where the chickenpox rash is most concentrated. The disease is caused by a reactivation of the chickenpox virus that has been dormant in certain nerves following an episode of chickenpox. Exactly how or why this reactivation occurs is not clear; however, it is believed that the reactivation is triggered when the immune system becomes weakened as in the examples described above.

Early signs of shingles are often vague and can easily be mistaken for other illnesses. The condition may begin with **fever** and malaise (a vague feeling of weakness or discomfort). Within two to four days, severe pain, **itching**, and numbness/tingling (paresthesia) or extreme sensitivity to touch (hyperesthesia) can develop, usually on the trunk and occasionally on the arms and legs. Pain may be continuous or intermittent, usually lasting from one to four weeks. It may occur at the time of the eruption, but can precede the eruption by days, occasionally making the diagnosis difficult. Signs and symptoms may include the following:

- itching, tingling, or severe burning pain
- red patches that develop into blisters
- grouped, dense, deep, small blisters that ooze and crust
- swollen lymph nodes

Immunocompromised patients usually have a more severe course that is frequently prolonged for weeks to months. They develop shingles frequently and the infection can spread to the skin, lungs, liver, gastrointestinal tract, brain, or other vital organs.

Potentially serious complications can result from herpes zoster. Many individuals continue to experience persistent pain long after the blisters heal. This pain, called postherpetic neuralgia, can be severe and debilitating. Postherpetic neuralgia can persist for months or years after the lesions have disappeared.

Other complications include a secondary bacterial infection, and rarely, potentially fatal inflammation of the brain (encephalitis) and the spread of an infection throughout the body. These rare, but extremely serious, complications are more likely to occur in those individuals who have weakened immune systems (immunocompromised).

Causes

Herpes zoster has been reported in patients with many different types of cancer. However, the cancers that affect an individual's immune system, such as leukemia or **lymphoma**, are the types that place people at particular risk. Herpes zoster is also a particular problem after the various forms of cancer therapy. A study performed in 1998 looked at 766 episodes of herpes zoster infection at a large cancer center from 1972 to 1980. The highest risk of infection was present among patients with lymphoma and leukemia. In those who received radiation treatment and then developed herpes zoster, half of them developed this within seven months. They developed zoster on the area of their body where the radiation was given. This study showed that a period of months can pass before developing zoster as a consequence of radiation. In those who developed zoster after being treated with chemotherapy, half of them developed zoster within a month.

A study in 1999 looked at 215 consecutive patients who had received high-dose chemotherapy and autologous stem cell rescue to help determine what the incidence and severity of herpes zoster infection was. Herpes zoster was developed in 40 people. Over 80% of these infections occurred within six months of receiving the autologous stem cell rescue. Similar rates of herpes zoster have been seen in patients who received bone marrow transplants. A 1996 study looked at 107 children who had received bone marrow transplants for various malignancies. Thirty-three percent of these children developed herpes zoster. Approximately 90% of the cases developed within one year from the time of bone marrow transplant.

Treatment

Shingles almost always resolves spontaneously and may not require any treatment except for the relief of symptoms. In most people, the condition clears on its own in one or two weeks and seldom recurs. The antiviral drugs acyclovir, valacyclovir, and famciclovir can be used to treat shingles. These drugs may shorten the course of the illness. Their use results in more rapid healing of the blisters when drug therapy is started within 72 hours of the onset of the rash. In fact, the earlier the

drugs are administered, the better, because early cases can sometimes be stopped. If taken later, these drugs are less effective but may still lessen the pain. Antiviral drug treatment does not seem to reduce the incidence of postherpetic neuralgia, but recent studies suggest famciclovir may cut the duration of postherpetic neuralgia in half. Side effects of typical oral doses of these antiviral drugs are minor with headache and nausea reported by 8%–20% of patients. Severely immunocompromised individuals, such as those with cancer, may require intravenous administration of antiviral drugs. Preventive administration of acyclovir to seropositive patients (people who have evidence in their blood of past infection with varicella) who undergo leukemia induction or bone marrow transplant not only effectively prevents herpes zoster recurrence but also reduces the severity of chemotherapy-induced **mucositis**. Therefore, acyclovir prophylaxis should be considered in seropositive patients, especially if they have had a recurrence during previous chemotherapy cycles.

Alternative and complementary therapies

Cool, wet compresses may help reduce pain. If there are blisters or crusting, applying compresses made with diluted vinegar will make the patient more comfortable. The patient can mix one-quarter cup of white vinegar in two quarts of lukewarm water, and use the compress twice each day for ten minutes. The patient should stop using the compresses when the blisters have dried up.

Soothing baths and lotions such as colloidal oatmeal baths, starch baths or lotions, and calamine lotion may help to relieve itching and discomfort. The skin should be kept clean, and contaminated items should not be reused. While the lesions continue to ooze, the person should be isolated to prevent infecting other susceptible individuals.

Later, when the crusts and scabs are separating, the skin may become dry, tight, and cracked. If that happens, the patient can rub on a small amount of plain petroleum jelly three or four times a day.

There are non-medical methods of prevention and treatment that may speed recovery. For example, getting lots of rest, eating a healthy diet, exercising regularly, and minimizing stress are always helpful in preventing disease. Supplementation with vitamin B_{12} during the first one to two days and continued supplementation with vitamin B complex, high levels of vitamin C with bioflavonoids, and calcium are recommended to boost the immune system. Herbal antivirals such as echinacea can be effective in fighting infection and boosting the immune system. Patients should consult their physician before taking supplements.

Although no single alternative approach, technique, or remedy has yet been proven to reduce the pain, there are a few options that may be helpful. For example, topical applications of lemon balm (*Melissa officinalis*), licorice (*Glycyrrhiza glabra*), or peppermint (*Mentha piperita*) may reduce pain and blistering. Homeopathic remedies include *Rhus toxicodendron* for blisters, *Mezereum* and *Arsenicum album* for pain, and *Ranunculus* for itching. Practitioners of Eastern medicine recommend self-hypnosis, acupressure, and acupuncture to alleviate pain. All of these or similar alternative therapies should be discussed with the treating physician before using.

See also Antiviral therapy.

Resources

BOOKS

Goldman, L., and D. Ausiello, eds. *Cecil Textbook of Medicine.* 24th ed. Philadelphia: Saunders, 2012.

PERIODICALS

Chiu HF, B. K. Chen, and C. Y. Yang. "Herpes Zoster and Subsequent Risk of Cancer: A Population-Based Study." *Journal of Epidemiology* 23, no. 3 (2013): 205–10.

David Greenberg, MD

Hexalen *see* **Altretamine**

Hickmann lines *see* **Vascular access**

Histamine 2 antagonists

Definition

Histamine 2 antagonists are drugs that block the production of acid in the stomach.

Purpose

Histamine 2 antagonists are used to treat the precancerous condition of **Barrett's esophagus**. They are also used to treat **Zollinger-Ellison syndrome** and **multiple endocrine neoplasia**, rare cancerous conditions in which the stomach makes too much acid, and to prevent the development of gastric (stomach) and duodenal (upper part of the small intestine) ulcers.

Description

Histamine 2 blockers are familiar to most people as the over-the-counter heartburn medications Tagamet (cimetidine), Pepcid (famotidine), and Zantac

---

(ranitidine). Axid (nizatidine) is less well known. These drugs also come in prescription strengths. Histamine 2 blockers work by reducing the amount of acid the stomach produces.

The esophagus is a tube 10–13 inches long and about 1 inch wide that carries food from the mouth to the stomach. Normally, the esophagus is lined with cells that are similar to skin cells and look smooth and pinkish-white.

The stomach makes acid to help digest food. A different type of cell that is resistant to acid lines the stomach. These cells look red and velvety. At the place where the esophagus meets the stomach, there is a ring of muscle called a sphincter that normally keeps acid stomach juices from backflowing into the esophagus. When this sphincter is not working correctly, stomach acid enters the bottom portion of the esophagus. This backflow is called reflux or heartburn. When reflux occurs frequently over an extended period of time, it is called gastroesophageal reflux disease (GERD).

Barrett's esophagus is a precancerous condition in which normal cells lining the esophagus are repeatedly exposed to stomach acid and are replaced with abnormal cells that, in some people, develop into a type of **cancer** of the esophagus called **adenocarcinoma**. Histamine 2 blockers are given to reduce acid in the stomach and eliminate exposure of the esophageal cells to acid.

Histamine 2 blockers are also used to treat two rare cancerous conditions: multiple endocrine neoplasia (MEN) and Zollinger-Ellison syndrome, both of which can cause the stomach to produce too much acid. In MEN, an inherited form of cancer, tumors form in more than one gland. Depending on which glands are affected, the stomach may be stimulated to produce excess acid. In Zollinger-Ellison syndrome, a tumor in the digestive tract secretes a hormone called gastrin that stimulates the production of stomach acid. These tumors are malignant (cancerous) in 50%–65% of people with Zollinger-Ellison syndrome.

Histamine 2 blockers are sometimes given in advance of **chemotherapy** to help reduce the gastrointestinal side effects of chemotherapy drugs. Cimetidine was the first histamine 2 blocker approved by the United States Food and Drug Administration (FDA) in 1976.

Recommended dosage

Recommended dose varies depending on how much stomach acid is produced. Histamine 2 blockers are available in low doses without a prescription and in higher doses with a prescription. They are available in tablet, chewable tablet, liquid, and injectable liquid form. In 2004, the FDA also approved a 25 mg effervescent tablet form of ranitidine (Zantac 25 Efferdose). If histamine 2 inhibitors are unsuccessful in controlling acid reflux, proton pump inhibitors (Prevacid, Prilosec) are usually given as an alternative.

Precautions

People who have trouble with heartburn should stay away from acidic foods such as orange, grapefruit, and tomato juice; coffee; and carbonated drinks (sodas) because these all increase stomach acid. Waiting at least two hours after eating before lying down, avoiding smoking, limiting drinking of alcohol, losing excess weight, and avoiding wearing tight-fitting clothes are other ways to prevent heartburn. Although animal studies show that histamine 2 blockers appear to be safe during pregnancy, these drugs pass into breast milk and should not be taken by nursing mothers.

Side effects

Histamine 2 blockers have few side effects. These drugs are excreted by the kidney, and may slow the excretion of other drugs excreted by the kidney. People with reduced kidney function may need a reduced dose of histamine 2 blockers.

Rare cases of irregular heart rhythms and high blood pressure have been reported when histamine 2 blockers are given intravenously (IV, injected directly into a vein). Mild **diarrhea** has been reported by some people taking these drugs.

Interactions

Histamine 2 blockers are reported to have few interactions with other drugs. However, because they reduce the level of acid in the stomach, they may inhibit the uptake of drugs such as ketoconazole that depend on an acid environment in the stomach to work. These drugs should be administered at least two hours before histamine 2 blockers are taken. Prior to starting any over-the-counter medications, herbal medications, or new medications, patients should notify their physician and check with their pharmacists for any potential drug interactions.

Resources

WEBSITES

Micromedex. "Histamine H2 Antagonist (Oral Route, Injection Route, Intravenous Route)." MayoClinic.com. http://www. mayoclinic.org/drugs-supplements/histamine-h2-antagonist-oral-route-injection-route-intravenous-route/description/DRG-20068584 (accessed December 4, 2014).

Tish Davidson, AM

HIV-related cancers *see* **AIDS-related cancers**

Hodgkin lymphoma

Definition

Hodgkin **lymphoma** is a rare **cancer** of the lymphatic system, an important part of the body's immune system.

Description

Hodgkin lymphoma, also called Hodgkin disease, was first described in 1832 by Thomas Hodgkin, a British physician. Hodgkin clearly differentiated this disease from the much more common non-Hodgkin lymphomas, showing that Hodgkin lymphoma was localized, diagnosed early, and was without extranodal (outside the lymph nodes) involvement, whereas **non-Hodgkin lymphoma** was typically diagnosed late and was widespread throughout the lymph system with extranodal involvement. Prior to 1970, few individuals survived Hodgkin lymphoma, but now the majority of individuals who develop this cancer can be cured.

The lymphatic system

The lymphatic system is the part of the body's immune system that functions in fighting disease and producing blood cells. It includes lymph or lymphatic fluid that circulates through the system; the lymph vessels and nodes that contain the lymphatic fluid; and the spleen, bone marrow, and thymus. The narrow lymphatic vessels carry lymphatic fluid throughout the body. The lymph nodes are small organs or glands that filter the lymphatic fluid and trap foreign substances, including viruses and bacteria that have invaded the body and cancer cells that have developed within the body.

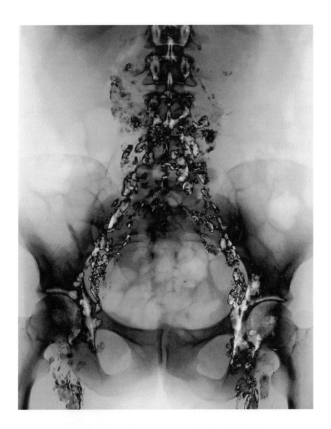

X-ray revealing growths caused by Hodgkin lymphoma (shown in blue). *(Zephyr/Science Source)*

The spleen, in the upper left abdomen, removes old cells and debris from circulating blood, filters the blood, and destroys old cells. As a result of its activity, it stores a quantity of blood at any given time. The bone marrow, the tissue inside the bones, produces new red and white blood cells.

Lymphocytes are white blood cells that recognize and destroy disease-causing organisms. Lymphocytes of many types are produced in the lymph nodes, spleen, and bone marrow. They circulate throughout the body in the blood and lymphatic fluid. Clusters of immune cells also exist in major organs as a safety network, prepared to respond to invading organisms or abnormal cells.

Hodgkin lymphoma

Hodgkin lymphoma is a malignancy of the antibody-producing cells (B-cell lymphocytes) of the lymphatic system that undergo transformation and develop into specific cells called Reed-Sternberg cells, named for the doctors who first identified them. Uncontrolled growth of these cells usually begins in a single lymph node and progresses slowly and predictably to spread via the lymphatic vessels from one group of lymph nodes, to the next in an orderly manner. Sometimes the abnormal cells invade organs adjacent to the lymph nodes, but involvement outside the lymph system is less common

in Hodgkin lymphoma than in non-Hodgkin lymphoma. If the cancer cells do spread into the bloodstream, the disease can reach almost any site in the body and advanced cases may involve the spleen, liver, bone marrow, or lungs. Because Hodgkin lymphoma is typically diagnosed early, early treatment prevents spreading (**metastasis**) of this type in a majority of cases.

Different subtypes of Hodgkin lymphoma include:

• nodular sclerosis, the classic Hodgkin lymphoma (30%–60% of cases)

• mixed cellularity (20%–40% of cases)

• nodular lymphocyte predominant (5%–10% of cases)

• lymphocyte depleted (less than 5% of cases)

• lymphocyte predominant (about 3% of cases)

Risk factors

A family history of Hodgkin lymphoma and the presence of the Epstein-Barr virus are associated with an increased risk for developing Hodgkin lymphoma. Individuals with acquired immunodeficiency syndrome (AIDS) also are particularly susceptible. Otherwise few risk factors are associated with the disease.

Special concerns

Follow-up examinations continue for many years following treatment for Hodgkin lymphoma. Women who have had chest irradiation must have frequent mammograms and clinical and breast self-examinations for early detection of breast cancer. Frequent physical exams and chest x-rays may help to detect lung or thyroid cancer. Treatment with mantle field radiation causes hyperthyroidism, which may require thyroid medication and annual thyroid function tests.

Individuals with Hodgkin lymphoma do not have normal immune system function. Susceptibility to infection also can be intensified by chemotherapy, radiation, and removal of the spleen. Therefore, vaccinations and prompt treatment of infections are exceptionally important for people with Hodgkin lymphoma.

Demographics

The American Cancer Society estimated that 9,100 new cases of Hodgkin lymphoma would be diagnosed in the United States in 2014—affecting about 3,900 females and 5,200 males in a male-to-female ratio of 1.4:1, including in children. About 1,180 patients die of the disease annually.

Hodgkin disease can occur at any age but is rarely diagnosed before age 10. Approximately 10%–15% of cases are in children and young teens under age 17. The

KEY TERMS

Antibody—An immune system protein that recognizes a specific foreign molecule (antigen) on the surface of cells.

Biopsy—The removal of a small sample of tissue for pathologic examination under a microscope; used for the diagnosis of cancer and to check for infection.

Bone marrow—Tissue inside the bones that produces red and white blood cells.

Chemotherapy—Treatment with various combinations of cytotoxic chemicals or drugs that destroy cells or affect cellular activity, particularly applied for the treatment of cancer and autoimmune diseases.

Epstein-Barr virus (EBV)—A common virus that infects immune cells and is responsible for causing mononucleosis.

Interferon—A potent immune-defense protein produced by viral-infected cells; used as an anticancer and antiviral drug.

Interleukins—A family of potent immune-defense molecules; used in various clinical therapies.

Laparotomy—A surgical incision of the abdomen.

Leukapheresis—A technique that uses a machine to remove stem cells from the blood; the cells are frozen and then returned to the patient following treatment that has destroyed the bone marrow.

Lymph nodes—Small round glands, located throughout the body and containing lymphocytes that remove foreign organisms and debris from the lymphatic fluid.

Lymphatic system—The vessels, lymph nodes, and organs, including the bone marrow, spleen, and thymus, that produce and carry white blood cells to fight disease.

Lymphocyte—White blood cells that produce antibodies and other agents for fighting disease.

PBSCT—Peripheral blood stem cell transplant; a method for replacing blood-forming cells that are destroyed by cancer treatment.

Radiotherapy—Disease treatment involving exposure to x-rays or other types of radiation.

Reed-Sternberg cells—An abnormal binuclear lymphocyte that is characteristic of Hodgkin disease.

Spleen—An organ of the lymphatic system, on the left side of the abdomen near the stomach; it produces and stores lymphocytes, filters the blood, and destroys old blood cells.

Splenectomy—Surgical removal of the spleen.

Staging—The use of various diagnostic methods to accurately determine the extent of disease; used to select the appropriate type and amount of treatment and to predict the outcome of treatment.

Stem cells—The cells from which all blood cells are derived.

Thymus—An organ of the lymphatic system, located behind the breast bone, that produces the T lymphocytes of the immune system.

Thyroid—A gland in the throat that produces hormones that regulate growth and metabolism.

---

majority of cases develop in early adulthood (ages 15–40) and another peak occurs in people aged 50–60.

Causes and symptoms

The cause of Hodgkin lymphoma is not known. It is suspected that interaction between an individual's genetic makeup, environmental exposure (e.g., occupations such as woodworking), a history of infection (e.g., **Epstein-Barr virus** infection, *Mycobacterium tuberculosis*, herpes virus, or HIV), or toxic agents (e.g., prior treatment with **phenytoin**, radiation, or **chemotherapy**) may be responsible. Immune system deficiencies also may increase risk, including congenital immunodeficiency disorders or deficiencies resulting from taking immunosuppressive drugs for treatment of certain autoimmune diseases (e.g., rheumatoid arthritis,

lupus erythematosis, celiac sprue) or post-transplant immunosuppression to avoid organ rejection.

Painless, swollen lymph glands in the neck, under the arms, or in the groin are the most common early symptom of Hodgkin lymphoma, although as many as 75% of individuals diagnosed with Hodgkin lymphoma do not have any typical symptoms. Other early symptoms of Hodgkin lymphoma may be constitutional (multiple symptoms that affect the whole body) similar to those of the flu:

- fevers, night sweats, chills
- fatigue
- loss of appetite (anorexia)
- weight loss
- itching

- pain after drinking alcoholic beverages
- swelling of one or more lymph nodes

Sudden or emergency symptoms of more advanced Hodgkin lymphoma that has already spread through the lymphatic system include:

- sudden high fever
- loss of bladder and/or bowel control
- enlarged liver and/or spleen
- numbness in the arms and legs and loss of strength

As lymph nodes swell with the presence of tumor masses, they may compress other nearby structures, causing a variety of symptoms:

- pain due to pressure on nerve roots
- loss of function in muscle groups served by compressed nerves
- coughing or shortness of breath due to compression of the windpipe and/or airways by swollen lymph nodes in the chest
- kidney failure from compression of the ureters, the tubes that carry urine from the kidneys to the bladder
- swelling in the face, neck, or legs due to pressure on veins
- paralysis in the legs due to pressure on the spinal cord

As Hodgkin lymphoma progresses, the immune system becomes less effective at fighting infection. The disease is noted for a slowly progressive defect in T-cell activity that may lead to bacterial, viral, and fungal infections and, in advanced disease, may lead to systemic infection in the blood (sepsis).

Diagnosis

As with many forms of cancer, diagnosis of Hodgkin lymphoma has two major components:

- identification of the specific cells that cause Hodgkin lymphoma in order to confirm the diagnosis
- staging of the disease to determine whether the disease is localized or has spread (metastasized) throughout the lymphatic system or outside the lymphatic system

The initial diagnosis of Hodgkin lymphoma often results from abnormalities noted in a chest x-ray that was performed because of nonspecific symptoms. A detailed medical history will be taken to review symptoms, history of previous illnesses, medications and procedures, and family medical history. A complete physical examination will be performed, especially to check for swollen lymph nodes throughout the body, as well as laboratory tests of the blood and urine (complete blood count, alkaline phosphatase, lactic dehydrogenase, liver function tests, albumin, calcium, blood urea nitrogen, and creatinine); an immunohistochemical evaluation; a chest x-ray; **computed tomography** (CT) scans of chest, abdomen, and pelvis; and **lymph node biopsy**. Sometimes a **bone marrow biopsy** will also be done. **Positron emission tomography** (PET) scans will likely be done for disease staging and **magnetic resonance imaging** (MRI) will be done if symptoms of nerve compression are present.

Lymph node biopsy

The size, tenderness, firmness, and location of swollen lymph nodes are determined during physical examination and correlated with any signs of infection. If **antibiotics** are given, lymph nodes that do not shrink after treatment may be a cause for concern. The lymph nodes that are most often affected by Hodgkin lymphoma include those of the neck, above the collarbone, under the arms, and in the chest above the diaphragm.

Diagnosis of Hodgkin lymphoma requires either the removal of an entire enlarged lymph node (an excisional **biopsy**) or an incisional biopsy, in which only a small part of a large tumor is removed. These require a surgical procedure and, if the node is near the skin, a local anesthetic will be used. However, if it is inside the chest or abdomen, laparoscopic surgery will be performed and general anesthesia is required.

The sample of biopsied tissue is prepared on a glass slide, stained and examined under a microscope. Giant cells with two nuclei (binuclear) called Reed-Sternberg cells must be present to confirm a diagnosis of Hodgkin lymphoma. Normal cells have only one nucleus (the organelle within the cell that contains the genetic material). Affected lymph nodes may contain only a few Reed-Sternberg cells and may be difficult to recognize, or more may be present in more widespread disease. Characteristics of other types of cells in the biopsied tissue help to diagnose the four subtypes of Hodgkin disease (nodular sclerosis, mixed-cellularity, lymphocyte-rich, lymphocyte-depleted) or rarely, a lymphocyte-predominant classification. Identification of certain proteins (antigens) on the surfaces of cancer cells or changes in the genetic make-up (DNA) of cells may be done to differentiate Hodgkin lymphoma from non-Hodgkin lymphoma.

A fine needle aspiration (FNA) biopsy, in which a thin needle and syringe are used to remove a small amount of fluid and bits of tissue from a tumor, has the advantage of not requiring surgery. An FNA may be performed prior to an excisional or incisional biopsy to see if the swelling is being caused by an infection or the metastasis of cancer from another organ. An excisional biopsy will still need to be performed to confirm the diagnosis.

Clinical staging

Clinical staging is part of the diagnostic workup but is also the basis for determining appropriate treatment and monitoring therapy once it begins. The presenting symptoms, results of physical examination and imaging tests (x-ray, CT, MRI, PET), and biopsies are sufficient to stage the disease and laparotomy (pathological staging) is usually not necessary. Cardiac and pulmonary function tests may be needed in some individuals to help determine therapy.

IMAGING. Imaging of the abdomen, chest, and pelvis is performed to identify areas of enlarged lymph nodes and abnormalities in the spleen or other organs. CT scanning uses a rotating x-ray beam to obtain multiple images of specific areas of the body, while MRI uses magnetic fields and radio waves to produce images. Chest **x-rays** also are taken to find enlarged nodes in the chest cavity. The various images may reveal rounded lumps called tumor nodules in the affected lymph nodes and other organs.

PET scans are extremely accurate in staging Hodgkin lymphoma or monitoring the effectiveness of therapy. A very low dose of radioactive glucose (a type of sugar) is injected into the body. The glucose travels to metabolically active sites, including cancerous regions that require large amounts of glucose. The PET scan detects the radioactivity and produces images of the entire body that are able to clearly distinguish between cancerous and non-cancerous tissues.

BONE MARROW BIOPSY. Anemia (a low red-blood-cell count and low hemoglobin) and iron deficiency, fevers, or **night sweats** are indications that Hodgkin disease may involve the bone marrow. In these cases, a **bone marrow aspiration and biopsy** may be ordered. For a bone marrow biopsy, a large needle is used to remove a narrow, cylindrical piece of bone. Alternatively, an aspiration may be used, in which a needle is used to remove small bits of bone marrow from the back of the hip or another large bone such as the sternum in the chest. This procedure helps to determine if the cancer has spread.

Treatment team

The cancer care team for Hodgkin lymphoma includes a medical oncologist (a physician specializing in cancer), oncology nurses, clinical laboratory technologists, and social workers. A surgeon performs the biopsies, as well as the laparotomy and **splenectomy** if required. Pathologists examine the biopsy specimens for the presence of Reed-Sternberg and other abnormal cells.

In the United States, most children with Hodgkin lymphoma are treated at children's cancer centers. Here, the treatment team includes a pediatric oncologist along with psychologists, child life specialists, nutritionists, and nurse educators.

Clinical staging

Staging of the disease is mainly done to decide on the most appropriate treatment course. Since most treatments for Hodgkin lymphoma have serious short- or long-term side effects, accurate staging is necessary so that physicians and patients can choose the least traumatic treatment approach to cure the disease. The staging system for Hodgkin disease is a modified Ann Arbor Staging Classification called the Cotswold System.

Hodgkin lymphoma is divided into four stages, with additional substages:

- Stage I: The disease is confined to one lymph node area.
- Stage IE: The disease extends from the one lymph node area to adjacent regions.
- Stage II: The disease is in two or more lymph node areas on one side of the diaphragm (the muscle below the lungs).
- Stage IIE: The disease extends to adjacent regions of at least one of the affected nodes.
- Stage III: The disease is in lymph node areas on both sides of the diaphragm.
- Stage IIIE/IIISE: The disease extends into adjacent areas or organs (IIIE) and/or the spleen (IIISE).
- Stage IV: The disease has spread from the lymphatic system to one or more other organs, such as the bone marrow, lungs, or liver.

Treatment for Hodgkin lymphoma depends both on the stage of the disease and whether or not symptoms are present. When treatment is underway, the presence of symptoms will correlate with the response to treatment. Stages of the disease are labeled with an A if no systemic symptoms are present. If one or more systemic symptoms are present, the stage is labeled with a B. These symptoms include:

- loss of more than 10% of body weight over the previous six months
- fevers above 100° F (37.8° C)
- drenching night sweats

Treatment

Chemotherapy

Chemotherapy is the mainstay of treatment for Hodgkin lymphoma. It typically utilizes a combination of drugs, each of which kills cancer cells in a different way. The drugs may be delivered together intravenously over a period of time or directly into a vein or muscle, or taken orally in pill or liquid form. Stages I and II are generally treated with a short-term chemotherapy regimen referred to as ABVD (Adriamycin or doxorubicin, **bleomycin, vincristine**, and **dacarbazine**). This may be accompanied with or followed by **radiation therapy** or a longer course of chemotherapy. This treatment regimen is curative for about 80% of patients.

Stages IIIA and IIIB are also treated with ABVD combination chemotherapy alone with good results. Cure rates of up to 80% have been achieved with this combination. Even patients with the more advanced stages IVA and IVB may receive ABVD, which is reported to achieve complete remission in 75%–80% of patients. Other drug combinations for these later stages include BEACOPP (bleomycin, **etoposide, doxorubicin, cyclophosphamide**, vincristine [Oncovin], **procarbazine**, and prednisone). Chemotherapy may continue for a longer time in advanced disease with metastases, and it may be combined with radiation.

The side effects of chemotherapy for Hodgkin lymphoma depend on the drug dosage and the length of time they are taken. Since these drugs target rapidly dividing cancer cells, they also affect the rapid growth of normal cells such as cells of the bone marrow, linings of the mouth and intestines, and hair follicles. Damage to bone marrow leads to anemia with **fatigue** and bruising, lower white blood cell counts, and lower resistance to infection. Damage to intestinal cells leads to a loss of appetite and associated **weight loss (anorexia)**, and **nausea and vomiting**. Mouth sores and hair loss **(alopecia)** also are common side effects of chemotherapy. These side effects disappear when the chemotherapy is discontinued. Drugs may be given that help to reduce or prevent the nausea and vomiting.

Chemotherapy for Hodgkin lymphoma may lead to long-term complications. The drugs may damage the heart, lungs, kidneys, and liver. In children, growth may be impeded. Some chemotherapy can cause sterility, so men may choose to have their sperm frozen prior to treatment. Women may stop ovulating and menstruating during chemotherapy. This may or may not be permanent.

Radiation therapy

Radiation therapy is sometimes used during or following chemotherapy but combined treatment is usually reserved for treating more advanced disease. External-beam radiation, a focused beam from an external machine, is used to irradiate only the affected lymph nodes. Specific types include involved-field radiation therapy (IFRT), involved-node radiation therapy, and involved-site radiation therapy (ISRT). ISRT is replacing IFRT as the standard method, as ISRT reduces the size of the radiation field so that noncancerous tissue is not exposed.

Since external-beam radiation damages healthy tissue near the cancer cells, the temporary side effects of radiotherapy can include sunburn-like skin damage, fatigue, nausea, and **diarrhea**. Other temporary side effects may include a sore throat and difficulty swallowing. Long-term side effects depend on the dose and the location of the radiation and the age of the patient. Since radiation of the ovaries causes permanent sterility (the inability to have children), the ovaries of girls and young women are protected during radiotherapy. Sometimes the ovaries are surgically moved from the region being irradiated, a process known as transposition of the ovaries or oophoropexy. Other fertility preservation techniques, such as semen cryopreservation and in vitro fertilization, may be an option for women who still wish to have children.

Children who are sexually mature when they develop Hodgkin lymphoma, and whose muscle and bone mass are almost completely developed, usually receive the same treatment as adults. Younger children usually are treated with chemotherapy, since radiation will adversely affect bone and muscle growth. However, radiation may be used in low dosages in combination with chemotherapy. The chemotherapy for children with Hodgkin lymphoma may include combinations of more drugs, such as the BEACOPP regimen.

The development of a secondary cancer is the most serious risk from radiation and chemotherapy treatment for Hodgkin lymphoma. In particular, there is a risk of developing leukemia, **breast cancer**, bone cancer, or **thyroid cancer**. Chemotherapy or chemotherapy in conjunction with radiotherapy increases the risk for acute leukemia, whereas other cancers (such as of the lung, breast, stomach, and head and neck region) are associated with the use of radiotherapy. However, researchers are finding that the distinction between leukemia and lymphoma is narrow and many clinical characteristics are similar. It was once thought that lymphoma was restricted to the lymphatic system and leukemia to the bone marrow, but this is not always true, which has spurred additional study.

Resistant, progressive, and recurrent Hodgkin lymphoma

During and following treatment, the original diagnostic tests for Hodgkin lymphoma are repeated to monitor the effects of therapy and to determine whether all traces of the cancer have been eliminated. The tests will also reveal clinical effects of the treatment. In resistant Hodgkin lymphoma, some cancer cells remain following treatment. If the cancer continues to spread during treatment, it is called progressive Hodgkin lymphoma. If the disease returns after treatment, it is known as recurrent Hodgkin lymphoma. It may recur in the area where it first started or elsewhere in the body. It may recur immediately after treatment or many years later.

Additional treatment is necessary with resistant or recurrent Hodgkin lymphoma. Chemotherapy with different drugs, or higher doses, may be used to treat recurrent disease. However, radiation to the same area is never repeated.

Bone marrow and peripheral blood stem cell transplantations

An autologous bone marrow and/or a peripheral blood **stem cell transplantation** (PBSCT) using cells from the patient being treated is often recommended for treating resistant or recurrent Hodgkin disease, particularly if the disease recurs within a few months of a chemotherapy-induced remission. The patient's bone marrow cells or peripheral blood stem cells (immature bone marrow cells found in the blood) are collected and frozen prior to high-dosage chemotherapy that will destroy bone marrow cells. A procedure called leukapheresis is used to collect the stem cells. After the patient has received the high-dosage chemotherapy, and possibly radiation, the bone marrow cells or stem cells that were removed prior to treatment are reinfused into the patient intravenously.

Immunologic therapies, also known as immunotherapies, biological therapies, or biological response modifier therapies, utilize substances that are normally produced by the immune system. These include interferon (an immune system protein), **monoclonal antibodies** (specially engineered antibodies), colony-stimulating (growth) factors (such as **filgrastim**), and vaccines. Many immunotherapies for Hodgkin lymphoma are experimental and available only through **clinical trials**.

Alternative and complementary therapies

Most complementary therapies for Hodgkin lymphoma are designed to stimulate the immune system to destroy cancer cells and repair normal cells that have been damaged by treatment. These therapies are used in conjunction with standard treatment.

Coenzyme Q10 (CoQ10) and polysaccharide K (PSK) are being evaluated for their ability to stimulate the immune system and protect healthy tissue, as well as possible anti cancer activities. Camphor, also known as 714-X; green tea; and hoxsey (which is a mixture of a number of substances) have been promoted as immune system enhancers. However, there is no evidence that they are effective against Hodgkin lymphoma.

Coping with cancer treatment

Sufficient rest and good nutrition are important for relieving the side effects of treatment for Hodgkin lymphoma. As strength returns, patients are advised to begin a weekly exercise routine. Support groups may be helpful in dealing with emotional problems that may arise during treatment.

Prognosis

Hodgkin lymphoma, particularly in children, is one of the most curable forms of cancer. Approximately 90% of individuals are cured of the disease after receiving various regimens of chemotherapy, sometimes with radiation.

The one-year relative survival rate following treatment for Hodgkin lymphoma is 93%. Relative survival rates do not include individuals who die of causes other than Hodgkin lymphoma. The five-year survival rate is 90%–95% for those with stage I or stage II disease, 85%–90% for those diagnosed with stage III, and approximately 80% for those diagnosed with stage IV disease. The 15-year relative survival rate is 63%. Approximately 75% of children are alive and cancer-free 20 years after the original diagnosis of Hodgkin lymphoma. Patients who do not have complete remission or have resistant or recurrent Hodgkin lymphoma have a poorer prognosis.

Acute myelocytic leukemia, an exceptionally serious cancer, may develop in as many as 2%–6% of individuals receiving certain types of treatment for Hodgkin lymphoma. Women under the age of 30 who are treated with radiation to the chest have a much higher risk for developing breast cancer. Both men and women are at higher risk for developing lung or thyroid cancers as a result of chest irradiation.

Individuals with the more common type of Hodgkin lymphoma known as nodular lymphocytic predominant have a 2% chance of developing non-Hodgkin lymphoma. This is associated with the mechanism of Hodgkin lymphoma itself and not a result of treatment.

Clinical trials

Many clinical trials for specific treatments of Hodgkin lymphoma are recruiting or planning to recruit participants. Most of these studies are investigating drugs (**gemcitabine**, bendamustine, panobinostat, lenalidomide) for treating resistant (refractory) or recurrent (relapsed) Hodgkin lymphoma in both children and adults. Some are aimed at specific stages or subtypes of Hodgkin lymphoma. Some trials are for previously treated individuals and others are for those who have not yet received treatment. Several cancer organizations help patients and their families find suitable clinical trials.

Genetic studies in children and adults with Hodgkin lymphoma are ongoing and quality-of-life studies in children who are undergoing treatment are also underway.

See also Amenorrhea; Bone marrow transplantation; Childhood cancers; Fertility and cancer; Imaging studies; Immune response; Immunohistochemistry.

Resources

BOOKS

Bartlett, Nancy L., Kelley V. Foyil. "Hodgkin Lymphoma." In *Abeloff's Clinical Oncology*, edited by Martin D. Abeloff. 5th ed. New York: W.B. Saunders, 2013.

Porter, Robert S., MD, and Justin L. Kaplan, MD, eds. "Hodgkin Lymphoma; Section 9, Hematology and Oncology." In *The Merck Manual of Diagnosis and Therapy*. 19th ed. Whitehouse Station, NJ: Merck Research Laboratories, 2011.

PERIODICALS

Mulvihill, David J., et al. "Involved-Nodal Radiation Therapy Leads to Lower Doses to Critical Organs-At-Risk Compared To Involved-Field Radiation Therapy." *Radiotherapy and Oncology* (July 28, 2014): e-pub ahead of print. http://dx.doi.org/10.1016/j.radonc.2014.06.018 (accessed August 14, 2014).

Specht, Lena, et al. "Modern Radiation Therapy for Hodgkin Lymphoma: Field and Dose Guidelines From the International Lymphoma Radiation Oncology Group (ILROG)." *International Journal of Radiation Oncology, Biology, Physics* 89, no. 4 (2014): 854–62. http://dx.doi.org/10.1016/j.ijrobp.2013.05.005 (accessed August 14, 2014).

Terenziani, M., et al. "Oophoropexy: A Relevant Role in Preservation of Ovarian Function After Pelvic Irradiation." *Fertility and Sterility* 91, no. 3 (2009): 935.e16–16. http://dx.doi.org/10.1016/j.fertnstert.2008.09.029 (accessed August 14, 2014).

WEBSITES

American Cancer Society. "How is Hodgkin Disease Diagnosed?" http://www.cancer.org/cancer/hodgkindisease/detailedguide/hodgkin-disease-diagnosis (accessed August 14, 2014).

American Cancer Society. "Radiation Therapy for Hodgkin Disease." http://www.cancer.org/cancer/hodgkindisease/detailedguide/hodgkin-disease-treating-radiation (accessed August 14, 2014).

Mayo Clinic staff. "Hodgkin's Lymphoma." Mayo Clinic. http://www.mayoclinic.org/diseases-conditions/hodgkins-lymphoma/basics/definition/CON-20030667 (accessed October 31, 2014).

National Cancer Institute. "Adult Hodgkin Lymphoma Treatment." http://www.cancer.gov/cancertopics/pdq/treatment/adulthodgkins/HealthProfessional/page1/AllPages (accessed August 14, 2014).

ORGANIZATIONS

American Cancer Society, 1599 Clifton Rd., NE, Atlanta, GA 30329, (404) 320-3333, (800) ACS-2345 (227-2345), http://www.cancer.org.

ClinicalTrials.gov, A service of the U.S. National Institutes of Health, 8600 Rockville Pike, Bethesda, MD 20894, http://clinicaltrials.gov.

The Leukemia and Lymphoma Society, 600 Third Avenue, New York, NY 10016, (914) 949-5213, (800) 955-4572, http://www.leukemia-lymphoma.org.

The Lymphoma Research Foundation of America, Inc., 8800 Venice Boulevard, Suite 207, Los Angeles, CA 90034, (310) 204-7040, http://www.lymphoma.org.

National Cancer Institute, Public Inquiries Office, Building 31, Room 10A31, 31 Center Drive, MSC 2580, Bethesda, MD 20892-2580, (800) 4-CANCER (422-6237), http://www.nci.nih.gov.

Rosalyn S. Carson-DeWitt, MD
Margaret Alic, PhD.
REVISED BY L. LEE CULVERT
REVIEWED BY MELINDA GRANGER OBERLEITNER,
RN, DNS, APRN, CNS

Home health services

Definition

Home health services refers to those healthcare services provided to the patient in his or her own home.

Description

Home health services can vary depending on the insurance coverage, but usually include nursing, **physical therapy**, occupational therapy, speech therapy, home health aides, social work, nutritional education, infusion therapy, blood drawing, and other laboratory services. Such services may also include bringing medical equipment into the home for patient use. Home health services do not provide around-the-clock care, but rely on the patient having other caregivers, such as family members, friends, or other community resources.

Home care services can be provided by many different organizations, such as the Visiting Nurses Association (VNA), home health agencies (which vary in the range of services provided), hospice organizations, providers of home medical equipment, and pharmacies with delivery services. Patients requiring a range of specialized services may find more continuity of care if one agency is able to provide all, or almost all, of the services they need. **Hospice care** is care provided to patients who are terminally ill. Most hospices care for their clients within the home. The goal of hospice is to help the client and their family deal with the physical, emotional, and spiritual issues associated with dying. Excellent **pain management** is a priority.

Nursing care

Skilled nursing care provides the backbone for home care. Visits may include wound and ostomy care; infusion therapy such as home **chemotherapy**, **antibiotics**, or home parenteral nutrition (HPN); patient and caregiver teaching; ongoing assessment of the client's physical and emotional condition and progress; pain control; psychological support; and supervision of home health aides. The nurse may function as a case manager and coordinate the various other services the client is receiving. The nurse assesses the home environment for safety and for appropriateness of continued home care.

Physical therapy

Physical therapists develop a plan for the client to restore (as much as possible) the physical condition lost following surgery or as a result of a decline due to the disease process. They also teach patients how to prevent further injury or deterioration and how to maintain gains made.

Occupational therapy

Occupational therapists assist patients in restoring or enhancing their ability to perform their tasks of daily living. Patients may need to learn how to use adaptive equipment such as a prosthesis. The goal is to achieve the highest level of functioning possible.

Speech therapy

Speech therapists work with clients who have difficulty swallowing or clearly communicating.

Home health aides

Home health aides function under the supervision of a registered nurse. They provide care with personal hygiene, such as bathing and dressing, feeding, and ambulating. They may assist a nurse in providing patient care. They may provide homemaking services and companionship, or those tasks may be covered by a homemaker or attendant.

Social work

Social workers may assist clients in accessing the services that are available to them based on their insurance, and in learning what community resources exist. They may also facilitate the referral process, and provide counseling and patient advocacy.

Nutritional education

Nutritionists and registered dieticians may educate clients on their nutritional needs, and on how to go about attaining them. They may also be involved if HPN is required.

Infusion therapy

Some patients may receive their chemotherapy or antibiotics at home, or may require infusion of liquid nutrition (HPN). While these services may be provided by a nurse, a separate agency or company may provide the equipment and products.

Laboratory work

Blood drawing and other laboratory services may be provided by a nurse, a phlebotomist, or a laboratory technician.

Home medical equipment

Following surgery or treatment in a hospital, patients may need the delivery and servicing of items such as special beds, wheelchairs, walkers, catheters, and wound care and ostomy supplies.

Volunteers

Volunteers may provide a range of assistance such as respite care for the primary caregiver(s), caring for the home, cooking, cleaning, emotional support, companionship, running errands, making telephone calls, child care, elder care, and providing transportation. They may come from the patient's circle of friends or religious organization, or from such agencies as Meals on Wheels.

Causes

Many individuals with conditions that do not necessitate care in a hospital setting often require short-term or long-term home care. They may need care to assist them in regaining their health similar to that prior to their illness, or may need ongoing care as their condition deteriorates due to metastatic disease. One trend that is gathering speed is an increase in home healthcare services as opposed to nursing home care.

Special concerns

Insurance coverage plays a major role in funding home health care. In organizing home care the patient must fully understand which services will be fully covered, covered but with a co-payment, or not covered at all. Insurance coverage may vary depending on whether the service provider is within a specified approved network. It must also be clear how often and for how long the services will be needed, and whether the insurance benefits cover the entire time period of anticipated care. The patient's safety must always remain a priority. The patient and the caregiver(s) may suffer from isolation and **depression**. Primary caregivers may become overwhelmed with caring for the patient, and there may come a point at which the level of care needed may no longer be able to be provided in the home setting. The health of the primary caregiver must periodically be assessed.

Treatment

Treatments provided in the home include wound and ostomy care; intravenous (IV) chemotherapy or antibiotics; HPN; and physical, occupational, and speech therapy.

Newer trends and future concerns

One trend in home health care is greater use of the telephone and Internet for contact between home healthcare workers and medical professionals, and for information gathering. The U.S. Department of Health and Human Services has sponsored a new website intended to help consumers as well as professionals make informed choices about home healthcare agencies. In addition, the growth of so-called telehealth systems has already had an impact on nursing education and practice in the home healthcare field. The field of telehealth is expected to continue to expand dramatically, as experts estimate that home health care is 10–15 years behind other fields in its use of computers.

Another trend is the growing emphasis on culturally sensitive home health care. In many cases, patients from minority ethnic groups and cultures are more comfortable being cared for in their homes by caregivers who share their background or have been trained to understand it than being sent to large urban nursing homes where they are isolated from familiar customs and language. Studies of the feasibility of home health care for Native Americans in remote locations are presently being conducted in Canada.

One worrisome concern for the future is the increasing difficulty of recruiting and retaining high-quality home healthcare workers in the United States and Canada. The aging of the general North American population coupled with the high turnover in the field of home health care poses a serious problem for policy makers.

Alternative and complementary therapies

Clients may contract to have home acupuncture or massage therapy. On their own they may engage in yoga, t'ai chi, meditation, guided imagery, visualization, or other stress-reducing techniques that help them better cope with their situation. They may also choose to investigate herbal supplements and medications; all supplemental medications should be approved by a physician before use.

Resources

BOOKS

Levin, Bernard. *American Cancer Society: Colorectal Cancer.* New York: Villard Books, 1999.

Runowicz, Carolyn D., Jeanne A. Petrek, and Ted S. Gansler. *American Cancer Society: Women and Cancer.* New York: Villard Books/Random House, 1999.

Teeley, Peter, and Philip Bashe. *The Complete Cancer Survival Guide.* New York: Doubleday, 2000.

PERIODICALS

Applebaum, R. A., S. A. Mehdizadeh, and J. K. Straker. "The Changing World of Long-Term Care: A State Perspective." *Journal of Aging and Social Policy* 16 (January 2004): 1–19.

Fermazin, M., M. O. Canady, P. R. Milmine, et al. "Home Health Compare: Web Site Offers Critical Information to Consumers, Professionals." *Lippincott's Case Management* 9 (March-April 2004): 89–95.

Hotson, K. E., S. M. Macdonald, and B. D. Martin. "Understanding Death and Dying in Select First Nations Communities in Northern Manitoba: Issues of Culture and Remote Service Delivery in Palliative Care." *International Journal of Circumpolar Health* 63 (March 2004): 25–38.

Lee, H., and M. Cameron. "Respite Care for People with Dementia and Their Carers." *Cochrane Database Systems Review.* February 2004: CD004396.

Stone, R. I. "The Direct Care Worker: The Third Rail of Home Care Policy." *Annual Review of Public Health* 25 (2004): 521–537.

Williams, K. "Preparing Nurses for Telehealth: A Home Health Care Example." *Medinfo.* 2004 (CD): 1998.

WEBSITES

American Cancer Society. "Home Care Agencies." http://www.cancer.org/treatment/findingandpayingfortreatment/choosingyourtreatmentteam/homecareagencies/index (accessed December 4, 2014).

National Cancer Institute. "Home Care for Cancer Patients." http://www.cancer.gov/cancertopics/factsheet/support/home-care (accessed December 4, 2014).

ORGANIZATIONS

American Cancer Society, 250 Williams St. NW, Atlanta, GA 30303, (800) 227-2345, http://www.cancer.org.

National Association for Home Care & Hospice, 228 Seventh St. SE, Washington, DC 20003, (202) 547-7424, Fax: (202) 547-3540, http://www.nahc.org.

National Cancer Institute, 9609 Medical Center Dr., BG 9609 MSC 9760, Bethesda, MD 20892-9760, (800) 4-CANCER (422-6237), http://www.cancer.gov.

Visiting Nurse Associations of America, 2121 Crystal Dr., Ste. 750, Arlington, VA 22202, (571) 527-1520, (888) 866-8773, Fax: (571) 527-1521, vnaa@vnaa.org, http://vnaa.org.

Esther Csapo Rastegari, RN, BSN, EdM
Rebecca J. Frey, PhD.

Horner syndrome

Description

William Edmonds Horner (1793–1853) first described a small muscle at the angle of the eyelid (tensor tarsi) as well as a description of an ingenious operation to correct problems with the lower lid in 1824 in the *American Journal of the Medical Sciences*. Since that time, his name has been associated with the syndrome of a small, regular pupil; drooping of the eyelid on the same side; and occasional loss of sweat formation on the forehead of the affected eye. In appearance, it occurs on one side of the face with a sinking in of the eyeball (enophthalmos), drooping upper eyelid (ptosis), slight elevation of the lower lid, excessive contraction of the pupil of the eye (miosis), narrowing of the eyelid, and an absence of facial sweat on the affected side (anhidrosis). Other symptoms may include a variation in color of the iris and changes in the consistency of tears.

Causes

Horner syndrome is caused by damage or interruption of the sympathetic nerve to the eye. There are two major divisions of the nervous system: the voluntary (conscious control) and involuntary (without conscious control). The involuntary (autonomic nervous system) has two divisions: sympathetic and parasympathetic nervous systems. Under normal conditions, there is a fine balance between sympathetic and parasympathetic stimulation. If an individual is threatened by a situation, the pupils dilate, blood is shifted to the muscles, and the heart beats faster as the person prepares to fight or flee. This is sympathetic stimulation. The eye has both sympathetic (responds to challenges) and parasympathetic (slows the body down) innervation. The nerve that carries the sympathetic innervation travels down the spinal cord from the brain (hypothalamus), emerges in the chest cavity, and then finds it way up the neck along with the carotid artery and jugular vein through the middle ear and into the eye. If these sympathetic impulses were blocked, the eye would have an overbalance of parasympathetic supply, which would result in a constriction of the pupil, relaxation of all the muscles around the eye, and a sinking of the eye into the orbit— Horner syndrome. Thus, damage that occurs anywhere along the course of this nerve's route from the brain to the eye can evoke this syndrome.

If the syndrome exists from birth (congenital), it is typically noted around the age of two years with the presence of a variation in the color of the iris and the lack of a crease in the drooping eye. Since eye color is completed by the age of two, a variation in color is an uncommon finding in Horner syndrome acquired later in life.

The common causes of acquired Horner syndrome include aortic dissection (a tear in the wall of the aorta to create a false channel where blood becomes trapped), carotid dissection, tuberculosis, Pancoast tumor (a tumor in the upper end of the lung), **brain tumors**, spinal cord injury in the neck, trauma to the cervical or thoracic portions of the spinal cord, cluster migraine headache, vertebrae destruction or collapse, compression of the spinal cord by enlarged lymph nodes, and neck or thyroid surgery.

The diagnosis and localization of this disorder is made with the use of pharmacological testing by an ophthalmologist. The physician places drops of a 10% liquid cocaine into the eyes, blocking the parasympathetic nerves so the sympathetic nervous system can be evaluated. After thirty minutes, the dilation of the pupils is noted and a Horner pupil dilates poorly. A positive cocaine test does not, however, localize the area of the damage. After waiting for 48 hours, other medications are used to determine where the nerve interruption occurs. This solution routinely has been hydroxyamphetamine bromide. However, it has not been routinely available and in 2004, a study reported that a phenylephrine solution works as well. An individual's urine can test positive for cocaine up to two days following the initial test.

Treatment

Treatment for congenital cases

Children who are diagnosed with Horner syndrome of a congenital origin may undergo surgical correction to strengthen the muscle of the eyelid and give it an appearance similar to the unaffected eye. The surgery improves the appearance of the child but does not alleviate the syndrome. For these cases a plastic surgeon may be preferred. Occasionally Horner syndrome may be seen in a newborn with a **neuroblastoma** (tumor originating from nerve cells). This is almost always a sign of a localized tumor and is associated with a relatively good prognosis. In these cases, a neurologist may be consulted for treatment since their specialty is the nervous system.

Treatment for acquired cases

The treatment for acquired Horner syndrome depends upon the cause and is focused toward eliminating the disease that produces the syndrome. Frequently, there is no treatment that improves or reverses the condition, but recognition of the signs and symptoms is extremely important for early diagnosis and treatment. Early detection of the syndrome may facilitate treatment related to those caused by tumors as they can be removed before extensive damage is done. Causes related to an interruption in nerve transmission once the nerve leaves the spinal cord are usually related to blood circulation and are easier to treat. Any numbness or paralysis on one side of the body means the problem is within the spinal cord or brain and is more difficult to treat. Some acquired Horner may be corrected slightly by plastic surgery for appearance changes.

Alternative and complementary therapies

Acupuncture may be utilized to enhance disruptions in nerve transmissions and herbs or supplements that improve circulation may benefit some cases of acquired syndrome. These herbs and supplements would include Ginkgo biloba and vitamin E. As with any complementary treatment, patients should notify their physician of any herbal or over-the-counter medications they are taking.

Resources

BOOKS

Jarvis, Carolyn. *Physical Examination and Health Assessment.* Philadelphia: W.B. Saunders Company, 2000.

PERIODICALS

Danesh-Meyer, H.V., P. Savino, and R. Sergott. "The Correlation of Phenylephrine 1% with Hydroxyamphetamine 1% in Horner's Syndrome." *British Journal of Ophthalmology* April 2004: 592–594.

WEBSITES

Handbook of Ocular Disease Management. (cited July 6, 2005). http://www.revoptom.com.

Linda K. Bennington, CNS, MSN
Teresa G. Odle

Hospice care

Definition

Hospice care is palliative care given to individuals who are terminally ill with an expected survival of six months or less. The focus of hospice care is on meeting the physical, emotional, and spiritual needs of the dying individual, while fostering the highest quality of life possible. Although certain treatments or medications are given, the emphasis is on the patient's comfort rather than cure.

Description

Hospice services provide palliative care to individuals with a life expectancy of six months or less. Most hospice care is provided in the home, but also may take place in a hospice center or a hospice/palliative care unit

within an acute care or long-term care facility. Almost all **cancer** centers have a palliative care unit for cancer patients who are in an advanced stage and no longer receiving treatment. Requesting hospice care may be the first indication that individuals, or their families, acknowledge that their conditions are not treatable. It may be the first time they have to deal with their pending deaths as a reality that may take place within a few months. The emotional journey necessary to address these issues can take time, and therefore may delay the transfer from cancer treatment to hospice care.

The focus of hospice is not on treatment, but on pain and symptom management, comfort measures, supporting the family, and trying to provide the best quality of life for the time remaining. Hospice adopts the philosophy that although some terminally ill patients may no longer receive treatment, they still require and deserve care. Sometimes, when patients transfer to hospice care, they are less anxious and begin to feel better even without continued treatment.

Hospice care is interdisciplinary in nature, providing the services of physicians; psychologists; nurses; healthcare aides; social workers; and physical, speech, or occupational therapists. Addressing the spiritual needs of the hospice client is a fundamental aspect of hospice care. Clergy or spiritual guides of the patient's choice are available as needed. Home hospice care relies on the family and friends of the patient to provide most of the daily care. Nursing and other services are provided daily or weekly, with 24-hour, 7-days-a-week on-call access.

Hospice care was first established in the United States in 1974 in Branford, Connecticut. The Branford hospice was patterned on St. Christopher's Hospice in London, which was established by Dame Cicely Saunders in 1967. In 1969, the book *On Death and Dying*, by Dr. Elizabeth Kubler-Ross, identified five emotional stages that a terminally ill person experiences. In the book, Dr. Kubler-Ross addressed the importance of patients having a role in the decisions affecting the quality of their life and death. In 1972, she testified at the first U.S. Senate national hearing on dying with dignity.

Deciding on hospice care is a choice made by someone who is terminally ill. To be eligible, the patient's physician needs to document that survival is predicted to be six months or less. Should the patient recover, and the prognosis change, the relationship with hospice is terminated, but can be reestablished if needed at a later date. Not all patients will choose hospice. If only home hospice care is available, individuals who would be eligible may decide that hospice is not a good choice for them. Reasons for not choosing home hospice include:

• The patient lives alone, with little or no family support available.

• The patient has a need for 24-hour nursing care.

• The patient has family, but they are unable to provide the supportive care required.

• The patient is concerned about being a burden to the caregiver.

• The patient feels more secure in a hospital environment.

Hospice has been slow to adopt videophones, an aspect of telemedicine, to help care for patients who receive hospice care at home. Neither nurses nor hospice agencies have yet fully endorsed the videophones or provided them for patients. However, telemedicine has been shown to supplement face-to-face visits by nurses and provide an additional tool to help nurses work with family caregivers and patients and to be available for support between visits.

Ethnically and culturally sensitive hospice care is sometimes available. While hospice services in the United States and Canada were used disproportionately

QUESTIONS TO ASK YOUR DOCTOR

• What is my prognosis?

• What choices do I have to manage my pain and other symptoms?

• What level of symptom management can I expect to receive?

• What types of care, conventional or complementary, might improve my quality of life during the time I have left?

• Will my insurance cover the care you suggest?

• If I choose hospice care, how will that affect my relationship with my doctors and treatment team?

• What kind of support is there for my family until I die and afterwards?

by Caucasians before 2004, some cities and institutions have developed more culturally sensitive programs. One innovative Native American hospice program is working well delivering palliative care at the Pueblo of Zuni in New Mexico. The Zuni program combines tribal-based home health care with inpatient care at an Indian Health Service (IHS) hospital.

Treatment

Hospice provides palliative care; curative treatments are discontinued. However, hospice places great importance on minimizing or alleviating pain and symptoms such as loss of appetite, **fatigue**, weakness, fluid retention, constipation, difficulty breathing, confusion, nausea, vomiting, cough, and dry or sore mouth. For many people with advanced cancer, fatigue may be the worst symptom. Research has shown that a tailored exercise program or forms of **physical therapy** can increase activity tolerance without increasing fatigue. In addition, hospice patients have reported an increase in quality of life and decreased anxiety. Many hospice patients have breakthrough pain in addition to their chronic pain. Research has shown that an indwelling subcutaneous needle for delivery of pain medications provided pain control in 88% of patients whose pain was not well controlled with oral medications. Chronic pain requires continuous pain relief such as that provided with a pump or patch. Patients who previously received **chemotherapy** may have a port through which pain medication such as morphine may be administered continuously around the clock or as needed.

Night respite service is an additional hospice service offered by volunteers or home health caregivers. This overnight service allows the patient's family caregiver a few hours or a weekend away from direct patient care. Night respite care in a hospice setting involves trained aides who care for the patient in his or her home overnight, thus allowing other family members to catch up on necessary sleep. Studies indicate that many patients as well as family members feel that night respite care is a good option that allows patients to remain at home rather than being transferred to an inpatient hospice.

Because time is limited for patients receiving hospice care, patients and their caregivers, whether family or professional, are advised to respond swiftly concerning areas of dissatisfaction, such as the quality of care being provided or insufficient symptom management.

Complementary therapies

Dealing with issues surrounding death may be addressed through talking with others; writing in a journal; or creative expression such as painting, writing poetry, or composing music. Meditation may be beneficial to some patients. Gentle body movement practices such as t'ai chi or yoga may be helpful, depending on the patient's activity tolerance.

Special concerns

Some issues that patients express concern over when nearing the end of life include:

- remaining mentally aware

- feeling as though they are a burden on family and caregivers

- having funeral arrangements planned

- helping other patients in similar circumstances

- finding spiritual peace

- looking toward freedom from pain

- talking about and coming to terms with the meaning of death

Resources

BOOKS

Teeley, Peter and Philip Bashe. *The Complete Cancer Survival Guide*. New York: Doubleday, 2000.

PERIODICALS

Dean, S., K. Libby, W. J. McAuley, and J. Van Nostrand. "Access to bereavement services in hospice." *Omega* 69 (January 2014): 79–92.

Finke, B., T. Bowannie, and J. Kitzes. "Palliative Care in the Pueblo of Zuni." *Journal of Palliative Medicine* 7 (February 2004): 135–143.

Kristjanson, L. J., K. Cousins, K. White, et al. "Evaluation of a Night Respite Community Palliative Care Service." *International Journal of Palliative Nursing* 10 (February 2004): 84–90.

Lyke, J., and M. Colon. "Practical Recommendations for Ethnically and Racially Sensitive Hospice Services." *American Journal of Hospice and Palliative Care* 21 (March-April 2004): 131–133.

Quest, T. E., C. A. Marco, and A. R. Derse. "Hospice and palliative medicine: new subspecialty, new opportunities." *Annals of Emergency Medicine* 54 (July 2009): 94–102.

Strand, J. J., J. K. Mandel, and K. M. Swetz. "The growth of palliative care." *Minnesota Medicine* 97 (June 2014): 39–43.

Whitten, P., B. Holtz, E. Meyer, and S. Nazione. "Telehospice: reasons for slow adoption in home hospice care." *Journal of Telemedicine and Telecare* 15 (April 2009): 187–190.

ORGANIZATIONS

American Academy of Hospice and Palliative Medicine (AAHPM), 8735 W. Higgins Rd., Ste. 300, Chicago, IL 60631, (847) 375-4712, Fax: (847) 375-6475, info@aahpm.org, http://aahpm.org.

American Cancer Society, 250 Williams St. NW, Atlanta, GA 30303, (800) 227-2345, http://www.cancer.org.

Hospice Foundation of America, 1710 Rhode Island Ave. NW, Suite 400, Washington, DC 20036, (202) 457-5811, (800) 854-3402, http://hospicefoundation.org.

National Association for Home Care & Hospice, 228 Seventh St. SE, Washington, DC 20003, (202) 547-7424, Fax: (202) 547-3540, http://www.nahc.org.

National Cancer Institute, 9609 Medical Center Dr., BG 9609 MSC 9760, Bethesda, MD 20892-9760, (800) 4-CANCER (422-6237), http://www.cancer.gov.

L. Lee Culvert
Esther Csapo Rastegari, RN, BSN, EdM
Rebecca J. Frey, PhD.

HPV *see* **Human papillomavirus**

Human growth factors

Definition

Human growth factors are compounds made by the body that function to regulate cell division and cell survival. Some growth factors are also produced in the laboratory by genetic engineering and are used in biological therapy.

Description

Human tumors express large amounts of growth factors and their receptors. A tumor will not grow beyond the size of a pinhead without new blood vessels to supply oxygen and nutrients. Growth factors are significant because they can induce **angiogenesis**, the formation of blood vessels around a tumor. These growth factors also encourage cell proliferation, differentiation, and migration on the surfaces of the endothelial cells—cells found inside the lining of blood vessels. Of the approximately 20 proteins that activate endothelial cell growth, two growth factors in particular, vascular endothelial growth factor (VEGF) and basic fibroblast growth factor (bFGF), are expressed by many tumors and appear important in contributing to tumor growth and promoting tumor spread throughout the body. Several compounds that block VEGF or its receptor are now in **clinical trials**.

See also Angiogenesis inhibitors.

Crystal Heather Kaczkowski, MSc

Human papillomavirus

Definition

Human papillomavirus or human papilloma virus—commonly called HPV—is a large group of related viruses that infect the skin and mucous membranes. While some types of HPV cause common warts on various parts of the body, more than 40 types are sexually transmitted infections (STIs) of the male and female genitals, anus, mouth, and throat. Some of these HPV types can cause cervical and other cancers.

Description

There are more than 150 known types of HPV that can cause different types of warts on various parts of the body, including sexually transmitted genital warts in the pubic area and between the thighs. Most HPV infections, including most sexually transmitted HPVs, do not cause symptoms or health problems, and 90% disappear on their own within two years, especially in children. However, persistent infection with some types of HPV can cause **cervical cancer** and less common but serious cancers of the vulva, vagina, penis, anus, and oropharynx. HPV is also associated with a threefold increased risk for **esophageal cancer**.

Sexually transmitted HPVs that preferentially infect the mucosal surfaces of the genitals are classified into low-risk and high-risk or oncogenic types. Soft genital warts, which are quite common, are usually caused by low-risk HPV types 6 and 11. They do not cause **cancer**. Although high-risk HPV types do not usually cause cancer, they are associated with an increased risk for the development of precancerous lesions and, if untreated, the possible development of cervical and other cancers. Type 16 is the most common high-risk HPV. Infection with high-risk HPV is common in adolescents and women in their 20s, and abnormal cervical cells containing high-risk HPV types are most often observed in Pap smears of women over age 30. Most of these infections disappear on their own in one or two years, although such transient infections may cause temporary abnormalities in cervical cells. Persistent high-risk HPV infections can lead to more serious cell abnormalities and lesions that, if untreated, may progress to cancer. About 10% of women with high-risk HPV in their cervical tissues will develop long-lasting infections that put them at risk for cervical cancer.

HPV vaccination coverage among U.S. adolescents 13–17 years

Year	Girls		Boys	
	% Initiated (≥1 dose)	% Completed	% Initiated (≥1 dose)	% Completed
2011	53.0	34.8	8.3	1.3
2012	53.8	33.4	20.8	6.8
2013	57.3	37.6	34.6	13.9

SOURCE: Stokley, Shannon, et al., "Human Papillomavirus Vaccination Coverage Among Adolescents, 2007–2013, and Postlicensure Vaccine Safety Monitoring, 2006–2014—United States," *Morbidity and Mortality Weekly Report (MMWR)* 63, no. 29 (July 25, 2014). Available online at: http://www.cdc.gov/mmwr/preview/mmwrhtml/mm6329a3.htm.

Table listing HPV vaccination rates among U.S. adolescents from 2011 to 2013. (*Table by Lumina Datamatics Ltd. © 2015 Cengage Learning®.*)

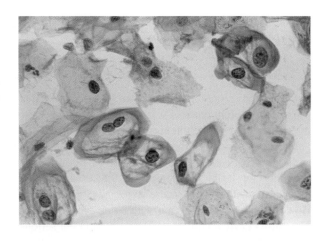

Light micrograph of cervical cells infected with human papillomavirus (HPV). HPV has been associated with the development of cervical cancer, as well as some oral cancers. *(SPL/Science Source)*

High-risk sexually transmitted HPV causes about 5% of all cancers worldwide, including essentially all cervical cancers, 90% of anal cancers, and 40% of vaginal and vulvar cancers. There are at least 12 high-risk HPV types, but types 16 and 18 cause about 70% of cervical cancers and almost half of vaginal, vulvar, and penile cancers. More than half of oropharyngeal cancers and about 85% of anal cancers are associated with HPV-16. Colorectal cancer, which is much more common than **anal cancer**, is not caused by HPV.

Demographics

Genital HPV is the most common STI in the United States. Most sexually active people become infected with at least one type of genital HPV at some point. In 2013, about 79 million Americans—primarily those in their late teens and early 20s—were infected, and about 14 million Americans are newly infected each year. At any given time, 42.5% of women have a genital HPV infection. Fewer than 7% of adults have oral HPV infections.

Each year in the United States, HPV causes about 19,000 cancers in women and about 8,000 cancers in men, including an estimated:

• 10,300 cervical cancers in women and 4,000 deaths

• 2,100 vulvar cancers

• 500 vaginal cancers

• 2,800 anal cancers in women

• 1,500 anal cancers in men

• 400–600 penile cancers

• 1,700 oropharyngeal (back of the throat) cancers in women and 5,600–6,700 in men

Between 2000 and 2013, there was an increase in some uncommon sexually transmitted HPV-related cancers, including anal cancer, cancer of the vulva, and some types of throat cancer. The incidence of HPV-associated cancers of the oropharynx—the middle part of the throat including the soft palate, base of the tongue, and tonsils—has increased over the past three decades, particularly in heterosexual, middle-aged men. HPV now accounts for 70% of such cancers, up from 16% in the 1980s. It has been predicted that HPV will be responsible for more oropharyngeal cancers than cervical cancers in the United States by 2020.

Risk factors

Young people under the age of 25 appear to be more susceptible to HPV. Others at greater risk for sexually transmitted HPV include:

• people who have multiple sexual partners or are in a sexual relationship with someone with multiple partners

• homosexual and bisexual men

• people with HIV/AIDS or other diseases that weaken the immune system

• people taking immunosuppressive drugs

High-risk HPV infections that last for many years increase the risk of cancer. A weakened immune system, chronic inflammation, and smoking also increase the risk of HPV-associated cancer. The use of oral contraceptives for longer than five years appears to increase the risk of HPV-related precancerous cervical lesions, and having numerous children may increase the risk of cervical cancer. Men who have sex with other men are at approximately 17-fold greater risk for anal cancer than men who have sex only with women. Poor oral hygiene increases the risk of **oropharyngeal cancer**.

Causes and symptoms

Genital HPV strains are very contagious and readily transmitted through skin contact during vaginal, oral, or anal sex. Since HPV infection does not usually cause symptoms, most people are unaware that they are infected and can transmit the virus to their sexual partners.

HPV enters the body through small breaks in the skin surface or in mucous membranes lining the genitals. The virus infects epithelial cells—the layers of cells that cover the external and internal surfaces of the body, including the skin, genitals, anus, and throat. Since HPV does not appear to enter the bloodstream, infection is restricted to a small area. In most cases, the body's immune system recognizes and destroys infected cells within a few weeks. In some people, however, HPV remains dormant in a lower skin layer for a period ranging from a few weeks to three years. As these cells mature and move to the surface, the virus begins to replicate (make copies of itself). The virus particles affect the shape of the cells, causing warts or precancerous changes. High-risk HPV may produce two proteins that interfere with normal cell functioning, causing them to avoid cell death and grow out of control. Persistently infected growing cells may develop mutations that promote more cell growth, leading to a high-grade lesion and possibly eventual tumor formation. An estimated 2%–5% of women have abnormal Pap smears due to HPV at some point in their lives, which, if untreated, increases the risk of cervical cancer. However, among high-grade cervical lesions, 50% or fewer develop into invasive cervical cancer.

It is not known why most high-risk HPV infections are of short duration, whereas a small percentage persist and eventually cause cancerous transformations. Other factors may be involved in HPV-associated precancerous changes and cancers. For example, tobacco and alcohol may contribute to HPV-associated oropharyngeal cancers. Viruses other than HPV may also be involved in some HPV-associated cancers.

Genital HPV infections in women can be transmitted to an infant's respiratory tract during childbirth, leading to a rare disorder called juvenile-onset recurrent respiratory papillomatosis (JO-RRP). Although JO-RRP can be life-threatening, it rarely develops into cancer.

HPV-associated cancers typically take 10–30 years to develop following initial infection. Precancerous changes in the female cervix are flat growths that cannot be seen or felt by the woman. Symptoms of anal cancer may include bleeding, pain, or discharge from the anus; swollen lymph nodes in the anal or groin areas; or changes in bowel habits. Anal cancer sometimes has no symptoms. Early signs of cancer of the penis may include color changes, thickening of the skin, tissue growths, or sores. Symptoms of oropharyngeal cancer may include constant sore throat or ear pain, constant coughing, pain or difficulty swallowing or breathing, **weight loss**, hoarseness or voice changes, or a lump or mass in the neck.

Diagnosis

Examination

Diagnosis of HPV-associated cancers depends on the type of cancer.

Tests

Women should be periodically screened for cellular abnormalities in their cervical tissue. The most common

---

KEY TERMS

Cervical intraepithelial neoplasia (CIN)—A precancerous condition in which abnormal cells grow on the cervix, but do not extend into the deeper layers of tissue.

Cervix—The narrow neck or outlet of a woman's uterus.

Colposcopy—The visual examination of the vagina and cervix using a magnifying instrument.

Cryosurgery (or cryotherapy)—Tissue destruction by freezing, as with liquid nitrogen.

Herd immunity—Community immunity; disease protection for nonimmune or unvaccinated individuals that is conferred by the prevailing immunity within a population due to widespread vaccination coverage.

Lesion—An injured, diseased, or damaged area of tissue.

Oropharynx—The portion of the pharynx (the tube between the mouth and esophagus) that is below the soft palate and above the epiglottis and continuous with the mouth.

Pap test—A screening test for cervical cancer devised by Georgios Papanikolaou (1883–1962) in the 1940s.

Sexually transmitted infection (STI)—An infection, such as HPV, that is transmitted through sexual activity.

---

test is the Pap smear, devised by Greek physician Georgios Papanikolaou in the 1940s. Cells are removed from the outer surface of the cervix with a small spatula, smeared on a slide, and examined in a laboratory for abnormalities. Some experts recommend that gay, bisexual, and HIV-positive men have annual anal Pap tests.

In some cases, the cytologist or pathologist examining a Pap smear reports a "borderline" result, in which it is unclear whether observed abnormalities are due to early precancerous changes or to inflammation caused by some other infectious agent or irritant. If abnormal or questionable cells are identified from a Pap smear, the cells may be tested for high-risk HPV. The available tests are approved by the U.S. Food and Drug Administration (FDA) for women with abnormal Pap results, or as a cervical cancer screen in conjunction with a **Pap test** for women over 30. The most common test detects DNA from several high-risk HPV types, but does not identify the specific type. Other available tests:

- are specific for types 16 and 18 DNA that cause most HPV-associated cancers
- detect DNA from several high-risk HPVs and identify types 16 or 18
- detect RNA from the most common high-risk types

Procedures

Colposcopy is used to examine the cervix for precancerous lesions. Endoscopic procedures may be used for diagnosing other types of cancer.

Treatment

Traditional

Low-grade precancerous changes observed on Pap smears are not usually treated because they generally disappear on their own without developing into cancer. Follow-up Pap smears ensure that the tissues have returned to normal. If Pap results indicate cancer or a higher-grade precancerous condition, the cancer or precancerous lesion is removed by excisional or ablative therapy. Excised cervical tissue may be examined to confirm the diagnosis or tested for the presence of high-risk HPV types. Cervical treatments include:

- cryosurgery to destroy the tissue by freezing
- a loop electrosurgical excision procedure (LEEP) or electrocauterization that removes the tissue using a hot wire loop
- surgical conization with a scalpel and/or laser vaporization conization that removes a cone-shaped section of tissue from the cervix and cervical canal

HPV-associated precancerous lesions of the vagina, vulva, penis, or anus may be treated with:

- excisional surgery
- cryosurgery with liquid nitrogen
- electrosurgery that dries the tissue with an electric needle and then scrapes it off with a sharp instrument called a curette
- laser surgery

Other HPV-associated cancers are generally treated similarly to non-HPV-associated cancers, depending on the type and stage. However, research indicates that HPV-positive oropharyngeal cancers may require less intensive treatment than HPV-negative oropharyngeal cancers.

Drugs

HPV-associated precancerous lesions of the vagina, vulva, penis, or anus may be treated with topical

QUESTIONS TO ASK YOUR DOCTOR

- Should I have HPV testing in addition to my regular Pap smear?
- Should I have an HPV test if my Pap smear results are abnormal?
- Based upon my Pap smear results and HPV testing, when should I have my next Pap smear?
- Should I get the HPV vaccine?
- Should I have my daughters and sons vaccinated against HPV?

chemicals or drugs. Higher-stage HPV-associated cancers may require **chemotherapy**.

Prognosis

Cervical cancer precursors, termed cervical intraepithelial neoplasia (CIN), when identified early before they become invasive, can almost always be completely removed by minor surgery, essentially curing the cancer before it develops. However, eradication of HPV is not always 100% effective, and the incidence of latent or recurrent infection is high. Thus, safe sex practices are essential for decreasing the risk of becoming reinfected or infecting others.

Prevention

Safe sex practices decrease the risk of being infected or reinfected with HPV, as well as the risk of transmitting the virus to partners. Measures that reduce the risk of infection include:

- abstaining from all skin-to-skin oral, anal, and genital contact
- reducing the number of sexual partners or having sex only with an uninfected partner in a monogamous relationship
- always using latex condoms, although HPV can infect areas not covered by a condom

Vaccines

Vaccination against HPV could prevent approximately 21,000 cancers annually in the United States. There are two vaccines—Gardasil and Cervarix—that effectively protect against HPV types 16 and 18 that cause most cervical and HPV-associated vulvar, vaginal, and anal cancers, as well as precancerous lesions.

Gardasil also protects against HPV types 6 and 11 that cause most cases of genital warts, and a 2013 study indicated that it protects against HPV-associated throat cancer contracted through oral sex. Because sexually transmitted HPV is so widespread and the vaccines do not cure an existing infection, they are most effective when administered before an individual becomes sexually active. Gardasil is administered as a series of three shots over a six-month period. It is recommended for all 11- and 12-year-old girls and for girls and women aged 13–26 who have not had all three doses. Gardasil is also recommended for all boys aged 11 or 12 and men aged 21 and younger who have not had all three doses. It protects men from genital warts and anal cancer and may also protect against other HPV-related cancers. It is safe for men through age 26, but is more effective at a younger age.

Since the introduction of the HPV vaccine in 2006, studies have reported a 56% reduction in infections with HPV types 16 and 18 among teenage girls in the United States. In Australia, there was a 59% reduction in cases of genital warts among females aged 12–26 within two years of launching an HPV vaccination program. Although only one-third of American girls aged 13–17—and far fewer boys—have been fully vaccinated, there has been a 39% reduction in genital warts among unvaccinated heterosexual men. This is explained by "herd immunity," as well as the unexpected effectiveness of a partial dosage of the vaccine, since about half of teenage girls have received at least one dose.

Vaccination rates are particularly low in the southern United States. In other countries, even developing nations such as Rwanda, vaccination rates are above 80%. In 2010, 44% of American parents reported that they would not have their daughters vaccinated. In addition to unfounded concerns about vaccine safety, some parents worried that the vaccine encourages sexual promiscuity. Although the vaccine is expensive, with full implementation of the Affordable Care Act, insurance providers will cover the full cost. An 80% vaccination rate in the United States would prevent 50,000 eventual cervical cancers.

Resources

BOOKS

Bringle, Jennifer. *Young Women and the HPV Vaccine*. New York: Rosen, 2012.

Defenbaugh, Nicole, and Kimberly N. Kline. "Gendered Construction of HPV: A Post-Structuralist Critique of Gardasil." In *Challenging Images of Women in the Media: Reinventing Women's Lives*, Theresa Carilli and Jane Campbell, eds. Lanham, MD: Lexington Books, 2012.

Dizon, Don S., Ashley R. Stuckey, and Michael L. Krychman. *Dx/Rx: Human Papilloma Virus*. Sudbury, MA: Jones & Bartlett Learning, 2012.

Garland, Suzanne M. "Human Papillomavirus (HPV)." In *Sexually Transmitted Diseases*, Richard H. Beigi, ed. Hoboken, NJ: Wiley-Blackwell, 2012.

Herrero, Rolando. "HPV and Cervical Cancer." In *Cancer Epidemiology: Low- and Middle-Income Countries and Special Populations*, Amr Soliman, David Schottenfeld, and Paolo Boffetta, eds. New York: Oxford University, 2013.

Langwith, Jacqueline. *HPV*. Detroit: Gale, Cengage Learning, 2013.

Pfister, Herbert. *Prophylaxis and Early Detection of HPV-Related Neoplasia*. New York: Karger, 2012.

Sutton, Amy L. *Sexually Transmitted Diseases Sourcebook*, 5th ed. Detroit: Omnigraphics, 2013.

Watkins, Heidi. *Sexually Transmitted Infections*. Detroit: Greenhaven, 2012.

PERIODICALS

Bakalar, Nicholas. "Patterns: Some Cancers Linked to HPV on the Rise." *New York Times* (January 15, 2013): D6.

Grabiel, Marlee, et al. "HPV and HPV Vaccines: The Knowledge Levels, Opinions, and Behavior of Parents." *Journal of Community Health* 38, no. 6 (December 2013): 1015–1021.

Kester, Laura M., et al. "A National Study of HPV Vaccination of Adolescent Girls: Rates, Predictors, and Reasons for Non-Vaccination." *Maternal and Child Health Journal* 17, no. 5 (July 2013): 879–885.

Marchand, Erica, Beth A. Glenn, and Roshan Bastani. "HPV Vaccination and Sexual Behavior in a Community College Sample." *Journal of Community Health* 38, no. 6 (December 2013): 1010–1014.

Martin, Timothy W. "HPV Cases in Teens Plunge—Infections Fall 56% in Girls, but CDC Says Vaccination Rate Is Still Too Low." *Wall Street Journal* (June 20, 2013): A6.

Morin, Monte. "HPV Vaccination Rates Lagging." *Los Angeles Times* (July 29, 2013): A12.

Tavernise, Sabrina. "Vaccine Is Credited in Steep Fall of HPV Infection in Teenagers." *New York Times* (June 20, 2013): A6.

Walden, Rachel. "What You Need to Know About the HPV Vaccine." *Women's Health Activist* 38, no. 4 (July/August 2013): 11.

Zhang, Wen Jie, et al. "The Case for Semi-Mandatory HPV Vaccination in China." *Nature Biotechnology* 31, no. 7 (July 2013): 590–591.

WEBSITES

American Sexual Health Association. "HPV." http://www.ashasexualhealth.org/stdsstis/hpv/ (accessed January 29, 2015).

Centers for Disease Control and Prevention. "Genital HPV Infection—Fact Sheet." Sexually Transmitted Diseases (STDs). July 25, 2013. http://www.cdc.gov/std/HPV/STDFact-HPV.htm (accessed August 27, 2014).

Centers for Disease Control and Prevention. "HPV and Men—Fact Sheet." Sexually Transmitted Diseases (STDs). February 23, 2012. http://www.cdc.gov/std/hpv/STDFact-HPV-and-men.htm (accessed August 27, 2014).

Gearhart, Peter A. "Human Papillomavirus." Medscape Reference. August 26, 2013. http://emedicine.medscape.com/article/219110-overview#showall (accessed August 27, 2014).

"HPV and Cancer." National Cancer Institute. March 15, 2012. http://www.cancer.gov/cancertopics/factsheet/Risk/HPV (accessed August 27, 2014).

"Human Papillomavirus (HPV)." Centers for Disease Control and Prevention. February 1, 2013. http://www.cdc.gov/hpv (accessed August 27, 2014).

Mayo Clinic Staff. "HPV Infection." Mayo Clinic. March 12, 2013. http://www.mayoclinic.com/health/hpv-infection/DS00906 (accessed August 27, 2014).

ORGANIZATIONS

American Congress of Obstetricians and Gynecologists, PO Box 70620, Washington, DC 20024-9998, (202) 638-5577, (800) 673-8444, http://www.acog.org.

American Sexual Health Association, PO Box 13827, Research Triangle Park, NC 27709, (919) 361-8400, Fax: (919) 361-8425, info@ashastd.org, http://www.ashasexualhealth.org.

Centers for Disease Control and Prevention, 1600 Clifton Road, Atlanta, GA 30333, (800) CDC-INFO (232-4636), cdcinfo@cdc.gov, http://www.cdc.gov.

National Cancer Institute, 6116 Executive Boulevard, Suite 300, Bethesda, MD 20892-8322, (800) 4-CANCER (422-6237), http://www.cancer.gov.

U.S. Food and Drug Administration, 10903 New Hampshire Avenue, Silver Spring, MD 20993-0002, (888) INFO-FDA (463-6332), http://www.fda.gov.

Warren Maltzman, PhD.
REVISED BY MARGARET ALIC, PhD.
REVIEWED BY MELINDA GRANGER OBERLEITNER, RN, DNS, APRN, CNS

Hycamtin *see* **Topotecan**

Hydrea *see* **Hydroxyurea**

Hydrocodone *see* **Opioids**

Hydrocortisone *see* **Corticosteroids**

Hydromorphone *see* **Opioids**

Hydroxyurea

Definition

Hydroxyurea, also known by its trade name Hydrea, is an antineoplastic agent, meaning it is used to treat **cancer**. It is taken orally.

KEY TERMS

Mucositis—A painful inflammation of the mucous membranes.

Mutagen—An agent capable of causing DNA changes.

Myelosuppression—Diminished bone marrow activity resulting in decreased red blood cells, white blood cells, and platelets.

Plateletpheresis—A procedure in which platelets are removed from whole blood.

Purpose

Hydroxyurea is used to treat the following conditions:

- Melanoma.
- Chronic myelocytic leukemia that is resistant to other therapies.
- Ovarian cancer that is recurrent, metastatic, or inoperable.
- Squamous cell carcinoma of the head and neck, excluding the lip. (In this case, hydroxyurea is given with radiation therapy.)
- Sickle cell anemia.
- Other: Hydroxyurea has shown promise in the management of thrombocytosis, a condition in which platelet levels are abnormally high.

Description

Hydroxyurea belongs to antimetabolites, a group of compounds that interfere with the production of nucleic acids. Hydroxyurea exerts its anticancer activity by inhibiting ribonucleotide reductase, an enzyme required for DNA synthesis. When used in conjunction with **radiation therapy**, the effectiveness of hydroxyurea increases because it also inhibits the ability of cells damaged by radiation to repair themselves.

Recommended dosage

Hydroxyurea dosages are calculated based on a person's weight as milligrams per kilogram (mg/kg). Doctors will usually use whichever value is lowest—the patient's actual weight or the patient's ideal weight—to calculate dosages. The drug is not given if white blood cell levels drop below 2500 mm^3, or if red blood cell levels drop below 100,000 mm^3. Usually, bone marrow recovery is rapid, and few doses are missed.

Hydroxyurea is usually given for six weeks before its effectiveness can be adequately evaluated.

Hydroxyurea is administered in a capsule form, each containing 500 mg of the drug. If a patient is unable to swallow the capsule, its contents can be dissolved in a glass of water and swallowed immediately. The drug will not completely dissolve in water. Dosages have not been established for children in part because the cancers for which hydroxyurea is useful do not normally occur in that age group.

In the treatment of solid tumors, such as ovarian cancers, patients are usually given 80 mg/kg once every three days. Alternatively, a dose of 20–30 mg/kg may be given every day.

In **head and neck cancers** also treated with radiation, 80 mg/kg of hydroxyurea is given once every three days. The drug should be started a week before radiation therapy begins, and should continue for some time after radiation therapy.

When it is used to treat resistant **chronic myelocytic leukemia**, hydroxyurea is given in the dosage of 20–30 mg/kg once a day.

In thrombocytosis, doses of 15–30 mg/kg taken once a day are usually effective. Platelet levels return to a normal level within two to six weeks of therapy. In more severe cases, doses of 1.5–3.0 grams per day have been given with plateletpheresis, a procedure that removes platelets from the blood.

Precautions

This drug should not be administered to a person who has had a previous allergic reaction to it. Liver and kidney function should be evaluated prior to, and during, treatment. The drug may interfere with certain lab tests. For example, creatinine levels may be elevated. Patients taking hydroxyurea should stay well-hydrated, drinking up to 12 glasses per day of water or other fluids.

Hydroxyurea is potentially mutagenic, meaning that it causes mutations in DNA. Patients taking the drug should discuss the potential effects on their future conception plans. Hydroxyurea should not be administered to pregnant women, and women taking the drug should use birth control methods to prevent pregnancy. Hydroxyurea is excreted in breast milk; therefore, women taking the drug should not breast-feed.

Side effects

Hydroxyurea and radiation therapy each cause adverse side effects. When they are used together, the incidence and severity of side effects may increase.

Bone marrow suppression is the major side effect of hyroxyurea therapy, and may develop within two days of the first dose. Blood tests are performed routinely to monitor for changes. Usually, leukopenia (decreased white blood cells) develops first. Reduced red blood cells and platelets can also occur, but generally not as frequently. If **anemia** develops, it should be corrected with whole blood transfusions. Hydroxyurea causes red blood cell abnormalities that are not severe and that do not reduce the red blood cell survival time.

Gastrointestinal symptoms are not as common as **myelosuppression** and are usually mild. These symptoms may include nausea, vomiting, **diarrhea**, and constipation. Usually, medications can control **nausea and vomiting**. **Mucositis**, a painful swelling of the mucous membranes, may also develop, especially if the patient is undergoing radiation treatment to the head and neck. Mucositis can be managed with medicated mouthwashes, good oral hygiene, and hydration to keep the mouth moist.

Headache and dizziness may occur. With long-term use, skin changes, such as hyperpigmentation of the skin and nails, have also been reported.

Hydroxyurea has also been linked to leg ulcers. Studies suggest that leg ulcers have been reported mainly in older patients who might be at an increased risk. There have also been reports of hydroxyurea causing leg ulceration when it is used in psoriasis for a prolonged period.

Interactions

Patients at risk for bone marrow suppression should inform their doctor about all medications they are taking, both prescription and nonprescription. Many over-the-counter medications contain aspirin, which acts as a blood thinner, increasing the potential for bleeding. Patients with reduced platelets should not take aspirin.

Resources

BOOKS

Chu, Edward, and Vincent T. DeVita Jr. *Physicians' Cancer Chemotherapy Drug Manual 2014*. Burlington, MA: Jones & Bartlett Learning, 2014.

WEBSITES

American Cancer Society. "Hydroxyurea." http://www.cancer.org/treatment/treatmentsandsideeffects/guidetocancerdrugs/hydroxyurea (accessed November 4, 2014).

Leukemia & Lymphoma Society. "Hydroxyurea." http://www.lls.org/diseaseinformation/managingyourcancer/treatmentnextsteps/typesoftreatment/chemotherapyotherdrugtherapies/drugs/hydroxyurea (accessed November 4, 2014).

ORGANIZATIONS

U.S. Food and Drug Administration, 10903 New Hampshire Ave., Silver Spring, MD 20993, (888) INFO-FDA (463-6332), http://www.fda.gov.

Tamara Brown, RN

Hypercalcemia

Description

Hypercalcemia is an abnormally high level of calcium in the blood, usually more than 10.5 milligrams per deciliter of blood. It is the most common life-threatening metabolic disorder associated with **cancer**.

Calcium plays an important role in the development and maintenance of bones in the body. It is also needed in tooth formation and is important in other body functions. As much as 99% of the body's calcium is stored in bone tissue. A healthy person experiences a constant turnover of calcium as bone tissue is built and reshaped. The remaining 1% of the body's calcium circulates in the blood and other body fluids. Calcium in the blood plays an important role in the control of many body functions, including blood clotting, transmission of nerve impulses, muscle contraction, and other metabolic activities.

Cancer-caused hypercalcemia produces a disruption in the body's ability to maintain a normal level of calcium. This abnormally high level of calcium in the blood develops because of increased bone breakdown and release of calcium from the bone. The disorder occurs in approximately 10%-20% of all cancer cases. The most common cancers associated with hypercalcemia are breast, prostate, and lung cancer, as well as **multiple myeloma** or other tumors with extensive **metastasis** to the bone. It may also occur in patients with head and neck cancer, **cancer of unknown primary**, **lymphoma**, leukemia, **kidney cancer**, and gastrointestinal cancer. Hypercalcemia most commonly develops as a late complication of cancer, and its appearance constitutes an emergency.

Several clinical symptoms are associated with cancer-related hypercalcemia. Symptoms may appear gradually and often look like signs of other cancers and diseases. The symptoms of hypercalcemia are not only related to the elevated level of calcium in the blood, but—more importantly—to how rapidly the hypercalcemia develops. The severity of the symptoms is often dependent upon factors such as previous cancer treatment, reactions to medications, or other illnesses a patient may have. Most patients do not experience all of the symptoms of hypercalcemia, and some may not have any signs at all. Rapid diagnosis of hypercalcemia may be complicated because the symptoms are often nonspecific and are easily ascribed to other factors. These symptoms include:

- decreased muscle tone and muscle weakness
- delirium, disorientation, incoherent speech, and psychotic symptoms such as hallucinations and delusion
- constipation
- fatigue
- poor appetite, nausea and/or vomiting
- frequency of urination and increased thirst
- pain

Causes

The fundamental cause of cancer-related hypercalcemia is increased movement of calcium out of the bones and into the bloodstream, and secondarily, an inadequate ability of the kidneys to get rid of higher calcium levels. Normally, healthy kidneys are able to filter out large amounts of calcium from the blood, getting rid of the excess that is unneeded by the body and keeping the amount of the calcium the body does need. However, the high levels of calcium in the body caused by cancer-related hypercalcemia may cause the kidneys to become overworked, thus making them unable to excrete the excess. Another problem is that some tumors produce a substance that may cause the kidneys to get rid of too little calcium.

Two types of cancer-caused hypercalcemia have been identified: osteolytic and humoral. Osteolytic occurs because of direct bone destruction by a primary or metastatic tumor. Humoral is caused by certain factors secreted by malignant cells, which ultimately cause calcium loss from the bones. Certain types of hormonal therapy may precipitate hypercalcemia and the use of some diuretics may contribute to the disorder.

Because immobility causes an increase in the loss of calcium from bone, cancer patients who are weak and spend most of their time in bed are more prone to hypercalcemia. Cancer patients are often dehydrated because they take in inadequate amounts of food and fluids and often suffer from **nausea and vomiting**. Dehydration reduces the ability of the kidneys to remove excess calcium from the body, and therefore is another contributing factor in the development of hypercalcemia in cancer patients.

Treatment

Individuals at risk for developing hypercalcemia may be the first to recognize symptoms, such as **fatigue**. The patient and family should be aware of the signs and symptoms so that a health care professional can be notified as early as possible should they occur. Patients can take several preventative measures like ensuring adequate fluid intake, controlling nausea and vomiting, maintaining the highest possible mobility, and avoiding drugs that affect the functioning of the kidneys. This includes avoiding those medications containing calcium, vitamin D, or vitamin A. Since absorption of calcium is usually decreased in individuals with hypercalcemia, dietary calcium restriction is unnecessary.

The mortality rate for untreated hypercalcemia is quite high. Early diagnosis and prompt treatment are essential. The magnitude of hypercalcemia and the severity of symptoms is usually the basis for determining what type of treatment is indicated.

For those patients who have mild hypercalcemia, are experiencing no symptoms, and have cancer that is responsive to treatment, giving intravenous fluids and observing the patient may be all that is necessary to treat the condition. If the patient is experiencing symptoms or has a cancer that is expected to respond poorly to treatment, then medication to treat the hypercalcemia should be initiated. Additional treatment focuses on controlling nausea and vomiting, encouraging activity, and avoiding any medication that causes drowsiness.

In treating moderate or severe hypercalcemia, replacing fluids is the first treatment intervention. Though providing fluid replacement will not restore normal calcium levels in all patients, it is still the most important initial step. Improvement in mental status and nausea and vomiting is usually apparent within 24 hours for most patients. However, rehydration is only a temporary measure. If the cancer is not treated, then drugs that will help to control the hypercalcemia are necessary. Many drugs are used to treat hypercalcemia, including **calcitonin**, **plicamycin** (formerly mithramycin), **gallium nitrate**, and **bisphosphonates**. Bisphosphonates are some of the most effective drugs for controlling hypercalcemia. Loop diuretics like furosemide are often given because they help to increase the excretion of excess serum calcium. For severe hypercalcemia that is complicated by kidney failure, dialysis is an option. Because of the large amounts of intravenous fluids given to treat hypercalcemia, the health care team will carefully observe for any signs of overhydration or other electrolyte imbalances.

The severity of hypercalcemia determines the amount of treatment necessary. Severe hypercalcemia should be treated immediately and aggressively. Less severe hypercalcemia should be treated according to the symptoms. A positive response to the treatment is exhibited by the disappearance of the symptoms and a decreased level of calcium in the blood. Mild hypercalcemia does not usually need to be treated aggressively. After calcium levels return to normal, urine and blood should continue to be checked often to make certain the treatment is still working.

Alternative and complementary therapies

There are no known proven alternative treatments for cancer-related hypercalcemia. Some of the medications used are more effective than others, and the patient and family should discuss which ones are the most appropriate for the patient's needs.

Hypercalcemia usually develops as a late complication of cancer, and its appearance is very serious. The outlook is often quite grim. However, it is not clear if death occurs because of the hypercalcemia crisis or because of the advanced cancer. Because hypercalcemia is often a complication that occurs in the final stages of cancer, the decision to treat it depends upon the overall goals of treatment determined by the patient, family, and physician. The natural course of untreated hypercalcemia will progress to loss of consciousness and coma. Some patients may prefer this at the end of life rather than have unrelieved suffering and/or untreatable symptoms. It is therefore important for the patient and caregivers to discuss what supportive care measures are wanted.

Resources

WEBSITES

U.S. National Library of Medicine. "Hypercalcemia." MedlinePlus. http://www.nlm.nih.gov/medlineplus/ency/article/000365.htm (accessed December 15, 2014).

ORGANIZATIONS

National Cancer Institute, 9609 Medical Center Dr., BG 9609 MSC 9760, Bethesda, MD 20892-9760, (800) 4-CANCER (422-6237), http://www.cancer.gov.

Deanna Swartout-Corbeil, RN

Hypercoagulable states *see*
Hypercoagulation disorders

Hypercoagulation disorders

Description

Hypercoagulation disorders (or hypercoagulable states or disorders) cause an increased tendency for clotting of the blood. In normal hemostasis (the stoppage of bleeding), clots form at the site of the blood vessel's injury. However, in hypercoagulation disorders, the clots can develop in circulating blood. This may put a patient at risk for obstruction of veins and arteries (phlebitis, thrombosis, or thrombophlebitis). The hypercoagulable state and thrombophlebitis are common in cases of **cancer** involving solid tumors such as pancreatic, breast, ovarian, and **prostate cancer**.

Hypercoagulation disorders can cause clots throughout the body's blood vessels, a condition known as thromboembolic disease. Thromboembolic disease can lead to infarction (death of tissue as a result of blocked blood supply to the tissue). Other serious results of hypercoagulation make this a dangerous condition. Clotting (thrombosis) in the veins and arteries leading to the lungs can prevent blood flow, causing sudden and severe loss of breath and chest pain. These clots, called pulmonary embolisms, are potentially fatal. Clots in the blood vessels of the brain can result in a stroke, and clots in the heart's blood vessels can result in a heart attack.

Symptoms of hypercoagulation disorders include swelling or discoloration of the limbs, pain or tenderness of the skin, visible obstructions in the surface veins, and ulcers of the lower parts of the legs.

The diagnosis of hypercoagulation disorders is completed with a combination of physical examination, **imaging studies**, and blood tests. The presence of deep clots can be determined using Doppler ultrasound examination, special x-ray techniques called venography or arteriography (in which a solution is injected into the blood vessel to aid in imaging), or a specific type of blood pressure test called plethysmography. There are a number of blood tests that can determine the presence or absence of proteins, clotting factors, and platelet counts in the blood. Among the tests used to detect hypercoagulation is the Antithrombin III assay. Protein C and Protein S concentrations can be diagnosed with immunoassay or plasma antigen level tests.

Causes

Hypercoagulation disorders are associated with cancer of the pancreas. About half of patients with **pancreatic cancer** experience incidence of thrombosis. Approximately 10% of patients with pancreatic cancer develop a specific type of hypercoagulation disorder known as migratory thrombophlebitis, or Trousseau's syndrome. In Trousseau's syndrome, the blood vessels become inflamed and clots in the blood vessels spontaneously appear and disappear. Other types of cancer may also result in hypercoagulation disorders.

In order for blood coagulation to occur, platelets (small, round fragments in the blood) help contract blood vessels to lessen blood loss and also to help plug damaged blood vessels. The conversion of platelets into actual clots is a complicated process involving proteins that are identified clotting factors. The factors are carried in the plasma, or liquid portion, of the blood. Proteins C and S are two of the clotting factors that are present in the plasma to help regulate or activate parts of the clotting process. It is believed that pancreatic tumors produce chemicals that promote clotting, or coagulation, of the blood (procoagulants), or that they activate platelet function. It is also possible that tumors interfere with the functions of proteins C and S.

Treatment

The treatment for patients with hypercoagulation disorders varies depending upon the severity of the clotting and the other conditions it may have caused. Medications may include blood thinners (anticoagulants) such as **heparin** and **warfarin**, which prevent the formation of new blood clots; antiplatelet drugs such as aspirin; or thrombolytic drugs to dissolve existing clots. Pain medications and nonsteroidal anti-inflammatory medications may be given to reduce pain and swelling. **Antibiotics** will be prescribed if infection has occurred.

Resources

BOOKS

Deloughery, Thomas G. *Hemostasis and Thrombosis*. Georgetown, TX: Landes Bioscience, 1999.

Goodnight, Scott H., and William E. Goodnight. *Disorders of Hemostasis and Thrombosis*. 2nd ed. New York: McGraw-Hill, 2000.

WEBSITES

American Academy of Family Physicians. "Hypercoagulation." FamilyDoctor.org. http://familydoctor.org/familydoctor/en/diseases-conditions/hypercoagulation.html (accessed December 4, 2014).

ORGANIZATIONS

National Heart, Lung, and Blood Institute, 31 Center Dr. MSC 2486, Bldg. 31, Rm. 5A52, Bethesda, MD 20892, (301) 592-8573, nhlbiinfo@nhlbi.nih.gov, http://www.nhlbi.nih.gov.

National Hemophilia Foundation, 116 W. 32nd St., 11th Fl., New York, NY 10001, (212) 328-3700, Fax: (212) 328-3777, https://www.hemophilia.org.

Paul A. Johnson, EdM

Hyperthermia

Definition

Hyperthermia refers to the use of heat to treat various cancers on and inside the body. It is also called hyperthermia therapy or thermotherapy.

Hyperthermia therapy for **cancer** should not be confused with heat therapy, which is a treatment that involves the application of mild heat from heating pads or warm compresses to localized areas of the body to relieve muscle and joint pain or stiffness. Hyperthermia therapy is specifically intended to kill or weaken tumors rather than to temporarily relieve discomfort caused by arthritis, sprains and strains, or similar conditions. It can be applied to a very small area (local hyperthermia), an entire limb or organ (regional hyperthermia), or the patient's entire body (whole-body hyperthermia).

Purpose

The purpose of hyperthermia is to shrink and hopefully destroy cancerous tissues without harming noncancerous cells. It can be used to treat cancer in many areas of the body, including the brain, thyroid, lung, breast, and prostate. It is thought that high temperatures, up to 106 degrees Fahrenheit, can help shrink cancerous tumors. Hyperthermia is starting to be more widely used because it does not usually have severe side effects like such other forms of cancer treatment as radiation or **chemotherapy**. In most instances, hyperthermia is used at the same time with other forms of cancer therapy.

Demographics

Although hyperthermia treatment was considered an experimental form of cancer therapy in the 1980s, its proponents believe that the treatment has been accepted by many physicians, and that use of hyperthermia will increase as more cancer centers install the high-tech equipment necessary for regional and whole-body hyperthermia. Cancer care centers offering whole-body treatment are limited in number; however, there are several in larger cities across the United States that offer local hyperthermia. In general, hyperthermia is used more often in Europe as an adjuvant treatment for cancer than in North America.

The American Cancer Society has acknowledged that hyperthermia can make the cancer cells of some cancers more responsive to treatment, but still considers the treatment experimental, especially in whole-body form. The Cancer Treatment Centers of America (CTCA), however, lists local hyperthermia as a conventional treatment under the larger heading of **radiation therapy**. The **National Cancer Institute** (NCI) sponsors ongoing **clinical trials** of hyperthermia in cancer treatment; there were eight active trials as of late 2014. The types of cancer being studied in these trials included **liver cancer**, **adrenocortical carcinoma**, **ovarian cancer**, and uterine cancer.

Precautions

Patients who have extensive **metastasis** (spreading of the cancer throughout their body) are not considered the best candidates for hyperthermia, although they can receive whole-body treatment. Patients must be free of major infections and able to tolerate the high temperatures of the treatment. Caution must be used when areas of the body are heated with such external heat sources as heating pads to avoid potentially dangerous burns.

Other types of patients who should be treated cautiously with hyperthermia include:

• Pregnant women.

• People who are anemic.

• People known to be sensitive to high temperatures.

• Diabetics.

• People with tuberculosis.

• People with seizure disorders.

Description

Hyperthermia can be used on the body from very small areas of the body to the entire body itself. Local hyperthermia refers to heating just one area of the body, usually where the tumor is located. The heat is applied for about an hour. Heat can be applied from outside the body using microwaves or high-frequency radio waves. Heat can be applied from inside the body or even inside the tumor itself by the use of thin heated wires, small tubes filled with hot water, implanted microwave antennae, or radiofrequency electrodes. Some cancer centers use ultrasound to produce heat within the tumor. Ultrasound is more easily focused than other energy modalities, and can be applied to tumors located on the skin surface or up to 3 inches (8 cm) inside the body.

If heat is used to treat an entire organ or limb, it is referred to as regional hyperthermia. High-energy magnets or other devices that produce high energy, and thus heat, are placed over the larger areas to be heated. Magnetic fluid hyperthermia involves the injection of a fluid containing magnetic nanoparticles directly into the malignant tumor. When the nanoparticles are placed in an alternating magnetic field with frequencies similar to FM radio signals, they generate heat and destroy the tumors.

Another method of regional hyperthermia is the use of perfusion. Hyperthermia perfusion is a technique that uses the patient's own blood; the blood is removed, heated outside the body, then pumped back into the area that contains the cancer. A warmed solution containing **anticancer drugs** may also be used as part of perfusion hyperthermia. One form of perfusion hyperthermia that is used to treat abdominal cancers is called continuous hyperthermic peritoneal perfusion or CHPP. Performed during open surgery, this procedure involves the circulation of heated anticancer drugs through the abdominal cavity to raise the temperature of the internal organs to 106–108°F (41–42°C).

For treatment of cancers that have spread throughout the body, whole-body hyperthermia can be considered. Various methods are used to heat up a patient's entire body, including warm water or electric blankets, hot wax, or thermal chambers that are very much like incubators used to warm newborn babies, except much larger.

Origins

Hyperthermia has a long history; the earliest report of heat treatment to cure systemic disease is found in the writings of Hippocrates (c. 400 BC). A century before Hippocrates, another Greek philosopher/physician named Parmenides (520–450 BC) thought that an artificially induced **fever** could cure any disease. In ancient India, practitioners of Ayurveda used regional and whole-body hyperthermia to treat various disorders. In North America in more recent times, many Native American tribes used sweat lodges for healing rituals or to purify warriors wounded in battle.

The use of heat as a cancer treatment in scientific medicine dates from the nineteenth century. A German physician reported in 1866 that a patient with a neck **sarcoma** was cured of the tumor after surviving a high fever. In 1893, a Swedish gynecologist named Westermark experimented with fevers induced by bacterial toxins and the use of a coil filled with hot water to treat uterine tumors. No controlled studies were conducted at the time, however, and reports of successful cancer treatment using heat were considered anecdotal.

Interest in heat as a possible treatment for cancer declined in the early twentieth century but rose again in the 1960s when some researchers working with cancer cells in mice thought that the malignant cells might be more sensitive to heat than normal cells. Unfortunately, later studies demonstrated that cancer cells are not necessarily more sensitive to heat by itself than normal cells. Doctors presently think that hyperthermia is effective only in combination with radiotherapy or chemotherapy.

Preparation

Patients should be prepared for hyperthermia by an explanation of the specific technique that is to be used and what to expect during and after the procedure. In most cases, the patient will be given a local anesthetic when temperature probes are inserted to monitor the heat levels in the part of the body being treated. **Radiofrequency ablation** or perfusion of the peritoneal cavity usually requires general anesthesia.

Aftercare

Patients will usually need to rest afterward. Those who have had general anesthesia will need to be monitored during recovery. Patients who have had whole-body hyperthermia may need aftercare for **nausea and vomiting**. Patients who have had perfusion hyperthermia may need aftercare for tissue swelling or bleeding.

Risks

The major risks of hyperthermia use are pain and external burns. Heat applied directly to the skin can cause minor discomfort to significant pain, especially when high temperatures are used. Blistering and actual burning of the skin can also occur at higher temperatures, although with careful application of the instrument or device, these side effects are very rare. Many cancer centers use **magnetic resonance imaging** (MRI) not only to locate the tumor, but to guide the application of hyperthermia to the cancerous cells.

Risks associated with perfusion hyperthermia include swollen tissues, blood clots, and bleeding; these side effects are usually temporary, however. Risks associated with whole-body hyperthermia include nausea, vomiting, and **diarrhea**. Rare side effects with whole-body hyperthermia include heart and vascular disorders.

Results

The goal of hyperthermia is to control the growth and shrink hyperthermia-sensitive tumors. As stated earlier, hyperthermia can also be used to help sensitize tumors to such other cancer treatment modalities as radiation and chemotherapy. While hyperthermia is considered effective in shrinking tumors or making them more sensitive to other therapies, there is little evidence that it extends patients' survival time. It does, however, improve their quality of life, as several European studies have reported.

QUESTIONS TO ASK YOUR DOCTOR

- Should I consider hyperthermia as an adjuvant therapy?
- What is your opinion of hyperthermia?
- What type of hyperthermia would you recommend?
- Can you recommend a cancer center with the necessary equipment and experience in this form of treatment?
- Should I consider participation in a clinical trial of hyperthermia as an adjunctive treatment for my type of cancer?
- What are the risks of hyperthermia?

Abnormal results

Hyperthermia has fewer severe side effects than radiation therapy or chemotherapy. As noted above, tissue swelling and bleeding may be temporary side effects in some patients, while some experience nausea and other gastrointestinal disturbances following whole-body hyperthermia. Such side effects as pain and burning from external heat sources can be minimized with careful application of the heat.

Healthcare team roles

Hyperthermia usually requires at least two doctors to administer, an oncologist and a radiologist. An anesthesiologist will be needed if the specific procedure requires the patient to be under general anesthesia. Nursing staff are required to monitor patients for vital signs and possible side effects during the recovery period.

Alternatives

Radiofrequency ablation (RFA) is used more frequently than perfusion or whole-body hyperthermia to deliver heat to malignant tumors. RFA makes use of a special probe inserted directly into a tumor that uses radiofrequency waves to heat the tumor above 122°F (50°C), a temperature that is high enough to kill the tumor cells. This is a higher temperature level than can be used with hyperthermia. In addition to its ability to actually kill malignant cells, RFA has the additional advantage of targeting malignant tumors precisely with minimal risk to nearby healthy tissue.

Research and general acceptance

While radiofrequency ablation is a proven mainstream alternative to regional or whole-body hyperthermia, one type of hyperthermia therapy that is not only unproven but potentially dangerous is intracellular hyperthermia, also called 2-4-dinitrophenol or DNP therapy. DNP is an organic substance injected directly into the body to cause an artificial fever. There is no evidence that dinitrophenol is effective in treating cancer; moreover, some patients have died as a result of DNP injections.

Caregiver concerns

Hyperthermia is administered in a clinic or hospital rather than at home. Caregivers should, however, monitor patients who have received whole-body hyperthermia after they return home for possible side effects.

Resources

BOOKS

Ades, Terri, et al., editors. *American Cancer Society Complete Guide to Complementary and Alternative Cancer Therapies*. 2nd ed. Atlanta, GA: American Cancer Society, 2009.

Baronzio, Gian Franco, and E. Dieter Hager, eds. *Hyperthermia in Cancer Treatment: A Primer*. New York: Springer, 2006.

Niederhuber, John E., et al. *Abeloff's Clinical Oncology*. 5th ed. Philadelphia: Elsevier/Saunders, 2014.

PERIODICALS

Curley, Steven A., et al. "The Effects of Non-Invasive Radiofrequency Treatment and Hyperthermia on Malignant and Nonmalignant Cells." *International Journal of Environmental Research and Public Health* 11, no. 9 (2014): 9142–53. http://dx.doi.org/10.3390/ijerph110909142 (accessed October 24, 2014).

Januszewski, Adam, and Justin Stebbing. "Hyperthermia in Cancer: Is It Coming of Age?" *The Lancet Oncology* 15, no. 6 (2014): 565–66. http://dx.doi.org/10.1016/S1470-2045(14)70207-4 (accessed October 24, 2014).

Silvio, Dutz, and Rudolf Hergt. "Magnetic Particle Hyperthermia—A Promising Tumour Therapy." *Nanotechnology* 25, no. 45 (2014): e-pub ahead of print. http://dx.doi.org/10.1088/0957-4484/25/45/452001 (accessed October 24, 2014).

WEBSITES

American Cancer Society. "Hyperthermia to Treat Cancer." http://www.cancer.org/treatment/treatmentsandsideeffects/treatmenttypes/hyperthermia (accessed October 24, 2014).

Cancer Treatment Centers of America. "Hyperthermia." http://www.cancercenter.com/treatments/hyperthermia (accessed October 24, 2014).

National Cancer Institute. "Hyperthermia in Cancer Treatment." http://www.cancer.gov/cancertopics/factsheet/Therapy/hyperthermia (accessed October 24, 2014).

ORGANIZATIONS

American Cancer Society, 250 Williams St. NW, Atlanta, GA 30303, (800) 227-2345, http://www.cancer.org.

Cancer Treatment Centers of America, (800) 615-3055, http://www.cancercenter.com.

International Clinical Hyperthermia Society (ICHS), inforequest@hyperthermia-ichs.org, http://www.hyperthermia-ichs.org.

National Cancer Institute, 9609 Medical Center Dr., BG 9609 MSC 9760, Bethesda, MD 20892-9760, (800) 4-CANCER (422-6237), http://www.cancer.gov.

National Center for Complementary and Alternative Medicine, 9000 Rockville Pike, Bethesda, MD 20892, (888) 644-6226, TTY: (866) 464-3615, http://nccam.nih.gov.

Edward R. Rosick, DO, MPH
Rebecca J. Frey, PhD.

Hypocalcemia

Definition

Hypocalcemia is a type of electrolyte disturbance in which the level of calcium in the blood is too low. It occurs when the concentration of free calcium ions in the blood falls below 4.0 mg/dL (dL = a deciliter or one-tenth of a liter, about 3.4 fluid ounces). The normal concentration of free calcium ions in the blood serum is 4.0–6.0 mg/dL. Hypocalcemia can be caused by a range of conditions or disorders that either decrease the entry of calcium into the blood or increase the loss of calcium from the blood.

Demographics

It is difficult to estimate the frequency of hypocalcemia in the general population because many people, particularly those with mild forms of the disorder, have no noticeable symptoms. Studies of hospitalized patients admitted to intensive care units have indicated that 15%–50%% have hypocalcemia.

Hypocalcemia can affect persons of any age, depending on the disorder or condition causing the imbalance. As far as is known, both sexes and all races are equally likely to develop hypocalcemia.

Description

Calcium is an important mineral for maintaining human health. It is not only a component of bones and teeth, but is also essential for normal blood clotting and necessary for normal muscle and nerve functioning. In the human body, 99% of the total calcium is in the bones and teeth, and 1% is in the blood plasma.

The calcium ion (Ca^{2+}) has two positive charges. In bone, calcium ions occur as a complex with phosphate to form crystals of calcium phosphate. In the bloodstream, calcium ions also occur in complexes, and here calcium is found combined with proteins and various nutrients. However, in the bloodstream, calcium also occurs in a free form. Normally, about 47% of the calcium in the blood plasma is free, while 53% occurs in a complexed form.

Although all of the calcium in the bloodstream serves a useful purpose, only the concentration of free calcium ions has a direct influence on the functioning of our nerves and muscles. For this reason, the measurement of the concentration of free calcium is more important in the diagnosis of disease than measuring the level of total calcium or of complexed calcium. The level of total calcium in the blood serum is normally 8.5–10.5 mg/dL, while the level of free calcium is normally 4–5 mg/dl.

Risk factors

Risk factors for hypocalcemia include:

- history of kidney disorders
- history of thyroid disorders
- poor nutrition, especially vitamin D deficiency
- eating disorders
- alcoholism
- diagnosis of breast or prostate cancer
- being treated with chemotherapy for cancer
- heavy use of laxatives or other medications containing magnesium
- pancreatitis
- treatment for heavy metal poisoning
- DiGeorge syndrome and other congenital disorders characterized by failure of the parathyroid gland to develop normally

Causes and symptoms

Causes

Hypocalcemia has several different possible causes. It can be caused by hypoparathyroidism, by failure to produce 1,25-dihydroxyvitamin D, by low levels of plasma magnesium, or by failure to get adequate amounts of calcium or vitamin D in the diet. Hypoparathyroidism involves the failure of the parathyroid gland to make parathyroid hormone. In some cases, hypoparathyroidism results from surgical removal of the parathyroid gland or from genetic disorders that affect the normal development of the parathyroid gland.

Parathyroid hormone controls and maintains plasma calcium levels. The hormone exerts its effect on the kidneys, where it triggers the synthesis of 1,25-dihydroxyvitamin D. Thus, hypocalcemia can be independently caused by damage to the parathyroid gland or to the kidneys. 1,25-dihydroxyvitamin D stimulates the uptake of calcium from the diet and the mobilization of calcium from the bone. Bone mobilization refers to the natural process by which the body dissolves part of the bone in the skeleton in order to maintain or raise the levels of plasma calcium ions.

Low plasma magnesium levels (hypomagnesemia) can result in hypocalcemia. Hypomagnesemia can occur with alcoholism or with diseases characterized by an inability to properly absorb fat. Magnesium is required for parathyroid hormone to play its part in maintaining plasma calcium levels. For this reason, any disease that results in lowered plasma magnesium levels may also cause hypocalcemia.

Hypocalcemia may also result from the consumption of toxic levels of phosphate. Phosphate is a constituent of certain enema formulas. An enema is a solution that is used to cleanse the intestines via a catheter or tube inserted into the rectum. Cases of hypocalcemia have been documented in which people swallowed enema formulas or an enema had been administered to an infant.

Other causes of hypocalcemia include:

- Cancers that metastasize (spread) from other organs to the bone and destroy the bone. The most likely cancers of this type are breast cancer and prostate cancer.
- Certain cancer chemotherapy drugs, particularly cisplatin, leucovorin, and 5-fluorouracil.
- Severe pancreatitis (inflammation of the pancreas).
- Chelation therapy. Chelation therapy involves the use of such chemicals as EDTA to treat heavy metal poisoning. The chelating agent binds to the mercury, lead, or other heavy metal and enables the body to excrete the toxic substance safely. Hypocalcemia is a side effect of chelation therapy, however.
- Hungry bone syndrome. Hungry bone syndrome is a disorder that develops in some patients after surgical removal of the parathyroid gland.
- Sepsis (whole-body inflammatory response to severe infection).
- Toxic shock syndrome.

Symptoms

Symptoms of severe hypocalcemia include numbness or tingling around the mouth or in the feet and hands, as well as muscle spasms in the face, feet, and hands. These involuntary muscle spasms are called tetany. Hypocalcemia can also result in **depression**, memory loss, or hallucinations. Severe hypocalcemia occurs when serum free calcium is under 3 mg/dL. Chronic and moderate hypocalcemia can result in cataracts (damage to the eyes). In this case, the term "chronic" means lasting one year or longer.

Diagnosis

Hypocalcemia is frequently asymptomatic. When suspected, it is diagnosed by taking a careful patient history, a physical examination, and a sample of blood serum. The blood is tested for the concentration of free calcium using a calcium-sensitive electrode. Hypocalcemia has several causes; hence a full diagnosis requires assessment of the parathyroid gland, kidneys, and plasma magnesium concentration.

The patient should be asked about a history of eating disorders, vitamin deficiencies, treatment for alcoholism, kidney or liver problems, disorders of the pancreas or digestive tract, thyroid or parathyroid disorders, recent neck or bowel surgery, or epilepsy.

Examination

Physical examination of a patient with suspected hypocalcemia includes an examination of the patient's skin, mouth, and hair. Patients with hypocalcemia often have dry skin, brittle hair and nails, teeth in bad condition, skin rashes or **itching** skin, and cataracts in the eye. If the patient has a disorder of the parathyroid gland, they may also be shorter than average, have a round "moon" face, and possibly have intellectual impairments.

The doctor may hear wheezing or rattling noises when listening to the patient's breathing. An electrocardiogram (EKG) may indicate some irregularities in heart rhythm.

The patient may complain of muscle cramps or spasms, intestinal cramping, difficulty swallowing, coughing spells, facial twitching, general aching sensations in the muscles, numbness in fingers or toes, or tingling sensations.

In severe hypocalcemia, the patient may have such neurological symptoms as seizures, hallucinations, and confusion.

Tests

The doctor will usually order blood tests to evaluate the level of calcium and other electrolytes (particularly magnesium and phosphate levels) in the blood as well as tests of liver and kidney function. The level of parathyroid hormone will be checked by means of an antibody-mediated radioimmunoassay. The doctor will also order an EKG if one was not performed in the office in order to evaluate abnormal heart rhythms.

Two diagnostic tests that may be performed are the Chvostek and Trousseau tests. In the Chvostek test, the doctor taps over the facial nerve along the jawline about an inch in front of the ear. A patient with hypocalcemia will develop twitching at the corner of the mouth, the nose, the eye, and the other facial muscles. In the Trousseau test, a blood pressure cuff is placed on the patient's arm and inflated above the level of the systolic pressure for three minutes. A patient with hypocalcemia will develop spasms in the hand and forearm and the wrist will flex upward.

Treatment

Traditional

The method chosen for treatment depends on the exact cause and on the severity of the hypocalcemia. Mild hypocalcemia may require nothing more than a thorough office examination and laboratory testing. Severe hypocalcemia requires admission to the hospital for supportive care and immediate injection of calcium ions, usually in the form of calcium gluconate. In severe cases, emergency room physicians will need to consult one or more specialists, including surgeons, neurologists, oncologists, dietitians, internists, endocrinologists, and toxicologists.

Drugs

Oral calcium supplements are prescribed for long-term treatment (non-emergency) of hypocalcemia. The oral supplements may take the form of calcium carbonate, calcium chloride, calcium lactate, or calcium gluconate. Where hypocalcemia results from kidney failure, treatment includes injections of 1,25-dihydroxyvitamin D. Oral vitamin D supplements can increase gastrointestinal absorption of calcium. Where hypocalcemia results from hypoparathyroidism, treatment may include oral calcium, 1,25-dihydroxyvitamin D, or other drugs. Where low serum magnesium levels occur concurrently with hypocalcemia, the magnesium deficiency must be corrected to effectively treat the hypocalcemia.

Prognosis

The prognosis for hypocalcemia from simple dietary deficiencies is excellent. In most cases, however, the prognosis depends on the disorder or condition causing the hypocalcemia. Patients with alcoholism or eating disorders may need psychiatric intervention as well as

medical treatment in order to recover fully. Severe symptomatic hypocalcemia can result in seizures, low blood pressure that does not respond to fluid, and irregular heart rhythms. In a few cases, cardiovascular collapse brought on by hypocalcemia has resulted in death.

Prevention

The first and most obvious way to help prevent hypocalcemia is to ensure that adequate amounts of calcium and vitamin D are consumed each day, either in the diet or as supplements. Hypocalcemia that may occur with damage to the parathyroid gland or to the kidneys cannot be prevented. Hypocalcemia resulting from overuse of enemas can be prevented by reducing enema usage. Hypocalcemia resulting from magnesium deficiency tends to occur in chronic alcoholics, and this type of hypocalcemia can be prevented by reducing alcohol consumption and increasing the intake of healthful food.

Resources

BOOKS

Fiebach, Nicholas H., et al, eds. *Principles of Ambulatory Medicine*. Philadelphia: Lippincott Williams and Wilkins, 2007.

Kleerekoper, Michael, Ethel S. Siris, and Michael McClung, eds. *The Bone and Mineral Manual: A Practical Guide*, 2nd ed. Burlington, MA: Elsevier Academic Press, 2005.

PERIODICALS

Ferron, M., and G. Karsenty. "The Gutsy Side of Bone." *Cell Metabolism* 10 (July 2009): 7–8.

Zhou, P., and M. Markowitz. "Hypocalcemia in Infants and Children." *Pediatrics in Review* 30 (May 2009): 190–92.

WEBSITES

Lewis, James L. III. "Hypocalcemia." *Merck Manual*. http://www.merckmanuals.com/professional/endocrine_and_metabolic_disorders/electrolyte_disorders/hypocalcemia.html (accessed November 4, 2014).

The Scott Hamilton CARES Initiative. "Hypocalcemia (Low Calcium)." Chemocare.com. http://chemocare.com/chemotherapy/side-effects/hypocalcemia-low-calcium.aspx (accessed November 4, 2014).

ORGANIZATIONS

American Association of Clinical Endocrinologists (AACE), 245 Riverside Ave., Suite 200, Jacksonville, FL 32202, 904-353-7878, http://www.aace.com.

American College of Emergency Physicians, 1125 Executive Cir., Irving, TX 75038-2522, (972) 550-0911, (800) 798-1822, Fax: (972) 580-2816, membership@acep.org, http://www.acep.org.

American Society for Nutrition (ASN), 9650 Rockville Pike, Bethesda, MD 20814, 301-634-7050, Fax: 301-634-7892, info@nutrition.org, http://www.nutrition.org.

National Toxicology Program (NTP), P.O. Box 12233, MD K2-03, Research Triangle Park, NC 27709, 919-541-0530, http://ntp.niehs.nih.gov.

U.S. Food and Drug Administration, 10903 New Hampshire Ave., Silver Spring, MD 20993, (888) INFO-FDA (463-6332), http://www.fda.gov.

Tom Brody, PhD.
Rebecca J. Frey, PhD.

I

Ibritumomab

Definition

Ibritumomab is a monoclonal antibody radioimmunotherapy used to treat **non-Hodgkin lymphoma** (NHL).

Purpose

Ibritumomab is used to treat individuals with low grade follicular NHL that has failed to respond or that has stopped responding to the drug **rituximab** (Rituxan).

NHL is a **cancer** that arises in the organs of the lymph system. It is the most common type of **lymphoma** in the United States. The lymph system is important in creating and transporting blood cells called lymphocytes that fight infection throughout the body. The major organs of the lymph system are the spleen, thymus, tonsils, and bone marrow. These organs produce several different kinds of cells that fight infection. The major ones are called T-cells and B-cells. Ibritumomab specifically targets both mature and immature B-cells.

In NHL, abnormal (cancerous) lymphocytes grow out of control. So many of these abnormal lymphocytes develop that they prevent other immune system cells and blood vessel from forming. There are several types of NHL. One form is called follicular lymphoma. In this form, the cancerous cells clump together. They may grow quickly, in which case the disease is called a high-grade lymphoma, or they may grow slowly, in which case the cancer is called low-grade lymphoma.

Standard treatments for NHL include **chemotherapy**, **radiation therapy**, stem cell therapy, and a newer form of therapy called biologic therapy. Biologic therapy uses the biopharmaceutical rituximab. Ibritumomab is used in patients with low-grade B-cell NHL who have failed to respond or who have relapsed after standard treatment.

Description

Ibritumomab, which is also called ibritumomab tiuxetan, is manufactured in the United States and sold under the brand name Zevalin by Biogen Idec. It was approved for use in February 2002 and was the first radioimmunotherapy approved by the United States Food and Drug Administration (FDA). Generic substitutes are not available, and currently there is only one American manufacturer.

Radioimmunotherapy is a form of biologic therapy that combines a protein that attaches to the target cell with a small dose of radioactive material that disrupts and kills the cell. Unique proteins called antigens exist on the surface of every cell. The body monitors these proteins, and when it recognizes a cell as foreign or defective, it creates other antigen-specific proteins called antibodies to attach to the unwanted cells and disable them. With NHL, this system of protection fails and defective cancerous cells are allowed to continue growing.

Ibritumomab is an antibody made of mouse (murine) protein that comes from Chinese hamster ovary cells. It binds with a protein called CD20 that is found on the surface of both normal and malignant B-cells. Ibritumomab alone does not kill B-cells, so it is bound to a radioactive material, either indium-111 (In-111) or yttrium-90 (Y-90). The role of ibritumomab is to deliver the radioactive material to specific target cells and bind it there. The radioactive rays given off by In-111 or Y-90 disrupt the cell's functions, resulting in cell death. This therapy kills both healthy and cancerous B-cells.

Recommended dosage

Ibritumomab is given only in a two-step cycle in conjunction with another nonradioactive monoclonal antibody called rituximab. Rituximab attacks the same B-cells as ibritumomab but does not deliver a dose of radioactive material to the cell. The two-step cycle of administration of ibritumomab is intended to occur only once.

KEY TERMS

Anaphylactic shock—A whole-body allergic reaction that is often fatal.

Malignant—Cancerous.

Neutrophil—A type of blood cell important to fighting infection.

Non-Hodgkin lymphoma—A cancer of the lymph system that causes the accumulation of large numbers of defective (cancerous) immune system cells.

Platelet—A tiny disk-shaped structure found in blood that has no nucleus and plays an important role in blood clotting.

Radioimmunotherapy—A treatment in which a radioactive material is delivered to specific cells by using a protein that binds to the surface of the target cells.

The material needed for the therapeutic administration of ibritumomab is sold under the name Zevalin. The ibritumomab carrier antibody is mixed with the radioactive material by the physician shortly before use.

Step 1 includes a single dose of rituximab. The dose is determined by the patient's body size. Rituximab is infused slowly into a vein while the physician watches for hypersensitivity reactions. Within four hours following administration of rituximab, a single dose of 5.0 milliCuries (mCi) ibritumomab tiuxetan that contains the radioactive material In-111 is injected intravenously (IV) over a period of 10 minutes.

Step 2 follows seven to nine days after Step 1. The patient is given another IV dose of rituximab, again based on body size. Within four hours following the rituximab, the patient is injected with a dose of radioactive ibritumomab Y-90. This dose is also based on body size up to a total maximum allowable dose of 32.0 mCi. This completes the active part of the therapy, but patients must continue to have their blood count monitored for several months, as the therapy continues to kill cells for weeks.

Precautions

People who are allergic to any type of mouse (murine) protein, rituximab, yttrium chloride, or indium chloride should not use this therapy. Ibritumomab can cause harm to the developing fetus and should not be used by pregnant women. Women should use birth control for 12 months after receiving this therapy. It has not been established whether this therapy is safe to use in breastfeeding women. A pediatric dose has not been established.

Zevalin is radioactive when it is being administered, and care should be taken to minimize exposure of patients and health care providers.

Side effects

Side effects are many and varied. Serious but rare side effects include:

- potentially fatal infusion hypersensitivity reactions, usually to the first dose of rituximab, that can cause low blood pressure, difficulty breathing, heart attack, and anaphylactic shock
- severe drop in platelet count (thrombocytopenia) or neutrophil count (neutropenia); uncontrolled bleeding
- development of secondary malignancies that arise from the therapy

More common but less serious side effects include:

- susceptibility to infections; fever or chills
- nausea, vomiting, diarrhea, black, tarry stools
- loss of appetite
- anemia
- joint pain
- dizziness
- increased cough or hoarseness
- rash, swelling, or puffiness around the face and neck

Interactions

It is important to tell the physician about all prescription medications, over-the counter medications, and herbal or alternative remedies that are being taken before treatment with Zevalin is begun. No formal drug interaction studies have been completed; however, Zevalin therapy does interfere with blood clotting and should not be used while individuals are taking blood thinners such as **warfarin** (Coumadin) or clopidogrel bisulfate (Plavix). Individuals who have a very low platelet count may not be able to use this therapy.

Individuals should not be vaccinated with a live virus vaccine prior to or soon after receiving this therapy. The interaction of live virus vaccines and this therapy has not been investigated, but it is recommended that individuals receiving ibritumomab avoid people who have recently been vaccinated with live virus oral polio vaccine.

Resources

BOOKS

Chu, Edward, and Vincent T. DeVita, Jr. *Physicians' Cancer Chemotherapy Drug Manual 2014.* Burlington, MA: Jones & Bartlett Learning, 2014.

WEBSITES

American Cancer Society. "Y 90 Ibritumomab Tiuxetan." http://www.cancer.org/treatment/treatmentsandsideeffects/guidetocancerdrugs/ibritumomab-tiuxetan (accessed November 4, 2014).

National Cancer Institute. "Ibritumomab Tiuxetan." http://www.cancer.gov/cancertopics/druginfo/ibritumomabtiuxetan (accessed November 4, 2014).

ORGANIZATIONS

U.S. Food and Drug Administration, 10903 New Hampshire Ave., Silver Spring, MD 20993, (888) INFO-FDA (463-6332), http://www.fda.gov.

Tish Davidson, A. M.

Idarubicin

Definition

Idarubicin (Idamycin) is a medication that kills **cancer** cells.

Purpose

Idarubicin is approved to treat only one single cancer, acute myelocytic leukemia (AML) in adults. Recent research suggests that using idarubicin rather than the more traditional **daunorubicin** in treating AML results in higher rates of complete remission (CR) and longer survival for patients. CR is the total elimination of all diseased cells detectable following therapy. The U.S. Food and Drug Administration (FDA) has not approved idarubicin as treatment for **acute lymphocytic leukemia** (ALL).

Much research involving idarubicin is now being conducted. Some of this has involved acute lymphocytic leukemia (ALL) as well as AML. For example, a recent study was conducted in patients with either AML or ALL who had received **bone marrow transplantation** and then relapsed. Patients received a combination of **cytarabine**, idarubicin, and **etoposide**, as well as a medicine called G-CSF (**filgrastim**). This treatment achieved a high CR rate in these patients.

Another recent study looked at the use of idarubicin in children with AML. All the children received cytarabine and etoposide. In addition, some of the

KEY TERMS

Bilirubin—A pigment produced when the liver processes waste products. A high bilirubin level causes yellowing of the skin.

Blasts—Immature cells.

Complete remission (CR)—The total elimination of all diseased cells detectable following therapy.

Necrosis—The sum of the morphological changes indicative of cell death. It may affect groups of cells or part of a structure or an organ.

children received idarubicin, while some received daunorubicin. Overall, patients in both groups fared equally well in terms of survival length. However, patients who had larger numbers of cells known as blasts (immature cells) tended to do better if they received idarubicin rather than daunorubicin. In addition, high-risk patients tended to do better with idarubicin than with daunorubicin. No subgroup of patients achieved better outcomes with daunorubicin than with idarubicin.

For older patients with acute nonlymphocytic leukemia, treatment with idarubicin is effective and has acceptable side effects. According to recent research from Italy, "There is growing interest in autologous **stem cell transplantation** (ASCT) for elderly patients with acute myeloid leukemia (AML)." While mortality and toxicity from ASCT have been reduced, relapse rate is still high.

Description

Idarubicin is an antibiotic, although doctors do not use this drug to attack infections. Its only use is to kill cancer cells. It does so by affecting how the DNA of cancer cells works.

Recommended dosage

In the treatment of AML, 12 mg of idarubicin per square meter may be given over a period of two to three days every three weeks in combination with other medications. Patients with liver problems may be given lower doses than other patients receive. Idarubicin is not typically given by mouth, as an insufficient amount of the medication would be transported through the stomach wall if this were done. Rather, this medication is usually administered through an intravenous (IV) procedure. During this time, it circulates widely throughout the body.

A new formulation of idarubicin has been developed that permits idarubicin to be taken orally. However, this formulation is currently available only in France and is used only in older patients who are not good candidates for intensive intravenous treatment. There is little information currently available on the effectiveness of this oral formulation. The studies that have been performed suggest that it is less effective than other formulations of idarubicin.

Precautions

Idarubicin may be associated with excessive toxicity in patients with congestive heart failure, liver function characterized by a high bilirubin level, or prior chest radiation to the heart.

Side effects

Like daunorubicin and **doxorubicin**, idarubicin may adversely affect the patient's heart. However, doctors are not certain how much of the drug it takes to cause such harm and, therefore, how to limit dosage so that such harm is not caused. However, idarubicin appears to be less likely to cause heart damage than similar drugs such as daunorubicin and doxorubicin. Another serious side effect that limits how much of the drug is given to patients is its potential adverse effect upon the bone marrow, where blood cells are produced.

Idarubicin may cause **nausea and vomiting**, baldness (**alopecia**), and stomach problems. In addition, idarubicin may cause blistering if extravasation occurs. Extravasation occurs when **chemotherapy** gets outside of the vein during infusion. If extravasation occurs, the drug may cause severe local pain, swelling, or tissue necrosis that may require plastic surgery.

Patients receiving idarubicin in conjunction with certain other **anticancer drugs** may develop a type of leukemia. However, this adverse effect is extremely rare.

In the few studies that have been conducted on the oral formulation of idarubicin, the most prominent side effects seen are low blood cell counts, nausea, vomiting, **diarrhea**, and alopecia.

Resources

BOOKS

Chu, Edward, and Vincent T. DeVita, Jr. *Physicians' Cancer Chemotherapy Drug Manual 2014*. Burlington, MA: Jones & Bartlett Learning, 2014.

WEBSITES

Cancer Research UK. "Idarubicin (Zavedos)." http://www.cancerresearchuk.org/about-cancer/cancers-in-general/treatment/cancer-drugs/idarubicin (accessed November 4, 2014).

The Scott Hamilton CARES Initiative. "Idarubicin." Chemocare.com. http://chemocare.com/chemotherapy/drug-info/idarubicin.aspx (accessed November 4, 2014).

ORGANIZATIONS

U.S. Food and Drug Administration, 10903 New Hampshire Ave., Silver Spring, MD 20993, (888) INFO-FDA (463-6332), http://www.fda.gov.

Bob Kirsch

IFEX *see* **Ifosfamide**

Ifosfamide

Definition

Ifosfamide is an anticancer (antineoplastic) agent classified as a nitrogen mustard alkylating agent. It also acts as a suppressor of the immune system. It is available under the brand name Ifex.

Purpose

Ifosfamide is approved by the U.S. Food and Drug Administration (FDA) to treat germ-cell **testicular cancer**. It is generally prescribed in combination with another medicine (**mesna**), which is used to prevent the bladder problems that may be caused by ifosfamide alone.

Ifosfamide also has activity against other cancers and is prescribed in practice for these **cancer** types:

• pancreatic cancer
• stomach cancer
• soft-tissue sarcoma
• Ewing sarcoma
• acute and chronic lymphocytic leukemia
• bladder cancer
• bone cancer
• breast cancer
• cervical cancer
• head and neck cancers
• lung cancer
• lymphomas
• neuroblastomas
• ovarian cancer
• Wilms tumor

Description

Ifosfamide chemically interferes with the synthesis of the genetic material (DNA and RNA) of cancer cells by cross-linking of DNA strands, which prevents these cells from being able to reproduce and continue the growth of the cancer.

Recommended dosage

Ifosfamide may be taken only as an injection into the vein. The dosage prescribed varies widely depending on the patient, the cancer being treated, and whether other medications are also being taken. Examples of common doses for adults are: 50 mg per kg per day, or 700–2,000 mg per square meter of body surface area for five days every three to four weeks. Another alternative regimen is 2,400 mg per square meter of body surface area for three days, or 5000 mg per square meter of body surface area as a single dose every three to four weeks. Examples of common dosing regimens for children are: 1,200 to 1,800 mg per square meter of body surface area per day for three to five days every 21 to 28 days; 5,000 mg per square meter of body surface area once every 21 to 28 days; or 3,000 mg per square meter of body surface area for two days every 21 to 28 days.

Precautions

Ifosfamide can cause an allergic reaction in some people. Patients with a prior allergic reaction to ifosfamide should not take this drug.

Ifosfamide should always be taken with plenty of fluids.

Ifosfamide can cause serious birth defects if either the man or the woman is taking this drug at the time of conception, or if the woman is taking this drug during pregnancy. Contraceptive measures should be taken by both men and women while on this drug. Because ifosfamide is easily passed from mother to child through breast milk, breastfeeding is not recommended during treatment.

Ifosfamide suppresses the immune system, and its excretion from the body is dependent on a normally functioning kidney and liver. For these reasons, it is important that the prescribing physician is aware of any of the following preexisting medical conditions:

• a current case of or recent exposure to chickenpox
• herpes zoster (shingles)
• all current infections
• kidney disease
• liver disease

Also, because ifosfamide is such a potent immunosuppressant, patients taking this drug must exercise extreme caution to avoid contracting any new infections.

Side effects

Inflammation and irritation of the bladder causing blood in the urine is the most common and severe side effect of ifosfamide. However, this side effect can be prevented and controlled with the administration of the bladder protectant drug mesna, and by vigorous hydration with intravenous fluids before, during, and after **chemotherapy**. Patients should also urinate frequently (at least every 2 hours) to enhance removal of the drug from the body, and drink 2 to 3 liters of fluids a day for 2 to 3 days after discontinuation of the chemotherapy.

Other common side effects of ifosfamide are:

• confusion
• hallucinations
• drowsiness
• dizziness
• temporary hair loss (alopecia)
• increased susceptibility to infection
• increased risk of bleeding (due to a decrease in the number of platelets involved in the clotting process)
• nausea and vomiting (can be prevented with prescribed antiemetics)

Less common side effects include:

• increased coloration (pigmentation) of the skin and fingernails
• loss of appetite (anorexia)
• diarrhea
• nasal stuffiness
• skin rash, itching, or hives

A doctor should be consulted immediately if the patient experiences any of these side effects:

• painful or difficult urination
• increase in frequency or feeling of urgency to urinate
• blood in the urine
• blood in the stool
• severe diarrhea

- mental status changes such as confusion, drowsiness, or hallucinations
- signs of infection such as cough, sore throat, fever and chills
- shortness of breath
- chest or abdominal pain
- pain in the lower back or sides
- unusual bleeding or bruising
- tiny red dots on the skin

Interactions

Ifosfamide should not be taken in combination with any prescription drug, over-the-counter drug, or herbal remedy without prior consultation with a physician. It should not be given together with live virus vaccines for measles, mumps, smallpox, polio, rubella, or influenza because of the patient's risk of developing a viral infection from the vaccine. It should not be given together with monoclonal antibodies because of the risk of serious infection.

Resources

BOOKS

Chu, Edward, and Vincent T. DeVita, Jr. *Physicians' Cancer Chemotherapy Drug Manual 2014.* Burlington, MA: Jones & Bartlett Learning, 2014.

WEBSITES

American Cancer Society. "Ifosfamide." http://www.cancer.org/treatment/treatmentsandsideeffects/guidetocancerdrugs/ifosfamide (accessed November 4, 2014).

Macmillan Cancer Support. "Ifosfamide (Mitoxana®)." Chemocare.com. http://www.macmillan.org.uk/Cancerinformation/Cancertreatment/Treatmenttypes/Chemotherapy/Individualdrugs/Ifosfamide.aspx (accessed November 4, 2014).

ORGANIZATIONS

U.S. Food and Drug Administration, 10903 New Hampshire Ave., Silver Spring, MD 20993, (888) INFO-FDA (463-6332), http://www.fda.gov.

Paul A. Johnson, Ed.M.

Imaging studies

Definition

Imaging studies are tests performed with a variety of techniques that produce pictures of the interior of a patient's body. They have become indispensable tools in **cancer** screening, detection, and treatment.

Description

Imaging tests are performed using sound waves, radioactive particles, magnetic fields, or x-rays that are detected and converted into images after passing through body tissues. Dyes are sometimes used with x-ray tests as contrasting agents to enhance visualization of organs or tissues that cannot be seen as clearly with conventional x-rays. The operating principle of the various techniques is based on the fact that rays and particles interact differently with various types of tissues, especially in the presence of cancerous growths. In this way, the interior of the body becomes visible, and digital pictures of normal structure and function as well as of abnormalities can be developed.

Imaging tests differ from endoscopic tests, which are carried out with a flexible lighted piece of tubing connected to a viewing lens or camera.

Screening refers to the use of imaging studies to detect cancer in its early stages. Screening is performed in patients who have no obvious cancer symptoms. Imaging studies are also used to locate tumors in patients who have symptoms, and to distinguish between benign growths or cancerous tumors. They are also used to determine the extent of a cancer and indicate whether a treatment is shrinking a tumor or eliminating cancer cells. As such, imaging studies represent crucial tools for cancer diagnosis and management.

Major imaging techniques

Computed tomography scan (CT scan)

Computed tomography scans show a cross-section of a part of the body. In this technique, a thin beam is used to produce a series of exposures detected at different angles. The exposures are fed into a computer, which yields a single image much like a slice of the organ or body part being scanned. A dye is often injected into the patient to improve contrast and obtain sharper images than those obtained with x-rays. CT images can be reconstructed into three-dimensional or four-dimensional planes. A four-dimensional image is one that displays the movement of the target organ or tissue as well as its length, width, and depth.

Magnetic resonance imaging (MRI)

Magnetic resonance imaging also produces cross-sectional images of the body using powerful magnetic fields rather than radiation. MRI is especially useful to detect and locate cancers of the liver and the central nervous system, which occur in the brain or the spinal cord. It uses a cylinder housing a magnet. The patient lies on a platform inside the scanner. The magnetic field aligns hydrogen atoms present in the tissue being scanned in a given direction. Following a burst of

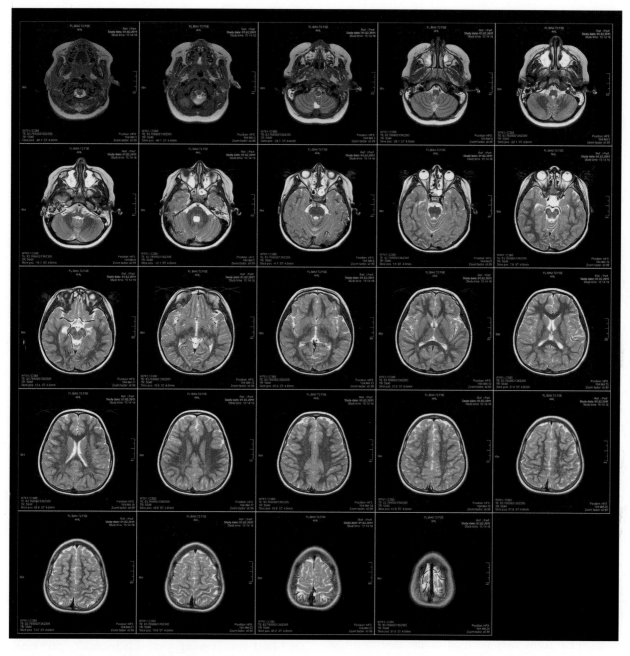

Magnetic resonance imaging (MRI) scans of the brain. *(Kondor83/Shutterstock.com)*

radio-frequency radiation, the atoms flip back to their original orientation while emitting signals that are fed into a computer for conversion to two-, three-, or four-dimensional images. Contrast agents can also be injected to produce clearer images of certain tissues, organs, or substances in the body.

Mammography

Mammography is an x-ray examination of the breast. It is often used as a screening tool to detect breast abnormalities and cancers before they can be felt. Mammograms (the image produced) use a special x-ray machine. The breast is compressed between two plates to allow the low-level x-ray radiation to penetrate the breast tissue evenly.

Nuclear scan

Nuclear scans, also called radionuclide imaging or scintigraphy, use substances called tracers or radionuclides that release low levels of radioactivity. The test is based on the principle that the tracers will be absorbed to different degrees by different tissues, thus allowing doctors to distinguish between normal and cancerous tissues. Common **nuclear medicine scans** for cancer patients include bone scans; liver, spleen, and thyroid scans are also frequently performed.

Position emission tomography (PET)

Positron emission tomography uses a form of sugar that contains a radioactive atom that emits particles called positrons. The positrons are absorbed to different extents by cells according to their metabolic rates. PET scans are especially useful for brain imaging studies, and are widely used to assess the spread of cancers in the lungs. PET scans may be used in the assessment or monitoring of a number of other cancers.

PET-CT

In recent years, manufacturers have discovered techniques for combining imaging methods so that the best qualities of each are fused to benefit the study of cancer and other diseases. Many centers now have PET-CT, which combines PET and CT images into one image; the information about tumor anatomy from the CT scan is combined with information about tumor sugar or glucose uptake from the PET scan. In most instances, a single piece of equipment is used to obtain both images. Soon, doctors hope to be able to merge PET and MRI images.

Ultrasound

Also called sonography or **ultrasonography**, ultrasound uses high-frequency sound waves and echoes to create images on a monitor. Because it uses no radiation, ultrasound may be chosen as an alternative to x-rays or CT for pregnant women or children. Usually, however, ultrasound has precise purposes and is useful in evaluating pain, swelling, and infection. Often, doctors use ultrasound first to help determine whether a mass might be solid or filled with fluid, which means it is more likely a cyst, and not a cancerous tumor. Ultrasound also can create three-dimensional and four-dimensional images and help provide measurements of masses.

X-rays

X-rays produce shallow images of certain specific organs or tissues. X-rays are a form of high-energy radiation; tissues of the body can absorb it to varying degrees. For example, bones absorb less radiation than soft tissue. After passing through the body, the x-rays are directed on to a film or cassette where the dense tissue appears as a white shadow, thus providing contrast with the soft tissue, which produces a darker impression on the image. X-rays produce a single image.

Chest x-rays are used to detect lung and bronchial cancers and also to evaluate a patient's symptoms, such as shortness of breath. Other types of x-rays such as abdominal x-rays, may also be ordered to assess a patient's symptoms but are not used to screen for cancer.

X-rays with dye studies

Dye studies are usually performed by injecting the contrast agent in to the patient's circulatory system or the target organ. These studies are used to produce angiograms, cystograms, myelograms, lymphangiograms and fistulograms.

ANGIOGRAM. An angiogram is an examination of the blood vessels using x-rays. It is usually performed with an intravenous injection of fluorescent dye followed by multiframe photography, a technique known as fluoroscopy. The doctor inserts a small tube (catheter) into the blood vessel and then injects the dye that makes the vessels visible within the x-ray image.

CYSTOGRAM. A cystogram is a scan of the bladder and ureters. The ureters are passages that lead from the kidneys to the bladder. A catheter is inserted into the bladder and a radioactive material called a radioisotope is introduced into the bladder. An oral cholecystogram (OCG) is an x-ray examination of the gallbladder, the organ that helps release bile into the small intestine for the digestion of fats. The gallbladder is difficult to visualize with conventional x-ray pictures, and special tablets are ingested by mouth to enhance contrast.

MYELOGRAM. A myelogram is an x-ray of the spine and spinal cord. The spinal cord is the nerve tissue enclosed in the vertebral column that runs from the bottom of the brain to halfway down the back. During a myelogram, x-ray dye is injected into the spinal fluid and mixes with it, flowing around the spinal cord, which can then be seen and recorded on x-ray film.

LYMPHANGIOGRAM. A lymphangiogram is an x-ray of the lymphatic system that also uses dye to enhance contrast. It is used to screen for lymph node involvement in cancer.

FISTULOGRAM. A fistula is an abnormal passage within body tissue. For example, a fistula may connect two organs inside the body that are not normally connected. A fistula may also lead from an internal organ inside the body to the surface outside. Examples include: between the skin and the bowel (enterocutaneous fistula) and between the stomach and the colon (gastrocolic fistula). A fistulogram is an x-ray examination of this abnormal passage. The contrasting agent is injected directly into the fistula so that it will show up clearly on x-ray pictures.

Fluoroscopy

Fluoroscopy is one of the oldest areas of diagnostic radiology. It is similar to x-ray in that a small dose of x-rays is directed through a body part but the x-ray beam is controlled in pulses to create a sequence of images. The fluoroscope provides images of internal body parts as they move, much like a movie. The body part and its motion can be seen on a monitor, which allows the radiologist to capture a single image during the examination.

During fluoroscopy, the patient is placed between the x-ray source and the monitor. The live images generated by the x-ray source strike the image-intensifying tube and allow doctors to see the size, shape, and structure of a patient's internal structures. Because the radiation is blocked more effectively by dense tissue, such as that of a tumor, the result is a dark shadow of the tumor on the screen against a light background. Most fluoroscopy devices include television or video cameras attached to the image-intensifier tube. The camera output can be digitized and sent through a computer for image enhancement.

In fluoroscopic studies, the radiologist can either insert an intravenous (IV) catheter (hollow tube inserted into blood vessels or into an organ) to **biopsy** a tumor, or can use a contrast agent to visualize the organ or area of interest. The contrast agent allows the image to be viewed more clearly. Contrast agents may be introduced into the patient's body by injection, swallowing, or an enema. Fluoroscopic exams include the following types of tests: barium swallow, **barium enema**, and intravenous pyelography (also called **intravenous urography**).

BARIUM SWALLOW. Barium studies are used to diagnose gastrointestinal (GI) diseases. The patient drinks a chalky milkshake-like concoction containing barium, which coats the esophagus and stomach. The barium absorbs the x-rays so that the lining of the upper digestive tract can be clearly seen. In barium x-rays, fluoroscopy allows the physician to see the movement of the intestines as the barium moves through them.

BARIUM ENEMA. In a lower GI series, the patient receives a barium enema that coats the intestines and rectum. A gap in the image in the stomach or small intestine might indicate an ulcer, and bubbles in the normally smooth large intestinal lining may be abnormal growths.

INTRAVENOUS PYELOGRAPHY (IVP). Pyelography, also called urography, consists of several x-rays of the entire urinary system, including the kidneys, ureter, bladder and urethra. A contrast agent is injected through a vein to make the organs visible for the x-rays.

See also Screening test; Ultrasonography.

Resources

BOOKS

Abeloff, M. D., et al. *Clinical Oncology.* 5th ed. New York: Churchill Livingstone, 2014.

Grainger, R. G., et al. *Grainger & Allison's Diagnostic Radiology: A Textbook of Medical Imaging.* 6th ed. Philadelphia: Saunders, 2015.

Mettler, F. A. *Essentials of Radiology.* 3rd ed. Philadelphia: Saunders, 2013.

Niederhuber, J. E., et al. *Clinical Oncology.* 5th ed. Philadelphia: Elsevier, 2014.

PERIODICALS

Frassica, F. J., J. A. Khanna, and E. F. McCarthy. "The Role of MR Imaging in Soft Tissue Tumor Evaluation: Perspective of the Orthopedic Oncologist and Musculoskeletal Pathologist." *Magnetic Resonance Imaging Clinics of North America* 8 (November 2000): 915-27.

Hopper, K. D., K. Singapuri, and A. Finkel. "Body CT and Oncologic Imaging." *Radiology* 215 (April 2000): 27-40.

Jain, P., and A. C. Arroliga. "Spiral CT for Lung Cancer Screening: Is It Ready for Prime Time?" *Cleveland Clinical Journal of Medicine* 68 (January 2001): 74-81.

Pomper, M. G., and J. D. Port. "New Techniques in MR Imaging of Brain Tumors." *Magnetic Resonance Imaging Clinics of North America* 8 (November 2000): 691-713.

Roelcke, U., and K. L. Leenders. "PET in Neuro-oncology." *Journal of Cancer Research and Clinical Oncology* 127 (January 2001): 2-8.

WEBSITES

American Cancer Society. "Imaging (Radiology) Tests." http://www.cancer.org/acs/groups/cid/documents/webcontent/003177-pdf.pdf (accessed December 2, 2014).

ORGANIZATIONS

National Cancer Institute, 9609 Medical Center Drive, Bethesda, MD 20892, (800) 422-6237, http://www.cancer.gov.

Radiological Society of North America, 820 Jorie Blvd, Oak Brook, IL 60523, (630) 571-2670, (800) 381-6660, Fax: (630) 571-7837, http://www.rsna.org/Patients.aspx.

Monique Laberge, PhD.
REVISED BY TERESA G. ODLE

Imatinib mesylate

Definition

Imatinib mesylate is an enzyme inhibitor used for **cancer** therapy. Imatinib mesylate is also known as STI571 and is sold under the brand name Gleevec. It was given the name STI571 during early development. STI stands for signal transduction inhibitor.

Purpose

Imatinib mesylate was first approved by the U.S. Food and Drug Administration (FDA) in 1993 to treat a rare cancer called chronic myeloid leukemia (CML). (CML is also called chronic myelogenous leukemia or chronic myelocytic leukemia.) As of 2014, the drug was

approved to treat leukemia and gastrointestinal stromal tumors (GIST), a type of tumor that forms most often in the walls of the stomach or small intestine. In 2013, the FDA approved the use of imatinib for treating children who have a specific type of acute lymphoblastic leukemia that is Philadelphia chromosome-positive. In this type of leukemia, which can come on suddenly and be life-threatening, part of a chromosome moves to another chromosome, an abnormality known as translocation.

Description

Imatinib mesylate is the first drug of its kind developed. It fights cancer by turning off an enzyme called tyrosine kinase, which causes CML cells to multiply at an abnormal rate. Its function is different from that of most other cancer drugs because it specifically targets an enzyme that allows the growth of CML cells. Imatinib has been shown to significantly reduce the number of cancer cells in the blood and bone marrow of treated patients.

Patients who are diagnosed with CML in the three phases of disease can be treated with imatinib mesylate.

KEY TERMS

CYP3A4—An enzyme that is predominately responsible for the metabolism of imatinib mesylate.

Enzyme—Any protein that acts as a catalyst, increasing the rate of a chemical reaction.

Kinase—A type of enzyme that catalyzes the transfer of phosphate groups to other molecules.

Leukemia—A type of cancer in which the bone marrow produces an excessive number of abnormal (leukemic) white blood cells. White blood cells protect the body against infection, but the abnormal cells suppress the production of normal white blood cells.

Tumor—An abnormal mass of tissue that serves no purpose. Tumors may be either benign (noncancerous) or malignant (cancerous).

Tyrosine—A nonessential amino acid. Amino acids are the building blocks of protein. They are the raw materials used by the body to make protein. Tyrosine is labeled nonessential because when this amino acid is lacking in the diet, it can be manufactured by the body.

Chronic myeloid leukemia appears to respond within one to three months following administration of this drug.

Recommended dosage

A doctor experienced in the treatment of patients with CML should initiate therapy.

To minimize the risk of gastrointestinal irritation, imatinib mesylate should be taken with food and a large glass of water. The recommended dosage varies according to clinical circumstances and stage of disease, but generally ranges between 300 and 600 mg per day. As long as the patient continues to benefit, treatment should be continued.

Precautions

Studies have not been performed with imatinib mesylate to determine whether it is a carcinogen (cancer causing); therefore, it is not known whether this drug may cause mutations or have cancer-causing effects.

Side effects

Commonly reported side effects include: **nausea and vomiting**, muscle cramps, edema (water retention), skin rash, **diarrhea**, heartburn, and headache. Serious side effects occur less frequently, but if they occur may include severe edema liver toxicity, and the potential for bleeding, especially in the elderly.

Interactions

Imatinib mesylate interacts with many other drugs. In some cases, side effects may be increased because imatinib mesylate might increase blood levels of certain drugs. Alternatively, imatinib mesylate may decrease blood levels of the drugs, thus reducing their effectiveness. In addition, the blood levels of imatinib mesylate may rise or fall because of other drugs. Therefore, the side effects of imatinib mesylate may be increased or its effectiveness may be reduced. Patients must discuss all of their medications with their doctor due to many potential drug-drug interactions.

CYP3A4 is an enzyme that is predominately responsible for the metabolism of imatinib mesylate. The following drugs or families of drugs may interact with imatinib mesylate:

- Inhibitors of the CYP3A4 family, including ketoconazole, itraconazole, and erythromycin.
- Co-medications that induce CYP3A4, including dexamethasone, phenytoin, carbamazepine, rifampin, phenobarbital, or St. John's wort. No formal studies have been conducted on these medications and imatinib mesylate together.

QUESTIONS TO ASK YOUR DOCTOR

- What should I do if I forget a dose?
- Which side effects might indicate a serious reaction or problem?
- I have high blood pressure; will that affect my taking the drug?
- How can I prevent edema while taking imatinib?

- CYP3A4 substrates, such as cyclosporine or pimozide.
- CYP3A4-metabolized drugs, such as certain HMG-CoA reductase inhibitors, triazolo-benzodiazepines, and dihydropyridine calcium channel blockers.
- Warfarin. Patients needing anticoagulant therapy while taking imatinib mesylate should be prescribed low-molecular weight or standard heparin.

This list does not include all possible interactions. Patients must inform their doctors of any drugs they are taking to avoid drug interactions.

Investigators have also evaluated the effect of St. John's wort (an herb used to treat mild-to-moderate **depression**) on the pharmacokinetics of imatinib. Studies showed that the administration of St. John's wort along with imatinib mesylate reduced absorption and increased elimination of imatinib, reducing drug exposure by as much as 42%. Since the clinical efficacy of imatinib is dependent on drug dose and concentration, interaction with St. John's wort could result in a loss of therapeutic effect. Therefore, the concurrent use of St. John's wort and imatinib should be avoided.

See also Low molecular weight heparins.

Resources

WEBSITES

"FDA Approves Gleevec for Children With Acute Lymphoblastic Leukemia." US Food and Drug Administration. http://www.fda.gov/NewsEvents/Newsroom/Press Announcements/ucm336868.htm (accessed October 10, 2014).

"General Information About Gastrointestinal Stromal Tumors." National Cancer Institute. http://www.cancer.gov/cancertopics/pdq/treatment/gist/Patient (accessed October 10, 2014).

"Gleevec." Novartis. http://www.gleevec.com/index.jsp?user-track.filter_applied=true&NovaId=4029462118440539469 (accessed October 10, 2014).

Crystal Heather Kaczkowski, MSc

Revised by Teresa G. Odle

Immune globulin

Definition

Immune globulin is a concentrated solution of antibodies pooled from donated blood, which is sometimes given to **cancer** patients whose own immune systems are either not working or are suppressed as a side effect of treatment. Immune globulin can also be called gamma globulin; in the United States some of the brand names are Gamimune, Gammagard, Gammar-P, Iveegam, Polygam, Sandoglobulin, and Venoglobulin.

Purpose

A healthy human body produces proteins called antibodies that act to destroy microorganisms (bacteria and viruses) that invade the body. Some cancer patients, due to the illness itself or side effects of treatment, become depleted of these proteins and therefore susceptible to serious infections. Immune globulin is given to these patients to restore their body's immunity. The use of immune globulin in this way is also called passive immunization. For example, immune globulin is given to bone marrow transplant recipients to prevent the development of severe bacterial infections while their own immune systems are not functioning, and **chronic lymphocytic leukemia** patients (of the type whose antibody-producing cells are the malignant cells) are given immune globulin to prevent the recurrent infections these patients sometimes suffer. Use in this disorder also allows the use of aggressive **chemotherapy** that will destroy the patient's own cancerous antibody-producing cells.

Immune globulin is also used to treat other diseases such as Lambert-Eaton myasthenic syndrome, a rare neurological disorder that sometimes occurs in association with **small cell lung cancer**. Also called Eaton-Lambert syndrome, it is an autoimmune disease in which a patient's own antibodies attack nerve cells. The use of immune globulin appears to cause the body to reduce its own production of antibody, thereby relieving the symptoms of the neurological disorder.

Description

Immune globulin primarily consists of antibody proteins of the type called IgG or gamma, although the solution may contain small amounts of other antibody types as well as sugars, proteins, and salt.

It is produced by pooling donated blood from at least 1,000 people who have been tested to be free of blood-borne diseases like HIV or hepatitis. The antibody proteins are then separated out of the whole blood, and the pH of the immune globulin solution is adjusted to match the normal

pH of blood. The preparation is also treated to remove any contaminants, including infectious bacteria or viruses.

Recommended dosage

The dose of immune globulin used varies with the specific problem that it is being used for. When immune globulin is used in patients with Eaton-Lambert syndrome, the effective dose is usually about 1 g/kg of body weight/day. (One gram equals 0.035274 ounce; one kilogram equals 2.2046 pounds.) When used to counteract immuno-deficiency, the dose is designed to produce an antibody level that stays at an effective threshold over a period of time.

When immune globulin is given to bone marrow transplant recipients, it is usually begun at the time of the transplant and continued for 100 days thereafter, with the objective of maintaining the level of IgG in the patient's blood above 400 mg per deciliter. (A deciliter equals 3.38 fluid ounces.) In patients with chronic lymphocytic leukemia (B-cell type), the target threshold for antibodies in the patient's blood is usually about 600 mg/dL. Although the amount required to maintain these levels varies from patient to patient (because different patients metabolize the drug at different rates) a dose between 10 and 200 mg/kg of body weight, given every 3-4 weeks, is usually sufficient.

Immune globulin is usually given intravenously, although intramuscular shots are available.

Precautions

Some people may have experienced severe reactions, including allergy-type reactions, to other antibody preparations. Generally, these people should not be given intravenous immune globulin. Patients with deficiency of antibody

IgA specifically should also avoid the use of immune globulin. People with a tendency to form blood clots or those with kidney problems should also avoid the use of this product, especially if elderly. While many pregnant women have been treated with immune globulin for different problems that have occurred during their pregnancies, because the method of action and specific effects on the fetus are not completely understood, pregnant women should avoid the use of immune globulin unless it is clearly necessary. Any patient who is given immune globulin should be watched carefully, and epinephrine should be kept available in case a severe allergic reaction is experienced. Immune globulin made to be given through intramuscular injection should never be administered intravenously.

Side effects

Administration of intramuscular immune globulin may result in tenderness, swelling, and possibly hives at the site of the injection.

Intravenous immune globulin may cause more severe reactions related to rapid introduction into the circulatory system. Possible side effects include headache, backache, aching muscles, **fever**, low blood pressure, and chest pain. More commonly, fever accompanied by chills or **nausea and vomiting** may be experienced. If these side effects occur, they are usually related to the immune globulin being administered too rapidly. If the rate of infusion is reduced, or if the infusion is stopped temporarily, negative effects will generally disappear. Rare but potentially serious side effects have included kidney failure and aseptic meningitis.

Interactions

Use of immune globulin may reduce the effectiveness of vaccinations (for example, measles, mumps, and rubella) for a few months following the use of the immune globulin preparation. Patients who have been given immune globulin should notify their doctors before any vaccinations are given. In addition, in some situations patients may need to have antibody levels measured to determine whether they have had a previous infection with a specific microorganism. Use of immune globulin can create the false impression of prior exposure to the organism due to the donated antibodies in the blood. Patients receiving immune globulin should use aspirin, ibuprofen, and acetaminophen with caution, as these medications increase the risk of kidney problems in patients receiving immune globulin.

See also Immunologic therapies

Resources

BOOKS

Edmunds, Marilyn Winterton. *Introduction to Clinical Pharmacology*. 7th ed. St. Louis, MO: Elsevier/Mosby, 2013.

WEBSITES

Dartmouth-Hitchcock Norris Cotton Cancer Center Health Encyclopedia. "Immune Globulin (Intravenous) (IGIV)." http://www.cancer.dartmouth.edu/pf/health_encyclopedia/d01133a1 (accessed December 2, 2014).

Wendy Wippel, M.S.

Immune response

Definition

The ability of any given cell in the body to recognize itself as part of the body and not as a foreign tissue or infectious agent (described as distinguishing self from nonself) is called the immune response. All normal cells in the body are recognized as self. Any microorganism (for example, a foreign body or tumor) that invades or attacks the cells is recognized as nonself—or foreign—requiring the immune system to mount a combat against the alien entity.

Immune system

The human immune system comprises two subsystems: the innate immune system, which is the body's first line of defense against infection and responds to disease organisms in a nonspecific manner; and the adaptive (or acquired) immune system, which consists of highly specialized cells and processes that respond to specific pathogens, including malignant tumors. The acquired immune system adapts to each new microbe it encounters and strengthens its specific responses during each subsequent encounter. This immunological memory is the basis of vaccination as a strategy for enhancing the body's immunity to specific diseases.

The acquired immune system comprises a network of immune cells generated in the bone marrow stem cells. A stem cell is a cell whose daughter cells may develop into other types of cells. From stem cells different types of immune cells originate that can handle specific immune functions.

Phagocytes (cell eaters) serve as the first line of defense, engulfing dead cells, debris, viruses, and bacteria. Macrophages are an important type of phagocyte, often presenting the antigen—which is usually a foreign protein—to other immune cells and thus are also called antigen-presenting cells (APCs). T and B lymphocytes, important immune-system cells, are also capable of recognizing the antigen and becoming activated. T lymphocytes are classified into two subtypes: killer T cells (also called cytotoxic T cells) and helper T cells. The primary response of the human immune system to cancerous tumors is to destroy the abnormal cells using killer T cells, sometimes with the assistance of helper T cells.

Killer T cells recognize and kill the infected or malignant cells that contain the antigen or the foreign protein. Helper T cells release cytokines (chemical messengers) upon activation that either directly destroy the tumor or stimulate other cells to kill the target (tumor). B lymphocytes produce antibodies after recognizing the antigens. The antibodies, which help protect the body from the antigen, are normally specific to that particular antigen. In cases of malignant tumors, the specific antibodies attach to the tumor cells and, through various mechanisms, impair the functions of the tumor, ultimately leading to the death of the **cancer** cells.

In addition to these lymphocytes, natural killer (NK) cells perform the task of eliminating foreign cells. Natural killer cells differ from killer T cells in that they target tumor cells and do not have to recognize an antigen before activation. These cells have been shown to be potentially useful in treating cancer.

Immune system and cancer

The acquired immune system serves as one of the primary defenses against cancer. When normal tissue becomes a tumor or cancerous tissue, new antigens develop on the surface of the tumor cells. These antigens send a signal to such immune cells as the cytotoxic T lymphocytes, NK cells, and macrophages, which in turn directly kill the tumor cells or release substances like cytokines that bring about tumor cell death. Thus under normal circumstances, the immune system provides continued surveillance and eliminates cells that might become malignant. Tumors can, however, survive by hiding or disguising their tumor antigens, or by producing substances that allow suppressor T cells (cells that block cytotoxic or killer T cells that would normally attack the tumor) to proliferate (multiply).

Adoptive T cell transfer is an experimental form of cancer treatment that seeks to enhance the natural cancer-fighting ability of a patient's T cells. One form of transfer therapy involves collecting cytotoxic T cells that have invaded the patient's tumor; growing the cells with the greatest anticancer activity in large numbers in the laboratory; depleting the patient's other white blood cells with **chemotherapy**; and infusing the laboratory-grown tumor-killing lymphocytes into the patient's blood. Adoptive T cell transfer has been used to treat metastatic **melanoma**, and is being used in **clinical trials** to treat colorectal cancer.

KEY TERMS

Adaptive immune system—A subsystem of the immune system that comprises highly specialized cells and processes that inhibit the growth of disease organisms. It is also known as the acquired immune system.

Antibody—A large protein molecule used by the immune system to identify and neutralize bacteria and viruses.

Antigen—Any substance that produces an adaptive immune response. Antigens are sometimes called antibody generators.

Cytokines—A broad category of small proteins that are important in cell signaling. They include interleukins and interferons, among others.

Innate immune system—The subsystem of the immune system comprised of cells and mechanisms that defend the body against infection in an immediate but nonspecific fashion.

Interferons—Proteins made and released by host cells in response to the presence of bacteria, viruses, parasites, or tumor cells.

Interleukins—A group of cytokines that were first discovered as the products of white blood cells (leukocytes), although it is now known that some are produced by other body cells.

Lymphocyte—A general term for three types of white blood cells: B cells, T cells, and natural killer (NK) cells.

Macrophage—A type of phagocyte that engulfs and digests cancer cells as well as bacteria and other microbes.

Phagocyte—A specialized white blood cell that protects the body by ingesting bacteria, foreign particles, and dead or dying cells.

Stem cell—An undifferentiated cell that can differentiate into specialized cells or divide through mitosis to form more stem cells.

Biological response modifiers in cancer therapy

Researchers have been working on stimulating the cells of the acquired immune system during cancer therapy with substances broadly classified as **biological response modifiers** or BRMs. Cytokines are one such substance. These are proteins that are predominantly released by immune cells upon activation or stimulation.

During the 1990s, the number of cytokines identified increased enormously and the functions associated with them are of immense potential in diagnostics and immune therapy. Cytokines include the **interferons** and interleukins, among others. Some of the key cytokines that have proven therapeutic value in cancer are interleukin-2 (IL-2), interferon gamma, and interleukin-12 (IL-12). Cytokines are normally injected directly into cancer patients during therapy; however, there are other cases in which a cancer patient's own lymphocytes are modified under laboratory conditions and injected back into the patient. Examples of these are lymphokine-activated killer (LAK) cells and tumor-infiltrating lymphocytes (TILs). These modified cells are capable of devouring cancer cells.

Immunoprevention of cancer

Immunotherapy is emerging as one of the management strategies for cancer. Although established tumors or large masses of tumor do not respond well to immunotherapy, there is clinical evidence that suggests that patients with minimal residual cancer cells (a few cells left after other forms of cancer treatment) are potential candidates for effective immunotherapy. In these cases immunotherapy often results in a prolonged tumor-free period of survival. Thus immune responses can be manipulated to prevent recurrence, even though they do not destroy large tumors. In addition, cancer immunotherapy combined with **radiation therapy** shows promise in treating solid malignancies. Based on results of immunotherapy trials, most immune therapies are geared toward designing such immunoprotective products as **cancer vaccines**.

Cancer vaccines

There are two basic types of cancer vaccines as of 2014: prophylactic, administered to prevent or lower the risk of specific cancers; and therapeutic, intended to treat the cancer. Cancer vaccines can be made with whole inactivated tumor cells, or with fragments or cell surface substances (called cell-surface antigens) present in the tumors. Because vaccines are less toxic than some other cancer therapies, they are being tested in clinical trials in combination with other forms of cancer therapy such as chemotherapy, radiation therapy, and hormonal therapy. In addition to the whole-cell or antigen vaccines, biological response modifiers like cytokines serve as substances that boost immune response in cancer patients.

Because cancer vaccines are still under clinical evaluation, caution should be exercised when choosing them as a mode of therapy. As of 2014, there were three FDA-approved prophylactic cancer vaccines: a vaccine for

hepatitis B virus (HBV), which can cause **liver cancer** in chronically infected people; and two vaccines against **human papillomavirus** (HPV) types 6, 11, 16, and 18. HPV infection is associated with cancers of the cervix, vulva, vagina, anus, penis, and oropharynx. In 2010, the FDA also approved one cancer treatment vaccine, **sipuleucel-T**, to treat men with metastatic **prostate cancer**. The results to date of treatment with this vaccine amount to a modest extension of the patient's life. More effective treatment vaccines for cancer will require further research into the complex interactions between vaccines and the human immune system.

The patient's cancer care team will provide further insight on whether cancer vaccine or cytokine therapy will be beneficial after they assess the patient's stage and the various modes of treatments available.

Resources

BOOKS

Curiel, Tyler J., ed. *Cancer Immunotherapy: Paradigms, Practice and Promise*. New York: Springer, 2013.

Morrow, John W., ed. *Vaccinology: Principles and Practice*. Chichester, UK: Wiley-Blackwell, 2012.

Pecorino, Lauren. *Molecular Biology of Cancer: Mechanisms, Targets, and Therapeutics*, 3rd ed. New York: Oxford University Press, 2012.

Prendergast, George, and Elizabeth M. Jaffee, eds. *Cancer Immunotherapy: Immune Suppression and Tumor Growth*, 2nd ed. Boston, MA: Elsevier/Academic Press, 2013.

PERIODICALS

Bae, J., N.C. Munshi, and K.C. Anderson. "Immunotherapy Strategies in Multiple Myeloma." *Hematology/Oncology Clinics of North America* 28 (October 2014): 927–943.

Girotti, M.R., et al. "No Longer an Untreatable Disease: How Targeted and Immunotherapies Have Changed the Management of Melanoma Patients." *Molecular Oncology* 8 (September 12, 2014): 1140–1158.

Harris, T.J., and C.G. Drake. "Primer on Tumor Immunology and Cancer Immunotherapy." *Journal for Immunotherapy of Cancer* 1 (July 29, 2013): 12.

Kalos, M., and C.H. June. "Adoptive T Cell Transfer for Cancer Immunotherapy in the Era of Synthetic Biology." *Immunity* 39 (July 25, 2013): 49–60.

Kono, K. "Current Status of Cancer Immunotherapy." *Journal of Stem Cells and Regenerative Medicine* 10 (April 30, 2014): 6–13.

Naidoo, J., D.B. Page, and J.D. Wolchok. "Immune Modulation for Cancer Therapy." *British Journal of Cancer*, September 11, 2014 [E-publication ahead of print].

Petrizzo, A., et al. "Systems Vaccinology for Cancer Vaccine Development." *Expert Review of Vaccines* 13 (June 2014): 711–719.

Tang, C., et al. "Combining Radiation and Immunotherapy: A New Systemic Therapy for Solid Tumors?" *Cancer Immunology Research* 2 (September 2014): 831–838.

Woller, N., et al. "Oncolytic Viruses as Anticancer Vaccines." *Frontiers in Oncology* 4 (July 21, 2014): 188.

WEBSITES

American Cancer Society (ACS). "Cancer Immunotherapy." http://www.cancer.org/acs/groups/cid/documents/webcontent/003013-pdf.pdf (accessed September 9, 2014).

BreastCancer.org. "Understanding Your Immune System." http://www.breastcancer.org/tips/immune (accessed September 9, 2014).

Cancer Research UK. "The Immune System and Cancer." http://www.cancerresearchuk.org/about-cancer/what-is-cancer/body-systems-and-cancer/the-immune-system-and-cancer (accessed January 29, 2015).

National Cancer Institute (NCI). "Fact Sheet: Biological Therapies for Cancer." http://www.cancer.gov/cancertopics/factsheet/Therapy/biological (accessed August 22, 2014).

National Cancer Institute (NCI). "Fact Sheet: Cancer Vaccines."http://www.cancer.gov/cancertopics/factsheet/Therapy/cancer-vaccines (accessed August 22, 2014).

ORGANIZATIONS

American Cancer Society (ACS), 250 Williams Street NW, Atlanta, GA 30303, (800) 227-2345, http://www.cancer.org/aboutus/howwehelpyou/app/contact-us.aspx, http://www.cancer.org/index.

American Society of Clinical Oncology (ASCO), 2318 Mill Road, Suite 800, Alexandria, VA 22314, (571) 483-1300, (888) 651-3038, Fax: (571) 366-9537, contactus@cancer.net, http://www.asco.org.

Food and Drug Administration (FDA), 10903 New Hampshire Avenue, Silver Spring, MD 20993, (888) INFO-FDA (463-6332), http://www.fda.gov/AboutFDA/ContactFDA/default.htm, http://www.fda.gov/default.htm.

National Cancer Institute (NCI), BG 9609 MSC 9760, 9609 Medical Center Drive, Bethesda, MD 20892-9760, (800) 4-CANCER (422-6237), http://www.cancer.gov/global/contact/email-us, http://www.cancer.gov.

Society for Immunotherapy of Cancer (SITC), 555 East Wells Street, Suite 1100, Milwaukee, WI 53202-3823, (414) 271-2456, Fax: (414) 276-3349, info@sitcancer.org, http://www.sitcancer.org/about-sitc.

Kausalya Santhanam, PhD.

REVISED BY REBECCA J. FREY, PhD.

Immunoelectrophoresis

Definition

Immunoelectrophoresis, also called gamma globulin electrophoresis or immunoglobulin electrophoresis, is a method of determining the blood levels of three major

---

KEY TERMS

Antibody—A protein manufactured by the white blood cells to neutralize an antigen in the body. In some cases, excessive formation of antibodies leads to illness, allergy, or autoimmune disorders.

Antigen—A substance that can cause an immune response resulting in production of an antibody as part of the body's defense against infection and disease. Many antigens are foreign proteins not found naturally in the body, and include germs, toxins, and tissues from another person used in organ transplantation.

Autoimmune disorder—A condition in which antibodies are formed against the body's own tissues, as in some forms of arthritis.

---

immunoglobulins: immunoglobulin M (IgM), immunoglobulin G (IgG), and immunoglobulin A (IgA).

Purpose

Immunoelectrophoresis is a powerful analytical technique with high resolving power as it combines separation of antigens by electrophoresis with immunodiffusion against an antiserum. The increased resolution is beneficial in the immunological examination of serum proteins. Immunoelectrophoresis aids in the diagnosis and evaluation of the therapeutic response in many disease states affecting the immune system. It is usually requested when a different type of electrophoresis, called a serum **protein electrophoresis**, has indicated a rise at the immunoglobulin level. Immunoelectrophoresis is also used frequently to diagnose **multiple myeloma**, a disease affecting the bone marrow.

Precautions

Drugs that may cause increased immunoglobulin levels include therapeutic gamma globulin, hydralazine, isoniazid, **phenytoin** (Dilantin), procainamide, oral contraceptives, methadone, steroids, and tetanus toxoid and antitoxin. The laboratory should be notified if the patient has received any vaccinations or immunizations in the six months before the test. This precaution is required mainly because prior immunizations lead to increased immunoglobulin levels, resulting in false positive results.

It should be noted that because immunoelectrophoresis is not quantitative, it is being replaced by a procedure called immunofixation, which is more sensitive and easier to interpret.

Description

Serum proteins separate in agar gels under the influence of an electric field into albumin, alpha 1, alpha 2, and beta and gamma globulins. Immunoelectrophoresis is performed by placing serum on a slide containing a gel designed specifically for the test. An electric current is then passed through the gel, and immunoglobulins, which contain an electric charge, migrate through the gel according to the difference in their individual electric charges. Antiserum is placed alongside the slide to identify the specific type of immunoglobulin present. The results are used to identify different disease entities, and to aid in monitoring the course of the disease and the therapeutic response of the patient with such conditions as immune deficiencies, autoimmune disease, chronic infections, chronic viral infections, intrauterine fetal infections, multiple **myeloma**, and monoclonal gammopathy of undetermined significance.

There are five classes of antibodies: IgM, IgG, IgA, IgE, and IgD.

IgM is produced upon initial exposure to an antigen. For example, when a person receives the first tetanus vaccination, antitetanus antibodies of the IgM class are produced 10 to 14 days later. IgM is abundant in the blood but is not normally present in organs or tissues. IgM is primarily responsible for ABO blood grouping and rheumatoid factor, yet is involved in the immunologic reaction to other infections, such as hepatitis. Since IgM does not cross the placenta, an elevation of this immunoglobulin in the newborn indicates an intrauterine infection like rubella, cytomegalovirus (CMV), or a sexually transmitted disease (STD).

IgG is the most prevalent type of antibody, comprising approximately 75% of the serum immunoglobulins. IgG is produced upon subsequent exposure to an antigen. As an example, after receiving a second tetanus shot, or booster, a person produces IgG antibodies in five to seven days. IgG is present in both the blood and tissues, and is the only antibody to cross the placenta from the mother to the fetus. Maternal IgG protects the newborn for the first months of life until the infant's immune system produces its own antibodies.

IgA constitutes approximately 15% of the immunoglobulins within the body. Although it is found to some degree in the blood, it is present primarily in the secretions of the respiratory and gastrointestinal tract, in saliva, colostrum (the yellowish fluid produced by the breasts during late pregnancy and the first few days after childbirth), and in tears. IgA plays an important role in defending the body against invasion of germs through the mucous membrane-lined organs.

IgE is the antibody that causes acute allergic reactions; it is measured to detect allergic conditions. IgD, which constitutes the smallest portion of the immunoglobulins, is rarely evaluated or detected, and its function is not well understood.

Preparation

This test requires a blood sample.

Aftercare

Because this test is ordered when either very low or very high levels of immunoglobulins are suspected, the patient should be alert for any signs of infection after the test, including **fever**, chills, rash, or skin ulcers. Any **bone pain** or tenderness should also be immediately reported to the physician.

Risks

Risks for this test are minimal, but may include slight bleeding from the blood-drawing site, fainting or feeling lightheaded after venipuncture, or bruising.

Results

Reference ranges vary from laboratory to laboratory and depend upon the method used. For adults, normal values are usually found within the following ranges (1 mg = approximately 0.000035 oz. and 1 dL = approximately 0.33 fluid oz.):

- IgM: 60–290 mg/dL
- IgG: 700–1,800 mg/dL
- IgA: 70–440 mg/dL

Abnormal results

Increased IgM levels can indicate **Waldenström macroglobulinemia**, a malignancy caused by secretion of IgM at high levels by malignant lymphoplasma cells. Increased IgM levels can also indicate chronic infections, such as hepatitis or mononucleosis, and autoimmune diseases, like rheumatoid arthritis.

Decreased IgM levels can be indicative of AIDS, immunosuppression caused by certain drugs like steroids or dextran, or leukemia.

Increased levels of IgG can indicate chronic liver disease, autoimmune diseases, hyperimmunization reactions, or certain chronic infections, such as tuberculosis or sarcoidosis.

Decreased levels of IgG can indicate Wiskott-Aldrich syndrome, a genetic deficiency caused by inadequate synthesis of IgG and other immunoglobulins. Decreased IgG can also be seen with AIDS and leukemia.

Increased levels of IgA can indicate chronic liver disease, chronic infections, or inflammatory bowel disease.

Decreased levels of IgA can be found in ataxia, a condition affecting balance and gait, limb or eye movements, speech, and telangiectasia, an increase in the size and number of the small blood vessels in an area of skin, causing redness. Decreased IgA levels are also seen in conditions of low blood protein (hypoproteinemia), and drug immunosuppression.

Resources

BOOKS

Fischbach, Frances T. *A Manual of Laboratory and Diagnostic Tests.* 9th ed. Philadelphia: Wolters Kluwer Health, 2015.

Pagana, Kathleen D., and Timothy J. Pagana. *Mosby's Manual of Diagnostic and Laboratory Tests.* 5th ed. St. Louis: Elsevier/Mosby, 2014.

Janis O. Flores

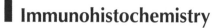

Immunohistochemistry

Definition

Immunohistochemistry (IHC) is a method for identifying and analyzing cell types based on the binding of antibodies to specific components (antigens) of the cells. It is sometimes referred to as immunocytochemistry or immunophenotyping.

Purpose

IHC is used to distinguish between benign (non-cancerous) and malignant (cancerous) tumors, diagnose the type of **cancer**, guide treatment, and indicate the prognosis. It is also used to detect and evaluate residual cancer cells that may remain after treatment. IHC is used especially in the diagnosis and classification of leukemias and lymphomas. It is also used to determine whether breast or other cancers are HER2-positive, meaning that the cancer cells have excess levels of a protein called human epidermal growth factor receptor 2 (HER2) that promotes cancer cell growth. About 20% of breast cancers are HER2-positive and can be treated with antibodies that target HER2, kill the cells, and decrease the risk of recurrence. IHC can also determine the amount of HER2 present in a sample. **Carcinoma** of unknown primary origin is cancer that has metastasized (spread to other parts of the body), but the site of the original tumor and the type of cancer cell is not known. In such cases, IHC may be used to identify cell types by characteristic markers on the

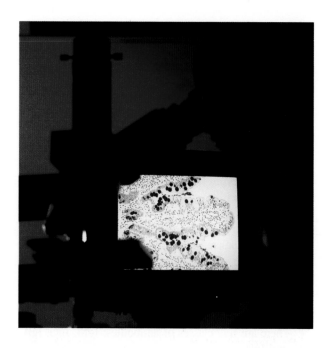

Researcher examining the human intestine through the use of immunohistochemistry. The screen shows a sample of the intestine. Antibodies are created to identify specific proteins on the intestinal cells, indicated by the black dots. *(Colin Cuthbert/Science Source)*

cell surfaces. In certain cases, IHC is also used to detect and classify antibodies.

Description

IHC requires a sample of tissue or bone marrow from a **biopsy**. Sometimes it is performed on a blood sample withdrawn from a vein in the arm or another fluid sample. The sample is usually examined fresh, but frozen or chemically preserved material can also be used. The tissue sample is sliced extremely thin—approximately one cell in thickness. The sample is fixed onto a glass slide. Tumor cells have characteristic markers called antigens on their cell surfaces that can be used to help identify the specific cell type. Antibodies against these specific antigens bind to the cells on the slide. Excess antibody is washed away. The antibodies that remain bound to the cells have labels that either fluoresce (glow), or undergo a color reaction that makes them visible under a microscope. The pathologist is able to see the cells containing the specifically labeled tumor antigens.

The antibodies used in IHC are manufactured in the laboratory. There are hundreds of antibodies available for a wide variety of antigens that are important for diagnosing cancer types by IHC. Many antibodies react with only one or a few types of cancer cells, so it is often necessary to test several different antibodies. In addition

KEY TERMS

Antibody—A protein produced by the immune system that binds to a specific antigen.

Antigen—Any protein that elicits a unique immune response.

Biopsy—A sample of tissue taken from a tumor for immunohistochemistry examination.

Carcinoembryonic antigen (CEA)—A fetal protein that is present in the blood of patients with some forms of cancer, such as breast or digestive system cancers.

HER2—Human epidermal growth factor receptor 2, which is overproduced in HER2-positive breast cancers and can be detected by immunohistochemistry.

Histology—The study of tissues.

Immunophenotyping—Immunohistochemistry or flow cytometry to identify cell types using antibodies.

Leukemia—An acute or chronic cancer of white blood cells classified according to the type of white blood cell that is overproduced.

Lymphoma—Cancer of the lymphatic tissue.

Prostate-specific antigen (PSA)—A prostate protein that can be detected by immunohistochemistry; PSA levels in blood tend to be proportional to the prostate cancer stage.

to determining whether a tumor is benign or malignant, antibody reactions can help determine the origin of the tumor, whether it is growing rapidly, and whether it is a type of tumor that responds well to a particular treatment. IHC is also useful for identifying cancer cells when there are only a few present in a sample. IHC results are used in conjunction with the appearance of the cells, the location of the cancer, and patient information to classify the cancer and select the most appropriate treatment.

IHC is used to detect cell types present in an inappropriate part of the body; for example, prostate cells in a lymph node. IHC on a **lymph node biopsy** can help determine whether the cancer started in a lymph node—meaning it is a lymphoma—or whether it migrated to the lymph node from elsewhere in the body, which could indicate metastatic cancer. IHC may also be used to assess the level of maturity of the tumor cells, which can help determine their origin. Proteins involved in the replication of genetic material and cell growth may be present in greater amounts; for example, antibodies

against the antigen Ki-67 are used to evaluate malignant melanomas, breast carcinomas, and non-Hodgkin lymphomas. Hormone receptors may also be examined. The presence of receptors for estrogen and/or progesterone indicates a good prognosis for **breast cancer** patients, because such cancers can be treated with medications that prevent these receptors from growing in response to female hormones. IHC may also be used to assess the levels of tumor suppressor proteins.

IHC can be particularly useful for diagnosing **lymphoma**. Biopsy tissue from a swollen lymph node may contain a large number of immune system white blood cells (lymphocytes), but there are normally many different kinds of lymphocytes present. IHC indicating that the lymphocytes are mostly of one type suggests that they are all derived from a single abnormal cell, which indicates lymphoma.

Preparation

The physician will choose the type of sample for IHC based on the type of tumor. For a solid tumor, a biopsy may remove a portion of the tumor for examination. A biopsy sample can also be taken from a tumor that has been surgically removed. The patient will be informed about preparations for a biopsy or surgery. If IHC is performed on a routine blood sample, no additional preparation is required.

Aftercare

Aftercare depends on the type of sample collection. A blood draw requires no particular aftercare, whereas major surgery may require a great deal of aftercare.

Risks

Risks associated with IHC are those associated with the sample collection process, either a biopsy or blood draw. The only other risk is the possibility that the test may yield inconclusive results.

Results

With normal IHC results, the cells in the sample appear normal. The cells will have a high level of maturity and be located only at sites appropriate to their cell type. For example, analysis of a lymph node will reveal various types and proportions of lymphocytes that are normally found in a lymph node, rather than cell types normally found in the breast. Furthermore, the cells will show no increase in specific cancer-associated antigens.

Abnormal results

An abnormal IHC result might consist of cells that appear immature or poorly differentiated, or that are located in a tissue inappropriate to their cell type. The presence and amount of a particular antigen, such as Ki-67, carcinoembryonic antigen (CEA), or prostate-specific antigen (PSA) may be reported. In such cases, the abnormal results may be reported in comparison with standard normal values or ranges that help the physician determine the type of cancer, appropriate treatment, and prognosis.

See also Receptor analysis; Tumor markers.

Resources

BOOKS

Abeloff, M. D., et al. *Clinical Oncology.* 5th ed. New York: Churchill Livingstone, 2014.

Dabbs, David J. *Breast Pathology.* Philadelphia: Elsevier/Saunders, 2012.

Goldman, L., and D. Ausiello, eds. *Cecil Textbook of Internal Medicine.* 24th ed. Philadelphia: Saunders, 2012.

Hicks, David G., and Susan Carole Lester. *Diagnostic Pathology: Breast.* Salt Lake City, UT: Amirsys, 2012.

Kim, Minseok S., Seyong Kwon, and Je-Kyun Park. "Breast Cancer Diagnostics Using Microfluidic Multiplexed Immunohistochemistry." In *Microfluidic Diagnostics: Methods and Protocols,* edited by Gareth Jenkins and Colin D. Mansfield. New York: Humana, 2013.

McPherson, R. A., et al. *Henry's Clinical Diagnosis and Management By Laboratory Methods.* 22nd ed. Philadelphia: Saunders, 2011.

Niederhuber, J. E., et al. *Clinical Oncology.* 5th ed. Philadelphia: Elsevier, 2014.

Nikiforov, Yuri, Paul W. Biddinger, and Lester D. R. Thompson. *Diagnostic Pathology and Molecular Genetics of the Thyroid.* 2nd ed. Philadelphia: Wolters Kluwer Health/Lippincott Williams & Wilkins, 2012.

Putnam, Angelica R. *Diagnostic Pathology: Pediatric Neoplasms.* Salt Lake City, UT: Amirsys, 2012.

WEBSITES

"Immunophenotyping." Lab Tests Online. December 3, 2012. http://labtestsonline.org/understanding/analytes/immunophenotyping/tab/glance (accessed August 14, 2014).

"Testing Biopsy and Cytology Specimens for Cancer." American Cancer Society. March 7, 2013. http://www.cancer.org/acs/groups/cid/documents/webcontent/003185-pdf.pdf (accessed August 11, 2014).

ORGANIZATIONS

American Cancer Society, 250 Williams Street NW, Atlanta, GA 30303, (800) 227-2345, http://www.cancer.org.

Racquel Baert, M.S.
Margaret Alic, PhD.

Immunotherapy

Definition

Immunotherapy, also called immune therapy or immunologic therapy, treats **cancer** using medications that stimulate the body's natural **immune response**.

Purpose

Immunotherapy is used to improve the immune system's natural ability to fight cancer and other diseases. These drugs may also be used to help the immune system recover from the reduced ability to fight infection (immunosuppression) that results from cancer treatments such as **chemotherapy** or **radiation therapy**.

Description

Greater understanding of the interactions between tumors and the immune system have led to the development of immune therapies as standard treatment for many types of cancer. The drugs that have been developed for immune-based cancer treatment work in several ways: some enhance the immune system's antitumor response by increasing specialized white blood cells called T cells to attack tumor cells; some target new blood vessels that carry oxygen and nutrients to tumor cells to stop cancer cells from growing and multiplying; and other drugs may block natural regulatory processes of the immune system that would normally result in reduced immune response (immune tolerance). Sometimes certain immunologic drugs are combined with chemotherapy to enhance effectiveness. Newer immune therapy includes therapeutic vaccinations against substances on the surface of cancer cells called tumor-associated antigens. Vaccines may be used with chemotherapy for certain cancers, and some vaccines may be used alone to halt disease progression without the toxic reactions associated with chemotherapy.

Most drugs used in immune therapy for cancer are synthetic versions of immune system components produced naturally in the body. In their natural forms, these substances help defend the body against disease. Several different types of immune therapies are approved for use, including **monoclonal antibodies**, which are synthetic (laboratory-created) versions of immune system proteins; cytokines, including interleukins, colony-stimulating factors, and **interferons**, which have a more generalized effect in boosting the immune system; and vaccines called targeted T-cell-based vaccines, which trigger an immune response directed specifically against the cancer cells. Specific drugs in these classes include the following:

- Trastuzumab (Herceptin) is a monoclonal antibody against a specific type of protein called HER2. This protein is found on the surfaces of cancer cells in breast and stomach tumors. The drug binds to the proteins to prevent them from becoming active. This monoclonal antibody is also given by injection.

- Ibritumomab tiuxetan (Zevalin) is a radioactive protein that reacts with the CD20 antigen, another protein found on specialized lymphocytes known as B cells. The drug carries radioactivity directly to cancerous B cells in diseases such as non-Hodgkin lymphoma.

- Chemolabeled monoclonal antibodies, proteins with chemotherapy drugs attached to them, include brentuximab vedotin (Adcetris), which is used to treat cases of Hodgkin lymphoma and anaplastic large cell lymphoma that have failed to respond to other therapies. Ado-trastuzumab emtansine (Kadcyla) is a chemolabeled monoclonal antibody that is used to treat advanced breast cancer.

- Denileukin diftitox (Ontak) is an immune system protein called interleukin-2 (IL-2), which attaches to certain cells with the CD25 antigen on their surfaces. It is used to treat a skin lymphoma known as cutaneous T-cell lymphoma.

- Aldesleukin (Proleukin) is a synthetic form of interleukin-2 that helps to increase the types and functions of specialized white blood cells that fight cancer. Aldesleukin is administered to patients with kidney cancer and skin cancer (melanoma) that have spread (metastasized) to other parts of the body.

- Filgrastim (Neupogen) and sargramostim (Leukine) are synthetic versions of natural substances called granulocyte-macrophage colony-stimulating factors, which encourage the bone marrow to make new specialized white cells called T cells.

- Other colony-stimulating factors include epoetin (Epogen, Procrit), a synthetic version of human erythropoietin, which stimulates the bone marrow to make new red blood cells, and thrombopoietin, which stimulates the production of tiny disk-shaped cells called platelets that are critical components of blood clotting.

- Interferons produced naturally or in a laboratory boost the ability of immune cells to attack cancer cells, helping the body resist infections and cancer. Interferons (IFN) are designated by Greek letters, including IFN-alfa, IFN-beta, and IFN-gamma. However, only the alfa interferons are used to treat cancer. Synthetic interferons include recombinant interferon alfa-2a, recombinant interferon alfa-2b, interferon alfa-n1, and interferon alfa-n3. Alfa interferons are approved for use in treating hairy cell leukemia, chronic myelogenous leukemia, follicular non-Hodgkin lymphoma, cutaneous T-cell lymphoma, kidney cancer, malignant melanoma, and Kaposi sarcoma, a type of cancer associated with HIV infection.

- Cancer vaccines are being developed for the treatment of cancer but are not yet widely used. Sipuleucel-T (Provenge) is a dendritic cell vaccine that has been approved for treating advanced prostate cancer that has not responded to hormone therapies. So far, it is the only approved therapeutic vaccine. The vaccine is created by removing specific immune cells from a prostate cancer patient; stimulating them in the laboratory to mature into dendritic cells; and then injecting these dendritic cells back into the patient, where they trigger other immune cells to attack the cancer cells. Although the vaccine does not cure advanced prostate cancer, it does prolong life. Vaccines are being studied for their effectiveness in treating a wide range of cancers, including brain tumors, cancers of the breast, cervix, colon, kidneys, lungs, pancreas, and prostate as well as lymphoma and melanoma.

Recommended dosage

For most immunotherapy, dosage will be determined individually based on the patient's weight, cancer stage, and other treatments being administered. The recommended dosage will also depend on the type of immunotherapy. Monoclonal antibodies and cytokines are injected intramuscularly or intravenously. Cytokines also may be injected under the skin. Some types of immunotherapy are administered only in a hospital under physician supervision so that the patient can be monitored carefully for unwanted effects. Patients who are taking drugs at home will be instructed in the correct dosage as well as how to take and store the drugs. Drugs that are delivered by injection will be administered by a home health nurse or cancer care provider.

Side effects

Drugs used for immune therapy may have side effects but they are generally less severe than those associated with chemotherapy drugs.

Monoclonal antibodies

Monoclonal antibodies are proteins that sometimes cause symptoms of an allergic reaction such as rashes, **fever**, chills, weakness, headache, **nausea and vomiting**, **diarrhea**, and low blood pressure.

Interleukins

Side effects of interleukins like **aldesleukin** are usually temporary and do not require medical attention unless they are bothersome. These include dry skin; an itchy or burning rash or redness followed by peeling of the skin; loss of appetite; and flu-like symptoms, including chills, fever, **fatigue**, and confusion. Weight gain can also occur and some patients experience nausea and vomiting or diarrhea. Medications can be used to treat resulting low blood pressure. Some people experience dizziness, unusual fatigue, or drowsiness while taking IL-2 drugs. Patients taking these drugs are advised not to drive, use heavy machinery, or do anything else that requires full alertness until they have determined how the drugs affect them.

Interferons

Adverse effects of interferons may include flu-like symptoms as well as loss of appetite, skin rashes, and thinning hair. Fatigue may be the prevailing symptom, and may persist long after treatment has been discontinued.

Colony-stimulating factors

The typical adverse effects of colony-stimulating factors include headache, joint or muscle pain, and skin rash or **itching**. These effects tend to disappear as the body adjusts to the medicine, and medical treatment is not required unless they continue or if they interfere with normal activities. Patients may also experience mild pain in the lower back or hips in the first few days of treatment with colony-stimulating factors. This side effect results from stimulation of the bone marrow and is not cause for concern. It usually disappears within a few days. If the pain is intense or causes severe discomfort, a painkiller may be prescribed.

Epoetin may cause flu-like symptoms such as muscle aches, **bone pain**, fever, chills, shivering, and sweating within a few hours after its administration. These symptoms usually disappear within 12 hours and typically do not require medical attention unless they persist or are severe. Some patients may also develop diarrhea, nausea and vomiting, and fatigue or weakness.

Cancer vaccines

The known adverse effects of vaccines that have been used to treat cancer include fever, chills, fatigue, nausea, and headache. A few patients who received **sipuleucel-T** vaccine for **prostate cancer** treatment experienced difficulty breathing and high blood pressure. However, vaccines are being studied and the full range of adverse effects has not yet been measured or confirmed.

Precautions

Monoclonal antibodies

The monoclonal antibody **bevacizumab** targets the VEGF protein that is involved in blood vessel growth within a tumor. It can raise blood pressure or result in bleeding, poor wound healing, blood clots, and kidney damage.

Interleukins

IL-2 drugs such as aldesleukin may temporarily increase the patient's risk of infection. It can also reduce the number of platelets in the blood, interfering with the blood's ability to clot. More serious complications of IL-2 drugs include the development of an abnormal heartbeat, chest pain, or other heart problems. IL-2 drugs are therefore administered in the hospital so that heart function can be monitored closely.

Interferons

Interferons, like interleukins, can temporarily increase the risk of infection and lower the number of platelets in the blood, which can lead to clotting problems. Interferons can also intensify the effects of alcohol and other drugs, including antihistamines, over-the-counter cold medicines, allergy medications, sleep aids, anticonvulsants, tranquilizers, some pain relievers, and muscle relaxants that slow down the central nervous system. Interferons may intensify the effects of anesthetics, including local anesthetics used in dental procedures. As with other cytokines, interferons can result in a low blood count and increased risk of developing infection. Rarely, long-term effects involve nerve damage, including in the brain and spinal cord.

Interferons can worsen some medical conditions, including heart disease, kidney disease, liver disease, lung disease, diabetes, bleeding problems, and certain psychiatric disorders. In people who have overactive immune systems, these drugs can even increase the activity of the immune system. People who have shingles or chickenpox, or who have recently been exposed to chickenpox, may have an increased risk of developing severe problems in other parts of the body while taking interferons. People with a history of seizures or associated mental disorders may also be at risk if they take interferons.

Interferons can cause changes in the menstrual cycles of young women. Young women are advised to discuss this possibility with their physicians. Women who are pregnant or who might become pregnant are advised to discuss with their physicians the safety of taking these drugs during pregnancy. Women who are breast feeding might need to stop while taking this medicine. It is not yet known whether interferons pass into breast milk; however, because of the chance of serious side effects to the baby, women are advised not to breast feed while taking interferons.

Colony-stimulating factors

Although colony-stimulating factors help restore the body's natural defenses by increasing the production of white blood cells by the bone marrow, the process takes time. During treatment, these drugs will also reduce the body's ability to fight infections. Prompt treatment for infections is important, especially while taking these medications. Patients taking colony-stimulating factors are advised to call their physician at the first signs of illness or infection, such as sore throat, fever, or chills. In addition, patients with kidney disease, liver disease, or conditions related to inflammation or immune system disorders may find that colony-stimulating factors worsen their diseases or disorders. Epoetin in particular appears to be associated with a greater risk of side effects in people with high blood pressure, disorders of the heart or blood vessels, or a history of blood clots. People with heart disease are more likely to experience such adverse effects as water retention and irregular heart rhythm while taking these drugs. The risk of shortness of breath is increased in patients with lung disease. In addition, epoetin may not work properly in people who have bone disorders or sickle cell **anemia**. Epoetin can also cause seizures in people with seizure disorders. People taking epoetin should not drive, operate heavy machinery, or engage in activities that could be dangerous to themselves or others in the event of a seizure.

Women taking the colony-stimulating factor epoetin who are or might become pregnant are advised to check with their physicians for the most up-to-date information on the safety of taking this medicine during pregnancy. This drug helps the body make new red blood cells, but it is not effective unless there are adequate iron stores in the body. Iron supplements may be recommended by the physician to maintain the body's iron supply.

Immunosuppressive effects

Complications associated with the immunosuppressive effects of immune therapy can be reduced by following these general guidelines:

- Avoid contact with people who have infectious diseases.
- Be alert to such signs of infection as fever, chills, sore throat, pain in the lower back or side, cough, hoarseness, or painful or difficult urination. Patients are advised to call their physicians immediately if such symptoms occur.
- Be alert to such signs of bleeding problems as black or tarry stools, tiny red spots on the skin, blood in the urine or stools, or any other unusual bleeding or bruising.
- Take care to avoid cuts or other injuries, particularly when using knives, razors, nail clippers, and other sharp objects. Patients are advised to consult the dentist for the best ways to clean the teeth and mouth without injuring the gums. In addition, patients are advised to check with their physician before dental procedures.
- Wash hands frequently, and avoid touching the eyes or inside of the nose unless the hands have just been washed.

General precautions

Regular appointments with the doctor are necessary during immunotherapy treatment. These checkups give the physician the opportunity to determine whether the medication is working and to monitor the patient for unwanted side effects. Patients who experience unusual reactions to the drugs used in immunotherapy are advised to inform their doctors before resuming the drugs. Any allergies to foods, dyes, preservatives, or other substances should also be reported.

The development of any significant side effects of immunotherapy should be brought to a physician's attention as soon as possible, including:

- dizziness
- drowsiness
- confusion
- difficulty thinking or concentrating
- agitation
- depression
- nausea and vomiting
- diarrhea

- sores in the mouth and on the lips
- tingling of hands or feet
- decrease in urination
- unexplained weight gain of 5 lb. (2 kg) or more
- swelling of the face, fingers, lower legs, ankles, or feet
- nervousness
- sleep problems
- numbness or tingling in the fingers, toes, and face

Interactions

Some combinations of drugs can increase or decrease the effects of one or both drugs, or increase the likelihood of adverse effects. Patients who receive immunotherapy are advised to inform their physician about all other medications they are taking, including over-the-counter medicines and herbal remedies.

Clinical trials

Drugs in **clinical trials** include some that target immune system checkpoints. The function of immune system checkpoints is to keep disease-fighting cells from attacking normal cells in the body. Cancer cells often find a way to bypass these checkpoints in order to avoid attack by the immune system. CTLA-4, PD-1 and PDL1 are important checkpoint molecules found on T cells of the immune system. A drug called ipilimumab (Yervoy), approved by the FDA in 2011, stimulates the immune system in general. Other drugs are being developed that are reported to boost the immune system in a more specific way than ipilimumab. The drug nivolumab has been used to help shrink melanomas, kidney cancers, and non-small cell lung cancers. Large clinical trials are under way to continue studying this drug and determine whether it works best alone or in combination with other treatments.

Tumor-infiltrating lymphocytes (TILs) are T-cell lymphocytes that are found deep inside some tumors. They can be taken from tumor samples and multiplied in the laboratory by treating them with an interleukin-2 (IL-2) drug. When given back to the patient, the cells become active cancer cell fighters. TILs are being tested in clinical trials in patients with **melanoma**, **kidney cancer**, **ovarian cancer**, and some other cancers. The **National Cancer Institute** (NCI) reports that the early results of clinical trials show promise for TILs although the tumor-infiltrating lymphocytes cannot be obtained from tumors in all patients.

Clinical trials for these novel drugs are ongoing. The NCI lists many clinical trials across the United States, including studies of immunostimulatory agents and other immune therapies. The NCI and other cancer organizations may be contacted to help patients and their families locate clinical trials.

Additional research

IMMUNOPREVENTION. Immunoprevention is a treatment that has been proposed as a form of cancer therapy. There are two types of immunoprevention: active and passive. Treatment that involves such immune molecules as cytokines (interleukins, interferons, and colony-stimulating factors), which are prepared synthetically, or other immune molecules that are not produced by patients themselves, including monoclonal antibodies, are called passive immunotherapy. Newer cytokines and monoclonal antibodies are in development that promise to improve safety profiles and effectiveness with fewer adverse side effects. The newer monoclonal antibodies are being attached to drugs and other substances to increase their power. **Cancer vaccines** now in development are a form of active immunotherapy, and studies are under way that involve the application of vaccines to overcome the ability of cancer cells to protect themselves against immune system activity.

KEY TERMS

Bone marrow—Soft tissue that fills the hollow centers of bones. Blood cells and platelets are produced in the bone marrow.

Chemotherapy—Treatment of an illness with chemical agents. The term is usually used to describe the treatment of cancer with drugs.

Hepatitis—Inflammation of the liver caused by a virus, chemical, or drug.

Immune response—The body's natural protective reaction against disease and infection.

Immune system—The system that protects the body against disease and infection through immune responses.

Inflammation—Pain, redness, swelling, and heat that develop in response to injury or illness.

Seizure—A sudden attack, spasm, or convulsion.

Shingles—A disease caused by the herpes zoster virus—the same virus that causes chickenpox. Symptoms of shingles include pain and blisters along one nerve, usually on the face, chest, stomach, or back.

Sickle cell anemia—An inherited disorder in which red blood cells contain an abnormal form of hemoglobin, an iron-bearing protein that carries oxygen to organs throughout the body.

QUESTIONS TO ASK YOUR DOCTOR

- Will immunotherapy help treat my cancer?
- Which type of immune therapy drug is best for my type of cancer?
- Will I take this drug alone or with chemotherapy or radiation?
- Will I take the drug orally or by injection?
- Will I need to be hospitalized when I receive the drug?
- What are the possible side effects?
- How long will I need to take this drug?

CANCER VACCINES. Advances in immune therapies have helped to spur the exploration of vaccines for specific types of cancer. Vaccines can be administered along with other substances called adjuvants to boost immune system activity and promote vaccine effectiveness. Tumor cell vaccines are autologous vaccines, which are vaccines derived from the cells of a specific patient that were removed during surgery. The cells are then prepared in the laboratory to become more suitable targets for the vaccine. They are returned to the patient by injection, when they become vulnerable to the immune system cells. Antigen vaccines use only one protein-based antigen from cancer cells instead of whole-tumor cells, but the process of producing the vaccine is similar. The difference is that antigen vaccines are specific for a type of cancer, but they are allogeneic vaccines, meaning that they are not made for a specific patient and can be given to anyone with that type of cancer. Vector vaccines are a third type of vaccine that uses special delivery systems called vectors to deliver antigens to the body; the vectors can be viruses, bacteria, yeast cells, or other structures. When they deliver antigens, vector vaccines trigger an immune system response. Vaccines are a form of active immune therapy because they elicit an immune response from the patient's body. Cancer vaccines may be made from whole-tumor cells or from substances or fragments of tumor cells known as antigens. Vaccines currently in development are being tested for effectiveness in treating **brain tumors**, cancers of the breast, cervix, colon, kidneys, lungs, pancreas, and prostate as well as **lymphoma** and melanoma, among others.

ADOPTIVE IMMUNOTHERAPY. Adoptive immunotherapy involves stimulating T cells by exposing them to tumor antigens. These modified cells are cultivated in the laboratory and then injected into patients. Since the cells taken from a different person for this purpose are likely rejected, patients serve both as donor and recipient of their own T cells. Chimeric antigen receptor (CAR) T-cell therapy is an example of adoptive immunotherapy. In this treatment, cancer-fighting T-cells are removed from a patient, stimulated to multiply in the laboratory, and then infused back into the patient. The T-cells will seek out the cancer cells and attack them. Adoptive immunotherapy is particularly effective in patients who have received massive doses of radiation and chemotherapy. In such patients, this form of immune therapy results in immunosuppression (a weakened immune system), making them more vulnerable to the development of infections.

Resources

BOOKS

Prendergast, George C., and Elizabeth M. Jaffee, eds. *Cancer Immunotherapy: Immune Suppression and Tumor Growth.* 2nd ed. San Diego: Academic Press/Elsevier, 2013.

Wilson, Billie Ann, Margaret T. Shannon, and Kelly Shields. *Pearson Nurse's Drug Guide 2013.* Upper Saddle River, NJ: Prentice Hall, 2012.

PERIODICALS

Dougan, M., and G. Dranoff. "Immune Therapy for Cancer." *Annual Review of Immunology* 27 (2009): 83–117.

Dubsky, P. C., and G. Curigliano. "Immunotherapy in Breast Cancer—Towards a New Understanding of Both Tumor and Host." *Breast Care* 7, no. 4 (2012): 258–60. http://dx.doi.org/10.1159/000342629 (accessed August 7, 2013).

WEBSITES

American Cancer Society. "Immunotherapy." http://www.cancer.org/treatment/treatmentsandsideeffects/treatmenttypes/immunotherapy/index (accessed August 7, 2013).

ORGANIZATIONS

American Cancer Society, 250 Williams St. NW, Atlanta, GA 30303, (800) 227-2345, http://www.cancer.org.

American Society of Health-System Pharmacists, 7272 Wisconsin Ave., Bethesda, MD 20814, (301) 664-8700, (866) 279-0681, custserv@ashp.org, http://www.ashp.org.

National Cancer Institute, 6116 Executive Blvd., Ste. 300, Bethesda, MD 20892-8322, (800) 4-CANCER (422-6237), http://cancer.gov.

U.S. Food and Drug Administration, 10903 New Hampshire Ave., Silver Spring, MD 20993, (888) INFO-FDA (463-6332), http://www.fda.gov.

Nancy Ross-Flanigan
REVISED BY RENEE LAUX, MS
REVISED BY L. LEE CULVERT
REVIEWED BY MARIANNE VAHEY, MD

Implantable subcutaneous ports *see* **Vascular access**

Imuran *see* **Azathioprine**

Incontinence, cancer-related

Definition

Cancer-related incontinence is the inability to control bladder or bowel function (or both) as a result of the direct effects of **cancer** on the body or the effects of various forms of cancer therapy. In some patients, cancer-related incontinence can be easily treated and controlled, but requires specialized consultation and treatment in others.

Demographics

The demographics of urinary and fecal incontinence vary widely according to the type of cancer and the treatments for it. One study reported that about 35% of women treated for cancers of the female reproductive system developed urinary incontinence, while another found that 80% of women treated for cancer of the uterus with **radiation therapy** developed urinary incontinence. Between 50 and 80% of patients receiving **irinotecan** (Camptosar), a drug given to treat **colon cancer**, develop severe **diarrhea** and fecal incontinence. About 99% of patients given opioid drugs to relieve pain develop constipation, which can lead to fecal incontinence if untreated.

Description

Incontinence is the loss of normal control of the bowel or bladder. Incontinence can involve the involuntary voiding of urine (urinary incontinence) or of stool and gas (fecal or bowel incontinence). There are several types of urinary incontinence. Those most frequently seen as side effects of cancer include overflow incontinence, urge incontinence, and stress incontinence. In rare cases incontinence occurs as the result of cancer, but more commonly it is a side effect of treatment.

Because the subjects of bowel and bladder control are perceived as socially unacceptable, those affected with incontinence often feel ashamed or embarrassed by the problem. Instead of seeking medical attention, these individuals try to hide the problem or manage it themselves. For this reason, incontinence is sometimes referred to as "the silent affliction." The psychological effects of incontinence include low self-esteem, social withdrawal and isolation, and **depression**. In most cases incontinence can be successfully treated, so affected individuals should discuss the problem with a doctor.

Risk factors

Risk factors for cancer-related incontinence include:

- Previous history of irritable bowel syndrome, Crohn's disease, diabetes, or multiple sclerosis.
- Being diagnosed with Alzheimer's or Parkinson's disease in addition to the cancer.
- In women, previous history of childbirth by vaginal delivery.
- In men, diagnosis of and treatment for prostate cancer.
- Any cancer treatment that involves surgical removal of part of the digestive tract.
- Radiation therapy to the stomach or abdomen as part of cancer treatment.
- Cancers that arise in or spread to the brain and spinal cord.
- Anticancer drugs that affect the nervous system.
- Pain relievers that contain opium or opium derivatives. These drugs include fentanyl, morphine, codeine, oxycodone, tramadol, and dextropropoxyphene. Opioids can cause constipation that can lead in turn to fecal incontinence.

Causes and symptoms

Incontinence can result from damage to the muscles, nerves, or structures of the body parts involved in the control of voiding. Complex systems of hollow organs (such as the bladder) and tube-shaped structures (such as the rectum and urethra) work together to store and release waste. Special muscles, including sphincters, are especially important in maintaining the tight seals that hold in waste. When physical damage to muscle or organ structure occurs, the system can no longer maintain these tight seals, and waste can leak out.

Nerves carry messages between the brain and the bowel and bladder systems. Injury to these nerves or the related part of the brain interferes with the delivery of these messages, which can prevent the body from recognizing the signals telling it when to void. Without these signals and messages, an individual cannot coordinate the brain with the bowel and bladder systems, and incontinence results.

Several types of cancer and its treatments are associated with incontinence. Usually, it is the treatment of cancer that causes incontinence rather than the cancer itself. Fecal incontinence frequently results from **anticancer drugs** that cause either diarrhea or constipation. Anticancer drugs that can cause constipation include the vinca alkaloids, oxaliplatins, taxanes, and **thalidomide**. Drugs that can cause diarrhea include the fluoropyrimidines, doxorubicin, **cisplatin**, and irinotecan; in one study, 80% of cancer patients receiving these drugs developed severe diarrhea.

Prostate cancer

The treatment of **prostate cancer** is one of the most common causes of cancer-related urinary incontinence, largely because the prostate is located so closely to the nerves, muscles, and structures involved in urine control. Surgical removal of the prostate, or **prostatectomy**, carries the highest risk of urinary incontinence as a side effect; the risk from radiation therapy is somewhat lower. The incontinence (typically stress or urge incontinence) is often temporary, but in a small percentage of men it may be long lasting.

Prostate cancer itself seldom causes incontinence. However, this depends on the location and size of the cancer; a large cancerous prostate can interfere with the flow of urine and result in overflow incontinence.

Bladder cancer

Incontinence is only occasionally the direct result of **bladder cancer**, but it is a common side effect of some treatments. For early-stage cancer in which treatment does not require the bladder to be removed, incontinence almost never occurs. But removal of the bladder and surrounding structures is often necessary to treat more advanced cancer. This surgery requires creation of an artificial system for storing and releasing urine and carries a risk of long-term incontinence.

Colon cancer and rectal cancer

Muscles in the anal and rectal region largely control bowel evacuation, with the colon storing stool and gas. When these regions are removed or damaged during cancer treatment, or if injury to the related nerves occurs, fecal incontinence can result. Fecal incontinence is most commonly a side effect of surgery. Weakening of bowel muscles or damaging of nerves by radiation therapy can also cause incontinence, but this type is more likely to be mild and temporary, and will often improve as these areas heal. However, in some patients, radiation causes permanent and severe fecal incontinence; this condition is known as radiation **enteritis**.

Other causes

Loss of voluntary bowel and bladder control is less commonly associated with other cancers of the genital and urinary systems, mainly as a side effect of treatment. Incontinence can also result from cancer or treatment damage in the brain and spinal cord. Other cancers indirectly cause incontinence; for example, constant coughing from lung cancer can lead to stress incontinence. Incontinence can be a side effect of certain other medications.

Diagnosis

The diagnosis of incontinence is usually obvious on the basis of the patient's treatment history and reported symptoms.

Treatment

Traditional

The method of treatment depends on the cause and type of incontinence. Surgical treatment is usually reserved for severe or long-lasting incontinence. An artificial pouch for storing urine or stool can be placed inside the body as a substitute for a removed bladder, colon, or rectum. Placement of an artificial sphincter successfully treats other cases. For mild or temporary incontinence, treatment may include medications, dietary changes, muscle-strengthening exercises, or behavioral training, such as establishing a time pattern for voiding. A small group of patients, however, requires a permanent **colostomy** or **urostomy**.

Electrical stimulation therapy, which targets involved muscles with low-current electricity, can be used to treat either urinary or fecal incontinence. Biofeedback uses electronic or mechanical devices to improve bladder or bowel control by teaching an individual how to recognize and respond to certain body signals.

Embarrassment may lead some people to manage the symptoms of incontinence themselves by wearing absorbent pads to prevent the soiling of their clothes. However, many treatments exist to successfully restore or improve control of bowel and bladder function, so individuals experiencing incontinence should speak to a doctor or nurse.

Cancer patients who have difficulty with frequent or occasional incontinence may find the following tips helpful:

- Always use the bathroom before leaving home.
- Always carry a backpack or tote containing cleansing towelettes and a change of underwear.
- Locate public restrooms before the need to use them is urgent.
- If the problem is specifically fecal incontinence, try taking an oral fecal deodorant. Over-the-counter products approved by the U.S. Food and Drug Administration (FDA) include Devrom and Nullo. These products work by reducing the number of odor-causing bacteria in stool.
- Wear disposable undergarments or sanitary pads if an episode of incontinence seems likely.

Drugs

Constipation caused by cancer therapy can be treated by one or more stimulant **laxatives**, stool softeners, lubricant laxatives, or agents that increase the bulk of the stools. Patients whose constipation is caused by opioid pain relievers can be given a drug called methylnaltrexone (Relistor), which will relieve the constipation without affecting the patient's pain control.

Diarrhea caused by cancer treatment can be treated by giving the patient loperamide, a drug that slows down intestinal motility. Other medications include octreotide (Sandostatin) and absorbent materials like pectin or methylcellulose, which absorb excess liquid in the digestive tract.

Alternative

Good results for cancer-related fecal incontinence have been reported for biofeedback training, although the subject is still being researched. In successful cases, patients regain complete control over defecation, or at least improve their control, by learning to contract the external part of the anal sphincter whenever stools enter the rectum.

Home remedies

In some cases, patients with fecal incontinence related to cancer treatment may be helped by eating small frequent meals and avoiding certain foods. The most frequent offenders include milk and dairy products, spicy foods, alcohol, caffeine-containing foods and beverages (including coffee, tea, and cola), certain fruit juices, gas-forming foods and beverages, high-fiber foods, and high-fat foods.

Prognosis

Success in treating cancer-related incontinence depends on the location of the cancer and the methods used to treat it. In most cases the patient can obtain at least partial relief. When incontinence remains a problem despite medical treatment, disposable underwear and other commercial incontinence products are available to make life easier. Doctors and nurses can offer advice on coping with incontinence, and people should never be embarrassed about seeking their assistance. Counseling and information are also available from support groups.

Prevention

Incontinence related to cancer or cancer treatment is difficult to prevent, in part because researchers do not understand as of 2014 why some patients become incontinent with cancer or cancer therapy and others do not.

Resources

BOOKS

Airley, Rachel. *Cancer Chemotherapy*. Hoboken, NJ: Wiley-Blackwell, 2009.

DeAngelis, Lisa M., and Jerome B. Posner. *Neurologic Complications of Cancer*, 2nd ed. New York: Oxford University Press, 2009.

Klingele, Christopher J., and Paul M. Pettit, eds. *Mayo Clinic on Managing Incontinence*. 2nd ed. Rochester, MN: Mayo Clinic, 2013.

Leupold, Nancy E., and James J. Scubba, eds. *Meeting the Challenges of Oral and Head and Neck Cancer: A Survivor's Guide*. San Diego, CA: Plural Publishing, 2008.

McKay, Judith, and Tamera Schacher. *The Chemotherapy Survival Guide: Everything You Need to Know to Get through Treatment*, 3rd ed. Oakland, CA: New Harbinger Publications, 2009.

Perry, Michael P., ed. *The Chemotherapy Source Book*. Philadelphia: Wolters Kluwer Health/Lippincott Williams and Wilkins, 2008.

PERIODICALS

Bartlett, L., et al. "Impact of Fecal Incontinence on Quality of Life." *World Journal of Gastroenterology* 15 (July 14, 2009): 3276–82.

Chamlou, R., et al. "Long-term Results of Intersphincteric Resection for Low Rectal Cancer." *Annals of Surgery* 246 (December 2007): 916–921.

Lange, M.M., and C. J. van de Velde. "Faecal and Urinary Incontinence after Multimodality Treatment of Rectal Cancer." *PLoS Medicine* 5 (October 7, 2008): 202.

Muehlbauer, P. M., et al. "Putting Evidence into Practice: Evidence-based Interventions to Prevent, Manage, and Treat Chemotherapy- and Radiotherapy-induced Diarrhea." *Clinical Journal of Oncology Nursing* 13 (June 2009): 336–41.

Parsons, B. A., et al. "Prostate Cancer and Urinary Incontinence." *Maturitas* 63 (August 20, 2009): 323–28.

OTHER

National Cancer Institute (NCI). *Managing Chemotherapy Side Effects: Urination Changes.* http://www.cancer.gov/cancertopics/coping/chemo-side-effects/urination.pdf

WEBSITES

American Cancer Society (ACS). "Managing Incontinence for Men With Cancer." http://www.cancer.org/treatment/treatmentsandsideeffects/physicalsideeffects/managing-incontinence-for-men-with-cancer (accessed November 4, 2014).

National Cancer Institute (NCI). "Gastrointestinal Complications (PDQ®). http://www.cancer.gov/cancertopics/pdq/supportivecare/gastrointestinalcomplications/Patient (accessed December 18, 2014).

ORGANIZATIONS

American Cancer Society, 250 Williams St. NW, Atlanta, GA 30303, (800) 227-2345, http://www.cancer.org.

American College of Gastroenterology, 6400 Goldsboro Rd., Ste. 200, Bethesda, MD 20817, (301) 263-9000, http://gi.org.

American Society of Clinical Oncology (ASCO), 2318 Mill Rd., Ste. 800, Alexandria, VA 22314, (571) 483-1300, (888) 651-3038, contactus@cancer.net, http://www.asco.org.

National Association for Continence (NAFC), PO Box 1019, Charleston, SC 29402, (843) 419-5309, (800) BLADDER (252-3337), Fax: (843) 352-2563, memberservices@nafc.org, http://www.nafc.org.

National Cancer Institute, 9609 Medical Center Dr., BG 9609 MSC 9760, Bethesda, MD 20892-9760, (800) 4-CANCER (422-6237), http://www.cancer.gov.

National Institute of Diabetes and Digestive and Kidney Diseases (NIDDK),Bethesda, MD 20892-2560, (301) 496-3583, http://www.niddk.nih.gov.

International Foundation for Functional Gastrointestinal Disorders (IFFGD), P.O. Box 170864, MilwaukeeWI53217-8076, 414-964-1799, Fax: 414-964-7176, iffgd@iffgd.org, http://www.iffgd.org.

Stefanie B.N. Dugan, M.S.
REVISED BY REBECCA J. FREY, PhD.

Infection and sepsis

Definition

In its most general sense, an infection represents the body's reaction to the rapid growth of a foreign organism, such as a bacterium. The infecting organism multiplies by effectively robbing the body of necessary nutrition, which compromises the body's health. Sepsis occurs when the infection spreads throughout the entire body and affects multiple organ systems. The English word *sepsis* comes from the Greek word for putrefaction or decay.

In 1992, the American College of Chest Physicians and the Society of Critical Care Medicine clarified sepsis syndromes by listing them in order of severity:

- Sepsis: the presence of a systemic inflammatory response syndrome (SIRS) in the setting of an infection.
- Severe sepsis: infection with evidence of end-organ dysfunction as a result of hypoperfusion (inadequate blood supply to tissues and organs).
- Septic shock: severe sepsis with persistent low blood pressure despite fluid resuscitation and resulting tissue hypoperfusion.

Description

Infection is characterized by an inflammatory response to the presence of foreign microorganisms in the body. This response may include **fever**, chills, redness, swelling, and/or pus formation. The most common cause of illness and death in patients with **cancer** is infection. Patients with cancer who are treated with **chemotherapy**, **radiation therapy**, and/or surgery are at increased risk of developing infection. Mortality from infection in cancer patients decreased during the late 1900s due to the development of new types of **antibiotics**, the use of hematopoietic growth factors (HGFs), which activate proliferation (multiplication) and maturation of blood cell lines. In addition, the prophylactic (preventive) use of antifungal and antiviral agents became more common at that time. In order to fight infection, the body needs blood cell lines, which markedly decrease with chemotherapy, commonly used to treat cancer. Most infections in cancer patients result from foreign bacteria; however, the most serious infections usually result from fungi.

If left untreated, or if inadequately treated, infection can progress to sepsis. Vital sign changes that may indicate sepsis include a temperature of greater than 38 degrees Celsius (100.4° Fahrenheit) or less than 36°C (96.8°F), heart rate greater than 90 beats per minutes, and respiratory rate greater than 20 breaths per minute.

Risk factors

Risk factors for infection and sepsis include:

- weakened immune system
- hospitalization—many infections are acquired during a hospital stay
- surgery, dental work, catheter or pacemaker insertion; placement of a prosthesis or artificial joint; or other procedures that involve cutting into or injuring tissue
- concurrent HIV infection
- treatment for cancer
- homelessness
- poor personal hygiene
- treatment for severe burns—like cancer patients, burn patients are highly susceptible to infections

- age below 1 year or over 35 years
- pregnancy
- minority ethnicity
- history of lung disease—the lungs are the single most common site of the initial infection leading to sepsis
- using injected drugs of abuse
- abnormalities of the heart valves

Demographics

Sepsis affects about 3 in every 1,000 Americans each year; severe sepsis accounts for 500,000–750,000 cases each year in Canada and the United States, with 200,000 deaths. As of 2014, it was the tenth most common cause of death in the United States. Sepsis occurs in 1%–2% of all hospitalizations and accounts for as much as 25% of ICU bed utilization. About half of all patients with sepsis require hospitalization in an intensive care setting. About 60% of cases of severe sepsis occur in patients over the age of 65. There are several reasons that the numbers for sepsis are high:

- the growing proportion of elderly in the general population; more efficient diagnosis of severe disease
- a sharp rise in the number of invasive procedures and organ transplants
- increased use of immunosuppressive agents and chemotherapy in cancer patients
- increased use of indwelling lines and devices in hospitalized patients
- a rise in such chronic diseases as end-stage renal disease and HIV infection
- an increased frequency of multidrug-resistant organisms

The incidence rate of sepsis in cancer patients in North America is estimated at 45%. Mortality rates from sepsis in cancer patients exceed 30%. Although the incidence of sepsis in cancer patients has increased by 2% per year since the early 2000s, a study conducted at three university-associated cancer centers reported in 2014 that mortality rates were declining. Lung cancer patients are at highest risk of dying from sepsis.

Causes and symptoms

Causes

There are many reasons that cancer patients are prone to infection. For example, certain cancers interfere with the body's immune system response, which increases the likelihood of infection. These cancer types include acute leukemia, **chronic lymphocytic leukemia**, **multiple myeloma**, **Hodgkin lymphoma**, and **non-Hodgkin lymphoma**. Certain therapies used to treat cancer also compromise the immune system that normally fights infection. These therapies include chemotherapy (which interrupts bone marrow production of white blood cells, red blood cells, and platelets), radiation therapy, **bone marrow transplantation**, and treatments using **corticosteroids**.

Some cancer patients experience protein-calorie malnutrition, which suppresses the immune system and increases the risk of infection. Many cancer patients develop infections from procedures that puncture the skin, which allows the introduction of microorganisms into the body. These procedures include venipunctures, biopsies, insertion of urinary catheters, and use of long-term central venous catheters, all of which are common during the course of cancer treatment. Infection rates associated with long-term central venous catheter use in cancer patients are estimated to be as high as 60%. Once a patient's immune system is severely compromised, infection can result from food sources, plants, and even the air a patient breathes.

Myelosuppression is the term used to describe the decrease in numbers of circulating white blood cells (WBC), red blood cells (RBC), and platelets. Myelosuppression is often a side effect of chemotherapy and/or radiation therapy. Blood counts usually begin to fall one to three weeks after treatment with chemotherapy, depending upon the type of chemotherapy and the blood cell type involved. The counts generally begin to recover to normal levels within two to three weeks. The neutrophil, a component of the white blood cells, is the body's first line of defense against bacteria-caused infection. **Neutropenia** indicates a decrease in the number of neutrophils. Neutropenia is the single greatest predictor of infection in patients with cancer. Three key factors help predict a patient's chances of infection in the event of myelosuppression. These factors include: 1) the degree of neutropenia, i.e., as the neutrophil count falls, the likelihood of infection increases; 2) the duration of the neutropenia, i.e., the longer a patient is neutropenic, the greater the likelihood of infection; and 3) the rate at which neutropenia develops—the more rapid the development, the greater the risk of infection.

Bacterial infections in cancer patients develop quickly, especially in the neutropenic patient, and account for 85–90% of the microorganisms associated with neutropenia accompanied by fever. The most serious episodes occur from infections attributed to such gram-negative organisms as *Enterobacteriaceae* or *Pseudomonas aeruginosa*. However, infections from such gram-positive organisms as *Staphylococcus, Streptococcus, Corynebacteria,* and *Clostridia* have increased in the 2000s, probably due to the increased use of implanted central venous catheters and prophylactic antibiotics (to which these organisms develop an immunity). Listeriosis, a severe bacterial infection caused by *Listeria monocytogenes*, is another infection on the increase in cancer patients. Listeriosis has become a common complication of bone marrow transplantation since the early 2000s as well as a frequent cause of patient death.

Other organisms that cause infections in the immunocompromised cancer patient include such herpesviruses as **herpes simplex** virus 1 and 2 (HSV-1, HSV-2), varicella zoster virus (VZV), cytomegalovirus (CMV), and **Epstein-Barr virus** (EBV). Sources of secondary infections include the fungus *Candida albicans*. Common causes of secondary infection in severely immunosuppressed patients include CMV and the filamentous fungus *Aspergillus*. Aspergillosis is an increasingly common and often fatal infection in patients with hematologic (blood-related) cancers.

The symptoms of sepsis are not the result of bacteria or other pathogens themselves. Instead, sepsis is the systemic consequence of the body's release of certain chemicals in response to an infectious agent like bacteria or fungi. The incidence of sepsis and septic shock increases when the patient remains neutropenic for longer than seven days. Other factors that put the cancer patient at high risk for the development of sepsis include infection with a gram-negative organism, presence of a central venous catheter, history of prior infection, malnutrition, history of frequent hospitalization, increased age of patient, and concurrent (at the same time) presence of such other diseases as diabetes, cardiovascular, gastrointestinal, hepatic, pulmonary, and/or renal disease. Sites of infection that most often lead to sepsis include infection of the lungs, invasive lines, and urinary tract.

Symptoms

Sepsis appears with both local and systemic symptoms that involve the neurologic, endocrine, immunologic, and cardiovascular systems. Signs of sepsis and septic shock include changes in blood pressure, heart rate, and respiratory rate, among others. If left untreated, the patient can progress to septic shock, which may result in death even if the shock episode is treated. Factors that appear to increase the patient's chances of survival include rapid admission to an intensive care unit and aggressive treatment with antibiotics.

Diagnosis

The diagnosis of sepsis is based on the following criteria:

- Temperature above 101°F or below 96°F.
- Heart rate above 90 beats per minute (bpm).
- Respiration faster than 20 breaths per minute.
- WBC higher than 12,000/mm^3 or lower than 4,000/mm^3.
- Low blood pressure: lower than 90 mmHg, or a reduction of 40 mmHg or more from the patient's baseline blood pressure.
- Hypoxemia, or low blood oxygen levels.
- Increased levels of lactate in the plasma.
- Abnormalities in platelet count.
- Altered mental status: delirium, confusion, anxiety, and/or agitation.
- Reduced output of urine (oliguria).

All of these criteria do not need to be present to diagnose severe sepsis or septic shock.

Examination

In addition to abnormalities in the patient's vital signs, the doctor may also observe changes in mental status or the condition of the patient's skin. In the early stages of septic shock, the patient's skin is often warm to the touch; in later stages, the skin may become clammy and cool to the touch and develop a pale, grayish, or mottled color. The doctor will listen to the patient's breathing for evidence of fluid accumulation in the lungs. If the infection appears to be localized, or limited to one location on the body, the doctor will look for redness, swelling, pain, or a discharge at that location.

Tests

Standard laboratory tests for infection and suspected sepsis include:

- a complete blood cell count (CBC) and a blood chemistry panel
- blood coagulation studies
- measurement of hemoglobin levels
- cultures of bodily fluids such as blood, sputum, urine, and/or cerebrospinal fluid (CSF) to identify the organism causing the infection
- liver function tests
- urinalysis and a urine culture
- a test of the patient's sputum if pneumonia is suspected

The patient's procalcitonin level may also be tested; this test helps distinguish sepsis from other noninfectious conditions that produce similar symptoms. Procalcitonin is a precursor of the hormone **calcitonin**, which regulates calcium levels in the blood. Procalcitonin levels are virtually undetectable in the blood of healthy persons but rise to measurable levels in persons with severe bacterial infections.

Imaging tests are ordered as appropriate according to the location of the infection. They may include chest x-rays, abdominal ultrasounds, CT or MRI imaging, or x-ray studies of the extremities when soft-tissue infections are suspected. An EKG is often conducted to check for abnormal heart rhythms.

Procedures

Patients with severe sepsis or septic shock are usually intubated to keep the airway open. Other procedures that may be performed include lumbar punctures (spinal tap) if meningitis is suspected; placement of urinary catheters to monitor the patient's urine output; and surgical drainage of any abscesses.

Treatment

Sepsis is a medical emergency and is usually treated in an intensive care unit (ICU). Treatment includes maintenance of ventilation, oxygenation, fluid volume, and cardiac output as well as administration of antibiotics and **nutritional support**. Patients may be placed on a mechanical ventilator to assist with breathing or given supplemental oxygen if needed. Speed of treatment is essential; antibiotics should be administered within an hour of diagnosis. Several studies have indicated that every hour of delay in the administration of appropriate antibiotic therapy is associated with a 7% rise in mortality.

Drugs

Empiric antibiotic therapy is the mainstay of treatment for infection in the cancer patient. Empiric therapy involves the initiation of antibiotic therapy prior to the identification of the infecting organism. In order to target the widest range of possible infectious agents, the first line of defense is a broad-spectrum antibiotic, one that is effective against both gram-negative and gram-positive organisms. Commonly used agents include aminoglycosides, fluoroquinolones, third-generation cephalosporins, glycopeptides, and such beta-lactams as penicillins, cephalosporins, carbapenems, and monobactams.

Empiric **antifungal therapy** is initiated 5–7 days after empiric antibiotic therapy has been initiated if the patient remains febrile (with a fever). Antiviral agents may be administered if there is evidence of a viral infection. The Infectious Diseases Society of America (IDSA) recommends a minimum of five to seven days additional treatment with parenteral (introduced in other ways than intestinal absorption) antibiotic therapy once

the fever returns to a normal level. Continued monitoring of bacterial and fungal culture results is essential to enable precise tailoring of the antibiotic therapy to the specific infectious agent.

If untreated, a neutropenic patient with fever can progress quickly to sepsis. The patient may also progress to septic shock with inadequate empiric antibiotic therapy. Infection with gram-negative bacteria is the most common cause of septic shock in cancer patients.

In addition to antibiotics, corticosteroids may be administered to reduce inflammation; vasopressors are sometimes used to restore normal blood pressure. The vasopressor used most often is norepinephrine, although dopamine or vasopressin may be administered in specific situations.

Surgery

Some conditions will not respond to standard antibiotic treatment until the source of the infection is surgically removed; these include soft-tissue abscesses, infected catheters or prosthetic devices, and necrotizing fasciitis. The surgeon may also remove damaged or dead tissue.

Prognosis

Reports of the mortality rate for severe sepsis and septic shock range from 20% to 50%. The most detailed recent study reports a death rate of 30%. Other studies claim that between 20% and 35% of patients with severe sepsis and 40–60% of patients with septic shock die within 30 days of hospital admission. Risk factors for mortality with infection and sepsis include delayed antibiotic treatment; male sex; age over 50 years; the presence of two or more concurrent illnesses; altered mental status; and in-hospital acquisition of the infection.

Prevention

Strategies that prevent or minimize infection in the neutropenic patient include:

• Identification of patients at highest risk of infection.

• Avoidance by health care workers of practices known to increase colonization of microorganisms.

• Use of as few invasive procedures as possible.

• Vaccination of susceptible individuals against influenza and pneumonia.

Cancer patients at risk of neutropenia may also benefit from treatment with two new hematopoietic growth factors, pegfilgrastim (Neulasta) and darbepoetin alfa (Aranesp). These drugs appear effective in reducing the risk of opportunistic infections in cancer patients and improving their overall quality of life.

QUESTIONS TO ASK YOUR DOCTOR

- What is causing the infection?

- What antibiotics will you prescribe? What are their possible side effects?

- What is the normal course of this illness? When can I expect to feel better?

- Can I transmit this infection to others?

- What complications might occur from this type of infection? How might I prevent complications?

- Will treatment for the infection interfere with cancer therapy?

- Has the infection progressed to sepsis or severe sepsis?

Specific interventions in the hospital setting that can be used to prevent or minimize infection include:

• Scrupulous handwashing by patient, staff, and visitors.

• Good personal and oral hygiene by the patient.

• Ambulation (movement).

• Aggressive efforts to promote lung expansion.

• Elimination of uncooked fruits and vegetables from the diet.

• Removal of plants and other sources of stagnant water from the patient's room.

• Minimizing the number of outside visitors and avoiding those with signs of infection.

In addition, hospitalized patients should be assessed at least every four hours; samples should be collected and subjected to laboratory analysis to determine risk for and presence of neutropenia.

The administration of hematopoietic growth factors (HGFs) has gained favor in recent years, because it seems to lessen the duration of neutropenia, thereby decreasing the period of maximum risk of infection. HGFs work by activating the production and maturation of RBCs, WBCs, and platelet cell lines. Specific HGFs stimulate the production and maturation of aggressive neutrophils and macrophages, which act to destroy pathogens (bacteria or viruses that cause infection or disease).

Resources

BOOKS

Khardori, Nancy, ed. *Sepsis: Diagnosis, Management and Health Outcomes.* Hauppauge, NY: Nova Science Publishers, 2014.

Mancini, Nicasio. *Sepsis: Diagnostic Methods and Protocols.* New York: Springer, 2014.

Yealy, Donald M., and Clifton W. Callaway, eds. *Emergency Department Critical Care.* New York: Oxford University Press, 2013.

PERIODICALS

Debiane, L., et al. "The Utility of Proadrenomedullin and Procalcitonin in Comparison to C-Reactive Protein as Predictors of Sepsis and Bloodstream Infections in Critically Ill Patients With Cancer." *Critical Care Medicine*, July 31, 2014 [E-publication ahead of print].

Dellinger, R.P., et al. "Surviving Sepsis Campaign: International Guidelines for Management of Severe Sepsis and Septic Shock: 2012." *Critical Care Medicine* 41 (February 2013): 580–637.

Friend, K.E., et al. "Procalcitonin Elevation Suggests a Septic Source." *American Surgeon* 80 (September 2014): 906–909.

Marin, M., et al. "Bloodstream Infections in Patients with Solid Tumors: Epidemiology, Antibiotic Therapy, and Outcomes in 528 Episodes in a Single Cancer Center." *Medicine (Baltimore)* 93 (May 2014): 142–149.

Mokart, D., et al. "Neutropenic Cancer Patients with Severe Sepsis: Need for Antibiotics in the First Hour." *Intensive Care Medicine* 40 (August 2014): 1173–1174.

Rolston, K.V. "Neutropenic Fever and Sepsis: Evaluation and Management." *Cancer Treatment and Research* 161 (2014): 181–202.

Sammon, J.D., et al. "Sepsis after Major Cancer Surgery." *Journal of Surgical Research*, July 24, 2014 [E-publication ahead of print].

Soares, M., et al. "Intensive Care in Patients with Lung Cancer: A Multinational Study." *Annals of Oncology* 25 (September 2014): 1829–1835.

Starr, M.E., and H. Saito. "Sepsis in Old Age: Review of Human and Animal Studies." *Aging and Disease* 6 (April 1, 2014): 126–136.

White, L., and M. Ybarra. "Neutropenic Fever." *Emergency Medicine Clinics of North America* 32 (August 2014): 549–561.

WEBSITES

Cleveland Clinic Disease Management Program. "Sepsis." http://www.clevelandclinicmeded.com/medicalpubs/diseasemanagement/infectious-disease/sepsis (accessed September 3, 2014).

Kalil, Andre. "Septic Shock." Medscape Reference. http://emedicine.medscape.com/article/168402-overview (accessed September 2, 2014).

Lab Tests Online. "Sepsis." http://labtestsonline.org/understanding/conditions/sepsis (accessed September 2, 2014).

Mayo Clinic. "Sepsis." http://www.mayoclinic.org/diseases-conditions/sepsis/basics/definition/con-20031900 (accessed September 2, 2014).

MedlinePlus. "Sepsis." http://www.nlm.nih.gov/medlineplus/ency/article/000666.htm (accessed September 2, 2014).

ORGANIZATIONS

American College of Emergency Physicians (ACEP), P.O. Box 619911, Dallas, TX 75261-9911, (972) 550-0911, (800) 798-1822, Fax: (972) 580-2816, http://www.acep.org.

Centers for Disease Control and Prevention (CDC), 1600 Clifton Rd., Atlanta, GA 30333, (800) 232-4636, http://wwwn.cdc.gov/dcs/RequestForm.aspx, http://www.cdc.gov.

Infectious Diseases Society of America (IDSA), 1300 Wilson Blvd., Suite 300, Arlington, VA 22209, (703) 299-0200, Fax: (703) 299-0204, http://www.idsociety.org/Index.aspx.

National Cancer Institute (NCI), BG 9609 MSC 9760, 9609 Medical Center Drive, Bethesda, MD 20892-9760, (800) 4-CANCER (422-6237), http://www.cancer.gov/global/contact/email-us, http://www.cancer.gov.

Melinda Granger Oberleitner, R.N., D.N.S.
Rebecca J. Frey, PhD.

Infertility *see* **Fertility issues**

Intensity-modulated radiation therapy

Definition

Intensity-modulated **radiation therapy** is a form of radiation therapy that uses a computer to deliver precise three-dimensional doses of x-rays to a tumor to treat **cancer**. It is the second-generation version of three-dimensional conformal radiation therapy (3-D CRT) and has been in use since 1998.

Purpose

As a newer form of radiation therapy, intensity-modulated radiation therapy (IMRT) offers special treatment options for cancer patients. When a patient has cancer, he or she may have radiation therapy to destroy the tumor or cancerous cells. The radiation therapy may be the only treatment prescribed, or it may be part of a regimen that includes surgery and/or **chemotherapy**.

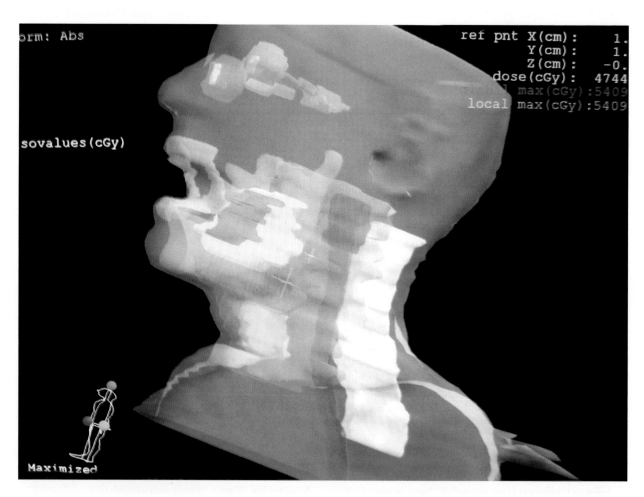

Intensity-modulated radiation therapy for neck cancer. *(S. Needell/Custom Medical Stock Photo)*

KEY TERMS

Ionizing radiation—Energy that is strong enough to remove an electron from an atom. It is used for diagnostic x-rays and for radiation therapy.

Neutropenia—An abnormally low number of neutrophils (a type of white blood cell) in the blood.

Recur, recurrence—Referring to cancer that reappears after initial treatment and the passage of time.

Thrombocytopenia—The medical term for low levels of platelets in the blood (below 50,000 platelets per microliter).

The radiation aimed at the cancerous cells sometimes destroys nearby healthy cells. IMRT is an advanced treatment method that allows physicians to target the cancer so precisely that healthy tissue receives little to no radiation, even when the tumor surrounds a vital organ. This feature makes IMRT a good choice for many cancer patients, particularly those with small tumors, brain and spinal cord tumors, **prostate cancer**, cancer of the head and neck, bone cancer, **gastrointestinal cancers**, and for those who have previously received radiation treatments. Research continues about expanding use of IMRT for a number of cancers; **clinical trials** are under way around the world.

Description

Physicians have used radiation to treat cancer for more than 100 years. The damaging effects of x-rays can destroy cancerous cells in the body and help rid the patient of the pain or related spread and complications of some cancers. For some patients, radiation therapy is the first-choice treatment; for others the treatment is used following surgery or chemotherapy or at the same time as chemotherapy. Radiation therapy is also sometimes called radiotherapy.

The goal of radiation therapy is to destroy as many cancer cells as possible while limiting damage to nearby healthy tissue. To accomplish this task, complicated dose measurements are calculated based on information gathered by studying the tumor before radiation treatment begins. Today, physicians use such imaging modalities as **computed tomography** (CT) or **magnetic resonance imaging** (MRI) to produce three-dimensional models to better pinpoint the tumor. Planning radiation treatments in three dimensions allows physicians to target the radiation beams at the tumor's height, width, and depth.

This technique is called 3-D conformal radiation therapy or 3D CRT; it was introduced commercially in 1989.

As noted above, IMRT is a newer type of 3-D conformal radiation therapy that uses beams of varying intensities. By doing so, the beams can strike the tumor from three dimensions and can also deliver varying doses simultaneously to small areas of tissue. This capacity allows more individualized targeting of the tumor than in the past, so that the radiation oncologist (a physician who specializes in using radiation to treat cancer) can plan higher doses to the tumor and lower doses to nearby tissues. Insurance companies consider IMRT a valuable treatment for many cancers because it is so effective.

Tomotherapy is a form of IMRT that delivers the radiation dose by rotating the beams over a small slice of tissue.

Most IMRT procedures are performed in a cancer center, radiation oncology physician office or outpatient facility, or in a hospital. The radiation oncologist oversees the patient's plan, working closely with a team of professionals. A medical physicist has special training in radiation physics and the operation and repair of radiology and radiation therapy equipment. The physicist also may help develop the patient's treatment plan. A medical dosimetrist works under the direction of the radiation oncologist and medical physicist to calculate the radiation dose. IMRT treatments are usually performed by a radiation therapist, a specially trained technologist who positions the patient and runs the equipment. A radiation oncology nurse may also help manage care, side effects, and explain the treatments.

A medical linear accelerator or LINAC is the machine that actually delivers the IMRT. It is about the size of a small car, about 10 feet high and 15 feet long. The patient may hear noises or smell odors from the equipment but will not feel the radiation itself. The LINAC uses microwave technology similar to that used in airport radar installations. The room in which the LINAC is situated is lined with lead and concrete walls to limit radiation exposure to anyone outside the treatment room; the radiation therapist must leave the treatment room to operate the machine.

As the treatment begins, the patient is positioned on a treatment table in a precise location that has been planned ahead during simulation sessions. A special molding or other device may be applied to restrict movement during the procedure. The radiation therapist is able to observe the patient throughout the procedure through a window or closed-circuit television. The therapist may reposition the patient during the procedure. A treatment session usually lasts about 15 to 30 minutes. The procedure is usually painless, but the therapist can halt treatment if the patient experiences discomfort. The number of treatments a patient undergoes depends on the type and stage of cancer. Some patients receive daily treatments over the span of several weeks.

Precautions

Whenever a patient is considered for radiation therapy, physicians weigh the risks and benefits of the procedure. IMRT, like any external radiation therapy procedure, introduces x-rays (ionizing radiation) to the patient's skin, tissues, and organs near the treatment area. Some patients are not candidates for this treatment. Patients who receive IMRT must visit the radiation oncology facility frequently for the prescribed treatment plan and follow instructions exactly to deal with radiation side effects. However, the accuracy of IMRT allows some patients who may not have been candidates for radiation therapy under older, less precise methods to undergo radiation treatment for their disease. IMRT delivers radiation to the intended target precisely, thus sparing surrounding organs and tissues. Patients should discuss all risks and benefits of IMRT with their oncology treatment team.

Preparation

Before beginning IMRT treatment, the radiation oncologist and treatment team must pinpoint the precise location of the tumor (anatomical position). This need for precision may require the patient to have several **imaging studies** in addition to those used for initial diagnosis. Computed tomography (CT), **positron emission tomography** (PET) scans, and magnetic resonance imaging (MRI) can be used to provide three-dimensional information for the IMRT system. These imaging visits and the resulting work of the treatment team are called treatment simulation. The patient may also visit the radiation therapy facility prior to treatment for a planning session. In this session, a special device is sometimes molded that enables the patient to maintain an exact treatment position. A mark or tattoo with colored ink may be applied to help align and target the equipment once treatment begins.

Aftercare

The radiation oncologist, radiation therapist, or radiation oncology nurse will provide instructions on IMRT aftercare. Because some effects of radiation therapy do not appear until several treatments have been completed, these instructions may vary throughout the course of treatment. The most common side effects of external radiation therapy are **fatigue** and skin changes.

People undergoing radiation therapy who become fatigued may need to modify their activities. The treatment team is available for advice about fatigue and its effects as well as care for skin conditions that result from treatment.

Risks

Radiation therapy includes risk of radiation damage to normal tissues or organs near the area being targeted. However, IMRT treatment is more precise than other external radiation therapy procedures. Since doses are calculated by FDA-approved software, the risk of dose miscalculation is minimal. IMRT facilities are carefully regulated to ensure the correct dose is delivered to the precise location on the correct patient.

Radiation therapy may also result in low levels of white blood cells and platelets, conditions known as **neutropenia** and **thrombocytopenia** respectively. White blood cells help fight infection and platelets help blood clot. Radiation therapy sometimes causes hair loss (**alopecia**), although the hair typically grows back.

Some recent research suggests that IMRT increases a patient's risk of a second cancer, defined as a new cancer that appears after treatment for the original cancer has been completed.

Results

After completion of IMRT treatments, cancer cells should stop dividing and growing, which slows tumor growth. Often, cancer cells completely die and the tumor shrinks or disappears. With IMRT, radiation damage to the normal, healthy tissues around the tumor is minimized and incidence of side effects is reduced.

Abnormal results

The treatment might not eliminate cancer cells entirely. A cancer might still partially remain or recur at a later date. Physicians usually follow up with imaging studies to monitor treatment progress and set up a future schedule of checkups for cancer recurrence.

Resources

BOOKS

Halperin, Edward C., Carlos A. Perez, and Luther W. Brady, eds. *Perez and Brady's Principles and Practice of Radiation Oncology.* 5th ed. Philadelphia, PA: Wolters Kluwer Health/Lippincott Williams and Wilkins, 2008.

Khan, Faiz M., and John P. Gibbons. *The Physics of Radiation Therapy.* 5th ed. Philadelphia, PA: Lippincott Williams and Wilkins/Wolters Kluwer, 2014.

Lee, Nancy Y., and Jiade J. Lu, eds. *Target Volume Delineation and Field Setup: A Practical Guide for Conformal and Intensity-modulated Radiation Therapy.* Heidelberg, Germany: Springer, 2013.

PERIODICALS

Fontenot, J.D. "Evaluation of a Novel Secondary Check Tool for Intensity-modulated Radiotherapy Treatment Planning." *Journal of Applied Clinical Medical Physics* 15 (September 8, 2014): 4990.

Gandhi, A.K., et al. "Early Clinical Outcomes and Toxicity of Intensity-modulated Versus Conventional Pelvic Radiation Therapy for Locally Advanced Cervix Carcinoma: A Prospective Randomized Study." *International Journal of Radiation Oncology, Biology, Physics* 87 (November 1, 2013): 542–548.

Liu, G.F., et al. "Clinical Outcomes for Gastric Cancer Following Adjuvant Chemoradiation Utilizing Intensity-modulated Versus Three-dimensional Conformal Radiotherapy." *PLoS One* 9 (January 9, 2014): e82642.

Riou, O., et al. "Implementing Intensity-modulated Radiotherapy to the Prostate Bed: Dosimetric Study and Early Clinical Results." *Medical Dosimetry* 38 (Summer 2013): 117–121.

Spiotto, M.T., and R.R. Weichselbaum. "Comparison of 3D Conformal Radiotherapy and Intensity-modulated Radiotherapy With or Without Simultaneous Integrated Boost during Concurrent Chemoradiation for Locally Advanced Head and Neck Cancers." *PLoS One* 9 (April 8, 2014): e94456.

WEBSITES

American College of Radiology (ACR). "Intensity-Modulated Radiation Therapy (IMRT)." Page includes a 7-1/2-minute video about IMRT. http://www.radiologyinfo.org/en/info.cfm?pg=imrt (accessed September 5, 2014).

International RadioSurgery Association (IRSA). "IMRT." http://www.irsa.org/imrt.html (accessed September 6, 2014).

Mayo Clinic. "Intensity-modulated Radiation Therapy." http://www.mayoclinic.org/tests-procedures/intensity-modulated-radiation-therapy/basics/definition/PRC-20013330 (accessed September 4, 2014).

Penn Medicine: Radiation Oncology. "Intensity-Modulated Radiation Therapy (IMRT)." http://www.pennmedicine.

org/radiation-oncology/patient-care/treatments/intensity-modulated-radiation-therapy-imrt (accessed September 5, 2014).

ORGANIZATIONS

American College of Radiology (ACR), 1891 Preston White Dr., Reston, VA 20191, (703) 648-8900, info@acr.org, http://www.acr.org.

American Society for Radiology and Oncology (formerly the American Society for Therapeutic Radiology and Oncology), 8280 Willow Oaks Corporate Drive, Suite 500, Fairfax, VA 22031, (703) 502-1550, (800) 962-7876, Fax: (703) 502-7852, https://www.astro.org.

International RadioSurgery Association (IRSA), P.O. Box 5186, Harrisburg, PA 17110, (717) 260-9808, http://www.irsa.org/ContactIrsa.html, http://www.irsa.org.

Teresa G. Odle

REVISED BY REBECCA J. FREY, PhD.

Interferons

Definition

Interferons are in a class of naturally occurring small proteins or glycoproteins called cytokines. They are produced by white blood cells called leucocytes and T lymphocytes (T cells) and by fibroblasts, as part of an **immune response** to infection or other biological stimuli. Interferons are synthesized or produced through genetic engineering for use as **immunotherapy** medications in the treatment of viral infections, **cancer**, and multiple sclerosis (MS).

Purpose

The first interferon was discovered in 1957 as an immune-system agent that was produced in response to viral infection and interfered with the production of new viral particles—hence the name *interferon*. Recombinant DNA technology has since been adapted to produce interferons for research and drug treatments. Interferons attach to specific receptors on the surfaces of cell membranes, where they have a variety of effects on the immune system, including the stimulation and inhibition of enzymes, inhibition of cell proliferation, and enhancement of macrophage and T-lymphocyte activities.

There are several different classes of interferons, including alfa, beta, gamma, tau, and omega. These classes are further broken into subclasses designated with Arabic numerals and letters. Alfa and beta interferons are type I interferons that are produced by white blood cells and fibroblasts (a type of connective-tissue cell). Gamma interferon is a type II interferon produced by T cells when they are activated by infection or another stimulus.

Alfa interferons are used to treat viral infections and cancer:

• Interferon alfacon-1 is a synthetic interferon used to treat chronic hepatitis C infection. It binds to the same receptor that binds the hepatitis C virus, thereby preventing the virus from entering and infecting host cells.

• Interferons alfa-2a and alfa-2b are used to treat both cancer and viral infections.

• Peginterferon (also called pegylated interferon) is interferon alfa combined with polyethylene glycol (PEG), which keeps the interferon active longer. Peginterferon alfa-2a and alfa-2b are used to prevent further liver damage in patients with chronic hepatitis C infections, often in combination with the antiviral drug ribavirin. Peginterferon alfa-2a is also used to treat chronic hepatitis B infections.

• Interferon alfa-n3 is used to treat recurring or refractory genital or venereal warts.

In cancer immunotherapy, alfa interferons activate tumor-specific cytotoxic T lymphocytes that destroy tumor cells, although the molecular details of this activity remain unclear. Interferons may cause antigens on the exposed tumor surface to more readily stimulate the immune system's T-cell response. Tumor growth may also be slowed by interferon-mediated damage to the blood cells that nourish the tumor. Alfa interferons are used to treat **hairy cell leukemia**, malignant **melanoma**, and **Kaposi sarcoma**, an AIDS-related cancer. Alfa interferons are used off-label to treat many other cancers, including kidney and bladder cancers, **chronic myelocytic leukemia**, carcinoid tumors, **non-Hodgkin lymphoma**, **ovarian cancer**, and skin cancers. Alfa interferons may be combined with other chemotherapeutic drugs such as **doxorubicin**.

Interferons beta-1a and beta-1b are used to decrease the number of symptomatic episodes or flare-ups of MS and to slow the progression of the disease in patients with relapsing-remitting MS. Interferon does not help patients with chronic progressive MS, in which symptoms are always present. MS is an autoimmune disease in which the body's own immune system demyelinates the myelin sheaths enclosing nerve cells. Demyelination causes malfunctions in the transmission of impulses from nerve to nerve and from nerve to muscle. Interferon beta-1a is in a class of medications called immunomodulators, but it is not known exactly how it decreases MS flare-ups.

Interferon beta-1b is a synthetic version of a human protein that is in a class of medications known as biologic response modifiers. It enhances T-cell activity while simultaneously reducing the production of inflammatory cytokines. Interferon beta-1b also retards the exposure of antigens on the surfaces of cells, thereby reducing the immune response to the antigen and slowing the appearance of lymphocytes in the central nervous system. This dampening of the immune response can reduce both symptomatic episodes of MS and damage to neurons in the brain. In 2006 the U.S. Food and Drug Administration (FDA) extended approval of interferon beta 1-b for use in patients who are at high risk of developing MS.

Interferon gamma-1b is a synthetic version of a naturally occurring interferon. It is used to treat chronic granulomatous disease, an inherited immune-system disorder.

Description

There are no generic forms of interferon. Interferons are always administered by injection, usually by the patient or caregiver. They cannot be taken by mouth because they are destroyed by stomach acids. The injections can be either intramuscular (IM; into a muscle) or subcutaneous (SC). SC injections are made under the skin between the fat layer and the muscle, often in the abdomen, thigh, buttocks, or upper arm—anywhere that there is a fat layer between the skin and muscle, except around the waist or near the navel. Each injection is given at a different site from the previous one, because side effects at the injection site are common. Injections are always on the same day(s) of the week at approximately the same time of day, usually late afternoon or evening before bedtime, so that the worst side effects occur during sleep.

U.S. brand names

• Infergen (interferon alfacon-1, SC injection) supplied as a 30-microgram (mcg) per milliliter (mL) solution of 0.3 or 0.5 mL

• Roferon-A (interferon alfa-2a, recombinant)

• Intron A (interferon alfa-2b, recombinant)

• Pegasys (peginterferon alfa-2a), for SC injection, supplied in a 1.2 mL solution vial of 180 mcg per mL or a pre-filled syringe with 180 mcg in 0.5 mL

• PEG-Intron (peginterferon alfa-2b), for SC injection, supplied as powder in a vial to which solution is added or as a single-dose injection pen

• Alferon N (interferon alfa-n3) supplied as a 1 mL 5-million-unit solution

• Avonex (interferon beta-1a, IM injection) supplied as a liquid in a pre-filled syringe or as a powder in a single-use vial that is mixed into a solution

- Rebif (interferon beta-1a, SC injection) supplied in 22 mcg pre-filled syringes
- Betaseron (interferon beta-1b, SC injection) supplied with pre-filled syringes to which the medication is added; also available in an autoinjector
- Actimmune (interferon gamma-1b)

Canadian brand names

- Infergen (alfacon-1)
- Alferon N (alfa-n3)
- Pegasys (peginterferon alfa-2a)
- PEG-Intron (peginterferon alfa-2b)
- Avonex (beta-1a)
- Betaseron (beta-1b)

International brand names

- Infergen, Inferax (alfacon-1)
- Pegintron, ViraferonPeg (peginterferon alfa-2b)

Recommended dosage

- Interferon alfacon-1 is injected three times per week at 9 mcg per dose for 24 weeks. For patients who do not respond or have relapsed, the dosage may be increased to 15 mcg for six months.
- Dosages of interferons alfa-2a and -2b depend on various factors including the condition being treated, the patient's weight, and other medications that are being administered. They are generally injected daily for 10–24 weeks during what is called the induction period. During the following maintenance period, the drug is injected once every three weeks. Treatment usually continues for at least six months.
- The usual adult dosage of peginterferon alfa-2a is 180 mcg (less if side effects are severe) once per week for 24 or 48 weeks, injected into the abdomen or thigh.
- Peginterferon alfa-2b is injected once per week at a dosage that depends on body weight. Treatment usually continues for one year.
- Interferon alfa-n3 (0.05 mL; 250,000 units) is injected into each wart twice weekly for a maximum of eight weeks. The treatment is not repeated for at least three months.
- The usual dosage of interferon beta-1a is 30–44 mcg. Avonex is injected once per week. Rebif is injected three times per week, with at least 48 hours between injections. The initial dosage of Rebif is usually 8.8 mcg, gradually increased to 44 mcg over a four-week period.

- Interferon beta-1b is usually injected every other day at an initial dose of 62.5 mcg, gradually increased over six weeks to 250 mcg.
- Interferon gamma-1b is SC injected three times per week.

Precautions

Interferons can reduce the number of white blood cells in the body, causing increased susceptibility to infection. Patients on interferon should avoid contact with people who have infections, and should consult their physicians immediately if they believe they are developing an infection. Patients should take care not to cut themselves, should not touch their eyes or inside of their nose with unwashed hands, and should take care when brushing their teeth so as not to cause bleeding. Patients are often advised to drink extra water to avoid low blood pressure. Patients on interferon beta should have periodic liver function tests.

Pediatric

Most interferon treatments have not been studied for safety in children under age 18. However, beta interferon is approved for treating MS in children.

Geriatric

Although interferon treatment has not been studied in elderly patients, they may require lower dosages.

Pregnant or breastfeeding

Alpha interferons have not been shown to cause problems in fetuses. The fetal effects of beta interferons are unknown and they are not approved for use during pregnancy. Women of childbearing potential should use reliable birth control while on beta interferon. The FDA has required interferon manufacturers to develop pregnancy registers to monitor the outcomes in women who have become unintentionally pregnant while receiving beta interferon. Because it is not known whether interferons cross into breast milk, women should not breastfeed while undergoing interferon treatment.

Other conditions and allergies

The following conditions may be exacerbated by interferons:

- bleeding problems
- depression or other mental problems
- convulsions
- diabetes mellitus
- heart disease

• heart attack

• liver disease

• kidney disease

• lung disease

• an overactive immune system

Patients who have had or are at risk for seizures, as well as those with heart disorders such as angina, congestive heart failure, or an irregular heartbeat, should be closely monitored following interferon injection. Before receiving an interferon injection, patients should notify their doctors if they are allergic to immunoglobulins or egg whites.

Side effects

The side effects of interferon treatment vary from the uncomfortable to the severe. The most common side effects of interferons are general flu-like symptoms including:

• headache

• loss of appetite

• nausea and vomiting

• fatigue

• fever

• chills

• sweating

• muscle aches

• an unusual metallic taste in the mouth

• irritability

These symptoms tend to diminish with time. Physicians may suggest taking acetaminophen (e.g., Tylenol) or ibuprofen (e.g., Advil) before each dosage.

Interferons sometimes cause serious side effects from their actions on the central nervous system. Since most side effects are dose-dependent, severe side effects may require dosage modification. Symptoms of central nervous system side effects include:

• difficulty concentrating

• confusion

• mental depression

• nervousness

• numbness or tingling in the fingers, toes, and face Although uncommon, patients who are already clinically depressed may develop suicidal feelings during interferon treatment.

Other side effects may include:

• infection, swelling, inflammation, bruising, or necrosis (cell death) at the site of injection

---

QUESTIONS TO ASK YOUR DOCTOR

• How should I store this medication?

• How do I administer this medication?

• Will interferon interact with any of my other medications?

• What should I do if I miss a dose?

• What side effects can I expect?

• When should I contact my doctor about side effects?

• menstrual cycle changes in women

• liver and thyroid malfunction

• decreases in platelets and red and white blood cells

• a variety of other—sometimes very serious—side effects, depending on the specific interferon

Other conditions and allergies

Interferon induces an allergic reaction in some people. However, the massive and sometimes fatal allergic reaction termed anaphylaxis is rare with interferons.

Interactions

Interferons can interact with a variety of other medications, in some cases increasing their effects. Interferons should not be combined with any other medications except under a physician's supervision.

Most medications that interact with alfa interferons are those that affect the central nervous system, including:

• antihistamines

• sedatives

• tranquilizers

• sleeping medications

• prescription pain medicines

• seizure medications

• muscle relaxants

• narcotics

• barbiturates

Other drugs that may interact with interferons include:

• warfarin

• clozapine, an antipsychotic

- theophylline
- prednisone

Alfa interferons can increase the effects of alcohol. Alcohol can worsen the side effects of beta interferons. During interferon treatment, alcohol should be consumed only with the physician's consent. Alcohol should never be consumed by patients with hepatitis.

Resources

BOOKS

Pitha, Paula M. *Interferon: The 50th Anniversary.* New York: Springer, 2007.

Plotnikoff, Nicholas P. *Cytokines: Stress and Immunity,* 2nd ed. Boca Raton, FL: CRC/Taylor & Francis, 2007.

Stephensen, Frank Harold. *DNA: How the Biotech Revolution Is Changing the Way We Fight Disease.* Amherst, NY: Prometheus Books, 2007.

Thomas, Joe H., and Adrian Roberts, eds. *Interferons: Characterization, Mechanism of Action and Clinical Applications.* Hauppauge, NY: Nova Biomedical, 2012.

PERIODICALS

Coghlan, Andy. "Cheap Drug Dodges Big Pharma Patents." *New Scientist* 193, no. 2585 (January 6–12, 2007): 14.

Cooper, Chet. "MS in Children." *Ability Magazine* 2007, no. 5 (2007): 56–61.

Criscuolo, Domenico. "A Place for Proteins." *Applied Clinical Trials* (May 2009): 6–8.

WEBSITES

"Biological Therapies for Cancer." National Cancer Institute. http://www.cancer.gov/cancertopics/factsheet/Therapy/biological (accessed November 4, 2014).

"Interferons, Alfa." American Cancer Society. http://www.cancer.org/treatment/treatmentsandsideeffects/guidetocancerdrugs/interferons-alfa (accessed November 4, 2014).

ORGANIZATIONS

American Cancer Society, 250 Williams St. NW, Atlanta, GA 30303, (800) 227-2345, http://www.cancer.org.

National Cancer Institute, 9609 Medical Center Dr., BG 9609 MSC 9760, Bethesda, MD 20892-9760, (800) 4-CANCER (422-6237), http://www.cancer.gov.

National Digestive Diseases Information Clearinghouse, 2 Information Way, Bethesda, MD 20892-3570, (800) 891-5389, TTY: (866) 569-1162, Fax: (703) 738-4929, nddic@info.niddk.nih.gov, http://www.digestive.niddk.nih.gov.

National Multiple Sclerosis Society, 733 Third Avenue, New York, NY 10017, (800) 344-4867, http://www.nationalmssociety.org.

U.S. Food and Drug Administration, 10903 New Hampshire Ave., Silver Spring, MD 20993, (888) INFO-FDA (463-6332), http://www.fda.gov.

Sally C. McFarlane-Parrott
Brian Douglas Hoyle, PhD.
Margaret Alic, PhD.

Interleukin 2

Definition

Interleukin-2 (IL-2) is a protein produced naturally in the body in very small amounts. It is produced by a type of white blood cell called a T-lymphocyte and acts as part of the immune system by helping white blood cells work. **Aldesleukin** is a biological response modifier, a synthetic form of interleukin-2.

Purpose

Interleukin-2 (IL-2) is a naturally occurring chemical called a cytokine produced by certain cells of the immune system. It is also manufactured and administered as a drug to augment immune responses. While it is approved by the U.S. Food and Drug Administration (FDA) only for the treatment of **kidney cancer**, it is also used in the treatment of HIV and AIDS. Inhaled interleukin-2 may halt disease progression in patients with kidney **cancer** that has spread to the lungs. Aldesleukin, a synthetic version of interleukin-2, is used to treat cancer of the kidney and **skin cancer** that has spread to other parts of the body.

Aldesleukin is approved by the United States Food and Drug Administration (FDA) for treatment of metastatic malignant **melanoma** (skin cancer that has spread to other parts of the body), and metastatic renal cell **carcinoma** (kidney cancer that has spread to other parts of the body). It has also been used in combination with other drugs in treatment of AIDS and **cutaneous t-cell lymphoma**.

Description

The kidneys are a pair of bean-shaped organs located on the sides of the spine. The kidneys filter the blood and eliminate waste in the urine through a complex system of filtration tubules. All the blood in the body passes through the kidneys approximately twenty times an hour. Renal cell cancer (RCC) is an uncommon form of cancer that is most often characterized by the presence of cancer cells in the lining of the filtration tubules of the kidney. Advanced (metastatic) RCC refers to cancer that has spread outside the kidneys to other locations in the body. The only agent approved for metastatic RCC is high-dose Proleukin (interleukin-2). One site of cancer spread in metastatic RCC is the lungs, referred to as pulmonary **metastasis**.

Recommended dosage

IL-2 is usually administered by injection into a vein, but can also be injected under the skin (subcutaneous injection). It can be given in a hospital or clinic setting by a healthcare professional and is sometimes given at home. The dosage depends on the height and weight of the patient. It is given as an infusion for 15 minutes every eight hours for up to five days followed by nine days without the drug and then another five-day cycle of infusion. Up to four subsequent maintenance cycles of IL-2 can be given with four-week intervals without the drug to patients who have responded favorably to the treatment. About 15% of patients respond to treatment. It is difficult to estimate the cost of IL-2 treatment since the dose and number of treatment cycles given varies according to patients' individual responses; however, the cost is quite high, perhaps as much as $2,000 for one cycle. A six-cycle regimen of IL-2 may cost about $14,100. Because of the high cost and low effectiveness of interleukin-2, it is often not covered by insurance plans, especially HMOs. It is covered by Medicare if given in a hospital.

Precautions

IL-2 is highly toxic and usually makes patients feel generally unwell. Any side effects should be reported to a physician, but the course of medicine should continue even though the patient feels ill, unless the physician or healthcare professional tells the patient to stop. While using aldesleukin, IL-2 patients will be more susceptible to infection. They should avoid people with colds, flu, and bronchitis. They should not have any vaccinations without their IL-2 prescriber's approval, and they should avoid anyone who has recently had an oral polio vaccine. Patients should drink several glasses of water a day to help reduce possible kidney problems.

Aldesleukin should not be used by lactating mothers. It should also be avoided in patients with the following conditions:

- acute S-T segment elevation myocardial infarction (STEMI)
- angina pectoris
- atrial fibrillation
- bacterial infection
- bradycardia
- capillary leak syndrome
- coma
- epilepsy
- fungal infections
- impaired cognition
- intestinal perforation
- ischemic bowel disease
- neoplasm metastatic to the central nervous system
- organ transplantation
- pericardial tamponade
- protozoal infection
- pulmonary disease
- renal failure
- supraventricular tachycardia
- toxic psychosis
- ventricular tachycardia
- viral infection

The drug should be avoided or used with extreme care in patients with the following:

- arthritis
- bone marrow depression
- bullous pemphigoid
- cerebral arteritis
- cholecystitis
- Crohn's disease
- diabetes mellitus
- disease of liver
- glomerulonephritis
- myasthenia gravis
- psychotic disorder
- renal disease
- scleroderma thyroiditis
- untreated hypothyroidism

The drug should be avoided by people who have the following conditions:

- chickenpox (including recent exposure)
- herpes zoster (shingles)

- heart disease
- immune system problems
- liver disease
- lung disease
- psoriasis
- underactive thyroid
- infection
- kidney disease
- mental problems
- history of seizures

Side effects

When IL-2 is given by intravenous infusion, the most common side effect is called capillary leak syndrome. This condition causes weight gain, swelling, low blood pressure, and other problems. At lower doses, people taking IL-2 get flu-like symptoms, including **fever** and muscle aches. Because IL-2 stimulates the immune system, it can make some immune disorders get worse, including arthritis, psoriasis, and diabetes. It can also reduce the number of neutrophils, a particular type of infection-fighting cell, and can cause low levels of thyroid.

When IL-2 is given by subcutaneous injection, the side effects are usually milder than with intravenous infusions. There is the added side effect of irritation at the site of the injection. Side effects show up from two to six hours after injection of IL-2 and disappear quickly after the end of each cycle. IL-2 can cause mood changes, including irritability, insomnia, confusion, or **depression**. These can continue for several days after IL-2 is stopped.

Interleukin-2 has a number of other side effects. More common ones include fever or chills, shortness of breath, agitation, confusion, **diarrhea**, dizziness, drowsiness, mental depression, **nausea and vomiting**, sores in the mouth and on the lips, tingling of hands or feet, unusual decrease in urination, unusual tiredness, a weight gain of five to ten pounds or more, **anemia**, heart problems, kidney problems, liver problems, low blood pressure, low platelet counts in blood, low white blood cell counts, other blood problems, underactive thyroid, dry skin, loss of appetite, skin rash or redness with burning or **itching** followed by peeling, and an unusual feeling of general discomfort or illness.

Less common problems include black and tarry stools, skin blisters, blood in the urine, bloody vomit, chest pain, cough or hoarseness, lower back or side pain, painful or difficult urination, pinpoint red spots on the skin, severe stomach pain, unusual bleeding or bruising, bloating and mild stomach pain, blurred or double vision, faintness, fast or irregular heartbeat, loss of taste, rapid

breathing, redness, swelling, and soreness of the tongue, trouble in speaking, yellow eyes and skin, constipation, headache, joint pain, and muscle pain.

Rare problems include changes in menstrual periods, clumsiness, coldness, convulsions, listlessness, muscle aches, pain or redness at site of injection, sudden inability to move, swelling in the front of the neck, swelling of the feet or lower legs, and weakness.

Interactions

Interleukin-2 can adversely interact with the anti-cancer drug **dacarbazine** and hormones such as prednisone or cortisone.

Resources

BOOKS

Chu, Edward, and Vincent T. DeVita, Jr. *Physicians' Cancer Chemotherapy Drug Manual 2014.* Burlington, MA: Jones & Bartlett Learning, 2014.

WEBSITES

American Cancer Society. "Interleukin-2 (Aldesleukin)." http://www.cancer.org/treatment/treatmentsandsideeffects/guidetocancerdrugs/interleukin-2 (accessed October 29, 2014).

The Scott Hamilton CARES Initiative. "Interleukin-2." Chemocare.com. http://chemocare.com/chemotherapy/drug-info/interleukin-2.aspx (accessed November 4, 2014).

ORGANIZATIONS

U.S. Food and Drug Administration, 10903 New Hampshire Ave., Silver Spring, MD 20993, (888) INFO-FDA (463-6332), http://www.fda.gov.

Ken R. Wells

Intimacy *see* **Sexual issues for cancer patients**

Intraocular melanoma *see* **Melanoma**

Intrathecal chemotherapy

Definition

Intrathecal **chemotherapy** is a method of administration in which the chemotherapy drugs and other drugs are introduced directly into the cerebrospinal fluid.

Purpose

Intrathecal chemotherapy is used primarily to treat leukemias and lymphomas. The chemotherapy drugs are injected directly into the cerebrospinal fluid (CSF), which is the fluid that surrounds the brain and the spinal cord. Intrathecal chemotherapy is used to kill **cancer** cells that have entered the CSF, but it is not used as a therapy if tumors have begun to grow on the spinal cord or brain. Intrathecal chemotherapy frequently is used in the treatment of leukemias.

Precautions

Intrathecal chemotherapy is not appropriate for everyone. Chemotherapy drugs can cause serious side effects. Women who are pregnant or breastfeeding should discuss risks and alternatives with their doctors.

Description

Intrathecal chemotherapy introduces chemotherapy drugs directly in the cerebrospinal fluid to kill cancer cells that exist there. To introduce the chemotherapy drugs into the CSF, two methods are commonly used. The first, called **lumbar puncture** (sometimes called a spinal tap), injects the chemotherapy drugs into the spinal column. The second introduces the drugs directly into the fluid around the brain using a device called a **Ommaya reservoir**.

Regular chemotherapy procedures such as giving chemotherapy by mouth or intravenously, usually are not effective for killing cancer cells that exist in the CSF. This is because most chemotherapy drugs cannot move past the blood-brain barrier. The blood-brain barrier is made up of special, very tightly packed cells that allow some small molecules, such as oxygen, through but do not allow larger molecules to pass into the CSF. This barrier helps to protect the brain from bacteria, viruses, and other cells and molecules that may be harmful to it. Unfortunately, the blood-brain barrier also restricts the passage of most chemotherapy drugs. Therefore, to get chemotherapy drugs into the CSF, they must be injected directly.

Lumbar puncture

The lumbar puncture procedure introduces chemotherapy drugs directly into the fluid surrounding the spinal cord. To begin the procedure, the patient usually lies face down on a table, and a small area of back above the spine is treated with local anesthetic. A small device called a stopcock is then inserted into the spinal column. The stopcock allows for the injection of chemotherapy drugs and the removal of CSF without repeated punctures. A small needle is inserted through the stopcock into the spinal column. Some of the CSF may be withdrawn for diagnostic tests or for use in flushing the stopcock after the injection of the chemotherapy drugs. The chemotherapy drugs are then injected through

the stopcock, and the stopcock is flushed and removed. After removal of the stopcock, the area around the puncture site is cleaned and bandaged.

Ommaya reservoir

The Ommaya reservoir is used to introduce chemotherapy drugs directly into the fluid surrounding the brain. An Ommaya reservoir is a small plastic dome-shaped device that has a catheter (thin tube) attached to it. The placement of the Ommaya reservoir requires a surgical procedure. An area of hair is shaved, and then a small hole is made in the skull into which the reservoir is placed. The reservoir is very small and remains in place throughout the duration of chemotherapy treatment. It allows the doctor to remove fluid samples for testing or introduce chemotherapy drugs without requiring a new surgical incision in the skull each time. To perform intrathecal chemotherapy, a very small needle is inserted into the Ommaya reservoir, and the chemotherapy drugs are injected into the fluid surrounding the brain.

Preparation

Each patient is given individual instructions on how to prepare for the intrathecal chemotherapy by his or her cancer care team. Patients may be advised not to eat any solid foods for three or more hours before the procedure. Patients may also be advised to drink plenty of clear liquids. In some cases, CSF is removed during the procedure, and good hydration can help the body replace the fluid more quickly.

Some patients may be given antinausea drugs before the procedure. **Nausea and vomiting** are common side-effects of chemotherapy, and taking anti-nausea drugs before the procedure can help reduce the severity of these problems and in some cases prevent them altogether.

Some patients may be asked to stop taking specific medications a day or more before the procedure. Anti-coagulants like **warfarin** (Coumadin) and aspirin may increase the risk of bleeding during and after the procedure, so patients may be instructed to stop taking the medications several days before the procedure. The cancer care team should provide an individualized set of instructions about which medications should be stopped and when they can be started again. Patients should never stop taking medications without consulting their physician.

Aftercare

After the procedure the patient may be instructed to lie flat on his or her stomach for up to eight hours. This position helps to reduce the side effects of the lumbar puncture, and can help the chemotherapy drugs to distribute evenly throughout the CSF. Activities may need to be limited for 24 hours after the procedure.

Risks

Women who are pregnant should talk to their doctors carefully about the risks and benefits of intrathecal chemotherapy, as the chemotherapy drugs can pose a significant risk to the fetus. Women who are breastfeeding should talk to their doctors about alternatives to breastfeeding, as chemotherapy drugs may pass to the nursing infant through the breast milk.

The risks of intrathecal chemotherapy differ depending on the type and amount of chemotherapy drug being used. Risks include bleeding, soreness, and infection at the injection site, dizziness, nausea or vomiting, and **fatigue**. Headaches are a relatively common side effect of lumbar punctures. In some cases the headaches can be severe, although they usually resolve within hours after the procedure. Lying prone (flat and face-down) and drinking plenty of fluids can help reduce this risk. If the headache is very severe or does not resolve in a few hours, patients should alert their doctors.

Chemotherapy commonly causes hair loss, dryness of the mouth and throat, and sores in the mouth. It also frequently causes intestinal problems that can cause **diarrhea** and upset stomach. Decreased interest in sex, hormone changes, and kidney and bladder irritation are also common side effects. Individuals undergoing chemotherapy are also at increased risk of infection because chemotherapy drugs kill many beneficial immune system cells that are needed to combat infection as well as killing cancer cells.

Results

Results of intrathecal chemotherapy vary. Each person's body reacts to chemotherapy differently, and each type of cancer is different. Results can depend on the stage of the cancer, the type of chemotherapy drug used, any health problems the patient has in addition to cancer, and a variety of other factors. Patients should ask their physician and cancer care team about the expected results for their specific situation.

Health care team roles

Intrathecal chemotherapy is administered by a hematologist (doctor who specializes in treating diseases of the blood) or an oncologist (doctor who specializes in treating cancer). The doctor may be assisted by another doctor during the procedure. One or more nurses may assist by helping to prepare the patient, administering local anesthetic, and providing other assistance. The

QUESTIONS TO ASK YOUR DOCTOR

- Are there certain side effects for which I am especially at risk?
- Will I have to lie still after the procedure? For how long?
- How often and for how long will I need intrathecal chemotherapy?
- How long should I expect the procedure to take?
- Can I eat and drink normally before the procedure?
- Are there any medications I should stop taking before the procedure?

chemotherapy drugs are mixed by a pharmacist with specialized knowledge of chemotherapy drugs.

Caregiver concerns

Intrathecal chemotherapy affects different people in different ways. Some individuals may have few or no side effects from the treatment, but many individuals will feel tired, sore, and/or nauseated after the procedure.

If the intrathecal chemotherapy is being given on an outpatient basis, the patient will need someone to help him or her get home after treatment. If the car ride home is very long, the patient may need to lie as flat as possible in the car to help reduce side effects from the lumbar puncture and to help the chemotherapy drugs spread correctly. The patient may vomit on the way home; caregivers should be prepared for this.

During a course of chemotherapy treatment patients often feel nauseated; foods that were once enjoyed may seem unappealing. Caregivers may want to organize friends and loved ones to help provide nutritious high-calorie meals and snacks.

Helping with housework, childcare, errands, and chores can be a great way to help an individual undergoing intrathecal chemotherapy. Individuals undergoing chemotherapy are often very tired, and juggling chemotherapy with other responsibilities can be overwhelming.

Resources

BOOKS

Aryan, Henry E. *Spinal Tumors: A Treatment Guide for Patients and Family.* Sudbury, MA: Jones and Bartlett Publishers, 2010.

McKay, Judith, and Tamera Schacher. *The Chemotherapy Survival Guide: Everything You Need to Know to Get Through Treatment*. 3rd ed. Oakland, CA: New Harbinger Publications, 2009.

Perry, Michael C., ed. *The Chemotherapy Source Book*. 5th ed. Philadelphia: Wolters Kluwer Health/Lippincott Williams and Wilkins, 2012.

Polovich, M., LeFebvre, K.B., and Olsen, M., eds. *Chemotherapy and Biotherapy Guidelines and Recommendations for Practice*. 4th edition. Pittsburgh, PA: Oncology Nursing Society, 2014.

ORGANIZATIONS

American Cancer Society, 250 Williams St. NW, Atlanta, GA 30303, (800) 227-2345, http://www.cancer.org.

National Cancer Institute, 9609 Medical Center Dr., BG 9609 MSC 9760, Bethesda, MD 20892-9760, (800) 4-CANCER (422-6237), http://www.cancer.gov.

Tish Davidson, AM

Intravenous urography

Definition

Intravenous urography is a test that x-rays the urinary system using intravenous dye for diagnostic purposes.

The kidneys excrete the dye into the urine. X-rays can then create pictures of every structure (kidney, renal pelvis, ureter, bladder, urethra) through which the urine passes.

The procedure has several variations and many names:

- Intravenous pyelography (IVP).
- Urography.
- Excretory urography.
- Pyelography.
- Antegrade pyelography differentiates this procedure from retrograde pyelography, which injects dye into the lower end of the system, therefore flowing backward or retrograde.
- Nephrotomography is somewhat different in that the x-rays are taken by a moving x-ray source onto a film moving in the opposite direction. By accurately coordinating the movement, all but a single plane of tissue is blurred, and that plane is seen without overlying shadows.

Every method available gives good pictures of this system, and the question becomes one of choosing

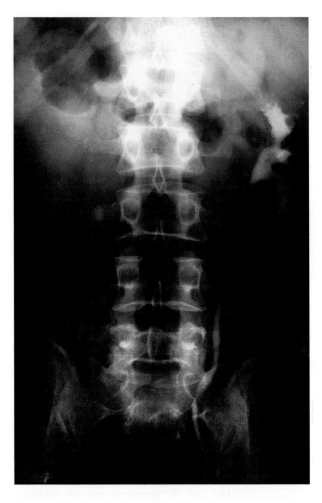

Intravenous urography showing contrast in the distal ureter. The ureter is the narrow tube shown at the lower right of the image, and the dye has traveled from the kidney (above) and is traveling to the bladder. *(CMSP/Custom Medical Stock Photo)*

among many excellent alternatives. Each condition has special requirements, while each technique has distinctive benefits and drawbacks.

- Nuclear medicine scans rely on the radiation given off by certain atoms. Chemicals containing such atoms are injected into the bloodstream. They reach the kidneys, where images are constructed by measuring the radiation emitted. The radiation is no more dangerous than standard x-rays. The images require considerable training to interpret, but unique information (e.g., blood flow, kidney function, etc.) is often available using this technology. Different chemicals can concentrate the radiation in different types of tissue. This technique may require several days for the chemical to concentrate at its destination. It also requires a special detector to create the image.

- Ultrasound is a quick, safe, simple, and inexpensive way to obtain views of internal organs. Although less detailed than other methods, it may be sufficient, especially to detect obstructions.

- Retrograde pyelography is better able to define problems in the lower parts of the system and is the only way to get x-rays if the kidneys are not working well. Dye is usually injected through an instrument (cystoscope) passed into the bladder through the urethra.

- A computed tomography scan (CT or CAT scanning) uses the same kind of radiation used in x-rays, but it collects information by computer in such a way that three-dimensional images can be constructed, eliminating interference from nearby structures. CT scanning requires a special apparatus but often gives better information on masses within the kidney.

- Magnetic resonance imaging (MRI) uses magnetic fields and radiofrequency signals instead of ionizing radiation to create computerized images. This form of energy is entirely safe as long as the patient does not have any implanted metal such as artificial joints, aneurysm clips, etc. The technique is far more versatile than CT scanning as it can not only demonstrate masses but also look at the blood vessels. However, MRI requires special apparatus and, because of the powerful magnets needed, even a special, separate building. It is quite expensive and only occasionally is its degree of detail required.

Purpose

IVP will provide information concerning most diseases of the kidneys, ureters, and bladder. The procedure is comprised of two phases. First, it requires a functioning kidney to filter the dye from the blood into the urine. The time required for the dye to appear on x-rays correlates accurately with kidney function. The second phase gives detailed anatomical images of the urinary tract. Within the first few minutes the dye "lights up" the kidneys, a phase called the nephrogram. Subsequent pictures follow the dye downward through the ureters and into the bladder. A final film taken after urinating reveals how well the bladder empties.

IVPs are most often done to assess structural abnormalities or obstruction to urine flow. If kidney function is at issue, more films are taken sooner to catch the earliest phase of the process.

- Stones, tumors, and congenital malformations account for many of the findings.
- Kidney cysts and cancers can be seen.
- Displacement of a kidney or ureter suggests a space-occupying lesion (like a cancer of the colon, rectum, or gynecological organs) pushing it out of the way.
- Defective valves where the ureters enter the bladder will often show up.
- Bladder cancers and other abnormalities are often outlined by the dye in the bladder.
- An enlarged prostate gland will show up as incomplete bladder emptying and a bump at the bottom of the bladder.

Precautions

The only serious complication of an IVP is allergy to the iodine-containing dye that is used. Such an allergy is rare, but it can be dramatic and even lethal. Emergency measures taken immediately are usually effective.

Description

IVPs are usually done in the morning. In the x-ray suite, the patient undresses and lies down. There are two methods of injecting the dye. An intravenous line can be established through which the dye is consistently fed through the body during the procedure. The other method is to give the dye all at once through a needle that is immediately withdrawn. X-rays are taken until the dye has reached the bladder, an interval of half an hour or less. The patient is asked to empty the bladder before one last x-ray. A compression device (a wide belt containing two balloons that can be inflated) may be used to keep the contrast material in the kidneys. The patient needs to urinate after the compression device is removed. Another picture is taken after the bladder is emptied to see how empty the bladder is.

In the past, of the many ways to obtain images of the urinary system, the intravenous injection of a contrast agent has been considered the best. Recent studies are showing, however, that while intravenous urography is a useful technique, there may be other imaging techniques, such as B-mode ultrasound, Doppler ultrasound, renal scintigraphy with angiotensin-converting enzyme inhibitors, intravenous and intraarterial catheter **angiography**, computed tomographic angiography, and magnetic resonance angiography, that are better or less costly.

Preparation

Emptying the bowel with **laxatives** or enemas prevents bowel shadows from obscuring the details of the urinary system. An empty stomach prevents the complication of vomiting, a rare effect of the contrast agent. Therefore, the night before the IVP the patient is asked to evacuate the bowels and to drink sparingly.

Preparation for infants and children depends on the age of the infant or child.

Aftercare

Feeling weak, nauseous, and/or lightheaded for a short time after the procedure is a possibility.

Risks

Allergy to the contrast agent is the only risk. Anyone with a possible iodine allergy, a previous reaction to x-ray dye, or an allergy to shellfish must be particularly careful to inform the x-ray personnel.

Exposure to x-ray radiation should be noted. Most experts agree that the risk of exposure to low levels of radiation is minor compared to the benefits. Pregnant women and children are more sensitive to the risks of x-rays.

Results

X-ray images of the kidney and bladder structures appear normal.

Abnormal results

An abnormal intravenous urography result may indicate kidney disease, a birth defect, tumor, kidney stone, and/or inflammation caused by infections.

Resources

BOOKS

Ballinger, Philip W., and Eugene D. Frank. *Merrill's Atlas of Radiographic Positions and Radiologic Procedures*. 10th ed. St. Louis: Mosby 2003.

PERIODICALS

Aitchson, F., and A. Page. "Diagnostic Imaging of Renal Artery Stenosis" *Journal of Human Hypertension* September 1999: 595–603.

Dalla-Palma, L. "What is Left of I.V. Urography?" *European Radiology* March 2001: 931–939.

Hession, P., et al. "Intravenous Urography in Urinary Tract Surveillance in Carcinoma of the Bladder." *Clinical Radiology* July 1999: 465–467.

Little, M. A., et al. "The Diagnostic Yield of Intravenous Urography." *Nephrology Dialysis Transplantation* February 2000: 200–204.

WEBSITES

RadiologyInfo.org. "Intravenous Pyelogram (IVP)." http://www.radiologyinfo.org/en/info.cfm?pg=ivp (accessed December 3, 2014).

ORGANIZATIONS

American Cancer Society, 250 Williams St. NW, Atlanta, GA 30303, (800) 227-2345, http://www.cancer.org.

Kidney Cancer Association, PO Box 803338, Chicago, IL 60680-3338, (847) 332-1051, (800) 850-9132, office@kidneycancer.org, http://www.kidneycancer.org.

National Cancer Institute, 9609 Medical Center Dr., BG 9609 MSC 9760, Bethesda, MD 20892-9760, (800) 4-CANCER (422-6237), http://www.cancer.gov.

National Kidney Foundation, 30 E. 33rd St., New York, NY 10016, (800) 622-9010, info@kidney.org, http://www.kidney.org.

J. Ricker Polsdorfer, MD
Laura Ruth, PhD.

Investigational drugs

Definition

Investigational drugs refers to drugs that have received FDA approval for human testing, including those drugs still undergoing **clinical trials**, but are not approved for marketing to the general public.

Description

Investigational drugs represent interesting and novel new agents in the fight against **cancer**. These agents include **chemotherapy** designed to treat specific cancers, to provide palliative therapy for pain and symptoms, and to reduce invasive cancers in high-risk patients. The challenge faced by private and commercial investigators is to reduce the lag time in bringing an investigational drug to market without compromising drug quality or patient safety. The guidelines that insure the correct procedures are being followed in the process of drug development and approval fall under the direction of the U.S. Food and Drug Administration (FDA).

At present, the cycle of investigational drug research and development, to clinical trials, to FDA approval can easily cover a period of 10–12 years. Under exceptional circumstances, provisions can be made for patient use of investigational drugs under the guidance of specially trained and registered oncologists. These specific investigational drugs are classified as Group C drugs, and have demonstrated a high level of reproducible activity in preclinical testing. There is also the route of accelerated FDA approval for some investigational drugs. Accelerated approval relies on specific indicators that suggest that a particular investigational drug is likely to have beneficial effects before the benefits have been clinically verified. All investigational drugs that have been granted accelerated approval must undergo follow-up testing in order to receive final FDA approval. Some researchers are presently working on a format to combine traditional clinical testing of investigational drugs with a global database of drug information. This integrated system would give FDA monitoring agencies and healthcare providers access to the most comprehensive source of archived data available on investigational drugs. This combined approach is another attempt to reduce approval time for investigational drugs and make these agents available to the cancer patient for treatment.

Resources

PERIODICALS

DiMasi, J. A., et al. "Clinical Approval Success Rates for Investigational Cancer Drugs." *Clinical Pharmacology and Therapeutics* 94, no. 3 (2013): 329–35.

WEBSITES

American Cancer Society. "Compassionate Drug Use." http://www.cancer.org/treatment/treatmentsandsideeffects/clinicaltrials/compassionate-drug-use (accessed November 4, 2014).

National Cancer Institute. "Access to Investigational Drugs." http://www.cancer.gov/cancertopics/factsheet/Therapy/investigational-drug-access (accessed November 4, 2014).

ORGANIZATIONS

U.S. Food and Drug Administration, 10903 New Hampshire Ave., Silver Spring, MD 20993, (888) INFO-FDA (463-6332), http://www.fda.gov.

Jane Taylor-Jones, Research Associate, M.S.

Iressa *see* **Gefitinib**

Irinotecan

Definition

Irinotecan is a drug used to treat certain types of **cancer**. Irinotecan, also known as CPT-11, is available under the trade name Camptosar, and may also be referred to as irinotecan hydrochloride or camptothecin-11.

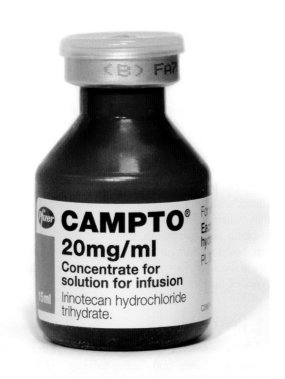

Vial of irinotecan, used to treat colon cancer. *(Dr. P. Marazzi/Science Source)*

KEY TERMS

Alkaloid—A class of nitrogen-containing compounds occurring in plants.

Anorexia—Loss of appetite.

Apoptosis—An active process in which a cell dies due to a chemical signal. Programmed cell death.

Diuretic—An agent that increases the amount of urine the body produces.

Inflammation—A response to injury, irritation, or illness characterized by redness, pain, swelling, and heat.

Metastatis—Spread of a disease from the organ or tissue of origin to other parts of the body.

Purpose

Irinotecan is an antineoplastic agent used to treat cancer. A primary use of the drug is treatment of colon or rectal cancers that have recurred or progressed while the patient was on 5-FU (**fluorouracil**) therapy. Irinotecan also can be given as first-line therapy with 5-FU and **leucovorin** for patients with metastatic colon or **rectal cancer**. Other uses for irinotecan include treatment of **small cell lung cancer**, non-small cell lung cancer, **ovarian cancer**, **stomach cancer**, **breast cancer**, **pancreatic cancer**, leukemia, **lymphoma**, and **cervical cancer**.

Several studies showed some potential uses for irinotecan. One reported that a combination of irinotecan and **docetaxel** can help patients with **esophageal cancer** who have been extensively pretreated with **cisplatin**. Weekly use of irinotecan has shown preliminary results in treating patients with nonsmall cell lung cancer with minimal side effects. Another study reported that when used in combination with cancer drugs cisplatin and **epirubicin**, irinotecan might have promising broad antitumor activity. In the future, irinotecan might be used in combination therapies to treat many types of tumors.

Description

Irinotecan is a synthetic derivative of the naturally occurring compound camptothecin. Camptothecin belongs to a group of chemicals called alkaloids and is extracted from plants such as *Camptotheca acuminata*. Camptothecin was initially investigated as a chemotherapeutic agent due to its anticancer activity in laboratory studies. The chemical structure and biological action of irinotecan is similar to that of camptothecin and **topotecan**.

Irinotecan inhibits the normal functioning of the enzyme topoisomerase I. The normal role of topoisomerase I is to aid in the replication, recombination, and repair of deoxyribonucleic acid (DNA). Higher levels of topoisomerase I have been found in certain cancer tumors compared to healthy tissue. Inhibiting topoisomerase I causes DNA damage. This damage leads to apoptosis, or programmed cell death.

Recommended dosage

Patients should be carefully monitored during irinotecan treatment for toxicity. Irinotecan is given at a dose of 125 mg per square meter of body surface area per week for four weeks, followed by a two week rest period. Other dosing schedules include 100 mg per square meter of body surface area per day for three days every three weeks, 100–115 mg per square meter of body surface area per week, or 200–350 mg per square meter of body surface area every three weeks. The drug is administered through the vein over a 90-minute period. The initial dose of irinotecan may be adjusted downward depending on patient tolerance of the toxic side effects of irinotecan.

Treatment may be continued as long as intolerable side effects do not develop and patients continue to benefit from the treatment.

Precautions

Irinotecan should be used only under the supervision of a physician experienced in the use of cancer chemotherapeutic agents. Special caution, especially in those 65 years and older, should be taken to monitor the toxic effects of irinotecan, particularly **diarrhea**, nausea, and vomiting. Because irinotecan is administered intravenously, the site of infusion should be monitored for signs of inflammation. Should inflammation occur, flushing the site with sterile water and applying ice are recommended. Irinotecan may cause **nausea and vomiting**, and premedication with antiemetic agents is recommended.

Neither the effects of irinotecan in patients with significant liver dysfunction nor the safety of irinotecan in children have been established. Irinotecan should not be administered to pregnant women. Women of childbearing age are advised not to become pregnant during treatment with this drug.

Side effects

Early- or late-onset diarrhea are common side effects of irinotecan. Late-onset diarrhea, occurring more than 24 hours after irinotecan administration, can be life-threatening and should be treated promptly. Patients should immediately report diarrhea to their physician. Patients can also take the antidiarrheal drug loperamide as prescribed by their physician at the first sign of diarrhea. Suppression of bone marrow function is another serious side effect commonly observed in this treatment. Additional side effects, including nausea, vomiting, **anorexia** (loss of appetite), pain, **fatigue**, and hair loss (**alopecia**) may occur.

Interactions

Irradiation treatment during the course of irinotecan treatment is not recommended. Patients who have received prior pelvic or abdominal irradiation treatment should notify their physician. Since irinotecan may cause diarrhea, the use of **laxatives** should be avoided. The use of diuretics should be closely monitored. The adverse side effects caused by irinotecan may be increased by other **antineoplastic agents** having similar adverse effects and should generally be avoided.

Resources

PERIODICALS

"Cisplatin, Irinotecan, and Epirubicin Have Promising Broad Antitumor Activity." *Cancer Weekly* October 14, 2003:12.

"Irinotecan and Docetaxel Shows Some Activity in Extensively Pretreated Patients." *Clinical Trials Week* October 13, 2003: 25.

"Weekly Irinotecan Showed Antitumoral Activity and Minimum Toxicity in NSCCLC." *Clinical Trials Week* October 13, 2003: 25.

WEBSITES

American Cancer Society. "Guide to Cancer Drugs: Irinotecan." http://www.cancer.org/treatment/treatmentsandside effects/guidetocancerdrugs/irinotecan (accessed December 3, 2014).

Marc Scanio
Teresa G. Odle

Islet cell carcinoma *see* **Pancreatic cancer, endocrine**

Itching

Description

Itching, also called pruritus, is an unpleasant sensation of the skin that causes a person to scratch or rub the area to find relief. Itching can be confined to one spot (localized) or over the whole body (generalized).

Severe scratching can injure the skin causing redness, bumps, and scratches. Injured skin is prone to infection.

Itching can profoundly affect quality of life. It can torment the patient and cause discomfort, stress, loss of sleep, concentration difficulty, and constant concern.

Causes

The biology underlying itching is not fully understood. It is believed that itching results from the interactions of several different chemical messengers. Although itching and pain sensations were at one time thought to be sent along the same nerve pathways, researchers reported the discovery in 2003 of itch-specific nerve pathways. Nerve endings that are specifically sensitive to itching have been named pruriceptors.

Research into itching has been helped by the recent invention of a mechanical device called the Matcher, which electrically stimulates the patient's left hand. When the intensity of the stimulation equals the intensity of itching that the patient is experiencing elsewhere in the body, the patient stops the stimulation and the device automatically records the measurement. The Matcher was found to be sensitive to immediate changes in the patient's perception of itching as well as reliable in its measurements.

Itching is associated with a variety of factors including skin diseases, blood diseases, emotions, and drug reactions as well as **cancer** and cancer treatments. Itching can be a symptom of cancer, including **Hodgkin lymphoma**, **non-Hodgkin lymphoma**, leukemia, **Bowen disease**, **multiple myeloma**, central nervous system (brain and spinal cord) tumors, **germ cell tumors**, and invasive squamous cell **carcinoma**. The buildup of toxins in the blood, caused by kidney, gallbladder, and liver disease, can cause itching. Cancer treatments that are associated with itching are: **radiation therapy**, **chemotherapy**, and **biological response modifiers** (drugs that improve the patient's immune system). Skin reactions are more severe when both chemotherapy and radiation therapy are used. Patients treated with **bone marrow transplantation** may develop itching resulting from graft-versus-host disease. Itching can be caused by infection.

General medications that may be used by cancer patients can cause itching. Itching can be caused by drug reactions from **antibiotics**, **corticosteroids**, hormones, and pain relievers (analgesics).

Itching can be a sign that the patient is very sensitive to a particular chemotherapy drug. Chemotherapy drugs and biological response modifiers that can cause itching include:

- allopurinol
- aminoglutethimide

- bleomycin
- carmustine
- chlorambucil
- cyclophosphamide
- cytarabine
- daunorubicin
- doxorubicin
- hydroxyurea
- idarubicin
- interleukin (aldesleukin)
- mechlorethamine
- megestrol acetate
- mitomycin-C
- tamoxifen
- topiramate

Itching commonly occurs during radiation therapy. Parts of the body that are particularly sensitive to radiation are the underarms, groin, abdomen, breasts, buttocks, and skin around the genitals (perineum) and anus (perianal). Itching is usually caused by skin dryness when the oil (sebaceous) glands are damaged by the radiation. Radiation also causes skin darkening, redness, and skin shedding, which can all cause itching.

Itching caused by cancer usually disappears once the cancer is in remission or cured. Chemotherapy-induced itching usually disappears within 30 to 90 minutes after the drug has been administered. Itching caused by radiation therapy will resolve once the injured skin has healed.

Treatment

There are three aspects to the treatment of itching: managing the underlying cancer, maintaining skin health, and relief of itching.

Patients should avoid the particular substances or situations that cause or worsen their itching. Also, patients can take measures to maintain skin health. Suggestions include:

- taking short baths in warm water
- using mild soaps and rinsing well
- applying bath oil or moisturizing cream after bathing
- avoiding use of cosmetics, perfumes, deodorants, and starch-based powders
- avoiding wool and other harsh fabrics
- using mild laundry detergents and rinsing thoroughly
- avoiding use of dryer anti-static sheets
- wearing loose-fitting cotton clothing

- avoiding high-friction garments such as belts, pantyhose, and bras
- maintaining a cool environment with a 30% to 40% humidity level
- using cotton rather than polyester sheets
- avoiding vigorous exercise (if sweating causes itching)
- avoiding skin products that are scented or contain alcohol or menthol

To reduce skin injury caused by scratching, the patient should keep fingernails short, wear soft cotton mittens and socks at night, and keep the hands clean. Gently rubbing the skin around the itch or applying pressure or vibration to the itchy spot may reduce itching. Using a soft infant toothbrush to gently stroke the itchy area may relieve itching. Itching may also be relieved by applying a cool washcloth or ice to the itchy area.

The most effective way to relieve itching is to treat the underlying disease. Sometimes itching disappears as soon as a tumor is treated or removed.

Itching may be relieved by applying any of a variety of different products to the skin. The patient may need to try several before the most effective one is found. The patient's physician should be consulted before any anti-itch products are used. Topical treatments include:

- Corticosteroids, such as hydrocortisone, reduce inflammation and itching.
- Calamine lotions can cool and soothe itchy skin. These products can be drying, which may be helpful for weeping or oozing rashes.
- Antihistamine creams stop itching that is associated with the chemical messenger histamine.
- Moisturizers treat dry skin, which helps to relieve itching. Moisturizers that are recommended to cancer patients include brand names Alpha Keri, Aquaphor, Eucerin, Lubriderm, Nivea, Prax, and Sarna. Moisturizers should be applied after bathing and at least two or three times daily.
- Gels that contain a numbing agent (e.g., lidocaine) can be used on some parts of the body.

Itching may be treated with whole-body medications. Some of these systemic treatments include:

- antihistamines
- tricyclic antidepressants
- sedatives or tranquilizers
- such selective serotonin reuptake inhibitors as paroxetine (Paxil) and sertraline (Zoloft)
- binding agents (such as cholestyramine, which relieves itching associated with kidney or liver disease).

- aspirin

- cimetidine

Alternative and complementary therapies

A well-balanced diet that includes carbohydrates, fats, minerals, proteins, **vitamins**, and liquids will help to maintain skin health. Capsules that contain eicosapentaenoic acid, which is obtained from herring, mackerel, or salmon, may help to reduce itching. Vitamin A plays an important role in skin health. Vitamin E (capsules or ointment) may reduce itching. Patients should check with their treating physician before using supplements.

Homeopathy has been reported to be effective in treating systemic itching associated with hemodialysis.

Baths containing oil with milk or oatmeal are effective at relieving localized itching. Evening primrose oil may soothe itching and may be as effective as corticosteroids. Calendula cream may relieve short-term itching. Other herbal treatments that have been recently reported to relieve itching include sangre de drago, a preparation made with sap from a South American tree; and a mixture of honey, olive oil, and beeswax.

Distraction, music therapy, relaxation techniques, and visualization may be useful in relieving itching. Ultraviolet light therapy may relieve itching associated with conditions of the skin, kidneys, blood, and gallbladder. There are some reports of the use of acupuncture and transcutaneous electrical nerve stimulators (TENS) to relieve itching.

Resources

BOOKS

Beers, Mark H., MD, and Robert Berkow, MD, editors. "Pruritus." In *The Merck Manual of Diagnosis and Therapy*. Whitehouse Station, NJ: Merck Research Laboratories, 2007.

PERIODICALS

Al-Waili, N. S. "Topical Application of Natural Honey, Beeswax and Olive Oil Mixture for Atopic Dermatitis or Psoriasis: Partially Controlled, Single-Blinded Study." *Complementary Therapies in Medicine* 11 (December 2003): 226–234.

Browning, J., B. Combes, and M. J. Mayo. "Long-Term Efficacy of Sertraline as a Treatment for Cholestatic Pruritus in Patients with Primary Biliary Cirrhosis." *American Journal of Gastroenterology* 98 (December 2003): 2736–2741.

Cavalcanti, A. M., L. M. Rocha, R. Carillo, Jr., et al. "Effects of Homeopathic Treatment on Pruritus of Haemodialysis Patients: A Randomised Placebo- Controlled Double-Blind Trial." *Homeopathy* 92 (October 2003): 177–181.

Ikoma, A., R. Rukwied, S. Stander, et al. "Neurophysiology of Pruritus: Interaction of Itch and Pain." *Archives of Dermatology* 139 (November 2003): 1475–1478.

Jones. K. "Review of Sangre de Drago (*Croton lechleri*)—A South American Tree Sap in the Treatment of Diarrhea, Inflammation, Insect Bites, Viral Infections, and Wounds: Traditional Uses to Clinical Research." *Journal of Alternative and Complementary Medicine* 9 (December 2003): 877–896.

Ochoa, J. G. "Pruritus, a Rare but Troublesome Adverse Reaction of Topiramate." *Seizure* 12 (October 2003): 516–518.

Stener-Victorin, E., T. Lundeberg, J. Kowalski, et al. "Perceptual Matching for Assessment of itch; Reliability and Responsiveness Analyzed by a Rank-Invariant Statistical Method." *Journal of Investigative Dermatology* 121 (December 2003): 1301–1305.

Zylicz, Z., M. Krajnik, A. A. Sorge, and M. Costantini. "Paroxetine in the Treatment of Severe Non- Dermatological Pruritus: A Randomized, Controlled Trial." *Journal of Pain and Symptom Management* 26 (December 2003): 1105–1112.

WEBSITES

Butler, David F. "Pruritus and Systemic Disease." Medscape Reference. http://emedicine.medscape.com/article/ 1098029-overview (accessed December 3, 2014).

Belinda Rowland, PhD.

Rebecca J. Frey, PhD.

Itraconazole *see* **Antifungal therapy**

IVP *see* **Intravenous urography**

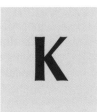

K

Kadcyla *see* **Ado-trastuzumab emtansine**

Kaposi sarcoma

Definition

Kaposi **sarcoma** (KS) is a **cancer** of the skin, mucous membranes, and blood vessels; it is the most common form of cancer in AIDS patients. It was named for Dr. Moritz Kaposi (1837–1902), a Hungarian dermatologist who first described it in 1872. All patients who have KS also have human herpesvirus 8.

Description

Kaposi sarcoma develops in many different sites on the patient's skin or internal organs and is characterized by bleeding. The lesions (areas of diseased or damaged skin) are usually round or elliptical in shape and a quarter of an inch to an inch in size, The purple or brownish color of the lesions results from blood leaking out of

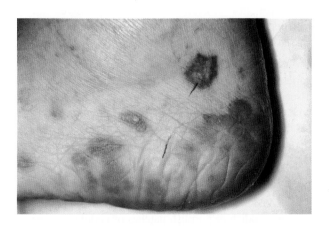

Purple-colored (violaceous) plaques of Kaposi sarcoma on the heel and side of the foot. *(Centers for Disease Control and Prevention)*

capillaries (small blood vessels) in the skin. In KS, the capillaries begin to grow too rapidly and irregularly, which causes them to become leaky and eventually break. The lesions themselves may become enlarged and bleed, or cause the mucous membranes of the patient's internal organs to bleed.

There are three types of KS lesions, defined by their appearance:

- Nodular. These are reddish-purple in color but are sometimes surrounded by a border of yellowish or brown pigment. Nodular lesions may appear to be dark brown rather than purple in patients with dark skin.
- Infiltrating. Infiltrating lesions may be large or have a raised surface. They typically grow downward under the skin.
- Lymphatic. These lesions are found in the lymph nodes and may be confused with other causes of swollen lymph nodes.

KS is classified into five types:

- Classic KS. This form of KS is sometimes called indolent KS because it is slow to develop. Classical KS is most commonly found in men between 50 and 70 years of age and of Italian or Eastern European Jewish descent.
- African (endemic) KS. This form of the disease appears in both an indolent and an aggressive form in native populations in equatorial Africa. It accounts for almost 10% of all cancers in central Africa, affecting both adults and children. In children, the condition is particularly aggressive.
- Immunosuppressive or transplant-related KS. The third form of KS occurs in organ transplant patients who have received drugs to suppress their immune systems, usually prednisone and azathioprine. This form of KS is sometimes called iatrogenic KS, which means that it is caused unintentionally by medical treatment.
- Epidemic KS. Epidemic KS was first reported in 1981 as part of the AIDS epidemic. Most cases of KS in the

KEY TERMS

Angiogenesis—The formation of blood vessels.

Cryotherapy—A form of treatment that involves freezing KS lesions with liquid nitrogen.

Disseminated—Widely distributed or spread. Epidemic KS almost always develops into a disseminated form, in which the disease spreads throughout the patient's body.

Highly active antiretroviral therapy (HAART)—A form of drug-combination treatment for HIV infection introduced in 1998. Most HAART regimens are combinations of three or four drugs, usually nucleoside analogs and protease inhibitors.

Iatrogenic—Caused unintentionally by medical treatment. Immunosuppressive treatment-related KS is sometimes called iatrogenic KS.

Immunosuppressive—Any form of treatment that inhibits the body's normal immune response.

Indolent—Relatively inactive or slow-spreading. Classic KS is usually an indolent disease.

Liposomes—Artificial sacs composed of fatty substances that are used to coat or encapsulate an inner core containing another drug. Some drugs used to treat epidemic KS are given in the form of liposomes.

Opportunistic infections (OI)—Diseases caused by organisms that multiply to the point of producing symptoms only when the body's immune system is impaired.

Systemic—Affecting the entire body in general instead of being confined to a local area or organ.

United States are of this type and are diagnosed in people who are infected with HIV.

• KS in HIV-negative men who have sex with men. This form of KS occurs in homosexual men who do not develop HIV infection. It is an indolent form of the disease that primarily affects the patient's skin.

Demographics

Kaposi sarcoma was rare in the United States before the HIV/AIDS epidemic, affecting only about two people per million in the United States. By the early 1990s, there were nearly 50 cases per one million Americans. Early on, AIDS patients had a one in two chance of developing KS. Improved therapy for HIV, however, has helped decrease rates of KS in AIDS patients. Currently, the condition occurs in about six out of every million people in the United States. In the United States, it is still very closely associated with HIV-AIDS. In Africa, KS occurs at a rate of nearly 38 per 100,000 men and 20 per 100,000 women. About 1 in 200 transplant recipients in the United States develops KS.

Causes and symptoms

Causes

HUMAN HERPES VIRUS 8. The human herpesvirus 8 (HHV-8), which is sometimes called KS-associated herpesvirus (KSHV), is now known as the cause of KS. Fragments of the HHV-8 genome were first detected in 1994 using a technique based on polymerase chain reaction (PCR) analysis. HHV-8 belongs to a group of herpesviruses called rhadinoviruses, and is the first herpesvirus of this subtype to be found in humans. HHV-8 is, however, closely related to the human herpesvirus called **Epstein-Barr virus** (EBV). EBV is known to cause infectious mononucleosis as well as tumors of the lymphatic system and may be involved in other malignancies, including the African form of Burkitt **lymphoma**, **Hodgkin lymphoma**, and **nasopharyngeal cancer**.

HHV-8 has been found in tissue samples from patients with all types of KS. Most people who have HHV-8 do not develop Kaposi sarcoma, but those who have other risk factors for the disease are at risk of KS because of the HHV-8 virus. A weakened immune system, one effect of HIV/AIDS, is a major risk factor for KS.

IMMUNOSUPPRESSION. In addition to organ transplant patients receiving immunosuppressive drugs, patients who are taking high-dose **corticosteroids** are also at increased risk of developing KS.

GENETIC FACTORS. The role of genetic factors in KS varies across its five types. Classic KS is the only form associated with specific ethnic groups. In addition, patients with classic KS and immunosuppressive treatment-related KS have a higher incidence of a genetically determined immune factor called HLA-DR.

Symptoms

CLASSIC KS. The symptoms of classic KS include one or more reddish or purplish patches or nodules on one or both legs, often on the ankles or soles of the feet. The lesions slowly enlarge over a period of 10–15 years, with additional lesions sometimes developing. It is rare for classic KS to involve the patient's internal organs, although bleeding from the digestive tract sometimes occurs. About 34% of patients with classic KS eventually develop **non-Hodgkin lymphoma** or another primary cancer.

AFRICAN KS. The symptoms of the indolent form of African KS resemble those of classic KS. The aggressive form, however, produces tumors that may penetrate the tissue underneath the patient's skin, and even the underlying bone.

EPIDEMIC KS. Epidemic KS has more varied presentations than the four other types of KS. Its onset is usually, though not always, marked by the appearance of widespread lesions at many different points on the patient's skin and in the mouth. Most HIV-infected patients who develop KS skin and mouth lesions feel healthy and have no systemic symptoms. On the other hand, KS may affect the patient's lymph nodes or gastrointestinal tract prior to causing skin lesions.

Patients with epidemic KS almost always develop disseminated (widespread) disease. The illness progresses from a few localized lesions to lymph node involvement and further spread to other organs. Disseminated KS is defined by the appearance of one or more of the following: a count of 25 or more external lesions; the appearance of 10 or more new lesions per month; and the appearance of visible lesions in the patient's lungs or stomach lining.

In some cases, disseminated KS causes painful swelling (edema) of the patient's feet and lower legs. The lesions may also cause the surrounding skin to ulcerate or develop secondary infections. The spread of KS to the lungs, called pleuropulmonary KS, usually occurs at a late stage of the disease. KS involvement of the lungs causes bleeding, coughing, shortness of breath, and eventual respiratory failure. Most patients who die directly of KS die from its pleuropulmonary form.

Diagnosis

Physical examination and patient history

The diagnosis of any form of KS requires a careful examination of all areas of the patient's skin. Even though the characteristic lesions of classic KS appear most frequently on the legs, all forms of KS can produce lesions on any area of the skin. An experienced doctor, who may be a dermatologist, an internist, or a primary care physician, can make a tentative diagnosis of KS on the basis of the external appearance of the skin lesions (size, shape, color, and location on the face or body), particularly when they are accompanied by evidence of lymph node involvement, internal bleeding, and other

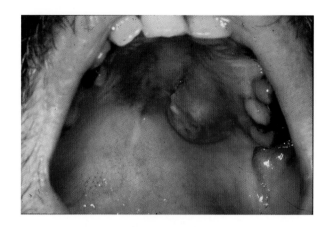

Kaposi sarcoma inside the mouth. The tumor is toward the back of the mouth, to the right. *(Wellcome Image Library/ Custom Medical Stock Photography)*

symptoms associated with disseminated KS. The doctor may touch or press on the lesions to see whether they turn pale (blanch); KS plaques and nodules do not blanch under fingertip pressure. In addition, KS lesions are not painful when they first appear.

Other signs of KS may appear on the soft palate or the membranes covering the eye (conjunctivae). In addition, the doctor will press on the patient's abdomen to detect any masses in the liver or spleen.

A thorough history is necessary to determine whether the patient's ethnic background, lifestyle, or medical history places him or her in a high-risk category for KS, including exposure to the HHV-8 virus.

Biopsy

A definitive diagnosis of KS requires a **skin biopsy** in order to rule out bacillary angiomatosis, a bacterial infection caused by the bacillus, *Bartonella henselae*. Collecting a tissue sample for a **biopsy** is not difficult if the patient has skin lesions, but can be complicated if the nodules are primarily internal. An endoscopy of the upper end of the digestive tract may be performed in order to obtain a tissue sample from an internal KS lesion.

Under the microscope, an AIDS-related KS lesion will show an unusually large number of spindle-shaped cells mixed together with small capillaries. The origin of the spindle-shaped cells is still unknown. The tumor cells in a KS lesion resemble smooth muscle cells or fibroblasts, which are cells that help to form the fibers in normal connective tissue.

If the patient's lymph nodes are enlarged, a biopsy may be performed to rule out other causes of swollen lymph nodes.

Other tests

Other diagnostic tests may be performed if the patient appears to have disseminated KS. These tests include:

- Chest x-ray. A radiograph of the patient's lungs will show patchy areas of involved tissue.

- Gallium scan. The results will be negative in KS.

- Bronchoscopy. This procedure allows the doctor to examine the patient's bronchial pathways for visible KS lesions. It is not, however, useful for obtaining tissue samples for biopsy.

- Endoscopy. Examination of the patient's stomach allows the doctor to examine the mucous lining for KS lesions as well as to obtain a tissue sample.

Treatment team

KS patients may receive treatment for skin lesions from a dermatologist or radiation therapist as well as treatment for lung or lymphatic involvement from internists or primary care practitioners. A surgeon may be called upon to remove lesions in the digestive tract if they are bleeding or blocking the passage of food. Patients also may receive treatment from oncologists, doctors who specialize in cancer treatment, and from infectious disease specialists. Children with KS may be treated by pediatricians or by primary care physicians who specialize in treating AIDS patients.

Clinical staging

Several staging systems have been proposed for KS, which does not fit into the typical **tumor staging** system used for most cancers. Most doctors treating patients with AIDS-related KS use the AIDS Clinical Trials Group staging system.

AIDS Clinical Trials Group (ACTG) staging system

The ACTG Oncology Committee published a staging system for epidemic KS in 1989. This system is reevaluated regularly and changed as needed. It is based on three criteria: extent of tumor; condition of the patient's immune system; and presence of systemic illness:

- Tumor (T): Good risk (0) is a tumor limited to the skin and/or lymph nodes and/or minimal oral disease (limited to the palate). Poor risk (1) is any of the following: edema associated with the tumor; widespread KS in the mouth; KS in the digestive tract; KS in the lungs.

- Immune system (I): Good risk (0) is a CD4 cell count greater than 150 per cubic millimeter. Poor risk (1) is a CD4 cell count lower than 150 per cubic millimeter.

- Systemic illness (S): Good risk (0) is no history of opportunistic infections (OI) or thrush; no "B" symptoms (unexplained fever, night sweats, diarrhea, weight loss greater than 10%); performance status above 70 on the Karnofsky scale. Poor risk (1) is any of the following: history of OI or thrush; presence of "B" symptoms; Karnofsky score lower than 70; and other HIV-related illnesses.

Treatment

The most important treatment for KS is controlling immune system deficiency and related infections such as HHV-8 or HIV. By using treatments such as highly active antiretroviral therapy (HAART) to control HIV infection, fewer patients develop KS and doctors can better control widespread KS. Treatment of local KS lesions depends on the type of the disease.

Classic KS

Radiation therapy is usually quite effective if the patient has small lesions or lesions limited to a small area of skin. Low-voltage photon radiation or electron beam therapy gives good results. Surgical removal of small lesions is sometimes performed, but the lesions are likely to recur. The best results are obtained from surgical treatment when many small lesions are removed over a period of years.

For widespread skin disease, radiation treatment with electron beam therapy is recommended. Classic KS has not often been treated with **chemotherapy** in the United States, but some researchers report that treatment with **vinblastine** or **vincristine** has been effective. Disease that has spread to the lymph nodes or digestive tract is treated with a combination of chemotherapy and radiation.

Immunosuppressive treatment-related KS

The standard pattern of therapy for this form of KS begins with discontinuing the immunosuppressive medications if they are not essential to the patient's care. Treatment of the KS itself may include radiation therapy if the disease is limited to the skin, or single- or multiple-drug chemotherapy.

Epidemic KS

There is no cure for epidemic KS, but the use of HAART has changed the clinical course of the disease and should be the first step in treatment of epidemic KS. Local treatment is aimed at reducing the size of skin lesions and alleviating the discomfort of open ulcers or swollen tissue in the legs. There are no data that indicate that treatment prolongs the survival of patients with epidemic KS.

Small KS lesions respond very well to radiation treatment. They can also be removed surgically or treated with **cryotherapy**, a technique that uses liquid nitrogen to freeze the lesion. Lesions inside the mouth (on the palate) can be treated with injections of vinblastine. In addition, the patient may be given topical alitretinoin (Panretin gel), which is applied directly to the lesions. Alitretinoin received FDA approval for treating KS in 1999.

Systemic treatments for epidemic KS consist of various combinations of anticancer drugs and interferon alpha. The effectiveness of systemic treatments ranges from 50% for high-dose therapy with interferon alpha to 80% for certain chemotherapy combinations. The drawbacks of systemic treatment include the toxicity of these drugs and their many side effects. Interferon alpha can be given only to adult patients with relatively intact immune systems and no signs of lymphatic involvement. Many patients with weakened immune systems cannot tolerate chemotherapy. The side effects of systemic chemotherapy include hair loss (**alopecia**), **nausea and vomiting**, **fatigue**, **diarrhea**, headaches, loss of appetite (**anorexia**), allergic reactions, back pain, abdominal pain, and increased sweating.

As of fall 2014, experimental treatments for KS include a topical drug called imiquimod (Aldara), which might regulate the immune system and shrink KS skin lesions. Researchers are testing the use of **angiogenesis inhibitors**, which can be sent to the area of KS lesions and block their blood supply so that they will stop growing and eventually die. Other cancer treatments are being studied in clinical trials for use in managing KS.

Alternative and complementary therapies

SHARK CARTILAGE. Some people claim that shark cartilage can help patients with KS. Shark cartilage products are widely available in the United States as over-the-counter (OTC) preparations that do not require FDA approval. Although shark cartilage is probably safe, there are no scientific studies proving its effectiveness in managing symptoms or growth of KS lesions.

The side effects of treatment with shark cartilage include mild-to-moderate nausea, vomiting, abdominal cramps, constipation, low blood pressure, abnormally high levels of blood calcium (**hypercalcemia**), and generalized weakness.

OTHER ALTERNATIVE THERAPIES. Other alternative treatments for KS are aimed almost completely at

---

QUESTIONS TO ASK YOUR DOCTOR

- What can I do to prevent more lesions from appearing?
- What is the best treatment for my type of KS that has the least severe side effects?
- Is there anything I can do to minimize the appearance of the lesions before and after treatment?
- Are there support services available?

---

epidemic KS. Most are based on assumptions that AIDS patients have had their immune systems weakened by such environmental toxins as lead and radioactive materials or by psychological stress generated by societal disapproval of homosexuality. Naturopaths would add such lifestyle stresses as the use of tobacco and alcohol as well as poor sleep patterns and nutritional deficiencies. Homeopaths believe that AIDS is the product of hereditary predispositions to disease called miasms, specifically two miasms related to syphilis and gonorrhea respectively.

Alternative topical treatments for the skin lesions of AIDS-related KS include homeopathic preparations made from periwinkle, **mistletoe**, or phytolacca (poke root). Other alternative skin preparations include a selenium solution made from aloe gels, selenium, and tincture of silica; a mixture of aloe vera and dried kelp (seaweed); and a mixture of aloe vera, tea tree oil, and tincture of St. John's wort. Alternative treatments for KS lesions on the internal organs include a mixture of warm wine and Yunnan Paiyao powder, a Chinese patent medicine made from ginseng; castor oil packs; or a three- to seven-day grape fast repeated every 120 days.

Alternative systemic treatments for AIDS-related KS include:

- Naturopathic remedies: High doses of vitamin C, zinc, echinacea, or goldenseal to improve immune function; or preparations of astragalis, osha root, or licorice to suppress the HIV virus.

- Homeopathic remedies: These include a homeopathic preparation of cyclosporine and another made from a dilution of dead typhoid virus.

- Ozone therapy: Isolated reports from Europe and the United States attest to remission of AIDS-related KS several months after treatment with ozone given via rectal insufflation.

Alternative treatments aimed at improving the quality of life for KS patients include Reiki, reflexology, meditation, and chromatherapy.

There is no compelling scientific evidence for alternative therapies, and all patients who have KS should discuss their use with their treatment team before proceeding.

Coping with cancer treatment

Studies of treatment side effects in patients with epidemic KS are complicated by the difficulty of distinguishing between side effects caused by treatment aimed at HIV and those caused by treatment for KS. Common problems related to KS treatment include damage to the bone marrow, hair loss, and nerve damage from medications.

Other treatment-related issues include **weight loss** due to poor appetite and swelling of body tissues from fluid retention. Patients may receive nutritional counseling, medications to stimulate the appetite, and radiation treatment or diuretics to reduce the level of fluid in the tissues.

Prognosis

The prognosis of KS varies depending on its form. Patients with classic KS often survive for many years after diagnosis; death is often caused by another cancer, such as non-Hodgkin lymphoma, rather than the KS itself. Current research suggests that the overall five-year survival rate is about 72%. The aggressive form of African KS has the poorest prognosis. Patients with immunosuppressive treatment-related KS have variable prognoses; in many cases, however, the KS goes into remission once the immune-suppressing drug is discontinued. The prognosis of patients with epidemic KS also varies depending on the patient's general level of health. As a rule, patients whose KS has spread to the lungs have the poorest prognosis.

Clinical trials

In fall 2014, there were 12 active clinical trials for KS, including a comparison of chemotherapy regimens as additions to HAART and evaluation of an inhibitor to block the growth of KS tumor cells. Updated information about the content of and patient participation in clinical trials can be obtained at the web site of the **National Cancer Institute**: http://cancertrials.nci.nih.gov.

Prevention

The only known preventive strategy for reducing one's risk for epidemic KS is abstinence from intercourse or modification of sexual habits. Homosexual or bisexual males can reduce their risk of developing KS by avoiding passive anal intercourse. Women can reduce their risk by avoiding vaginal or anal intercourse with bisexual males.

Organ transplant patients who are at increased risk of developing KS as a result of taking prednisone or other immunosuppressive drugs should consult their primary physician about possible changes in dosage.

Special concerns

The two special concerns most likely to arise with epidemic KS are social isolation from the appearance of KS lesions on the patient's face, and spiritual or psychological concerns related to the tumor's connection to AIDS and homosexuality. There are many local and regional support groups for cancer patients that can help patients deal with concerns about appearance. With regard to religious/spiritual issues, most major Christian and Jewish bodies in the United States and Canada have task forces or working groups dealing with AIDS-related concerns. The National Catholic AIDS Network (NCAN) maintains an information database and web site (http://www.ncan.org) and accepts call-in referrals at (707) 874-3031.

See also AIDS-related cancers.

Resources

BOOKS

Abeloff, M. D., et al. *Clinical Oncology*. 5th ed. New York: Churchill Livingstone, 2014.

Acton, Ashton, ed. *HIV/AIDS and Kaposi Sarcoma: New Insights for the Healthcare Professional*. Atlanta: ScholarlyEditions, 2013.

Niederhuber, J. E., et al. *Clinical Oncology*. 5th ed. Philadelphia: Elsevier, 2014.

PERIODICALS

Gramolelli, Silvia, and Thomas F. Schulze. "The Role of Kaposi Sarcoma-Associated Herpesvirus in the Pathogenesis of Kaposi Sarcoma." *Journal of Pathology* (September 12, 2014): e-pub ahead of print. http://dx.doi.org/10.1002/path.4441 (accessed October 30, 2014).

Rashidghamat, E., et al. "Kaposi Sarcoma in HIV-Negative Men Who Have Sex with Men." *British Journal of Dermatology* (September 26, 2014): e-pub ahead of print. http://dx.doi.org/10.1111/bjd.13102 (accessed October 30, 2014).

WEBSITES

American Cancer Society. "Kaposi Sarcoma." http://www.cancer.org/cancer/kaposisarcoma (accessed October 30, 2014).

MedlinePlus. "Kaposi's Sarcoma." U.S. National Library of Medicine, National Institutes of Health. http://www.nlm.nih.gov/medlineplus/kaposissarcoma.html (accessed October 30, 2014).

National Cancer Institute. "Kaposi Sarcoma Treatment (PDQ®)." http://www.cancer.gov/cancertopics/pdq/treatment/kaposis/Patient (accessed October 30, 2014).

ORGANIZATIONS

American Cancer Society, 250 Williams St. NW, Atlanta, GA 30303, (800) 227-2345, http://www.cancer.org.

National Cancer Institute, 9609 Medical Center Dr., BG 9609 MSC 9760, Bethesda, MD 20892-9760, (800) 4-CANCER (422-6237), http://www.cancer.gov.

San Francisco AIDS Foundation, 1035 Market Street, Suite 400, San Francisco, CA 94103, (415) 487-3000, http://sfaf.org.

Rebecca J. Frey, PhD.
REVISED BY TERESA G. ODLE

Ketoconazole *see* **Antifungal therapy**

Ki67

Definition

Ki67 is a protein molecule that can be easily detected in growing cells in order to gain an understanding of the rate at which the cells within a tumor are growing.

Purpose

Detection of Ki67 is carried out on biopsies, samples of tumor tissue. The goal of this assay is to evaluate an important characteristic of the cells within the tumor, namely the percentage of tumor cells that are actively dividing and giving rise to more **cancer** cells. The number obtained through this examination is termed the S-phase, growth, or proliferative fraction. This information can play an important part in deciding the best treatment for a cancer patient.

Precautions

This test is performed on tissue or cells that have been removed during the initial surgery or diagnostic procedure used to determine the precise nature of the cancer. It usually does not require any new surgery or blood draw from the patient and so does not entail any additional precautions for the patient.

Description

Cancer is a group of diseases characterized by abnormal, or neoplastic, cellular growth in particular tissues. In many instances this growth is abnormal because cells are growing more rapidly than is normal.

This unregulated growth is how a tumor is formed. A tumor is more or less a collection of cells that grow more rapidly than the surrounding normal tissue. Most importantly, this difference in growth rate is central to the way in which many cancer drugs, termed cytotoxic agents, work. The ability of these drugs to eliminate cancer cells depends on their ability to kill cells that are actively proliferating but do less damage to cells that are not actively dividing. This characteristic makes it useful to know how actively the cells in tumor are growing compared to the surrounding tissue. The measurement of Ki67 is one of the most common ways to measure the growth fraction of tumor cells. This molecule can be detected only in the nucleus of actively growing cells.

Analysis of Ki67 in tumors is accomplished by a pathologist who examines a piece of the tumor tissue using special techniques. The technique used is termed immunocytochemistry. This analysis involves the preparation of a histologic section, a very thin piece of tumor tissue placed on a glass microscope slide. These kinds of tissue sections are used in the diagnosis of cancer. In the case of Ki67 assays, the section is incubated with antibodies that react with the Ki67 molecule, and then treated with special reagents that cause a color to appear where antibody has bound. In this way, when the pathologist looks at the section using a microscope, the fraction of growing cells whose nuclei are stained for Ki67 can be determined for the tumor cells and compared with normal tissue. In some instances, depending on the particular type of cancer, the pathologist might consider it more appropriate to use a different technique to assess the growth fraction of a specific tumor or leukemia.

Preparation, Aftercare, and Risks

Because this test is performed on tissue or cells that had been removed during an initial **biopsy** or other diagnostic procedure, and because no new surgery or sample is required, no additional recommendations regarding preparation, aftercare, or risks are necessary.

Results

The proliferative or growth fraction as determined by Ki67 analysis is interpreted in view of what is normal for the tissue in which the tumor has been found or from which it originated. In the case of certain types of tissue—for example, brain—there is little cellular growth in normal tissue. In other cases, such as breast tissue or the cells that line the colon, cellular growth is a normal part of the function of that tissue. The significance of an increased proliferative fraction is interpreted in light of the experience of the oncologist as well as the knowledge and experience of other clinicians as reported in the medical literature. The Ki67 result, often termed the Ki67 labeling index, can be used in some cases as a prognostic indicator for some cancers. For example, for **brain tumors**, such as astrocytomas and glioblastomas, a high Ki67 labeling index is one factor that predicts a poor prognosis. For breast tumors, the clinician will consider the proliferative fraction in conjunction with other factors such as patient age, results of receptor assays, and whether there is evidence of spread of the disease to lymph nodes or other sites within the body. The value of Ki67 is not as firmly established for other cancers, such as bladder or **pituitary tumors**.

Resources

PERIODICALS

Chassevent, A., et al. "S-Phase Fraction and DNA Ploidy in 633 T1T2 Breast Cancers: A Standardized Flow Cytometric Study." *Clinical Cancer Research* 7 (2001): 909-17.

WEBSITES

Dr. Susan Love Research Foundation. "What Is Ki-67?" http://www.dslrf.org/breastcancer/content.asp?L2=3&L3=7&PID=&sid=132&cid=1487 (accessed December 1, 2014).

Warren Maltzman, PhD.

Kidney cancer

Definition

Kidney **cancer**, also called renal cancer, is a disease in which the cells in certain kidney tissues start to grow uncontrollably and form tumors. Renal cell **carcinoma** (RCC), an **adenocarcinoma** of the kidneys also referred to as hypernephroma, occurs in epithelial cells that line the kidneys. It is the most common type of kidney cancer, accounting for 90%–95% of all malignant kidney tumors. **Transitional cell carcinoma** is a less common type of kidney cancer. **Wilms tumor** is a rapidly developing cancer of the kidney most often found in children under four years of age.

Description

The kidneys are a pair of organs shaped like kidney beans that lie on either side of the spine just above the waist. Inside each kidney are tiny tubes (tubules) that filter and clean the blood, taking out the waste products and making urine. The urine made by the kidney passes into the bladder through a tube called the ureter. Urine is held in the bladder until it is discharged from the body. RCC generally develops in the lining of the tubules that filter and clean the blood. Cancer that develops in the central portion of the kidney (where the urine is collected and drained into the ureters) is known as transitional cell carcinoma of the renal pelvis. Transitional cell cancer is similar to RCC, but accounts for less than 5% of kidney tumors. Wilms tumor is the most common type of childhood kidney cancer and is distinct from kidney cancer in adults.

Demographics

Kidney cancer accounts for approximately 2–3% of all cancers. In the United States, kidney cancer is the tenth most common cancer in both men and women. The incidence was increasing in the 1990s, but has leveled off since 1995. Increases may have been due to advanced imaging by which more cases were detected rather than an actual increase in the number of people affected. The American Cancer Society estimates that 83,920 Americans will be diagnosed with kidney cancer in 2014, including 39,140 men and 24,780 women. About 13,860 of these people will die from the disease (8,900 men and 4,960 women). RCC accounts for 90–95% of malignant neoplasms that originate in the kidney.

Kidney cancer occurs most often in men aged 45 and older; it is seldom diagnosed in people younger than 45. The median age at diagnosis is 64. RCC occurs twice as often in men as in women, which is believed to be related

KEY TERMS

Biopsy—The surgical removal and microscopic examination of living tissue for diagnostic purposes.

Bone scan—An x-ray study in which patients are given an intravenous injection of a small amount of a radioactive material that travels in the blood. When it reaches the bones, it can be detected by x-ray to provide an image of their internal structure.

Chemotherapy—Treatment with anticancer drugs.

Computed tomography (CT) scan—A medical procedure in which a series of x-ray images are made and combined by a computer to form detailed pictures of areas inside the body.

Cryoablation—A technique for removing diseased tissue by destroying it with extreme cold.

Hematuria—Blood in the urine.

Immunotherapy—Treatment of cancer by stimulating the body's immune defense system.

Intravenous pyelogram (IVP)—A procedure in which dye injected into a vein in the arm travels through the body and concentrates in the urine for discharge. When an x-ray is taken, the dye highlights the kidneys, ureters, and urinary bladder, which reveals any abnormalities of the urinary tract.

Magnetic resonance imaging (MRI)—A diagnostic imaging procedure in which images of body organs can be created using a magnet linked to a computer; it measures the response of body tissues to high-frequency radio waves in the magnetic field.

Nephrectomy—A surgical procedure performed to remove a kidney.

Primary tumor—A cancer's origin or location of initial growth.

Radiation therapy—Treatment with high-energy radiation from x-ray machines, cobalt, radium, or other sources.

Renal ultrasound—A painless and noninvasive diagnostic imaging procedure that bounces high frequency sound waves off the kidneys to produce precise images of areas inside the kidney (sonograms).

---

to men's smoking more than women and the greater exposure of men to cancer-causing chemicals in the workplace. Rates of RCC are somewhat higher among African Americans, Native Americans, and Native Alaskans than among Caucasians.

Wilms tumor typically affects children aged three to four and seldom occurs in children older than age five.

Causes and symptoms

The precise causes of kidney cancer are unknown, but many risk factors are associated with the disease. The risk factors listed from greatest to smallest include:

- von Hippel-Lindau disease
- chronic dialysis
- obesity
- tobacco use
- first-degree relative with kidney cancer
- hypertension
- occupational exposure to dry cleaning solvents
- use of diuretics (non-hypertension use)
- trichloroethylene exposure
- heavy phenacetin use
- polycystic kidney disease
- cadmium exposure
- arsenic exposure
- asbestos exposure

Certain rare inherited conditions are associated with developing RCC; therefore, genetic causes are being investigated. **Von Hippel-Lindau disease**, which is caused by mutations in the *VHL* gene, and certain hereditary forms of RCC (i.e., papillary RCC and leiomyoma-RCC), which are linked to changes in the *FH* gene, are associated with an increased risk of developing other tumors, especially RCC. Birt-Hogg Dubé (BHD) syndrome also increases the risk of developing RCC.

Symptoms typically appear late when the tumor is large and has already spread outside the kidneys. Earlier detection of a renal tumor often occurs when abdominal imaging scans are performed for another reason. The most common symptom of kidney cancer is blood in the urine (hematuria). Other symptoms include painful urination, pain in the lower back or on the sides, abdominal pain, a lump or hard mass that can be felt in the kidney area, unexplained **weight loss**, **fever**, weakness, **fatigue**, and sometimes high blood pressure (hypertension).

Diagnosis

Diagnosis of kidney cancer begins with taking a thorough medical history and performing a complete physical examination in which the doctor will probe (palpate) the abdomen for lumps or masses. However, small kidney tumors cannot usually be felt because the kidneys lie too deep within the body. A routine urinalysis will be done to look for blood in the urine, a common sign of kidney cancer. Blood tests, including renal function and liver function tests, will be ordered to check for changes in body chemistries caused by substances released by tumors. Laboratory tests may show abnormal levels of iron in the blood. Either a low red blood cell count (**anemia**) or a high red blood cell count (erythrocytosis) may accompany kidney cancer. High calcium levels are a common finding.

Diagnostic imaging tests will be performed to examine the renal system closely. **Computed tomography** (CT) and **magnetic resonance imaging** (MRI) are the main imaging modalities used to evaluate the kidneys and the surrounding organs. These techniques reveal abnormalities such as lesions or tumor masses, both solid and cystic types. The scans will also determine whether the tumor has spread outside the kidney (**metastasis**) to renal veins or other organs in the abdomen. Renal ultrasound may also be done to detect the presence of tumors, even the smallest ones. It is a painless and noninvasive diagnostic imaging procedure in which sound waves are used to form an image of the kidneys. An intravenous urogram (IVU) is sometimes performed as well. However, ultrasound and IVU provide less detailed information about tumor characteristics and spreading than do CT and MRI. Contrast enhanced ultrasound, noted for its use in diagnosing **liver cancer**, is being investigated for its ability to provide more detailed images of renal masses.

Three-dimensional CT, CT **angiography**, or MRI angiography may be done to examine the renal veins and arteries prior to a patient receiving surgery. If laboratory tests have revealed an elevated alkaline phosphatase level and/or the patient complains of **bone pain**, a bone scan may be ordered to rule out spread to the bones. A chest x-ray is usually taken to rule out metastasis to the lungs. If the chest x-ray is abnormal, a chest CT will be done.

A kidney **biopsy** is performed to confirm the diagnosis of kidney cancer by identifying characteristic cell types. The imaging techniques are not always able to tell whether tumors are benign or malignant, so cancer cells must be identified in the kidney tissue. During the biopsy procedure, a small piece of tissue is removed from the tumor, sometimes with needle biopsy and sometimes

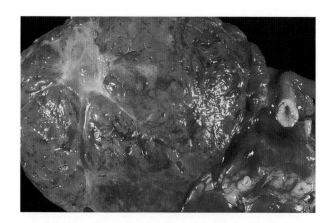

An extracted cancerous kidney. *(Riedlinger/Custom Medical Stock Photo)*

during surgery, and is then examined under a microscope. The biopsy will give information about the type of tumor, the type of cells involved, and whether the tumor is localized or has spread to nearby or distant structures (**tumor staging**).

Clinical staging

Staging guidelines for RCC are provided by the American Joint Commission on Cancer (AJCC) using four stages with TNM classification (T=tumor, N=node metastasis, M=distant metastasis) as follows (2.5 cm equals approximately 1 in.):

- Stage I: Primary tumor measures 7 cm or less in greatest dimension (T1) and is limited to the kidney, with no lymph node involvement (N0) and no metastases (M0).

- Stage II: Primary tumor is larger than 7 cm in greatest dimension (T2) and is limited to the kidney, with no lymph node involvement (N0) and no metastases (M0).

- Stage III: Primary tumor measures from 5–10 cm and may extend into major renal veins or invade perinephric tissues, but not beyond the Gerota fascia (a layer of connective tissue encapsulating the kidneys) or into the adrenal glands (T3a); may extend into vena cava (T3b,c). There may be metastasis in a single lymph node (N1) but not into distant structures (M0).

- Stage IV: Primary tumor is of any size (any T) and invades beyond the Gerota fascia with metastasis in more than one lymph node (any N). Metastasis to distant structures in the body (M1) is present.

Treatment

Treatment is determined according to the clinical condition of the patient and the location, size, and extent of the tumor as well as the patient's age and medical

QUESTIONS TO ASK YOUR DOCTOR

- What should I expect from undergoing a biopsy?
- What type of kidney cancer do I have?
- What is the stage of the disease?
- What are the treatment choices? Which do you recommend? Why?
- What are the risks and possible side effects of each treatment?
- What are the chances that the treatment will be successful?
- What new treatments are being studied in clinical trials?
- How long will treatment last?
- Will I have to stay in the hospital?
- Will treatment affect my normal activities? If so, for how long?
- What is the treatment likely to cost?

history. Surgical treatment is applied for early stages of RCC and palliative treatment for advanced RCC. Palliative care is advised when cure is not possible and the main goal is to maintain the patient's comfort by treating symptoms only. Experimental therapies may be applied for some patients through **clinical trials**.

The primary treatment for stages I to III of kidney cancer that has not spread to other parts of the body is surgical removal of the diseased kidney, the adrenal gland, perirenal fat, and the Gerota fascia (radical **nephrectomy**). Because most cancers affect only one kidney, the patient can function well with the remaining one. Sometimes the lymph nodes surrounding the kidney are also removed. Partial nephrectomy, called nephron-sparing surgery, removes only part of the diseased kidney along with the tumor. This procedure is performed either when the tumor is exceptionally small (less than 4 to 7 cm) or when it is not possible to remove the entire kidney (e.g., when the patient has only one kidney or when both kidneys have tumors). Nephrectomy can also be applied for stage IV cancers in conjunction with palliative treatment. Removing the tumor has proven to provide palliation and may even prolong the life of a patient with advanced kidney cancer. Other palliative measures may include tumor embolization and external beam radiation. **Radiation therapy** has been shown to alleviate pain and bleeding, especially when the cancer is inoperable. It is also applied for stage IV kidney cancer when bone

metastasis is present. However, radiation has not proven to be effective in destroying kidney tumor cells and is not often combined with surgery as a primary treatment for kidney cancer.

Radical nephrectomy is performed either as an open procedure or as a laparoscopic procedure, with comparable results, although recovery is faster with laparoscopic surgery. Laparoscopic techniques have made it possible for surgeons to remove small tumors while sparing the rest of the kidney. Most tumors removed by **laparoscopy** are 4 cm (1.6 in.) in size or smaller. Laparoscopy also allows the surgeon to remove small tumors with cryoablation (destroying the tumor by freezing it) rather than cutting. However, nonsurgical destruction of renal tumors using freezing (cryosurgery) or thermal energy (radiofrequency ablation) is not performed as a primary treatment due to the lack of long-term information about safety and effectiveness.

Certain **anticancer drugs** (**chemotherapy**) applied in the treatment of kidney cancer have been shown to reduce tumor size and prolong life in some patients with advanced tumors. Good responses have been seen with **sunitinib**, **sorafenib**, axitinib, **bevacizumab**, and pazopanib. Interferon alfa-2b (IL-2), an immunologic therapy (**immunotherapy**) that uses the immune system to help eradicate the cancer, also has been used effectively, but results are not long lasting in the majority of patients. Experimental therapies include **stem cell transplantation**, interleukins, antiangiogenesis therapy and vaccine therapy. Clinical trials are ongoing for some of these treatments, as well as for new combinations of chemotherapy agents.

Alternative and complementary therapies

Several healing philosophies, approaches, and therapies may be used as supplemental or instead of traditional treatments. These treatments may have varying effectiveness in boosting the immune system and/or treating a tumor. The efficacy of each treatment also varies from person to person. None of the treatments, however, have demonstrated safety or effectiveness on a consistent basis. Patients should research such treatments for any potential dangers and notify their physician before utilizing them.

Coping with cancer treatment

Side effects of treatment, nutrition, emotional well-being, and other complications are all parts of coping with cancer. The possible side effects of cancer treatments include:

- constipation
- diarrhea

- confusion or delirium
- fatigue
- fever, chills, sweats
- nausea and vomiting
- mouth sores, dry mouth, bleeding gums
- pruritus (itching)
- changes in sexuality
- sleep disorders
- pain

Anxiety, **depression**, feelings of loss, post-traumatic stress disorder, loss of sexual desire, and **substance abuse** are all possible emotional side effects. Getting essential nutrients before, during, and after treatments can also be of concern.

Prognosis

Advances in renal imaging techniques and more precise staging guidelines have contributed to increased incidental detection of early-stage RCC when the tumor is localized, that is, confined to the kidney. Therefore, the chances of a surgical cure are good for people whose kidney cancer is in stages I through III. Patients in stage IV will undergo palliative surgery and have treatments such as radiation and drug therapies that may increase their life expectancy even with metastases. Five-year survival rates range from 81% in people with stage 1 kidney cancer to 8% in people with stage IV metastatic kidney cancer. The prognosis is poorer for patients with metastatic or recurrent RCC.

Clinical trials

The **National Cancer Institute** (NCI) lists many clinical trials in place across the United States that are studying new types of chemotherapy with new drugs and drug combinations, biological and immunological therapies, ways of combining various types of treatment for kidney cancer, side effect reduction, and improving quality of life. Immunostimulatory agents and gene-therapy techniques that modify tumor cells, antiangiogenesis compounds, cyclin-dependent kinase inhibitors, and differentiating agents are all being investigated as target therapies. One may consult http://clinicaltrials.gov and a doctor for a list of kidney cancer clinical trials. The NCI and other cancer organizations will also help patients and their families locate clinical trials.

Prevention

The exact cause of kidney cancer is not known, so it is not possible to prevent all cases. However, because a strong association between kidney cancer and tobacco use has been shown, avoiding tobacco is the best way to lower one's risk of developing this cancer. Avoiding known risk factors or using care when working with cancer-causing agents such as asbestos and cadmium may reduce the risk of developing kidney cancer. Maintaining optimum health by eating a well-balanced diet, avoiding stress, and exercising regularly may also help prevent kidney cancer.

Resources

BOOKS

Edge, S. B., et al. *AJCC Cancer Staging Manual.* 7th ed. New York: Springer, 2010.

Porter, Robert S., and Justin L. Kaplan, eds. "Renal Cell Carcinoma (Hypernephroma; Adenocarcinoma of the Kidney), Section 17: Genitourinary Disorders." In *The Merck Manual of Diagnosis and Therapy*, 19th ed. Whitehouse Station, NJ: Merck Research Laboratories, 2011, 2472.

PERIODICALS

Gupta, S., V. Parsa, L. K. Heilbrun, D. W. Smith, et al. "Safety and Efficacy of Molecularly Targeted Agents in Patients with Metastatic Kidney Cancer with Renal Dysfunction." *Anticancer Drugs* 22 (September 2011): 794–800.

Ignee, A., B. Straub, G. Schuessler, C. F. Dietrich. "Contrast Enhanced Ultrasound of Renal Masses." *World Journal of Radiology* 2 (January 2010): 15–31.

WEBSITES

Kidney Cancer Association. "About Kidney Cancer." http://www.kidneycancer.org/knowledge/learn/about-kidney-cancer (accessed January 29, 2015).

ORGANIZATIONS

American Cancer Society, 1599 Clifton Rd. NE, Atlanta, GA 30329, (800) 227-2345, http://www.cancer.org.

American Urological Association, 1120 N. Charles St., Baltimore, MD 21201, (410) 727-1100, http://www.auanet.org.

Cancer Research Institute, 681 Fifth Ave., New York, NY 10022, (800) 992-2623, http://www.cancerresearch.org.

Kidney Cancer Association, PO Box 803338, Chicago, IL 60680-3338, (847) 332-1051, (800) 850-9132, office@kidneycancer.org, http://www.kidneycancer.org.

National Cancer Institute (NCI), 9000 Rockville Pike, Building 31, Room 10A16, Bethesda, MD 20892, (800) 422-6237, http://www.nci.nih.gov.

National Kidney Foundation, 30 East 33rd St., New York, NY 10016, (800) 622-9010 http://www.kidney.org.

Lata Cherath, PhD.
Rebecca Frey, PhD.
REVISED BY L. LEE CULVERT

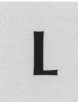

L

Lactulose *see* **Laxatives**

Lambert-Eaton myasthenic syndrome

Definition

Lambert-Eaton myasthenic syndrome (LEMS), sometimes called Eaton-Lambert syndrome, is a rare disorder affecting the muscles and nerves. LEMS is known to be associated with small-cell lung **cancer**. It may also be associated with such cancers as **lymphoma**, **non-Hodgkin lymphoma**, T-cell leukemia, non-small-cell lung cancer, **prostate cancer**, and **thymoma**. LEMS was first identified in 1956 by a team of three American neurologists, Lee Eaton, Edward Lambert, and Edward Rooke.

Demographics

LEMS is a rare disorder; the number of people affected by it is at best an estimate. Various figures that have been given are that 400 people in the United States have the disorder at any one time. This figure does not include patients with LEMS who do not have cancer. About half of patients diagnosed with LEMS do not have cancer; this form of LEMS is called idiopathic LEMS, which means that its origin is unknown.

Another estimate is that LEMS affects 3% of patients with small-cell lung cancer (SCLC), or about 4 people in every million. Between 50% and 70% of patients diagnosed with LEMS have an identifiable cancer of some type, the vast majority having SCLC. LEMS has also been associated with non-SCLC, lymphosarcoma, malignant thymoma, or **carcinoma** of the breast, stomach, colon, prostate, bladder, kidney, or gallbladder.

Description

LEMS is a disorder characterized by muscular weakness and **fatigue** caused by a disruption of electrical impulses between the nerves and muscle cells. The disruption in turn results from an autoimmune process.

About half of all cases of LEMS are associated with cancer, particularly small-cell lung cancer (SCLC). The other half of cases have no known cause and are called idiopathic LEMS. The disorder is typically slow in onset; it usually begins with a dry mouth and some weakness or aching in the legs, progressing to difficulty swallowing or holding up the head, problems in focusing the eyes, and general fatigue. LEMS chiefly affects the patient's quality of life and ability to carry out everyday activities; patients with cancer-associated LEMS usually die from the cancer, not the muscle syndrome.

Risk factors

Risk factors for LEMS include:

- Being diagnosed with SCLC or another type of cancer.
- Age. LEMS is more common in middle-aged and older adults than in children and adolescents. The average age at diagnosis is 60 years.
- Sex. LEMS is slightly more common in men than in women. It is most likely to be diagnosed in men over 40.
- Having another autoimmune disorder.
- Smoking. All patients with SCLC diagnosed with LEMS have been found to be heavy smokers.

Causes and symptoms

Causes

The symptoms of LEMS are the result of an insufficient release of a neurotransmitter called acetylcholine at the junctions between the nerves and muscle cells. Acetylcholine is a chemical that passes signals from the nerve cells to the muscles in order for the muscles to move. The decreased level of acetylcholine causes a muscle reaction to the nerve signal that is lower than normal. The underlying cause of the lower-than-normal neurotransmitter release seen in LEMS patients is believed to be related to a disorder of the immune system (an autoimmune reaction). This autoimmune reaction is caused by antibodies produced by the patient in response to small-cell lung cancer or one of the other cancers associated with LEMS.

Since continued use of the muscles may lead to a buildup of acetylcholine to normal levels, symptoms of LEMS can often be lessened or alleviated by using the affected muscles. **Myasthenia gravis** (MG), another disorder that has symptoms similar to LEMS, is caused by a blockage of neurotransmitters by antibodies. Symptoms of myasthenia gravis do not improve with continued muscle use. The improvement in symptoms that is observable in LEMS patients often helps to differentiate LEMS from myasthenia gravis. In contrast to MG, the symptoms of LEMS tend to be worse in the morning and improve toward evening with exercise and nerve stimulation. In addition, LEMS usually does not affect the muscles that control breathing as severely as MG does.

LEMS is made worse by neuromuscular blocking agents used during surgery; certain **antibiotics**, such as the aminoglycosides and fluoroquinolones; magnesium; calcium channel blockers; and iodinated intravenous contrast agents used in medical imaging.

Symptoms

The symptoms of LEMS in cancer patients typically begin 2–4 years before the cancer is diagnosed. The primary symptom is muscular weakness or paralysis that varies in intensity and location throughout the body. Other symptoms of LEMS include tingling sensations in the skin, double vision, difficulty maintaining a steady gaze, and dry mouth or difficulty in swallowing.

The first signs of LEMS tend to be a dry mouth and weakness or soreness in the legs. Some patients also complain of a metallic taste in the mouth as well as dryness. Later symptoms of LEMS include:

- changes in vision
- weakened posture and muscle tone
- difficulty in chewing or swallowing
- difficulty in climbing stairs
- difficulty in lifting simple objects
- speech impairment
- impotence in men
- a drooping head
- fatigue
- and/or a need to use the hands to get up from a sitting or lying position

Diagnosis

LEMS is often misdiagnosed as myasthenia gravis because of the similarities between the symptoms of these two disorders. The diagnosis is usually made by a combination of chest **x-rays** (to detect lung cancer), blood tests for antibodies to the calcium channels at the ends of nerve fibers, and electrical stimulation tests. An increased response of muscle fibers to very high frequencies of electrical stimulation indicates LEMS rather than MS.

If the doctor does not find a tumor within the first two years after the onset of the patient's symptoms, the patient probably has idiopathic LEMS.

Examination

The doctor may notice drooping eyelids, a dry mouth, and weakness when the patient is asked to stand up. The patient's reflexes will be weaker than normal, and the muscles may appear smaller than usual or wasted.

Treatment

Traditional

The goal of treatment for LEMS patients is to improve muscle strength while also treating the cancer or other underlying disorder that is causing LEMS.

When possible, patients affected with LEMS should undergo a **physical therapy** program that is tailored to their health status and abilities. This program may include stretching and flexibility maneuvers as well as light strength and cardiovascular exercises. Symptoms of LEMS tend to be aggravated by prolonged exercise, so any physical therapy undertaken should be relatively short in duration.

Some LEMS patients are not able to undertake physical therapy because of their current state of health. In these cases, plasmapheresis (also called plasma exchange), a procedure in which blood plasma is removed from the patient and replaced, may be recommended. This procedure can be effective in a majority of LEMS patients.

Heat appears to worsen the symptoms of LEMS; patients typically feel much worse in hot weather and when they are running a **fever**. The doctor will usually advise the patient to take lukewarm rather than hot showers or baths.

Drugs

Medications that suppress the **immune response** or that suppress the antibodies responsible for the muscle weakness have also been shown to improve LEMS symptoms in some patients. These medications include high-dose intravenous immunoglobulin, **azathioprine**, and steroid drugs like prednisone. Another type of drug that has been shown to be beneficial is drugs that improve the transmission of nerve impulses to the muscles. These drugs include di-amino pyridine (DAP) and pyridostigmine bromide (Mestinon).

Alternative and complementary therapies

Yoga and other stretching exercises may be effective treatments for alleviating the physical symptoms of LEMS patients. Some LEMS patients also report improvement of symptoms after deep body massage or hydrotherapy.

Prognosis

The most important prognostic factor for LEMS patients diagnosed with cancer is the prognosis of the cancer. People with idiopathic LEMS have a better prognosis than those with cancer; however, recovery of muscle strength varies from patient to patient. In general, patients whose symptoms progress more rapidly have a worse prognosis.

Prevention

There is no way to prevent LEMS because its underlying cause is unknown.

Resources

BOOKS

Benatar, Michael. *Neuromuscular Disease: Evidence and Analysis in Clinical Neurology.* Totowa, NJ: Humana Press, 2006.

Engel, Andrew G., ed. *Myasthenia Gravis and Myasthenic Disorders.* 2nd ed. New York: Oxford University Press, 2012.

Kalman, Bernadette, and Thomas H. Brannagan III. *Neuroimmunology in Clinical Practice.* Malden, MA: Blackwell Publishing, 2008.

PERIODICALS

Titulaer, M. J., et al. "Screening for Small-cell Lung Cancer: A Follow-up Study of Patients with Lambert-Eaton Myasthenic Syndrome." *Journal of Clinical Oncology* 26 (September 10, 2008): 4276–81.

Weimer, M. B., and J. Wong. "Lambert-Eaton Myasthenic Syndrome." *Current Treatment Options in Neurology* 11 (March 2009): 77–84.

Wirtz, P.W., et al. "Efficacy of 3,4-diaminopyridine and Pyridostigmine in the Treatment of Lambert-Eaton Myasthenic Syndrome: A Randomized, Double-blind, Placebo-controlled, Crossover Study." *Clinical Pharmacology and Therapeutics* 86 (July 2009): 44–48.

WEBSITES

A.D.A.M. Medical Encyclopedia. "Lambert-Eaton Syndrome." MedlinePlus. http://www.nlm.nih.gov/medlineplus/ency/article/000710.htm (accessed November 4, 2014).

National Institute of Neurological Disorders and Stroke (NINDS). "Lambert-Eaton Myasthenic Syndrome Information Page." http://www.ninds.nih.gov/disorders/lambert_eaton/lambert_eaton.htm (accessed November 4, 2014).

ORGANIZATIONS

American Academy of Neurology, 201 Chicago Ave., Minneapolis, MN 55415, (612) 928-6000, (800) 879-1960, Fax: (612) 454-2746, memberservices@aan.com, https://www.aan.com.

American Physical Therapy Association (APTA), 1111 North Fairfax Street, Alexandria, VA 22314-1488, 703-684-APTA (2782), 800-999-APTA (2782), Fax: 703-684-7343, http://www.apta.org//AM/Template.cfm?Section=Home.

National Institute of Neurological Disorders and Stroke (NINDS), NIH Neurological Institute, PO Box 5801, Bethesda, MD 20824, (301) 496-5751, (800) 352-9424, http://www.ninds.nih.gov.

National Organization for Rare Disorders (NORD), P.O. Box 1968, Danbury, CT 06813-1968, 203-744-0100, 800-999-NORD, Fax: 203-798-2291, http://www.rarediseases.org.

Paul A. Johnson, Ed.M.
Rebecca J. Frey, PhD.

Lanvis *see* **Thioguanine**

Laparoscopy

Definition

Laparoscopy, sometimes also called laparoscopic (LAP) surgery, is a minimally invasive procedure that uses a thin, lighted tube (laparoscope) to visualize internal

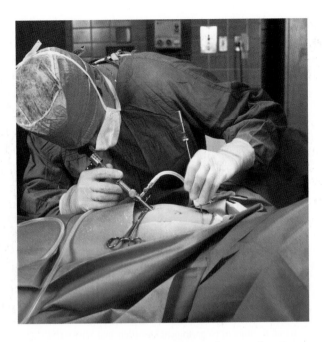

This surgeon is performing a laparoscopic procedure on a patient. In laparoscopy, instruments are inserted through several small cuts instead of making one large incision. (SOUTHERN ILL UNIV/Science Source)

organs. Laparoscopy is most commonly used during surgery on the abdominal and pelvic organs but may also be used for surgery of the thoracic cavity, head, or neck. In addition, tissue samples can be collected for **biopsy** using laparoscopy, and malignancies may be treated using laparoscopic techniques combined with other therapies. Laparoscopic surgery is preferred over open surgery for several types of procedures because it is minimally invasive and associated with fewer complications.

Purpose

Laparoscopy is performed to examine the abdominal and pelvic organs to diagnose certain conditions. It can also be used to perform surgery. Laparoscopy is commonly used in gynecology to examine the outside of the uterus, the fallopian tubes, and the ovaries—particularly in pelvic pain cases in which the underlying cause cannot be determined using diagnostic imaging (ultrasound and **computed tomography**). Examples of gynecologic conditions diagnosed using laparoscopy include endometriosis, ectopic pregnancy, ovarian cysts, pelvic inflammatory disease (PID), infertility, and **cancer**. Laparoscopy is used in general surgery to examine the abdominal organs, including the gallbladder, bile ducts, liver, appendix, and intestines.

Cancer staging

Laparoscopy can be used in determining the spread of certain cancers. It is sometimes combined with ultrasound. Although laparoscopy is a useful staging tool, its use depends on a variety of factors that are considered for each patient. Types of cancers where laparoscopy may be used to determine the spread of the disease include:

- liver cancer
- gallbladder cancer
- pancreatic cancer
- esophageal and stomach cancers
- Hodgkin lymphoma (may include splenectomy, or removal of the spleen).
- prostate cancer

Cancer treatment

Laparoscopy is sometimes used as part of a palliative cancer treatment. This type of treatment is not a cure but can often lessen the symptoms. An example is the feeding tube, which cancer patients may need if they are unable to take in food by mouth. The feeding tube provides nutrition directly into the stomach. Inserting the tube with a laparoscopy saves the patient the ordeal of open surgery.

Description

Laparoscopy is typically performed in the hospital under general anesthesia, although some laparoscopic procedures can be performed using local anesthetic agents. Once under anesthesia, a urinary catheter is inserted into the patient's bladder for urine collection. To begin the procedure, a small incision is made just below the navel, and a cannula or trocar is inserted into the incision to accommodate the insertion of the laparoscope. Other incisions may be made in the abdomen to allow the insertion of additional laparoscopic instrumentation. A laparoscopic insufflation device is used to inflate the abdomen with carbon dioxide gas to create a space in which the laparoscopic surgeon can maneuver the instruments. After the laparoscopic diagnosis and treatment are completed, the laparoscope, cannula, and other instrumentation are removed, and the incision is sutured and bandaged.

Laparoscopes have integral cameras for transmitting images during the procedure, and these are available in various sizes depending upon the type of procedure performed. The images from the laparoscope are transmitted to a viewing monitor that the surgeon uses to visualize the internal anatomy and guide any surgical procedure. Video and photographic equipment are also used to document the surgery and may be used postoperatively to explain the results of the procedure to the patient.

Robotic systems are available to assist with laparoscopy. A robotic arm attached to the operating table may be used to hold and position the laparoscope. This reduces unintentional camera movement that can occur when a surgical assistant holds the laparoscope. The surgeon controls the robotic arm movement by foot pedal with voice-activated command or with a handheld control panel.

Microlaparoscopy has become more common over the past few years. The procedure involves the use of smaller laparoscopes—2 millimeters (mm), compared to sizes from 5 mm to 10 mm for hospital laparoscopy—with the patient undergoing local anesthesia with conscious sedation in a physician's office. Video and photographic equipment may be used.

Laparoscopy has been explored in combination with other therapies for the treatment of certain types of malignancies, including pelvic and aortic **lymph node dissection**, **ovarian cancer**, and early **cervical cancer**. Laparoscopic **radiofrequency ablation** is a technique whereby laparoscopy assists in the delivery of radiofrequency probes that distribute pulses to a tumor site. The pulses generate heat in malignant tumor cells and destroy them.

The introduction of items such as temperature-controlled instruments, surgical instruments with greater rotation and articulation, improved imaging systems, and multiple robotic devices will expand the utility of laparoscopic techniques in the future. The skills of surgeons will be enhanced as well, with further development of training simulators and computer technology.

Preparation

Before undergoing laparoscopic surgery, the patient should be prepared by the doctor for the procedure both psychologically and physically. It is very important that the patient receives realistic counseling before surgery and prior to giving informed consent. This counseling includes discussion about further open abdominal surgery (laparotomy) that may be required during laparoscopic surgery, information about potential complications during surgery, and the possible need for blood transfusions. In the case of diagnostic laparoscopy for chronic pelvic pain, the procedure may simply indicate that all organs are normal, and the patient should be prepared for this possibility. The surgery may be explained using pictures, models, videos, and movies. It is especially important for the patient to be able to ask questions and express concerns. It may be helpful for the patient to have a family member or friend present during discussions with the doctor to help take notes.

There is usually a presurgical examination two weeks before the surgery to gather a medical history and obtain blood and urine samples for laboratory testing. It is important that the patient inform the doctor completely about any prior surgeries, medical conditions, or medications taken on a regular basis, including **nonsteroidal anti-inflammatory drugs** (NSAIDs), such as aspirin; other over-the-counter medications; and **vitamins** and supplements. Patients taking blood thinners like **warfarin** (Coumadin) should never adjust their medication themselves and should speak with their prescribing doctors regarding their upcoming surgery. If a tubal dye study is planned during the procedure, the patient may also be required to provide information on menstrual history. For some procedures, an autologous blood donation may be suggested prior to the surgery to replace any blood lost during the procedure. Chest **x-rays** may also be required. For some obese patients, **weight loss** may be necessary prior to surgery.

Immediately before surgery, there are several preoperative steps that the patient may be advised to take. The patient should shower at least 24 hours prior to the surgery and gently but thoroughly cleanse the umbilicus (belly button) with antibacterial soap and water using a cotton-tipped swab. Because laparoscopy requires general anesthesia in most cases, the patient may be asked to eat lightly 24 hours prior to surgery and fast at least 12 hours prior to surgery. Bowel cleansing with a laxative may also be required, which allows it to be more easily visualized and to prevent complications in the unlikely event of bowel injury. People with diabetes or hypoglycemia may wish to schedule their procedures early in the morning to avoid low blood sugar reactions. The patient should follow the directions of the hospital staff, arriving early on the day of surgery to sign paperwork and be screened by the anesthesiology staff. The patient will be asked questions regarding current medications and dosages, allergies to medication, previous experiences with anesthesia (that is, allergic reactions, and previous experiences regarding time-to-consciousness), and other topics. It is often helpful for the patient to make a list of this information beforehand so that it can be retrieved easily when requested by the hospital staff.

Aftercare

Following laparoscopy, patients are required to remain in a recovery area until the immediate effects of anesthesia subside and normal voiding is accomplished (especially if a urinary catheter was used during the surgery). Vital signs are monitored to ensure that there are no reactions to anesthesia or internal injuries present. There may be some nausea and/or vomiting, which may be reduced by the use of the anesthetic propofol for healthy patients undergoing elective procedures such as tubal ligation, diagnostic laparoscopy, or hernia repair. Laparoscopy is usually an outpatient procedure and patients are discharged from the recovery area within a few hours after the procedure. For elderly patients and patients with other medical conditions, recovery may be slower. Patients with more serious medical conditions or patients undergoing emergency laparoscopy may be required to stay overnight or longer.

Once patients are discharged, they will receive instructions regarding activity level, medications, post-operative dietary modifications, and possible side effects of the procedure. It may be helpful to have a friend or family member present when these instructions are given, as the aftereffects of anesthesia may cause some temporary confusion. Postoperative instructions may include information on when to resume normal activities such as bathing, housework, and driving. Depending on the nature of the laparoscopic procedure and the patient's medical condition, daily activity may be restricted for a few days and strenuous activity restricted for several days to weeks. Pain-relieving medications and **antibiotics** may be prescribed for several days postoperatively.

Patients will be instructed to watch for signs of a urinary tract infection (UTI) or unusual pain; either may indicate organ injury. It is important to understand the difference between normal discomfort and pain, because pain may indicate a problem. Patients may also experience an elevated temperature and occasionally a condition known as postlaparoscopy syndrome; this condition is similar in appearance to peritonitis (marked by abdominal pain, constipation, vomiting, and **fever**) that disappears shortly after surgery without antibiotics. Any postoperative symptoms that cause concern for the patient should be discussed with the doctor so that any fears can be alleviated. Due to the aftereffects of anesthesia, patients should not drive themselves home.

It is advisable for someone to stay with the patient for a few hours following the procedure in case complications arise. Injury to an organ might not be readily apparent for several days after the procedure. The physical signs that should be watched for and reported immediately include:

• fever and chills

• abdominal distention

• vomiting

• difficulty urinating

• sharp and unusual pain in the abdomen or bowel

• redness at the incision site, which indicates infection

• discharge from any places where tubes were inserted or incisions were made

Additional complications may include a urinary tract infection (resulting from catheterization) and minor infection of the incision site. Abdominal distention or a pain in the flank may indicate an injury to the ureter. Additional testing may be required if a complication is suspected.

Risks

Complications may be associated with the laparoscopy procedure in general or may be specific to the type of operation that is performed. Patients should consult with their doctors regarding the types of risks that are specific for their procedures. The most serious complication that can occur during laparoscopy is laceration of a major abdominal blood vessel resulting from improper positioning, inadequate insufflation (inflation) of the abdomen, abnormal pelvic anatomy, and too much force exerted during scope insertion. Thin patients with well-developed abdominal muscles are at higher risk, because the aorta may be only an inch or so below the skin. Obese patients are also at higher risk because more forceful and deeper needle and scope penetration is required. During laparoscopy, there is also a risk of bleeding from blood vessels, and adhesions may require repair by open surgery if bleeding cannot be stopped using laparoscopic instrumentation. In laparoscopic procedures that use electrosurgical devices, burns to the incision site are possible due to passage of electrical current through the laparoscope caused by a fault or malfunction in the equipment.

Complications related to insufflation of the abdominal cavity include gas inadvertently entering a blood vessel and causing an embolism, pneumothorax, or subcutaneous emphysema. One common but not serious side effect of insufflation is pain in the shoulder and upper chest area for a day or two following the procedure.

Any abdominal surgery, including laparoscopy, carries the risk of unintentional organ injury (punctures and perforations). For example, the bowel, bladder, ureters, or fallopian tubes may be injured during the laparoscopic procedure. Many times these injuries are unavoidable due to the patient's anatomy or medical condition. Patients at higher risk of bowel injury include those with chronic bowel disease, PID, a history of previous abdominal surgery, or severe endometriosis. Some types of laparoscopic procedures carry a higher risk of organ injury. For instance, during laparoscopic removal of endometriosis adhesions or ovaries, the

KEY TERMS

Ascites—Accumulation of fluid in the abdominal cavity.

Autologous blood donation—Donation of the patient's own blood, made several weeks before elective surgery.

Cannula—A small, flexible tube.

Cholecystitis—Inflammation of the gallbladder, often diagnosed using laparoscopy.

Conscious sedation—A level of sedation during which the patient remains awake but relaxed.

Electrosurgical device—A medical device that uses electrical current to cauterize or coagulate tissue during surgical procedures.

Embolism—Blockage of an artery by a clot, air or gas, or foreign material. Gas embolism may occur as a result of insufflation of the abdominal cavity during laparoscopy.

Endometriosis—A disease involving occurrence of endometrial tissue (lining of the uterus) outside the uterus in the abdominal cavity.

Hysterectomy—Surgical removal of the uterus; often performed laparoscopically.

Insufflation—Inflation of the abdominal cavity using carbon dioxide; performed prior to laparoscopy to give the surgeon space to maneuver surgical equipment.

Oophorectomy—Surgical removal of the ovaries.

Pneumothorax—Air or gas in the pleural space (lung area) that may occur as a complication of laparoscopy and insufflation.

Subcutaneous emphysema—A pathologic accumulation of air underneath the skin resulting from improper insufflation technique.

Trocar—A small sharp instrument used to puncture the abdomen at the beginning of the laparoscopic procedure.

QUESTIONS TO ASK YOUR DOCTOR

- Will this surgery be covered by my insurance? Will any postsurgical care that I require also be covered?
- What must I do to prepare for the surgery? Are there any restrictions on diet, fluid intake, or other measures?
- Are there any medications that should be stopped prior to the surgery?
- Does my medical history pose any potential problems that need to be considered before undergoing this procedure?
- What aftereffects can I expect?
- Are there any postsurgical symptoms that might indicate a complication that I should report, and to whom should these questions be directed? What postsurgical symptoms should be considered normal and how might discomfort be relieved?
- What is the expected recovery period from this procedure?
- What special care or self-care is required following this surgery?

Results

In diagnostic laparoscopy, the surgeon will be able to see signs of a disease or condition immediately, and can either treat the condition surgically or proceed with appropriate medical management. In diagnostic laparoscopy, tissue biopsies may be taken in questionable areas, and the laboratory results will determine the course of treatment. In therapeutic laparoscopy, the surgeon performs a procedure that rectifies a known medical problem, such as hernia repair or appendix removal. Because laparoscopy is minimally invasive compared to open surgery, patients may experience less trauma and postoperative discomfort, have fewer procedural complications, have a shorter hospital stay, and return more quickly to daily activities. The results will vary, however, depending on the patients's condition and type of treatment.

Alternatives

The alternatives to laparoscopy vary, depending on the medical condition being treated. Laparotomy (open abdominal surgery with larger incision) may be pursued

ureters may be injured due to their proximity to each other.

Several clinical studies have shown that the complication rate during laparoscopy is associated with inadequate surgeon experience. Surgeons who are more experienced in laparoscopic procedures have fewer complications than those performing their first 100 cases.

when further visualization is needed to treat the condition. For female patients with pelvic masses, transvaginal sonography may be a helpful technique in obtaining information about whether such masses are malignant, assisting in the choice between laparoscopy or laparotomy.

Health care team roles

Laparoscopy may be performed by a gynecologist, general surgeon, thoracic surgeon, gastroenterologist, or other physician, depending upon the patient's condition. An anesthesiologist or other specifically trained anesthesia personnel, such as a certified registered nurse anesthetist, is required during the procedure to administer general and/or local anesthesia and to perform patient monitoring. Nurses and surgical technicians/assistants are needed during the procedure to assist with scope positioning, camera operation, video system adjustments and image recording, and laparoscopic instrumentation.

Resources

BOOKS

Falcone, Tommaso, and William W. Hurd, eds. *Clinical Reproductive Medicine and Surgery: A Practical Guide.* New York: Springer, 2013.

Gabbe, Steven G., et al., eds. *Obstetrics: Normal and Problem Pregnancies.* Philadelphia: Elsevier/Saunders, 2012.

Lentz, Gretchen M., et al. *Comprehensive Gynecology.* Philadelphia: Mosby Elsevier, 2013.

Nussbaum, Michael S., ed. *Gastric Surgery.* Philadelphia: Wolters Kluwer Health/Lippincott Williams & Wilkins, 2013.

Tinelli, Andrea, ed. *Laparoscopic Entry: Traditional Methods, New Insights, and Novel Approaches.* London: Springer, 2012.

PERIODICALS

Di, Baoshan, et al. "Laparoscopic versus Open Surgery for Colon Cancer: A Meta-Analysis of 5-Year Follow-Up Outcomes." *Surgical Oncology* 22, no. 3 (2013): e39–43. http://dx.doi.org/10.1016/j.suronc.2013.03.002 (accessed October 3, 2014).

Muniraj, T., and P. Barve. "Laparoscopic Staging and Surgical Treatment of Pancreatic Cancer." *North American Journal of Medical Sciences* 5, no. 1 (2013): 1–9 http://dx.doi.org/10.4103/1947-2714.106183 (accessed August 18, 2014).

Singla, Anand, et al. "Is the Growth in Laparoscopic Surgery Reproducible with More Complex Procedures?" *Surgery* 146, no. 2 (2009): 367–74. http://dx.doi.org/10.1016/j.surg.2009.06.006 (accessed October 3, 2014).

Varela, J. E., and N. T. Nguyen. "Disparities in Access to Basic Laparoscopic Surgery at U.S. Academic Medical Centers." National Center for Biotechnology Information. (April 25, 2011). http://dx.doi.org/10.1007/s00464-010-1345-y (accessed October 3, 2014).

WEBSITES

A.D.A.M. Medical Encyclopedia. "Diagnostic Laparoscopy." MedlinePlus. http://www.nlm.nih.gov/medlineplus/ency/article/003918.htm (accessed October 3, 2014).

Ballehaninna, Umashankar K. "Exploratory Laparoscopy." Medscape Reference. http://emedicine.medscape.com/article/1829816-overview (accessed October 3, 2014).

Cleveland Clinic. "Diagnostic Laparoscopy." http://my.clevelandclinic.org/services/laparoscopic_diagnostics/hic_diagnostic_laparoscopy.aspx (accessed October 3, 2014).

Society of American Gastrointestinal Endoscopic Surgeons. "Diagnostic Laparoscopy Patient Information from SAGES." http://www.sages.org/publications/patient-information/patient-information-for-diagnostic-laparoscopy-from-sages (accessed October 3, 2014).

ORGANIZATIONS

American Congress of Obstetricians and Gynecologists, 409 12th St. SW, Washington, DC 20024-2188, (202) 638-5577, (800) 673-8444, resources@acog.org, http://www.acog.org.

Society of American Gastrointestinal Endoscopic Surgeons (SAGES), 11300 West Olympic Blvd., Ste. 600, Los Angeles, CA 90064, (310) 437-0544, Fax: (310) 437-0585, webmaster@sages.org, http://www.sages.org.

Society of Laparoendoscopic Surgeons, 7330 SW 62nd Pl., Ste. 410, Miami, FL 33143-4825, (305) 665-9959, Info@SLS.org, http://www.sls.org.

Jennifer E. Sisk, MA
Jill Granger, MS
REVISED BY WILLIAM A. ATKINS, BB, BS, MBA

Lapatinib

Definition

Lapatinib (Tykerb) is an anticancer drug designed to treat **cancer** of the breast. Lapatinib inhibits tumor cellular signaling by antagonizing a signaling pathway effecting tumor cell development. The tumor cells lapatinib is used against have a receptor on their cell surface called the human epidermal growth factor receptor type 2 (HER2).

Purpose

Lapatinib is used to treat advanced or metastatic **breast cancer** that has high levels of the growth factor receptor HER2 on the tumor cell surface. Lapatinib is used in patients who have received prior therapy with an anthracycline, a taxane, or **trastuzumab** and now need a new agent to treat their cancer.

KEY TERMS

Cytochrome P450—Enzymes present in the liver that metabolize drugs.

Epilepsy—Neurological disorder characterized by recurrent seizures.

Metastasis—The process by which cancer spreads from its original site to other parts of the body.

QT prolongation—Potentially dangerous heart condition that affects the rhythm of the heart beat and alters the ECG reading of the heart.

Receptor tyrosine kinase—Cell surface receptors that interact with growth factors and hormones to affect the normal life cycle of a cell.

Tuberculosis—Potentially fatal infectious disease that commonly affects the lungs, is highly contagious, and is caused by an organism known as *Mycobacterium tuberculosis*.

Description

Lapatinib is an anticancer drug that acts on receptor tyrosine kinases to inhibit the growth of tumors. Receptor tyrosine kinases are receptors for growth factors that are a natural part of cell development and necessary for normal cell growth. When tyrosine kinase receptors are activated, they initiate chemical signals that tell the cell how to grow and develop. Normal tyrosine kinase receptors turn on and off as needed for usual amounts of growth. However, when cells have constantly activated tyrosine kinase receptors, it can lead to abnormal growth and cancer. Drugs like lapatinib inhibit these overly active tyrosine kinase receptors.

Lapatinib is an inhibitor of two growth factor receptors, HER2 and epidermal growth factor receptor (EGFR). Both receptors are tyrosine kinases. Lapatinib is used in combination with the drug **capecitabine** for the treatment of advanced or metastatic HER2 breast cancer. The combination of capecitabine and lapatinib has an additive anticancer effect.

Lapatinib is manufactured by GlaxoSmithKline under the trade name Tykerb. It is sold under the trade name Tyverb in the European Union. Studies have shown that lapatinib is an effective drug, affecting both time to tumor progression and progression-free survival. The term *time to tumor progression* describes a period of time from when disease is diagnosed (or treated) until the disease starts to get worse. *Progression-free survival* describes the length of time during and after treatment in which a patient is living with a disease that does not get worse. Both time to tumor progression and progression-free survival may be used in a clinical study or trial to help find out how well a new treatment works. In studies done on lapatinib, patients receiving lapatinib in combination with capecitabine had a longer median time to tumor progression and a longer median progression-free survival than those receiving placebo or capecitabine alone.

Recommended dosage

Lapatinib is taken as an oral medication once a day. Lapatinib should not be taken with food and must be administered at least one hour apart from meals (one hour before or after meals). Lapatinib may be given in combination with capecitabine. The usual adult dose of lapatinib is 1.25 g per day. If a dose is missed, the patient should seek the advice of the physician and not double the next dose. It is important that the medication not be taken more than once daily. In patients with severe liver impairment, the dose of lapatinib may need to be reduced to 750 mg a day. Treatment with lapatinib is continued until disease progression occurs or until unacceptable levels of toxicity occur, whichever comes first.

Precautions

Lapatinib is not recommended for use in pregnant women. Birth control is recommended while using this drug. Lapatinib is a pregnancy Category D drug. Category D describes drugs in which there is evidence of potential human fetal risk based on adverse reaction data from investigational or marketing experience or studies in humans, but potential benefits may warrant use of the drug in pregnant women despite potential risks. For Category D drugs, medical necessity must be great enough to warrant risking harm to the fetus. Lapatinib is both a teratogen and lethal to fetuses in animal studies. Lapatinib is contraindicated for use in breast-feeding women. Lapatinib is used only in adults, as safety for use in patients less than 18 years of age has not been established. Lapatinib is absorbed through the skin and lungs if inhaled in powder form. Women who are pregnant or who may become pregnant should not handle lapatinib or breathe the dust from the tablets.

Lapatinib may cause a heart condition that affects the rhythm of the heartbeat known as QT prolongation. Sometimes QT prolongation can cause a serious cardiac condition that includes a fast and irregular heartbeat with severe dizziness and fainting. The risk of developing QT prolongation syndrome may be increased if the patient is taking other drugs that also affect the rhythm of the heart, or if the patient has cardiac problems. Low blood levels of potassium or magnesium may also increase risk of QT prolongation. Lapatinib toxicity may cause other adverse side effects affecting heart function, and multiple other medical heart conditions may result from use of lapatinib.

Lapatinib may not be suitable for patients with a history of certain types of heart failure. Caution must be used for lapatinib treatment in patients with liver disease or impairment. The liver is responsible for metabolizing lapatinib into inactive compounds. If this metabolism is impaired, higher levels of lapatinib in the bloodstream may cause toxicity. Patients with liver impairment may need a lower dose for treatment. Caution may be needed in patients with kidney impairment, as safety and effectiveness has not been fully established in this group of patients.

Side effects

Lapatinib is used when the medical benefit is judged to be greater than the risk of side effects. The most frequent side effects of lapatinib treatment are **diarrhea**, dry skin, rash, upset stomach, **fatigue**, diarrhea, nausea, and vomiting. Lapatinib also commonly causes hand-foot syndrome, caused by leakage of lapatinib out of small blood vessels in the hands and feet. During some types of **chemotherapy**, small amounts of medication in the bloodstream leak out of capillaries in the palms of the hands and the soles of the feet. Drug leakage is increased by heat exposure or friction. The result is redness, tenderness, and sometimes peeling of the skin of the palms and soles. The appearance of sunburn, numbness, and tingling may develop, and may interfere with the activity level of the patient.

Less commonly, lapatinib therapy may cause insomnia, body aches, and inflammation of the tissue lining the inside of the mouth. Lapatinib may cause abnormal liver function test results, liver disease, difficulty breathing, lung disease and inflammation, heart failure, and the heart condition called prolonged QT interval.

Interactions

Patients should advise their doctor of any and all medications or supplements they are taking before using lapatinib. Lapatinib interacts with many other drugs. Some drug interactions may make lapatinib unsuitable for use, while others may be monitored and attempted.

Lapatinib may have dangerous additive effects with other drugs that also cause QT prolongation. Drugs that interact with lapatinib in this way include amiodarone, dofetilide, pimozide, procainamide, quinidine, sotalol, and macrolide **antibiotics** such as erythromycin.

Lapatinib is metabolized by a set of liver enzymes known as cytochrome P450 (CYP-450) subtype 3A4.

QUESTIONS TO ASK YOUR DOCTOR

- How long must I take this drug before you can tell whether it helps me?
- How often must I have blood work and other laboratory tests done to check the effect the drug is having?
- Is this drug safe to take with the other drugs that I am currently taking?
- What side effects should I watch for? When should I call the doctor about them?
- Are there any clinical trials of this drug combined with other therapies that might benefit me?

Drugs that induce, or activate these enzymes increase the metabolism of lapatinib. This side effect results in lower levels of therapeutic lapatinib, thereby negatively affecting treatment of cancer. For this reason drugs that induce CYP-450 subtype 3A4 may not be used with lapatinib. This includes some antiepileptic drugs, such as **carbamazepine**; some anti-inflammatory drugs, such as **dexamethasone**; anti-tuberculosis drugs such as rifampin; and the herb St. John's wort.

Drugs that act to inhibit the action of CYP-450 subtype 3A4 may cause undesired increased levels of lapatinib in the body. This side effect could lead to toxic doses. Some examples are antibiotics such as clarithromycin, antifungal drugs such as ketoconazole, antiviral drugs such as indinavir, antidepressants such as fluoxetine, and some cardiac agents, such as verapamil. Grapefruit juice may also increase the amount of lapatinib in the body. Patients should avoid drinking grapefruit juice or eating grapefruit while taking lapatinib.

Resources

BOOKS

Brunton, Laurence, Bruce Chabner, and Bjorn Knollman. *Goodman and Gilman's The Pharmacological Basis of Therapeutics.* 12th ed. New York: McGraw-Hill Medical Publishing, 2012.

WEBSITES

American Cancer Society. "Lapatinib." http://www.cancer.org/treatment/treatmentsandsideeffects/guidetocancerdrugs/lapatinib (accessed November 4, 2014).

ORGANIZATIONS

National Cancer Institute, 9609 Medical Center Dr., BG 9609 MSC 9760, Bethesda, MD 20892-9760, (800) 4-CANCER (422-6237), http://www.cancer.gov.

U.S. Food and Drug Administration, 10903 New Hampshire Ave., Silver Spring, MD 20993, (888) INFO-FDA (463-6332), http://www.fda.gov.

Maria Basile, PhD.

Laryngeal cancer

Definition

Laryngeal **cancer** is cancer of the larynx or voice box.

Description

The larynx is located where the throat divides into the esophagus and the trachea. The esophagus is the tube that takes food to the stomach. The trachea, or windpipe, carries air to the lungs. The area where the larynx is located is sometimes called the Adam's apple.

The larynx has two main functions. It contains the vocal cords, cartilage, and small muscles that make up the voice box. When a person speaks, small muscles tighten the vocal cords, narrowing the distance between them. As air is exhaled past the tightened vocal cords, it creates sounds that are formed into speech by the mouth, lips, and tongue.

The second function of the larynx is to allow air to enter the trachea and to keep food, saliva, and foreign material from entering the lungs. A flap of tissue called the epiglottis covers the trachea each time a person swallows. This flap keeps foreign material from entering the lungs. When a person is not swallowing, the epiglottis

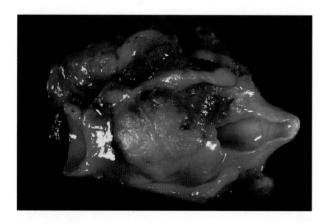

An extracted tumor found on the larynx. *(Gage/Custom Medical Stock Photo)*

retracts, allowing air to flow into the trachea. During treatment for cancer of the larynx, both of these functions may be lost.

Cancers of the larynx develop slowly. About 95% of these cancers develop from thin, flat cells similar to skin cells called squamous epithelial cells. These cells line the larynx. Gradually, the squamous epithelial cells begin to change and are replaced with abnormal cells. These abnormal cells are not cancerous but are premalignant cells that have the potential to develop into cancer. This condition is called dysplasia. Most people with dysplasia never develop cancer. The condition simply goes away without treatment, especially if the person with dysplasia stops smoking and drinking alcohol.

The larynx is made up of three parts, the glottis, the supraglottis, and the subglottis. Cancer can start in any of these regions. Treatment and survival rates depend on which parts of the larynx are affected and whether the cancer has spread to neighboring areas of the neck or distant parts of the body.

The glottis is the middle part of the larynx. It contains the vocal cords. Cancers that develop on the vocal cords are often diagnosed very early because even small vocal cord tumors cause hoarseness. In addition, the vocal cords have no connection to the lymphatic system, which means that cancers on the vocal cord do not spread easily. When confined to the vocal cords without any involvement of other parts of the larynx, the cure rate for this cancer is 75–95%.

The supraglottis is the area above the vocal cords. It contains the epiglottis, which protects the trachea from foreign materials. Cancers that develop in this region are usually not found as early as cancers of the glottis because the symptoms are less obvious. The supraglottal region has many connections to the lymphatic system, so cancers in this region tend to spread easily to the lymph nodes and may spread to other parts of the body (lymph nodes are small bean-shaped structures found throughout the body; they produce and store infection-fighting cells). In 25–50% of people with cancer in the supraglottal region, the cancer has already spread to the lymph nodes by the time they are diagnosed. Because of this, survival rates are lower than for cancers that involve only the glottis.

The subglottis is the region below the vocal cords. Cancer starting in the subglottis region is rare. When it does, it is usually detected only after it has spread to the vocal cords, where it causes obvious symptoms such as hoarseness. Because the cancer has already begun to spread by the time it is detected, survival rates are generally lower than for cancers in other parts of the larynx. Infection with **human papillomavirus** (HPV) is also a risk factor.

KEY TERMS

Dysplasia—Any abnormal change in size, shape, development, or organization of adult epithelial cells.

Human papillomaviruses (HPV)—A family of viruses that cause common warts of the hands and feet, as well as lesions and warts in the genital and vaginal area. More than 50 types of HPV have been identified, some of which are linked to cancerous and precancerous conditions.

Lymph—Clear, slightly yellow fluid carried by a network of thin tubes to every part of the body. Cells that fight infection are carried in the lymph.

Lymph nodes—Small bean-shaped collections of tissue found in a lymph vessel. They produce cells and proteins that fight infection and also filter lymph. Nodes are sometimes called lymph glands.

Lymphatic system—Primary defense against infection in the body. The lymphatic system consists of tissues, organs, and channels (similar to veins) that produce, store, and transport lymph and white blood cells to fight infection.

Malignant—Cancerous. Cells that tend to reproduce without normal controls on growth to form tumors or invade other tissues.

Metastasis—Spread of cells from the original site of the cancer to other parts of the body where secondary tumors are formed.

Monoclonal antibodies—Genetically engineered antibodies that are created in large numbers in the laboratory from a single immune cell; thus, they are all identical. They are useful in treating cancer because they bind to a specific site on the target cell and destroy it.

Demographics

The American Cancer Society predicted that 12,630 new cases of cancer of the larynx would be diagnosed in the United States in 2014 and about 3,610 people would die that year from the disease. Laryngeal cancer is between four and five times more common in men than in women. Almost all men who develop laryngeal cancer are over age 55. Laryngeal cancer is about 50% more common among African American men than among other Americans.

It is thought that older men are more likely to develop laryngeal cancer than women because the two main risk factors for the disease are lifetime habits of smoking and alcohol abuse. Men tend to smoke and drink more than women, and more African American men are heavy smokers compared to men of other races in the United States. As smoking becomes more prevalent among women, it seems likely that cases of laryngeal cancer in females will increase; however, smoking rates have begun to decline in the United States, and it is possible that the incidence of laryngeal cancer will likewise decline.

Causes and symptoms

Laryngeal cancer develops when the normal cells lining the larynx are replaced with abnormal cells (dysplasia) that become malignant and reproduce to form tumors. The development of dysplasia is strongly linked to lifelong habits of smoking and heavy use of alcohol. The more a person smokes, the greater the risk of developing laryngeal cancer. It is unusual for someone who does not smoke or drink to develop cancer of the larynx. Occasionally, however, people who inhale asbestos particles, wood dust, paint, or industrial chemical fumes over a long period develop the disease.

The symptoms of laryngeal cancer depend on the location of the tumor. Tumors on the vocal cords are rarely painful, but cause hoarseness. Anyone who is continually hoarse for more than two weeks or who has a cough that does not go away should see a doctor.

Tumors in the supraglottal region above the vocal cords often cause more varied but less obvious symptoms. These include:

• persistent sore throat

• pain when swallowing

• difficulty swallowing or frequent choking on food

• bad breath

• lumps in the neck

• persistent ear pain (called referred pain; the source of the pain is not the ear)

• change in voice quality

Tumors that begin below the vocal cords are rare, but may cause noisy or difficult breathing. All these symptoms can also be caused by other cancers as well as by less serious illnesses. However, if these symptoms persist, it is important to see a doctor and discover their cause; the earlier cancer treatment begins, the more successful it is.

QUESTIONS TO ASK YOUR DOCTOR

- What stage is my cancer, and what exactly does that mean?

- What are possible treatments for my cancer?

- How long will my treatment last?

- What are some of the changes in my activities that will occur because of my treatment?

- What is daily life like after a laryngectomy?

- How will I speak?

- I've heard about clinical trials using radiation and drugs to treat cancer of the larynx. Where can I find out more about these trials?

- What changes in my lifestyle can I make to help improve my chances of beating this cancer?

- How often will I have to have checkups?

- What is the likelihood that I will survive this cancer?

- Can you suggest any support groups that would be helpful to me or my family?

Diagnosis

On the first visit to a doctor for symptoms that suggest laryngeal cancer, the doctor takes a complete medical history, including family history of cancer and lifestyle information about smoking and alcohol use. The doctor also completes a physical examination, paying special attention to the neck region for lumps, tenderness, or swelling.

The next step is examination by an otolaryngologist, or ear, nose, and throat (ENT) specialist. This doctor also performs a physical examination, but in addition also looks inside the throat at the level of the larynx. Initially, the doctor may spray a local anesthetic on the back of the throat to prevent gagging, then use a long-handled mirror to look at the larynx and vocal cords. This examination is done in the doctor's office. It may cause gagging but is usually painless.

A more extensive examination involves a **laryngoscopy**. In a laryngoscopy, a lighted fiberoptic tube called a laryngoscope that contains a tiny camera is inserted through the patient's nose and mouth and snaked down the throat so that the doctor can see the larynx and surrounding area. This procedure can be completed with a sedative and local anesthetic in a doctor's office. More often, the procedure is done in an outpatient surgery clinic or hospital under general anesthesia. This examination allows the doctor to use tiny clips on the end of the laryngoscope to take biopsies (tissue samples) of any areas that look abnormal.

Laryngoscopies are usually painless and take about one hour. Some people complain of a scratchy throat after the procedure. Because laryngoscopies are done under sedation, patients should not drive immediately after the procedure and should have someone available to take them home. Laryngoscopy is a standard procedure that is covered by insurance.

The locations of the samples taken during the laryngoscopy are recorded, and the samples are then sent to the laboratory to be examined under the microscope by a pathologist who specializes in diagnosing diseases through cell samples and laboratory tests. It may take several days to get the results. Based on the findings of the pathologist, cancer can be diagnosed and staged.

Once cancer is diagnosed, other tests will be done to help determine the exact size and location of the tumors. This information is helpful in determining the most appropriate treatments. These tests may include:

- Endoscopy. Similar to a laryngoscopy, this test is done when it appears that cancer may have spread to other areas, such as the esophagus or trachea.

- Computed tomography (CT or CAT) scan. Using x-ray images taken from several angles and computer modeling, CT scans allow parts of the body to be seen in cross section. This imaging helps locate and size the tumors, and provides information on whether they can be surgically removed.

- Magnetic resonance imaging (MRI). MRI uses magnets and radio waves to create more detailed cross-sectional scans than computed tomography. This detailed information is needed if surgery is planned.

- Barium swallow. Barium is a substance that, unlike soft tissue, shows up on x-rays. Swallowed barium coats the throat and allows x-ray pictures to be made of the tissues lining the throat.

- Chest x-ray. Done to determine whether cancer has spread to the lungs. Because most people with laryngeal cancer are smokers, the risk of lung cancer or emphysema is high.

- Fine-needle aspiration (FNA) biopsy. If lumps on the neck are found, a thin needle is inserted into the lump and some cells are removed for analysis by the pathologist.

- Additional blood and urine tests. These tests do not diagnose cancer, but help to determine the patient's general health and provide information to determine which cancer treatments are most appropriate.

Treatment team

An otolaryngologist and an oncologist (cancer specialist) generally lead the treatment team. They are supported by radiologists to interpret CT and MRI scans, a head and neck surgeon, and nurses with special training in assisting cancer patients.

A speech pathologist is often involved in treatment, both before surgery to discuss various options for communication if the larynx is removed, and after surgery to teach alternate forms of voice communication. A social worker, psychologist, or family counselor may help both the patient and the family meet the changes and challenges brought on by living with laryngeal cancer.

At any point in the process, the patient may want a second opinion from another doctor in the same specialty. This is a common practice and does not indicate a lack of faith in the original doctor but simply a desire for more information. Some insurance companies require a second opinion before surgery.

Clinical staging

Once cancer of the larynx is discovered, additional tests will determine whether cancer cells have spread to other parts of the body. This process is called staging. Knowing the stage of the disease is necessary to plan treatment. In cancer of the larynx, the definitions of the early stages depend on where the cancer started.

Stage I

The cancer is limited to the area where it started and has not spread to lymph nodes in the immediate area or to other parts of the body. The exact definition of stage I depends on where the cancer started, as follows:

- Supraglottis: The cancer is limited to one area of the supraglottis and the vocal cords can move normally.

- Glottis: The cancer is limited to the vocal cords and the vocal cords can move normally.

- Subglottis: The cancer has not spread beyond the subglottis.

Stage II

The cancer is limited to the larynx and has not spread to lymph nodes in the area or to other parts of the body. The exact definition of stage II depends on where the cancer started, as follows:

- Supraglottis: The cancer appears in more than one area of the supraglottis, but the vocal cords can move normally.

- Glottis: The cancer has spread to the supraglottis or the subglottis or both. The vocal cords may or may not be able to move normally.

- Subglottis: The cancer has spread to the vocal cords, which may or may not be able to move normally.

Stage III

Either of the following may be true:

- The cancer has not spread beyond the larynx but the vocal cords cannot move normally, or the cancer has spread to tissues next to the larynx.

- The cancer has spread to one lymph node on the same side of the neck as the cancer, and the lymph node measures no more than 3 centimeters (just over 1 inch).

Stage IV

Any of the following may be true:

- The cancer has spread to tissues around the larynx, such as the pharynx or the tissues in the neck. The lymph nodes in the area may or may not contain cancer.

- The cancer has spread to more than one lymph node on the same side of the neck as the cancer, to lymph nodes on one or both sides of the neck, or to any lymph node that measures more than 6 centimeters (over 2 inches).

- The cancer has spread to other parts of the body.

Recurrent

Recurrent disease means that the cancer has come back (recurred) after treatment. It may recur in the larynx or in another part of the body.

Treatment

Treatment is based on the stage of the cancer as well as its location and the health of the individual. Generally, there are four types of treatments for cancer of the larynx. These are surgery, radiation, **chemotherapy**, and targeted therapy. They can be used alone or in combination according to the stage of the cancer. It helps to have a second opinion once the cancer has been staged to evaluate treatment options.

Surgery

The goal of surgery is to remove the tissue that contains malignant cells. There are several common surgeries to treat laryngeal cancer.

Stage III and stage IV cancers are usually treated with total **laryngectomy**. The entire larynx is removed. Sometimes other tissues around the larynx are also removed. A total laryngectomy involves the removal of the vocal cords. Alternate methods of voice communication must be learned with the help of a speech pathologist.

Smaller tumors are sometimes treated by partial laryngectomy. The goal is to remove the cancer but save as much of the larynx (and corresponding speech capability) as possible. Very small tumors or cancer in situ are sometimes successfully treated with laser excision surgery. In this surgery, a narrowly targeted beam of light from a laser is used to remove the cancer.

Advanced cancer (Stages III and IV) that has spread to the lymph nodes often requires an operation called a neck dissection. The goal of a neck dissection is to remove the lymph nodes and prevent the cancer from spreading. There are several forms of neck dissection. A **radical neck dissection** is the operation that removes the most tissue.

Several other operations may be performed for laryngeal cancer. A tracheotomy is a surgical procedure in which an artificial opening is made in the trachea (windpipe) to allow air into the lungs. This operation is necessary when the larynx is totally removed. A **gastrectomy** tube is a feeding tube placed through skin and directly into the stomach. It is used to give nutrition to people who cannot swallow or whose esophagus is blocked by a tumor. People who have a total laryngectomy usually do not need a gastrectomy tube as long as their esophagus remains intact.

Radiation

Radiation therapy uses high-energy rays, such as x-rays or gamma rays, to kill cancer cells. The advantage of radiation therapy is that it preserves the larynx and the ability to speak. The disadvantage is that it may not kill all the cancer cells. Radiation therapy can be used alone in early-stage cancers or in combination with surgery. Sometimes the plan is made to try radiation first; if it fails to cure the cancer, surgery still remains an option. Often, radiation therapy is used after surgery for advanced cancers to kill any cells the surgeon may have missed.

There are two types of radiation therapy. External beam radiation therapy focuses rays from outside the body on the cancerous tissue. This is the most common type of radiation therapy used to treat laryngeal cancer. With internal radiation therapy, also called brachytherapy, radioactive materials are placed directly in the cancerous tissue. This type of radiation therapy is a much less common treatment for laryngeal cancer.

External radiation therapy is administered in doses called fractions. A common treatment involves giving fractions five days a week for seven weeks. **Clinical trials** are under way to determine the benefits of accelerating the delivery of fractions (accelerated fractionation) or dividing fractions into smaller doses given more than once a day (hyperfractionation). Side effects of radiation therapy include dry mouth, sore throat, hoarseness, skin problems, trouble swallowing, and diminished ability to taste.

Chemotherapy

Chemotherapy is the use of drugs to kill cancer cells. Unlike radiation therapy, which targets a specific tissue, chemotherapy drugs are either taken by mouth or intravenously (through a vein) and circulate throughout the body. They are used mainly to treat advanced laryngeal cancer that is inoperable or that has metastasized to a distant site. Chemotherapy is often used after surgery or in combination with radiation therapy. Clinical trials are under way to determine the best combination of treatments for advanced cancer.

The two most common chemotherapy drugs used to treat laryngeal cancer are **cisplatin** and 5-fluorouracil (5-FU or **fluorouracil**). There are many side effects associated with chemotherapy drugs, including **nausea and vomiting**, loss of appetite (**anorexia**), hair loss (**alopecia**), **diarrhea**, and mouth sores. Chemotherapy can also damage the blood-producing cells of the bone marrow, which can result in low blood cell counts, increased chance of infection, and abnormal bleeding or bruising.

Targeted therapy

Targeted therapy is treatment with **monoclonal antibodies** that attack the specific protein produced by cancer cells. These antibodies are produced in large numbers in the laboratory and then infused into the patient's blood. They target a specific protein on the surface of the cancer cell and destroy it. Targeted therapy will not cure cancer, but it will slow the growth and decrease the number of cancer cells. Targeted therapies are often used along with chemotherapy for the most effective results.

Alternative and complementary therapies

Alternative and complementary therapies range from herbal remedies, vitamin supplements, and special diets to spiritual practices, acupuncture, massage, and similar treatments. When these therapies are used in addition to conventional medicine, they are called complementary therapies. When they are used instead of conventional medicine, they are called alternative therapies.

Complementary or alternative therapies are widely used by people with cancer. No specific alternative therapies have been directed toward laryngeal cancer. However, good nutrition and activities that reduce stress and promote a positive view of life have no unwanted side effects and appear beneficial in boosting the ability of the immune system to fight cancer.

Unlike traditional pharmaceuticals, complementary and alternative therapies are not evaluated by the United States Food and Drug Administration (FDA) for either safety or effectiveness. These therapies may have interactions with traditional pharmaceuticals. Patients should be wary of "miracle cures" and notify their doctors if they are using herbal remedies, vitamin supplements or other unprescribed treatments because these remedies may interact in harmful ways with other drugs the individual is taking. Alternative and experimental treatments are not normally covered by insurance.

Coping with cancer treatment

Cancer treatment, even when successful, has many unwanted side effects. In laryngeal cancer, the primary side effects are the loss of speech due to total laryngectomy and the need to breathe through a hole in the neck called a stoma. Several alternative methods of sound production, both mechanical and learned, are available, and should be discussed with a speech pathologist. Support groups also exist for people who have had their larynx removed. Coping with speech loss and care of the stoma is discussed more extensively in the laryngectomy entry.

Chemotherapy is accompanied by many unwanted side effects, most of which disappear once the chemotherapy ends. For example, hair will regrow, and until it does, a wig can be used. Medications are available to treat nausea and vomiting. Side effects such as dry skin are treated symptomatically.

Prognosis

Cure rates and survival rates can predict group outcomes, but can never precisely predict the outcome for a single individual. However, the earlier laryngeal cancer is discovered and treated, the more likely it will be cured.

Cancers found in stage 0 and stage 1 have a 75–95% cure rate depending on the site. Late-stage cancers that have metastasized have a very poor survival rate, with intermediate stages falling somewhere in between. People who have had laryngeal cancer are at greatest risk of recurrence (having cancer come back), especially in the head and neck, during the first two to three years after treatment. Check-ups during the first year are needed every other month, and four times a year during the second year. It is rare for laryngeal cancer to recur after five years of being cancer-free.

Clinical trials

Clinical trials are government-regulated studies of new treatments and techniques that may prove beneficial in diagnosing or treating a disease. Participation is always voluntary and at no cost to the participant. Clinical trials are conducted in three phases. Phase 1 tests the safety of the treatment and looks for harmful side effects. Phase 2 tests the effectiveness of the treatment. Phase 3 compares the treatment to other treatments available for the same condition.

The selection of clinical trials under way changes frequently. Patients and their families can search for new trials on the **National Cancer Institute** website at http://www.cancer.gov/clinicaltrials/search.

Prevention

By far, the most effective way to prevent laryngeal cancer is to not smoke. Smokers who quit smoking also significantly decrease the risk of developing the disease. Other ways to prevent laryngeal cancer include limiting the use of alcohol, eating a well-balanced diet, seeking treatment for prolonged heartburn, and avoiding inhaling asbestos and chemical fumes. Vaccination against HPV may also provide some protection against the development of throat cancers, although its main purpose is to prevent **cervical cancer** in women and genital warts in men and women.

Special concerns

Diagnosis with cancer is traumatic. Not only is one's health affected, one's whole life suddenly revolves around trips to the doctor for cancer treatment and adjusting to the side effects of these treatments. This process is stressful for both the cancer patient and family members. It is not unusual for family members to feel resentment about the changes that occur in the family, and then feel guilty about that resentment.

The loss of voice because of laryngeal surgery may be the most traumatic effect of laryngeal cancer. Losing the ability to communicate easily with others can be isolating. Support groups and psychological counseling is helpful for both the cancer patient and family members. Many national organizations that support cancer education can provide information on in-person or online support and education groups.

Resources

BOOKS

National Cancer Institute, ed. Gale Schoenle. *Cancer of the Larynx - Enhanced Edition: Learn What Is Cause, Risk Factors, Symptoms, Diagnosis, Treatment and Health Care* MedHealth, 2012 (e-book only).

WEBSITES

American Cancer Society. "Laryngeal and Hypopharyngeal Cancer." http://www.cancer.org/cancer/laryngealandhypopharyngealcancer/detailedguide/index (accessed June 8, 2014).

Johnson, Jonas T. "Malignant Tumors of the Larynx." Medscape Reference. http://emedicine.medscape.com/article/848592-overview (accessed June 8, 2014).

"Throat Cancer." MedlinePlus. http://www.nlm.nih.gov/medlineplus/throatcancer.html (accessed June 8, 2014).

ORGANIZATIONS

American Academy of Otolaryngology—Head and Neck Surgery, 1650 Diagonal Road, Alexandria, VA 22314-2857, (703) 836-4444.

American Cancer Society, 1599 Clifton Rd., NE, Atlanta, GA 30329, (404) 320-3333, (800) ACS-2345, http://www.cancer.org.

National Cancer Institute, BG 9609 MSC 9760, 9609 Medical Center Drive, Bethesda, MD 20892-9760, (800) 4-CANCER; TTY: (800) 332-8615, http://www.cancer.gov.

Tish Davidson, AM
REVISED BY MELINDA G. OBERLEITNER, DNS, RN

Laryngeal nerve palsy

Description

Laryngeal nerve palsy is damage to the recurrent laryngeal nerve (or less commonly the vagus nerve) that results in paralysis of the larynx (voice box). Paralysis may be temporary or permanent. Damage to the recurrent laryngeal nerve is most likely to occur during surgery on the thyroid gland to treat **cancer** of the thyroid. Laryngeal nerve palsy is also called recurrent laryngeal nerve damage.

The vagus nerve is one of 12 cranial nerves that connect the brain to other organs in the body. It runs from the brain to the large intestine. In the neck, the vagus nerve gives off a paired branch nerve called the recurrent laryngeal nerve. The recurrent laryngeal nerves lie in grooves along either side of the trachea (windpipe) between the trachea and the thyroid gland.

The recurrent laryngeal nerve controls movement of the larynx. The larynx is located where the throat divides into the esophagus, a tube that takes food to the stomach, and the trachea (windpipe) that carries air to the lungs. The larynx contains the apparatus for voice production: the vocal cords, and the muscles and ligaments that move the vocal cords. It also controls the flow of air into the lungs. When the recurrent laryngeal nerve is damaged, the movements of the larynx are reduced. This reduction causes vocal weakness, hoarseness, or sometimes the complete loss of voice. The changes may be temporary or permanent. In rare life-threatening cases of damage, the larynx is paralyzed to the extent that air cannot enter the lungs.

Causes

Laryngeal nerve palsy is an uncommon side effect of surgery to remove the thyroid gland (thyroidectomy). It occurs in 1–2% of operations for total thyroidectomy to treat cancer, and less often when only part of the thyroid is removed. Damage can occur to either one or both branches of the nerve, and it can be temporary or permanent. Most people experience only transient laryngeal nerve palsy and recover their normal voice within a few weeks.

Laryngeal nerve palsy can also occur from causes unrelated to thyroid surgery. These include damage to either the vagus nerve or the laryngeal nerve due to tumors in the neck and chest or disorders in the chest such as aortic aneurysms. Both tumors and aneurysms press on the nerve, and the pressure causes damage.

Treatment

Once the recurrent laryngeal nerve is damaged, there is no specific treatment to heal it. With time, most cases of recurrent laryngeal palsy improve on their own. In the event of severe damage, the larynx may be so paralyzed that air cannot flow past it into the lungs. When this happens, an emergency tracheotomy must be performed to save the patient's life. A tracheotomy is a surgical procedure to make an artificial opening in the trachea (windpipe) to allow air to bypass the larynx and enter the lungs. If paralysis of the larynx is temporary, the tracheotomy opening can be surgically closed when it is no longer needed.

Some normal variation in the location of the recurrent laryngeal nerve occurs among individuals. Occasionally the nerves are not located exactly where the surgeon expects to find them. Choosing a board-certified head and neck surgeon who has had extensive experience with thyroid operations is the best way to prevent laryngeal nerve palsy.

Alternative and complementary therapies

There are no alternative or complementary therapies to heal laryngeal nerve palsy. The passage of time alone restores speech to most people. Some alternatives for artificial speech exist for people whose loss of speech is permanent.

See also Laryngectomy.

Resources

PERIODICALS

Bures, C., et al. "Late-onset Palsy of the Recurrent Laryngeal Nerve after Thyroid Surgery." *British Journal of Surgery* 101 (November 2014): 1556–1559.

Harti, Dana M., and Daniel F. Brasnu. "Recurrent Laryngeal Nerve Paralysis: Current Concepts and Treatment." *Ear, Nose and Throat Journal* 79, no. 12 (December 2000): 918.

WEBSITES

Grebe, Werner, M.D. "Thyroid Operations." *EndocrineWeb. com.* [cited July 19, 2009]. http://www.endocrineweb.com/surthyroid.html.

University of Virginia Health System. "Surgical Tutorial: Surgical Approach for a Thyroid Mass." *University of Virginia Health System, Department of Surgery.* [cited July 19, 2009]. http://hsc.virginia.edu/surgery/tutorial-surgthyroid.html.

Tish Davidson, AM

Laryngectomy

Definition

A laryngectomy is the partial or complete surgical removal of the voice box (larynx).

Purpose

Because of its location, the voice box, or larynx, plays a critical role in breathing, swallowing, and speaking. The larynx is located above the windpipe (trachea) and in front of the food pipe (esophagus). It contains two small bands of muscle called the vocal cords that close to prevent food from entering the lungs and vibrate to produce the voice. If **cancer** of the larynx develops, a laryngectomy is performed to remove tumors or cancerous tissue. In rare cases, the procedure may also be performed when the larynx is badly damaged by gunshot, automobile injuries, or other traumatic accidents.

Description

Laryngectomies may be total or partial. In a total laryngectomy, the entire larynx is removed. If the cancer has spread to other surrounding structures in the neck, such as the lymph nodes, they are removed at the same time. If the tumor is small, a partial laryngectomy is performed, in which only a part of the larynx, usually one vocal chord, is removed. Partial laryngectomies are also often performed in conjunction with other cancer treatments, such as **radiation therapy** or **chemotherapy**.

During a laryngectomy, the surgeon removes the larynx through an incision in the neck. The procedure also requires the surgeon to perform a tracheotomy, because air can no longer flow into the lungs. He or she makes an artificial opening called a stoma in the front of the neck. The upper portion of the trachea is brought to the stoma and secured, making a permanent alternate pathway for air to reach the lungs. The connection between the throat and the esophagus is not normally affected, so after healing, the person whose larynx has been removed can eat normally.

Preparation

A laryngectomy is performed after cancer of the larynx has been diagnosed by a series of tests that allow the otolaryngologist (a physician often called an ear, nose and throat, or ENT specialist) to examine the throat and take tissue samples (biopsies) to confirm and stage the cancer. People need to be in good general health to undergo a laryngectomy, and will have standard preoperative blood work and tests to make sure they are able to safely withstand the operation.

As with any surgical procedure, the patient is required to sign a consent form after the procedure is thoroughly explained. Blood and urine studies, along with a chest x-ray and EKG, may be ordered as required. If a total laryngectomy is planned, the patient meets with a speech pathologist for discussion of postoperative expectations and support.

Aftercare

A person undergoing a laryngectomy spends several days in intensive care (ICU) and receives intravenous (IV) fluids and medication. As with any major surgery, blood pressure, pulse, and respiration are monitored regularly. The patient is encouraged to turn, cough, and breathe deeply to help mobilize secretions in the lungs. One or more drains are usually inserted in the neck to remove any fluids that collect. These drains are removed after several days.

It takes two to three weeks for the tissues of the throat to heal. During this time, the patient cannot swallow food and must receive nutrition through a tube inserted through the nose and down the throat into the stomach. Normal speech is also no longer possible; patients are instructed in alternate means of vocal communication by a speech pathologist.

When air is drawn in normally through the nose, it is warmed and moistened before it reaches the lungs. When air is drawn in through the stoma, it does not have the opportunity to be warmed and humidified. In order to keep the stoma from drying out and becoming crusty, patients are encouraged to breathe artificially humidified air. The stoma is usually covered with a light cloth to keep it clean and to keep unwanted particles from accidentally entering the lungs. Care of the stoma is extremely important, because it is the person's only way to get air to the lungs. After a laryngectomy, a healthcare professional will teach the patient and his or her caregivers how to care for the stoma.

There are three main methods of vocalizing after a total laryngectomy. In esophageal speech, patients learn how to "swallow" air down into the esophagus and create sounds by releasing the air. Tracheoesophageal speech diverts air through a hole in the trachea made by the surgeon. The air then passes through an implanted artificial voice box. The third method involves using a hand-held electronic device that translates vibrations into sounds. The choice of vocalization method depends on several factors including the age and health of the patient, and whether other parts of the mouth, such as the tongue, have also been removed (**glossectomy**).

Risks

Laryngectomy is often successful in curing early-stage cancers; however, it requires major lifestyle changes, and there is a risk of severe psychological stress from unsuccessful adaptations. Patients must learn new ways of speaking, and they must be constantly concerned about the care of their stoma. Serious problems can occur if water or other foreign material enters the lungs through an unprotected stoma. Also, women who undergo partial laryngectomy or who learn some types of artificial speech will have a deep voice similar to that of a man. For some women, this change presents psychological challenges. As with any major operation, there is a risk of infection. Infection is of

QUESTIONS TO ASK YOUR DOCTOR

- Is laryngectomy my only viable treatment option?
- How will drinking and eating be affected?
- How will I talk without my larynx?
- How will my breathing be affected?
- What about my usual activities?
- Is there a support group in the area that can assist me after surgery?
- How long will it be until I can verbally communicate? What are my options?
- What is the risk of recurrent cancer?

particular concern to patients who have chosen to have a voice prosthesis implanted and is one of the major reasons for having to remove the device.

Results

Ideally, removal of the larynx will remove all cancerous material. The person will recover from the operation, make the necessary lifestyle adjustments, and return to an active life.

Alternatives

Radiation and chemotherapy are two alternative forms of treatment. Radiation therapy uses high-energy rays (such as **x-rays**) to kill or shrink cancer cells. Chemotherapy uses drugs to kill cancer cells. The drugs are usually delivered into a vein or by mouth. Once the drugs enter the bloodstream, they spread throughout the body to the cancer site.

Health care team roles

A laryngectomy is usually performed by an otolaryngologist in a hospital operating room. In cases of trauma to the throat, the procedure may be performed by an emergency room physician.

Resources

BOOKS

Flint, Paul F., et al. *Cumming's Otolaryngology: Head and Neck Surgery*. 5th ed. rev. Philadelphia: Mosby/Elsevier, 2010.

Niederhuber, John E., et al. *Abeloff's Clinical Oncology*. 5th ed. Philadelphia: Saunders/Elsevier, 2013.

PERIODICALS

Basheeth, N., et al. "Hypocalcaemia after Total Laryngectomy: Incidence and Risk Factors." *The Laryngoscope* (October 1, 2013): e-pub ahead of print. http://dx.doi.org/10.1002/lary.24429 (accessed October 3, 2014).

Lagier, A., et al. "The Influence of Age on Postoperative Complications after Total Laryngectomy or Pharyngolaryngectomy." *European Journal of Surgical Oncology (EJSO)* (September 17, 2013): e-pub ahead of print. http://dx.doi.org/10.1016/j.ejso.2013.09.010 (accessed October 3, 2014).

WEBSITES

A.D.A.M. Medical Encyclopedia. "Laryngectomy." MedlinePlus. http://www.nlm.nih.gov/medlineplus/ency/article/007398.htm (accessed October 3, 2014).

American Cancer Society. "What Are the Key Statistics about Laryngeal and Hypopharyngeal Cancers?" http://www.cancer.org/cancer/laryngealandhypopharyngealcancer/detailedguide/laryngeal-and-hypopharyngeal-cancer-key-statistics (accessed October 3, 2014).

National Cancer Institute. "Laryngeal Cancer Treatment (PDQ®)." http://www.cancer.gov/cancertopics/pdq/treatment/laryngeal/Patient (accessed October 3, 2014).

National Cancer Institute. "Throat (Laryngeal and Pharyngeal) Cancer." http://www.cancer.gov/cancertopics/types/throat (accessed October 3, 2014).

University of Pittsburgh Medical Center. "Total Laryngectomy." http://www.upmc.com/patients-visitors/education/cancer/Pages/total-laryngectomy.aspx (accessed January 29, 2015).

ORGANIZATIONS

American Academy of Otolaryngology—Head and Neck Surgery, 1650 Diagonal Rd., Alexandria, VA 22314-2857, (703) 836-4444, http://www.entnet.org.

American Cancer Society, 250 Williams St. NW, Atlanta, GA 30303, (800) 227-2345, http://www.cancer.org.

International Association of Laryngectomees (IAL), 925B Peachtree St., NE Ste. 316, Atlanta, GA 30309, (866) 425-3678, http://www.theial.com.

National Cancer Institute, 6116 Executive Blvd., Ste. 300, Bethesda, MD 20892-8322, (800) 4-CANCER (422-6237), http://cancer.gov.

National Institute on Deafness and Other Communication Disorders (NIDCD), NIDCD Office of Health Communication and Public Liaison, 31 Center Dr., MSC 2320, Bethesda, MD 20892-2320, (301) 496-7243, (800) 241-1044, TTY: (800) 241-1055, nidcdinfo@nidcd.nih.gov, http://www.nidcd.nih.gov.

Kathleen Dredge Wright
Tish Davidson, AM
Monique Laberge, PhD.
REVISED BY ROSALYN CARSON-DEWITT, MD

Laryngoscopy

Definition

Laryngoscopy refers to a procedure used to view the inside of the larynx (the voice box).

Description

The purpose and advantage of seeing inside the larynx is to detect tumors, foreign bodies, nerve or structural injury, or other abnormalities. Two methods allow the larynx to be seen directly during the examination. In one, a flexible tube with a fiber-optic device is threaded through the nasal passage and down into the throat. The other method uses a rigid viewing tube passed directly from the mouth through the throat and into the larynx. A light and lens affixed to the endoscope are used in both methods. The endoscopic tube may also be equipped to suction debris or remove material for **biopsy**. **Bronchoscopy** is a similar but more extensive procedure in which the tube is passed through the larynx and down into the trachea and bronchi.

Preparation

Laryngoscopy is done in the hospital with a local anesthetic spray to minimize discomfort and suppress the gag reflex. Patients are requested not to eat for several hours before the examination.

Aftercare

If the throat is sore, soothing liquids or lozenges may help relieve any temporary discomfort.

Risks

This procedure carries no serious risks, although the patient may experience soreness in the throat or cough up small amounts of blood until the irritation subsides.

Results

A normal result is the absence of signs of disease or damage.

Abnormal results

An abnormal finding, such as a tumor or an object lodged in the tissue, would either be removed or identified for further medical attention.

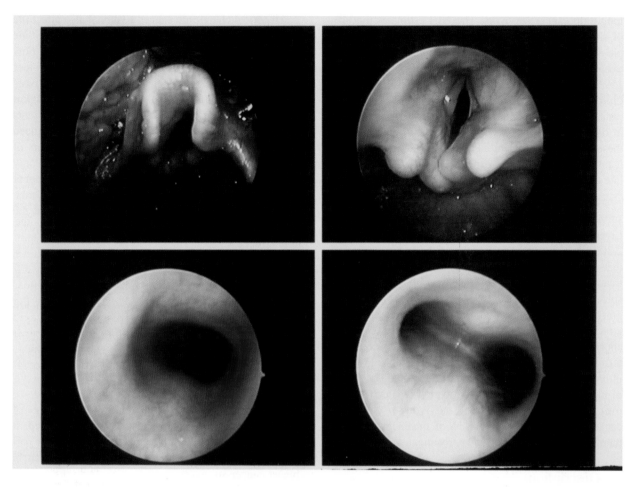

In a laryngoscopy, a tube (laryngoscope) is inserted through the mouth to visualize the larynx. Images show the epiglottis, vocal cords, and interior of the trachea and bronchus. *(CMSP/Custom Medical Stock Photo)*

KEY TERMS

Endoscope—A tube that is inserted into a hollow organ permitting a physician to see inside it.

Resources

WEBSITES

A.D.A.M. Medical Encyclopedia. "Laryngoscopy." Medline-Plus. http://www.nlm.nih.gov/medlineplus/ency/article/007507.htm (accessed November 4, 2014).

Canadian Cancer Society. "Laryngoscopy." http://www.cancer.ca/en/cancer-information/diagnosis-and-treatment/tests-and-procedures/laryngoscopy/?region=on (accessed November 4, 2014).

Jill S. Lasker

L-asparaginase *see* **Asparaginase**

Late effects of cancer treatment

Definition

In general, a late effect of any disease is defined as a condition or symptom that appears once the acute phase of a disease has ended and the disease has been treated. Late effects may be direct, a result of the original disease, or indirect, a consequence of the therapies that were used to treat the disease. With regard to **cancer** in particular, the **National Cancer Institute** (NCI) defines a late effect as "A health problem that occurs months or years after a disease is diagnosed or after treatment has ended . . . [It] may be caused by cancer or cancer treatment [and] may include physical, mental, and social problems and second cancers."

Demographics

Late effects of cancer therapy have become an issue in recent years due to the sheer increase in the numbers of long-term cancer survivors. The NCI estimates that 4% of the American population—about 14.5 million people—have survived for 5 years or longer after cancer treatment, with 41% having lived 10 years or longer, and 15% having lived 20 years or more. With regard to **childhood cancers**, 270,000 survivors of childhood cancer reside in the United States as of 2014, or about 1 in 640 young people. By any standard of measurement, these survivors represent a sizable population of Americans who have already experienced or may anticipate late effects of cancer treatment.

Recent studies indicate that a majority of cancer survivors report late symptoms of treatment. The Livestrong Foundation conducted a survey in 2006 of 2,300 adult respondents. Results of the survey indicated that 91% reported at least one physical late effect of treatment; 95% reported at least one emotional or spiritual late effect; and 75% reported at least one practical concern (education, finances, etc.) related to late effects. The most common physical late effects experienced by the survivors were **fatigue** (59%); cognitive difficulties (55%); and problems with sexuality and intimacy (46%). A group of researchers at the University of Florida College of Medicine reported in late 2013 that over 80% of a group of 1,660 survivors of childhood cancer suffered from late effects of treatment, some of them as much as 30 years after treatment.

Description

Late effects are a major concern of cancer survivors. They may arise months or even years after cancer treatment has ended, and are usually evaluated and treated during the third or long-term stage of cancer survivorship. It is, however, difficult to generalize about either the severity or the type of late effects experienced by survivors; some have almost no late effects and can return to their previous level of function while others experience severe disability that lasts for years. The American Cancer Society (ACS) noted in 2013 that the following groups of survivors are at increased risk of severe late effects:

• people who were treated with more aggressive or intensive cancer therapies

• people who were diagnosed in childhood or adolescence

• people from groups with lower socioeconomic status

• people of African American or Hispanic ethnicity

The ACS also found that those diagnosed at younger ages tended to have more severe emotional effects while those diagnosed when they were older tended to have more severe physical effects.

Historical changes in cancer treatment also affect the nature of late effects of this group of diseases. Some treatments that were standard before the 1990s are now obsolete, but survivors who were treated under the older protocols may experience late effects that survivors treated more recently do not. An example is **Hodgkin lymphoma**. Spleen removal was common in patients with this disease prior to 1988. Patients without a spleen are at increased risk of infection. Currently, survivors of Hodgkin **lymphoma** have their spleens removed only when needed for palliative therapy. Since cancer treatment has progressed a great deal in recent years, many late effects are still unknown. It is likely that the profile of late effects of cancer treatment will change over the next decade.

Causes and late effects

Late effects of cancer treatment are usually categorized by type of therapy:

Surgery

Late effects of surgery may include:

• Lymphedema. Lymphedema refers to swelling of tissues in areas where lymph nodes were removed; it is caused by the buildup of lymphatic fluid in that part of the body. Lymphedema is particularly common in breast cancer survivors.

• Infertility. Men who have had lymph nodes removed near the kidneys, bladder, rectum, or testicles may be unable to father children. Women who have had a complete hysterectomy and oophorectomy cannot bear children.

• Nutritional imbalances or digestive problems. These are most common in survivors of stomach or colon cancer, or surgery on the throat or oral cavity affecting the ability to swallow.

• Phantom limb pain. Phantom limb pain, the painful sensation that an amputated limb is still attached to the body, may be experienced by survivors who have had limbs removed to treat cancers of the bone or soft tissue.

• Psychological and emotional distress. Distress often follows surgery that disfigures the face or neck, requires amputation, or otherwise affects the survivor's body image.

Radiation therapy

Radiation therapy is known to produce more late effects than surgery:

- Increased risk of second cancers. A second cancer is a different primary cancer that occurs at least two months after cancer therapy ends.
- Cataracts in the eye.
- Dental problems: gum loss and tooth decay.
- Bone loss and osteoporosis.
- Heart problems.
- Intestinal disorders.
- Infertility.
- Lung disease.
- Hypothyroidism.
- Memory loss and difficulty thinking clearly. Sometimes referred to as "chemo brain," this condition can also occur as a late effect of radiation therapy.

Chemotherapy

Late effects of **chemotherapy** are also more numerous than those resulting from surgery. They include all the late effects of radiation therapy plus:

- Infertility in women.
- Chronic pain.
- Liver disorders.
- Early menopause in women.
- Bone, joint, and soft tissue disorders.
- Increased risk of stroke.
- Peripheral neuropathy: tingling or burning sensations in the extremities resulting from nerve damage.
- Chronic diarrhea.
- Weight gain. This late effect is found most often in breast cancer survivors.
- Muscle weakness.

Each type of cancer therapy may result in late emotional effects, including fear of cancer recurrence, anxiety, **depression**, impotence or loss of interest in sex, or posttraumatic stress disorder (PTSD). About 10% of cancer survivors meet the criteria for major depressive disorder and another 20% meet the criteria for PTSD. And although most cancer patients recover a normal level of energy after treatment ends, between 17% and 26% of survivors report persistent fatigue as a late effect of therapy.

Special populations

As noted earlier, the profile of late effects is different for younger survivors of cancer therapy from those of persons treated as adults. Two major factors are responsible for the difference: first, younger survivors are treated while they are still growing; second, younger survivors have a longer period of survivorship following treatment, which allows more time for late effects to appear. The risk of developing late effects increases over time.

Children and adolescents

Late effects in children and adolescents vary according to the child's sex; age at diagnosis and treatment; family history of cancer (if any); and the child's health problems prior to cancer diagnosis. Since late effects in this age group are a major concern, parents might consider treatment and follow-up at a specialized children's cancer center if possible. Late effects that appear frequently among survivors of childhood cancer include:

- Increased risk of second cancers. Survivors of childhood cancers have a higher risk of second cancers than adult survivors.
- Increased risk of stroke, damaged blood vessels, and heart attacks. These are most common in survivors of childhood leukemias, lymphomas, brain tumors, and head and neck cancers.
- Short stature resulting from delayed or stunted growth of the long bones.
- Obesity, delayed puberty, and infertility.
- Loss of vision and/or hearing.
- Memory problems and learning disorders; difficulty in learning to read, write, or do simple arithmetic.
- Increased risk of suicidal thoughts and attempted suicide compared to survivors of adult cancer.
- Increased risk of seizures, problems with hand-eye coordination, chronic headaches, or loss of bladder and bowel control.
- Social withdrawal, difficulty forming relationships, delayed dating, marriage, and family formation.
- Missing or improperly formed teeth; incompletely formed jawbone.
- Increased risk of gallstones, liver failure, and type 2 diabetes.
- Increased risk of thyroid disorders (hyperthyroidism or hypothyroidism).

Young adults

Young adult cancer survivors (defined as persons between the ages of 20 and 39) experience late effects from treatment similar to those of children. The effects are usually less severe because most of their physical and intellectual growth is completed before diagnosis and treatment. Young adult survivors are at greatest risk of late effects in body systems that were not fully mature at the time of diagnosis. They also face major financial challenges related to insurance coverage, as Medicaid coverage of children with cancer ends at age 18 or 21, depending on the state. According to the ACS, the most common late effects in young adult survivors are:

- Difficulties with completing post-high school education or job training and finding employment.

- Loss of fertility in both women and men. In some cases, it may be possible to store the young adult's eggs or sperm prior to cancer treatment.

- Increased risk of second cancers.

- Disorders of the heart, lungs, liver, or kidneys.

- Hearing or vision problems.

- Hormone deficiencies.

- Chronic pain or swelling in various parts of the body. The ACS recommends that young adult survivors consult the Children's Oncology Group (COG), which has extensive experience in treating younger survivors, and download the COG's guidelines for long-term follow-up at the link provided below.

Coping with late effects

Cancer survivors need ongoing follow-up care, including regular checkups, recommendations for a healthy recovery, and in some cases, regular screenings for **second cancers**. A newer approach to improved long-term care of cancer survivors is the survivorship care plan or SCP. SCPs were first introduced in 2007 on the recommendation of the Institute of Medicine. A survivorship care plan includes a comprehensive summary of the patient's cancer treatment, with information about the survivor's primary cancer, stage, and date of diagnosis; the specific therapies administered and their dates; complications (if any); and supplemental therapies provided (**physical therapy**, psychotherapy, etc.). The SCP includes a detailed plan for follow-up care, including who will perform the tests and screenings and where those will occur; signs or symptoms of cancer recurrence that the survivor should be aware of; a list of possible late effects and their symptoms; and specific recommendations for lifestyle changes if needed.

Survivors coping with late effects of cancer treatment often benefit from supportive care, which may include mental health services, support groups, financial counseling, or palliative treatments for chronic pain or other late physical effects. Others find the use of complementary and alternative (CAM) treatments helpful for relieving insomnia, lowering emotional stress levels, assisting with **pain management**, and strengthening immune function. The National Center for Complementary and Alternative Medicine (NCCAM) reported in 2011 that cancer survivors are more likely than the general public to use CAM approaches, and that 65% of

---

KEY TERMS

Chemo brain—A term used to describe problems with memory, concentration, or thinking clearly following chemotherapy.

Late effect—In general, a condition or symptom that appears after the acute phase of a disease has run its course. The late effect may be caused directly by the original disease or indirectly by treatments for the disease.

Lymphedema—A condition that occurs when lymph nodes under the arm are removed by surgery or damaged by radiation therapy as part of breast cancer treatment. Fluid build-up in the affected area results in pain and sometimes partial loss of arm function.

Peripheral neuropathy—Spontaneous tingling or burning sensations in the extremities, or muscle twitching or muscle weakness due to nerve damage resulting from cancer therapy.

Protocol—A detailed written plan for a medical treatment, procedure, or clinical study.

Second cancer—A different primary cancer that occurs at least two months after cancer treatment ends. Second cancers may occur months or years after treatment for a first cancer has concluded.

Supportive care—In regard to cancer, the prevention or management of the adverse effects of cancer and cancer treatment.

Survivorship care plan (SCP)—The record of a patient's cancer history and recommendations for follow-up care. It details the responsibilities of all care providers, whether cancer-related, primary care, or psychosocial. The SCP is intended to improve the survivor's care coordination and avoid duplication of resources.

---

survivors used at least one CAM treatment during recovery from cancer treatment. The CAM approaches used most often by long-term cancer survivors were prayer and meditation (61%); deep breathing and other relaxation techniques (44%); and **vitamins** and nutritional supplements (40%).

Prevention

As of 2014, there is no known way to prevent late effects of cancer therapy, partly because of the wide variation in types of treatment received, body parts affected, and responses to therapy. Also, the long-term

QUESTIONS TO ASK YOUR DOCTOR

- Can you help me draw up a survivorship care plan?
- Which late effects of my treatment am I at greatest risk of developing?
- Which signs or symptoms of late effects should I watch for?
- Should I consult any specialists for screening or treatment of late effects?
- Am I at significant risk of a second cancer?
- What lifestyle changes do you recommend to help me maintain a healthy recovery?
- Where can I go for help with anxiety or depression?

effects of newer cancer therapies are still unknown. Doctors are able to predict a survivor's risk of some late effects if they have complete records of treatments and the dates of administration.

Resources

BOOKS

Berger, Ann M., John L. Shuster, Jr., and Jamie Von Roenn, eds. *Principles and Practice of Palliative Care and Supportive Oncology.* 4th ed. Philadelphia, PA: Wolters Kluwer Health/Lippincott Williams and Wilkins, 2013.

Institute of Medicine (IOM). *Implementing Cancer Survivorship Care Planning: Workshop Summary.* Washington, DC: National Academies Press, 2007. Available online free of charge at http://books.nap.edu/openbook.php?record_id=11739.

[No author listed]. *Alert—Late Adverse Effects of Cancer Treatment.* New York: Springer, 2013.

Olver, Ian N., ed. *The MASCC Textbook of Cancer Supportive Care and Survivorship.* New York: Springer, 2011.

PERIODICALS

Brinkman, T.M., et al. "Suicide Ideation and Associated Mortality in Adult Survivors of Childhood Cancer." *Cancer* 120 (January 15, 2014): 271–277.

D'Agostino, N.M., and K. Edelstein. "Psychosocial Challenges and Resource Needs of Young Adult Cancer Survivors: Implications for Program Development." *Journal of Psychosocial Oncology* 31 (December 2013): 585–600.

Effinger, K.E., et al. "Oral and Dental Late Effects in Survivors of Childhood Cancer: A Children's Oncology Group Report." *Supportive Care in Cancer* 22 (July 2014): 2009–2019.

Fernbach, A., et al. "Evidence-Based Recommendations for Fertility Preservation Options for Inclusion in Treatment Protocols for Pediatric and Adolescent Patients Diagnosed with Cancer." *Journal of Pediatric Oncology Nursing* 31 (May 5, 2014): 211–222.

Hoekstra, R.A., M.J. Heins, and J.C. Korevaar. "Health Care Needs of Cancer Survivors in General Practice: A Systematic Review." *BMC Family Practice* 15 (May 13, 2014): 94.

Huang, I.C., et al. "Association between the Prevalence of Symptoms and Health-related Quality of Life in Adult Survivors of Childhood Cancer: A Report from the St. Jude Lifetime Cohort Study." *Journal of Clinical Oncology* 31 (November 20, 2013): 4242–4251.

Mao, J.J., et al. "Complementary and Alternative Medicine Use Among Cancer Survivors: A Population-based Study." *Journal of Cancer Survivorship* 5 (March 2011): 8–17.

Treanor, C.J., and M. Donnelly. "The Late Effects of Cancer and Cancer Treatment: A Rapid Review." *Journal of Community and Supportive Oncology* 12 (April 2014): 137–148.

Ward, E., et al. "Childhood and Adolescent Cancer Statistics, 2014." *CA: A Cancer Journal for Clinicians* 64 (March-April 2014): 83–103.

WEBSITES

American Cancer Society (ACS). "Cancer Treatment and Survivorship: Facts and Figures 2012–2013." http://www.cancer.org/acs/groups/content/@epidemiologysurveilance/documents/document/acspc-033876.pdf (accessed July 28, 2014).

American Cancer Society (ACS). "Late and Long-term Effects of Cancer Treatment in Young Adults." http://www.cancer.org/cancer/cancerinyoungadults/detailedguide/cancer-in-young-adults-treating-late-effects (accessed July 27, 2014).

Cancer.Net. "Long-term Side Effects of Cancer Treatment." http://www.cancer.net/survivorship/long-term-side-effects-cancer-treatment (accessed July 26, 2014).

Children's Oncology Group (COG). "Long-Term Follow-up Guidelines, version 3.0." http://www.survivorshipguidelines.org (accessed July 28, 2014).

Livestrong Foundation. "Late Effects of Cancer Treatment." http://www.livestrong.org/we-can-help/healthy-living-after-treatment/late-effects-of-cancer-treatment (accessed July 27, 2014).

Mayo Clinic. "Cancer Survivors: Late Effects of Cancer Treatment." http://www.mayoclinic.org/diseases-conditions/cancer/in-depth/cancer-survivor/ART-20045524 (accessed July 26, 2014).

National Cancer Institute (NCI). "Late Effects of Treatment for Childhood Cancer (PDQ)." http://www.cancer.gov/cancertopics/pdq/treatment/lateeffects/Patient/page1/AllPages (accessed July 27, 2014).

Nemours Foundation. "Late Effects of Cancer and Cancer Treatment." http://kidshealth.org/parent/_cancer_center/cancer_basics/late_effects.html (accessed July 27, 2014).

Susan G. Komen. "Late Effects of Breast Cancer Treatment." http://ww5.komen.org/BreastCancer/LateEffects.html (accessed July 27, 2014).

ORGANIZATIONS

American Cancer Society (ACS), 250 Williams Street NW, Atlanta, GA 30303, (800) 227-2345, http://www.cancer.org/aboutus/howwehelpyou/app/contact-us.aspx, http://www.cancer.org/index.

American Society of Clinical Oncology (ASCO), 2318 Mill Road, Suite 800, Alexandria, VA 22314, (571) 483-1300, (888) 651-3038, Fax: (571) 366-9537, contactus@cancer.net, http://www.asco.org.

Children's Oncology Group (COG), 222 E. Huntington Drive, Suite 100, Monrovia, CA 91016, (626) 447-0064, Fax: (626) 445-4334, HelpDesk@childrensoncologygroup.org, http://www.childrensoncologygroup.org.

Multinational Association of Supportive Care in Cancer (MASCC), c/o Åge Schultz, Herredsvejen 2, Hillerød, Denmark DK-3400, +45 48 20-7022, Fax: +45 48 21-7022, aschultz@mascc.org, http://www.mascc.org.

National Cancer Institute (NCI) Office of Cancer Survivorship, BG 9609 MSC 9760, 9609 Medical Center Drive, Bethesda, MD 20892-9760, (240) 276-6690, http://www.cancer.gov/global/contact/email-us, http://cancercontrol.cancer.gov/ocs/index.html.

National Comprehensive Cancer Network (NCCN), 275 Commerce Drive, Suite 300, Fort Washington, PA 19034, (215) 690-0300, Fax: (215) 690-0280, http://www.nccn.org.

Susan G. Komen, 5005 LBJ Freeway, Suite 250, Dallas, TX 75244, (877) 465-6636, http://ww5.komen.org/Contact.aspx, http://ww5.komen.org.

Rebecca J. Frey, PhD.

Laxatives

Definition

A laxative is a drug that helps relieve constipation.

Purpose

Laxatives are used to prevent or treat constipation. They are also used to prepare the bowel for an examination or surgical procedure.

Description

Laxatives work in different ways: by stimulating colon movement, adding bulk to the contents of the colon, or drawing fluid or fat into the intestine. Some laxatives work by combining these functions. Most primary care physicians recommend that patients try the bulk-producing laxatives first before taking saline or stimulant laxatives.

Bisacodyl

Bisacodyl is a nonprescription stimulant laxative. It reduces short-term constipation and is also used to prepare the colon or rectum for an examination or surgical procedure. The drug works by stimulating colon movement (peristalsis); constipation is usually relieved within 15 minutes to one hour after administration of the suppository form and in 6 to 12 hours after taking the drug orally.

Calcium polycarbophil

Calcium polycarbophil is a nonprescription bulk-forming laxative that is used to reduce both constipation and **diarrhea**. It draws water to the intestine, enlarging the size of the colon and thereby stimulating movement. It reduces diarrhea by removing extra water from the stool. This drug should relieve constipation in 12 to 24 hours and have maximum effect in three days. Colitis patients should see a reduction in diarrhea within one week.

Docusate calcium/docusate sodium

Docusate, a nonprescription laxative, helps a patient avoid constipation by softening the stool. It works by increasing the penetration of fluids into the stool by emulsifying feces, water and fat. Docusate prevents constipation and softens bowel movements and fecal impactions. This laxative should relieve constipation within one to three days.

Lactulose

Lactulose, a prescription laxative, reduces constipation and lowers blood ammonia levels. It works by drawing fluid into the intestine, raising the amount of water in the stool, and preventing the colon from absorbing ammonia. It is used to help people who suffer from chronic constipation.

Psyllium

Psyllium is a nonprescription bulk-forming laxative that reduces both constipation and diarrhea. It mixes with water to form a gel-like mass that can pass easily passed through the colon. Constipation is relieved in 12 to 24 hours and maximum relief is achieved after several days.

Senna/senokot

Senna/senokot is a nonprescription laxative that reduces constipation by promoting colon movement. It is used to treat bouts of constipation and to prepare the colon for an examination or surgical procedure. This laxative reduces constipation in eight to 10 hours.

New and investigational treatments for constipation

Some newer options for the treatment of chronic constipation are being developed by various groups of researchers. These include such alternative therapies as biofeedback; newer drugs like tegaserod (Zelnorm) and prucalopride (Resolor), which stimulate peristalsis; a nerve growth factor known as neurotrophin-3; and electrical stimulation of the colon.

Recommended dosage

Laxatives may be taken by mouth or rectally (suppository or enema).

Bisacodyl

- Adults or children over 12 years: 5–15 mg taken by mouth in morning or afternoon (up to 30 mg for surgical or exam preparation).
- Adult (rectal): 10 mg.
- Children age 2 to 11 years: 10 mg rectally as single dose.
- Children over three years: 5–10 mg by mouth as single dose.
- Children under two years: 5 mg rectally as single dose.

Calcium polycarbophil

- Adult: 1 g by mouth every day, up to four times a day as needed (not to exceed 6 g by mouth in a 24-hour time period).
- Children age 6 to 12 years: 500 mg by mouth twice a day as needed (not to exceed 3 g in a 24-hour time period).

- Children age 3 to 6 years: 500 mg twice a day by mouth, as needed (not to exceed 1.5 g in a 24-hour time period).

Docusate

- Adult (docusate sodium): 50–300 mg by mouth per day.
- Adult (docusate calcium or docusate potassium): 240 mg by mouth as needed.
- Adult (docusate sodium enema): 5 mL.
- Children over 12 years (docusate sodium enema): 2 mL.
- Children age 6 to 12 years (docusate sodium): 40–120 mg by mouth per day.
- Children age 3 to 6 years (docusate sodium): 20–60 mg by mouth per day.
- Children under 3 years (docusate sodium): 10–40 mg by mouth every day.

Lactulose

CONSTIPATION.
- Adult: 15–60 mL by mouth every day.
- Children: 7.5 mL by mouth every day.

ENCEPHALOPATHY.
- Adult: 20–30 g three or four times a day until stools become soft. Retention enema: 30–45 mL in 100 mL of fluid.
- Infants and children: Parents should follow the physician's directions for infants and children with encephalopathy.

Psyllium

- Adult: 1–2 teaspoons mixed in 8 ounces of water two or three times a day by mouth, followed by 8 ounces water; or one packet in 8 ounces water two or three times a day, followed by 8 ounces of water.
- Children over 6 years: 1 teaspoon mixed in 4 ounces of water at bedtime.

Senna/senokot

- Adult (Senokot): 1 to 8 tablets taken by mouth per day or 1/2–4 teaspoons of granules mixed in water or juice.
- Adult (rectal suppository): 1 to 2 at bedtime.
- Adult (syrup): 1–4 teaspoons at bedtime.
- Adult (Black Draught): 3/4 ounce dissolved in 2.5 ounces liquid, given between 2 P.M. and 4 P.M. on the day prior to a medical exam or procedure.
- Children: Parents should ask their doctor as dosage is based on weight. Black Draught is not to be used by children.

• Children age 1 month to 1 year (Senokot): 1.25–2.5 mL of syrup at bedtime.

Precautions

The doctor should be informed of any prior allergic drug reaction, especially prior reactions to any laxatives. Pregnancy is also a concern. Animal studies have shown laxatives to have adverse effects on pregnancy, but no human studies regarding pregnancy are currently available. These drugs are given in pregnancy only after the risks to the fetus have been taken under consideration. Nursing mothers should use caution and consult their doctors before receiving these drugs.

Bisacodyl should not be administered to patients with rectal fissures, abdominal pain, nausea, vomiting, appendicitis, abdominal surgery, ulcerated hemorrhoids, acute hepatitis, fecal impaction, or blockage in the biliary tract. Calcium polycarbophil should not be given to anyone with a gastrointestinal blockage (obstruction).

Both psyllium and docusate calcium/docusate sodium should be avoided by patients with intestinal blockage, fecal impaction, or **nausea and vomiting**. Lactulose should be avoided by patients who are elderly, have diabetes mellitus, eat a low-galactose diet, or whose general health is poor.

Senna/senokot is inadvisable for patients with congestive heart failure, gastrointestinal bleeding, intestinal blockage, abdominal pain, nausea and vomiting, appendicitis, or prior abdominal surgery.

The American College of Toxicology states that cathartics should *not* be used as a means of clearing poisons from the digestive tract of a poisoning victim. Although some physicians have administered these laxatives along with activated charcoal in order to reduce the body's absorption of the poison, this treatment is no longer recommended.

Side effects

Laxatives may have side effects. Some, such as nausea and vomiting, are more common than others. Side effects related to specific laxatives are described in this section. With repeated use, people may become dependent on laxatives. All side effects should be reported to a doctor.

Bisacodyl

Common side effects:

• nausea

• vomiting

• loss of appetite (anorexia)

• cramps

Less common side effects:

• muscle weakness

• diarrhea

• electrolyte changes

• rectal burning (when suppositories are used).

Life-threatening:

• severe muscle spasms (tetany)

Calcium polycarbophil

Side effects may include:

• abdominal bloating (distention)

• gas

• laxative dependency

Life-threatening:

• gastrointestinal obstruction

Docusate calcium/docusate sodium

Side effects include:

• bitter taste in the mouth

• irritated throat

• nausea

• cramps

• diarrhea

• loss of appetite

• rash

Lactulose

Common side effects include:

• nausea

• vomiting

• loss of appetite

• abdominal cramping

• bloating

• belching

• diarrhea

Psyllium

Common side effects include:

• nausea

• vomiting

• loss of appetite

• diarrhea

Less common side effects include:

• abdominal cramping

• blockage of the esophagus or intestine

Senna/senokot

Common side effects include:

• nausea

• vomiting

• loss of appetite

• abdominal cramping

Less common side effects include:

• diarrhea

• gas

• urine that is pink-red or brown-black in color

• abnormal electrolyte levels

Life-threatening:

• Severe muscle spasms (tetany)

Interactions

Laxatives may interact with other drugs. Sometimes the laxative can interfere with proper absorption of another drug. A patient must notify the doctor or pharmacist if he or she is already taking any medications so that the proper laxative can be selected or prescribed. Specific drug interactions are:

• Bisacodyl: Antacids, H2 blockers, and some herbal remedies (lily of the valley, pheasant's eye, squill).

• Calcium polycarbophil: lowers the absorption of tetracycline.

• Docusate calcium/docusate sodium: Increases the absorption of mineral oil if taken together with Haley's M-O, Kondremul, or other preparations containing mineral oil.

• Lactulose: Neomycin and other laxatives.

• Psyllium: Cardiac glycosides, oral anticoagulants, and salicylates.

• Senna/senokot: Disulfiram should never be taken with this drug. Also, senna/senokot lowers the absorption of other drugs taken by mouth.

Resources

BOOKS

Beers, Mark H., MD, and Robert Berkow, MD, editors. "Diarrhea and Constipation." In The *Merck Manual of Diagnosis and Therapy*. Whitehouse Station, NJ: Merck Research Laboratories, 2007.

Karch, A. M. *Lippincott's Nursing Drug Guide*. Springhouse, PA: Lippincott Williams & Wilkins, 2003.

PERIODICALS

DiPalma, J. A. "Current Treatment Options for Chronic Constipation." *Reviews in Gastroenterological Disorders*4, Supplement 2 (2004): S34–S42.

Newton, G. D., W. S. Pray, and N. G. Popovich. "New OTC Drugs and Devices 2003: A Selective Review." *Journal of the American Pharmaceutical Association* 44 (March-April 2004): 211–225.

Paré, P., and R.N. Fedorak. "Systematic Review of Stimulant and Nonstimulant Laxatives for the Treatment of Constipation." *Canadian Journal of Gastroenterology and Hepatology* 28 (November 2014): 549–557.

"Position Paper: Cathartics." *Journal of Toxicology: Clinical Toxicology* 42 (March 2004): 243–253.

Schiller, L. R. "New and Emerging Treatment Options for Chronic Constipation." *Reviews in Gastroenterological Disorders* 4, Supplement 2 (2004): S43–S51.

Talley, N. J. "Management of Chronic Constipation." *Reviews in Gastroenterological Disorders* 4 (Winter 2004): 18–24.

ORGANIZATIONS

ASHP (formerly the American Society of Health-System Pharmacists), 7272 Wisconsin Ave., Bethesda, MD 20814, (301) 664-8700, (866) 279-0681, custserv@ashp.org, http://www.ashp.org.

National Digestive Diseases Information Clearinghouse, 2 Information Way, Bethesda, MD 20892-3570, (800) 891-5389, TTY: (866) 569-1162, Fax: (703) 738-4929, nddic@info.niddk.nih.gov, http://www.digestive.niddk.nih.gov.

U.S. Food and Drug Administration, 10903 New Hampshire Ave., Silver Spring, MD 20993, (888) INFO-FDA (463-6332), http://www.fda.gov.

Rhonda Cloos, R.N.
Rebecca J. Frey, PhD.

Leiomyosarcoma

Definition

Leiomyosarcoma is a **cancer** that consists of smooth muscle cells and small-cell **sarcoma** tumor. The cancer begins in smooth muscle cells that grow uncontrollably and form tumors.

Description

Leiomyosarcomas can originate in any organ that contains smooth muscle but are also sometimes found in the walls of the stomach, large and small intestines, esophagus, uterus, or deep within the abdomen (retroperitoneal). Smooth-muscle cancers are quite rare: less

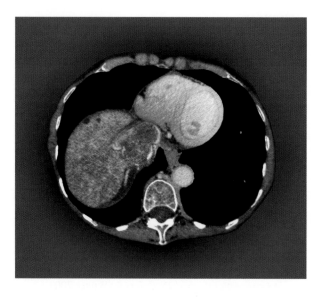

Computed tomography (CT) scan of the heart revealing a leiomyosarcoma, shown in purple. *(ZEPHYR/Science Photo Library)*

than 1% of all cancers are leiomyosarcomas. Very rarely, leiomyosarcomas begin in blood vessels or the skin.

Most leiomyosarcomas are found in the stomach. The second most common site is the small bowel, followed by the colon, rectum, and esophagus.

Demographics

Leiomyosarcomas rarely occur in the breast and uterus. Uterine sarcomas comprise less than 1% of gynecological malignancies and 2–5% of all uterine malignancies. They affect only 0.1% of women of childbearing age who have tumors of the uterus. Less than 2% of tumors in women over age 60 who are undergoing hysterectomy are leiomyosarcomas.

Causes and symptoms

The exact causes of leiomyosarcomas are unknown, although they are associated with certain genetic and environmental risk factors. Some inherited conditions may increase the risk of leiomyosarcoma. High-dose radiation exposure, such as radiotherapy used to treat other types of cancer, has also been linked to leiomyosarcoma. It is possible that exposure to certain chemical herbicides may increase the risk of sarcomas, but this association is not proven.

Because leiomyosarcomas can occur in any location, the symptoms vary according to the site of the tumor. When a leiomyosarcoma begins in an organ in the abdomen, such as the stomach or small bowel, a large lump or mass may be evident upon physical examination.

When a leiomyosarcoma affects a blood vessel, the flow of blood to the body part supplied by the artery may be blocked. Symptoms may include:

- painless lump or mass
- painful swelling
- abdominal pain
- weight loss
- nausea and vomiting

Diagnosis

A leiomyosarcomas may be diagnosed when a patient discovers a lump or mass or swelling on a body part and visits the doctor. Others have symptoms related to the internal organ affected by the leiomyosarcoma. For example, a tumor in the stomach may cause nausea, feelings of fullness, internal bleeding, and **weight loss**. The patient's doctor will take a detailed medical history followed by a complete physical examination, with special attention to the suspicious symptom or body part.

Depending on the location of the tumor, the doctor may order **imaging studies** such as an x-ray, **computed tomography** (CT) scan, or **magnetic resonance imaging** (MRI) to help determine the size, shape, and exact location of the tumor. A **biopsy** of the tumor is needed to make the definitive diagnosis of leiomyosarcoma. The tissue sample is examined by a pathologist (specialist in the study of diseased tissue).

Types of biopsy

The type of biopsy depends on the tumor location. For some small tumors, the doctor may perform an excisional biopsy, removing the entire tumor and a margin of surrounding normal tissue. Most often, the doctor will perform an incisional biopsy, a procedure that involves cutting out only a small piece of the tumor to determine its type and grade.

Treatment team

Patients with leiomyosarcoma are usually cared for by a multidisciplinary team of health professionals. The patient's family or primary care doctor may refer the patient to other specialists, such as surgeons and oncologists (specialists in cancer medicine), radiologic technicians, nurses, and laboratory technicians. Depending on the tumor's location and treatment plan, patients may benefit from rehabilitation therapy with physical therapists and nutritional counseling from dieticians.

Biopsy—The surgical removal and microscopic examination of living tissue for diagnostic purposes.

Chemotherapy—Treatment of cancer with synthetic drugs that destroy the tumor, either by inhibiting the growth of cancerous cells or by killing them.

Oncologist—A doctor who specializes in cancer medicine.

Pathologist—A doctor who specializes in the diagnosis of disease by studying cells and tissues under a microscope.

Radiation therapy—Cancer treatment using high-energy radiation.

Stage—A term used to describe the size and extent of spread of cancer.

Clinical staging

Tumors are staged to determine how far the disease has advanced and to develop a treatment plan. Stage is determined by the size of the tumor, whether the tumor has spread to nearby lymph nodes, whether the tumor has spread elsewhere in the body, and what the cells look like microscopically. For leiomyosarcoma, doctors also consider whether the tumor is deep or superficial.

The pathologist classifies tumors as high grade or low grade by staining the tissue and examining it under a microscope. The cells in a high-grade tumor increase more rapidly, which makes these tumors more serious than low-grade tumors.

Tumors are staged using numbers I through IV. The higher the number, the further the tumor has advanced. Stage IV leiomyosarcomas either involve lymph nodes or have spread to distant parts of the body.

Treatment

Treatment for leiomyosarcoma varies according to the location of the tumor, its size and grade, and the extent of its spread. Treatment planning also takes into account the patient's age, medical history, and general health.

Leiomyosarcomas on the arms and legs may be treated by **amputation** (removal of the affected limb) or by limb-sparing surgery to remove the tumor only. These tumors may also be treated with **radiation therapy**, **chemotherapy**, or a combination.

Generally, tumors inside the abdomen are surgically removed. The site, size, and extent of the tumor determine the type of surgery performed. Leiomyosarcomas of organs in the abdomen may also be treated with radiation and chemotherapy.

As researchers learn more about the genes and cells underlying leiomyosarcoma and other soft tissue sarcomas, treatments improve. New targeted therapies, which attack precise molecules in cancer cells that support their growth while sparing healthy cells, are improving treatment of all cancers, including soft tissue cancers. A drug called **sunitinib** shows promise in slowing **soft tissue sarcoma** tumor growth. Other promising drugs block vessels that provide blood to sarcomas, thus slowing tumor growth. A drug called **bevacizumab** may help stop blood supply to some sarcomas.

Side effects

The surgical treatment of leiomyosarcoma carries risks related to the surgical site, such as loss of function resulting from amputation or from nerve and/or muscle loss. Risks include those associated with any surgical procedure, such as reactions to general anesthesia or infection after surgery.

The side effects of radiation therapy depend on the site being radiated. Radiation therapy can produce side effects such as **fatigue**, skin rashes, nausea, and **diarrhea**. Most of the side effects lessen or disappear completely once the radiation therapy is complete.

The side effects of chemotherapy vary according to the medication or combination of **anticancer drugs** used. Nausea, vomiting, **anemia**, lower resistance to infection, and hair loss (**alopecia**) are common side effects. Medication may alleviate the unpleasant side effects of chemotherapy.

Alternative and complementary therapies

Many patients explore alternative and complementary therapies to help to reduce the stress associated with illness, and improve immune function and overall comfort. While there is no evidence that these therapies specifically combat disease, activities such as biofeedback, relaxation, therapeutic touch, massage therapy, and guided imagery have been reported to enhance well-being.

Coping with cancer treatment

Fatigue is a common complaint during cancer treatment and recovery. Many patients benefit by learning how to conserve energy to accomplish their daily tasks. It is important to rest and take breaks from strenuous activities. It is often helpful to plan activities around times of day when energy is highest. Mild exercise; small, frequent nutritious snacks; and limiting physical and emotional stress also help to combat fatigue.

Depression, emotional distress, and anxiety associated with the disease and its treatment may respond to counseling from a mental health professional. Many cancer patients and their families find participation in mutual aid and group support programs helpful in relieving feelings of isolation and loneliness.

Prognosis

The outlook for patients with leiomyosarcoma varies. It depends on the location and size of the tumor, its type, and the extent of its spread. The prognosis is excellent for patients who have had small tumors located in or near the skin surgically removed. Their 5-year survival is greater than 90%. Among patients with leiomyosarcomas in organs in the abdomen, survival is most likely when the tumor has been completely removed. In general, high-grade tumors that have spread widely throughout the body are not associated with favorable survival rates. Patients with weakened immune systems also tend to have aggressive tumors and a poor prognosis.

Clinical trials

When patients have rare tumors such as leiomyosarcoma, a clinical trial often is the best option. Patients also might want to seek care, or a second opinion, from a cancer center that specializes in treatment of sarcomas. The **National Cancer Institute** (NCI) website lists current **clinical trials** at http://cancertrials.nci.nih.gov.

Prevention

Since the causes of leiomyosarcoma are not completely known, there are no recommendations for prevention. This type of cancer is thought to be linked to radiation exposure; however, high levels of radiation exposure are the result of therapy to treat other forms of cancer. Among families with an inherited tendency to develop soft tissue sarcomas, careful monitoring may help to ensure early diagnosis and treatment of the disease.

Special concerns

Leiomyosarcoma, like other cancer diagnoses, may produce a range of emotional responses. Education, counseling, and participation in support group programs may help to reduce feelings of fear, anxiety and hopelessness. For many patients suffering from spiritual distress, visits with clergy members and participation in organized prayer may offer comfort.

Resources

BOOKS

Abeloff, M. D., et al. *Clinical Oncology*. 5th ed. New York: Churchill Livingstone, 2014.

Niederhuber, J. E., et al. *Clinical Oncology*. 5th ed. Philadelphia: Elsevier, 2014.

WEBSITES

"An Introduction to Leiomyosarcoma of the Bone and Soft Tissue." The Liddy Shriver Sarcoma Initiative. http://sarcomahelp.org/leiomyosarcoma.html#tpm1_1 (accessed October 9, 2014).

"New Research and Treatments." National Leiomyosarcoma Foundation. http://www.nlmsf.org/what-is-lms/treatments/new-research-treatments (accessed October 9, 2014).

ORGANIZATIONS

American Cancer Society, 250 Williams St. NW, Atlanta, GA 30303, (800) 227-2345, http://www.cancer.org.

National Cancer Institute, 9609 Medical Center Drive, Bethesda, MD 20892, (800) 422-6237, http://www.cancer.gov.

Barbara Wexler, M.P.H.
REVISED BY TERESA G. ODLE

Leptomeningeal carcinomatosis *see* **Carcinomatous meningitis**

Letrozole *see* **Aromatase inhibitors**

Leucovorin

Definition

Leucovorin (also known as Wellcovorin and citrovorum factor or folinic acid) is a drug that can be used either to protect healthy cells from **chemotherapy** or to enhance the anticancer effect of chemotherapy.

Purpose

Leucovorin is most often used in **cancer** patients undergoing either **methotrexate** or **fluorouracil** chemotherapy. Methotrexate is used to treat a wide range of cancers, including **breast cancer**, **head and neck cancers**, **acute leukemias**, and Burkitt **lymphoma**. Fluorouracil is used in combination with leucovorin to treat colorectal cancer. When leucovorin and methotrexate are used together, this therapy often is called leucovorin rescue because leucovorin rescues healthy cells from the toxic effects of methotrexate. In patients with colorectal cancer, however, leucovorin increases the anticancer effect of fluorouracil.

Leucovorin also is used to treat megaloblastic **anemia**, a blood disorder in which red blood cells become larger than normal, and to treat accidental overdoses of drugs such as methotrexate.

Description

Leucovorin is a faster-acting and stronger form of **folic acid**, and has been used for several decades. Folic acid also is known as vitamin B_9, and is needed for the normal development of red blood cells. In humans, dietary folic acid must be reduced metabolically to tetrahydrofilic acid (THFA) to exert its vital biochemical functions. The coenzyme THFA and its subsequent other cofactors participate in many important reactions, including DNA synthesis.

Leucovorin rescue

Some chemotherapy drugs, such as methotrexate (Trexall), work by preventing cells from using folic acid. Methotrexate therapy causes cancer cells to develop a folic acid deficiency and die. However, normal cells also are affected by folic acid deficiency. As a result, patients treated with drugs such as methotrexate often develop blood disorders and other toxic side effects. When these patients are given leucovorin, it enters normal cells and rescues them from the toxic effects of methotrexate. Leucovorin cannot enter cancer cells, however, and they continue to be killed by methotrexate. Leucovorin also works by rescuing healthy cells in patients who take an accidental overdose of drugs similar to methotrexate.

Combination therapy

Patients with colorectal cancer frequently are treated with fluorouracil (Adrusil). Fluorouracil, commonly called 5-FU, is effective, but works for only a short time once it is in the body. Leucovorin enhances the effect of fluorouracil by increasing the time that it remains active. As a result, the combination of the two drugs produces a greater anticancer effect than fluorouracil alone.

Recommended dosage

Leucovorin can be given as an injection, intravenously, or as oral tablets. For rescue therapy, leucovorin usually is given intravenously or orally within 24 hours

of methotrexate treatment. Dosage varies from patient to patient. When used in combination with fluorouracil, leucovorin is given to the patient intravenously first, followed by fluorouracil treatment. To treat unintentional folic acid antagonist overdose, leucovorin is usually given intravenously as soon as possible after the overdose. Patients with megaloblastic anemia receive oral leucovorin.

Precautions

Patients with anemia or any type of blood disorder should tell their doctors. Leucovorin can treat only anemia caused by folic acid deficiency. Patients with other types of anemia should not take leucovorin. The effect of leucovorin on the fetus is not known, and it is not known whether the drug is found in breast milk. Leucovorin should therefore be used with caution during pregnancy and should not be used by women who are breastfeeding. Elderly patients treated with leucovorin and fluorouracil for advanced colorectal cancer are at greater risk of developing severe side effects.

Side effects

The vast majority of patients do not experience side effects from leucovorin therapy. Side effects are usually caused by the patient's chemotherapy rather than by leucovorin. In rare cases, however, some patients can develop allergic reactions to the drug. These include skin rash, hives, nausea and vomiting, and **itching**. In 2004, Swiss researchers found that oral desensitization may work in cases of severe allergic reaction to leucovorin.

Interactions

Patients should tell their doctors about any over-the-counter or prescription medication they are taking, particularly medications that can cause seizures. Using leucovorin together with sulfamethoxazole/trimethoprim (Bactrim) increases the risk of treatment failure. Leucovorin increases the effects of capecitabine, raising the patient's risk of anemia or bleeding disorders.

Resources

PERIODICALS

Cohen, I. J., and J. E. Wolff. "How Long Can Folinic Acid Rescue Be Delayed after High-Dose Methotrexate without Toxicity?" *Pediatric Blood and Cancer* 61 (January 2014): 7–10.

"Oral Desensitization May Work in Some Cases of Allergy to Leucovorin." *Drug Week* (November 14, 2003): 128.

Alison McTavish, M.Sc.

Teresa G. Odle

Leukapheresis *see* **Pheresis**

Leukemia *see* **Acute erythroblastic leukemia; Acute lymphocytic leukemia; Acute myelocytic leukemia; Chronic lymphocytic leukemia; Chronic myelocytic leukemia; Leukemias, acute; Leukemias, chronic**

Leukemias, acute

Definition

Acute leukemia is a type of **cancer** in which excessive numbers of abnormal white blood cells are produced in blood-forming tissue such as the bone marrow and released into the bloodstream. It arises from malignant transformation of white cells known as B-lymphocytes or T-lymphocytes, occurring at the stem cell level.

Description

Acute leukemias progress rapidly, while **chronic leukemias** progress more slowly, often over a period of years. Acute leukemia is classified by the type of white blood cell that undergoes malignant transformation. The most common of the acute leukemias are:

• Acute lymphoblastic leukemia (ALL) or acute lymphocytic leukemia, in which excessive numbers of lymphoblasts, or immature lymphocytes, are produced.

• Acute myeloblastic leukemia (AML), also known as acute myeloid leukemia and acute nonlymphocytic leukemia (ANLL), in which excessive numbers of immature myeloid cells are produced.

All leukemias are cancers of specific white blood cells produced in the lymphatic system, mainly in the bone marrow. Bone marrow is the spongy tissue found inside the large bones of the body. Besides the bone marrow, the lymphatic system includes the lymphatic vessels (tiny

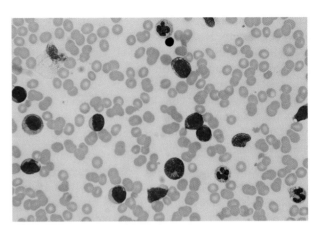

Acute myeloblastic leukemia, characterized by abnormal blood cells. (© *Mike Peres RBP SPAS/Custom Medical Stock Photo -- All rights reserved*)

tubes that branch like blood vessels into all parts of the body) and lymph nodes (pea-shaped organs that are found along the network of lymphatic vessels), which both carry lymph, a milky fluid containing specialized white cells that normally fight disease. Organs of the lymphatic system include the spleen in the upper abdomen, the thymus gland beneath the breastbone, and the tonsils in the throat. In leukemia, the malignant cells will circulate throughout the lymphatic system and in the blood and may infiltrate various organs, especially the liver, spleen, lymph nodes, central nervous system, kidneys, testicles, and ovaries.

The cells found in the blood include: red blood cells (RBCs) that carry oxygen and other materials such as iron to all tissues of the body; white blood cells (WBCs), which are a critical part of the immune system designed to fight infection; and platelets, which play an important role in blood coagulation. White blood cells are subdivided further into three main types: granulocytes (polymorphonuclear cells known as polys), monocytes, and lymphocytes.

The granulocytes, as their name suggests, contain particles (granules). These granules contain special proteins (enzymes) and several other substances that can break down chemicals and destroy microorganisms, including bacteria and viruses. Monocytes are also important in defending the body against invading pathogens. ANLL involves the monocytes and/or granulocytes.

Lymphocytes are of two primary types—T-lymphocytes and B-lymphocytes, each with different functions in the immune system. B cells protect the body by making antibodies against foreign substances or against antigens on the surface of cells. Antibodies are proteins that can attach to the surfaces of bacteria and viruses. This attachment signals other cell types to seek out and destroy the antibody-coated organisms. T cells protect the body against viruses. When a virus enters a cell, it produces certain proteins that are projected onto the surface of the infected cell. T cells recognize these proteins and make certain chemicals that are capable of destroying the virus-infected cells. In addition, T cells can destroy some types of cancer cells. Either T-lymphocytes or B-lymphocytes are involved in ALL, but in general, B-cell leukemias are more common.

Bone marrow makes stem cells, which are the precursors or early forms of the different blood cells. These stem cells mature through stages into RBCs, WBCs, or platelets. In acute leukemias, the maturation process of the white blood cells is interrupted. The immature cells (or "blasts"), transformed mainly by either genetic or viral sources, proliferate rapidly and begin to accumulate in various organs and tissues, thereby affecting their normal function. This uncontrolled proliferation of the immature cells in the bone marrow affects the production of the normal red blood cells and platelets as well. Essentially, in leukemia, the abnormal proliferation of the specific types of white rate of cells and their reduced rate of cell death (apoptosis) leads to the replacement of normal cells by the malignant cells.

Demographics

Leukemias account for 2% of all cancers. The incidence of acute leukemia is slightly higher among men than women. Although leukemia is the most common form of childhood cancer and accounts for one-third of all cancers in children, many more adults than children are diagnosed with leukemia. Half the cases of adult leukemia occur in people aged 60 or older. Chronic leukemia is diagnosed slightly more often than acute leukemia in adults. The American Cancer Society (ACS) estimates that approximately 52,380 new cases of all types of leukemia will be diagnosed in 2014 in the United States, and 24,000 people will die from the disease.

In adults, the most common type of leukemia is AML, which has several subtypes involving different cells (myeloid, myeloid-monocytic, monocytes, erythroid and megakaryocytic). In children, two-thirds of leukemia cases are **acute lymphocytic leukemia** (ALL), which is most prevalent in early childhood, with a peak incidence between the ages of two and four years. ALL represents about 26% of **childhood cancers** in children and 8% of cancers diagnosed in adolescents. Chronic leukemia is rare in children.

New cases of ALL diagnosed in 2014 are estimated to reach 6,020, affecting 2,670 children younger than age 14 and 410 adolescents aged 15–19. It is estimated that 1,440 children and adolescents will die of the disease in 2014.

ALL is more common among Caucasians than among African Americans, while acute myeloid leukemia (AML) affects both races equally. Acute promyelocytic leukemia (APL) is a subtype of AML that occurs in younger adults (average age 30) and particularly those of Hispanic descent. People with Jewish ancestry have a higher likelihood of developing leukemia.

Risk factors

Several risk factors have been identified as playing a role in the development of acute leukemia, including:

• exposure to ionizing radiation such as post-atomic bomb radiation
• exposure to medical radiation such as that used to treat cancer patients
• previous treatment with certain anticancer drugs (procarbazine, cyclophosphamide, melphalan, and etoposide or teniposide)
• previous infection with viruses such as human T-lymphotrophic virus and Epstein-Barr virus (present in mononucleosis)
• history of immunodeficiency disorders (HIV, AIDS), chronic myeloproliferative disorders, and disorders due to chromosomal translocations, like Down syndrome, Fanconi anemia, Bloom syndrome, ataxia-telangiectasia, and infantile X-linked agammaglobulinemia
• history of cigarette smoking
• exposure to certain toxic chemicals like benzene
• use of chloramphenicol, an antibiotic used to treat bacterial infections

Having a history of diseases that damage the bone marrow, such as aplastic **anemia**, or a history of cancers of the lymphatic system also increases the risk of developing acute leukemias.

Causes and symptoms

The precise cause of most leukemias is not known, but several explanations for the malignant transformation of cells have been suggested. The human T-cell leukemia virus (HTLV-I), a virus with similarities to the human immunodeficiency virus (HIV), is believed to be the causative agent of a rare form of ALL. The number of treatment-related cases of AML (individuals previously treated for cancer with **chemotherapy** and/or **radiation therapy**) is increasing, particularly among survivors of childhood and adolescent cancers such as **Hodgkin lymphoma, lymphoma, sarcoma, testicular cancer**, and **breast cancer**.

Genetic causes are also suggested, primarily changes in the location (translocation) of chromosomes in the nuclei of cells. For example, leukemic cells may have a normal number of chromosomes, but they may be abnormal in their forms. A specific abnormal chromosome called the Philadelphia (Ph) chromosome may be present, which is considered to be an unfavorable sign in ALL.

The most common presenting symptoms include anemia, infection, easy bruising, and bleeding (e.g., petechiae, or tiny red spots under the skin, nosebleeds, bleeding gums, and menstrual irregularity), which may appear only days or weeks before diagnosis. Other symptoms of leukemia are more vague and nonspecific. A patient may experience all or some of the following symptoms:

• weakness or chronic fatigue
• fever of unknown origin, chills and flu-like symptoms
• weight loss that is not due to dieting or exercise
• frequent bacterial or viral infections
• headaches
• skin rash
• nonspecific bone pain
• blood in urine or stools
• swollen and tender lymph nodes
• abdominal fullness
• night sweats
• more rarely, sores in the eyes or on the skin

The proliferation of cells may result in an enlarged spleen or liver, and these organs may be felt in the upper abdomen. In rare cases, the central nervous system will be affected and the patient will have headaches, vomiting, irritability, and possibly seizures.

Diagnosis

Examination

No screening tests are available for early detection of leukemias. If the doctor suspects leukemia, a thorough physical examination will be done to look for enlarged lymph nodes in the neck, underarm area, and pelvic region, as well as swollen gums, enlarged liver or spleen, bruises, or pinpoint red rashes all over the body. A careful personal and family history of previous illnesses and treatments received will also be taken.

Tests

A complete blood count with differential is usually the first test done; it will determine the numbers of red and white cells in the blood. Differential analysis of a blood smear will identify the percentages of different white cell types, mature and immature (blasts). The presence of a large percentage of blast cells may strongly suggest leukemia; however, the diagnosis must be confirmed by more specific tests and possibly gene studies. Urine tests will be ordered to check for microscopic amounts of blood in the urine.

Standard **imaging studies**, including chest x-ray, **computed tomography** scans (CT scans), and **magnetic resonance imaging** (MRI), may be performed to check whether the leukemic cells have invaded other areas of the body such as the bones, chest, kidneys, abdominal organs, or brain.

Sophisticated cytogenetic studies may be performed to examine the number and shape of chromosomes in the DNA of individual blast (immature) cells. Immunophenotyping of cells in the bone marrow will be done to identify specific cell types that may be associated with leukemia. This procedure involves removing a sample of bone marrow and applying various stains that will help a pathologist identify some of the proteins attached to the surface of the cells.

Procedures

A **bone marrow biopsy** may be taken by aspiration or needle to confirm the diagnosis of leukemia. During the **biopsy**, a cylindrical piece of bone and marrow is removed from a large bone like the hipbone or chest bone (sternum). These samples are sent to the pathology laboratory, where they are examined under a microscope by a hematologist, oncologist, or pathologist. Finding between 25%–95% blast cells in bone marrow confirms leukemia. Cytogenetics, immunophenotyping, and molecular biology will determine whether the blasts represent ALL or AML. In addition to the diagnostic biopsy, another biopsy will usually be performed during the treatment phase of the disease to see whether the leukemia is responding to therapy.

A spinal tap (**lumbar puncture**) is another procedure that the doctor may order to diagnose leukemia. In this procedure, a small needle is inserted into the spinal cavity in the lower back to withdraw a sample of cerebrospinal fluid that will be examined microscopically to look for leukemic cells.

Treatment

For a successful outcome, treatment for acute leukemia must begin as soon as possible. The goal of treatment is to arrest the leukemic disease process and induce remission. Leukemia treatment has two phases. The first phase is called induction therapy. As the name suggests, the primary aim of this phase of treatment is to reduce the number of leukemic cells and induce remission in the patient. Once the patient shows no obvious signs of leukemia (i.e., no leukemic cells are detected in blood tests and bone marrow biopsies), the patient is said to be in remission. The second phase of treatment is consolidation or maintenance therapy, and the goal is to kill any remaining cancer cells and to maintain the remission for as long as possible.

Chemotherapy is the primary treatment for leukemias. Sometimes **stem cell transplantation** is also performed. Surgery is not considered an option for treating leukemias, because bone marrow is the source of the abnormal cells and spreading is the result of malignant cells circulating in the body via the bloodstream and the lymphatic system.

Chemotherapy

Chemotherapy is the use of specific **anticancer drugs** to kill cancer cells. It is usually the treatment of choice in leukemia, and is used to relieve symptoms and achieve long-term remission. Generally, combination chemotherapy, in which multiple drugs are used simultaneously, is more efficient than using any single drug alone. Some drugs may be administered intravenously through a vein in the arm, while others may be given by mouth in the form of pills. If the cancer cells have invaded the brain, then chemotherapeutic drugs may be infused into the fluid that surrounds the brain through a needle in the brain or back (**intrathecal chemotherapy**).

Targeted therapies such as immunologic or biologic therapies, including the use of **monoclonal antibodies**, are increasingly used to treat acute leukemia by killing specific types of malignant cells without killing normal cells. For example, the monoclonal antibody, **rituximab** (Rituxan) may be used to treat adult ALL patients whose leukemic cells are positive for the CD20 antigen. Patients with Philadelphia-chromosome positive ALL and patients with AML may receive potent tyrosine kinase inhibitors such as imatinib (Gleevec), **dasatinib** (Sprycel), or **nilotinib** (Tasigna) to treat their leukemia. Many more such targeted therapies are in development.

Radiation

Radiation therapy, which involves the use of **x-rays** or other high-energy rays to kill cancer cells and shrink tumors, may be used in some cases. For acute leukemias, external (outside the body) radiation therapy is usually applied. If the leukemic cells have spread to the brain or other organs, radiation therapy may be directed to the involved organ system.

Prognosis

As with most cancers, the prognosis of leukemia depends on the patient's age, general health status, and response to therapy. Prognosis is fairly good for children and younger adults with ALL, and poorer among infants and elderly patients, or those with liver or kidney diseases and a WBC count higher than 25,000. Among children, more than 95% achieve remission and normal blood counts are restored, and in adults, 70%–90% achieve remission. The five-year survival rate is 75% in children, and 60%–88% will remain in remission after

---

---

five years, depending upon the cell type. Among adults, 30%–40% have disease-free survival for five years.

AML has only a slightly poorer prognosis than ALL, with remission induced in 50%–85% of patients. Twenty to forty percent of patients will have long-term disease-free survival, which can increase to as much as 50% in younger patients who have received intensive chemotherapy or stem cell transplantation. Patients with certain cytogenetic profiles have more favorable responses to therapy and improved rates of survival. If specific chromosomes are missing or karyotypes are abnormal, the risk of relapse is higher and prognosis can be markedly poorer.

Prevention

Many cancers can be prevented by changes in lifestyle or diet, which will reduce the risk factors. However, in leukemias, the main risk factors, such as chromosomal translocations and previous immunodeficiency or genetic disorders, are not modifiable, which makes prevention impossible. Avoiding exposure to tobacco smoke and toxic chemicals may help to reduce risk in some individuals. People who are at an increased risk of developing leukemia due to various types of exposure and preexisting conditions are advised to undergo periodic medical checkups and blood tests.

Resources

BOOKS

Appelbaum, Frederic R. "Acute Leukemia in Adults" In *Abeloff's Clinical Oncology.* 5th ed. Martin D. Abeloff, ed. New York: W. B. Saunders, 2013.

Campana, Daria and C. H. Pui. "Childhood Leukemia" In *Abeloff's Clinical Oncology*. 5th ed. Martin D. Abeloff, ed. New York: W. B. Saunders, 2013.

PERIODICALS

Brown, P., S. P. Hunger, F. O. Smith, W. L. Carroll, and G. H. Reaman. "Novel Targeted Drug Therapies for the Treatment of Childhood Acute Leukemia" *Expert Review of Hematology* 2 (2009): 145–58.

Ohanian, M., J. H. Cortes, and Jabbour E. Kantarjian. "Tyrosine Kinase Inhibitors in Acute and Chronic Leukemias." *Expert Opinion on Pharmacotherapy* 13 (2012): 927–938.

Pui, C. H., L. L. Robinson, and A. T. Look. "Acute Lymphoblastic Leukemia." *Lancet* 371 no. 9617 (March 22, 2008): 166–78.

WEBSITES

Leukemia & Lymphoma Society. "Cutaneous T-Cell Lymphoma Facts" http://www.lymphoma.org/content/nationalcontent/ resource center/freeeducationmaterials/lymphoma/pdf/ cutaneous (accessed August 9, 2014).

University of Pennsylvania Cancer Center. Oncolink. http:// cancer.med.upenn.edu (accessed August 9, 2014).

ORGANIZATIONS

American Cancer Society, 1599 Clifton Road, N.E., Atlanta, Georgia 30329, (800) 227-2345, http://www.cancer.org.

Cancer Research Institute, 681 Fifth Avenue, New York, NY 10022, (800) 992-2623, http://www.cancerresearch.org.

Leukemia & Lymphoma Society, 1311 Mamaroneck Ave., Ste. 310, White Plains, NY 10605, (914) 949-5213, Fax: (914) 949-6691, infocenter@lls.org, http://www.lls.org.

National Cancer Institute, Building 31, Room 10A31, 31 Center Drive, MSC 2580, Bethesda, MD 20892-2580, (800) 4-CANCER, http://www.nci.nih.gov.

Melinda Granger Oberleitner, RN, DNS, APRN, CNS
REVISED BY L. LEE CULVERT

Leukemias, chronic

Definition

Chronic leukemia is a type of **cancer** in which excessive numbers of abnormal white blood cells are produced in blood-forming tissue such as the bone marrow and released into the bloodstream. It usually begins slowly and progresses over a period of years, or it can have a long chronic phase that eventually becomes an accelerated phase with complications similar to those of acute leukemia. Chronic leukemia arises from the malignant transformation of specific white cells at the stem cell level.

Demographics

Leukemias account for about 2% of all cancers and occur in both sexes and in all ages. The incidence of leukemia is slightly higher among men than women. Although leukemia is the most common form of childhood cancer and accounts for one-third of all cancers in children, many more adults are actually diagnosed with leukemia. Half the cases of adult leukemia occur in people who are aged 60 or older. Chronic leukemia is diagnosed slightly more often than acute leukemia in adults and only rarely occurs in children. The American Cancer Society (ACS) estimates that approximately 52,380 new cases of leukemia of all kinds will be diagnosed in 2014 in the United States, and 24,000 people will die from the disease.

Chronic leukemias are named for the specific type of white blood cells (WBC) involved. **Chronic lymphocytic leukemia** (CLL), which involves lymphocytes, is by far the most common chronic type. **Chronic myelocytic leukemia** (CML), also called chronic granulocytic leukemia, chronic myelogenous leukemia, and chronic myeloid leukemia, involves myeloid cells called granulocytes. Lymphoid leukemias are significantly more common among Caucasians than among African Americans, while myeloid leukemias are only slightly more common in Caucasians.

The incidence of CLL increases with age. About eighty percent of cases of CLL are observed in patients who are age 60 or older, with an average age at diagnosis of 72 years. Rarely is CLL diagnosed in a patient who is younger than age 40 and it almost never occurs in children or adolescents. The American Cancer Society estimates that approximately 15,720 new cases of CLL will be diagnosed in 2014 and 4,600 Americans will die from the disease. Average lifetime risk of developing CLL is about 1 in 200. CLL affects both men and women. Among patients younger than 65, CLL is slightly more common in men but occurs equally between men and women among patients older than age 75. The incidence of CLL has increased significantly since the 1960s. However, many scientists attribute this increase to more reliable diagnosis than to the disease being more common than in the past. Fifty years ago, only one of ten CLL patients was diagnosed during the early phase. Today, half of all CLL patients are diagnosed in the early phase of the disease.

CML accounts for about 15% of all adult leukemias. The average lifetime risk of developing CML is about 1 in 588. Although CML can occur at any age, the average age at diagnosis is 64 years. It is rarely diagnosed before age 10. The American Cancer Society estimates about 5,980 new cases of CML will be diagnosed in the United

States in 2014, and about 810 people will die from the disease.

Description

As noted above, chronic leukemias are named for the type of white blood cell that undergoes malignant transformation. In CLL, mature-appearing abnormal white blood cells called lymphocytes, usually B-lymphocytes (only 2%–3% of cases involve T-cells), are produced. In CML, also known as chronic granulocytic leukemia (CGL), uncontrolled proliferation of white blood cells called granulocytes occurs. Although blasts, the hallmark of acute leukemia, are also present in chronic leukemia, it is primarily the T- or B-lymphocytes that undergo malignant transformation. Chronic leukemias typically progress slowly, with less rapid growth than acute leukemia, which progresses rapidly. However, CML has an accelerated phase that more closely resembles acute leukemia.

All leukemias are cancers of specific white blood cells produced in the lymphatic system, mainly in the bone marrow. Bone marrow is the spongy tissue found inside the large bones of the body. Besides the bone marrow, the lymphatic system includes the lymphatic vessels (tiny tubes that branch like blood vessels into all parts of the body) and lymph nodes (pea-shaped organs that are found along the network of lymphatic vessels), which both carry lymph, a milky fluid containing specialized white cells that normally fight disease. Organs of the lymphatic system also include the spleen in the upper abdomen, the thymus gland beneath the breastbone, and the tonsils in the throat. In leukemia, the malignant cells will circulate throughout the lymphatic system and in the blood and may infiltrate various organs, especially the liver, spleen, lymph nodes, central nervous system, kidneys, testicles, and ovaries.

The cells found in the blood include red blood cells (RBCs), which carry oxygen and other materials such as iron to all tissues of the body; white blood cells (WBCs), which are a critical part of the immune system designed to fight infection; and platelets, which play an important role in blood coagulation. White blood cells are subdivided further into three main types: granulocytes (polymorphonuclear cells known as polys), monocytes, and lymphocytes.

The granulocytes, as their name suggests, contain particles (granules). These granules contain special proteins (enzymes) and several other substances that can break down chemicals and destroy microorganisms, including bacteria and viruses.

Lymphocytes are of two primary types—T-lymphocytes and B-lymphocytes, each with different functions in the immune system. B-cells protect the body by making antibodies against foreign substances or against antigens on the surface of cells. Antibodies are proteins that can attach to the surfaces of bacteria and viruses. This attachment signals other cell types to seek out and destroy the antibody-coated organisms. T-cells protect the body against viruses. When a virus enters a cell, it produces certain proteins that are projected onto the surface of the infected cell. T-cells recognize these proteins and make certain chemicals that are capable of destroying the virus-infected cells. In addition, T-cells can destroy some types of cancer cells.

Bone marrow makes stem cells, which are the precursors or early forms of the different blood cells. These stem cells mature through stages into RBCs, WBCs, or platelets. In CLL, the specific B-cells undergo malignant transformation in the bone marrow, which spreads to the lymph nodes and organs of the lymph system, finally resulting in an enlarged spleen and liver, and reductions in the number of RBCs (**anemia**), WBCs (**neutropenia**), and platelets (**thrombocytopenia**). In CML, it is the translocation known as the Philadelphia chromosome that leads to excessive production of granulocytes, primarily in the bone marrow, but also in the spleen and liver. Other cells such as RBCs, monocytes, and even T-cells and B-cells are involved in the process. Normal stem cells, however, are retained, and can reemerge after the CML has been arrested.

Risk factors

Several established risk factors are related to the development of leukemias, including exposure to certain chemicals such as **benzene** and having hereditary gene mutations or chromosome translocations, especially the Philadelphia chromosome. Exposure to Agent Orange, an herbicide used in the Vietnam War, and long-term exposure to **pesticides** are reported to increase the risk of developing leukemia. A family history of leukemia also appears to be a risk factor. First-degree relatives (parents, siblings, and children) of CLL patients are two to four times more likely to be diagnosed with CLL than people who have no family history of CLL. Exposure to high-dose radiation, such as radiation from an atomic blast or nuclear reactor accident, increases the risk of leukemia. A higher incidence of leukemia has also been observed among people with immunodeficiency disorders such as HIV, chronic myeloproliferative disorders, and disorders due to chromosomal translocations like Down syndrome, **Fanconi anemia**, Bloom syndrome, ataxia-telangiectasia, and infantile X-linked agammaglobulinemia, which also may increase the risk of developing some form of leukemia.

Having a history of diseases that damage the bone marrow, such as aplastic anemia, or a history of cancers of the lymphatic system puts people at high risk of developing leukemias. Similarly, the use of anticancer medications, immunosuppressants, and the antibiotic chloramphenicol are also considered risk factors for developing leukemias.

Causes and symptoms

Causes

To date, the precise cause of most leukemias is not known, but several explanations for the malignant transformation of cells have been proposed. In about 95% of patients with CLL, specific CD+ B-lymphocytes undergo malignant transformation in the bone marrow, which spreads to the lymph nodes and other components of the lymph system. This transformation may be triggered by genetic causes or other causes associated with risk. Genetic causes primarily involve changes in the location (translocation) of chromosomes in the nuclei of cells. Although leukemic cells may have a normal number of chromosomes, they may be abnormal in their forms. Ninety-five percent of patients with CML have a chromosome translocation called the Philadelphia chromosome (Ph). The Ph chromosome develops when a piece of chromosome 9 that contains the cancer gene (oncogene) c-abl translocates to chromosome 22 and fuses to the gene BCR. This translocation forms BCR-ABL, a fusion gene that is important in the origination of CML.

Symptoms

The symptoms of chronic leukemia are generally vague and nonspecific, and are frequently overlooked until they are noticed on routine physical examination, especially when a routine blood test such as a complete blood count (CBC) is performed. A CBC may show unusually large numbers of a certain white cells, primarily lymphocytes and monocytes, in the blood. Chronic leukemias may exist for years without manifesting any symptoms at all, but can also develop symptoms similar to **acute leukemias**. Chronic myeloid leukemia in particular has a two- or three-stage progression: a chronic phase that can last for several years; an accelerated phase; and a terminal blastic phase, a malignant phase in which immature granulocytes are suddenly generated in huge numbers, producing symptoms similar to those of acute leukemia. In such cases, a patient may experience all or some of the following symptoms:

• weakness or chronic fatigue

• fever of unknown origin, chills, and flu-like symptoms

• unexplained weight loss

• frequent bacterial or viral infections

• viscous (sticky) blood (which slows down the supply to various organs)

• headache

• nonspecific bone pain

• easy bruising

• bleeding from gums or nose

• blood in urine or stools

• swollen and tender lymph nodes and/or spleen

• abdominal fullness

• night sweats

• petechiae, or tiny red spots under the skin

• priapism, or persistent, painful erection of the penis

• rarely, sores in the eyes or on the skin

Diagnosis

Examination

If leukemia is suspected based on symptoms or results of a blood count done for other reasons, a thorough physical examination will be conducted to look for enlarged lymph nodes in the neck, underarm area, and pelvic region. Swollen gums and an enlarged liver or spleen are other signs of chronic leukemia that may present on physical examination. A personal and family history of previous illnesses and treatments will also be taken.

Tests

A complete blood count with differential is usually the first test done; it will determine the numbers of red and white cells in the blood. Differential analysis of a blood smear will identify the percentages of different white cell types, mature and immature (blasts). The presence of a large percentage of blast cells may strongly suggest leukemia; however, the diagnosis must be confirmed by more specific tests and possibly gene studies. Urine tests will be ordered to check for microscopic amounts of blood in the urine.

Standard **imaging studies**, including chest x-ray, **computed tomography** scans (CT scans), and **magnetic resonance imaging** (MRI), may be performed to check whether the leukemic cells have invaded other areas of the body such as the bones, chest, kidneys, abdominal organs, or brain.

Sophisticated cytogenetic studies may be performed to examine the number and shape of chromosomes in the DNA of individual blast (immature) cells. The presence of the Philadelphia (Ph) chromosome is a crucial factor in the diagnosis of CML. Immunophenotyping of cells in the bone marrow will be done to identify specific cell types that may be associated with leukemia. This procedure involves removing a sample of bone marrow and applying various stains that will help a pathologist identify some of the proteins attached to the surface of the cells.

Procedures

A **bone marrow biopsy** may be taken by aspiration or needle to confirm the diagnosis of leukemia. During the **biopsy**, a cylindrical piece of bone and marrow is removed from a large bone like the hipbone or chest bone (sternum). These samples are sent to the pathology laboratory, where they are examined under a microscope by a hematologist, oncologist, or pathologist. In addition to the diagnostic biopsy, another biopsy will usually be performed during the treatment phase of the disease to see whether the leukemia is responding to therapy.

A spinal tap (**lumbar puncture**) is another procedure that the doctor may order to diagnose leukemia. In this procedure, a small needle is inserted into the spinal cavity in the lower back to withdraw a sample of cerebrospinal fluid that will be examined microscopically to look for leukemic cells.

Laboratory findings indicate whether a CML patient is in the chronic phase of the disease or has entered the accelerated phase. In the chronic phase, fewer than 10% of cells in the blood or marrow are blasts or immature cells. Once there are more than 10% but less than 20% of blasts detected in the blood or bone marrow, the patient is said to be in the accelerated phase of CML. When greater than 20% of blasts are detected in the blood or the bone marrow, the CML patient is said to be in the blast phase. Other names for this phase are acute phase or blast crisis, in which the disorder behaves like a more aggressive acute form of leukemia.

Some CLL patients will have a condition called hypogammaglobulinemia, which can be identified by certain blood tests. Immunoglobulins are important parts of the immune system that rid the body of infection. Patients with hypogammaglobulinemia have very low levels of immunoglobulins (IgG, IgA and others) and are less able to fight infection.

Standard imaging tests such as chest **x-rays**, computed tomography (CT) scans, and magnetic resonance imaging (MRI) may be used to determine whether malignant cells have invaded other areas of the body, such as the bones, chest, kidneys, abdomen, or brain.

Procedures

A bone marrow biopsy may be performed, during which a small piece of bone and marrow is removed, generally taken from the hipbone. A spinal tap (lumbar puncture) may also be done if central nervous system involvement is suspected. In this procedure, a small needle is inserted into the spinal cavity in the lower back to withdraw some cerebrospinal fluid and to look for leukemic cells.

Treatment

Treatment of CLL

Because the long-term prognosis for many patients with CLL is excellent, many patients (about one-third) receive no treatment at all at first. Many patients (about one-third) go for years before developing aggressive disease that requires treatment. Another third of patients will require immediate intervention at the time of diagnosis.

Treatment for CLL is typically initiated in a step-wise progression from the least invasive method of monitoring blood work and symptoms at regular intervals, known as watchful waiting, to treatment with **chemotherapy**, monoclonal antibody therapy, **corticosteroids** (for associated anemia and thrombocytopenia), and/or **stem cell transplantation**. Decisions to initiate treatment are based on the stage of disease, presence of symptoms, and disease activity.

Treatment of early-stage CLL is started only when one of the following conditions appears:

• Symptoms of the disease are growing worse, including a higher fever, weight loss, night sweats, and so forth.

• The spleen is enlarging, or enlargement of the spleen has become painful.

• Disease of the lymph nodes has become more severe.

• The condition of the bone marrow has deteriorated, and anemia and a marked reduction in the number of blood platelets is present.

• The population of malignant lymphocytes is growing rapidly.

• The patient is developing numerous bacterial infections due to reduced immunoglobulins.

Therapy for CLL usually starts with chemotherapy. Depending on the stage of the disease, single or multiple drugs may be given. Drugs commonly prescribed include **fludarabine**, **cladribine**, **chlorambucil**, and **cyclophosphamide**, or combinations of these drugs. The monoclonal antibody **rituximab** and/or cyclophosphamide have been used successfully for CML, with response rates up to 75%. Another monoclonal antibody, **alemtuzumab**, has had a 75%–80% response rate in patients not treated previously. Alemtuzumab may be used when patients are refractory to fludarabine-based regimens. Close monitoring for life-threatening infections is important with the use of alemtuzumab. It is being combined effectively with chemotherapy to completely clear bone marrow infiltration of malignant cells.

Another option for CLL patients is allogeneic stem cell transplantation. This option is typically reserved for patients younger than 65 years old because of the intensity of the conditioning regimen and the high risk of mortality.

Clinical trials are ongoing to evaluate the effectiveness of newer agents to treat CLL, including flavopiridol (Alvocidib) and lenalidomide (Revlimid).

Treatment of CML

In recent years, targeted therapy using tyrosine kinase inhibitors (TKi) has become the treatment of choice for CML. This is because the fusion gene *BCR-ABL* associated with the Philadelphia chromosome translocation is involved in the production of a specific tyrosine kinase. These drugs seem to work best for patients in the chronic phase of the disease, although they may also be effective for patients with more advanced disease. TKi drugs, including **imatinib mesylate** (Gleevec), which was the first approved TKi, and the newer **dasatinib** and **nilotinib**, have shown positive responses without relapse among newly diagnosed patients with Philadelphia chromosome-positive or *BCR-ABL*-positive-chronic phase CML. Side effects of these drugs may include **diarrhea**, nausea, **fatigue**, muscle pain, and skin rashes, as well as swelling around the eyes, feet, or abdomen. Differences in the toxicity profile of the different TKi drugs and the health status of patients determine the choice of a specific TKi agent.

Chemotherapy use in CML is now reserved for patients as part of treatment preceding stem cell transplantation. **Radiation therapy** is used only sparingly in the treatment of CML. It may be used to shrink an enlarged spleen, to treat pain caused by an increase in malignant cells in the bone marrow, or in low doses as pretreatment for stem cell transplantation.

Because of the demonstrated long-term effectiveness of targeted TKi drugs in sustaining remission in most CML patients, the role of stem cell transplantation is being reevaluated. The effectiveness of targeted TKi agents in treating both chronic and acute leukemias has spurred ongoing research to develop new drugs of this class with improved toxicity profiles, fewer side effects, and better patient outcomes.

The typical treatment protocol for CML by phase includes: chronic phase—treatment with TKi; accelerated phase—may include TKi, which has induced remission although it may not be long-term and chemotherapy may be used to induce remission prior to undergoing stem cell transplantation; blast phase—high dose TKi may be

---

QUESTIONS TO ASK YOUR DOCTOR

- What type of chronic leukemia do I have?
- How will the leukemia be treated?
- Can I receive treatment in my community, or should I consider receiving treatment in a specialized treatment center?
- How long will my treatment last?
- What side effects can I expect from the treatment?
- What is my long-term prognosis?

---

effective for patients who haven't been treated previously. The newer TKi drugs dasatinib and nilotinib may be more effective in this phase, but that is determined case by case. Patients who do not respond to a TKi drug may be considered for stem cell transplantation, which is more likely to be effective if remission of CML can be induced prior to transplantation. Treatment for CML is not known to be curative except after successful stem cell transplantation.

Prognosis

For many CLL patients, the prognosis is based on stage at diagnosis. Using the Binet and Rai staging systems criteria, patients staged as low-risk usually survive more than ten years. Patients staged as intermediate-risk usually survive about seven years. Patients staged as high-risk usually survive about two to five years. The average patient survives nine or more years after diagnosis.

CML prognosis has improved with the consistent use of TKi agents. With imatinib, more than 90% of patients survive five years after diagnosis of the chronic phase. Prior to the use of imatinib, the first TKi approved for CML, 5%–10% of patients died within two years of diagnosis and another 10%–15% died in each successive year. Most deaths from CML occur after a blast phase or accelerated phase. Ph chromosome-negative CML and chronic myelomonocytic leukemia have a poorer prognosis than Ph chromosome-positive CML.

Prevention

Because the risk factors for leukemia are not modifiable, there is no known way to prevent chronic leukemia. People who are at an increased risk of developing chronic leukemia because of proven exposure to radiation or Agent Orange, or long-term exposure to pesticides, and people with a family history of chronic leukemia, are advised to undergo periodic medical evaluations with accompanying blood tests.

Resources

BOOKS

Applebaum, Frederic R. "Chronic Lymphocytic Leukemia." In *Abeloff's Clinical Oncology*, 5th ed. Martin D. Abeloff, ed. New York: W.B. Saunders, 2013.

PERIODICALS

Cervantes, F., and M. Mauro. "Practical Management of Patients with Chronic Myeloid Leukemia." *Cancer* 117 (2011): 4343–4354.

Maddocks, K. J. and Lin, T. S. "Update in the Management of Chronic Lymphocytic Leukemia." *Journal of Hematology & Oncology* 2 (2009): 29.

Ohanian, M. J., H. Cortes, and Jabbour E. Kantarjian. "Tyrosine Kinase Inhibitors in Acute and Chronic Leukemias." *Expert Opinion on Pharmacotherapy* 13 (2012): 927–938.

WEBSITES

Leukemia & Lymphoma Society. "Cutaneous T-Cell Lymphoma Facts." http://www.lymphoma.org/content/nationalcontent/resource center/freeeducationmaterials/lymphoma/pdf/cutaneous (accessed August 11, 2014).

National Comprehensive Cancer Network: NCCN Practice Guidelines in Oncology. "Chronic Myelogenous Leukemia." http://www.nccn.org/professionals/physician_gls/PDF/cml.pdf (accessed August 11, 2014).

ORGANIZATIONS

American Cancer Society, 1599 Clifton Road, N.E., Atlanta, Georgia 30329, (800) 227-2345, http://www.cancer.org.

Cancer Research Institute, One Exchange Place, 55 Broadway, Suite 1802, New York, NY 10006, (800) 992-2623, http://www.cancerresearch.org.

Leukemia & Lymphoma Society, 1311 Mamaroneck Ave., Ste. 310, White Plains, NY 10605, (914) 949-5213, Fax: (914) 949-6691, infocenter@lls.org, http://www.lls.org.

National Cancer Institute, Building 31, Room 10A31, 31 Center Drive, MSC 2580, Bethesda, MD 20892-2580, (800) 4-CANCER, http://www.nci.nih.gov.

Melinda Granger Oberleitner, RN, DNS, APRN, CNS

REVISED BY L. LEE CULVERT

Leukeran *see* **Chlorambucil**

Leukine *see* **Sargramostim**

Leukoencephalopathy

Description

Leukoencephalopathy is a disease occurring primarily in the white matter of the brain that involves defects in

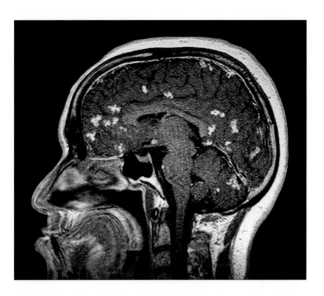

A magnetic resonance imaging (MRI) scan indicating leukoencephalopathy, characterized by several brain lesions (shown in white). *(Zephyr/Science Source)*

either the formation or the maintenance of the myelin sheath, a fatty coating that protects nerve cells. Leukoencephalopathy has several different forms and causes.

The symptoms of leukoencephalopathy reflect the mental deterioration that occurs as the myelin cover of nerve cells is eroded at multiple sites within the brain, leaving nerve cells exposed with no protective insulation. Patients may exhibit problems with speech and vision, loss of mental function, uncoordinated movements, and extreme weakness and **fatigue**. Patients may also have no desire to eat. The disease is usually progressive; patients continue to lose mental function, may also have seizures, and finally lapse into a coma before death. Some patients stabilize, however, although loss of neurologic function is usually irreversible.

Leukoencephalopathy as it relates to **cancer** patients is primarily associated with methotrexate chemotherapy, which is used in the treatment of many different types of cancer along with some other medications, including **cytarabine**, **fludarabine**, **carmustine** and **fluorouracil** in conjunction with **levamisole**. The disease may appear years after the administration of **methotrexate**. Although rare, the incidence of leukoencephalopathy is increasing as stronger drugs are developed and increased survival times allow time for the side effects of the treatments to appear.

A devastating type of leukoencephalopathy called multifocal, or disseminated, necrotizing leukoencephalopathy, has been shown to occur primarily when methotrexate or cytarabine therapy is used in conjunction with a large cumulative dose of whole-head irradiation. This disease is characterized by multiple sites of necrosis of the nerve cells in the white matter of the brain, involving both the myelin coating and the nerve cells themselves. Although some patients may stabilize, the course is usually progressive, with patients experiencing relentless mental deterioration and finally death.

Although leukoencephalopathy is primarily associated with methotrexate therapy, this disease has also been observed in association with other chemotherapeutic drugs (like intrathecal cytarabine), and has occasionally been reported in association with cancers that have not yet been treated.

Another particularly lethal type of leukoencephalopathy called progressive multifocal leukoencephalopathy (PML) is an opportunistic infection that occurs in cancer patients who experience long-term immunosuppression as a result of the cancer (as in leukemia or **lymphoma**) or as a result of **chemotherapy** or immunosuppressive drugs. PML results when, due to chronic immunosuppression, the JC virus, widely found in the kidneys of healthy people, becomes capable of entering the brain. The virus infects the cells that produce myelin and forms multiple sites of nerve cells in the brain that lack the protective fatty coating. For reasons that are not completely clear, PML has a rapid and devastating clinical course, with death occurring typically less than six months after diagnosis.

Causes

It is only relatively recently that longer survival times for cancer patients have enabled scientists to identify the association of leukoencephalopathy with intensive chemotherapy (particularly methotrexate), especially when combined with large doses of whole-head radiation. The causes of the neural degeneration observed are still not completely understood.

Most cases of leukoencephalopathy observed have occurred in patients who received methotrexate (either directly into the brain, through a tube in the skull, or intravenously) or who have received large doses of radiation to the head. Up to 50% of children who have received both treatments have developed necrotizing leukoencephalopathy, which differs from regular leukoencephalopathy in that the multiple sites of demyelinization also involve necrosis (the death of cells due to the degradative action of enzymes). Deterioration of the nerve tissue in necrotizing leukoencephalopathy appears to begin with the nerve and then spread into the myelin coating.

The method of action in PML is also not well understood. Long-term immunosuppression somehow appears to create an environment in which the JC virus that inhabits most healthy human kidneys can mutate into a form that gains access to the brain. When in the brain, the virus infects and kills the cells that produce the myelin that forms a protective coating around the nerve.

Treatment

Unfortunately, there is no cure for any form of leukoencephalopathy, and no treatments were approved as of 2014. Although some medications have shown some effect against the deterioration involved in this disease, those identified have been highly toxic themselves, and none so far have been effective enough to justify their use. The treatment of people with this disorder therefore tends to concentrate on alleviating discomfort.

Since there are no effective treatments, prevention must be emphasized. As the risks of certain treatment choices have become better defined, physicians must pursue careful treatment planning to produce optimal chance of tumor eradication while avoiding increased risk of the onset of a fatal and incurable side effect. The need for judicious treatment planning is especially true in children. The cases observed have largely occurred in children, which implies that the developing brain is at higher risk of developing treatment-associated leukoencephalopathy.

Alternative and complementary therapies

There are no commonly used alternative treatments, although because the disease is incurable, there is little risk in trying nontraditional medications. Complementary therapies (yoga, t'ai chi, etc.) that improve patient well being are appropriate if the patient finds them helpful.

Resources

BOOKS

Abeloff, Martin et al. *Abeloff's Clinical Oncology*. 5th New York: 5th ed. Philadelphia: Elsevier, 2014.

Mandell, Gerald, et al., eds. *Mandell, Douglas, and Bennett's Principles and Practice of Infectious Diseases*. 7th ed. Philadelphia: Churchill Livingstone/Elsevier, 2010.

WEBSITES

"Progressive Multifocal Leukoencephalopathy." *A Healthy Me.* [cited July 5, 2009]. http://www.ahealthyme.com/article/gale/100083914.

Wendy Wippel, M.Sc.

Leukotriene inhibitors

Definition

Leukotriene inhibitors are drugs used to treat asthma and allergy symptoms. Leukotrienes are fatty compounds that function as part of the immune system, and cause inflammation and constriction of the airways. Leukotriene inhibitors act to prevent this mechanism and open the airways to facilitate breathing. The three main leukotriene inhibitors are the drugs montelukast, zafirlukast, and zileuton.

Purpose

Leukotriene inhibitors are mainly used to treat chronic asthma as part of maintenance therapy. Maintenance therapy helps prevent acute asthma attacks and maintains a baseline of open airways. Leukotriene inhibitors are not used to treat acute asthma attacks, only prevent them from happening. Asthma induced by exercise may also be treated by leukotriene inhibitors. Allergy symptoms of sneezing, runny nose, and wheezing may be treated by leukotriene inhibitors.

Description

Leukotriene inhibitors are used to treat respiratory conditions that are caused by obstruction of the airways. Breathing involves the passage of air through the nose or mouth, down the trachea within the throat and into air passages called bronchi that lead into the lungs. Obstruction of the airways may be due to the constriction of the smooth muscle that lines the bronchi, causing a condition known as bronchospasm (spasm of the smooth muscle). Relaxation of the smooth muscle allows opening of the airway, thereby facilitating the breathing process. Leukotrienes are released by the body during an allergic reaction or in patients with asthma, and cause contraction of the bronchial airway smooth muscle as well as inflammation and mucus production. All these effects disrupt breathing and are ameliorated by leukotriene inhibitors.

Multiple leukotriene inhibitors are available, including the drugs montelukast, zafirlukast, and zileuton. Montelukast is manufactured by Merck under the trade name Singulair. Zafirlukast is manufactured by AstraZeneca Pharmaceuticals under the trade name Accolate. Zileuton is manufactured by Cornerstone Therapeutics under the trade name Zyflo. Leukotriene inhibitors specifically target the receptor for leukotrienes (body chemicals that induce inflammation) present on cell surfaces in the respiratory tract. Leukotriene inhibitors are a type of chemical receptor that sits on the outer membrane of cells present in the respiratory system. These receptors activate a sequence of cellular events known as a chemical cascade or signaling pathway. It is these signaling pathways that are responsible for many normal body functions. Drugs or natural chemicals that bind to and activate the receptor signaling pathway are known as receptor agonists. Drugs

KEY TERMS

Asthma—Disorder involving chronic inflammation in which the airways are narrowed in a reversible manner making it difficult to breathe normally, especially during acute exacerbations known as asthma attacks.

Bronchi—Airway passages in the respiratory system that conduct air into the lungs.

Bronchospasm—Spasm of the smooth muscles surrounding the bronchi causing constriction and obstructed airways.

Cytochrome P450—Enzymes present in the liver that metabolize drugs.

Phenylketonuria—Disorder of metabolism involving a deficiency in liver enzymes that metabolize the amino acid phenylalanine, causing it to accumulate and resulting in severe medical problems.

QT prolongation—Potentially dangerous heart condition that affects the rhythm of the heart beat and alters the ECG reading of the heart.

or natural chemicals that bind to the receptor and block them from creating a signaling pathway are known as receptor antagonists because they oppose the effects of that receptor. Leukotriene receptors bind leukotriene agonists to create signaling cascades that are a natural part of the **immune response** and create inflammation of the airways. In patients with asthma and allergies, this natural inflammatory process is excessive and creates uncomfortable symptoms. Leukotriene inhibitors antagonize the leukotriene receptor by binding and prevent the activation of signaling pathway for inflammation, restoring a normal balance.

Recommended dosage

The dose of montelukast used for asthma maintenance therapy or allergy symptoms is 10 mg taken orally in the evening. For asthma induced by exercise in patients who are not already on montelukast maintenance therapy, the dose is 10 mg, given at least two hours before exercise with a maximum dose of 10 mg per day. The same dose is used for both adults and children greater than 15 years of age. For children from 6 to 14 years of age a dose of 5 mg a day is used. For children from 1 to 5 years of age a dose of 4 mg a day is used, available as a chewable tablet or as powder that may be mixed with food. Montelukast is not appropriate for use in children less than 1 year of age.

The dose of zafirlukast used for asthma maintenance therapy is 20 mg taken orally twice a day. The maximum dose used is 40 mg per day. The same dose is used for both adults and children greater than 12 years of age. For children from 5 to 11 years of age, a dose of 10 mg twice a day is used. Doses are taken 1 hour before or 2 hours after meals. Zafirlukast is not appropriate for use in children less than 5 years of age.

The dose of zileuton used for asthma maintenance therapy is 1,200 mg taken orally twice a day. The maximum dose used is 2,400 mg per day. The same dose is used for both adults and children greater than 12 years of age. Doses are taken within an hour of meals. Zileuton is not appropriate for use in children less than 12 years of age.

Precautions

Leukotriene inhibitors are used as a part of asthma maintenance and are not effective for acute asthma attacks. However, treatment with leukotriene inhibitors is not stopped during acute asthma exacerbations when other drugs are necessary to treat the acute attack. Leukotriene inhibitors may not be appropriate for use in patients with existing liver disease, anxiety, **depression**, dream disorders, hallucinations, alcoholism, mood swings, or tremors. Use of leukotriene inhibitors during breastfeeding is not recommended.

Montelukast and zafirlukast are pregnancy category B drugs. Pregnancy category B drugs are drugs in which there is no evidence of fetal risk in studies done on animals and there are no studies done in pregnant women, or drugs in which there is evidence of fetal harm in animal studies but studies done in pregnant women have not shown risk. These drugs may be used during pregnancy as fetal harm is possible but unlikely. Zafirlukast is not approved for use in children less than five years of age. Montelukast is not approved for use in children less than 1 year of age. The chewable form of montelukast may not be appropriate for use in children with the metabolic disorder phenylketonuria.

Zafirlukast may cause a heart condition that affects the rhythm of the heartbeat known as QT prolongation. Sometimes QT prolongation can cause a serious cardiac condition that includes a fast and irregular heartbeat with severe dizziness and fainting. The risk of developing QT prolongation syndrome may be increased if the patient is taking other drugs that also affect the rhythm of the heart, or if the patient has cardiac problems. Low blood levels of potassium or magnesium may also increase the risk of QT prolongation.

Zileuton is a pregnancy Category C drug, and is used during pregnancy only when medically necessary. A

QUESTIONS TO ASK YOUR DOCTOR

- How long must I take this drug before you can tell whether it helps me?
- How often must I have blood work and other laboratory tests done to check the effect the drug is having?
- Is this drug safe to take with the other drugs that I am currently taking?
- What side effects should I watch for? When should I call the doctor about them?
- Are there any clinical trials of this drug combined with other therapies that might benefit me?

pregnancy Category C drug is one for which studies done in animals have shown potential harm to a fetus but there are not sufficient data in humans. If the potential benefits for the patient outweigh the potential risks to the fetus, the drug may be used during pregnancy. Zileuton is not approved for use in children less than 12 years of age. Use of zileuton in children may cause mood changes; patients in this age range should be monitored carefully. Use of zileuton in females older than 65 years of age may cause alterations in liver enzymes that need to be monitored.

Side effects

Leukotriene inhibitors generally have very few side effects and are well tolerated. Headaches are the most common symptom. Leukotriene inhibitors may be associated with the side effects of upset stomach, irritation of the nasal passages, dizziness, nausea, inflammation of the sinuses, sore throat, abdominal pain and cramping, vomiting, **diarrhea**, liver disease, muscle pain, rash, upper respiratory infections. Very rarely leukotriene inhibitors may cause aggressive behavior, anxiety, depression, dream disorders, hallucinations, insomnia, suicidal thoughts, and tremors. Montelukast and zafirlukast have been associated with the severe side effects of liver failure, alterations of the immune system, and inflammation of the blood vessels. Montelukast has been associated with bronchitis, weakness, and vision disturbances.

Interactions

Leukotriene inhibitors are metabolized by a set of liver enzymes known as cytochrome P450 (CYP450).

Multiple subtypes of CYP450 metabolize leukotriene inhibitors, with subtype 3A4 as the main metabolizer. Drugs that induce or activate these enzymes increase the metabolism of leukotriene inhibitors. This process results in lower levels of therapeutic leukotriene inhibitors, thereby negatively affecting treatment. For this reason drugs that induce CYP450 subtype 3A4 may not be used with leukotriene inhibitors. These drugs include some antiepileptic drugs, such as **carbamazepine**; some anti-inflammatory drugs, such as **dexamethasone**; anti-tuberculosis drugs such as rifampin; and the herb St. John's wort.

Drugs that act to inhibit the action of CYP450 subtype 3A4 may cause undesired increased levels of leukotriene inhibitors in the body. This action could lead to toxic doses. Some examples are **antibiotics** such as clarithromycin, antifungal drugs such as ketoconazole, antiviral drugs such as indinavir, antidepressants such as fluoxetine, and some cardiac agents, such as verapamil. Grapefruit juice may also increase the amount of leukotriene inhibitors in the body. Patients should avoid drinking grapefruit juice or eating grapefruit while taking leukotriene inhibitors.

Zafirlukast may have dangerous additive effects with other drugs that also cause QT prolongation. Drugs that interact with zafirlukast in this way include cisapride, amiodarone, dofetilide, pimozide, procainamide, quinidine, sotalol, and macrolide antibiotics such as erythromycin. Interactions with the blood thinning drug **warfarin** may increase the risk of bleeding.

Leukotriene inhibitors may also interact with other drugs to increase their toxicity. The dose of the bronchodilator theophylline should be reduced when initiating leukotriene inhibitor therapy to prevent toxicity. The blood pressure and cardiac drug propranolol and related compounds may cause toxicity when used with leukotriene inhibitors.

Resources

BOOKS

Brunton, Laurence L., et al., eds. *Goodman and Gilman's Pharmacological Basis of Therapeutics*. 12th ed. New York: McGraw-Hill, 2011.

Hamilton, Richard J., ed. *Tarascon Pharmacopoiea 2015*. Burlington, MA: Jones and Bartlett Learning, 2014.

ORGANIZATIONS

American Academy of Allergy, Asthma & Immunology, 555 E. Wells St., Ste. 1100, Milwaukee, WI 53202-3823, (414) 272-6071, http://www.aaaai.org.

Asthma and Allergy Foundation of America, 8201 Corporate Dr., Ste. 1000, Landover, MD 20785, (800) 7-ASTHMA (727-8462), info@aafa.org, http://aafa.org.

National Heart, Lung, and Blood Institute, 31 Center Dr. MSC 2486, Bldg. 31, Rm. 5A52, Bethesda, MD 20892, (301) 592-8573, nhlbiinfo@nhlbi.nih.gov, http://www.nhlbi.nih.gov.

U.S. Food and Drug Administration, 10903 New Hampshire Ave., Silver Spring, MD 20993, (888) INFO-FDA (463-6332), http://www.fda.gov.

Maria Basile, PhD.

Leuprolide acetate

Definition

Leuprolide acetate is a synthetic (human-made) hormone that acts similarly to the naturally occurring gonadotropin-releasing hormone (GnRH). It is available under the tradename Lupron.

Purpose

Leuprolide acetate is used primarily to counter the symptoms of advanced **prostate cancer** in men when surgery to remove the testes or estrogen therapy are not options or are unacceptable to the patient. It is often used to ease the pain and discomfort of women suffering from endometriosis, advanced **breast cancer**, or advanced **ovarian cancer**.

Two less common uses of this drug are the treatment of **anemia** caused by bleeding uterine fibroids, and the treatment of early-onset (precocious) puberty.

Description

Leuprolide acetate is a synthetic protein that mimics many of the actions of gonadotropin releasing hormone. In men, it decreases blood levels of the male hormone **testosterone**. In women, it decreases blood levels of the female hormone estrogen.

Recommended dosage

In men, there are three methods of dosing: daily injections, a monthly injection, or an annual implanted capsule. In the case of daily injections, 1 mg of leuprolide acetate is injected under the skin (subcutaneously). In the case of monthly injections, an implanted capsule that contains 7.5 mg of leuprolide acetate is injected into a muscle. In the case of an annual implanted capsule, the capsule contains 72 mg of leuprolide acetate. Both the monthly and the annual capsules are specially designed to slowly release the drug into the patient's bloodstream

KEY TERMS

Endometrial tissue—The tissue lining the uterus that is sloughed off during a woman's menstrual period.

Fibroid—A benign smooth muscle tumor of the uterus.

Gonadotropin-releasing hormone (GnRH)—A hormone produced in the brain that controls the release of other hormones that are responsible for reproductive function.

Prostate gland—A small gland in the male genitals that contributes to the production of seminal fluid.

over the specified time. The monthly capsule dissolves completely over the course of the month. The annual capsule must be removed after 12 months.

In the case of self-administered daily injections, a patient who misses a dose should take that dose as soon as it is noticed. However, if he or she does not remember until the next day, the missed dose should be skipped. Doses should not be doubled.

Precautions

People taking leuprolide acetate should not drive a car, cook, or engage in any activity that requires alertness until they have been taking the medication long enough to know how it affects them.

Leuprolide acetate may cause birth defects if taken during pregnancy, and may be passed to an infant via breast milk. Therefore, women who are pregnant or nursing should not take leuprolide acetate without first consulting their doctors.

Leuprolide acetate will also interfere with the chemical actions of birth control pills. For this reason, sexually active women who do not wish to become pregnant should use some form of birth control other than birth control pills.

Side effects

In patients of both sexes, common side effects of leuprolide acetate include:

- tumor flare, which manifests as bone pain (due to a temporary initial increase in testosterone/estrogen before its production is finally decreased)
- sweating accompanied by feelings of warmth (hot flashes)
- lack of energy (lethargy)

- depression or other mood changes
- headache
- enlargement of the breasts
- decreased sex drive

Other common side effects in women include:

- light, irregular vaginal bleeding
- no menstrual period
- pelvic pain
- vaginal dryness and/or itching
- emotional instability
- increase in facial or body hair
- deepening of the voice

Less common side effects in patients of either sex include:

- burning or itching at the site of the injection
- nausea and vomiting
- insomnia
- weight gain
- swollen feet or lower legs
- constipation

Other side effects in men can include impotence and decreased testicle size.

A doctor should be consulted immediately if the patient experiences any of the above symptoms.

Interactions

There are no known interactions of leuprolide acetate with any food or beverage. People taking leuprolide acetate should consult their physician before taking any other prescription drug, over-the-counter drug, or herbal remedy. People currently taking any other hormone or steroid-based medications should not take leuprolide acetate without first consulting their physician.

See also Endometrial cancer.

Paul A. Johnson, Ed.M.

Leustatin *see* **Cladribine**

Levamisole

Definition

Levamisole is used to treat **colon cancer**, specifically stage III colon **cancer**. Levamisole takes the full name of levamisole hydrochloride, and it is also known by the brand name Ergamisol.

Purpose

Levamisole is used to treat patients with stage III colon cancer after they have had surgery to remove the tumor, or as much of the tumor as possible. In stage III colon cancer, the cancer has spread to nearby lymph nodes. Levamisole is approved for use with **fluorouracil** (specifically, 5-fluorouracil), a drug that is thought to prevent cells from replicating by interfering with the manufacture of the hereditary material the cells carry. The use of levamisole with fluorouracil makes it an adjuvant therapy, or one that when used in conjunction with another drug seems to increase the defenses of the patient.

Description

Levamisole was first made by laboratory synthesis in 1966, and since then it has been used in veterinary medicine to eliminate intestinal, or lower gut, parasites in domestic animals. It was found to be an immunostimulant in 1972 and approved for use for colon cancer in 1990.

The drug seems to have a number of benefits for the patient. It increases the response of T cells, or cells belonging to the lymphatic system that can fight cancer cells. It also seems to increase the activity of cells that attack and destroy invading or cancer cells, including both monocytes and macrophages.

Because of the response levamisole induces in T cells, causing them to be more active, it falls into the category of drugs known as **biological response modifiers**.

Recommended dosage

The drug is given orally in tablet form. Tablets contain 50 milligrams of levamisole hydrochloride, and a standard dose is one tablet every eight hours for three days. Thereafter, the patient takes the same three-day course every two weeks for about a year.

Dosage must be adjusted according to the count of white blood cells and platelets in a patient's blood. In some cases, levamisole can be continued even when fluorouracil must be stopped.

Precautions

The drug can cause changes in the composition of the blood, which can be fatal. For example, agranulocytosis, also known as **neutropenia**, may develop. The condition refers to a drop in a kind of white blood cell known as neutrophils that are important in the defense

---

KEY TERMS

Adjuvant therapy—Addition of a drug or other treatment to a primary therapy.

Macrophage—Large cell-eating cell.

Monocyte—A specialized type of white blood cell that attacks other cells and acts as a phagocyte.

Neutrophil—A specialized type of white blood cell that attacks other cells and acts as a phagocyte.

Parasite—An organism that lives by taking its nourishment from another organism.

Phagocyte—Cell-eating cell.

T cell—A cell in the lymphatic system that contributes to immunity by directly attacking foreign bodies, such as bacteria and viruses.

---

against bacteria and fungi. Thus, the patient becomes more likely to get a bacterial or fungal infection.

Side effects

Nausea and vomiting, **diarrhea**, hair loss (**alopecia**), and changes in the composition of the white blood cells (such as neutropenia), are among the most common side effects.

Interactions

Levamisole often interacts with alcohol in the same way that the drug disulfiram, which is used to discourage alcohol consumption in alcoholics (alcohol deterrent), does. The reaction is extremely unpleasant, and alcohol use is best avoided when levamisole is being taken.

The drug also interacts with **warfarin**, which is often given to heart patients to reduce the chance of blood clots forming. Levamisole can interfere with the action of warfarin, allowing blood clots to form; therefore adjustments in the amount of warfarin heart patients take may be necessary if they are also taking levamisole.

Resources

BOOKS

Chu, Edward, and Vincent T. DeVita, Jr. *Physicians' Cancer Chemotherapy Drug Manual 2014*. Burlington, MA: Jones & Bartlett Learning, 2014.

WEBSITES

University of Pittsburgh Medical Center (UPMC). "Levamisole (Generic Name)." http://www.upmc.com/patients-visitors/

education/cancer-chemo/Pages/levamisole.aspx (accessed November 4, 2014).

Diane M. Calabrese

L-glutamine *see* **Glutamine**

Li-Fraumeni syndrome

Definition

Li-Fraumeni syndrome (LFS) is a genetic disorder caused by a hereditary mutation in a **cancer** susceptibility gene. Individuals with LFS have an increased risk of developing certain types of cancer, often at younger ages than is typically observed in the general population.

Description

Li-Fraumeni syndrome (LFS) was first described by Dr. Frederick Li and Dr. Joseph Fraumeni in 1969. It is caused by mutations in the *TP53* gene, located on chromosome 17. The types of mutations that cause LFS are known as hereditary mutations, and therefore can be inherited, or passed from a parent to a child.

Cancer risks

The *TP53* gene is a tumor suppressor gene. When an individual inherits a mutation in this type of gene from one of his or her parents, there is an increased risk for developing certain kinds of cancer. The most common kinds of cancer associated with LFS are sarcomas, or tumors that arise in connective tissues like bone or cartilage.

Females with LFS have an increased risk of developing **breast cancer**. Males and females may also be at risk of developing leukemia, **melanoma**, colon, pancreatic, and brain cancer. They may also develop adrenalcorticoid tumors, which form on the outer surface of the adrenal glands. These cancers often occur at younger ages than are typically observed in the general population, often before age 45.

Some individuals with LFS may develop certain cancers such as **brain tumors**, sarcomas, or adrenalcorticoid tumors in childhood. In addition, individuals with a mutation in the *TP53* gene have a higher risk of developing multiple primary cancers. For example, a person with LFS who develops a **sarcoma** at a young age and survives that cancer has an increased risk of developing a second or possibly even a third different kind of cancer.

Age of onset for cancers associated with Li-Fraumeni syndrome

Age of onset	Type of cancer
Infancy	Development of adrenocortical carcinoma
Under five years of age	Development of soft-tissue sarcomas
Childhood and young adulthood	Acute leukemias and brain tumors
Adolescence	Osteosarcomas
Twenties to thirties	Premenopausal breast cancer is common

Table listing the usual age at onset for cancers associated with Li-Fraumeni syndrome. *(Table by GGS Creative Resources. © Cengage Learning®.)*

Diagnosis

Genetic testing for mutations in the *TP53* gene is usually performed on a blood sample from the relative in the family who has had one of the cancers associated with LFS at a young age. One of the most effective ways to test for mutations in the *TP53* gene is by sequencing, a process whereby the chemical components of a patient's DNA is compared to that of DNA that is known to be normal. If the entire DNA code of the *TP53* gene is sequenced, it is believed that the majority (98%) of the (mutations) that are responsible for Li-Fraumeni syndrome can be identified. However, as the process of sequencing is a difficult and often time-consuming process, it is not always performed for every patient. Often, only specific areas of the *TP53* gene where there is most likely to be a mutation associated with LFS, are analyzed. The length of time to receive results depends on the extent of testing that is performed and the laboratory that is used.

Due to the fact that some of the cancers associated with LFS can occur at very young ages, there is a question as to whether genetic testing should be an option for at-risk children. Typically, genetic testing is not offered to anyone under the age of 18. However, because there are some screening options available for children with LFS, it is thought that the option of testing could not be denied if a parent thinks that it is important for his or her son or daughter's future health. Groups such as the National Society of Genetic Counselors are beginning to explore the issue of genetic testing in minors (those under age 18) for mutations in cancer susceptibility genes, especially if these minors would be at risk of developing **childhood cancers**.

It is important to understand the various categories of results associated with undergoing genetic testing for mutations in the *TP53* gene. A positive result indicates the presence of a genetic mutation that is known to be associated with an increased risk of developing the types

Adrenal glands—Structures located on top of the kidneys that secrete hormones.

Adrenocortical tumors—Cancers that arise on the outer surface of the adrenal glands.

Cancer—The process by which cells grow out of control and subsequently invade nearby cells and tissue.

Cancer susceptibility gene—The type of gene involved in cancer. If a mutation is identified in this type of gene it does not reveal whether a person has cancer, but rather whether an individual has an increased risk (is susceptible) of developing cancer (or develop cancer again) in the future.

Chromosome—Structures found in the center of a human cell on which genes are located.

Gene—Packages of DNA that control the growth, development, and normal function of the body.

Genetic counselor—A specially trained health care provider who helps individuals understand if a disease (such as cancer) is running in their family and their risk for inheriting this disease. Genetic counselors also discuss the benefits, risks and limitations of genetic testing with patients.

Leukemia—Cancer that arises in blood cells.

Mammogram—A screening test that uses x-rays to look at a woman's breasts for any abnormalities, such as cancer.

Mutation—An alteration in the number or order of the DNA sequence of a gene.

Penetrance—The likelihood that a person will develop a disease (such as cancer) if he or she has a mutation in a gene that increases the risk of developing that disorder.

Sarcoma—Cancer that occurs in connective tissue, such as cartilage or bone.

Sequencing—A method of performing genetic testing where the chemical order of a patient's DNA is compared to that of normal DNA.

Tumor suppressor genes—Genes that typically prevent cells from growing out of control and forming tumors that may be cancerous.

Ultrasound—A test that uses sound waves to examine organs in the body.

---

of cancer associated with LFS. Once this kind of mutation has been found in an individual, it is possible to test this person's relatives, such as the children, for the presence or absence of that particular mutation. Individuals who have a mutation in the *TP53* gene have a 50% chance of passing on this mutation to their children.

Even if a patient has a mutation in the *TP53* gene, it does not mean that he or she will definitely develop one of the cancers associated with Li-Fraumeni. However, the risk for those with the mutation is much higher than for someone in the general population. The likelihood that persons will develop cancer if they have a mutation in a cancer susceptibility gene like *TP53* is called penetrance.

If the first person tested within a family is not found to have an alteration in the *TP53* gene, his or her result is negative. Often this result is called indeterminate because a negative test result cannot completely rule out the possibility of hereditary cancer being present within a family. The interpretation of this type of result can be very complex. For example, a negative result may mean that the method used to detect mutations in the *TP53* gene may not be sensitive enough to identify all mutations. Additionally,

the mutation might be located in a part of the gene that is difficult to analyze. It may also mean that a person has a mutation in another cancer susceptibility gene that has not yet been discovered or is very rare. Finally, a negative result could mean that the person tested does not have an increased risk of developing cancer because of a mutation in a single cancer susceptibility gene.

Prevention

With the exception of screening for breast cancer, there are no effective means to screen for and/or prevent the cancers associated with Li-Fraumeni syndrome. However, researchers have developed some screening guidelines for those with LFS. For men and women, it is recommended that they undergo a thorough physical exam with their doctor every year. This examination should include skin and **colon cancer** screening along with a complete exam of the nervous system. Women should also undergo breast cancer screening, which consists of annual mammograms, breast self-exams, and breast exams by a physician or health care provider. Individuals with Li-Fraumeni syndrome may choose to undergo screening more often and at an earlier age than people in the general population.

For children with a *TP53* mutation, it is recommended that they also undergo a complete physical exam once a year by their physician. This examination should include an analysis of their urine and blood and an abdominal ultrasound.

Resources

BOOKS

Hainaut, Pierre, et al., eds. *P53 in the Clinics*. New York: Springer, 2013.

WEBSITES

U.S. National Library of Medicine. "Li-Fraumeni Syndrome." Genetics Home Reference. http://ghr.nlm.nih.gov/condition/li-fraumeni-syndrome (accessed December 4, 2014).

ORGANIZATIONS

American Cancer Society, 250 Williams St. NW, Atlanta, GA 30303, (800) 227-2345, http://www.cancer.org.

National Cancer Institute, 9609 Medical Center Dr., BG 9609 MSC 9760, Bethesda, MD 20892-9760, (800) 4-CANCER (422-6237), http://www.cancer.gov.

National Society of Genetic Counselors, 330 N. Wabash Ave., Ste. 2000, Chicago, IL 60611, (312) 321-6834, nsgc@nsgc.org, http://www.nsgc.org.

Tiffani A. DeMarco, M.S.

Limb salvage

Definition

Limb salvage surgery is a type of surgery primarily performed to remove bone and soft-tissue cancers occurring in limbs in order to avoid **amputation**.

Purpose

Limb salvage surgery is performed to remove **cancer** and avoid amputation, while preserving the patient's appearance and the greatest possible degree of function in the affected limb. The procedure is most commonly performed for bone tumors and bone sarcomas, but it is also performed for soft-tissue sarcomas affecting the extremities. This complex alternative to amputation is used to treat cancers that are slow to spread from the limb where they originate to other parts of the body, or that have not yet invaded soft tissue.

Twenty years ago, the standard of care for a patient with cancer in a limb was to amputate the affected extremity. Limb salvage surgery was an exception to the rule. Today, it is the exception that a patient loses a limb as part of cancer treatment. This advance is due to improvements in surgical technique, both resection and reconstruction; imaging methods, such as **computed tomography** (CT) scan and **magnetic resonance imaging** (MRI); and survival rates of patients treated with **chemotherapy**.

In recent years, limb salvage has been extended more and more to patients severely affected by chronic degenerative bone and joint diseases, such as those with rheumatoid arthritis, facing diabetic limb amputation, or with acute and chronic limb wounds.

Demographics

According to the **National Cancer Institute**, primary bone cancer is rare, with only 2,500 new cases diagnosed each year in the United States. More commonly, bones are the sites of tumors that result from the spread of other primary cancers—that is, from cancers that spread from other organs such as the breasts, lungs, and prostate. Bone cancers occur more frequently in children and young adults.

KEY TERMS

Resection—Removal of a part of an organ.

Sarcoma—A form of cancer that arises in supportive tissues such as bone, cartilage, fat, or muscle.

Description

Also called limb-sparing surgery, limb salvage involves removing the cancer and about an inch of healthy tissue surrounding it. If the bone is removed, it is replaced. The replacement can be made with synthetic metal rods or plates (prostheses), pieces of bone (grafts) taken from the patient's own body (autologous transplant), or pieces of bone removed from a donor body (cadaver) and frozen until needed for transplant (allograft). In time, transplanted bone grows into the patient's remaining bone. Chemotherapy, radiation, or a combination of both treatments may be used to shrink the tumor before surgery is performed.

Limb salvage is performed in three stages. Surgeons remove the cancer and a margin of healthy tissue, implant a prosthesis or bone graft (when necessary), and close the wound by transferring soft tissue and muscle from other parts of the patient's body to the surgical site. This treatment cures some cancers as successfully as amputation.

Surgical techniques

BONE TUMORS. Surgeons remove the malignant lesion and a cuff of normal tissue (wide excision) to cure low-grade tumors of bone or its components. To cure high-grade tumors, they also remove muscle, bone, and other tissues affected by the tumor (radical resection).

SOFT TISSUE SARCOMAS. Surgeons use limb-sparing surgery to treat about 80% of soft-tissue sarcomas affecting extremities. The surgery removes the tumor, lymph nodes, or tissues to which the cancer has spread, and at least 1 in. (2.5 cm) of healthy tissue on all sides of the tumor.

Radiation and/or chemotherapy may be administered before or after the operation. Radiation may also be administered during the operation by placing a special applicator against the surface from which the tumor has just been removed, and inserting tubes containing radioactive pellets at the site of the tumor. These tubes remain in place during the operation and are removed several days later.

To treat a **soft tissue sarcoma** that has spread to the patient's lung, the doctor may remove the original tumor, administer radiation or chemotherapy treatments to shrink the lung tumor, and surgically remove the lung tumor.

Limb salvage for children

Doctors may use expandable prostheses to perform limb-salvage surgery on children who have not stopped growing (skeletal immaturity). These devices may be adjusted without additional surgeries, but they may need to be replaced once children reach their full adult heights.

Preparation

Before deciding that limb salvage is appropriate for a particular patient, the treating doctor considers what type of cancer the patient has, the size and location of the tumor, how the illness has progressed, and the patient's age and general health.

After determining that limb salvage is appropriate for a particular patient, the doctor makes sure that the patient understands what the outcome of surgery is likely to be, that the implant may fail, and that additional surgery—even amputation—may be necessary.

Physical and occupational therapists help prepare the patient for surgery by introducing the muscle-strengthening, ambulation (walking), and range-of-motion (ROM) exercises that the patient will begin performing right after the operation.

Aftercare

During the five to ten days the patient remains in the hospital following surgery, nurses monitor sensation and blood flow in the affected extremity, and watch for signs that the patient may be developing **pneumonia**, pulmonary embolism, or deep-vein thrombosis.

The doctor prescribes broad-spectrum **antibiotics** for at least the first 48 hours after the operation, and often prescribes medication (prophylactic anticoagulants) and antiembolism stockings to prevent blood clots. A drainage tube placed in the wound for the first 24–48 hours prevents blood (hematoma) and fluid (seroma) from accumulating at the surgical site. As postoperative pain becomes less intense, mild narcotics or anti-inflammatory medications replace the epidural catheter or patient-controlled analgesic pump used to relieve pain immediately after the operation.

Exercise intervention

Limb salvage requires extensive surgical incisions, and patients who have these operations need extensive rehabilitation. The amount of bone removed and the type of reconstruction performed dictate how soon and how much the patient can exercise, but most patients begin muscle-strengthening, continuous passive motion (CPM), and ROM exercises the day after the operation and continue them for the next 12 months.

A patient who has had upper-limb surgery can use the opposite side of the body to perform hand and shoulder exercises. Patients should not do active elbow or shoulder exercises for two to eight weeks after having surgery involving the bone between the shoulder and elbow (humerus). Rehabilitation following lower-extremity limb salvage focuses on strengthening the muscles that straighten the legs (quadriceps), maintaining muscle tone, and gradually increasing weight-bearing ability so that the patient is able to stand on the affected limb within three months of the operation. A patient who has had lower-extremity surgery may have to learn a new way of walking (gait retraining) or wear a lift in one shoe.

Goals of rehabilitation

Physical and occupational therapy regimens are designed to help the patient move freely, function independently, and accept changes in **body image**. Even patients who look the same after surgery as they did previously may feel that the operation has altered their appearance.

Before a patient goes home from the hospital or rehabilitation center, the doctor decides whether the patient needs a walker, brace, cane, or other assistive device, and should make sure that the patient can climb stairs. Also, the doctor should emphasize the lifelong importance of preventing infection and give the patient written instructions about how to prevent and recognize infection, as well as what steps to take if infection does develop.

Risks

The major risks associated with limb salvage are: superficial or deep infection at the site of the surgery; loosening, shifting, or breakage of implants; rapid loss of blood flow or sensation in the affected limb; and severe blood loss and **anemia** from the surgery.

Postoperative infection is a serious problem. Chemotherapy or radiation can weaken the immune system, and extensive bone damage can occur before the infection is identified. Tissue may die (necrosis) if the surgeon used a large piece of tissue (flap) to close the wound. Necrosis is most likely to occur if the surgical site was treated with radiation before the operation. Treatment for postoperative infection involves removing the graft or implant, inserting drains at the infected site, and giving the patient oral or intravenous (IV) antibiotic

---

QUESTIONS TO ASK YOUR DOCTOR

- What are the possible complications involved in limb salvage surgery?
- How do I prepare for surgery?
- What type of anesthesia will be used?
- How is the surgery performed?
- How long will I be in the hospital?
- How many limb salvage surgeries do you perform in a year?
- Why do you think limb salvage will be successful in my case?
- How will I look and feel after the operation?
- Will I be able to enjoy my favorite sports and other activities after the operation?

---

therapy for as long as 12 months. Doctors may have to amputate the affected limb.

Results

A patient who has had limb salvage surgery will remain disease-free as long as a patient whose affected extremity has been amputated.

Salvaged limbs always function better than artificial ones. However, it takes a year for patients to learn to walk again following lower-extremity limb salvage, and patients who have undergone upper-extremity salvage must master new ways of using the affected arm or hand.

Successful surgery reduces the frequency and severity of patient falls and fractures that often result from disease-related changes in bone. Although successful surgery results in limbs that look and function very much like normal, healthy limbs, it is not unusual for patients to feel that their appearance has changed.

Some patients may also need additional surgery within five years of the first operation.

Morbidity and mortality rates

Orthopedic oncologists recognize that an operation to remove a tumor that spares the limb is associated with an incidence of tumor recurrence higher than that following an amputation. However, because there is no significant difference in overall survival rates, the increased rate of recurrence in patients who undergo limb salvage surgery is considered acceptable.

Alternatives

If the cancer's location makes it impossible to remove the malignancy without damaging or removing vital organs, essential nerves, or key blood vessels, or if it is impossible to reconstruct a limb that will function satisfactorily, salvage surgery may not be an appropriate treatment, and amputation of the limb becomes the only alternative treatment.

Health care team roles

Limb salvage surgery is performed in a hospital setting by experienced orthopedic surgeons with demonstrated expertise in limb salvage.

Resources

BOOKS

Lerner, A., et al. *Severe Injuries to the Limbs: Staged Treatment*. New York: Springer, 2007.

Veves, Aristidis, et al., eds. *The Diabetic Foot*. 2nd ed. Totowa, NJ: Humana Press, 2010.

Yarbro, Connie Henke, Debra Wujcik, and Barbara Holmes Gobel. *Cancer Nursing: Principles and Practice*. 7th ed. Sudbury, MA: Jones and Bartlett, 2011.

PERIODICALS

Frykberg, Robert G., et al. "Limb Salvage Using Advanced Technologies: A Case Report." *International Wound Journal* (February 21, 2013): e-pub ahead of print. http://dx.doi.org/10.1111/iwj.12050 (accessed October 3, 2014).

Hwang, John S., et al. "From Amputation to Limb Salvage Reconstruction: Evolution and Role of the Endoprosthesis in Musculoskeletal Oncology." *Journal of Orthopaedics and Traumatology* (September 22, 2013): e-pub ahead of print. http://dx.doi.org/10.1007/s10195-013-0265-8 (accessed October 3, 2014).

WEBSITES

American Academy of Orthopaedic Surgeons. "Bone Sarcoma in the Upper Extremity: Treatment Options Using Limb Salvage or Amputation." http://orthoinfo.aaos.org/topic.cfm?topic=A00092 (accessed October 3, 2014).

American Cancer Society. "Bone Cancer." http://www.cancer.org/cancer/bonecancer/index (accessed October 3, 2014).

Florida Hospital. "Limb Salvage Surgery." https://www.floridahospital.com/limb-salvage-surgery (accessed October 3, 2014).

ORGANIZATIONS

American Academy of Orthopaedic Surgeons (AAOS), 6300 N. River Rd., Rosemont, IL 60018-4262, (847) 823-7186, Fax: (847) 823-8125, pemr@aaos.org, http://www.aaos.org.

American Diabetes Association, 1701 North Beauregard St., Alexandria, VA 22311, (800) DIABETES (342-2383), AskADA@diabetes.org, http://www.diabetes.org.

International Society of Limb Salvage (ISOLS), c/o Vienna Medical Academy, Alser Strasse 4, Vienna, Austria 1090, +43 1 405 13 83, office@isols.info, http://isols.info.

Maureen Haggerty
Monique Laberge, PhD
REVISED BY LAURA JEAN CATALDO, RN, EdD

Lip cancer

Definition

A lip **cancer** is a malignant tumor, or neoplasm, that originates in the surface layer cells of the epithelial tissue in the upper or lower lip.

Description

The upper and lower lips are the well-defined red (often called vermilion) areas that surround the opening to the mouth. They contain muscles and special cells (receptors) that are sensitive to heat and cold and sensations of touch. The thin reddish line that separates the colored portion of the upper or lower lip from the surrounding facial skin is called the vermilion border. Largely taken for granted, the lips are important in identifying types of food to the brain and in getting food into the mouth. Lips also play a crucial role in speech.

A malignant tumor, or neoplasm, that originates in the cells of one of the lips is a cancer of the lip. Lip cancer almost always begins in the flat (squamous) epithelial cells. Epithelial cells form coverings (tissues) for the surfaces of the body. Skin, for example, has an outer layer of epithelial tissue. Almost 95% of cancers on

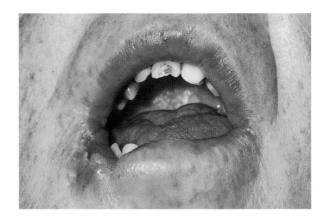

Squamous cell carcinoma on lip. *(English/Custom Medical Stock Photo)*

KEY TERMS

Biopsy—A procedure in which a tissue sample is taken from the body for examination.

Epithelial tissue—The collection of cells that cover the exterior and line the interior surfaces of the body.

Homograft—A graft made from tissue taken from a genetically nonidentical donor of the same species. It is also called an allograft.

Immunity—Ability to resist the effects of agents, such as bacteria and viruses, that cause disease.

Lymph node—A concentration of lymphatic tissue and part of the lymphatic system that collects fluid from around the cells and returns it to the blood vessels, and helps with the immune response.

Mohs surgery—A form of microscopically controlled surgery that allows for the precise removal of cancerous tissue. It is commonly used to treat various types of skin cancer, particularly in areas of the body where preserving as much tissue as possible is essential. Mohs surgery is also known as micrographic surgery.

Squamous cells—Flat epithelial cells, which usually make up the outer layer of epithelial tissue, the layer farthest away from the surface the epithelium covers.

Vermilion border—The thin line that divides the vermilion (reddish or reddish-orange)-colored portion of the upper or lower lip from the surrounding skin.

Xenograft—A graft made from tissue taken from a donor of another species.

the lower lip are squamous cell carcinomas or SCCs. Lip cancers usually look like chronic small lumps, ulcers, or scabby lesions, and are most likely to occur where the epithelium of the mucous membranes of the lower mouth joins the epithelium of the external skin. This area is called the mucocutaneous junction.

If a part of the lip is affected by cancer and must be removed by surgery, there will be significant changes in eating ability and speech function. The more lip tissue removed, the greater the disturbances in the patient's normal patterns of talking and eating.

Demographics

Lip cancer is decreasing as a subcategory of oral cancer in the developed world as of 2014, possibly as a result of declining use of tobacco products. Nine out of ten cases of lip cancer are diagnosed in people over the age of 45; the largest group of patients in the United States and Canada is Caucasian males over 50 years of age. Age, or the aging process, may contribute to the way the cancer develops. As a line of cells gets older, the genetic material in a cell loses some of its ability to repair itself. When the repair system is operating normally, damage to the genetic material, or DNA, caused by ultraviolet light from the sun is quickly weeded out. When the system fails, changes in the genetic material are kept, and they multiply when a cell divides.

If the genetic material cannot repair itself, damage caused by exposure to such environmental factors as sunlight and chemicals can quickly set in motion the uncontrolled growth of cells. A related factor is self-inflicted injury, such as the overuse of a toothpick or repeated lip biting. Self-inflicted damage to the tissues of the lip is most likely to lead to the emergence of a lip cancer when the patient has already weakened the oral mucosa by heavy smoking or the use of chewing tobacco.

The effects of factors that are known to cause lip cancer, such as smoking and exposure to sunlight, also add up as a person ages. Thus the combination of a breakdown in the repair system in the genetic material and the considerable periods of time (decades) over which a person is exposed to cancer agents probably causes lip cancers. However, as of 2014, researchers are still investigating exactly how lip cancers start.

Men are at greater risk of lip cancer than women. Depending on where they live, men are 3–13 times more likely to be diagnosed than women. This difference is thought to be related to the fact that more men than women work in outdoor occupations and are more likely to use tobacco or alcohol. In addition, the pigments in women's lipsticks offer some protection against sun exposure. Fair-skinned people are more likely to get lip cancer than those with dark skin. For reasons not yet understood, people in Asia have a much lower risk of lip cancer than those living on other continents. In many parts of Asia, lip cancer is extremely rare. In North America, nearly 13 out of 100,000 men will be diagnosed with lip cancer during their lifetime. In Australia, about 13.5 men per 100,000 will be diagnosed.

The frequency of lip cancer is often lumped together with oral cancer, although lip cancer is probably much more like **skin cancer** in origin. There are about 37,000 new diagnoses of mouth and lip cancer in the United States each year, but only about 0.6% of all new cancers are specifically cancers of the lip. The lower lip is 12 times more likely than the upper lip to develop cancer because of its greater exposure to sunlight; on the other hand, cancers of the upper lip are more aggressive than those of the lower lip.

Causes and symptoms

Exposure to sunlight and smoking, particularly pipe smoking, increases the risk of developing lip cancer. However, the way these factors do so is not completely understood as of 2014. Alcohol consumption is tied to **oral cancers** and may contribute to lip cancer as well.

Much of the evidence about the link between time spent in the sun and lip cancer comes from a look at those who are most likely to be diagnosed. Among them are farmers, golfers, professional tennis players, foresters, ranchers, field biologists, and others who spend long periods of time outdoors.

Lip cancer seems to share some properties with skin cancer in the way it originates. Yet several studies suggest that it takes more than exposure to sun to increase the risk of lip cancer. Viral infection is a risk factor, as is reduced immunity, which is a condition that may be caused by viral infection. A team of researchers in the Netherlands recently reported a link between liver transplants and a higher risk of lip and skin cancer following the transplant. The results are not unexpected. In this procedure, drugs are used to suppress, or lower, the activity of a recipient's immune system so that a donor organ will be accepted. Thus the immunity of the organ recipient is low, and lower immunity is linked to lip cancer.

Individuals with acquired immunodeficiency syndrome (AIDS) are at greater risk of lip cancer. People infected with **herpes simplex** viruses, human papillomaviruses (HPV), and other viruses may also be at greater risk.

Vitamin deficiency may also be a factor that contributes to lip cancer. The sorts of **vitamins** found in fruits and vegetables, particularly carotene, the substance the body uses to form vitamins A and C, seem to be important in preventing lip cancer.

In addition to lumps, open ulcers, or scabbed areas on the lip tissue, pain can also be a symptom of lip cancer, particularly pain in a lymph node near the affected part of the lip. This is a troubling symptom because it indicates that the cancer has metastasized (spread) beyond the lip.

Diagnosis

Cancer of the lip is often noticed by patients themselves when looking in the mirror while shaving, brushing the teeth, or applying makeup. Dentists also frequently identify a suspicious spot, sore, or lump on the lip. A good dental exam includes an examination of the lips and the mouth. X-ray and **biopsy** (the taking of a tissue sample for analysis) can be used to determine whether cancer is present. The doctor may also use laser light or a dye called toluidine blue to examine areas of suspicious tissue. Damaged tissue will look different from normal tissue under laser light. If toluidine blue is used, abnormal tissue will stain blue while normal tissue will not.

Because spots and sores on the lips can be short-lived, people should not be alarmed by every change that appears. When there is a change that lasts longer than three weeks, however, it should be investigated as soon as possible. If the next scheduled dental visit is several months away, a special appointment with the dentist or a dermatologist should be made. Dentists should tell their patients, particularly older adults, how to undertake a regular self-examination of the lips between check ups.

Treatment team

A physician who specializes in oncology, the study and treatment of cancer, will probably take the lead on treatment. An oral or maxillofacial surgeon will remove the cancer. Not all oncologists are surgeons, so it is likely that the team will include a medical oncologist, who coordinates treatment, as well as a surgical oncologist, who performs the surgery.

Because surgery on the lip can interfere with eating and talking, most teams include a nutritionist and a speech pathologist. Scars and alterations of facial features can produce changes in **body image**, and a psychiatrist or social worker may participate in the team to help a patient cope with such changes. It is possible that a dentist or oral surgeon will also play a role. Nurses who administer **chemotherapy** and monitor the status of patients will be involved, as will radiation technicians and a radiation oncologist. If reconstruction of a lip is necessary because of the amount of tissue removed or the size of the scar, a plastic surgeon will be added to the team.

Clinical staging

The ability to see a suspicious area on the lips and to detect lip cancer early combine to form the staging process. (One inch equals 2.5 cm.)

- Stage 0: There is no evidence of a cancerous tumor.

- Stage I: The cancer is less than 0.75 in. (2 cm) in diameter and has not spread.

- Stage II: The cancer is 0.75–1.5 in. (2–4 cm) in diameter and has not spread.

- Stage III: The cancer is either larger than 1.5 in. or has spread to a lymph node on the side of the neck that matches the primary location of the lip cancer. The lymph node is enlarged, but not much more than an inch.

- Stage IV: One or more of several changes has occurred. There may be a spread of cancer to the mouth or to the areas around the lip, more than one lymph node with cancer, or metastasis (spread) to other parts of the body.

Treatment

Early-stage lip cancers are typically removed by **Mohs surgery**. Also called micrographic surgery, Mohs surgery is a technique in which the tumor is removed in very thin slices. Each slice is examined by the surgeon under the microscope before the next slice is removed. The surgeon continues to remove these thin layers of tissue until cancer cells are no longer visible under the microscope.

Decisions about which method to use depend on many factors, but the size of the tumor and the tolerance a patient has for radiation or chemotherapy are particularly important. The larger the tumor, the more urgent is its removal. Smaller tumors can be treated with radiation or other methods in an effort to shrink them before surgery. In some cases, surgery might be avoided. For stage III cancer with lymph node involvement, the cancerous lymph nodes are also removed.

Chemotherapy may be used at any stage, but it is particularly important for stage IV cancer. In some cases, chemotherapy is used before surgery, just as radiation is, to try to eliminate the cancer without cutting, or at least to make it smaller before it is cut out (excised). After surgery, **radiation therapy** and chemotherapy are both used to treat patients with stage IV lip cancer, sometimes in combination.

There are many new and promising types of treatment for lip cancer. For example, heat kills some cancer cells, and a treatment known as **hyperthermia** uses heat to eliminate cancer in some patients.

Because lip cancers are well studied and often successfully treated, the best practices for dealing with the cancer or a suspected cancer are specific. In the case of how to extract and study tissue to determine whether a

suspicious growth is malignant (biopsy), size is an extremely useful guide.

It is possible to take tissue from a suspected lip cancer for examination, or biopsy, by simply piercing and extracting tissue with a large hollow needle. This technique is called a punch biopsy. However, the method is not recommended for any tumor that is thicker than about one-sixteenth of an inch. For thicker tumors, a tissue sample is better taken by cutting into the tumor; that is, making an incision.

The success with identifying lip cancer early and eliminating it means that it is not a major killer. Only four in 2.5 million people die from lip cancer each year, or about 112 individuals in the entire United States population. In contrast, cancers in the oral cavity, including the tongue, cause about 7,300 deaths in the United States each year.

Alternative and complementary therapies

Because there seems to be some link between a chronic absence of vitamins A and C in the diet and lip cancer, some complementary therapies promote taking massive amounts of the vitamins, or megavitamins. The value of such therapy has not been demonstrated as of 2014. In order to avoid possible side effects or harmful interactions with standard cancer treatment, patients should always notify their treatment team of any over-the-counter or herbal remedies that they are taking.

Patients being treated for lip cancer may benefit from some complementary therapies that promote relaxation and help to relieve stress. These include massage therapy, acupuncture, guided relaxation, and aromatherapy. Such forms of exercise as yoga and tai chi may also be helpful to some patients.

Coping with cancer treatment

The doctor and patient should discuss the need for a way to communicate if speech is impaired after surgery. A pad and pencil may be all that is needed for a short interval. If there will be a long period of speech difficulty, patients should be ready with additional means of communication, such as TYY telephone service.

A change in appearance after the removal of a lip cancer—particularly after a vermilionectomy (removal of the entire vermilion border)— can lead to concerns about body image, and social interactions may suffer. A support group can help. Discussions with a social worker, loved ones, or other patients who have undergone similar treatment can be of major benefit.

If a significant portion of lip is removed, speech therapy may be necessary to relearn how to make certain sounds. Scars and alterations of the lips usually can be reduced or hidden entirely with the techniques available from plastic surgery, so any alteration in appearance because of lip cancer is typically transient.

Reconstruction of the lip will help with appearance, but it might not make it easier to talk, especially if muscle tissue is removed during the surgery to eliminate the cancer. In many cases, the reconstruction process actually damages more muscle and sensory tissue. New methods of **reconstructive surgery** are being developed to avoid such an outcome. Some of these newer methods involve grafts of skin and muscle taken from the forearm or the area of the cheek near the angle of the jawbone. Other methods involve xenografts made from porcine (pig) tissue or homografts derived from human cadavers. In general, reconstruction of the lower lip is more difficult than reconstruction of the upper lip.

Appetite may be affected before, during, and after treatment. Before treatment, the presence of a tumor can interfere with the tasting of food, and food might not seem as appealing as it once did. During treatment, particularly radiation treatment, the area of the lips and mouth might be sore and make eating difficult. After treatment, a loss of sensation in the part of the lip affected can reduce appetite. A nutritionist or dietitian can help with supplements for those who experience significant **weight loss** and suffer loss of appetite.

Prognosis

The outlook for recovery from lip cancer is very good if it is diagnosed early; as of 2014, the 5-year survival rate for lip cancer was above 96% for Stage I cancers and 83% for Stage II cancers. For stage I and stage II cancers, surgery to remove the cancer or radiation treatment of the affected area is sometimes all that is required to produce a cure.

Clinical trials

The Cancer Information Service at the National Institutes of Health offers information about **clinical trials** that are looking for volunteers. There are no clinical trials exclusively for lip cancers as of mid-2014; however, of the 61 open trials presently registered with the National Institutes of Health, all of them group lip cancer together either with recurrent or advanced head and neck cancer, or with other cancers of the oral mucosa.

Prevention

The best preventive measures are minimizing sun exposure and avoiding the use of tobacco and alcohol. Eating plenty of fruits and vegetables is recommended as well. Even though the importance of fruits and vegetables is not proven to prevent lip cancer, overall, fruits and vegetables are demonstrated cancer-fighters. Any precaution that is taken against contracting human immunodeficiency virus (HIV), which causes AIDS, is also likely to reduce the chance of developing lip cancer—as are precautions taken to avoid contracting **human papillomavirus** (HPV).

Special concerns

Certain diseases can mimic a possible lip cancer. They must be ruled out if a suspicious spot is found. This is particularly true in areas where diseases that cause lesions, or sores, on the lips are found. One such disease is *histoplasmosis capsulatum*, which is caused by a fungus. It sometimes produces an ulcer or lesion on the lip that leads to suspicion of lip cancer.

Sometimes lip cancer cannot be cured. It may keep recurring. It may also metastasize, particularly to the lungs. But overall, lip cancer is considered highly curable. Talking openly with the physician in charge of care is important in order for the patient to understand the course of the disease and be prepared to make decisions about treatment options.

Resources

BOOKS

Cummings, Louise, ed. *The Cambridge Handbook of Communication Disorders*. Cambridge, UK: Cambridge University Press, 2014.

Wolk, Burrell H. *A Patient's Guide to Skin Cancer: What You Need to Know: Your Essential Guide to the Prevention, Early Detection, and Treatment of Skin and Lip Cancer*. Phoenix, AZ: Skin and Cancer Center of Arizona Publishing, 2010.

PERIODICALS

Aldelaimi, T. N., and A. A. Kahlil. "Lip Reconstruction Using Karapandzic Flap." *Journal of Craniofacial Surgery* 25 (March 2014): e136–e138.

Harirchian, S., and S. Baredes. "Use of AlloDerm in Primary Reconstruction after Resection of Squamous Cell Carcinoma of the Lip and Oral Commissure." *American Journal of Otolaryngology* 34 (September-October 2013): 611–613.

Kashyap, R. R., and R. S. Kashyap. "Self-inflicted Injury as a Potential Trigger for Carcinoma of Lip—A Case Report." *Gerodontology* 30 (September 2013): 236–238.

Lubek, J. E., and R. A. Ord. "Lip Reconstruction." *Oral and Maxillofacial Surgery Clinics of North America* 25 (May 2013): 203–214.

Pickert, A. J., and S. A. Nemeth Ochoa. "Use of Porcine Xenografts on Partial-thickness Vermilion Border and Mucosal Lower Lip Mohs Defects." *Dermatologic Surgery* 39 (June 2013): 948–950.

Schmults, C. D., et al. "Factors Predictive of Recurrence and Death from Cutaneous Squamous Cell Carcinoma: A 10-

year, Single-institution Cohort Study." *JAMA Dermatology* 149 (May 2013): 541–547.

Wollina, U. "Reconstruction of Medial Lower Lip Defects after Tumour Surgery: Modified Staircase Technique." *Journal of Cutaneous and Aesthetic Surgery* 6 (October 2013): 214–216.

WEBSITES

American Cancer Society (ACS). "Oral Cavity and Oropharyngeal Cancer." http://www.cancer.org/acs/groups/cid/documents/webcontent/003128-pdf.pdf (accessed August 10, 2014).

National Cancer Institute (NCI). "Oral Cancer." http://www.cancer.gov/cancertopics/types/oral (accessed August 10, 2014).

Scully, Crispian. "Cancers of the Oral Mucosa." Medscape Reference. http://emedicine.medscape.com/article/1075729-overview (accessed August 10, 2014).

Skin Cancer Foundation. "Lip Cancer: Not Uncommon, Often Overlooked." http://www.skincancer.org/skin-cancer-information/lip-cancer-not-uncommon (accessed August 10, 2014).

ORGANIZATIONS

American Academy of Facial Plastic and Reconstructive Surgery (AAFPRS), 310 South Henry Street, Alexandria, VA 22314, (703) 299-9291, Fax: (703) 299-8898, info@aafprs.org, http://www.aafprs.org.

American Cancer Society (ACS), 250 Williams Street NW, Atlanta, GA 30303, (800) 227-2345, http://www.cancer.org/aboutus/howwehelpyou/app/contact-us.aspx, http://www.cancer.org/index.

National Cancer Institute (NCI), BG 9609 MSC 9760, 9609 Medical Center Drive, Bethesda, MD 20892-9760, (800) 4-CANCER (422-6237), http://www.cancer.gov/global/contact/email-us, http://www.cancer.gov.

Skin Cancer Foundation, 149 Madison Avenue, Suite 901, New York, NY 10016, (212) 725-5176, http://www.skincancer.org/contact-us, http://www.skincancer.org.

Diane M. Calabrese, PhD
Rebecca J. Frey, PhD

Liver biopsy

Definition

A liver **biopsy** is a medical procedure performed to obtain a small piece of liver tissue for diagnostic testing. The sample is examined under a microscope by a pathologist, a doctor who specializes in the effects of disease on body tissues—in this case, to detect abnormalities of the liver. Liver biopsies are sometimes called percutaneous liver biopsies, because the tissue sample is obtained by going through the patient's skin. This is a useful diagnostic procedure with very low risk and little discomfort to the patient.

Purpose

A liver biopsy is usually done to evaluate the extent of damage that has occurred to the liver because of chronic and acute disease processes or toxic injury. Biopsies are often performed to identify abnormalities in liver tissues after other techniques have failed to yield clear results. In patients with chronic hepatitis C, liver biopsy may be used to assess the patient's prognosis and the likelihood of responding to antiviral treatment.

A liver biopsy may be ordered to diagnose or stage any of the following conditions or disorders:

- jaundice
- cirrhosis
- repeated abnormal results from liver function tests
- alcoholic liver disease
- unexplained swelling or enlargement of the liver (hepatomegaly)
- suspected drug-related liver damage like acetaminophen poisoning
- hemochromatosis, a condition of excess iron in the liver
- intrahepatic cholestasis, the buildup of bile in the liver
- hepatitis
- primary cancers of the liver, such as hepatomas, cholangiocarcinomas, and angiosarcomas
- metastatic cancers of the liver (more than 20 times as common in the United States as primary cancers)
- post-liver transplant to measure graft rejection
- fever of unknown origin
- suspected tuberculosis, sarcoidosis, or amyloidosis
- genetic disorders such as Wilson's disease (a disorder in which copper accumulates in the liver, brain, kidneys, and corneas)

Description

Percutaneous liver biopsy is sometimes called aspiration biopsy or fine-needle aspiration (FNA) because it is done with a hollow needle attached to a suction syringe. The special needles used to perform a liver biopsy are called Menghini or Jamshedi needles. The amount of specimen collected should be about 0.03–0.7 fluid ounces (1–2 cubic centimeters). In many cases, the biopsy is done by a radiologist, a doctor who specializes in **x-rays** and **imaging studies**. The radiologist will use **computed tomography** (CT) scan or ultrasound to guide the needle to the target site for the biopsy. Some ultrasound-guided biopsies are performed

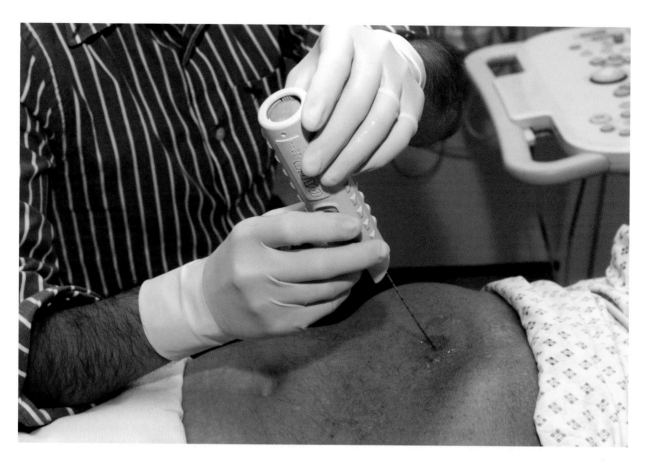

Doctor performing a percutaneous liver biopsy. *(P. Marazzi/Science Source)*

using a biopsy gun that has a spring mechanism that contains a cutting sheath. This type of procedure yields a greater amount of tissue.

An hour or so before the biopsy, the patient is given a sedative to aid in relaxation. The patient then lies back with the right elbow to the side and the right hand under the head. The patient must lie as still as possible during the procedure—a sensation resembling a pinch will occur in the right shoulder when the needle passes a certain nerve (the phrenic nerve), but the patient must remain motionless in spite of the momentary pain.

The doctor will mark a spot on the skin of the abdomen where the needle is to be inserted. The right side of the upper abdomen is thoroughly cleansed with an antiseptic solution, generally iodine. The patient is then given a local anesthetic at the biopsy site.

The doctor prepares the needle by drawing sterile saline solution into a syringe. The syringe is attached to the biopsy needle, which is inserted into the patient's chest wall. The doctor draws the plunger of the syringe back to create a vacuum. At this point, the patient is asked to take a deep breath and hold it. The needle is inserted into the liver and withdrawn quickly, usually

within two seconds or less. The negative pressure in the syringe draws or pulls a sample of liver tissue into the biopsy needle. As soon as the needle is withdrawn, the patient can breathe normally. This step takes only a few seconds. Pressure is applied at the biopsy site to stop any bleeding, and a bandage is placed over it. The liver tissue sample is placed in a cup with a 10% formalin solution and sent to the laboratory immediately. The entire procedure takes 10–15 minutes. Test results are usually available within a day.

Most patients experience minor discomfort during the procedure (up to 50% of patients) but not severe pain. According to a medical study of adult patients undergoing percutaneous liver biopsy, pain was most often described as mild to moderate (i.e., a rating of three on a scale of one to ten). Mild medications of a non aspirin type can be given after the biopsy if the pain persists for several hours.

Precautions

Some patients should not have percutaneous liver biopsies, including those with any of the following conditions:

KEY TERMS

Aspiration—The technique of removing a tissue sample for biopsy through a hollow needle attached to a suction syringe.

Bile—Liquid produced by the liver that is excreted into the intestine to aid in the digestion of fats.

Biliary—Relating to bile.

Biopsy—The surgical removal and microscopic examination of living tissue for diagnostic purposes.

Cirrhosis—A progressive disease of the liver characterized by the death of liver cells and their replacement with fibrous tissue.

Formalin—A clear solution of diluted formaldehyde that is used to preserve liver biopsy specimens until they can be examined in the laboratory.

Hepatitis—Inflammation of the liver caused by infection or toxic injury.

Jaundice—Also termed icterus; an increase in blood bile pigments that are deposited in the skin, eyes, deeper tissue, and excretions. The skin and whites of the eyes will appear yellow.

Menghini needle/Jamshedi needle—Special needles used to obtain a sample of liver tissue by aspiration.

Metastatic cancer—A cancer that has been transmitted through the body from a primary cancer site.

Percutaneous biopsy—A biopsy in which the needle is inserted and the sample removed through the skin.

Prothrombin test—A common test to measure the amount of time it takes for a patient's blood to clot; measurements are in seconds.

- a platelet count below 50,000

- a prothrombin test time greater than three seconds over the reference interval, indicating a possible clotting abnormality

- a liver tumor with a large number of veins

- a large amount of abdominal fluid (ascites)

- infection anywhere in the lungs, the lining of the chest or abdominal wall, the biliary tract, or the liver

- benign tumors (angiomas) of the liver, which consist mostly of enlarged or newly formed blood vessels and may bleed heavily

- biliary obstruction (bile may leak from the biopsy site and cause an infection of the abdominal cavity)

Preparation

Liver biopsies require some preparation. Because aspirin and ibuprofen (Advil, Motrin) are known to cause excessive bleeding by inhibiting platelets and impairing clotting function, patients should avoid taking any of these medications for at least a week before the biopsy. The doctor should check patients' records to see whether they are taking any other medications that may affect blood clotting. Both a platelet count (or complete blood count) and a prothrombin time (to assess how well the blood clots) are performed prior to the biopsy. These tests determine whether there is an abnormally high risk of uncontrolled bleeding from the biopsy site, which may contraindicate the procedure. Patients should limit food or drink for a period of four to eight hours before the biopsy.

Aftercare

Liver biopsies are now performed as outpatient procedures in most hospitals. Patients are asked to lie on their right sides for one hour and then to rest quietly for three more hours. At regular intervals, a nurse checks the patient's vital signs (pulse, temperature, breathing rate). If there are no complications, the patient is discharged, but will be asked to stay in an area that is within an hour from the hospital in case delayed bleeding occurs.

Patients should arrange to have a friend or relative take them home after discharge. Bed rest for a day is recommended, followed by a week of avoiding heavy work or strenuous exercise. The patient can immediately resume eating a normal diet.

Some mild soreness in the area of the biopsy is expected after the anesthetic wears off. Irritation of the muscle that lies over the liver can also cause mild discomfort in the shoulder for some patients. Acetaminophen can be taken for minor soreness, but aspirin and ibuprofen products are best avoided. The patient should, however, call the doctor if there is severe pain in the abdomen, chest, or shoulder; difficulty breathing; or persistent bleeding. These signs may indicate that there has been leakage of bile into the abdominal cavity, or that air has been introduced into the cavity around the lungs.

Risks

The complications associated with a liver biopsy are usually minor; most will occur in the first two hours following the procedure, and greater than 95% in the first 24 hours. The most significant risk is prolonged internal bleeding. Other complications from percutaneous liver biopsies include the leakage of bile or the introduction of air into the chest cavity (pneumothorax). There is also a small chance that an infection may occur. The risk that an internal organ such as the lung, gallbladder, or kidney might be punctured is decreased when using the ultrasound- or CT-guided procedure.

Results

After the biopsy, the liver sample is sent to the pathology laboratory and examined. A normal (negative) result finds no evidence of pathology in the tissue sample. It should be noted, however, that many diseases of the liver are concentrated in one area (focal) and not spread across the liver (diffuse); an abnormality may not be detected if the sample was taken from an unaffected site. If symptoms persist, the patient may need to undergo another biopsy.

The pathologist will perform a visual inspection of the sample to note any abnormalities in appearance. Carcinomas are white. In preparation for microscopic examination, the tissue is frozen and cut into thin sections, which are mounted on glass slides and stained with various dyes. In **liver cancer**, small dark malignant cells will be visible within the liver tissue. The pathologist also checks for the number of bile ducts and determines whether they are dilated. He or she also looks at the health of the small arteries and portal veins. Many different findings may be noted, and a differential diagnosis (one out of many possibilities) can often be made. In difficult cases, other laboratory tests will aid the clinician in determining the final diagnosis.

Alternatives

Liver biopsy is an invasive and sometimes painful procedure that is also expensive. In some instances, blood tests may provide enough information to health care providers to make an accurate diagnosis and therefore avoid a biopsy. Occasionally, a biopsy may be obtained using a laparoscope (an instrument inserted through the abdominal wall that allows the doctor to visualize the liver and obtain a sample) or during surgery if the patient is undergoing an operation on the abdomen. Imaging techniques (such as ultrasound) may also be employed during a liver biopsy in order to allow more accurate placement of the biopsy needle.

Health care team roles

The liver biopsy requires the skill of many clinicians, including the radiologist, hepatologist, and pathologist, to make the diagnosis. Nurses will assist the physician during the biopsy procedure and in caring for the patient after the procedure. Tissues are prepared for microscopic evaluation by a histologic technician in the pathology lab. The procedure is generally performed on an outpatient basis in a hospital.

QUESTIONS TO ASK YOUR DOCTOR

- Why is a biopsy indicated in my case?
- How many biopsies do you perform each year? What is your rate of complications?
- What will happen when I get the results?
- What alternatives are available to me?

Resources

BOOKS

Feldman, M., et al. *Sleisenger & Fordtran's Gastrointestinal and Liver Disease.* 9th ed. Philadelphia: Saunders/Elsevier, 2010.

PERIODICALS

Li, G. P., et al. "Fine Needle Aspirating and Cutting Is Superior to Tru-Cut Core Needle in Liver Biopsy." *Hepatobiliary & Pancreatic Diseases International* 12, no. 5 (2013): 508–11.

WEBSITES

American Cancer Society. "Liver Cancer." http://www.cancer.org/cancer/livercancer/index (accessed August 20, 2014).
Mayo Clinic staff. "Liver Biopsy." MayoClinic.com. http://www.mayoclinic.com/health/liver-biopsy/MY00949 (accessed August 20, 2014).
National Digestive Diseases Information Clearinghouse. "Liver Biopsy." National Institute of Diabetes and Digestive and Kidney Diseases. http://digestive.niddk.nih.gov/ddiseases/pubs/liverbiopsy (accessed August 20, 2014).

ORGANIZATIONS

American Cancer Society, 250 Williams St. NW, Atlanta, GA 30303, (800) 227-2345, http://www.cancer.org.
American Liver Foundation, 39 Broadway, Ste. 2700, New York, NY 10006, (212) 668-1000, (800) GO-LIVER (465-4837), Fax: (212) 483-8179, http://www.liverfoundation.org.

Jane E. Phillips, PhD
Stephanie Dionne Sherk
REVISED BY ROSALYN CARSON-DEWITT, MD

Liver cancer

Definition

Liver cancer is a relatively rare form of cancer, but it has a high mortality rate. Liver cancers can be classified into two types. They are either primary, when the cancer

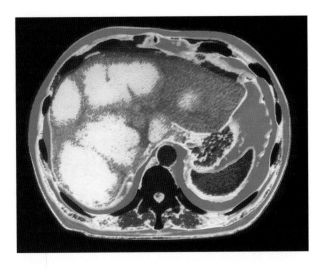

Computed tomography (CT) scan of a section of the abdomen showing liver cancer. The vertebra appears dark blue, the liver is large and appears light blue, and the light patches on the liver are the cancerous tumors. *(DPT CLINICAL RADIOLOGY SALSBURY HOSPITAL/Science Source)*

starts in the liver itself, or metastatic, when the cancer has spread to the liver from some other part of the body.

Description

Most liver cancers belong to one of two types: hepatocellular carcinomas (HCC), also called malignant hepatomas, which start in the liver tissue itself, and cholangiomas, or cholangiocarcinomas, which are cancers that develop in the bile ducts inside the liver. In the United States, 70%–75% of cases of primary liver cancers are HCC. In Africa and Asia, more than 90% of cases of primary liver **cancer** are HCC. Two rare types of primary liver cancer are mixed-cell tumors and Kupffer cell sarcomas.

One rare type of primary liver cancer, called a hepatoblastoma, usually occurs in children younger than four years of age. Unlike liver cancers in adults, hepatoblastomas have a good chance of being treated successfully. Approximately 70% of children with hepatoblastomas experience complete cures. If the tumor is detected early, the survival rate is over 90%.

Metastasis

The liver is a common site of **metastasis**. Because blood from all parts of the body must pass through the liver for filtration, cancer cells from other organs and tissues easily reach the liver, where they can lodge and grow into secondary tumors.

Demographics

Liver cancer in the United States represents about 2% of all malignancies and 4% of newly diagnosed cancers. Hepatocellular **carcinoma** (HCC) is much more common outside the United States, representing 10% to 50% of malignancies in Africa and parts of Asia. Rates of HCC in men are at least two to three times higher than for women, and in high-risk areas (East and Southeast Asia, sub-Saharan Africa), the rates are even higher.

According to the American Cancer Society, 33,190 people in the United States will be newly diagnosed with primary liver cancer in 2014, and 23,000 persons will die from the disease that year. The incidence of primary liver cancer has been rising in the United States and Canada since the mid-1990s, most likely as a result of the rising rate of hepatitis C infections. About 700,000 new cases of primary liver cancer are reported worldwide each year. Although uncommon in the United States and Canada, the disease is the leading cause of cancer deaths worldwide, causing about 600,000 deaths annually.

Causes and symptoms

Causes

The exact cause of primary liver cancer is still unknown. In adults, however, certain factors are known to place some individuals at higher risk of developing liver cancer. These factors include:

• Male sex.

• Age over 60 years

• Ethnicity: Asian Americans with cirrhosis have four times as great a chance of developing liver cancer as Caucasians with cirrhosis, and African Americans have twice the risk of Caucasians. In addition, Asians often develop liver cancer at much younger ages than either African Americans or Caucasians.

• Exposure to substances in the environment that may cause cancer (carcinogens): These include a substance produced by a mold that grows on rice and peanuts (aflatoxin); thorium dioxide, which was once used as a contrast dye for x-rays of the liver; vinyl chloride, used in manufacturing plastics; and cigarette smoke.

• Hereditary hemochromatosis: This is a disorder characterized by abnormally high levels of iron storage in the body. It often develops into cirrhosis.

• Cirrhosis: HCC appears to be a frequent complication of cirrhosis of the liver. Between 30% and 70% of HCC patients also have cirrhosis. It is estimated that a patient with cirrhosis has 40 times the chance of developing HCC than a person with a healthy liver.

KEY TERMS

Aflatoxin—A substance produced by molds that grow on rice and peanuts. Exposure to aflatoxin is thought to explain the high rates of primary liver cancer in Africa and parts of Asia.

Alpha-fetoprotein (AFP)—A protein in blood serum that is found in abnormally high concentrations in most patients with primary liver cancer.

Cirrhosis—A chronic degenerative disease of the liver, in which normal cells are replaced by fibrous tissue. Cirrhosis is a major risk factor for the later development of liver cancer.

Hepatitis—A viral disease characterized by inflammation of the liver cells (hepatocytes). People infected with hepatitis B or hepatitis C virus are at increased risk of developing liver cancer.

Metastatic—Referring to a cancer that has spread to an organ or tissue from a primary cancer located elsewhere in the body.

Radiofrequency ablation—A technique for removing a tumor by heating it with a radiofrequency current passed through a needle electrode.

- Exposure to hepatitis viruses B (HBV) and C (HCV): It is estimated that 80% of worldwide HCC is associated with chronic HBV infection. In Africa and most of Asia, exposure to hepatitis B is an important factor; in Japan and some Western countries, exposure to hepatitis C is connected with a higher risk of developing liver cancer. In the United States, nearly 25% of patients with liver cancer show evidence of HBV infection. Hepatitis is commonly found among intravenous drug abusers. The virus can be passed by sharing needles or engaging in sexual intercourse with an infected person. The increase in HCC incidence in the United States is thought to be due to increasing rates of HBV and HCV infections due to increased sexual promiscuity and illicit drug needle sharing.

Symptoms

The early symptoms of liver cancer are often vague and not unique to liver disorders. The long period between the beginning of the tumor's growth and the first signs of illness is the major reason why the disease has a high mortality rate. At the time of diagnosis, patients are often fatigued, with **fever**, abdominal pain, and loss of appetite (**anorexia**). They may look emaciated and generally ill. As the tumor enlarges, it stretches the

membrane surrounding the liver (the capsule), causing pain in the upper abdomen on the right side. The pain may extend into the back and shoulder. Some patients develop a collection of fluid known as **ascites** in the abdominal cavity. Others may show signs of bleeding into the digestive tract. In addition, the tumor may block the ducts of the liver or the gall bladder, leading to jaundice. In patients with jaundice, the whites of the eyes and the skin may turn yellow, and the urine becomes dark-colored.

Diagnosis

Physical examination

If the doctor suspects a diagnosis of liver cancer, he or she will check the patient's history for risk factors and pay close attention to the condition of the patient's abdomen during the physical examination. Masses or lumps in the liver and ascites can often be felt while the patient is lying flat on the examination table. The liver is usually swollen and hard in patients with liver cancer; it may be sore when the doctor presses on it. In some cases, the patient's spleen is also enlarged. The doctor may be able to hear an abnormal sound (bruit) or rubbing noise (friction rub) if he or she uses a stethoscope to listen to the blood vessels that lie near the liver. The noises are caused by the pressure of the tumor on the blood vessels.

Laboratory tests

Blood tests may be used to test liver function or to evaluate risk factors in the patient's history. Between 50% and 75% of primary liver cancer patients have abnormally high blood serum levels of a particular protein (alpha-fetoprotein or AFP). The AFP test, however, cannot be used by itself to confirm a diagnosis of liver cancer because cirrhosis or chronic hepatitis can also produce high alpha-fetoprotein levels. Tests for alkaline phosphatase, bilirubin, lactate dehydrogenase, and other chemicals indicate that the liver is not functioning normally. About 75% of patients with liver cancer show evidence of hepatitis infection. However, abnormal liver function test results are never specific for a diagnosis of liver cancer.

Imaging studies

Imaging studies are useful in locating specific areas of abnormal tissue in the liver. Liver tumors as small as an inch across can now be detected by ultrasound or **computed tomography** scan (CT scan). Imaging studies, however, cannot tell the difference between a hepatoma and other abnormal masses or lumps of tissue (nodules) in the liver. A sample of liver tissue for **biopsy** is needed to make the definitive diagnosis of a primary liver cancer. CT or ultrasound can be used to guide the doctor in selecting the best location for obtaining the biopsy sample.

Chest **x-rays** may be used to see whether the liver tumor is primary or has metastasized from the lungs.

Liver biopsy

Liver biopsy is considered to provide the definite diagnosis of liver cancer. A sample of the liver or tissue fluid is removed with a fine needle and is checked under a microscope for the presence of cancer cells. In about 70% of cases, the biopsy is positive for cancer. In most cases, there is little risk to the patient from the biopsy procedure. In about 0.4% of cases, however, the patient develops a fatal hemorrhage from the biopsy because some tumors are supplied with a large number of blood vessels and bleed very easily.

Laparoscopy

The doctor may also perform a **laparoscopy** to help in the diagnosis of liver cancer. First, the doctor makes a small cut in the patient's abdomen and inserts a small lighted tube called a laparoscope to view the area. A small piece of liver tissue is removed and examined under a microscope for the presence of cancer cells.

Clinical staging

The American Joint Committee on Cancer's TNM system is the primary method of staging liver cancer. This system assesses the size of the tumor (T), whether it has spread to the lymph nodes (N), and whether it has metastasized (M). Stage I cancers have only one tumor that has not yet grown into blood vessels or spread to other sites in the body. Stage II and III cancers consist of larger or multiple tumors that have penetrated nearby vessels or veins but have not yet spread to the lymph nodes or major organs. Stage IV cancers are the most serious and have begun to spread to other areas of the body.

Treatment

Treatment of liver cancer is based on several factors, including the type of cancer; stage (early or advanced); the location of other cancers in the patient's body (if present); the patient's age; and other coexisting diseases, including cirrhosis. For many patients, treatment of liver cancer is primarily intended to relieve the pain caused by the cancer but cannot cure it.

Surgery

Few liver cancers in adults can be cured by surgery because they are usually too advanced by the time they are discovered. If the cancer is contained within one lobe of the liver, and if the patient does not have cirrhosis, jaundice, or ascites, surgery is the best treatment option. Patients who can have their entire tumor removed have the best chance of survival, but unfortunately, very few patients fall into this group. If the entire visible tumor can be removed, about 25% of patients will be cured. The operation that is performed is called a partial hepatectomy, or partial removal of the liver. The surgeon will remove either an entire lobe of the liver (a **lobectomy**) or cut out the area around the tumor (a wedge resection).

Another technique that may be used for smaller tumors is laparoscopic **radiofrequency ablation** (RFA). RFA is a technique in which the surgeon places a special needle electrode in the tumor under guidance from MRI or CT scanning. When the electrode has been properly placed, a radiofrequency current is passed through it, heating the tumor and killing the cancer cells. RFA is most often used for tumors smaller than 4 centimeters (1.57 inches).

Chemotherapy

If the tumor cannot be removed by surgery, a technique known as **chemoembolization** may be used to administer **chemotherapy** directly to the tumor. A tube (catheter) is placed in the main artery of the liver and an implantable infusion pump is installed. The pump allows much higher concentrations of the cancer drug to be carried to the tumor than is possible with chemotherapy carried through the bloodstream. The drug that is used for infusion pump therapy is usually **floxuridine** (FUDR), given for 14-day periods alternating with 14-day rests. Systemic chemotherapy can also be used to treat liver cancer. The medications usually used are 5-fluorouracil (Adrucil, Efudex) or **methotrexate** (MTX, Trexall). Systemic chemotherapy does not, however, significantly lengthen the patient's survival time and has not been routinely used for patients diagnosed with advanced hepatocellular carcinoma.

Radiation therapy

Radiation therapy is the use of high-energy rays or x-rays to kill cancer cells or to shrink tumors, but because liver cancers are typically not sensitive to radiation, its use in liver cancer has traditionally been to give short-term relief from some of the symptoms. Newer techniques are under study, however, and are being used more frequently.

Targeted therapy

Targeted therapy uses drugs that target specific proteins that are found in cancer cells. They work differently from chemotherapy drugs and often have fewer or milder side effects. **Sorafenib** (Nexavar) is the targeted therapy drug of choice for liver cancer.

Liver transplantation

Removal of the entire liver (total hepatectomy) and liver transplantation can be used to treat liver cancer. However, there is a high risk of tumor recurrence and metastases after transplantation. In addition, most patients have cancer that is too far advanced at the time of diagnosis to benefit from liver transplantation.

Other therapies

Other therapeutic approaches that have been used or are being researched as treatments for liver cancer include:

- the injection of an alcohol-based agent directly into the tumor
- ultrasound-guided cryoablation, which uses liquid nitrogen (or a similar substance) to freeze the lesion
- immunotherapy or gene therapy

Alternative and complementary therapies

Many patients find that alternative and complementary therapies help to reduce the stress associated with illness, improve immune function, and boost spirits. While there is no clinical evidence that these therapies specifically combat disease, such activities as biofeedback, relaxation, therapeutic touch, massage therapy and guided imagery have no side effects and have been reported to enhance well-being.

Several other therapies are sometimes promoted as supplemental or replacement cancer treatments, but many of these therapies have not been the subject of safety and efficacy trials by the **National Cancer Institute** (NCI). The NCI has conducted trials on Cancell, laetrile, and some other alternative therapies and found no anticancer activity. These treatments have varying effectiveness and safety considerations. Patients using any alternative remedy should first consult their doctors in order to prevent harmful side effects or interactions with traditional cancer treatment.

Prognosis

Liver cancer has a very poor prognosis because it is often not diagnosed until it has metastasized. Fewer than 10% of patients survive three years after the initial diagnosis; the overall five-year survival rate for patients with HCC is around 4%. Most patients with primary liver cancer die within six months of diagnosis, usually from liver failure; fewer than 5% are cured of the disease.

Coping with cancer treatment

Side effects of treatment, nutrition, emotional well-being, and other issues are all parts of coping with cancer. There are many possible side effects for a cancer treatment, including:

- constipation
- delirium
- fatigue
- fever, chills, sweats
- nausea and vomiting
- mouth sores, dry mouth, bleeding gums
- pruritus (itching)
- affected sexuality
- sleep disorders

Anxiety, **depression**, feelings of loss, post traumatic stress disorder, affected sexuality, and **substance abuse** are all possible emotional side effects. Patients should seek out a support network to help them through treatment. Loss of appetite before, during, and after a treatment can also be of concern. Other complications of coping with cancer treatment include fever and pain.

Clinical trials

Clinical trials are government-regulated studies of new treatments and techniques that may prove beneficial in diagnosing or treating a disease. Participation is always voluntary and at no cost to the participant. Clinical trials are conducted in three phases. Phase 1 tests the safety of the treatment and looks for harmful side effects. Phase 2 tests the effectiveness of the treatment. Phase 3 compares the treatment to other treatments available for the same condition.

The selection of clinical trials under way changes frequently. Patients and their families can search for trials on liver cancer on the National Cancer Institute website at http://www.cancer.gov/clinicaltrials/search.

Prevention

Liver cancer is 75%–80% preventable. Current strategies focus on widespread vaccination for hepatitis B, early treatment of hereditary hemochromatosis (a metabolic disorder), and screening of high-risk patients with alpha-fetoprotein testing and ultrasound examinations.

Lifestyle factors that can be modified in order to prevent liver cancer include avoidance of exposure to toxic chemicals and foods harboring molds that produce aflatoxin. Most important, however, is avoidance of alcohol and drug abuse. Alcohol abuse is responsible for

60–75% of cases of cirrhosis, which is a major risk factor for eventual development of primary liver cancer. Hepatitis is a widespread disease among persons who abuse intravenous drugs.

See also Alcohol consumption; CT-guided biopsy; Hepatic arterial infusion; Immunotherapy.

Resources

BOOKS

Porter, Robert S. ed. "Primary Liver Cancer." In *The Merck Manual of Diagnosis and Therapy*, 19th ed. Whitehouse Station, NJ: Merck Research Laboratories, 2012.

WEBSITES

American Cancer Society. "How Is Liver Cancer Staged?" http://www.cancer.org/cancer/livercancer/detailedguide/liver-cancer-staging (accessed August 13, 2014).

American Cancer Society. "Liver Cancer." http://www.cancer.org/cancer/livercancer/detailedguide/index (accessed June 8, 2014).

Cicalesee, Luca. "Hepatocellular Carcinoma." May 30, 2014. http://emedicine.medscape.com/article/197319-overview (accessed June 8, 2014).

Johns Hopkins Medicine. "Chemoembolization." http://www.hopkinsmedicine.org/vascular/procedures/chemoembolization (accessed August 13, 2014).

"Liver Cancer." MedlinePlus May 8, 2014 http://www.nlm.nih.gov/medlineplus/livercancer.html (accessed June 8, 2014).

ORGANIZATIONS

American Cancer Society, 1599 Clifton Rd., NE, Atlanta, GA 30329, (404) 320-3333, (800) ACS-2345 (227-2345), http://www.cancer.org.

American Liver Foundation, 39 Broadway, Ste 2700, New York, NY 10006, (212) 668-1000, Fax: (212) 483-8179, http://www.liverfoundation.org.

National Cancer Institute, BG 9609 MSC 9760, 9609 Medical Center Drive, Bethesda, MD 20892-9760, (800) 4-CANCER (422-6237); TTY: (800) 332-8615, http://www.cancer.gov.

Rebecca J. Frey, PhD.
REVISED BY TISH DAVIDSON, AM
REVIEWED BY MELINDA GRANGER OBERLEITNER, RN, DNS, APRN, CNS

Liver scan *see* **Nuclear medicine scans**

Lobectomy

Definition

A lobectomy is the removal of a lobe of one of the organs, usually referring to the brain, the lung, or the liver.

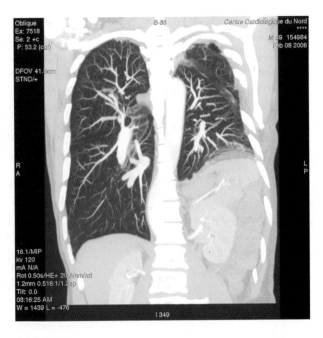

Scan showing a lung lobectomy; the bottom portion of the left lung (shown on the right side of the image) has been removed. *(BSIP SA/Alamy)*

Purpose

Lobectomies are usually performed to prevent the spread of **cancer** from one part of an organ to other parts of the same organ or to other parts of the body. Lobectomies also are performed on patients with severe seizure disorders (such as some forms of epilepsy) to prevent further seizures. However, there are differences in each of the three organs on which lobectomies may be performed.

Description

The brain

Each lobe of the brain performs a different function, and when part of the brain is removed, it does not grow back. However, other parts of the brain can take over some or all of the function of the missing part of the brain. Depending on the part of the brain removed, the effects may be quite severe or nearly nonexistent.

The most commonly referenced brain lobectomy in the medical literature is the removal of the temporal lobe. Temporal lobectomy usually is performed to prevent debilitating seizures. Seizures are commonly caused by temporal lobe epilepsy, but can also be caused by **brain tumors** in the temporal lobe. Thus, lobectomy of the temporal lobe in patients with a temporal lobe tumor reduces or eliminates seizures, and has the beneficial side effect of removing the tumor mass.

The lung

Lobectomies of the lung also are called pulmonary lobectomies. Each part of the lung performs the same function: it exchanges oxygen for carbon dioxide in the blood. There are many different lobes of the lung, however, and some lobes exchange more oxygen than others. Lobes of the lung do not regenerate after they are removed. Therefore, removal of a large portion of the lung may cause a person to need oxygen or ventilator support for the rest of his or her life. However, removal of a small portion of the lung may result in very little change to the patient's quality of life. A test (a quantitative ventilation/perfusion scan, or quantitative V/Q scan) may be used before surgery to help determine how much of the lung can safely be removed.

The outcome of lung lobectomies also depends on the general health of the entire lung; emphysema and smoking would have a negative impact on the health of a patient's lung. The surgeon may perform the surgery with video assistance and special tools to decrease pain and speed patient recovery following surgery.

The liver

A lobectomy of the liver is also called a hepatic lobectomy. The liver plays a major role in digestion, in

the transformation of food into energy, and in filtering and storing blood. It processes nutrients and drugs, produces bile, controls the level of glucose (sugar) in the blood, detoxifies blood, and regulates blood clotting. Unlike the brain and the lung, the liver may regrow, or regenerate, after part of the liver has been removed. In addition, since every part of the liver performs the same functions, the liver is the organ whose function is least likely to be severely affected by lobectomy in the long term because it regenerates. However, as the liver is central to the body's functions, removal of too much of the liver at once may result in coma or death.

Precautions

Brain lobectomies should not be performed unless the patient has been unable to control seizures through medication. Additionally, the seizures must be caused by a single, relatively small, localized part of the brain that can be resected without severe damage. Lung lobectomies should be performed only on patients with early-stage non-small cell **carcinoma** of the lung, or as part of a combination of therapies at later stages. Because even a complete removal of the tumor does not result in an overwhelming survival rate after five years, other therapies also may be considered. Small cell cancer of the lung does not respond to surgical intervention. Patients with liver disease that is too extensive may need a liver transplant rather than a liver lobectomy. Patients with blood clotting problems, either due to chemotherapeutic agents or for other reasons, should have these problems addressed before surgery.

Preparation

Before surgery, patients should not take aspirin or ibuprofen for one week. Patients also should consult their physician about any blood-thinning medications like **warfarin** (Coumadin). The night before surgery, patients will usually be asked not to eat or drink after a certain time.

Aftercare

Each surgery offers different aftercare challenges. Patients may need to be hospitalized for some time after the operation. Patients with portions of their brain removed may require rehabilitation of a physical, mental, or emotional nature depending on the portion of the brain that has been removed. Patients who have had portions of their lungs removed probably will require a tube in their chest to drain fluid, and may require a machine to help them breathe. They may require oxygen on either a temporary or permanent basis. Patients who have had hepatic lobectomies also may have drainage tubes and may have initial dietary restrictions. Physicians should be consulted for the specifics of aftercare in each individual situation.

Risks

Specific risks vary from surgery to surgery and should be discussed with a physician. In general, any surgery requiring a general anesthetic may uncommonly result in death. Improperly performed brain surgery may result in permanent brain damage. Depending on the surgeon and the size of the tissue removed, patients may be at risk of some types of brain damage. As previously mentioned, patients having part of a lung removed may have difficulty breathing and may require the use of oxygen. Patients also may experience infection (**pneumonia**), or blood clots. Liver resection (surgery) may result in the following complications: coma, slow return of normal bowel function, and biliary leakage.

Results

Most patients who undergo temporal lobectomy experience few or no seizures after surgery (some estimates range from about 70% to about 90% success rate). Unfortunately, lung lobectomy is not as successful. 50% of cancer patients with completely removable stage I non-small cell cancer of the lung survive five years after the procedure. If the cancer has progressed beyond this stage, or if the cancer is not completely removable, the chances for survival drop significantly. The results of liver resection vary. The possible outcomes of each surgical type should be discussed with the patient's physician. Generally, the less severe the cancer, and the less tissue that needs to be removed, the better the outcome.

Abnormal results

Abnormal results vary from operation to operation and should be discussed thoroughly with the patient's physician before surgery. Patients who undergo temporal lobectomy may on rare occasions die as a result of the operation (a complication in less than 1% of patients).

Patients also may have problems with their vision or problems with speech. Abnormal results from the removal of part of the lung could include pneumonia or blood clots (which may result in stroke, heart attack, or other problems) after the surgery. Also, a small percentage of patients undergoing lung lobectomy die during or soon after the surgery. The percentage of patients who suffer death varies from about 3–6% depending on the amount of lung tissue removed. Finally, abnormal outcomes from liver resection can include coma, death, and problems with liver function.

Resources

BOOKS

Skandalakis, Lee J., John E. Skandalakis, and Panajiotis N. Skandalakis. *Surgical Anatomy and Technique: A Pocket Manual.* 3rd ed. New York: Springer, 2009.

WEBSITES

Johns Hopkins Medicine. "Lobectomy." http://www.hopkins-medicine.org/healthlibrary/test_procedures/pulmonary/lobectomy_92,P07749/ (accessed November 4, 2014).

National Cancer Institute. "Non-Small Cell Lung Cancer Treatment (PDQ®)." http://www.cancer.gov/cancertopics/pdq/treatment/non-small-cell-lung/HealthProfessional/page7 (accessed November 4, 2014).

Michael Zuck, PhD.
Teresa G. Odle

Lomustine

Definition

Lomustine is one of the anticancer (antineoplastic) drugs in a class called alkylating agents. It is available under the brand name CeeNU. Another commonly used name is CCNU.

Purpose

Lomustine is primarily used to treat **brain tumors** and **Hodgkin lymphoma**, which is a type of **cancer** that affects the lymph nodes and spleen.

Description

Lomustine chemically interferes with the synthesis of the genetic material (DNA and RNA) of cancer cells, which prevents these cells from being able to reproduce and continue the growth of the cancer.

Antineoplastic—A drug that prevents the growth of a neoplasm by interfering with the maturation or proliferation of the cells of the neoplasm.

Hodgkin lymphoma—A disease characterized by enlargement of the lymph nodes and spleen.

Neoplasm—New abnormal growth of tissue.

Recommended dosage

Lomustine is taken orally (in pill form). The dosage is typically 100–130 mg per square meter of body surface area once every 6 weeks. Lomustine should be taken on an empty stomach just prior to bedtime to prevent possible nausea and/or vomiting. Patients should avoid alcohol one hour before and shortly after taking lomustine.

Precautions

Lomustine can cause an allergic reaction in some people. Patients with a prior allergic reaction to lomustine should not take this drug.

Lomustine can cause harm to the fetus if a woman is taking this drug during pregnancy. Women of childbearing potential should use appropriate contraceptive measures to prevent pregnancy while on lomustine. There have been reports of infertility in men taking this drug due to testicular damage.

It is not known whether lomustine is excreted in breast milk. Because of the potential of severe adverse effects, it is recommended that breastfeeding women should discuss with their physician the risk versus benefit of breastfeeding while taking lomustine.

Side effects

Common side effects of lomustine include nausea and/or vomiting, as well as an increased susceptibility to infection due to decreased production of the cells that fight infections. Patients should avoid crowds or exposure to any individuals who may have infections. Also, an increased risk of bleeding can occur due to decreased production of the platelets that are involved in the blood clotting process.

Less common side effects that may also occur include loss of appetite (**anorexia**), **diarrhea**, temporary hair loss (**alopecia**), and skin rash.

A doctor should be consulted immediately if the patient experiences any of the following effects:

- black, tarry or bloody stools
- blood in the urine
- confusion
- persistent cough
- fever and chills
- sore throat
- red spots on the skin
- shortness of breath
- unusual bleeding or bruising

Interactions

Lomustine should not be taken in combination with any prescription drug, over-the-counter drug, or herbal remedy without prior consultation with a physician. Lomustine should not be given together with any live virus vaccine or with any monoclonal antibody because of the increased risk of infection.

Resources

BOOKS

Chu, Edward, and Vincent T. DeVita, Jr. *Physicians' Cancer Chemotherapy Drug Manual 2014.* Burlington, MA: Jones & Bartlett Learning, 2014.

WEBSITES

American Cancer Society. "Lomustine." http://www.cancer. org/treatment/treatmentsandsideeffects/guidetocancer-drugs/lomustine (accessed November 4, 2014).

The Scott Hamilton CARES Initiative. "Lomustine." Chemocare.com. http://chemocare.com/chemotherapy/drug-info/Lomustine.aspx (accessed November 4, 2014).

Paul A. Johnson, Ed.M.

Loperamide *see* **Antidiarrheal agents**

Lorazepam

Definition

Lorazepam is a mild tranquilizer in the benzodiazepine class of drugs. It is used to treat anxiety, **nausea and vomiting**, insomnia, and seizures.

Purpose

Lorazepam is used:

- to treat anxiety
- to control muscle spasms that sometimes accompany severe pain

• to treat insomnia

• prior to the administration of chemotherapy to decrease the incidence of nausea and vomiting

• in combination with other drugs to help control nausea and vomiting associated with cancer treatment

• prior to surgery or other procedures to relieve anxiety, induce drowsiness and sedation, and reduce memories of the procedure

• in its injectable form, to control seizures

Description

Benzodiazepines depress the central nervous system primarily by enhancing the function of gamma-aminobutyric acid (GABA), a neurotransmitter that inhibits the transmission of nerve impulses in the brain and spinal cord. Lorazepam differs from other benzodiazepines, such as **diazepam** (Valium) and chlordiazepoxide (Librium), in that it is shorter-acting and does not accumulate in the body with repeated doses.

Lorazepam is available as 0.5 milligram (mg), 1 mg, and 2 mg tablets and in an intramuscular or intravenous injectable form. It is available as a generic drug.

U.S. brand names

• Ativan

• Lorazepam Intensol

Canadian brand names

• Ativan

• Apo-Lorazepam

• Novo-Lorazepam

• Nu-Loraz

• PMS-Lorazepam

• Riva-Lorazepam

International brand names

• Ativan

• Lorans

• Lorazepam

• Lorivan

• Sinestron

• Tavor

• Temesta

Recommended dosage

The lorazepam dosage is adjusted to the smallest dose that relieves symptoms. The usual recommended dosages are:

• 1–6 mg every 8–12 hours to relieve anxiety, with a maximum total daily dosage of 10 mg in two to three divided doses

• 0.05 mg per kilogram (kg) body weight every four to eight hours in infants and children for anxiety and sedation

• 2–4 mg at bedtime as a sleep aid

• 0.5–2 mg per day in divided doses for elderly or debilitated patients

• 0.5–1 mg every six to eight hours to control nausea and vomiting related to cancer or other medical treatments

• 2 mg 30 minutes prior to receiving chemotherapy and an additional 2 mg every four hours as needed to prevent stomach upset

• 0.05 mg per kg, up to 2 mg per intravenous dose, in children aged 2–15 prior to chemotherapy

• 2.5–5 mg prior to surgery

• 4 mg intravenously for seizures; increased to 8 mg in unresponsive patients

A missed dose should be taken as soon as possible, but two doses should not be taken at the same time. Lorazepam can be taken with or without food.

Precautions

Patients should not drive, operate machinery or appliances, or perform hazardous activities that require mental alertness until they have a sense of how lorazepam affects them. Lorazepam injection may impair performance and driving ability for 24–48 hours.

Lorazepam, like other drugs of this type, can cause physical and psychological dependence. It has a higher potential for dependence compared to other benzodiazepines and is generally prescribed for short-term use only (two to four weeks). Patients should not increase the dosage or frequency of this drug on their own, nor should they stop taking this medication suddenly. Instead, when stopping the drug, the dosage should gradually be decreased and then discontinued. Stopping lorazepam abruptly can cause agitation, irritability, insomnia, convulsions, and other withdrawal symptoms.

Pediatric

Lorazepam is not usually given to children under age 12. Children between the ages of 12 and 18 can be given oral lorazepam, although it is approved only as an antianxiety medication by the U.S. Food and Drug Administration (FDA) for those 18 and older. Intravenous lorazepam may be administered to children prior to **chemotherapy**.

Geriatric

Lorazepam injection may impair driving ability and performance for a longer period in older patients. The elderly dosage is normally lower, with a maximum initial dose of 2 mg.

Pregnant or breastfeeding

Pregnant women and those trying to become pregnant should not take lorazepam. This drug has been associated with fetal malformations when taken during the first three months of pregnancy. It can cause respiratory depression if administered near the time of delivery. Women should not breastfeed while taking lorazepam, since it passes into breast milk.

Other conditions and allergies

Lorazepam should not be used by patients with:

• narrow-angle glaucoma
• pre existing depression of the central nervous system
• severe uncontrolled pain
• severe low blood pressure
• allergies to benzodiazepines

Lorazepam should be used with caution in patients with:

• kidney or liver disease
• myasthenia gravis
• lung disease
• alcohol intoxication
• a history of drug or alcohol abuse

Side effects

Drowsiness and sleepiness are common and expected effects of lorazepam. Possible side effects include dizziness, unsteadiness, clumsiness, or weakness. Patients may have difficulty walking and be prone to falls for up to eight hours after receiving a lorazepam injection, so they should request assistance.

Less common side effects of lorazepam include:

• decreased sex drive
• nausea
• headache
• insomnia
• rash
• vomiting
• dry mouth
• constipation
• yellowing eyes

• vision changes
• hallucinations
• redness and pain at the injection site
• high or low blood pressure and partial blockage of the airways following injection

Serious side effects that require a physician's attention include:

• depression
• confusion
• agitation
• nightmares
• impaired coordination
• personality changes
• changes in urinary patterns
• chest pain
• heart palpitations

Symptoms of lorazepam overdose include:

• confusion
• coma
• slowed reflexes
• difficulty breathing

Geriatric

Patients over age 50 may experience greater and longer sedation after administration of lorazepam. These side effects may subside with continued use or dosage reduction.

Interactions

Alcohol and other central nervous system depressants can increase the drowsiness associated with lorazepam. Central nervous system depressants include some pain and over-the-counter (OTC) medications, as well as the herbs kava, St. John's wort, gotu kola, and valerian. Patients should check with their doctor before beginning any new medication, herb, or supplement. Alcohol should be avoided when taking lorazepam because the drug diminishes alcohol tolerance.

Lorazepam injection may impair driving ability and performance for a longer period in those taking other central nervous system depressants, including some pain medications. Patients should refrain from alcohol for 24–48 hours after a lorazepam injection. When injected, lorazepam may also interact with **scopolamine**, causing drowsiness, odd behavior, and hallucinations.

Resources

BOOKS

Breggin, Peter R. *Psychiatric Drug Withdrawal: A Guide for Prescribers, Therapists, Patients, and Their Families.* New York: Springer, 2013.

Hales, Robert E., et al. *What Your Patients Need To Know About Psychiatric Medications.* Washington, DC: American Psychiatric Publishing, 2007.

Toufexis, Donna, and Sayamwong E. Hammac. *Anti-Anxiety Drugs.* New York: Chelsea House Publishers, 2006.

PERIODICALS

Giersch, Anne, et al. "Impairment of Contrast Sensitivity in Long-Term Lorazepam Users." *Psychopharmacology* 186, no. 4 (July 2006): 594–600.

Hung, Yi-Yung, and Tiao-Lai Huang. "Lorazepam and Diazepam Rapidly Relieve Catatonic Features in Major Depression." *Clinical Neuropharmacology* 29, no. 3 (May–June 2006): 144–147.

Izaute, M., and E. Bacon. "Effects of the Amnesic Drug Lorazepam on Complete and Partial Information Retrieval and Monitoring Accuracy." *Psychopharmacology* 188, no. 4 (November 2006): 472–481.

Kamboj, Sunjeev K., and H. Valerie Curran. "Neutral and Emotional Episodic Memory: Global Impairment After Lorazepam or Scopolamine." *Psychopharmacology* 188, no. 4 (November 2006): 482–488.

Pomara, Nunzio, et al. "Dose-Dependent Retrograde Facilitation of Verbal Memory in Healthy Elderly After Acute Oral Lorazepam Administration." *Psychopharmacology* 185, no. 4 (May 2006): 487–494.

Yacoub, Adee, and Andrew Francis. "Neuroleptic Malignant Syndrome Induced by Atypical Neuroleptics and Responsive to Lorazepam." *Neuropsychiatric Disease and Treatment* 2, no. 2 (2006): 235–240.

WEBSITES

American Society of Health-System Pharmacists. "Lorazepam." *MedlinePlus.* http://www.nlm.nih.gov/medlineplus/druginfo/meds/a682053.html.

"Lorazepam." *University of Maryland Medical Center.* http://www.umm.edu/altmed/drugs/lorazepam-077600.htm

U.S. Food and Drug Administration. "Drug Details: Lorazepam." *Drugs@FDA.* http://www.accessdata.fda.gov/scripts/cder/drugsatfda/index.cfm?fuseaction=Search.DrugDetails.

ORGANIZATIONS

American Academy of Child & Adolescent Psychiatry, 3615 Wisconsin Avenue, NW, Washington, DC 20016-3007, (202) 966-7300, Fax: (202) 966-2891, http://www.aacap.org.

National Institute of Mental Health, 6001 Executive Boulevard, Room 8184, MSC 9663, Bethesda, MD 20892-9663, (301) 443-4513, (866) 615-6464, Fax: (301) 443-4279, nimhinfo@nih.gov, http://www.nimh.nih.gov.

U.S. Food and Drug Administration, 10903 New Hampshire Ave., Silver Spring, MD 20993, (888) INFO-FDA (463-6332), http://www.fda.gov.

Debra Wood, RN
Teresa G. Odle
Ajna Hamidovic, PharmD
Ruth A. Wienclaw, PhD
REVISED BY MARGARET ALIC, PhD

Loss of appetite *see* **Anorexia**

Low molecular weight heparins

Definition

Low molecular weight heparins (LMWHs) belong to a class of medications known as blood thinners. They are used to stop blood clots from forming and growing.

Purpose

LMWHs are used to prevent and treat blood clots in persons undergoing certain types of surgery, recent heart attack, severe chest pain caused by disease of heart vessels usually from fat deposits (unstable angina), and people who have blood clots in their veins (also known as deep vein thrombosis or DVT) or lungs (also known as pulmonary embolism or PE). As of 2014, there are eight drugs that belong to the class of LMWHs: bemiparin, nadroparin, reviparin, certoparin, parnaparin, enoxaparin, dalteparin, and tinzaparin. All eight have the same mechanism of action, but differ in their doses, structures, and Food and Drug Administration (FDA) indicated uses.

Many **cancer** patients can become prone to hypercoagulation, or overactive thickening and clotting of the blood. Hypercoagulation makes the patient more likely to experience deep vein thrombosis, possibly leading to death.

KEY TERMS

Deep vein thrombosis—Also known as DVT, a condition in which a blood clot (thrombus) formed in one part of the circulation, becomes detached and lodges at another point (usually in one of the veins of the legs or arms). People may feel pain, redness, and swelling at the site where the blood clot lodges.

Pulmonary embolism—Also known as PE, a condition in which a blood clot usually formed in of the leg veins becomes detached and lodges in the lung artery or one of its branches. Patients may cough up blood and experience trouble breathing. This condition is treated with blood thinning drugs such as LMWHs, heparin, or warfarin.

Description

LMWHs became available only in the mid-1990s, with enoxaparin (Lovenox) being the first and most studied drug in its class. Dalteparin (Fragmin) was the second LMWH to become available and tinzaparin (Innohep) was the third addition to this class. Nadroparin (Fraxiparine), certoparin (Embolex), bemiparin (Zibor), and the others were introduced in the early 2000s and are used more widely in Europe and Asia than in the United States. These medicines work by inhibiting certain clotting factors in the blood (Factor Xa and thrombin) and preventing blood clots from forming and enlarging.

LMWHs are closely related to **heparin**, which is one of the oldest blood thinners available. These drugs have an advantage over heparin in that they have longer duration in the body, more predictable effects after a given dose, require fewer blood tests to check for their effectiveness and side effects, and do not have to be given in the hospital setting only. LMWHs have been found to be safe and effective in blood clot prevention after general surgery, orthopedic surgery, neurosurgery, multiple trauma, hip fracture, certain types of stroke, unstable angina, heart attack and treatment DVT and PE. These drugs are usually given with **warfarin** (Coumadin) for treatment of blood clots and with aspirin for prevention of complications after heart attack or angina attack. Besides their use for blood clot prevention and treatment, there have been some research studies in animals and humans to suggest that they may prevent cancer by decreasing the blood supply needed for the tumor to grow. The effects of LMWHs on patients with cancer and blood clots are being investigated. The use of LMWH in cancer patients to prevent clots and improve the efficacy of some anticancer drugs for at least the first

3 to 6 months of long-term treatment has been recommended since 2007.

Recommended dosage

Administration

These medicines are given by injection beneath the skin (subcutaneous injection) and should not be injected directly into the vein or muscle. Injections can be given around the navel, upper thigh or buttock. The injection site should be changed daily. Massaging of the site before injection with an ice cube can decrease excessive bruising.

Doses and indications differ between three medicines. These drugs cannot be used interchangeably for one another.

Adults

PREVENTION OF BLOOD CLOTS AFTER ORTHOPEDIC SURGERY. The usual dose of tinzaparin is 50 units per kg daily starting two hours before surgery and continuing for 7–10 days. Doses of 75 units per kg per day have also been studied.

PREVENTION OF BLOOD CLOTS AFTER HIP OR KNEE REPLACEMENT SURGERY. Doses vary between different agents. The usual enoxaparin dose is 30 mg every 12 hours starting 12–24 hours after surgery in patients undergoing hip or knee surgery. Alternatively, 40 mg once a day with the first dose given approximately 12 hours before surgery can be used in patients undergoing hip replacement surgery. The average duration of the initial phase of treatment is 7–10 days (up to 14 days). After the initial phase, 40 mg once a day for three weeks is recommended.

For people undergoing hip replacement surgery, 5,000 units of dalteparin are given 10–14 hours before surgery, then 5,000 units 4–8 hours after surgery, followed by 5,000 units daily. The therapy is usually continued for five to ten days (up to 14 days). A physician should be consulted for alternative dosing regimens.

PREVENTION OF DVT IN PATIENTS AT HIGH RISK OF BLOOD CLOTS AFTER ABDOMINAL SURGERY. Enoxaparin is usually given at a dose of 40 mg once daily with the first dose given two hours before surgery for seven to ten days, up to 12 days.

In patients who are at moderate to high risk of blood clots, the usual dose of dalteparin is 2,500 units daily generally given for five to ten days. The first dose should be given one to two hours before surgery. In patients who are at high to very high risk of blood clots (those with cancer or history of DVT or PE) 5,000 units are given on the evening before surgery, followed by 5,000 units/day for five to ten days. A physician should be consulted for alternative dosing schedules.

Tinzaparin is usually dosed at 3,500 units daily starting two hours before surgery and continuing for seven to ten days.

TREATMENT OF DVT WITH OR WITHOUT PE. Enoxaparin doses of 1 mg per kg twice a day are given when people are treated at home. People who are treated in the hospital can be given 1 mg per kg twice a day or 1.5 mg per kg at the same time once a day. Warfarin is usually given to finish treatment and the two drugs overlap for about 72 hours until good response to warfarin is confirmed by blood tests.

Tinzaparin is usually dosed at 175 units per kg daily for six days or until good response to warfarin is confirmed by blood tests.

UNSTABLE ANGINA OR HEART ATTACK. In patients who are also getting aspirin, the usual dose of enoxaparin is 1 mg per kg every 12 hours for a minimum of two days (usually two to eight days).

The usual dose of dalteparin in people who are also getting aspirin is 120 units per kg (up to a maximum 10,000 units) every 12 hours. Treatment should continue until the patient is stable for five to eight days.

Children

TREATMENT OF DVT WITH OR WITHOUT PE. Children younger than two months of age should receive enoxaparin 1.5 mg per kg every 12 hours. Children older than two months of age should receive enoxaparin 1 mg per kg every 12 hours. A physician will do a blood test four to six hours after the dose to check for effectiveness.

PREVENTION OF BLOOD CLOTS. The usual dose of enoxaparin is 0.75 mg per kg every 12 hours for children younger than two months and 0.5 mg per kg every 12 hours for children older than two months of age. A physician will do a blood test four to six hours after the dose to check for effectiveness.

Precautions

The use of LMWHs should be avoided in persons undergoing any procedure involving spinal puncture or anesthesia. Using these medicines before these procedures has caused severe bruising and bleeding into the spine and can lead to paralysis.

The use of these medicines should be avoided in patients with allergies to LMWHs, heparin, or pork products; allergies to sulfites or benzyl alcohol; people with active major bleeding; and people with a history of heparin-induced low blood platelet count (also known as heparin-induced **thrombocytopenia** or HIT).

LMWHs should be used with caution in the following persons:

- people with bleeding disorders
- people with a history of recent stomach ulcers
- people who recently had brain, spine, or eye surgery
- people on other blood thinners (such as warfarin, aspirin, ibuprofen, naproxen) because of increased risk of bleeding
- people with kidney or liver disease (the dose of LMWHs may need to be decreased)
- breast-feeding mothers (it is not known whether these medicines cross into breast milk)
- women who are pregnant, unless benefits to the mother outweigh the risks to the baby

A doctor should be contacted immediately if any of these symptoms develop:

- tingling, weakness, numbness or pain
- blood in the urine or stool
- itching, swelling, skin rash, trouble breathing
- unusual bleeding or bruising

A physician may perform blood tests during therapy with LMWHs to prevent side effects. Blood tests to check for effectiveness of these medicines are usually not needed, except in children, people with kidney disease, and overweight persons.

Side effects

The most common side effects of LMWHs include irritation and pain at the injection site, easy bruising and bleeding, **fever**, increase in liver enzyme tests usually without symptoms, and allergic reactions. Severe painful erection sometimes requiring surgery has been reported with tinzaparin in some patients. LMWHs can lower platelet counts, which may necessitate discontinuation.

Interactions

LMWHs should be used with caution in people on other oral blood thinners (aspirin, non steroidal anti-inflammatory drugs, warfarin, and ticlopidine) because of increased risk of bleeding. If using both drugs together is necessary, the patients must be closely monitored.

Resources

BOOKS

Laposata, Michael. *Coagulation Disorders: Quality in Laboratory Diagnosis.* New York: Demos Medical Publishing, 2011.

PERIODICALS

"Low-molecular Weight Heparins May Interfere With Tumor Growth and Metastasis." *Drug Week* (July 2, 2004): 269.

Olga Bessmertny, Pharm.D.
Teresa G. Odle

Lumbar puncture

Definition

Lumbar puncture (LP, or spinal tap) is a diagnostic procedure performed to withdraw cerebrospinal fluid (CSF) from the spinal canal in the center of the spinal column. CSF is the clear watery liquid that protects the central nervous system in the spine from injury and cushions it from the surrounding bone structure. The fluid contains a variety of substances, including glucose (sugar), proteins, and white blood cells from the immune system. The fluid is analyzed to either confirm or rule out certain clinical conditions. It may also be performed as a therapeutic procedure to reduce pressure in the brain by removing excess spinal fluid.

Purpose

Lumbar puncture is used to diagnose malignancies, including certain types of brain **cancer** and leukemia, as well as other clinical conditions that affect the central nervous system such as meningitis or subarachnoid hemorrhage. In addition, it is sometimes used to confirm or rule out central nervous system conditions that may cause individuals to exhibit psychological or psychiatric symptoms.

Other clinical conditions diagnosed with lumbar puncture include:

- viral and bacterial meningitis

- syphilis, a sexually transmitted disease

- bleeding (hemorrhage) around the brain and spinal cord

- multiple sclerosis, a disease that affects the myelin coating of the nerve fibers of the brain and spinal cord

- Guillain-Barré syndrome, an inflammation of the nerves

Removing CSF may also be done as a therapeutic measure to reduce increased pressure in the brain (intracranial pressure). In addition, a lumbar puncture may be used to inject **chemotherapy** drugs or spinal

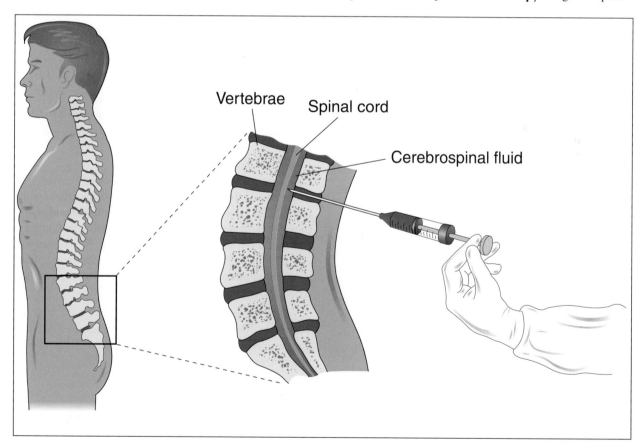

During a lumbar puncture, or spinal tap, the physician inserts a hollow thin needle in the space between two vertebrae in the lower back and slowly advances it toward the spine. Cerebrospinal fluid pressure is measured, and some fluid is withdrawn for laboratory analysis. *(Illustration by Electronic Illustrators Group. © Cengage Learning®.)*

Labels in illustration: Vertebrae, Spinal cord, Cerebrospinal fluid anesthesia directly into the CSF. This type of treatment is called intrathecal therapy.

Description

In a lumbar puncture, the lumbar spine in the curve of the lower back is used to obtain the CSF sample. The lumbar spine is the third, more flexible section of the spine below the cervical spine in the neck and the thoracic spine at the level of the lungs. The lower lumbar spine (usually between the vertebrae known as L4–5) is preferred because the spinal cord stops near L2, and a needle introduced below this level will miss the spinal cord and encounter only nerve roots. In rare instances, such as a spinal fluid blockage in the middle of the back, a doctor may perform a spinal tap in the cervical spine in the neck region.

A lumbar puncture takes about 15–30 minutes. Patients can undergo the test in a doctor's office, laboratory, or outpatient hospital setting. Depending on the patient's condition, it may require an inpatient hospital stay. If the patient has severe osteoarthritis of the spine, is extremely uncooperative, or obese, the spinal needle can be introduced using x-ray guidance.

In order to get an accurate sample of cerebrospinal fluid, the patient must be in the proper position. The spine must be curved to allow as much space as possible between the lower vertebrae (bones) of the spine to permit the doctor to insert a lumbar puncture needle between the vertebrae and withdraw a small amount of fluid. The most common position is for the patient to lie on the left or right side with the back at the edge of the exam table, head and chin bent down, knees drawn up to the chest, and arms clasped around the knees. Small infants and people who are obese may need to curve their spines in a sitting position. Studies have shown that the sitting flexed position is associated with greater success in obtaining CSF on the first attempt in infants younger than one year old. Adult patients are advised to consult with their doctors if they have any questions about their position because the procedure will be easier when the patient is comfortable and able to remain still during the entire procedure. If the patient is anxious or uncooperative, a short-acting sedative may be given.

During a lumbar puncture, the doctor drapes the patient's back with a sterile covering that has an opening over the puncture site. The skin in the area is cleaned with an antiseptic solution. Patients receive a local anesthetic to minimize any pain in the lower back. Then the doctor inserts a thin hollow needle into the space between two vertebrae of the lower back and slowly advances it through muscle ligaments (ligamentous tissues) toward the spine. A steady flow of clear

cerebrospinal fluid, normally the color of water, will begin to fill the needle as soon as it enters the spinal canal. The doctor measures the cerebrospinal fluid pressure with a special instrument called a manometer, and withdraws several vials of fluid for laboratory analysis. The amount of fluid collected depends on the type and number of tests needed to diagnose a particular medical disorder.

In some cases, if the needle hits bone or a blood vessel, or the patient reports sharp, unusual pain, the doctor may have to remove and reposition the needle to obtain an even flow of fluid.

Precautions

Lumbar puncture should be performed with extreme caution, and only if the physician believes that the benefits outweigh the risks. In most cases, lumbar puncture is safe and effective. However, some patients experience pain, difficulty urinating, infection, or leakage of cerebrospinal fluid from the puncture site after the procedure. A traumatic lumbar puncture is said to occur when a blood vessel is inadvertently ruptured during the procedure and leaks blood into the spinal fluid. If this rupture occurs as part of a diagnostic leukemia workup, there is the potential of contaminating the CSF specimen that has been removed with leukemia cells, causing a false positive test result. Patients, parents, and guardians are advised to talk with the physician ordering the lumbar puncture about possible complications associated with the procedure.

Preparation

Patients can go about their normal activities before having a lumbar puncture. Experts recommend that patients relax before the procedure to release any muscle tension, since the lumbar puncture needle must pass through muscle tissue before it reaches the spinal canal. A patient's level of relaxation before and during the procedure plays a critical role in the test's success. Relaxation may be difficult for patients who must face having frequent lumbar punctures, especially children with leukemia. In these cases, it is especially important for the child to receive psychological support before and after each procedure. Most children are sedated for lumbar punctures and seldom remember having the procedure done.

Aftercare

After the procedure, the doctor covers the site of the puncture with a sterile bandage. Patients must avoid sitting or standing, and remain lying down for as long as six hours after the lumbar puncture. Patients are encouraged to drink plenty of fluids to help prevent a lumbar puncture headache.

Risks

The most common side effect of lumbar puncture is a headache. This problem occurs in 10%–20% of adult patients and in up to 40% of children. It is caused by decreased CSF pressure related to a small leak of CSF through the puncture site. The headache pain is usually dull, although some people report a throbbing sensation. A stiff neck and nausea may accompany the headache. A lumbar puncture headache typically begins within a few hours to two days after the procedure and usually persists for a few days, but also may last several weeks or months. Research is still ongoing to find ways to alleviate the headache after lumbar puncture. In some cases, it can be prevented by lying flat for an hour after the lumbar puncture, and taking in more fluids for 24 hours after the procedure. Since an upright position worsens the pain, lying flat also helps control the pain, along with prescription or nonprescription analgesic medication, preferably one containing caffeine.

Some patients may also experience back pain. Headaches and backaches appear to be more common in adolescents than in younger children, and more common in girls than in boys.

In some circumstances, a lumbar puncture may lead to serious complications. For example, in people with blood clotting or bleeding disorders or who are on anticoagulant treatment, lumbar puncture may cause bleeding that can compress the spinal cord (spinal subdural hematoma). Although this is a rare complication of lumbar puncture, it warrants caution in some patients with cancer whose low platelet counts (**thrombocytopenia**) make them more susceptible to bleeding. Platelet transfusions are sometimes given to such patients prior to the procedure.

In rare cases, lumbar puncture in infants can lead to such complications as paraplegia. These complications are associated with the increased difficulty of avoiding certain parts of the spinal cord when performing lumbar puncture in infants as well as the smaller, less developed central nervous system in these patients.

If a patient has a large brain tumor or other mass in the brain, removal of CSF can cause pressure shifts within the brain (herniation). This alteration may in turn compress the brain stem and other vital structures, leading to irreversible brain damage or death. These problems may be avoided by checking blood coagulation parameters with laboratory tests prior to the procedure and by doing a **computed tomography** scan (CT) or **magnetic resonance imaging** (MRI) scan to make sure no tumor or mass is present. CT scans are usually done if the patient is over age 65, if previous seizures have occurred, or if other neurological signs are present. Lumbar puncture will not be performed if the cause of increased intracranial pressure is unknown, if there is an abnormal respiratory pattern, if hypertension or loss of consciousness are present, or if the spine has vertebral deformities such as scoliosis or kyphosis. A lumbar puncture will also not be performed at the site of a localized skin infection on the lower back to avoid introducing infection into the spinal column and CSF that could spread to the brain or spinal cord. It will also not be performed if any major infection is present that could result in systemic infection (sepsis).

Lumbar puncture has been shown to be less precise than some other methods in monitoring intracranial fluid pressure.

Chemotherapy

Patients who receive **anticancer drugs** through lumbar puncture sometimes experience **nausea and vomiting**. Intrathecal **methotrexate** can cause mouth sores. Some of these symptoms may be relieved by antinausea drugs prescribed by the physician.

QUESTIONS TO ASK YOUR DOCTOR

- Why should I have a lumbar puncture?
- What aftercare will be needed?
- Will lumbar puncture be used for chemotherapy, and if so, how often will I receive treatments?
- What are the risks for diagnostic procedures or treatments conducted through lumbar puncture?
- What techniques are suggested to relax patients, especially children, before and after a lumbar puncture?

Results

Normal CSF is clear and colorless. It may be straw or yellow-colored if there is excess protein, which may occur with cancer or inflammation. It may be cloudy in the presence of infection; blood-tinged if there was recent bleeding; or yellow to brown (xanthochromia) if caused by an older instance of bleeding.

A series of laboratory tests analyzes the CSF for a variety of substances to rule out cancer or other medical disorders of the central nervous system. The following are normal values for commonly tested substances:

- CSF pressure: 50–180 mm H_2O
- Glucose: 40–85 mg/dL
- Protein: 15–50 mg/dL
- Leukocytes (white blood cells) total less than 5 per mL
- Lymphocytes (a type of white blood cell): 60–70%
- Monocytes (a type of white blood cell): 30–50%
- Neutrophils (a type of white blood cell): none

No red blood cells, or fewer than 10, are found in a "negative" spinal tap. A "positive" spinal tap will have a red blood cell count of $100/mm^3$. Blood will not usually be found unless the needle passes through a blood vessel en route to the CSF. If this happens, more red blood cells will be found in the first tube collected than in the last.

Abnormal results

When a lumbar puncture is used as part of a diagnostic cancer workup, malignant cells may be found in the CSF, especially in **carcinomatous meningitis** or when a brain tumor is present, such as a **medulloblastoma**. Abnormal test result values in the pressure or any of the substances found in the cerebrospinal fluid may suggest a number of clinical conditions, including a tumor or spinal cord obstruction; hemorrhage in the

central nervous system; infection from bacterial, viral, or fungal microorganisms; or inflammation of the nerves. If there is a tumor in the meninges (membranes covering the brain and spinal cord), the CSF may have higher protein levels, lower glucose levels, and a mild increase in lymphocytes (pleocytosis). Patients will usually review the results of a cerebrospinal fluid analysis with their doctor and discuss treatment plans.

See also Acute lymphocytic leukemia; Brain and central nervous system tumors; Intrathecal chemotherapy.

Resources

BOOKS

Kasper, Dennis L. et al., eds. *Harrison's Principles of Internal Medicine*. 19th ed. New York: McGraw-Hill Education Medical, 2015.

PERIODICALS

Rusch, R., C. Schulta, L. Hughes, and J. S. Withycombe. "Evidence-Based Practice Recommendations to Prevent/ Manage Post-Lumbar Puncture Headaches in Pediatric Patients Receiving Intrathecal Chemotherapy." *Journal Of Pediatric Oncology Nursing* 21 (June 2014): 230–238.

Wright, B. L., J. T. Lai, and A. J. Sinclair. "Cerebrospinal Fluid and Lumbar Puncture: A Practical Review." *Journal of Neurology* 259 (August 2012): 1530–1545.

WEBSITES

Canadian Cancer Society. "Lumbar Puncture." http://www.cancer.ca/en/cancer-information/diagnosis-and-treatment/tests-and-procedures/lumbar-puncture/?region=on (accessed October 31, 2014).

Cancer Research UK. "Lumbar Puncture." http://www.cancer-researchuk.org/about-cancer/cancers-in-general/tests/lumbar-puncture (accessed October 31, 2014).

ORGANIZATIONS

American Academy of Neurology, 201 Chicago Ave., Minneapolis, MN 55415, (612) 928-6000, (800) 879-1960, Fax: (612) 454-2746, memberservices@aan.com, https://www.aan.com.

L. Lee Culvert
Martha Floberg Robbins
Rebecca J. Frey, PhD.

Lumpectomy

Definition

A lumpectomy is a type of surgery performed to treat **breast cancer**. It is called breast-conserving surgery as

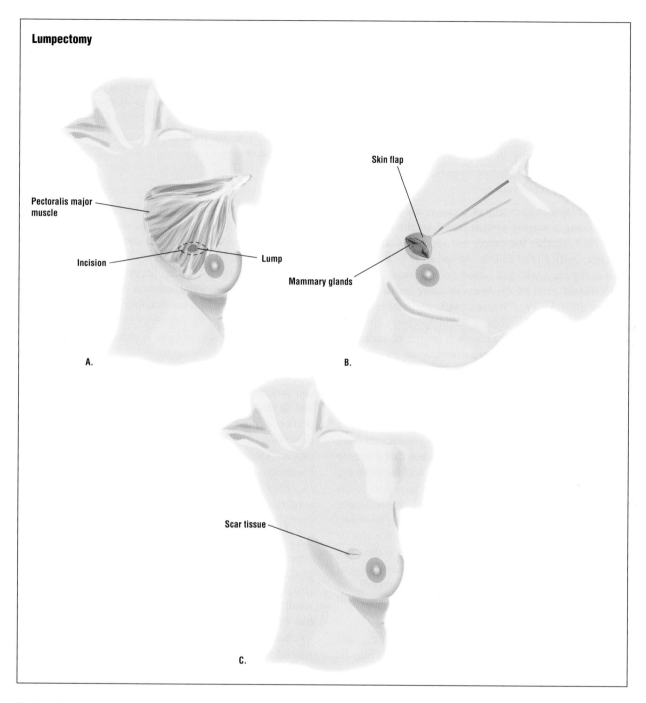

Lumpectomy

Pectoralis major muscle

Incision

Lump

A.

Skin flap

Mammary glands

B.

Scar tissue

C.

During a lumpectomy, a small incision is made around the area of the lump (A). The skin is pulled back and the tumor removed (B). The incision is closed (C). *(Illustration by GGS Information Services. © Cengage Learning®.)*

lumpectomy removes only the malignant tumor and a surrounding margin of normal breast tissue. Lymph nodes in the underarm area (axilla) also may be removed at the same time, using a procedure called **lymph node dissection**.

Purpose

Lumpectomy is a surgical treatment for newly diagnosed breast **cancer**. It is estimated that at least 50% of women with breast cancer are good candidates for this procedure. The location, size, and type of tumor are of primary importance when considering breast cancer surgery options. The size of the breast is another factor the surgeon considers when recommending surgery. The patient's psychological outlook, as well as her lifestyle and preferences, are also taken into account when considering treatment options. One of the advantages of lumpectomy is that less breast tissue is removed than in a **mastectomy**. A lumpectomy leaves the breast looking almost as it did before surgery, and the shape and nipple area are preserved.

The extent and severity of a cancer are evaluated or staged using a staging system based on the size of the tumor and whether the cancer has spread to other areas (metastasized). Breast cancer can spread to nearby areas, such as the chest wall and lymph nodes (Stages I and II), or to distant parts of the body or other organ systems (Stages III and IV). Women with early-stage breast cancer are the best candidates for lumpectomy. In most cases, patients will also undergo a course of **radiation therapy** after surgery. **Chemotherapy** or antiestrogen drugs might be prescribed to help prevent recurrence.

The 5-year survival rates for breast cancer by stage are 100% for stage I, 93% for stage II, 72% for stage III, and 22% for stage IV. Many patients will live much longer than 5 years, of course, and survival rates are improving as treatments improve. Studies that compare the survival rates of women who have had lumpectomy plus radiation therapy versus those who have had breast removal (mastectomy) show that overall survival rates are the same. Compared to mastectomy, however, lumpectomy is associated with a slightly higher risk of recurrence. The rate of spread to other organs is the same for both procedures. Studies indicate that dissection of axillary lymph nodes does not increase overall the disease-free survival in patients whose cancers are small and have not yet spread to the lymph nodes.

In some instances, women with later-stage breast cancer can opt for a lumpectomy. Chemotherapy may be administered before surgery to decrease tumor size and reduce the chance of spreading (**metastasis**).

Description

Lumpectomy is an imprecise term. Any amount of tissue, from 1%–50% of the breast tissue, might be removed and the procedure will still be termed a lumpectomy. However, much less breast tissue is removed than in a mastectomy. Breast conservation surgery is frequently used as a synonym for lumpectomy. Partial mastectomy, **quadrantectomy**, segmental excision, wide excision, and tylectomy are other less common terms for this procedure.

A lumpectomy is most often performed in a hospital setting (especially if lymph nodes are to be removed at the same time), but specialized outpatient facilities are sometimes preferred. The surgery is usually undertaken while the patient is under general anesthesia. Local anesthetic with additional sedation can be used on some patients. The tumor and surrounding margin of tissue are removed and sent to the pathology laboratory for staining and analysis. The surgical site is closed.

If axillary lymph nodes were not removed in a prior **biopsy**, a second incision is made in the armpit. The fat pad that contains lymph nodes is removed from this area and is also sent to the pathologist for analysis. This portion of the procedure is called an axillary lymph node dissection; it is critical for determining the stage of the cancer. Typically, 10 to 15 nodes are removed, but the number may vary. Surgical drains are often left in place in either location to prevent fluid accumulation. The surgery typically lasts from one to three hours.

The patient might stay in the hospital for one or two days or return home the same day. The length of stay generally depends on the extent of the surgery and the medical condition of the patient as well as physician and patient preferences. A woman usually goes home with a small bandage. The inner part of the surgical site usually has dissolvable stitches. The skin may be sutured or stitched, or the skin edges may be held together with a special thin, clear tape.

Precautions

Lumpectomy might not be performed if the tumor is too large or is located in an area where it might not be possible to remove it with a good cosmetic outcome. Sometimes several areas of cancer are found in one breast, so the tumor cannot be removed as a single lump. A cancer that has already attached itself to nearby structures such as the skin or the chest wall, might indicate the need for more extensive surgery. Sometimes lumpectomy is attempted, but the surgeon is unable to remove the tumor with a sufficient amount of normal tissue surrounding it. This situation is termed "persistently positive margins," or "lack of clear margins," referring to the margin of unaffected tissue around the tumor. Women who have had a previous lumpectomy and then a recurrence of the breast cancer are not considered good candidates for lumpectomy.

The need for radiation therapy after lumpectomy may make this surgery clinically unacceptable for some women. For instance, radiation therapy cannot be administered to pregnant women because it endangers the fetus. If radiation can be postponed until after delivery, pregnant women may undergo lumpectomy. Women with collagen vascular disease, such as lupus erythematosus or scleroderma, can experience scarring and damage to their connective tissue if exposed to radiation treatments. A woman who has already had therapeutic radiation to the chest area for other reasons should not receive additional radiation for breast cancer therapy.

Some women may choose to avoid lumpectomy for personal reasons. Some women may fear a recurrence of breast cancer and consider a lumpectomy too risky. Others feel uncomfortable with a breast that has had a cancer, and believe they will attain greater peace of mind with the entire breast removed. Some women choose more extensive surgery so that radiation will not be required. The frequency and duration of radiation treatments, usually five days a week for six weeks, might not be acceptable to some women due to financial or job-related constraints. Finally, in geographically isolated areas, a course of radiation therapy may require lengthy travel and time away from family and other responsibilities.

Preparation

Routine preoperative preparations, such as avoiding all food or drink the night before surgery, are typically required. Information about expected outcomes and potential complications are also part of the preparation for lumpectomy, as they are for any surgical procedure. It is especially important that women are informed about sensations they might experience after the operation to prevent their misinterpreting these sensations as signs of further cancer or poor healing.

If the tumor cannot be felt (not palpable), a pre operative localization procedure is needed. A fine wire or other device is placed at the tumor site, using x-ray or ultrasound imaging for guidance. This imaging is usually performed in the radiology department of a hospital. The woman is most often sitting up and awake, although some sedation might be administered.

Sometimes sentinel lymph node mapping and biopsy is performed prior to surgery, based on the notion that the presence of cancer cells in the first lymph node in the network that drains the affected area may predict whether the cancer has spread to the rest of the nodes. If this first, or sentinel, node is cancer-free, there is no need to look further and axillary lymph node dissection can be avoided.

Aftercare

After a lumpectomy, patients are usually cautioned not to lift anything that weighs more than five pounds until the wound heals. Other activities may be restricted (especially if the axillary lymph nodes were removed) according to individual needs. Pain is often sufficient to limit inappropriate motion. Women are usually instructed to wear a well-fitting support bra both day and night for approximately one week after surgery.

Pain is usually well controlled with prescribed medication. If it is not, the patient should contact the surgeon, as severe pain can signify a complication that requires medical attention. A return visit to the surgeon is typically scheduled about 10–14 days after the operation. Studies suggest that post-lumpectomy survival rates improve if women do not smoke.

Radiation therapy is usually started as soon as feasible after lumpectomy. Such other additional treatments as chemotherapy or hormone therapy might also be prescribed. The timing of these therapies is specific to individual patients.

Risks

A lumpectomy may cause loss of sensation in the breast. The size and shape of the breast may be altered by the removal of tissue, but the nipple area is usually preserved. Most adverse effects are related to the removal of lymph nodes. Approximately 2%–10% of patients develop lymphedema (swelling of the arm due to fluid accumulation) after axillary lymph node dissection. This swelling can range from mild to very severe. It can be treated with elastic bandages and specialized **physical therapy**, but it is a chronic condition requiring continuing care. Lymphedema can arise at any time, even years after surgery. A woman might experience decreased feeling in the back of her armpit and other sensations, including numbness, tingling, or increased skin sensitivity.

Other risks are similar to those associated with any surgical procedure. Risks include bleeding, infection, breast asymmetry, anesthesia reaction, or unexpected scarring. If lymph nodes have been removed, inflammation of the arm vein (phlebitis) can occur. Possible injury to the nerves controlling arm motion occurs only rarely.

Results

Lumpectomy is performed with the expectation that it will be the definitive surgical treatment for breast cancer. Other forms of therapy, especially radiation, are often prescribed as part of the total treatment plan. The expected outcome after lumpectomy and radiation is that breast cancer will not recur. Patients who have had whole-breast radiation after lumpectomy have a 5-year risk of local recurrence of only 1.5%. However, women who have had lumpectomies, particularly those who were young at the time of treatment, are advised to continue seeing their physicians for regular breast cancer check-ups to monitor for recurrence.

Abnormal results

An unforeseen outcome of lumpectomy can be recurrence of the breast cancer, either locally or distally (in a part of the body far from the original site). Recurrence may occur soon after lumpectomy or years after the procedure. For this reason, it is important that patients are closely monitored by their physicians. **Magnetic resonance imaging** (MRI) is considered highly accurate and specific in detecting recurrent cancer after lumpectomy. Women are advised to continue regular mammograms as well. While the scar tissue from lumpectomy and radiation therapy sometimes increase the discomfort of a mammogram, a special cushion is available that reduces discomfort in women who have had breast-conserving surgery.

Resources

BOOKS

Love, Susan M., with Karen Lindsey. *Dr. Susan Love's Breast Book*. 5th ed. Cambridge, MA: Perseus Publishing, 2010.

PERIODICALS

Agresti, R., et al. "Axillary Lymph Node Dissection Versus No Dissection in Patients with T1N0 Breast Cancer. A Randomized Clinical Trial." *Cancer* 120 (June 2014): 885–893.

Drukteinis, J.S., E.C. Gombos, and S. Raza, et al. "MR Imaging Assessment of the Breast after Breast Conservation Therapy: Distinguishing Benign from Malignant Lesions." *Radiographics* 32 (January-February 2012) 219–234.

Fisher, B., et al. "Twenty-year Follow-up of a Randomized Trial Comparing Total Mastectomy with Lumpectomy, and Lumpectomy Plus Irradiation for the Treatment of Invasive Breast Cancer." *New England Journal of Medicine* 347 (2002): 1223–1241.

Smith, S.L., P. T. Truong, L. Lu, M. Lesperance, and I.A. Olivotto. "Identification of Patients at Very Low Risk of Local Recurrence after Breast-conserving Surgery." *International Journal of Radiation Oncology, Biology, Physics* 89 (July 2014): 556–562.

ORGANIZATIONS

American Cancer Society, 250 Williams St. NW, Atlanta, GA 30303, (800) 227-2345, http://www.cancer.org.

Breastcancer.org, 7 E. Lancaster Ave., 3rd Fl., Ardmore, PA 19003, (610) 642-6550, Fax: (610) 642-6559, http://www.breastcancer.org.

National Cancer Institute, 9609 Medical Center Dr., BG 9609 MSC 9760, Bethesda, MD 20892-9760, (800) 4-CANCER (422-6237), http://www.cancer.gov.

L. Lee Culvert
Ellen S. Weber, M.S.N.
Teresa G. Odle

Lung biopsy

Definition

Lung **biopsy** is a procedure for obtaining a small sample of lung tissue for examination. The tissue is usually examined under a microscope and may be sent to a microbiological laboratory for culture. Microscopic examination is performed by a pathologist.

Purpose

A lung biopsy is usually performed to determine the cause of abnormalities such as nodules that appear on chest **x-rays**. It can confirm a diagnosis of **cancer**, especially if malignant cells are detected in the patient's

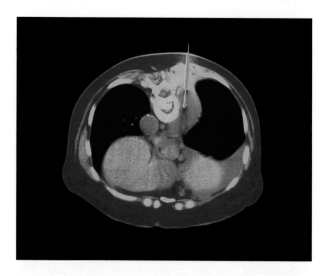

Computed tomography (CT) scan showing a lung biopsy taken by bronchoscope. The scope is shown in blue and is entering a tumor (shown in orange) that has formed on one of the lungs (shown in purple). *(Mehau Kulyk/Science Source)*

sputum or bronchial washing. In addition to evaluating lung tumors and their associated symptoms, lung biopsies may be used to diagnose lung infections, especially tuberculosis and Pneumocystis **pneumonia**, drug reactions, and chronic diseases of the lungs such as sarcoidosis and pulmonary fibrosis.

A lung biopsy can be used for treatment as well as diagnosis. **Bronchoscopy**, a type of lung biopsy performed with a long, flexible slender instrument called a bronchoscope, can be used to clear a patient's air passages of secretions and to remove airway blockages.

Demographics

Lung cancer accounts for more than a quarter of cancer-related deaths in the United States. According to the American Cancer Society, about 228,190 patients were newly diagnosed with lung cancer in 2013 (118,080 in men and 110,110 in women), with 159,480 deaths. Lung cancer kills more people than cancers of the breast, prostate, and colon combined. Cigarette smoking accounts for nearly 90% of cases of lung cancer in the United States.

Description

The right and left lungs are separated by the mediastinum, which contains the heart, trachea, lymph nodes, and esophagus. Lung biopsies sometimes involve **mediastinoscopy**.

Types of lung biopsies

Lung biopsies are performed using a variety of techniques, depending on where the abnormal tissue is located in the lung, the health and age of the patient, and the presence of lung disease. A bronchoscopy is ordered if a lesion identified on the x-ray seems to be located on the wall (periphery) of the chest. If the suspicious area lies close to the chest wall, a needle biopsy can be done. If both methods fail to diagnose the problem, an open lung biopsy may be performed. When there is a question about whether the lung cancer or suspicious mass has spread to the lymph nodes in the mediastinum, a mediastinoscopy is performed.

BRONCHOSCOPIC BIOPSY. During the bronchoscopy, a thin, lighted tube (bronchoscope) is passed from the nose or mouth down the windpipe (trachea) to the air passages (bronchi) leading to the lungs. Through the bronchoscope, the physician views the airways and is able to clear mucus from blocked airways and collect cells or tissue samples for laboratory analysis.

NEEDLE BIOPSY. During a needle biopsy procedure, the patient is mildly sedated but awake. He or she sits in a

---

KEY TERMS

Bronchoscopy—A medical procedure that enables the physician to see the breathing passages and the lungs through a hollow lighted tube.

Chest x-ray—Brief exposure of the chest to radiation to produce an image of the chest and its internal structures.

Endotracheal tube—A hollow tube inserted into the windpipe to administer anesthesia.

Lymph nodes—Small bean-shaped structures that serve as filters scattered along the lymphatic vessels. Lymph nodes trap bacteria or cancer cells that are traveling through the lymphatic system.

Malignant—Cancerous.

Mediastinoscopy—A procedure that allows the physician to see the organs in the mediastinal space using a thin lighted hollow tube (a mediastinoscope).

Mediastinum—The area between the lungs, bounded by the spine, breastbone, and diaphragm.

Pleural cavity—The space between the lungs and the chest wall.

Pneumothorax—A condition in which air or gas enters the pleura (area around the lungs) and causes a collapse of the lung.

Pulmonary nodule—Also called a lung nodule; a lesion surrounded by normal lung tissue. Nodules may be caused by bacteria, fungi, or a tumor (benign or cancerous).

Sputum—A mucus-rich secretion coughed up from the passageways (bronchial tubes) and the lungs.

Sputum cytology—A lab test in which a microscope is used to check for cancer cells in the sputum.

Thoracentesis—Removal of fluid from the pleural cavity.

---

chair with arms folded in front on a table. An x-ray technician uses a computerized axial tomography (CAT) scanner or a fluoroscope to identify the precise location of the suspicious areas. Markers are placed on the overlying skin to identify the biopsy site. The skin is thoroughly cleansed with an antiseptic solution, and a local anesthetic is injected to numb the area. The patient will feel a brief stinging sensation when the anesthetic is injected.

The physician makes a small incision, about half an inch (1.25 cm) in length. The patient is asked to take a deep breath and hold it while the physician inserts the biopsy needle through the incision into the lung tissue to be biopsied. The patient may feel pressure and a brief sharp pain when the needle touches the lung tissue. Most patients do not experience severe pain. The patient should refrain from coughing during the procedure. The needle is withdrawn when enough tissue has been obtained. Pressure is applied at the biopsy site and a sterile bandage is placed over the incision. A chest x-ray is performed immediately after the procedure to check for potential complications. The entire procedure takes 30–60 minutes.

OPEN BIOPSY. Open biopsies are performed in a hospital operating room under general anesthesia. Once the anesthesia has taken effect, the surgeon makes an incision over the lung area, a procedure called a **thoracotomy**. Some lung tissue is removed and the incision is closed with sutures. Chest tubes are placed with one end inside the lung and the other end protruding through the closed incision. Chest tubes are used to drain fluid and blood, and re-expand the lungs. The tubes are usually removed the day after the procedure. The entire procedure normally takes about an hour. A chest x-ray is performed immediately after the procedure to check for potential complications.

VIDEO-ASSISTED THORACOSCOPIC SURGERY. A minimally invasive technique, video-assisted thoraco-scopic surgery (VATS), can be used to biopsy lung and mediastinal lesions. VATS may be performed on select patients in place of open lung biopsy. While the patient is under general anesthesia, the surgeon makes several small incisions in the chest wall. A thoracoscope—a thin hollow lighted tube with a tiny video camera mounted on it—is inserted through one of the small incisions. The other incisions allow the surgeon to insert special instruments to retrieve tissue for biopsy.

MEDIASTINOSCOPY. This procedure is performed under general anesthesia. A 2–3 in. (5–8 cm) incision is made at the base of the neck. A thin hollow lighted tube called a mediastinoscope is inserted through the incision into the space between the right and the left lungs. The surgeon removes any lymph nodes or tissues that look abnormal. The mediastinoscope is then removed, and the incision is sutured and bandaged. A mediastinoscopy takes about an hour.

Diagnosis

Before scheduling a lung biopsy, the physician performs a careful evaluation of the patient's medical history and symptoms, and performs a physical examination. Chest x-rays and sputum **cytology** (examination of cells obtained from a deep-cough mucus sample) are other diagnostic tests that may be performed. An electrocardiogram (EKG) and laboratory tests may be performed before the procedure to check for blood clotting problems, **anemia**, and blood type, should a transfusion become necessary.

Preparation

During a preoperative appointment, usually scheduled within one to two weeks before the procedure, the patient receives information about what to expect during the procedure and the recovery period. During this appointment or just before the procedure, the patient usually meets with the physician (or physicians) performing the procedure (the pulmonologist, interventional radiologist, or thoracic surgeon).

A chest x-ray or CAT scan of the chest is used to identify the area to be biopsied.

About an hour before the biopsy procedure, the patient receives a sedative. Medication may also be given to dry up airway secretions. General anesthesia is not used for this procedure.

For at least 12 hours before the open biopsy, VATS, or mediastinoscopy procedures, the patient should not eat or drink anything. Prior to these procedures, an intravenous line is placed in the patient's arm to deliver medications or fluids as necessary. A hollow tube called an endotracheal tube is passed through the patient's mouth into the airway leading to the lungs. Its purpose is to deliver the general anesthetic. The chest area is cleansed with an antiseptic solution. In the mediastinoscopy procedure, the neck is also cleansed to prepare for the incision.

Smoking cessation

Patients who will undergo surgical diagnostic and treatment procedures should be encouraged to stop smoking and stop using tobacco products. The patient needs to make the commitment to be a nonsmoker after the procedure. Patients able to stop smoking several weeks before surgical procedures have fewer postoperative complications. The patient should ask a health care provider for more information if he or she needs help with **smoking cessation**.

Informed consent

Informed consent is an educational process between health care providers and patients. Before any procedure is performed, the patient is asked to sign a consent form. Prior to signing the form, the patient should understand the nature and purpose of the diagnostic procedure or treatment, its risks and benefits, and alternatives, including the option of not proceeding with the test or treatment. During the discussions, the health care providers should answer the patient's questions about the consent form or procedure.

Aftercare

Needle biopsy

Following a needle biopsy, the patient is allowed to rest comfortably. He or she may be required to lie flat for two hours following the procedure to prevent the risk of bleeding. The nurse checks the patient's status at two-hour intervals. If there are no complications after four hours, the patient can go home once he or she has received instructions about resuming normal activities. The patient should rest at home for a day or two before returning to regular activities, and should avoid strenuous activities for one week after the biopsy.

Open biopsy, VATS, or mediastinoscopy

After an open biopsy, VATS, or mediastinoscopy, the patient is taken to the recovery room for observation. The patient receives oxygen via a face mask or nasal cannula. If no complications develop, the patient is taken to a hospital room. Temperature, blood oxygen level, pulse, blood pressure, and respiration are monitored. Chest tubes remain in place after surgery to prevent the lungs from collapsing and to remove blood and fluids. The tubes are usually removed the day after the procedure.

The patient may experience some grogginess for a few hours after the procedure. He or she may have a sore throat from the endotracheal tube. The patient may also have some pain or discomfort at the incision site, which can be relieved by pain medication. It is common for patients to require some pain medication for up to two weeks following the procedure.

After receiving instructions about resuming normal activities and caring for the incision, the patient usually goes home the day after surgery. The patient should not drive while taking narcotic pain medication.

Patients may experience **fatigue** and muscle aches for a day or two because of the general anesthesia. The patient can gradually increase activities as tolerated. Walking is recommended. Sutures are usually removed after one to two weeks.

The physician should be notified immediately if the patient experiences extreme pain, light headedness, or difficulty breathing after the procedure. Sputum may be slightly bloody for a day or two after the procedure. Heavy or persistent bleeding requires evaluation by the physician.

Risks

Lung biopsies should not be performed on patients who have a bleeding disorder or abnormal blood clotting because of low platelet counts, or who have a prolonged prothrombin time (PT) or partial thromboplastin time (PTT). Platelets are small blood cells that play a role in the blood clotting process. PT and PTT measure how well blood is clotting. If clotting times are prolonged, it may be unsafe to perform a biopsy because of the risk of bleeding. If the platelet count is lower than 50,000/cubic mm, the patient may be given a platelet transfusion as a temporary relief measure, and a biopsy can then be performed.

In addition, lung biopsies should not be performed if other tests indicate that the patient has enlarged alveoli associated with emphysema, pulmonary hypertension, or enlargement of the right ventricle of the heart (cor pulmonale).

The normal risks of any surgical procedure include bleeding, infection, or pneumonia. The risk of these complications is higher in patients undergoing open biopsy procedures, as is the risk of pneumothorax (lung collapse). In rare cases, the lung collapses because of air that leaks in through the hole made by the biopsy needle. A chest x-ray is done immediately after the biopsy to detect the development of this potential complication. If a pneumothorax occurs, a chest tube is inserted into the pleural cavity to re-expand the lung. Signs of pneumothorax include shortness of breath, rapid heart rate, or blueness of the skin (a late sign). If the patient has any of these symptoms after being discharged from the hospital, he or she should call the health care provider or emergency services immediately.

Bronchoscopic biopsy

Bronchoscopy is generally safe, and complications are rare. If they do occur, complications may include spasms of the bronchial tubes that can impair breathing, irregular heart rhythms, or infections such as pneumonia.

Needle biopsy

Needle biopsy is associated with fewer risks than open biopsy because it does not involve general anesthesia. Some **hemoptysis** (coughing up blood) occurs in 5% of needle biopsies. Prolonged bleeding or infection may also occur, although these are very rare complications.

Open biopsy

Possible complications of an open biopsy include infection or pneumothorax. If the patient has very severe breathing problems before the biopsy, breathing may be further impaired following the operation. Patients with normal lung function prior to the biopsy have a very small risk of respiratory problems resulting from or following the procedure.

Mediastinoscopy

Complications due to mediastinoscopy are rare. Possible complications include pneumothorax or bleeding caused by damage to the blood vessels near the heart. Mediastinitis, or infection of the mediastinum, may develop. Injury to the esophagus or larynx may occur. If the nerves leading to the larynx are injured, the patient may be left with a permanently hoarse voice. All these complications are rare.

Results

Normal results indicate no evidence of infection in the lungs, no detection of lumps or nodules, and cells that are free from cancerous abnormalities.

Abnormal results of needle biopsy, VATS, and open biopsy may be associated with diseases other than cancer. Nodules in the lungs may be due to active infections, such as tuberculosis, or may be scars from a previous infection. In 33% of biopsies using a mediastinoscope, the biopsied lymph nodes prove to be cancerous. Abnormal results should always be considered in the context of the patient's medical history, physical examination, and other tests such as sputum examination and chest x-rays before a final diagnosis is made.

Morbidity and mortality rates

The risk of death from needle biopsy is rare. The risk of death from open biopsy is one in 3,000 cases. In mediastinoscopy, death occurs in fewer than one in 3,000 cases.

Alternatives

The type of alternative diagnostic procedures available depend upon each patient's diagnosis.

Some people may be eligible to participate in **clinical trials**, research programs conducted with patients to evaluate a new medical treatment, drug, or device. The purpose of clinical trials is to find new and improved methods of treating different diseases and special conditions. For more information on current clinical trials, visit the National Institutes of Health's ClinicalTrials website at http://www.clinicaltrials.gov or call (888) FIND-NLM (346-3656) or (301) 594- 5983.

The **National Cancer Institute** (NCI) has conducted a clinical trial to evaluate low-dose helical **computed tomography** for its effectiveness in screening

---

QUESTIONS TO ASK YOUR DOCTOR

- Why is the biopsy being performed?
- Are there any alternative options to having this procedure?
- What type of lung biopsy is recommended?
- Will I be awake during the procedure?
- How long will it take to recover?
- What types of adverse symptoms should I report after the biopsy?
- When will I find out the results?

---

for lung cancer. One study concluded that this test is more sensitive in detecting specific conditions related to lung cancer than other screening tests.

Health care team roles

Fiberoptic bronchoscopy is performed by pulmonologists, physician specialists in pulmonary medicine. CAT-guided needle biopsy is done by interventional radiologists, physician specialists in radiological procedures. Thoracic surgeons perform open biopsies and VATS. Specially trained nurses and x-ray and laboratory technicians assist during the procedures and provide pre- and postoperative education and supportive care.

The procedures are performed in an operating or procedure room in a hospital.

Resources

BOOKS

Mason, Robert J., et al. *Murray & Nadel's Textbook of Respiratory Medicine.* 5th ed. Philadelphia: Saunders/ Elsevier, 2010.

Niederhuber, John E., et al. *Abeloff's Clinical Oncology.* 5th ed. Philadelphia: Saunders/Elsevier, 2013.

PERIODICALS

Chang, C. H., et al. "The Utility of Surgical Lung Biopsy in Cancer Patients with Acute Respiratory Distress Syndrome." *Journal of Cardiothoracic Surgery* 8, no. 1 (2013): 128.

Dell'anna, A. M., and F. S. Taccone. "Lung Biopsy as Diagnostic Tool for Respiratory Failure Diagnosis in Hematological ICU Patients: Is It Time to Adopt It into Daily Practice?" *Minerva Anestesiologica* 79, no. 8 (2013): 829–31.

Nguyen, W., and K. C. Meyer. "Surgical Lung Biopsy for the Diagnosis of Interstitial Lung Disease: A Review of the

Literature and Recommendations for Optimizing Safety and Efficacy." *Sarcoidosis, Vasculitis, and Diffuse Lung Diseases* 30, no. 1 (2013): 3–16.

WEBSITES

American Cancer Society. "Lung Cancer." http://www.cancer.org/cancer/lungcancer/index (accessed October 3, 2014).

American Cancer Society. "What Are the Key Statistics about Lung Cancer?" http://www.cancer.org/cancer/lungcancer-non-smallcell/detailedguide/non-small-cell-lung-cancer-key-statistics (accessed October 3, 2014).

Lake Charles Memorial Health System. "Lung Biopsy." http://www.lcmh.com/Taxonomy/RelatedDocuments.aspx?sid=1&ContentTypeId=92&ContentID=P07750 (accessed October 3, 2014).

Radiological Society of North America. "Needle Biopsy of the Lung." RadiologyInfo.org. http://www.radiologyinfo.org/en/info.cfm?pg=nlungbiopl (accessed October 3, 2014).

ORGANIZATIONS

American Association for Respiratory Care, 9425 N. MacArthur Blvd. Ste. 100, Irving, TX 75063-4706, (972) 243-2272, info@aarc.org, http://www.aarc.org.

American Cancer Society, 250 Williams St. NW, Atlanta, GA 30303, (800) 227-2345, http://www.cancer.org.

American College of Chest Physicians, 3300 Dundee Rd., Northbrook, IL 60062-2348, (847) 498-1400, (800) 343-2227, Fax: (847) 498-5460, http://www.chestnet.org.

American Lung Association, 1301 Pennsylvania Ave. NW, Ste. 800, Washington, DC 20004, (202) 785-3355, (800) LUNG-USA (586-4872), http://www.lung.org.

American Thoracic Society, 25 Broadway, New York, NY 10004, (212) 315-8600, Fax: (212) 315-6498, atsinfo@thoracic.org, http://www.thoracic.org.

Cancer Research Institute, One Exchange Plz., 55 Broadway, Ste. 1802, New York, NY 10006, (212) 688-7515, (800) 99-CANCER (992-2623), http://cancerresearch.org.

National Cancer Institute, 6116 Executive Blvd., Ste. 300, Bethesda, MD 20892-8322, (800) 4-CANCER (422-6237), http://cancer.gov.

National Heart, Lung, and Blood Institute Information Center, PO Box 30105, Bethesda, MD 20824-0105, (301) 592-8573, Fax: (240) 629-3246, nhlbiinfo@nhlbi.nih.gov, http://www.nhlbi.nih.gov.

National Jewish Health's Lung Line, (800) 222-LUNG (222-5864), lungline@njhealth.org, http://www.nationaljewish.org/about/contact/lung-line.

National Lung Health Education Program, 18000 W. 105th St., Olathe, KS 66061, (913) 895-4631, info@nlhep.org, http://www.nlhep.org.

Pulmonary Paper, PO Box 877, Ormond Beach, FL 32175-0877, (800) 950-3698, info@pulmonarypaper.org, https://www.pulmonarypaper.org.

Barbara Wexler
Angela M. Costello
REVISED BY ROSALYN CARSON-DEWITT, MD

Lung cancer, non-small cell

Definition

Non-small cell lung **cancer** (NSCLC) is the most common type of lung cancer. In lung cancer, the cells of the lung tissues grow uncontrollably and form tumors, affecting lung function.

Description

There are two main types of lung cancer: small cell and non-small cell. Small cell lung cancers are shaped like oat grains and called oat-cell cancers; they are aggressive, spread rapidly, and represent about 15% of lung cancers. Non-small cell lung cancer represents almost 85% of all lung cancers.

The lungs

The lungs are located along with the heart in the chest cavity. The lungs are not simply hollow balloons, but have a very organized structure consisting of hollow tubes, blood vessels, and elastic tissue. The hollow tubes, called bronchi, are highly branched, becoming smaller and more numerous at each branching. They end in tiny sacs called alveoli that are made of elastic tissue. These sacs are where the oxygen a person inhales is taken up into the blood, and where carbon dioxide moves out of the blood to be exhaled.

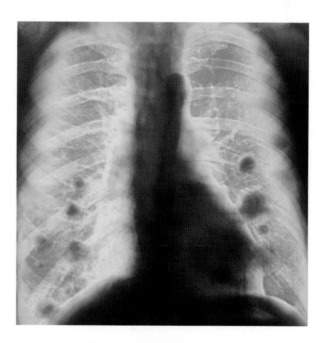

False-color chest x-ray showing evidence of cancerous masses (orange shadows) in both lungs. *(CNRI/Science Source)*

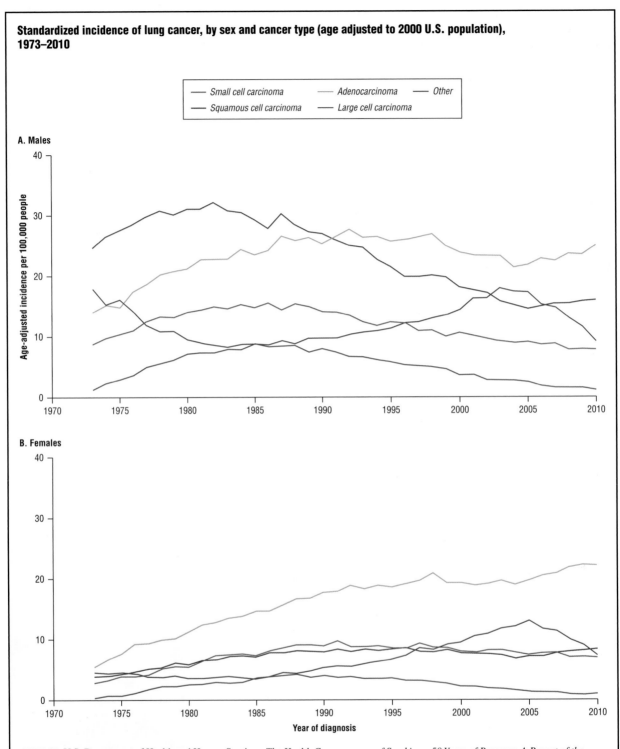

Standardized incidence of lung cancer, by sex and cancer type (age adjusted to 2000 U.S. population), 1973–2010

Legend:
— Small cell carcinoma — Adenocarcinoma — Other
— Squamous cell carcinoma — Large cell carcinoma

A. Males

Age-adjusted incidence per 100,000 people

B. Females

Year of diagnosis

SOURCE: U.S. Department of Health and Human Services, *The Health Consequences of Smoking—50 Years of Progress. A Report of the Surgeon General*, Atlanta, GA: U.S. Department of Health and Human Services, Centers for Disease Control and Prevention, National Center for Chronic Disease Prevention and Health Promotion, Office on Smoking and Health, 2014. Available online at: http://www.surgeongeneral.gov/library/reports/50-years-of-progress/full-report.pdf.

Line graph showing the incidence of lung cancer in the United States from 1973 to 2010. *(Graph by Lumina Datamatics Ltd. © 2015 Cengage Learning®.)*

Normal healthy lungs continually secrete mucus that not only keeps the lungs moist, but also protects the lungs by trapping foreign particles like dust and dirt. The interior of the lungs is covered with small hairlike structures called cilia. The cilia move in such a way that mucus is swept up out of the lungs and into the throat.

Lung cancer

Most NSCLCs start in the cells that line the bronchi, and can take years to develop. As they grow larger, they prevent the lungs from functioning normally. The tumor can reduce the capacity of the lungs or block the movement of air through the bronchi in the lungs. As a result, less oxygen gets into the blood and patients feel short of breath. Tumors may also block the normal upward movement of mucus into the throat. As a result, mucus builds up in the lungs and infection may develop behind the tumor. Once lung cancer has developed, it frequently spreads to other parts of the body.

The speed at which non-small cell tumors grow depends on the type of cells that make up the tumor. The following three types account for the vast majority of non-small cell tumors:

- Adenocarcinomas are the most common and often cause no symptoms. Frequently, they are not found until they are advanced. They account for between 35% and 40% of lung cancers and are the type of lung cancer most often seen in people who do not smoke.

- Squamous cell carcinomas usually produce symptoms because they are centrally located and block the lungs. They account for 25–30% of all lung cancers.

- Undifferentiated large cell and giant cell carcinomas tend to grow rapidly, and spread quickly to other parts of the body. They account for 10–15% of cancers.

Demographics

Lung cancers are decreasing in the United States, but increasing worldwide due to an increased use of tobacco. Worldwide, excluding **skin cancer**, lung cancer is the second most common cancer among both men and women and is the leading cause of cancer death in both sexes. It accounts for 1.6 million deaths each year.

In the United States, the American Cancer Society estimated that 224,210 new cases of lung cancer would be diagnosed in 2014, and about 159,260 people would die of the disease. Of these, about 10%–15% are small cell lung cancers. Although there are differences in mortality rates among ethnic groups, these differences are mainly due to differences in smoking habits. NSCLC is most common in people aged 60–80 years.

Causes and symptoms

Causes

Tobacco smoking accounts for 78% of all lung cancers in men and 90% in women. Giving up tobacco can prevent most lung cancers. Smoking marijuana **cigarettes** is considered another risk factor for cancer of the lung. Secondhand smoke also contributes to the development of lung cancer among nonsmokers.

Certain hazardous materials that people may be exposed to in their jobs have been shown to cause lung cancer. These include asbestos, coal products, and radioactive substances. Air pollution may also be a contributing factor. Exposure to radon, a colorless, odorless gas that sometimes accumulates in the basement of homes, may cause lung cancer in a small number of patients. In addition, patients whose lungs are scarred from other lung conditions may have an increased risk of developing lung cancer even if they do not smoke.

As the ability to decode gene sequences has improved, there are indications that certain genetic patterns, especially on chromosome 6, do not cause lung cancer but make the individual much more susceptible to its development.

Symptoms

Lung cancers tend to spread very early, and only 15% are detected in their early stages. The chances of early detection, however, can be improved by seeking medical care at once if any of the following symptoms appear:

- a cough that does not go away
- chest pain
- shortness of breath
- recurrent lung infections, such as bronchitis or pneumonia
- bloody or brown-colored saliva or phlegm (sputum)
- persistent hoarseness
- significant weight loss that is not due to dieting or vigorous exercise; fatigue and loss of appetite
- unexplained fever

Although these symptoms may be caused by diseases other than lung cancer, it is important to consult a doctor to rule out the possibility of lung cancer.

If lung cancer has spread to other organs, the individual may have other symptoms such as headaches, bone fractures, pain, bleeding, or blood clots.

Diagnosis

Physical examination and diagnostic tests

The doctor will first take a detailed medical history and assess risk factors. During a complete physical examination, the doctor will examine the patient's throat to rule out other possible causes of hoarseness or coughing, and will listen to the patient's breathing and chest sounds.

If the doctor has reason to suspect lung cancer, particularly if the patient has a history of heavy smoking or occupational exposure to irritating substances, a chest x-ray may be ordered to see whether there are any masses in the lungs. Special imaging techniques, such as **computed tomography** (CT) scans or **magnetic resonance imaging** (MRI), may provide more precise information about the size, shape, and location of any tumors.

Sputum analysis

Sputum analysis is a noninvasive test that involves microscopic examination of cells that are coughed up from the lungs. This test can diagnose at least 30% of lung cancers, even when tumors are not visible on chest **x-rays**. In addition, the test can detect cancer in its very early stages before it spreads to other regions. However, the sputum test does not provide any information about the location of the tumor.

Lung biopsy

Lung biopsy is the most definitive diagnostic tool for cancer. It can be performed in three different ways. **Bronchoscopy** involves the insertion of a slender lighted tube called a bronchoscope down the patient's throat and into the lungs. This test allows the doctor to see the tubes inside the lungs and to obtain samples of lung tissue. If a needle **biopsy** is to be performed, the location of the tumor is first identified using a computerized tomography (CT) scan or magnetic resonance imaging (MRI). The doctor then inserts a needle through the chest wall and collects a sample of tissue from the tumor. In the third procedure, known as surgical biopsy, the chest wall is opened and a part of the tumor, or all of it, is removed. A doctor who specializes in the study of diseased tissue (a pathologist) examines the tumor to identify the cancer's type and stage.

Clinical staging

Treatment for non-small cell lung cancer depends primarily on the stage of the cancer. Staging is a process that tells the doctor whether the cancer has spread and the extent of its spread. The most commonly used treatments are surgery, **radiation therapy**, and **chemotherapy**.

Non-small cell lung cancer has six stages:

- Occult carcinoma. Cancer cells have been found in the sputum, but no tumor has yet been found.
- Stage 0. A small group of cancerous cells have been found in one location.
- Stage I. The cancer is in the lung only and has not spread anywhere else.
- Stage II. The cancer has spread to nearby lymph nodes.
- Stage III. The cancer has spread to more distant lymph nodes and/or other parts of the chest, like the diaphragm.
- Stage IV. The cancer has spread to other parts of the body.

Treatment

Surgery

Surgery is the standard treatment for the earlier stages of non-small cell lung cancer. The surgeon will decide on the type of surgery, depending on how much of the lung is affected. There are three different types of surgical procedures:

• Wedge resection is the removal of a small part of the lung.

• Lobectomy is the removal of one lobe of the lung (the right lung has three lobes and the left lung has two lobes).

• Pneumonectomy is the removal of an entire lung.

Lung surgery is a major procedure; patients can expect to experience pain, weakness in the chest, and shortness of breath. Air and fluid collect in the chest after surgery. As a result, patients will need help to turn over, cough, and breathe deeply. Patients should be encouraged to perform these activities because they help get rid of the air and fluid and speed up recovery. It can take patients several months before they regain their energy and strength.

Radiotherapy

Patients whose cancer has progressed too far for surgery (Stages III and IV) may receive radiotherapy. Radiotherapy involves the use of high-energy rays to kill cancer cells. It is used either by itself or in combination with surgery or chemotherapy. The amount of radiation used depends on the size and the location of the tumor.

Radiation therapy may produce such side effects as tiredness, skin rashes, upset stomach, and **diarrhea**. Dry or sore throats, difficulty in swallowing, and loss of hair in the treated area are all minor side effects of radiation. These may disappear either during the course of the treatment or after the treatment is over.

Chemotherapy

Chemotherapy is also given to patients whose cancer has progressed too far for surgery. Chemotherapy is medication that is usually given intravenously to kill cancer cells. These drugs enter the bloodstream and travel to all parts of the body, killing cancer cells that have spread to different organs. Chemotherapy is used as the primary treatment for cancers that have spread beyond the lungs and cannot be removed by surgery. It can also be used in addition to surgery or radiation therapy.

Chemotherapy for NSCLC has made significant advances since the early 1980s in improving the patient's quality of life as well as length of survival. Cytotoxic (cell-killing) agents are typically combined with either **cisplatin** or **carboplatin** as first-line therapy for non-small cell lung cancer.

Newer drugs for lung cancer include gefitinib (Iressa) and **pemetrexed** (Alimta). The FDA approved gefitinib in May 2003 as a treatment for patients with NSCLC who have not responded to platinum-based or taxane chemotherapy. It is taken by mouth and works by inhibiting an enzyme involved in the growth of tumor cells. Pemetrexed, which is given by injection, was approved by the FDA in February 2004 for the treatment of **mesothelioma**, a type of lung cancer caused by exposure to asbestos fibers. However, the drug appears to be effective in treating other types of lung cancer as well. The FDA approved paclitaxel (Abraxane) in 2012 for advanced and metastatic lung cancer. In 2014, ceritinib (Zykadia) was approved for treatment of a subset of individuals with a specific genetic profile and resistance to certain other chemotherapy drugs. As of 2014, several drugs were available that targeted specific proteins produced by lung cancer cells, and others were under development.

Chemotherapy is also used as palliative treatment for non-small cell lung cancer. *Palliative* refers to any type of therapy that is given to relieve the symptoms of a disease, but not to cure it.

Alternative and complementary therapies

Many patients find that alternative and complementary therapies help to reduce the stress associated with illness, improve immune function, and boost spirits. While there is no clinical evidence that these therapies specifically combat disease, such activities as biofeedback, relaxation, therapeutic touch, massage therapy and guided imagery have no side effects and have been reported to enhance well-being.

Several other alternative therapies are sometimes offered as supplemental or replacement cancer treatments, but many of these therapies have not been the subject of safety and efficacy trials by the National Cancer Institute (NCI). The NCI has conducted trials on Cancell, laetrile, and some other alternative therapies and found no anticancer activity. These treatments have varying safety considerations, and some can cause harm. Patients using any alternative remedy should first consult with their doctors in order to prevent harmful side effects or interactions with traditional cancer treatment.

Coping with cancer treatment

The side effects associated with the treatment of non-small cell lung cancer can be severe. Patients should ask their doctors about medications to treat **nausea and vomiting**, and other side effects. It is particularly important to eat a nutritious diet and to drink plenty of fluids. In addition, most patients report feeling very tired and should get plenty of rest.

Patients should consider joining local support groups with people who are coping with the same experiences. Many people with cancer find they can share thoughts and feelings with group members that they do not feel comfortable sharing with friends or family. Support groups are also a good source of information about ways to cope with cancer.

Clinical trials

Clinical trials are government-regulated studies of new treatments and techniques that may prove beneficial in diagnosing or treating a disease. Participation is always voluntary and at no cost to the participant. Clinical trials are conducted in three phases. Phase 1 tests the safety of the treatment and looks for harmful side effects. Phase 2 tests the effectiveness of the treatment. Phase 3 compares the treatment to other treatments available for the same condition.

The selection of clinical trials under way changes frequently. Patients and their families can search for new trials on the **National Cancer Institute** website at http://www.cancer.gov/clinicaltrials/search. Patients diagnosed with non-small cell lung cancer should discuss participating in clinical trials with their doctor. There are many clinical trials currently under way that are investigating all different stages of the disease.

Prognosis

The prognosis for non-small cell lung cancer is better if the disease is found early, and removed surgically. According to the American Cancer Society, as of 2014, for patients whose disease is diagnosed in stage I, the five-year survival rate ranges from 30–49%. Up to 31% of stage II patients are alive after five years, but only about 10% of stage III patients live for five years, and the stage IV survival rate is only about 1%. Unfortunately, 85% of patients already have at least stage III cancer by the time they are diagnosed. Many of these patients have disease that is too advanced for surgery. Despite treatment with radiotherapy and chemotherapy, the five-year survival for patients with inoperable disease is extremely low.

Prevention

The best way to prevent lung cancer is not to start smoking or to quit smoking. **Secondhand smoke** from other people's tobacco should also be avoided.

QUESTIONS TO ASK YOUR DOCTOR

- What kinds of diagnostic studies will be required to ascertain the type and spread of this tumor?
- Could there be a genetic component to this tumor? Should other family members be tested?
- What types of treatments are available?
- What types of side effects from treatments can I expect? What are your recommendations to help me deal with those side effects?
- Am I eligible for any clinical trials? Would these be helpful to consider?
- Are there any lifestyle changes that I should make?
- What type of diet should I follow? Are there foods I should avoid?
- Should I avoid any medications?
- How often should I be checked after treatment has ended?
- Is there a support group that I can join to hear about other people's experiences with this disorder?

Appropriate precautions should be taken when working with cancer-causing substances (**carcinogens**). Testing houses for the presence of radon gas and removing asbestos from buildings have also been suggested as preventive strategies.

Resources

BOOKS

Jacob, Elliot. *Medifocus Guidebook on: Non-small Cell Lung Cancer.* Silver Spring, MD: MediFocus, 2012.

Schiller, Joan H. *100 Questions & Answers About Lung Cancer,* 3rd ed. Sudbury, MA: Jones & Bartlett Learning, 2014.

Zakowski, Maureen, Panos Fidias, Mark Socinski, and Jyoti Patel. *Non-Small Cell Lung Cancer: Across the Continuum of Care.* New York, NY: Asante Communications, 2012.

WEBSITES

American Cancer Society. "Lung Cancer (Non-small Cell)." http://www.cancer.org/cancer/lungcancer-non-smallcell/detailedguide/index (accessed September 25, 2014).

CancerCare. "Lung Cancer 101: What is Lung Cancer?" Lungcancer.org. http://www.lungcancer.org/find_information/publications/163-lung_cancer_101/265-what_is_lung_cancer (accessed September 25, 2014).

"Lung Cancer." MedlinePlus, June 6, 2014. http://www.nlm.
    nih.gov/medlineplus/lungcancer.html (accessed September
    25, 2014).
Tan, Winston. "Non-small Cell Lung Cancer." Medscape
    Reference. June 6, 2014 http://emedicine.medscape.com/
    article/279960-overview (accessed September 25, 2014).

ORGANIZATIONS

American Cancer Society, 1599 Clifton Rd., NE, Atlanta, GA
    30329, (404) 320-3333, (800) ACS-2345, http://www.
    cancer.org.
American Lung Association, 1301 Pennsylvania Ave. NW,
    Suite 800, Washington, DC 20001, (202) 758-3355, Fax:
    (202) 452-1805, (800) 548-8252, info@lungusa.org,
    http://www.lungusa.org.
CancerCare, 275 Seventh Ave., New York, NY 10001, (800)
    813-HOPE (4673), info@cancercare.org, http://www.can-
    cercare.org.
National Cancer Institute, BG 9609 MSC 9760, 9609 Medical
    Center Drive, Bethesda, MD 20892-9760, (800) 4-
    CANCER (422-6237), http://www.cancer.gov.

Lata Cherath, PhD
Rebecca J. Frey, PhD
REVISED BY TISH DAVIDSON, AM

Lung cancer, small cell

Definition

Small cell lung **cancer** (SCLC) is a disease in which the cells of the lung tissues grow uncontrollably and form tumors. SCLC is also called oat cell cancer or oat cell **carcinoma**.

Description

Lung cancer is divided into two main types: small cell lung cancer and **non-small cell lung cancer** (NSCLC). Small cell lung cancer is the less common of the two, accounting for only about 10–15% of all lung cancers. This type of lung cancer is very aggressive. It grows quickly and is more likely to spread to other organs in the body.

Along with the heart, the lungs are located in the chest cavity. They are not simply hollow balloons, but have a very organized structure consisting of hollow tubes, blood vessels, and elastic tissue. The hollow tubes, called bronchi, are multi-branched, becoming smaller and more numerous at each branching. They end in tiny sacs called alveoli that are made of elastic tissue. Oxygen is taken up into the blood and carbon dioxide moves out of the blood in the alveoli.

Normal healthy lungs continually secrete mucus that keeps the lungs moist and protects the lungs by trapping foreign particles such as inhaled dust and dirt. The interior of the lungs is covered with small hair-like structures called cilia. The cilia move in such a way that mucus is swept upward out of the lungs and into the throat.

Small cell lung tumors usually start in the central bronchi. They grow quickly and prevent the lungs from functioning at their full capacity. Tumors may block the movement of air through the bronchi in the lungs. As a result, less oxygen gets into the blood and patients feel short of breath. Tumors may also block the normal movement of mucus into the throat. As a result, mucus builds up in the lungs and infection may develop behind the tumor.

Demographics

Lung cancers are decreasing in the United States, but increasing worldwide due to an increased use of tobacco. Worldwide, excluding **skin cancer**, lung cancer is the second most common cancer among both men and women and is the leading cause of cancer death in both sexes. It accounts for 1.6 million deaths each year.

In the United States, the American Cancer Society estimated that 224,210 new cases of lung cancer would be diagnosed in 2014, and about 159,260 people would die of the disease. Of these, about 10–15% are small cell lung cancers. Although there are differences in mortality rates among ethnic groups, these differences are mainly due to differences in smoking habits. SCLC is most common in people aged 60–80 years.

Causes and symptoms

Causes

Tobacco smoking accounts for nearly 90% of all lung cancers. The risk of developing lung cancer is increased for smokers (pipe, cigarette, or cigar) who start at a young age, and for those who have smoked for a long time. The risk also increases as more tobacco is smoked, and when **cigarettes** with higher tar content are smoked. Smoking marijuana cigarettes is also a risk factor for lung cancer. These cigarettes have a higher tar content than tobacco cigarettes.

In addition, certain hazardous materials that people may be exposed to in their jobs have been shown to cause lung cancer. These include asbestos, coal products, and radioactive substances. Air pollution may also be a contributing factor. Exposure to radon, a colorless, odorless gas that sometimes accumulates in the basement of homes, may cause lung cancer in some patients. Exposure to secondhand smoke also increases risk. Also,

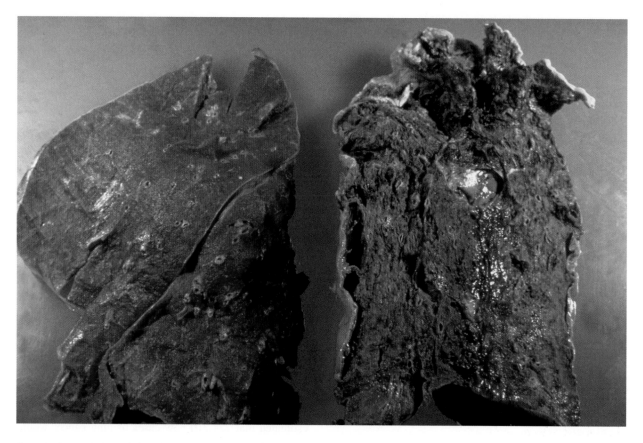

A normal lung (left) and the lung of a cigarette smoker (right). *(Arthur Glauberman/Science Source)*

patients whose lungs are scarred from other lung conditions or who are infected with the HIV virus may have an increased risk of developing lung cancer. Heavy smokers who use beta-carotene supplements are at higher risk as well.

Although the exact cause of lung cancer is not known, people with a family history of lung cancer appear to have a slightly higher risk of contracting the disease.

Symptoms

Small cell lung cancer is an aggressive disease that spreads quickly. Symptoms depend on the tumor's location within the lung, and on whether the cancer has spread to other parts of the body. More than 80% of small cell lung cancer patients have symptoms for only three months or less, and few cases are detected early.

The following symptoms are the most commonly reported by small cell lung cancer patients at the time of their diagnosis:

• a persistent cough

• chest pain

• shortness of breath and wheezing

• persistent hoarseness

• fatigue and loss of appetite

Although some patients may experience bloody sputum or phlegm, this symptom is more commonly seen in patients with other types of lung cancer.

Small cell tumors often press against a large blood vessel near the lungs called the superior vena cava (SVC), causing a condition known as SVC syndrome. This condition may cause individuals to retain water, cough, and have shortness of breath. Because small cell lung cancer often spreads quickly to the bones and central nervous system, individuals may also have **bone pain**, headaches, and seizures.

Small cell lung cancer can cause several hormonal disorders. About 40% of patients begin to secrete an antidiuretic hormone at the wrong time. This hormone causes the body to retain water, which may result in the patient's experiencing confusion, seizures, or coma. Less common are the development of **Cushing syndrome** and Lambert-Eaton syndrome. Symptoms of Cushing syndrome include obesity, severe **fatigue**, high blood pressure, backache, high blood sugar, easy bruising, and bluish-red stretch marks on the skin. Lambert-Eaton

KEY TERMS

Biopsy—A diagnostic procedure in which a tissue sample is removed from the body for examination.

Bronchi (singular, bronchus)—Two major airways that branch off the trachea and carry air to and from the lungs.

Bronchoscope—A thin flexible lighted tube that is used to view the air passages in the lungs.

Bronchoscopy—A procedure in which a thin flexible lighted tube is threaded through the airways to view the air passages in the lungs.

Computed tomography (CT)—A radiographic technique in which multiple x-ray images assembled by a computer give a three-dimensional image of a structure.

Lymph—Clear, slightly yellow fluid carried by a network of thin tubes to every part of the body. Cells that fight infection are carried in the lymph.

Lymph nodes—Small bean-shaped collections of tissue found in a lymph vessel. They produce cells and proteins that fight infection, and also filter lymph. Nodes are sometimes called lymph glands.

Lymphatic system—Primary defense against infection in the body. The lymphatic system consists of tissues, organs, and channels (similar to veins) that produce, store, and transport lymph and white blood cells to fight infection.

Magnetic resonance imaging (MRI)—Magnetic fields and radio frequency waves are used to image internal structures of the body.

Metastatic cancer—A cancer that has spread to an organ or tissue from a primary cancer located elsewhere in the body.

syndrome is a neuromuscular disorder (not hormonal) that causes muscle weakness, fatigue, and a tingling sensation on the skin. All these conditions usually diminish if the lung tumor is successfully treated.

Diagnosis

If lung cancer is suspected, the doctor will take a detailed medical and lifestyle history, including smoking, that checks both symptoms and risk factors. During a complete physical examination, the doctor will examine the patient's throat to rule out other possible causes of hoarseness or coughing, and listen to the patient's breathing and the sounds made when the patient's chest and upper back are tapped.

A chest x-ray will be ordered if lung cancer is suspected to check for masses in the lungs. Special imaging techniques such as **computed tomography (CT)** scans or **magnetic resonance imaging** (MRI), may provide more precise information about the size, shape, and location of any tumors.

Sputum analysis involves microscopic examination of the cells that are either coughed up from the lungs or are collected through a special instrument called a bronchoscope. The test looks for cancer cells. The sputum test does not, however, provide any information about the location of the tumor and must be followed by other tests.

Lung biopsy is the most definitive diagnostic tool for cancer. It can be performed in several different ways. The doctor can perform a **bronchoscopy**, which involves the insertion of a slender lighted tube called a bronchoscope down the patient's throat and into the lungs. In addition to viewing the passageways of the lungs, the doctor can use the bronchoscope to obtain samples of the lung tissue. In another procedure known as a needle **biopsy**, the location of the tumor is first identified using a CT scan or MRI. The doctor then inserts a needle through the chest wall and collects a sample of tissue from the tumor. In the third procedure, known as surgical biopsy, the chest wall is opened up and a part or all of the tumor is removed for examination.

Clinical staging

Unlike other types of lung cancer, the staging of small cell lung cancer is relatively simple. This is because approximately 70% of patients already have metastatic cancer when they are diagnosed, and small differences in the amount of tumor found in the lungs do not change the prognosis. To establish where the cancer has spread, various tests may be performed, including **bone marrow aspiration and biopsy**, CT scans of the chest and abdomen, MRI scans of the brain, and radionuclide bone scans. All these tests determine the extent to which the cancer has spread. Once the stage is determined, doctors decide on a course of treatment and have a better idea of the patient's prognosis.

Small cell lung cancer is usually divided into two stages: limited and extensive. Limited-stage cancer is found in one lung only and in lymph nodes close to the lung. Extensive-stage cancer has spread beyond the lungs to other parts of the body. If the cancer returns after being previously treated, it is referred to as recurrent. Alternate staging systems use a four-stage system with stage I having small tumors that do not affect the lungs or bronchi and that have not spread, and stage IV having cancer in both lungs and cancer spread to other organs.

Without treatment, small cell lung cancer has the most aggressive clinical course of any type of pulmonary tumor, with median survival from diagnosis of only 2–4 months. Compared to other cell types of lung cancer, small cell lung cancer has a greater tendency to be widely disseminated (spread) by the time of diagnosis, but it is much more responsive to **chemotherapy** and irradiation.

Treatment

Treatment of small cell lung cancer depends on whether the patient has limited, extensive, or recurrent disease. Treatment usually involves radiotherapy and chemotherapy. Surgery is rarely used for this type of lung cancer because the tumor is usually too far advanced.

Patients with limited-stage disease are usually treated with chemotherapy. Combinations of two or more drugs have a better effect than treatment with a single drug. Up to 90% of patients with this stage of disease respond to chemotherapy. The chemotherapy most commonly prescribed is a combination of the drugs **etoposide** (Vepesid) and **cisplatin** (Platinol) or **carboplatin**, although cisplatin in combination with other drugs is also used. Combining chemotherapy with chest radiotherapy and/or occasionally surgery has also prolonged survival for limited-stage patients.

In addition to chest radiotherapy, some patients are also treated with **radiation therapy** to the brain, even if no cancer is found there. This treatment, called prophylactic cranial irradiation (PCI), is given to prevent tumors from forming in the brain.

Combinations of different chemotherapy agents are also used for treating extensive-stage small cell lung cancer. However, compared with limited-stage patients, the percentage of extensive-stage patients who respond to therapy is lower. Commonly used drug combinations include etoposide and cisplatin, cisplatin and **irinotecan**, or carboplatin and irinotecan. Targeted radiation therapy may help improve outcomes even further in patients who respond well to chemotherapy treatment; as of 2014, this approach was being studied in **clinical trials**. Radiation therapy is also used for the palliative (pain relief) treatment of symptoms of metastatic lung cancer, particularly brain and bone tumors.

Patients who have recurrent small cell lung cancer often become resistant to chemotherapy. These patients are treated with palliative radiotherapy. Their doctor may also recommend that they take part in a clinical trial of a new therapy, as different chemotherapy agents may be available.

Alternative and complementary therapies

Many patients find that alternative and complementary therapies help to reduce the stress associated with illness, improve immune function, and boost spirits. While there is no clinical evidence that these therapies specifically combat disease, such activities as biofeedback, relaxation, therapeutic touch, massage therapy and guided imagery have no side effects and have been reported to enhance well-being.

Several other healing therapies are sometimes used as supplemental or replacement cancer treatments, such as antineoplastons, Cancell, cartilage (bovine and shark), laetrile, and **mistletoe**. Many of these therapies have not been the subject of safety and efficacy trials by the National Cancer Institute (NCI). The NCI has conducted trials on Cancell, laetrile, and some other alternative therapies and found no anticancer activity. These treatments have varying degrees of effectiveness and safety considerations. Patients using any alternative remedy should first consult their doctors in order to prevent harmful side effects or interactions with traditional cancer treatment.

Coping with cancer treatment

The side effects associated with treatment of small cell lung cancer can be severe. Patients should ask their doctor about medications to treat **nausea and vomiting** and other side effects. It is particularly important to eat a nutritious diet and to drink plenty of fluids. In addition, most patients report feeling very tired and should get plenty of rest.

Prognosis

Small cell lung cancer is a very aggressive disease. Without treatment, limited-stage patients will survive for three to six months, while extensive-stage patients will survive six to 12 weeks. However, small cell lung cancer is much more responsive to chemotherapy and radiation therapy than other types of lung cancer. Among patients treated with chemotherapy, 70–90% have a major response to treatment.

Survival in patients responding to therapy is four to five times longer than in patients without treatment. In addition, two years after the start of therapy, about 10% of patients remain free of disease. In general, women tend to have a better prognosis than men. Patients whose disease has spread to the central nervous system or liver have a much worse prognosis. Although the overall survival at five years is 5%–10% (with a 31% five-year survival rate for treated small cell lung cancer in patients with stage I disease, and a 2% survival rate for patients in stage IV), survival is higher in patients with limited stage disease. About 70% of patients who are disease-free after

QUESTIONS TO ASK YOUR DOCTOR

- What kinds of diagnostic studies will be required to ascertain the type and spread of this tumor?
- Could there be a genetic component to this tumor? Should other family members be tested?
- What types of treatments are available?
- What types of side effects from treatments can I expect? What are your recommendations to help me deal with those side effects?
- Am I eligible for any clinical trials? Would these be helpful to consider?
- Are there any lifestyle changes that I should make?
- What type of diet should I follow? Are there foods I should avoid?
- Should I avoid any medications?
- How often should I be checked after treatment has ended?
- Is there a support group that I can join to hear about other people's experiences with this disorder?

two years do not relapse. After five to ten disease-free years, relapses are rare.

Clinical trials

Clinical trials are government-regulated studies of new treatments and techniques that may prove beneficial in diagnosing or treating a disease. Participation is always voluntary and at no cost to the participant. Clinical trials are conducted in three phases. Phase 1 tests the safety of the treatment and looks for harmful side effects. Phase 2 tests the effectiveness of the treatment. Phase 3 compares the treatment to other treatments available for the same condition.

The selection of clinical trials underway changes frequently. Patients and their families can search for new trials on the **National Cancer Institute** website at http://www.cancer.gov/clinicaltrials/search.

Prevention

The best way to prevent lung cancer is to not start smoking or quit smoking. **Secondhand smoke** from other people's tobacco should also be avoided. Appropriate precautions should be taken when working with substances that can cause cancer (**carcinogens**). Testing houses for the presence of radon gas and removing asbestos from buildings have also been suggested as preventive strategies.

Resources

BOOKS

Jacob, Elliot. *Medifocus Guidebook on: Small Cell Lung Cancer.* Silver Spring, MD: MediFocus, 2012.

Schiller, Joan H. *100 Questions & Answers About Lung Cancer,* 3rd ed. Sudbury, MA: Jones & Bartlett Learning, 2014.

PERIODICALS

Yee, Don, et al. "Clinical Trial of Post-Chemotherapy Consolidation Thoracic Radiotherapy for Extensive-Stage Small Cell Lung Cancer." *Radiotherapy and Oncology* 102, no. 2 (2012): 234–238. http://dx.doi.org/10.1016/j.radonc.2011.08.042 (accessed September 24, 2014).

WEBSITES

American Cancer Society. "Lung Cancer (Small Cell)." http://www.cancer.org/cancer/lungcancer-smallcell/detailed-guide/index (accessed September 24, 2014).

"Lung Cancer." MedlinePlus, June 6, 2014. http://www.nlm.nih.gov/medlineplus/lungcancer.html (accessed September 24, 2014).

Tan, Winston. "Small Cell Lung Cancer." Medscape Reference, March 26, 2014. http://emedicine.medscape.com/article/280104-overview (accessed September 24, 2014).

ORGANIZATIONS

American Cancer Society, 1599 Clifton Rd., NE, Atlanta, GA 30329, (404) 320-3333, (800) ACS-2345, http://www.cancer.org.

American Lung Association, 1301 Pennsylvania Ave. NW, Suite 800, Washington, DC 20001, (202) 758-3355, Fax: (202) 452-1805, (800) 548-8252, info@lungusa.org, http://www.lungusa.org.

National Cancer Institute, BG 9609 MSC 9760, 9609 Medical Center Drive, Bethesda, MD 20892-9760, (800) 4-CANCER (422-6237), http://www.cancer.gov.

Lata Cherath, PhD
Alison McTavish, MSc
REVISED BY TISH DAVIDSON, AM

Lung carcinoid tumors *see* **Carcinoid tumors, lung**

Lung metastasis *see* **Metastasis; Lung cancer, non-small cell; Lung cancer, small cell**

Lung surgery *see* **Pneumonectomy; Thoracotomy; Lobectomy**

Lupron *see* **Leuprolide acetate**

Lymph node angiogram *see* **Lymphangiography**

Lymph node biopsy

Definition

A lymph node **biopsy** is a procedure in which all or part of a lymph node is removed and examined to determine whether **cancer** exists within the node.

Purpose

The lymphatic system is part of the body's primary defense against infection. It consists of the spleen, tonsils, thymus, lymph nodes, lymph vessels, and the clear, slightly yellow fluid called lymph. These components produce and transport white blood cells called lymphocytes and macrophages that rid the body of infection. The lymphatic system is also involved in the production of antibodies. Antibodies are proteins that fight bacteria, viruses, and other foreign materials that enter the body.

The lymph vessels are similar to veins, except rather than carrying blood, they circulate lymph to tissues in the body. Lymph nodes comprise about 600 small bean-shaped collections of tissue found along the lymph vessel. They produce cells and proteins that fight infection and clean and filter lymph. Lymph nodes are sometimes called lymph glands, although they are not true glands. When someone describes swollen glands, he or she is actually describing enlarged lymph nodes.

Normal lymph nodes are no larger than 0.5 in. (1.3 cm) in diameter and are difficult to feel. However, lymph nodes can enlarge to greater than 2.5 in. (6 cm) and become sore. Most often the swelling results from infection, but it is sometimes the result of cancer.

Cancers can metastasize (spread) through the lymphatic system from the site of the original tumor to distant parts of the body where secondary tumors are formed. The purpose of a lymph node biopsy is to determine the cause of the swelling and/or whether the cancer has begun to spread through the lymphatic system. This information is important in staging the cancer and devising a treatment plan.

Precautions

Pregnant women should inform their doctors about their pregnancy before a lymph node biopsy, although pregnancy will not affect the results.

Description

There are three kinds of lymph node biopsy. **Sentinel lymph node mapping** and biopsy is a technique that involves testing the sentinel, or first one

KEY TERMS

Lymph nodes—Small bean-shaped organs located throughout the lymphatic system. The lymph nodes store special cells that trap cancer cells or bacteria that are traveling through the body in lymph. Also called lymph glands.

Lymphocytes—Small white blood cells that carry out the activities of the immune system; they number about 1 trillion.

Malignant—Cancerous. Cancer cells reproduce without normal controls on growth and form tumors or invade other tissues.

Spleen—An organ located to the left of the stomach that acts as a reservoir for blood cells and produces lymphocytes and other products involved in fighting infection.

Thymus—An organ near the base of the neck that produces cells that fight infection. After puberty it declines in size and function.

Tonsils—Small masses of tissue at the back of the throat.

of a series of lymph nodes that receive drainage from a cancer site. It is most often used for **breast cancer** and **melanoma**. Fine-needle aspiration (FNA) biopsy, often just called needle biopsy, is performed when the lymph node of interest is near the surface of the body. A hematologist (a doctor who specializes in blood diseases) usually performs the test. In FNA biopsy, a needle is inserted through the skin and into the lymph node and a sample of tissue is drawn from the node. This material is preserved and sent to the laboratory for examination.

Although needle biopsies are performed less frequently on lymph nodes than are sentinel or open biopsies, needle biopsies are minimally invasive, requiring only a local anesthetic. Needle biopsies generally take less than half an hour with minimal pain following the procedure. The disadvantage of this procedure is that an existing cancer may not be detected in the small sample removed, making this procedure less precise than an open biopsy.

Open lymph node biopsy is performed by a surgeon, typically with the patient under sedation. In some cases, general anesthesia is administered. The surgeon makes a small cut and removes either the entire lymph node or a slice of tissue and then sends the sample to the laboratory for examination. Results from both types of biopsies require several days.

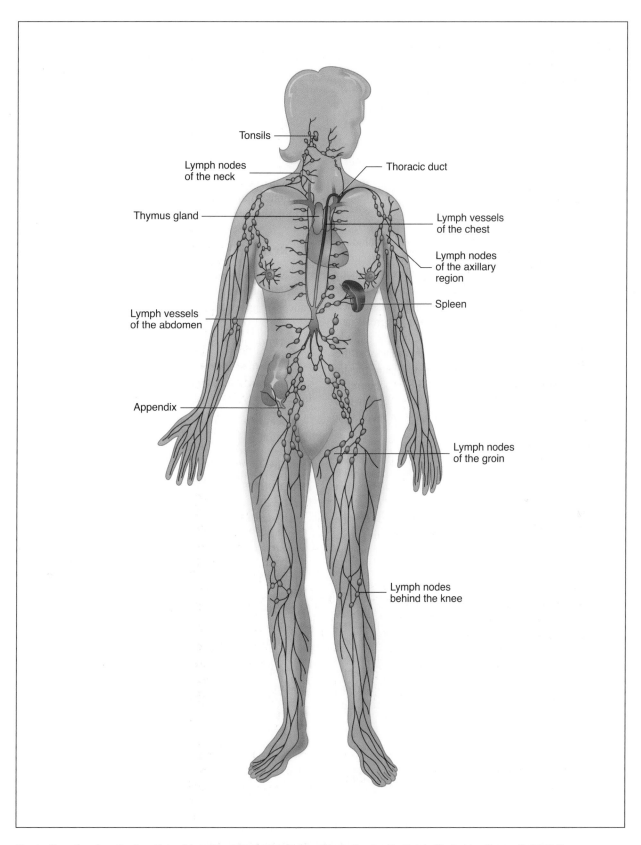

Tonsils

Lymph nodes
of the neck

Thymus gland

Lymph vessels
of the abdomen

Appendix

Thoracic duct

Lymph vessels
of the chest

Lymph nodes
of the axillary
region

Spleen

Lymph nodes
of the groin

Lymph nodes
behind the knee

Illustration showing the location of lymph nodes in the body. *(Illustration by Electronic Illustrators Group. © 2015 Cengage Learning®.)*

Advantages of open lymph node biopsy include a larger tissue sample, which permits more accurate identification of a cancer, and the ability to reach nodes that are deep inside the body. Surgery to remove a cancer will often include removal of nearby lymph nodes, which are then examined to determine the cancer's spread and tumor stage. Disadvantages of open node biopsy include a longer recovery time; more prolonged soreness at the biopsy site; and the use of more potent anesthesia, increasing the risks to the patient. The procedure is performed in a hospital or outpatient surgery center and takes about an hour, with additional time to recover if general anesthesia is administered.

The decision about which biopsy to perform depends on the type and location of a suspicious tumor or known cancer, along with other guidelines based on agreement of experts or evidence from **clinical trials**. For example, 2014 guidelines recommend that lymph nodes under the arm should not be removed in a woman with a diagnosis of breast cancer with no spread of the cancer to the sentinel lymph nodes.

Preparation

A needle biopsy requires no particular preparation. General health should be evaluated with standard preoperative blood and other tests prior to an open biopsy. The doctor should be informed about the patient's medications (prescription, nonprescription, or herbal) as well as past bleeding problems or allergies to medication or anesthesia.

Aftercare

A needle biopsy requires little aftercare other than a bandage to keep the biopsy site clean. Patients who have general anesthesia for an open biopsy often feel drowsy and tired for several days following the procedure, and they should arrange for someone to drive them home after the procedure. The incision site must be kept clean and dry, and a follow-up visit to check on healing is usually necessary. Patients who have biopsies in some areas, such as breast cancer patients who have an open or sentinel biopsy of the lymph nodes under the arm, will need to limit lifting or other physical activity for a period of time following the procedure.

Risks

There are few risks associated with lymph node biopsy. The main risks are excessive bleeding (usually only in people with blood disorders) and allergic reactions to anesthesia, which are rare. Occasionally the biopsy site becomes infected.

Results

Normal lymph nodes are small and flat. When examined under the microscope, they show no signs of cancer or infection.

Abnormal results

Abnormal lymph nodes are usually enlarged and contain cancerous (malignant) cells or show signs of infection.

See also Lymph node dissection; Radical neck dissection.

Resources

PERIODICALS

Verheuvel, N.C., et al. "The Role of Ultrasound-Guided Lymph Node Biopsy in Axillary Staging of Invasive Breast Cancer in the Post-ACOSOG Z0011 Trial Era." *Annals of Surgical Oncology* (September 10, 2014): e-pub ahead of print. http://dx.doi.org/10.1245/s10434-014-4071-1 (accessed October 23, 2014).

WEBSITES

Duke Cancer Institute. "Lymph Node Biopsy." Duke School of Medicine, Duke University. http://cancer.dukemedicine.org/cancer/health_library/care_guides/treatment_instructions/lymphnodebiopsy (accessed October 23, 2014).

Goldberg, Kristen. "ASCO Guideline for Sentinel Node Biopsy in Early Stage Breast Cancer; Evidence Supports Use of This Less Invasive Diagnostic in More Patients." http://www.asco.org/press-center/asco-updates-guideline-sentinel-node-biopsy-early-stage-breast-cancer-evidence-supports (accessed August 8, 2014).

ORGANIZATIONS

American Cancer Society, 250 Williams St. NW, Atlanta, GA 30303, (800) 227-2345, http://www.cancer.org.

American Society of Clinical Oncology, 2318 Mill Rd., Ste. 800, Alexandria, VA 22314, (571) 483-1300, (888) 651-3038, contactus@cancer.net, http://www.asco.org.

National Cancer Institute, 9609 Medical Center Dr., BG 9609 MSC 9760, Bethesda, MD 20892-9760, (800) 4-CANCER (422-6237), http://www.cancer.gov.

Tish Davidson, AM
REVISED BY TERESA G. ODLE

Lymph node dissection

Definition

Lymph node dissection (lymphadenectomy) is the surgical removal of one or more lymph nodes to assess the spread of **cancer** through the lymphatic system. If cancer cells are discovered, additional lymph nodes might be removed. Regional lymph node dissection removes some of the nodes in the tumor area. Radical lymph node dissection removes all of the lymph nodes in the area of the tumor.

Purpose

The lymphatic system is the body's primary defense against infection. It consists of the spleen, tonsils, thymus, lymph nodes, lymph vessels, and the clear, slightly yellow fluid called lymph. These components produce and transport cells and proteins that help rid the body of infection. Many types of cancer may spread to nearby lymph nodes and then throughout the lymphatic system to other parts of the body.

The lymph vessels are similar to veins, but instead of carrying blood, they circulate lymph fluid to tissues in the body. About 600 small bean-shaped tissue formations

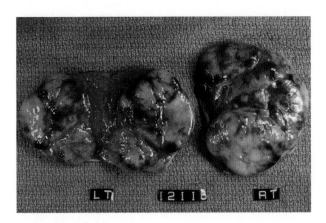

Diseased lymph nodes. *(O.J. Staats MD/Custom Medical Stock Photo)*

called lymph nodes are located along the lymph vessels. These nodes produce lymph and the cells and proteins that fight infection. They also clean and filter foreign and toxic cells, like bacteria or cancer cells, from the lymph fluid. Cancer cells can break off from the original tumor and spread (metastasize) through the lymphatic system to distant parts of the body, where secondary tumors may form.

Lymph node dissection is performed both to determine the extent of spread (**metastasis**) of the cancer cells and to remove lymph nodes that already contain cancer cells. Lymph node dissection is sometimes performed following **biopsy** of a sentinel lymph node (the lymph node nearest the tumor) when results indicate spread of the cancer. Lymph node dissection is performed for many types of cancers, including cancers of the head and neck, breast, prostate, testes, bladder, colon, and lung.

About 200 lymph nodes are located in the head and neck and another 30 to 50 in the underarm area. More are located in the groin area. Swollen lymph nodes are sometimes referred to as swollen glands, even though they are not true glands. Although lymph nodes are typically no larger than 0.5 inches (1.3 cm) in diameter and are difficult to feel, they can increase in size to greater than 2.5 inches (6 cm) if they trap bacteria or cancer cells. Most often, hot and painful swollen nodes are caused by trapped bacteria. Swollen lymph nodes caused by cancer are usually painless.

Precautions

This surgical procedure is unlikely to be performed if the cancer has already metastasized to another site, as removing the lymph nodes has not been shown to contain the cancer. In this case, external beam radiation might be applied to treat the affected nodes. As with any surgery, pregnant women should inform their doctors about their pregnancy before undergoing a lymph node dissection.

Description

Lymph node dissection is usually performed by a surgeon in a hospital setting under general anesthesia. Once an incision is made, the tissue is pulled back and the lymph nodes are revealed. The location of the original cancer guides the surgeon to the lymph nodes that must be removed. Samples of lymph node tissue are sent to the laboratory for pathologic examination. The presence of malignant cells in the excised nodes is an indication that the cancer has spread beyond the original site; further therapy can then be recommended.

QUESTIONS TO ASK YOUR DOCTOR

- How is it determined which lymph nodes should be removed?
- How should I prepare for this procedure?
- What precautions can I take to help prevent lymphedema?
- How will lymph node dissection affect my daily life?
- Will anything besides lymph nodes be removed?
- About how long is the expected hospital stay?
- Will removal of my lymph nodes increase my chance of infection?

KEY TERMS

Computed tomography (CT or CAT) scan—CT employs x-rays taken from many angles and computer modeling to determine the size and location of tumors and provide information about the possibility of their surgical removal.

Magnetic resonance imaging (MRI)—MRI uses magnets and radio waves to create detailed cross-sectional pictures of the interior of the body.

Malignant—Cancerous. Cancer cells reproduce without normal controls on growth and begin to form tumors and invade other tissues.

Metastasis—The spread of cells from the original site of the cancer to other parts of the body where secondary tumors are formed.

Preparation

Diagnostic imaging or **lymph node biopsy** may be performed before the operation to determine the location of the cancer and the nodes that should be removed. These tests might include **sentinel lymph node biopsy**, CT (**computed tomography**) scans, and MRI scans. In addition, standard pre operative blood tests, including liver function tests, are performed. The patient will meet with an anesthesiologist before the operation and is advised to notify the anesthesiologist about drug allergies and prescribed medication (prescription, nonprescription, or herbal).

Aftercare

The length of the hospital stay after lymph node dissection depends first on whether the lymphadenectomy was performed during the surgery to remove the primary tumor. If lymph node dissection takes place after the cancer surgery, the hospital stay depends on the number of lymph nodes removed and their locations. Drains are inserted under the skin to remove the fluid that accumulates after the lymph node removal; most patients return home with the drains still in place. Some patients leave the day of or the day following the procedure.

The most common adverse effect of lymph node dissection is accumulation of lymph fluid that causes swelling, a condition known as lymphedema. Patients are advised to report signs of swelling to their doctors. Swelling may indicate the presence of a new tumor that is blocking a lymph vessel or the development of lymphedema after lymph node dissection. Treatment for lymphedema in people with cancer varies from treatment of lymphedema that results from other causes.

In cancer patients, it is essential to alleviate swelling and avoid spreading cancer cells to other parts of the body. For that reason, an oncologist (cancer specialist) is often consulted before treatment begins.

Risks

People who have had lymph nodes removed are at increased risk of the development of lymphedema, which can occur in any part of the body where lymph accumulates in abnormal quantities. When the amount of fluid exceeds the capacity of the lymph system to move it through the body, it leaks into the tissues, resulting in swelling. Removing lymph nodes and lymph vessels through lymph node dissection increases the likelihood that the capacity of the lymph transport system will be exceeded.

Lymphedema may occur days or weeks after lymph node dissection. **Radiation therapy** also increases the chance of developing lymphedema, so patients receiving radiation therapy following lymph node dissection are at greatest risk of experiencing this side effect. Lymphedema slows healing; causes skin and tissue damage; and, when left untreated, can result in the development of hard or fibrous tissue. People with lymphedema are also at risk for repeated infection because pools of lymph in the tissues permit bacteria to grow. In severe cases, untreated lymphedema can develop into a rare form of cancer called lymphangiosarcoma.

Lymph node dissection includes risks similar to those for all major surgery: potential bleeding, infection, and allergic reactions to anesthesia.

Results

Normal lymph nodes are small and flat and display no cancer cells when the lymph tissue is stained and examined under the microscope.

Abnormal results

Abnormal lymph nodes are enlarged and show cancer cells when the lymph tissue is stained and examined under the microscope.

See also Radical neck dissection.

Resources

BOOKS

Pazdur, Richard, Lawrence D. Wagman, Kevin A. Camphausen, and William J. Hoskins, eds. "Principles of Surgical Oncology." *Cancer Management: A Multidisciplinary Approach.* 13th ed. Norwalk, CT: BM Medica, 2010.

PERIODICALS

Agresti, R., et al. "Axillary Lymph Node Dissection Versus No Dissection in Patients with T1N0 Breast Cancer: A Randomized Clinical Trial." *Cancer* 120 (June 2014): 885–893.

Bernet, L. and R. Cano. "Metastatic Sentinel Node and Axillary Lymphadenectomy Revisited." *Glandular Surgery* 1 (May 2012): 7–8.

WEBSITES

Breastcancer.org. "Lymph Node Dissection: What to Expect." http://www.breastcancer.org/treatment/surgery/lymph_node_removal/dissection_expectations (accessed October 30, 2014).

University of Michigan Health System. "Lymph Node Dissection." http://surgery.med.umich.edu/plastic/patient/forms/instructions/lymphnodedissection_postop.shtml (accessed October 30, 2014).

ORGANIZATIONS

American Cancer Society, 250 Williams St. NW, Atlanta, GA 30303, (800) 227-2345, http://www.cancer.org.

National Cancer Institute, 9609 Medical Center Dr., BG 9609 MSC 9760, Bethesda, MD 20892-9760, (800) 4-CANCER (422-6237), http://www.cancer.gov.

National Lymphedema Network, 225 Bush Street, Suite 357, San Francisco, CA 94104, (415) 908-3681, (800) 541-3259, Fax: (415) 908-3813, nln@lymphnet.org, http://lymphnet.org.

REVISED BY TISH DAVIDSON, AM
L. Lee Culvert

REVIEWED BY MARIANNE VAHEY, MD

Lymphangiogram *see*
Lymphangiography

Lymphangiography

Definition

Lymphangiography, also called fluorescence lymphangiography and x-ray lymphography, is a diagnostic procedure in which **x-rays** (angiograms) are taken after the injection of a radioactive oil-based contrast medium (a substance that highlights the tissue or organ of interest) to visualize the lymphatic vessels, lymph nodes, and the circulation of lymphatic fluid.

Purpose

The lymphatic system is the body's primary defense against infection. It consists of the spleen, tonsils, thymus, lymph nodes, lymph vessels, and a clear, slightly yellow fluid called lymph. These components produce and transport cells and proteins that help rid the body of infection. Many types of **cancer** can spread to

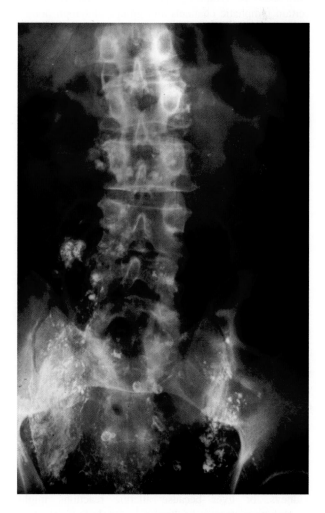

False-color lymphangiogram of the abdomen of a person suffering from lymphoma. *(MEHAU KULYK/Science Source)*

nearby lymph nodes and then throughout the lymphatic system to other parts of the body. Lymphangiography is used to:

- diagnose the presence or spread of tumors, lymphatic cancer (lymphoma), and other cancers

- distinguish primary lymphedema (swelling in a limb that arises from missing or impaired lymphatic vessels) from secondary lymphedema (swelling caused by damaged lymph vessels or after lymph node removal)

- localize tumors for surgical removal

- assess the effectiveness of chemotherapy and radiation therapy in treating problems associated with metastatic (spreading) cancer

Although the results of lymphangiography are considered reliable, additional tests, **imaging studies**, and clinical observations are necessary to establish a precise diagnosis. Used alone, lymphangiography misses tumors in about 20% of cases. One of the major drawbacks of lymphangiography is its failure to fill certain lymphatic channels and groups of lymph nodes, which may result from infection, injury, or tumor spread. When this filling failure occurs, certain segments of the lymphatic system in the abdomen and pelvis cannot be visualized; thus metastatic disease can be neither confirmed nor ruled out.

Conventional x-ray lymphangiography with an iodine oil-based contrast agent is used for the staging of urologic, gynecologic, and testicular malignancies.

From the 1930s until the 1990s, x-ray lymphangiography with oil-based contrast agents was the standard imaging technique applied to assess the lymphatic system. It is still used, especially to diagnose Hodgkin and **non-Hodgkin lymphoma**. Some malignant lesions in lymph nodes of normal size can be visualized more readily with x-ray lymphangiography than with CT scans. However, technical innovations in nuclear diagnostics and computer imaging have largely replaced x-ray lymphangiography with simpler, less invasive, and more reliable studies to visualize the lymphatic system, including **positron emission tomography** (PET), isotope lymphography (lymphangioscintigraphy), color Doppler ultrasound, and **magnetic resonance imaging** lymphangiography.

Precautions

Some patients may have adverse reactions to the contrast medium. Lymphangiography is usually not administered to patients with diseases of the lungs, heart, kidneys, or liver because allergic reactions might exacerbate symptoms of these diseases. Individuals with allergies to shellfish, iodine, or dye used in other

QUESTIONS TO ASK YOUR DOCTOR

- What is the purpose of the test?
- How long will the test take?
- Will I be sedated or receive anesthesia before the test?
- Is there anything special I should do before the test?
- May I drive myself home after the test?
- When will I get the results?

diagnostic tests are sometimes prescribed steroids or antihistamines before the test to decrease the risk of allergic reactions.

Description

Lymphangiography can be performed as an inpatient or outpatient procedure depending upon the patient's condition. A sedative might be given to help the patient relax. After the skin of each foot is cleaned with an antiseptic, a blue indicator dye (which identifies the lymph nodes but does not show up on x-rays) is injected between the first, second, and third toes of each foot. It takes about 15 to 30 minutes for the dye to spread into the lymphatic system. The thin bluish lines that appear on the top of each foot delineate the lymphatic vessels. Next, a local anesthetic is injected and a small incision is made into one of the larger blue lines in each foot. A needle or catheter (a thin flexible tube) is inserted into a vessel in each foot and an oil-based radioactive contrast medium (such as ethiodol, an ethiodized oil, or lipiodol) is injected at a slow, steady rate. Dosage of the contrast agent is determined by the patient's weight. Although patients may notice a feeling of pressure as the contrast medium is injected, it is important that the patient remain still to avoid dislodging the needle. Once the contrast agent is injected, the catheter is removed and the incisions are stitched and bandaged.

A fluoroscope—an x-ray machine that allows continuous visualization of internal structures on a TV monitor—is used to monitor the progress of the contrast medium as it spreads in 60 to 90 minutes through the lymphatic system, traveling up the legs, into the groin, and along the back of the abdominal cavity. Then x-rays are taken of the legs, pelvis, abdomen, and chest areas. Additional x-rays are taken the following day.

After the procedure, the patient's skin, feces, and urine may display a bluish tint for two to three days until

KEY TERMS

Contrast medium—A substance that highlights the tissue or organ being filmed.

Lymph node—A small bean-shaped encapsulated body in the lymphatic system that produces white cells (lymphocytes) and filters foreign cells such as bacteria and cancer cells from lymphatic fluid.

Lymphoma—A type of cancer of the lymphatic system.

Metastasis—The spread of cancer cells from the primary site of a malignant tumor or lesion to a nearby or distant location in the body.

the marker dye disappears. However, the dye may stay in the body for up to two years, which actually allows additional imaging tests. The patient may also experience some discomfort behind the knees and in the groin area. A radiologist will review the lymphangiography results and will send a report to the doctor who ordered the test within a few hours if abnormalities are detected. If the results are normal, the results may take a few days.

For monitoring **breast cancer**, the blue dye and contrast agent may be combined to serve as a guide for surgeons to obtain a **biopsy** sample and determine whether or not the cancer has spread.

Preparation

No special preparation, including dietary and activity restrictions or limits on medication intake are generally needed before lymphangiography. However, some radiology facilities require a clear liquid diet for a specified period of time before the test. Patients are asked to empty their bladders before testing. A patient undergoing lymphangiography (or a close family member) must sign a consent form before the test is administered.

Aftercare

After the procedure, the patient's blood pressure, pulse, breathing status, and temperature are monitored at regular intervals until patients are considered stable. The patient is monitored for breathing complications, such as hoarseness or shortness of breath, chest pain, low blood pressure, low-grade **fever**, or the development of a bluish tint to the lips or nailbeds due to clotting of the dye.

Bedrest for at least 24 hours following the test is recommended, with feet elevated to help reduce swelling at the incision sites. The incision sites might be sore for several days; ice packs can be applied to these sites to reduce swelling. The patient is advised to inspect the incision sites for infection once home. Sterile dressings should remain in place for two days, and the incision sites should be kept dry until after the sutures are removed (7 to 10 days after the test).

Risks

Introduction of the needle or tube through the skin carries the risk of infection or bleeding. Allergic reaction—usually not serious— to the contrast medium can occur in some patients. There is also a slight risk of developing an oil embolism (obstruction of a blood vessel) due to the oil-based contrast medium. The contrast medium eventually seeps from the lymphatic channels into the general circulation, where it can travel to and lodge in the lungs.

X-rays expose the patient to radiation in this procedure. Although pregnant women and children are particularly sensitive to these risks, physicians might order the procedure when the benefits appear to outweigh the risks.

Results

Normal test results indicate no anatomical or functional abnormalities in the lymphatic system and normal circulation of lymphatic fluid.

Abnormal results

Abnormal results might indicate:

• Hodgkin or non-Hodgkin lymphoma, cancers of the lymphatic system

• inflammation

• metastatic cancer in the lymph nodes

• primary lymphedema

• retroperitoneal tumors (tumors lying outside the peritoneum—the membrane lining the abdominal cavity)

• trauma

• filariasis (a tropical disease caused by worms living in the lymphatic system)

Alternatives

High-resolution magnetic resonance lymphangiography might be performed instead of x-ray **angiography**, eliminating exposure to radiation. Interstitial MR lymphography is a safe and technically feasible procedure by which to observe the lymph nodes and lymphatic vessels, especially in patients with primary and secondary lymphedema.

New contrast agents are also being developed for use with new lymphatic imaging techniques, and studies show that diagnostic accuracy continues to improve.

Resources

BOOKS

Brant, William E., and Clyde A. Helms. "Lymphadenopathy." In *Fundamentals of Diagnostic Radiology*. 4th ed. Philadelphia: Lippincott Williams & Williams, 2012.

PERIODICALS

Liu, N., and Y. Zhang. "Magnetic Resonance Lymphangiography for the Study of Lymphatic System in Lymphedema." *Journal of Reconstructive Microsurgery* (July 2014): e-pub ahead of print. http://dx.doi.org/10.1055/s-0034-1384213 (accessed October 31, 2014).

WEBSITES

A.D.A.M. Medical Encyclopedia. "Lymphangiogram." MedlinePlus. http://www.nlm.nih.gov/medlineplus/ency/article/003798.htm (accessed October 31, 2014).

ORGANIZATIONS

American College of Radiology, 1891 Preston White Dr., Reston, VA 20191, (703) 648-8900, info@acr.org, http://www.acr.org.

Lymphoma Research Foundation, 115 Broadway, Suite 1301, New York, NY 10006, (212) 349-2910, Fax: (212) 349-2886, LRF@lymphoma.org, http://www.lymphoma.org.

Genevieve Slomski, PhD
REVISED BY L. LEE CULVERT
REVIEWED BY MARIANNE VAHEY, MD

Lymphocyte immune globulin

Definition

Lymphocyte **immune globulin** is a drug used to suppress the immune system. Lymphocyte immune globulin is also known by the generic name antithymocyte globulin (ATG) and the brand names Atgam and Thymoglobulin. Atgam first received FDA approval in 1981 and Thymoglobulin in 1999.

Purpose

Lymphocyte immune globulin is used to treat aplastic **anemia** and to prevent rejections during **bone marrow transplantation**. This drug has also been used experimentally to treat advanced non-Hodgkin lymphomas and cutaneous T-cell lymphomas.

KEY TERMS

Adult respiratory distress syndrome (ARDS)—A lung disease characterized by widespread lung abnormalities, fluid in the lungs, shortness of breath, and low oxygen levels in the blood.

Antibodies—Proteins made by the immune system that attach to targeted molecules and cells.

Aplastic anemia—Failure of the bone marrow to make enough blood cells.

Blood cells—Cells found in the blood, including red blood cells that carry oxygen, white blood cells that fight infections, and platelets that help the blood to clot.

Bone marrow—A group of cells and molecules found in the centers of some bones. It makes all of the cells found in the blood, including the cells involved in immunity.

Graft-versus-host disease (GVHD)—A disease that develops when immune cells in transplanted bone marrow attack the body.

Immune system—The cells and organs that defend the body against infections.

Pulmonary edema—A disease characterized by excessive fluid in the lungs and difficulty breathing.

Sepsis—An infection that has spread into the blood.

Serum sickness—A type of allergic reaction against blood proteins. Serum sickness develops when the immune system makes antibodies against proteins that are not normally found in the body.

Skin test—A test used to diagnose allergies.

T lymphocyte or T cell—A type of white blood cell. Helper T cells aid other cells of the immune system, while cytotoxic T cells destroy abnormal body cells, including those that have been infected by a virus.

Thrombocytopenia—Too few platelets in the blood.

Description

This drug suppresses the immune system by slowing down T cells, cells critical in immunity. Without them, the immune system is essentially paralyzed. Lymphocyte immune globulin contains antibodies that attach to T cells and prevent them from working properly. This drug also decreases the number of T cells in the blood.

Lymphocyte immune globulin is made by vaccinating an animal with immature human T cells, then collecting the antibodies made against them. Atgam is made in horses and Thymoglobulin in rabbits.

Atgam is labeled for use only in kidney transplantation and aplastic anemia, and Thymoglobulin is specifically approved only for kidney transplantation. The effectiveness of either drug for treating aplastic anemia in **cancer** patients, however, is unknown.

Lymphocyte immune globulin is often used off-label to treat **graft-versus-host disease** (GVHD) after bone marrow transplantation. The drug has been beneficial for GVHD patients in some studies, but its effectiveness has not been conclusively demonstrated. In some **clinical trials**, it is also being used to prepare the patient's body for bone marrow transplantation. This drug produces short partial remissions of some lymphomas in published experiments.

Recommended dosage

The usual dose of Atgam in adults is 10–30 mg/kg (1 kilogram is 2.2 pounds). Doses of 5–25 mg/kg have been given to a few children. Thymoglobulin, which is about 10 times stronger, has a recommended dose of 1–1.5 mg/kg in adults. Typically these drugs are given daily or every other day for several days or weeks. They are injected into the blood over several hours under close supervision in the hospital or clinic.

Precautions

Patients should not take Atgam if they are allergic to horse proteins or Thymoglobulin if they are allergic to rabbit proteins. Patients should tell their doctors about any current or previous blood cell problems and about all their prescription and over-the-counter drugs.

Lymphocyte immune globulin can make infections more serious. Patients should check with their doctors if they have any symptoms of an infection, such as chills, **fever**, or sore throat. They should also avoid people with contagious diseases and anyone recently vaccinated with an oral polio vaccine. The drug decreases the effectiveness of vaccinations given just before or during treatment. Some types of vaccines are not safe to receive while taking this drug.

Lymphocyte immune globulin does not interact with any specific foods. However, patients should check with their doctor for specific recommendations for eating and drinking before the treatment.

Patients should be careful in planning their activities, as this drug can cause dizziness.

Side effects

Thymoglobulin and Atgam have very similar side effects. However, Thymoglobulin is approximately twice as likely to decrease the number of white blood cells and three times as likely to result in malaise. Dizziness is much more common with Atgam. Other numerous side effects caused by both drugs include:

- chills or fever in most patients
- risk of developing an infection, which has been seen in up to 30% of patients, and sepsis in approximately 10%
- risk of bleeding, due to thrombocytopenia (seen in 30–45% of patients)
- rarely, anemia or the destruction of white blood cells other than T cells
- pain, swelling, and redness where the drug is injected (minimized by injecting the drug into the faster-moving blood in a large vein)
- allergic reactions (Serious allergic reactions can cause difficulty breathing, swelling of the tongue, a drop in blood pressure, or pain in the chest, sides, or back. Severe allergic reactions are potentially life-threatening, but rare; milder allergic reactions can result in itching, hives, or rash. Skin tests are often done to predict the likelihood of an allergic reaction, but are not foolproof.)
- serum sickness, an immune reaction against the drug (can result in fever, chills, muscle and joint aches, rash, blurred vision, swollen lymph nodes, or kidney problems; serum sickness is common when lymphocyte immune globulin is used alone for aplastic anemia, but fairly rare when it is combined with other drugs that suppress immunity.)
- headaches, pain in the abdomen, diarrhea, nausea or vomiting, fluid retention, weakness, rapid heartbeats, or an abnormal increase in blood potassium (These side effects develop in more than one-fifth of all patients during treatment.)
- uncommon side effects such as kidney damage, high blood pressure, heart failure, lethargy, abnormal sensations like prickling in the skin, seizures, pulmonary edema, and adult respiratory distress syndrome
- risk of developing lymphoma or leukemia, if the immune system is greatly suppressed for a long time

Side effects in pregnant or nursing women

The effects of this drug on an unborn child are unknown. Doctors are not sure whether this drug enters breast milk.

Methods of preventing or reducing side effects

Drugs such as antihistamines, acetaminophen, and **corticosteroids** can prevent or decrease some side effects, including fevers, chills, and allergic reactions. **Antibiotics** may help to prevent infections.

Interactions

Combining this drug with other medications that suppress the immune system (including **chemotherapy**) can severely suppress immunity. Drugs that slow blood clotting, such as aspirin, can increase the risk of bleeding. Any drug that reduces the symptoms of an infection, including aspirin and acetaminophen, can increase the risk that a serious infection will go undetected.

See also Myelosuppression; Immune response; Infection and sepsis; Neuropathy.

Resources

WEBSITES

University of Pittsburgh Medical Center (UPMC). "Lymphocyte Immune Globulin." http://www.upmc.com/patients-visitors/education/cancer-chemo/Pages/lymphocyte-immune-globulin.aspx (accessed December 4, 2014).

Anna Rovid Spickler, D.V.M., PhD.

Lymphoma

Definition

Lymphoma is the name of a diverse group of cancers of the lymphatic system, a connecting network of glands, organs and vessels whose principal cell is the lymphocyte.

Description

When lymphoma occurs, cells in the lymphatic system grow abnormally. They divide too rapidly and grow without any order or control. Too much tissue is formed and tumors begin to grow. Because there is lymph tissue in many parts of the body, the **cancer** cells may involve the liver, spleen, or bone marrow.

Two general types of lymphoma are commonly recognized: Hodgkin disease or **Hodgkin lymphoma** (HD), and **Non-Hodgkin lymphoma** (NHL). The two are distinguished by cell type. These differ significantly in respect of their natural histories and their response to therapy. Hodgkin lymphoma tends to be primarily of nodal origin. Non-Hodgkin lymphomas, unlike HD, can spread beyond the lymphatic system.

See also AIDS-related cancers.

Kate Kretschmann

Lymphoplasmacytic lymphoma *see*
Waldenström macroglobulinemia

Lysodren *see* **Mitotane**

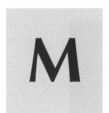

Magnetic resonance imaging

Definition

Magnetic resonance imaging (MRI) is a versatile medical imaging technology that uses strong magnets and pulses of radio waves to manipulate the natural magnetic properties of the body to produce highly refined images on the body's interior without surgery. MRI makes better images of organs and soft tissues than other scanning technologies. It is particularly useful for imaging the brain and spine, as well as the soft tissues of joints and the interior structure of bones. The entire body is visible to the technique, which poses few known health risks.

Purpose

MRI was developed in the 1980s. The latest additions to MRI technology are magnetic resonance **angiography** (MRA) and spectroscopy (MRS). MRA was developed to study blood flow, while MRS can identify the chemical composition of diseased tissue and produce color images of brain function. The many advantages of MRI include:

- Detail. MRI creates precise images of the body based on the varying proportions of magnetic elements in different tissues. Very minor fluctuations in chemical composition can be determined. MRI images have greater natural contrast than standard x-rays, computed tomography (CT) scans, or ultrasounds, all of which depend on the differing physical properties of tissues. This sensitivity lets MRI distinguish fine variations in tissues deep within the body. It is also particularly useful for spotting diseased tissues (tumors and other lesions) early in their development. Often, doctors prescribe an MRI scan to more fully investigate earlier findings of other imaging techniques.

- Scope. The entire body can be scanned, from head to toe and from the skin to the deepest recesses of the brain. Moreover, MRI scans are not obstructed by bone, gas, or body waste, which can hinder other imaging techniques. Nevertheless, MRI scans can be degraded by motion such as breathing, heartbeat, and normal bowel activity. The MRI process produces cross-sectional images of the body that are as sharp in the middle as on the edges, even of the brain through the skull. A close series of these two-dimensional images can provide a three-dimensional view of a targeted area.

- Safety. MRI does not depend on potentially harmful ionizing radiation, as do standard x-ray and CT scans. There are no known risks specific to the procedure, other than for people who might have metal objects (e.g., surgical screws, plates, unremoved shrapnel) in their bodies.

Doctors may prescribe an MRI scan for many different areas of the body, including:

- Brain and head. MRI technology was developed because of the need for brain imaging. It is one of the few imaging tools that can see through bone (the skull) and deliver high-quality pictures of the brain's delicate soft tissue structures. MRI may be needed for patients with symptoms of a brain tumor, stroke, or brain infection such as meningitis. MRI may also be used when cognitive and/or psychological symptoms suggest brain disease (e.g., Alzheimer's disease, Huntington's disease, multiple sclerosis), or when developmental delays suggest a birth defect. MRI can also provide pictures of the sinuses and other areas of the head beneath the face. Recent refinements in MRI technology may make this form of diagnostic imaging even more useful in evaluating patients with brain cancer, stroke, schizophrenia, or epilepsy. In particular, a new 3-D approach to MRI imaging known as diffusion tensor imaging (DTI) measures the flow of water within brain tissue, allowing the radiologist to tell where normal flow of fluid is disrupted and to distinguish more clearly between cancerous and normal brain tissue. The introduction of DTI has led to a technique known as fiber tracking, which allows the neurosurgeon

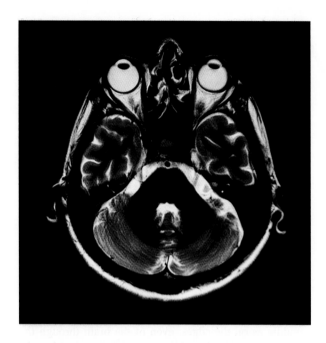

Magnetic resonance imaging (MRI) scan of the human brain. *(Mandritoiu/Shutterstock.com)*

to tell whether a space-occupying brain tumor has damaged or displaced the nerve pathways in the white matter of the brain. This information improves the surgeon's accuracy during the actual operation.

- Spine. Spinal problems can create a host of seemingly unrelated symptoms. MRIs are particularly useful for identifying and evaluating degenerated or herniated spinal discs. They can also be used to determine the condition of nerve tissue within the spinal cord.

- Joints. MRI scanning is most commonly used to diagnose and assess joint problems. MRI can provide clear images of the bone, cartilage, ligament, and tendon that make up a joint. MRI can be used to diagnose joint injuries due to sports, advancing age, or arthritis. MRI can also detect otherwise hidden tumors or infections within a joint and can be used to diagnose developmental joint abnormalities in children.

- Skeleton. The properties of MRI that allow it to see through the skull also allow it to view the inside of bones. It can be used to detect bone cancer, inspect bone marrow for leukemia and other diseases, assess bone loss (osteoporosis), and examine complex fractures.

- The rest of the body. While CT and ultrasound satisfy most chest, abdominal, and general body imaging needs, MRI scans may be needed in certain circumstances to provide better pictures or when repeated scanning is required. The progress of some therapies, such as liver cancer therapy, needs to be monitored, and

the effect of repeated x-ray exposure is a concern not encountered with MRI.

MRI is being used increasingly during operations, particularly those involving very small structures in the head and neck, as well as for preoperative assessment and planning. Intraoperative MRIs have been shown safe as well as feasible, and they improve the surgeon's ability to completely remove an entire tumor or other abnormality.

Description

In essence, MRI produces a map of hydrogen distribution in the body. Hydrogen is the simplest element known, is the most abundant element in biological tissue, and can be magnetized. It will align itself within a strong magnetic field, such as the needle of a compass. The earth's magnetic field is not strong enough to keep a person's hydrogen atoms pointing in the same direction, but the superconducting magnet of an MRI machine can. This makes up the "magnetic" part of an MRI.

Once a patient's hydrogen atoms have been aligned in the magnet, pulses of very specific radio wave frequencies are used to knock them back out of alignment. The hydrogen atoms alternately absorb and emit radio wave energy, vibrating back and forth between their resting (magnetized) state and their agitated (radio pulse) state. This is the "resonance" part of MRI.

The MRI equipment records the duration, strength, and source location of the signals emitted by the atoms as they relax and then translates the data into an image on a television monitor. The state of hydrogen in diseased tissue differs from healthy tissue of the same type, making MRI particularly good at identifying tumors and other lesions. In some cases, chemical agents such as gadolinium can be injected to improve the contrast between healthy and diseased tissue.

A single MRI exposure produces a two-dimensional image of a slice through the entire target area. A series of these image slices composes a virtual three-dimensional view of the area.

Magnetic resonance spectroscopy

Magnetic resonance spectroscopy (MRS) is different from MRI because MRS uses a continuous band of radio wave frequencies to excite hydrogen atoms in a variety of chemical compounds other than water. These compounds absorb and emit radio energy at characteristic frequencies, or spectra, that can be used to identify them. Generally, a color image is created by assigning a color to each distinctive spectral emission. This is the "spectroscopy" part of MRS. As of 2013, diagnostic MRS was available in only a limited number of research centers.

KEY TERMS

Angiography—Any of the different methods for investigating the condition of blood vessels, usually via a combination of radiological imaging and injections of chemical tracing and contrasting agents.

Diffusion tensor imaging (DTI)—A refinement of magnetic resonance imaging that allows the doctor to measure the flow of water and track the pathways of white matter in the brain. DTI is able to detect abnormalities in the brain that do not show up on standard MRI scans.

Gadolinium—A very rare metallic element useful for its sensitivity to electromagnetic resonance, among other things. Traces of it can be injected into the body to enhance the MRI pictures.

Hydrogen—The simplest, most common element known in the universe. It is composed of a single electron (negatively charged particle) circling a nucleus consisting of a single proton (positively charged particle). It is the nuclear proton of

hydrogen that makes MRI possible by reacting resonantly to radio waves while aligned in a magnetic field.

Ionizing radiation—Electromagnetic radiation that can damage living tissue by disrupting and destroying individual cells. All types of nuclear decay radiation (including x-rays) are potentially ionizing. Radio waves do not damage organic tissues they pass through.

Magnetic field—The three-dimensional area surrounding a magnet, in which its force is active. During MRI, the patient's body is permeated by the force field of a superconducting magnet.

Radio waves—Electromagnetic energy of the frequency range corresponding to that used in radio communications, usually 10,000–300 billion cycles per second. Radio waves are the same as visible light, x-rays, and all other types of electromagnetic radiation, but are of a higher frequency.

Doctors primarily use MRS to study the brain and related disorders, such as epilepsy, Alzheimer's disease, **brain tumors**, and the effects of drugs on brain growth and metabolism. The technique is also useful in evaluating metabolic disorders of the muscles and nervous system.

Magnetic resonance angiography

Magnetic resonance angiography (MRA) is another variation on standard MRI. MRA, like other types of angiography, looks specifically at fluid flow within the blood (vascular) system, but does so without the injection of dyes or radioactive tracers. Standard MRI cannot make a good picture of flowing blood, but MRA uses specific radio pulse sequences to capture usable signals. The technique is generally used in combination with MRI to obtain images that show both vascular structure and flow within the brain and head in cases of stroke, or when a blood clot or aneurysm is suspected.

MRI procedure

Regardless of the exact type of MRI planned, or area of the body targeted, the procedure involved is basically the same and takes place in a special MRI suite. The patient lies back on a narrow table and is made as comfortable as possible. Transmitters are positioned on the body and the cushioned table where the patient lies. The table then moves into a long tube that houses the

magnet. The tube is as long as an average adult lying down, and the tube is narrow and open at both ends. Once the area to be examined has been properly positioned, a radio pulse is applied. Then, a two-dimensional image corresponding to one slice through the area is made. The table then moves a fraction of an inch and the next image is made. Each image exposure takes several seconds and the entire exam will last anywhere from 30–90 minutes. During this time, the patient is not allowed to move. If the patient moves during the scan, the picture will not be clear.

Depending on the area to be imaged, the radio-wave transmitters are positioned in different locations.

• For the head and neck, a helmet similar to a hat is worn.

• For the spine, chest, and abdomen, the patient lies on the transmitters.

• For the knee, shoulder, or other joint, the transmitters are applied directly to the joint.

Additional probes monitor vital signs (e.g., pulse, respiration).

The MRI process is very noisy and confining. The patient hears a thumping sound for the duration of the procedure. Since the procedure is noisy, music supplied via earphones often is provided. Some patients become anxious or panic because they are in the small, enclosed tube. This is why vital signs are monitored. The patient and medical team also can communicate with each other.

If the chest or abdomen is to be imaged, the patient will be asked to hold his/her breath as each exposure is made. Other instructions may be given to the patient as needed. In many cases, the entire examination will be performed by an MRI operator who is not a doctor; however, the supervising radiologist should be available to consult as necessary during the exam, and will view and interpret the results some time later.

Given all its advantages, the MRI process is complex and costly. The process requires large, expensive, and complicated equipment; a highly trained operator; and a doctor specializing in radiology. Generally, MRI is prescribed only when serious symptoms and/or negative results from other tests indicate a need. Many times, another test is appropriate for the type of diagnosis needed.

Precautions

MRI scanning should not be used when there is the potential for an interaction between the strong MRI magnet and metal objects that might be embedded in a patient's body. The force of magnetic attraction on certain types of metal objects, including surgical steel, could move them within the body and cause serious injury. Metal may be embedded in a person's body for several reasons:

• People with implanted cardiac pacemakers, metal aneurysm clips, or who have had broken bones repaired with metal pins, screws, rods, or plates must tell their radiologist prior to having an MRI scan. In some cases (such as a metal rod in a reconstructed leg) the difficulty may be overcome.

• Patients must tell their doctors if they have bullet fragments or other metal pieces in their body from old wounds. The suspected presence of metal, whether from an old or recent wound, should be confirmed before scanning.

• People with significant work exposure to metal particles (e.g., working with a metal grinder) should discuss this with their doctor and radiologist. The patient may need pre-scan testing—usually a single x-ray of the eyes to see if any metal is present.

Chemical agents designed to improve the picture and/or allow for the imaging of blood or other fluid flow during MRA may be injected. In rare cases, patients may be allergic to or intolerant of these agents, and these patients should not receive them. If these chemical agents are to be used, patients should discuss any concerns they have with their doctor and radiologist.

The potential side effects of magnetic and electric fields on human health remain a source of debate. In particular, the possible effects on an unborn baby are not well known. Any woman who is or may be pregnant should carefully discuss this issue with her doctor and radiologist before undergoing a scan.

As with all medical imaging techniques, obesity greatly interferes with the quality of MRI.

Preparation

In some cases (such as for MRI brain scanning or an MRA), a chemical designed to increase image contrast may be given by the radiologist immediately before the exam. If a patient suffers from anxiety or claustrophobia, drugs may be given to help the patient relax.

The patient must remove all metal objects (watches, jewelry, eyeglasses, hair clips, etc.). Any magnetized objects (such as credit and bank machine cards, audio tapes, etc.) should be kept far away from the MRI equipment because they can be erased. Patients cannot bring their wallet or keys into the MRI machine. The patient may be asked to wear clothing without metal snaps, buckles, or zippers, unless a medical gown is worn during the procedure. The patient may be asked to remove any hair spray, hair gel, or cosmetics that may interfere with the scan.

Aftercare

No aftercare is necessary, unless the patient has received medication or had a reaction to a contrast agent. Normally, patients can immediately return to their daily activities. If the exam reveals a serious condition that requires more testing and/or treatment, appropriate information and counseling will be needed.

Risks

MRI poses no known health risks to the patient and produces no physical side effects. Again, the potential effects of MRI on an unborn baby are not well known. Any woman who is or may be pregnant, should carefully discuss this issue with her doctor and radiologist before undergoing a scan.

Results

A normal MRI, MRA, or MRS result is one that shows the patient's physical condition to fall within normal ranges for the target area scanned.

Abnormal results

Generally, MRI is prescribed only when serious symptoms and/or negative results from other tests indicate a need. There often exists strong evidence of a condition that the scan is designed to detect and assess.

QUESTIONS TO ASK YOUR DOCTOR

- Why am I having this MRI?
- Can I have an MRI if I am pregnant or breast-feeding?
- Will you be injecting a contrast medium for this MRI?
- Will I need someone to drive me home after the procedure or can I drive myself home?
- Will my insurance pay for this procedure?

Thus, the results will often be abnormal, confirming the earlier diagnosis. At that point, further testing and appropriate medical treatment is needed. For example, if the MRI indicates the presence of a brain tumor, an MRS may be prescribed to determine the type of tumor so that aggressive treatment can begin immediately without the need for a surgical **biopsy**.

Morbidity and mortality rates

Morbidity rates are minuscule. The most common problems are minor bleeding and bruising at the site of contrast injection. Since neither are reportable events, morbidity can only be estimated. Occasionally, an unknown allergy to seafood is discovered after injecting contrast. No deaths have been reported from MRI tests.

Alternatives

Alternatives to MRI include traditional **x-rays** and computed axial tomography (CT) scans. An alternative to traditional closed MRI is open MRI. In open MRI, the patient is positioned beneath the magnet, but the machine remains open on all four sides. This option is becoming more common and is helpful for patients who are claustrophobic or uncomfortable with closed MRI.

Resources

BOOKS
Westbrook, Catherine and Carolyn Kaut Roth. *MRI in Practice.* 4th ed. Malden, MA: Wiley-Blackwell, 2011.

WEBSITES
International Society for Magnetic Imaging in Medicine. "Information for Patients." http://www.ismrm.org/resources/information-for-patients (accessed October 3, 2014).

MedlinePlus. "MRI Scans." U.S. National Library of Medicine, National Institutes of Health. http://www.nlm.nih.gov/medlineplus/mriscans.html (accessed October 3, 2014).

Open MRI Centers. "What is an Open MRI?" http://open-mricenters.net/faq.php#faq_5 (accessed October 3, 2014).

U.S. Food and Drug Administration. "MRI (Magnetic Resonance Imaging)." http://www.fda.gov/Radiation-Emitting Products/RadiationEmittingProductsandProcedures/MedicalImaging/ucm200086.htm (accessed October 3, 2014).

ORGANIZATIONS
American College of Radiology, 1891 Preston White Dr., Reston, VA 20191, (703) 648-8900, info@acr.org, http://www.acr.org.

American Society of Radiologic Technologists (ASRT), 15000 Central Ave. SE, Albuquerque, NM 87123-3909, (505) 298-4500, (800) 444-2778, Fax: (505) 298-5063, memberservices@asrt.org, http://www.asrt.org.

International Society for Magnetic Resonance in Medicine, 2030 Addison St., 7th Fl., Berkeley, CA 94704, (510) 841-1899, Fax: (510) 841-2340, info@ismrm.org, http://www.ismrm.org.

Radiological Society of North America (RSNA), 820 Jorie Blvd, Oak Brook, IL 60523-2251, (630) 571-2670, (800) 381-6660, Fax: (630) 571-7837, http://www.rsna.org.

Kurt Richard Sternlof
L. Fleming Fallon, Jr., MD, DrPH
REVISED BY TISH DAVIDSON, AM

Male breast cancer

Definition

Male **breast cancer** is a malignant tumor that forms in a man's breast.

Description

Breast **cancer** is rare in men, but can be serious and fatal. Many people believe that only women can get breast cancer, but men have breast tissue that also can develop cancer. When men and women are born, they have a small amount of breast tissue with a few tubular passages called ducts located under the nipple and the area around the nipple (areola). By puberty, female sex hormones cause breast ducts to grow and milk glands to form at the ends of the ducts. But male hormones eventually prevent further breast tissue growth. Although male breast tissue still contains some ducts, it will have only a few or no lobules. Near the breasts of men and women are axillary lymph nodes. These are underarm small structures shaped like beans that collect cells from lymphatic vessels. Lymphatic vessels carry lymph, a clear fluid that contains fluid from tissues, cells from the immune system, and various waste products throughout the body. The axillary lymph nodes are important to breast cancer patients, as they play a role in the spread and staging of breast cancer.

Breast cancer is much more common in women, mostly because women have many more breast cells that can undergo cancerous changes and because women are exposed to the effects of female hormones.

Infiltrating ductal **carcinoma** is the most common type of breast cancer in men. It is a type of **adenocarcinoma**, or a cancer that occurs in glandular tissue. Infiltrating ductal carcinoma starts in a breast duct and spreads beyond the cells lining the ducts to other tissues in the breast. Once the cancer begins spreading into the breast, it can spread to other parts of the body. This distant spread is called **metastasis**. When breast cancer metastasizes to other areas of the body, it can cause serious, life-threatening consequences. For example, breast cancer might spread to the liver or lungs. About 80%–90% of all male breast cancers are infiltrating ductal carcinomas.

Ductal carcinoma in situ (DCIS) is not common; it accounts for about 10% of all male breast cancers. It also is an adenocarcinoma. In situ cancers remain in the immediate area where they began, so DCIS remains confined to the breast ducts and does not spread to the fatty tissues of the breast. This means that it is often found early. DCIS also may be called intraductal carcinoma.

Other types of breast cancer are very rare in men. Adenocarcinomas that are lobular (forming in the milk glands or lobules) only occur in about 2% of male breast cancer cases because men normally do not have milk gland tissues. Inflammatory breast cancer, a serious form of breast cancer in which the breast looks red and swollen and feels warm, also occurs rarely. Paget's disease of the nipple, a type of breast cancer that grows from the ducts beneath the nipple onto the nipple's surface, only accounts for about 1% of female breast cancers. Slightly more men have this form of breast cancer than women. Sometimes, Paget's disease is associated with another form of breast cancer. On rare occasions, men can develop basal cell carcinomas (BCCs) on the skin of the areola or the nipple itself. This type of cancer is usually found in elderly men with long histories of sun exposure; unfortunately, it is a very aggressive type of male breast cancer.

Although not a form of cancer, but a benign condition, gynecomastia is important to mention. It is the most common of all male breast disorders and can be associated with male breast cancer in a rare genetic condition called Klinefelter's syndrome. Men with Klinefelter's have one or more extra X chromosomes in

KEY TERMS

Areola—The pigmented area on the male or female breast that surrounds the nipple.

Axillary—Pertaining to the armpit. Axilla is the medical name for the armpit.

Brachytherapy—A form of radiation therapy in which small pellets of radioactive material are placed inside or near the area to be treated. It is also known as internal radiation therapy or sealed-source radiotherapy.

Gynecomastia—Benign enlargement of breast tissue in men. It may result from hormonal changes during puberty, the decline of testosterone production in older men, metabolic disorders, obesity, or Klinefelter's syndrome.

Klinefelter's syndrome—A genetic disorder in which a man has at least one extra X chromosome in addition to the normal XY karyotype. Some men with Klinefelter's may have three or even four X chromosomes. In addition to gynecomastia, men with Klinefelter's have smaller-than-normal testicles and are sterile.

Lymph node—One of a number of small, bean-shaped structures that run along the lymphatic system of vessels. The lymph nodes trap cancer cells, along with other cells and fluids.

Malignant—Causing worsening or death. Malignant tumors can invade other tissues and organs and spread to other areas of the body.

Orchiectomy—Surgical removal of the testicles. It is sometimes performed to lower androgen levels in patients with metastatic male breast cancer.

Targeted therapy—In cancer treatment, a type of drug therapy that blocks tumors by interfering with specific molecules that the cancer cells need for growth. Also called biologic therapy, targeted therapy is less harmful to normal cells than traditional chemotherapy.

addition to the normal XY sex chromosomes in a human male. Gynecomastia most often occurs in teenage boys when their hormones change during puberty. Older men also may experience the condition when their hormone balance changes as they age. Gynecomastia is an increase in the amount of breast tissue, or breast tissue enlargement. If a man has Klinefelter's syndrome, he can develop gynecomastia and an increased risk of breast cancer.

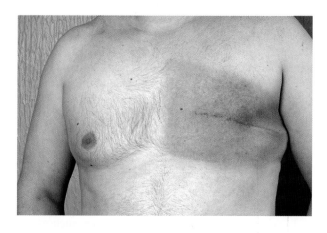

Breast cancer is more common in women but can occur in men. This man had his left breast removed after diagnosis of breast cancer. His skin is red due to burns from radiation therapy. *(Maria Platt-Evans/Science Source)*

Demographics

Breast cancer in men accounts for less than 1% of all breast cancers. Still, the American Cancer Society predicted that in 2014 about 2,360 American men were diagnosed with the disease and 430 men died. Although studies show the number of breast cancer cases in women has decreased in the United States and Europe since the 1960s, the number of breast cancer cases in men has remained stable since 1980.

Cancer of the male breast is rare in men younger than 35. The rate of increase in cases begins and steadily rises at age 50; the average age of patients with male breast cancer is between 60 and 70 years old, with a median age of 67 years (the average age for women is 63 years). Men often are diagnosed at a later stage than women; almost half of American men diagnosed with breast cancer are stage III or stage IV at the time of diagnosis.

Because cancer of the male breast is a comparatively rare malignancy, little is known as of 2014 as to whether race or ethnicity is a risk factor.

Causes and symptoms

Scientists do not know what causes most cases of male breast cancer; however, excellent progress is being made in genetic research and in understanding how genes instruct cells to grow, divide, and die. For example, researchers have now mapped all of the genes in the human body. Genes are part of the body's DNA, which is the chemical that instructs the cells. When DNA or genes carry defects (mutations), they activate changes in the cells, such as rapid cell division, that lead to cancer. Some genes, called tumor suppression genes, cause cells to die. Scientists have identified some genetic mutations

that are risk factors for breast cancer. In other cases, environmental, or outside, factors are thought to increase a man's risk of breast cancer.

Mutations in at least two versions of a tumor suppressor gene (**BRCA1 and BRCA2**) have been identified as causes of breast cancer in women. In men, the **BRCA2** mutation is considered responsible for about 15% of breast cancers. Men can inherit genes from either parent. Studies have shown that **BRCA1** also may increase a man's risk of breast cancer, but its role is less certain. These mutations have been shown to increase other cancers in men, including **prostate cancer**.

Several other factors also may cause male breast cancer. Some conditions, such as the liver disease cirrhosis, can cause an imbalance in a man's hormones, producing high levels of the female hormone estrogen, which can lead to breast cancer. Heavy drinking increases a man's risk of developing cirrhosis. Exposure to some substances, such as high amounts of radiation, may contribute to male breast cancer. Men who have been treated with estrogen as therapy for prostate cancer or who have taken estrogen prior to sex reassignment surgery have an increased risk of breast cancer, as do obese men. Obesity is a risk factor because fat cells in the body change androgens (male sex hormones) into estrogen. In addition, a **National Cancer Institute** study reported in 2014 that diabetes is also an independent risk factor for male breast cancer. Finally, injuries to the testicles, inflammation of the testicles due to mumps, or undescended testicles also increase a man's risk of breast cancer.

Many men do not realize they can develop breast cancer; they ignore the symptoms. The most common symptom is a mass, or lump in the chest area, particularly around the nipple. The lump will be firm, not tender or painful. Other signs that may warn of male breast cancer include:

• Skin dimpling or puckering

• Changes in the nipple, such as drawing inward (retraction)

• Nipple discharge of any kind

• Redness or scaling of the nipple or breast skin

• Abnormal swelling (or lump) of the breast, nipple, or chest muscle

• Prolonged rash or irritation of the nipple that may indicate Paget's disease

Diagnosis

Physicians follow the same steps for diagnosing breast cancer in men as in women, except that routine screening of breast cancer is not done in men. Once symptoms are noticed, however, physicians will proceed in the same way. The physician will conduct a thorough medical history and examination, including questions that may identify risk factors for breast cancer, such as male or female relatives with the disease. The medical history also helps gather details on possible symptoms for breast cancer.

The physician also performs a clinical breast examination. This helps the doctor locate and study a lump or suspicious area. The physician will feel (palpate) a mass to get an idea of its size, texture, likely location and relation to surrounding skin, muscles, and tissues. At this point, the physician will begin to look for signs that the cancer may have spread to other organs and to the lymph nodes. The physician will palpate lymph nodes and the liver, for instance, to see if they are enlarged.

The next step in diagnosis is usually a diagnostic mammogram. **Mammography** is an x-ray of the breast. Mammograms are performed by radiologic technologists who take special training in the procedure. Mammograms are evaluated by radiologists, physicians who receive medical training specifically in interpreting **x-rays**. If the initial mammogram shows suspicious findings, the radiologist may order magnification views to look more closely at the suspicious area. Mammograms can accurately show the tissue in the breast, even more so in men than women, because men do not have dense breasts or benign cysts in their breasts that interfere with the diagnosis.

The radiologist might also recommend an ultrasound to follow up on suspicious findings. Ultrasound is often used to image the breasts. Also known as sonography, the technique uses high-frequency sound waves to take pictures of organs and functions in the body. Sound wave echoes can be converted by computer to an image and displayed on a computer screen. Ultrasound does not use radiation. A technologist will perform the ultrasound and it will then be evaluated by the radiologist.

Biopsies, which involve removing a sample of tissue, are the only definite way to tell whether a mass is cancerous. At one time, surgical biopsies were the only option, requiring removal of all or a large portion of the lump in a complicated procedure. Today, fine-needle aspiration **biopsy** (FNAB) and core biopsies can be performed. In fine-needle aspiration biopsy, a thin needle is inserted to withdraw fluid from the mass. The physician may use ultrasound or other imaging guidance to locate the mass if necessary. The fluid is tested in a laboratory under a special microscope to determine whether it is cancerous.

A core biopsy is similar, but involves removing a small cylinder of tissue from the mass through a slightly larger needle. Core biopsy may require local anesthesia.

These biopsy techniques can usually be performed in a physician office or outpatient facility. The cells in biopsy samples help physicians determine if the lump is cancerous and the type of breast cancer. A tissue sample may also be used for assigning a grade to the cancer and to test for certain proteins and receptors that aid in treatment and prognosis decisions.

If there is discharge from the nipple, the fluid may also be collected and analyzed in a laboratory to see if cancer cells are present in the fluid.

Diagnosis of breast cancer spread may require additional tests. For example, a **computed tomography** (CT) scan may be ordered to check organs such as the liver or kidney for possible metastasized cancer. A chest x-ray can initially check for cancer spread to the lungs. Bone scans are nuclear medicine procedures that look for areas of diseased bone. **Magnetic resonance imaging** (MRI) has been increasingly used in recent years as a follow-up study to mammograms when findings are not clear. For metastatic breast cancer, however, an MRI is more likely to be ordered to check for cancer in the brain and spinal cord. **Positron emission tomography** (PET) scans also have become more common in recent years.

Clinical staging

After cancer has been definitively diagnosed, the next step is staging. Staging helps clarify details about the tumor, the adjacent and distant lymph nodes that may be affected, and the adjacent and distant organs that may be affected. This information helps determine what type of treatment is most appropriate.

The first step in staging may utilize a technique called **sentinel lymph node biopsy**. The sentinel node is the first one the cancer cells are likely to reach, so it is the first one checked for cancerous cells. Using a radioactive substance and blue dye injected into the area around the tumor, physicians can track the path of the cells and stage the cancer. This technique has been used for many years on women with breast cancer.

Cancer staging systems help physicians compare treatments and research and identify patients for **clinical trials**. Most of all, they help physicians determine treatment and prognosis for individual patients by describing how severe a patient's cancer is in relation to the primary tumor. The most common system used for cancer is the **American Joint Committee on Cancer** (AJCC) TNM system, which bases staging largely on the spread of the cancer. T stands for tumor and describes the tumor's size and spread locally, or within the breast and to nearby organs. The letter N stands for lymph nodes and describes the cancer's possible spread to and within the lymph node system. In some descriptions below, the cancer may have been found by sentinel node biopsy as microscopic disease in nodes that are in the breasts (rather than the armpits). For simplification, these findings have been grouped with the axillary lymph nodes. M stands for metastasis to note if the cancer has spread to distant organs. Further letters and numbers may follow these three letters to describe the number of lymph nodes involved, approximate tumor sizes, or other information. The following is a summary of breast cancer stages:

Stage 0: Tis, N0, M0: Ductal carcinoma in situ (DCIS). This is the earliest and least invasive form of breast cancer; the cancer cells are located within a duct and have not invaded surrounding fatty tissue.

Stage I: T1, N0, M0: The tumor is less than 0.75 in. in diameter (2 cm or less) and has not spread to lymph nodes or distant organs.

Stage IIA: T0, N1, M0/T2, N0, M0: No tumor is found; or the tumor is smaller than 0.75 in. (2 cm) and cancer is found in one to three axillary lymph nodes (even if no tumor is found); or the tumor is 0.75–2 in. (2–5 cm) in diameter but has not spread to the axillary lymph nodes. The cancer has not spread to distant organs.

Stage IIIB: T2, N1, M0/T3, N0, M0: The tumor is 0.75–2 in. (2–5 cm) in diameter and has spread to one to three axillary lymph nodes; or the tumor is larger than 2 in. (5 cm) has not grown into the chest wall or spread to the lymph nodes or distant organs.

Stage IIIA: T0-2, N2, M0/T3, N1, M0: The tumor is smaller than 2 in. (5 cm) in diameter and has spread to four to nine axillary lymph nodes; or the tumor is larger than 2 in. (5 cm) and has spread to one to nine axillary lymph nodes. The cancer has not spread to distant organs.

Stage IIIB: T4, N0-2, M0: The tumor has grown into the chest wall or the skin and may have spread to no lymph nodes or as many as nine lymph nodes. Cancer has not spread to distant sites.

Stage IIIC: T0-4, N3, M0: The tumor is any size, has spread to ten or more axillary lymph nodes or to one or more lymph nodes under or above the collarbone (clavicle) on the same side as the breast tumor. The cancer has not spread to distant organs.

Inflammatory breast cancer: Classified as stage III, unless it has spread to distant organs or lymph nodes not near the breast (which would classify it as Stage IV).

Stage IV: T0-4, N0-3, M1: Regardless of the tumor's size, the cancer has spread to such distant organs as the liver, bones, or lungs, or to lymph nodes far from the breast.

Treatment

If the axillary lymph nodes were identified as containing cancer at the time of the sentinel **lymph node biopsy**, they will be removed in an **axillary dissection**. Sometimes, this is done at the time of the biopsy.

For stage I, surgery often is the only treatment needed for men. Women often have lumpectomies, which remove as little surrounding breast tissue as possible, to preserve some of their breast shape. For men, this is less of a concern, and **mastectomy**, or surgical removal of the breast, is performed in 80% of all male breast cancers. Although lumpectomies are being performed more frequently in men, they do not appear to affect the rate of survival. Men with stage I tumors larger than 0.4 in. (1 cm) may receive additional (adjuvant) **chemotherapy**.

Men with stage II breast cancer also usually receive a mastectomy. If they have cancer in the lymph nodes, they probably will receive adjuvant therapy. Those with estrogen receptor-positive tumors (about 85% of male breast cancers) may receive hormone therapy with **tamoxifen**, a drug that blocks the estrogen receptor. If the cancer does not respond to tamoxifen, other anti-estrogen drugs like **toremifene** or fulvestrant may be tried. Other forms of hormone therapy for male breast cancer target androgens (male sex hormones), because most male breast cancers contain androgen receptors that cause the cancers to grow. Drugs that block androgen receptors include flutamide and bicalutamide. A surgical procedure that may be performed to lower the patient's androgen levels is **orchiectomy**, or surgical removal of the testicles, but this procedure is performed less frequently because of the availability of anti-androgen medications. Orchiectomy is most likely to be performed in patients with metastatic cancer of the male breast.

A newer form of drug therapy that may be given to stage II male breast cancer patients is targeted therapy (sometimes called biologic therapy), which blocks the growth of cancer cells by targeting specific molecules that the cancer cells need for growth and reproduction. Some male breast cancer cells carry a protein called HER2/neu on their surfaces that promote tumor growth. Drugs that target this protein include **trastuzumab**, pertuzumab, **ado-trastuzumab emtansine**, and **lapatinib**.

The treatment team may recommend adjuvant **radiation therapy** if the cancer has spread to nearby lymph nodes and/or to the skin. Radiation therapy is usually given to men in the form of external beam radiation therapy, although in some cases male breast cancer patients are treated with brachytherapy, a form of

QUESTIONS TO ASK YOUR DOCTOR

- What kinds of diagnostic studies will be required to ascertain the type and spread of this tumor?

- How far has my cancer advanced; what stage is it in?

- Could there be a genetic component to this tumor? Should other family members be tested?

- What types of treatments are available?

- What types of side effects from treatments can I expect? What are your recommendations to help me deal with those side effects?

- Am I eligible for any clinical trials? Would these be helpful to consider?

- Are there any lifestyle changes that I should make?

- How often should I be checked after treatment has ended?

- Is there a support group that I can join to hear about other people's experiences with this disease?

internal radiation therapy in which a catheter is inserted into the breast and small pellets containing radiative materials are placed in the catheter.

Stage III breast cancer requires mastectomy followed by adjuvant therapy with tamoxifen when hormones are involved. Most patients with stage III disease also will require chemotherapy and radiation therapy to the chest wall.

Men with stage IV breast cancer will require systemic therapy, or chemotherapy and perhaps hormonal therapy that works throughout the body to fight the cancer in the breast, as well as the cancer cells that have spread. Patients also may receive **immunotherapy** to help them fight infection following chemotherapy. Radiation and surgery may also be used to relieve symptoms of the primary cancer and areas where the cancer may have spread. The treatment team also may have to diagnose specific treatments for the metastatic cancers, depending on their sites.

If male breast cancer recurs in the breast or chest wall, it can be treated with surgical removal and followed by radiation therapy. An exception is recurrence in the same area, where additional radiation therapy can damage normal tissue. Recurrence of the cancer in distant sites is treated the same as metastases found at the time of diagnosis.

Alternative and complementary therapies

Many alternative and complementary therapies can help cancer patients relax and deal with pain, though none to date have been shown to treat or prevent male breast cancer. For example, traditional Chinese medicine offers therapies that stress the importance of balancing energy forces. Many studies also show that guided imagery, prayer, meditation, laughter, and a positive approach to cancer can help promote healing. Early studies have shown that soy and flaxseed may have some preventive properties for breast cancer; however, these trials have been conducted in women. When looking for these therapies, cancer support groups suggest asking for credible referrals and working with the medical treatment team to coordinate alternative and complementary care.

Prognosis

The prognosis of male breast cancer varies, depending on stage. Generally, prognosis is poorer for men than for women, because men tend to show up for diagnosis when their breast cancer has reached a later stage. The average five-year survival rate for stage I cancers is almost 100% as of 2014. For stage II, it is 91%. Stage III cancers carry an average five-year survival rate of 72%, and by stage IV, the rate drops to 20%.

Coping with cancer treatment

It is difficult for some men to accept and cope with a breast cancer diagnosis, since it is a relatively rare and unexpected disease for males. It is important that men work closely with their treatment team to talk about their concerns and to carefully follow all instructions for care. Support groups and family support are critical in coping with a breast cancer diagnosis.

Eating a nutritious diet, stopping the use of tobacco, and limiting the use of alcohol can help in recovery from breast cancer. Beginning a regular exercise program when the treatment team recommends also helps.

Clinical trials

Research was underway as of 2014 to test various targeted therapies and chemotherapy combinations for male breast cancer at different stages. Several clinical trials are also underway to investigate a vaccine for treating patients with metastatic breast cancer. The National Institutes of Health lists clinical trials by disease type, including those for which they are recruiting patients; there are 121 open studies for patients with male breast cancer as of mid-2014. Choosing to participate in a clinical trial is a decision that involves the patient, family, and treatment team.

Prevention

Some forms of male breast cancer cannot be prevented, but detecting the cancer at an early stage can prevent such serious complications as spread to distant organs. Men who have a history of breast cancer in their family should pay particular attention to the symptoms of breast cancer and seek immediate medical evaluation. Physicians may be able to test the blood of men with a family history for the presence of the *BRCA2* gene so they may more carefully watch for early signs of breast cancer. Avoiding exposure to radiation also may help prevent some male breast cancers. Other preventive measures include avoiding heavy drinking and keeping one's weight within the accepted guidelines for one's height.

Special concerns

Although more men are willing to see a doctor for a checkup about a breast abnormality (whether benign or malignant) than in the past, a 2014 study of 78 men assessed for disorders of the male breast found that the majority reported feelings of **depression**, anxiety, loss of masculinity, and embarrassment about their condition, even when the findings were benign. The authors suggest that men might benefit from breast assessment services tailored to their needs rather than being referred to services designed for women.

Resources

BOOKS

Foulkes, William D., and Kathleen A. Cooney, eds. *Male Reproductive Cancers: Epidemiology, Pathology and Genetics.* New York: Springer, 2010.

Johns, Alan, MD *The Lump: A Gynecologist's Journey with Male Breast Cancer.* Austin, TX: Live Oak Book Company, 2011.

Spar, Myles D., and George E. Muñoz, eds. *Integrative Men's Health.* New York: Oxford University Press, 2014.

PERIODICALS

Brinton, L. A., et al. "Anthropometric and Hormonal Risk Factors for Male Breast Cancer: Male Breast Cancer Pooling Project Results." *Journal of the National Cancer Institute* 106 (March 2014): djt465.

Cloyd, J. M., T. Hernandez-Boussard, and I. L. Wapnir. "Outcomes of Partial Mastectomy in Male Breast Cancer Patients: Analysis of SEER, 1983–2009." *Annals of Surgical Oncology* 20 (May 2013): 1545–1550.

Fields, E. C., et al. "Management of Male Breast Cancer in the United States: A Surveillance, Epidemiology and End Results Analysis." *International Journal of Radiation Oncology, Biology, Physics* 87 (November 15, 2013): 747–752.

Kalyani, R., et al. "Pigmented Basal Cell Carcinoma of Nipple and Areola in a Male Breast: A Case Report with Review of Literature." *International Journal of Biomedical Science* 10 (March 2014): 69–72.

Kipling, M., et al. "Psychological Impact of Male Breast Disorders: Literature Review and Survey Results." *Breast Care (Basel)* 9 (February 2014): 29–33.

Patten, D. K., L. K. Sharifi, and M. Fazel. "New Approaches in the Management of Male Breast Cancer." *Clinical Breast Cancer* 13 (October 2013): 309–314.

Zagouri, F., et al. "Fulvestrant and Male Breast Cancer: A Case Series." *Annals of Oncology* 24 (January 2013): 265–266.

OTHER

American Cancer Society (ACS). "Breast Cancer in Men." http://www.cancer.org/acs/groups/cid/documents/webcontent/003091-pdf.pdf (accessed August 10, 2014).

WEBSITES

National Cancer Institute (NCI). "Male Breast Cancer Treatment (PDQ)." http://www.cancer.gov/cancertopics/pdq/treatment/malebreast/HealthProfessional/page1/AllPages#1 (accessed August 10, 2014).

Susan G. Komen. "Breast Cancer in Men." http://ww5.komen.org/BreastCancer/BreastCancerinMen.html (accessed August 10, 2014).

WebMD. "Breast Cancer in Men." http://www.webmd.com/breast-cancer/guide/breast-cancer-men (accessed August 10, 2014).

ORGANIZATIONS

American Cancer Society (ACS), 250 Williams Street NW, Atlanta, GA 30303, (800) 227-2345, http://www.cancer.org/aboutus/howwehelpyou/app/contact-us.aspx, http://www.cancer.org/index.

National Cancer Institute (NCI), BG 9609 MSC 9760, 9609 Medical Center Drive, Bethesda, MD 20892-9760, (800) 4-CANCER (422-6237), http://www.cancer.gov/global/contact/email-us, http://www.cancer.gov/.

Office of Cancer Complementary and Alternative Medicine (OCCAM), 9609 Medical Center Dr., Room 5-W-136, Rockville, MD 20850, (240) 276-6595, Fax: (240) 276-7888, ncioccam1-r@mail.nih.gov, http://cam.cancer.gov/.

Susan G. Komen, 5005 LBJ Freeway, Suite 250, Dallas, TX 75244, (877) 465-6636, http://ww5.komen.org/.

Teresa G. Odle
REVISED BY REBECCA J. FREY, PHD

Malignant fibrous histiocytoma

Definition

Malignant fibrous histiocytoma (MFH), although rare, is the most common abnormal growth of soft tissue (**sarcoma**) in adults.

Description

MFH occurs as a painless mass most commonly in the skin, arms, legs, kidneys, or the pancreas. More rarely MFH may occur in the bones, heart, breasts, or inside the skull.

When MFHs spread (metastasize) to other organs, the most common site is the lung, but **metastasis** to local lymph nodes and to bone have also been reported.

MFHs tend to be slow growing and slow to metastasize.

Local recurrence of MFH after surgery to remove the initial tumor is common because MFHs grow along the fat layers that separate different layers of soft tissue. Often, an MFH is not completely removed because it has crossed, undetected, from one fat layer to another neighboring layer.

Demographics

MFHs are diagnosed in six of every one million people each year. MFHs can occur in people of any age, but they are extremely rare in children.

MFHs occur in a slightly higher frequency in Caucasians than in people of African descent or Asians. No relationship of MFHs appear to exist to any geographic region. Males are affected in slightly higher numbers than are females.

MFHs of the skin are seen almost exclusively in sun-exposed areas of the skin in elderly patients.

People affected with certain genetic diseases, such as neurofibromatosis, have a higher incidence of MFHs than unaffected people.

MFHs of the bone are seen almost exclusively in people who have a pre-existing skeletal disorder such as Paget disease or fibrous dysplasia of bone.

Causes and symptoms

The cause, or causes, of MFHs are not known. An elevated risk for the development of MFHs has been linked to the chemical phenoxyacetic acid found in herbicides; to chlorophenols found in wood preservatives; and to exposure to asbestos. People who have been exposed to high doses of radiation are also more prone to develop MFHs than the remainder of the population. Research is ongoing to determine if there is a genetic cause of MFHs.

The only direct symptom of MFHs is the presence of an abnormal mass, but some patients may also experience:

• abnormally high levels of a certain type of white blood cells (eosinophils) in the blood

• low blood sugar (hypoglycemia)

• fever

• abnormal liver function tests

Diagnosis

Prior to removal, MFHs are extremely difficult to distinguish from the other forms of **soft tissue sarcoma**. The definitive diagnosis of MFH usually occurs after a tumor has been surgically removed. This diagnosis is accomplished by conducting microscopic examinations on the tumor.

Treatment team

Treatment for MFHs is mostly surgical or observational. Surgeries to remove MFHs are generally performed by orthopedic surgeons. MFHs rarely require any chemotherapies or radiation therapies, however, when these treatments are called for they are directed by a medical oncologist and administered by health care personnel who specialize in these fields.

Clinical staging

MFHs are divided into three grades based on the appearance of the tissue within the tumor. Low grade tumors may closely resemble the surrounding normal tissue. Intermediate and high grade tumors may have little resemblance to normal tissue.

Additionally, MFHs are divided into two clinical stages based on size. Stage one MFHs are those tumors that are under 5 cm (2 in) in diameter. Stage two MFHs are those tumors larger than 5 cm (2 in) in diameter.

Treatment

A treatment plan is determined after the grade and stage of the tumor has been established. High and intermediate grade tumors generally, regardless of the stage, are surgically removed. Low grade, stage one, tumors may be observed for development to a higher grade or stage rather than removed if it is determined that the risks of anesthetic and surgery outweigh the risk of the tumor to the individual patient.

Stage one MFHs are generally removed by wide local excision. This technique involves the surgical removal of the tumor and an area of healthy surrounding tissue that is approximately the same size as the tumor itself.

Stage two MFHs require wide surgical excision with the removal of wider margins of healthy tissue than those margins removed in the excision of smaller tumors. In some instances, stage two MFHs may require **amputation**.

Post-operative treatment of MFH patients may include **chemotherapy** or **radiation therapy**, especially in cases of MFH of the bones and in cases of metastasis to the lungs.

In cases of large MFHs, the patient may undergo radiation treatments prior to surgery in an attempt to shrink the size of the tumor prior to excision.

Alternative and complementary therapies

There are no effective alternative treatments for MFHs other than surgical removal with or without chemotherapy or radiation treatments.

Prognosis

Overall survival from MFH is approximately 75% five-year disease-free survival. The prognosis is generally poorer if:

• the disease has metastasized to the lungs or bones
• complete tumor removal is not accomplished, or is not possible
• the patient is of an advanced age
• the tumor is large
• the location of the tumor is somewhere other than the arms or legs
• the tumor is located deep in the body, rather than superficially

Coping with cancer treatment

Most patients who undergo wide local excision to remove their tumors can resume their normal activities within a few days of the operation.

The loss of a limb may produce feelings of grief that are similar to that felt upon the death of a spouse or close family member. Patients who must undergo amputation to remove their **cancer** may require extended psychological care to help them to deal with this grief and to

---

QUESTIONS TO ASK YOUR DOCTOR

• Which type of MFH do I have?
• What is the size of my tumor?
• Will I require chemotherapy or radiation treatments to shrink my tumor prior to its removal?
• What is the likelihood of my type of MFH coming back?
• How often should I seek follow-up examinations?

---

help them develop a new, healthy, **body image**. These patients may also require extended **physical therapy** to learn to operate without the missing limb or to learn to use a prosthetic device.

Clinical trials

There were 21 **clinical trials** underway in late 2014 aimed at the treatment of MFHs and other soft tissue sarcomas. More information on these trials, including contact information, may be found by conducting a clinical trial search at the website of the **National Cancer Institute**: http://www.cancer.gov/clinicaltrials/search.

Prevention

Because the causes of MFHs are not known, there is no known prevention.

Special concerns

Repeat surgery may be necessary for MFHs because these tumors sometimes redevelop. Careful monitoring by the medical team will be required.

Resources

BOOKS
Brennan, Murry F., Cristina R. Antonescu, and Robert G. Maki. *Management of Soft Tissue Sarcoma*. New York: Springer, 2013.

WEBSITES
Dana-Farber Cancer Institute. "Malignant Fibrous Histiocytoma." http://www.dana-farber.org/Pediatric-Care/Treatment-and-Support/Malignant-Fibrous-Histiocytoma.aspx (accessed October 31, 2014).
National Cancer Institute. "General Information About Osteosarcoma and Malignant Fibrous Histiocytoma (MFH) of Bone." http://www.cancer.gov/cancertopics/pdq/treatment/osteosarcoma/HealthProfessional (accessed October 31, 2014).

ORGANIZATIONS

Sarcoma Alliance, 775 East Blithedale #334, Mill Valley, CA 94941, (415) 381-7236, Fax: (415) 381-7235, info@sarcomaalliance.org, http://sarcomaalliance.org.

Paul A. Johnson, EdM

Malignant melanoma *see* **Melanoma**

MALT lymphoma

Definition

MALT lymphomas are solid tumors that originate from cancerous growth of immune cells that are recruited to secretory tissue such as the gastrointestinal tract, salivary glands, lungs, and the thyroid gland.

Description

The digestive tract is generally not associated with lymphoid tissue, with the exception of small collections of lymphocytes such as Peyer's patches. A specific kind of white blood cell, B-lymphocytes, can accumulate in response to infections of the digestive tract and other secretory tissues, or as a result of autoimmune conditions such as Sjögren's syndrome. When the growth of these lymphocytes is maintained through continued infection or autoimmune disease, a malignant cell can arise and replace the normal lymphocytes. These lymphomas, derived from mucosa-associated lymphoid tissue (MALT), most commonly arise in the stomach. Their growth seems to be dependent upon continuous stimulation of the immune system by an infectious agent, such as *H. pylori*, or some other entity, termed an antigen, that the body recognizes as foreign. This antigen-driven growth permits these tumors to be treated by eliminating the stimulus that generated the original, normal **immune response**. In the stomach they are associated, in greater than 90% of all cases, with the bacteria called Helicobacter pylori (*H. pylori*). This bacteria is also associated with peptic stomach irritation, ulcers, and gastric **cancer**. MALT lymphomas are generally indolent, that is, they grow slowly and cause little in the way of symptoms. Those MALT lymphomas that arise in the stomach in response to *H. pylori* infections are generally successfully treated with **antibiotics**, which eliminate the bacteria.

Demographics

MALT lymphomas occur at a frequency of about 1.5 per 100,000 people per year in the United States and account for about 10% of all non-Hodgkin lymphomas. The frequency varies among different populations. For example, in parts of Italy the frequency of MALT lymphomas is as high as 13 per 100,000 people per year. This can in part be attributed to different rates of infection with *H. pylori*; however, other hereditary, dietary, or environmental factors are almost certainly involved.

Causes and symptoms

The majority of MALT lymphomas appear to be the result of infectious agents, most commonly *H. pylori* in the stomach. It is not known if infectious agents also cause MALT lymphomas outside of the stomach. In some cases, such as in the thyroid, MALT lymphomas seem to arise in patients who have autoimmune diseases, which make their immune systems treat their own tissue as foreign or antigenic. It is believed that there must be additional factors, in addition to infection or autoimmunity, that influence the development of MALT lymphomas. For example, in the United States, where infections with *H. pylori* are quite common, less than one in 30,000 people who have *H. pylori* in their stomachs develop MALT lymphomas. In addition, individuals who develop MALT lymphomas are more likely to develop other forms of cancer. This would suggest that there might be genetic factors predisposing individuals to develop MALT lymphomas or other tumors in response to environmental or infectious agents.

In general, patients have stomach pain, ulcers, or other localized symptoms, but rarely do they suffer from systemic complaints such as **fatigue** or **fever**.

Diagnosis

The indolent nature of most MALT lymphomas means that the majority of patients are diagnosed at early stages with relatively nonspecific symptoms. In the case of gastric MALT lymphomas, the physician will then have a gastroenterologist perform an endoscopy to examine the interior of the stomach. MALT lymphomas are then recognized as areas of inflammation or ulceration within the stomach. It is unusual for masses recognizable as tumors to be seen upon examination. Definitive diagnosis of MALT **lymphoma** requires a **biopsy**, in which a bit of tissue is removed from the stomach or other involved site. Examination of this tissue by a pathologist is the first step in distinguishing among the possible diagnoses of inflammation, indolent lymphoma, or a more aggressive form of cancer, such as gastric cancer or a rapidly growing **non-Hodgkin lymphoma**. The pathologist evaluates the type of lymphoid cells that are present in the biopsy to establish the nature of the lesion. In addition, it is essential that the pathologist determine whether or not the lymphoma has grown beyond the borders of the mucosa, which lines the stomach or other gland.

Treatment

The best staging system to employ for MALT lymphomas is still the subject of discussion. It is standard practice that patients presenting with MALT lymphomas should be evaluated in a similar manner to individuals with nodal lymphomas, the more common type of lymphoma that originates at sites within the lymphoid system. These procedures include a complete history and physical, blood tests, chest x-rays, and **bone marrow biopsy**. This evaluation will permit the oncologist to determine if the disease is localized or if it has spread to other sites within the body.

In general, the prognosis for patients with MALT lymphomas is good, with overall five-year survival rates that are greater than 80%. The features that are most closely related to the outlook for newly diagnosed individual patients are: whether the **primary site** is in the stomach or is extra-gastric; if the disease has spread beyond the initial location; and whether the histologic evaluation of the initial tumor biopsies is consistent with a low-grade, slowly growing lesion, as compared to a high-grade lesion that is more rapidly growing. In general, the histologic grade is the most important feature, with high-grade lesions requiring the most aggressive treatment.

Treatment of MALT lymphomas differs from that of most lymphomas. In the most common type of MALT lymphomas—low-grade lesions originating in the stomach—treatment with antibiotics to eliminate *H. pylori* leads to complete remissions in the majority of patients. The effectiveness of this treatment is indistinguishable from surgery, **chemotherapy**, **radiation therapy**, or a combination of surgery with drugs or irradiation. Approximately one-third of patients in this group have evidence of disseminated disease, where lymphoma cells are detected at sites in addition to the gastric mucosa. The response of these patients to antibiotic treatment is not significantly different from that for individuals with localized disease. For both groups a complete remission is achieved in about 75% of patients, who remain, on average, free of disease for about 5 years.

Clinical trials are underway and mostly concentrate upon optimizing treatment of gastric MALT lymphomas that involve *H. pylori*. The aspects of treatment being addressed are the most effective antibiotics and the use of antacids to modulate irritation in the stomach. These protocols have been designed to follow the natural

QUESTIONS TO ASK YOUR DOCTOR

- What kinds of diagnostic studies will be required to ascertain the type and spread of this tumor?
- Could there be a genetic component to this tumor? Should other family members be tested?
- What types of treatments are available?
- What types of side effects from treatments can I expect? What are your recommendations to help me deal with those side effects?
- Am I eligible for any clinical trials? Would these be helpful to consider?
- Are there any lifestyle changes that I should make?
- What type of diet should I follow? Are there foods I should avoid?
- Should I avoid any medications?
- How often should I be checked after treatment has ended?
- Is there a support group that I can join to hear about other people's experiences with this disease?

history of gastric lymphomas and to establish the biological features that predict treatment response to antibiotics and duration of remission.

Prognosis

Patients with MALT lymphomas arising outside of the digestive tract also have good prognoses. Effective treatment for these lymphomas has been achieved with local radiation, chemotherapy, and/or interferon. Surgery followed by chemotherapy or radiation is also effective with nongastrointestinal MALT lymphomas. Overall these patients have five-year survival rates greater than 90%.

While the outlook for patients with MALT lymphomas is good, difficulties in diagnosis and staging have left the optimal treatment a matter of continued study. This is an especially open question for those patients who fail to respond to antibiotic therapy, or whose disease recurs. It may be the case that in these patients, the MALT lymphoma may have already progressed to a point where high-grade lesions, not observed in the original biopsies, were resistant to the initial treatment. The best treatment for these patients remains to be established. In general, these patients are treated with chemotherapy in a similar manner to patients with other types of lymphoma. Given the success of antibiotics, and the good prognosis for gastric MALT lymphomas in general, no sufficient body of evidence exists to determine the best chemotherapy for patients who fail to achieve a complete and lasting remission upon initial treatment. At present, a chemotherapeutic regime designated CHOP includes the anti-cancer drugs **cyclophosphamide**, **doxorubicin**, **vincristine**, and prednisone. Similar drug combinations are being used for patients whose MALT lymphomas do not respond to antibiotic treatment.

Prevention

There are currently no commonly accepted means to prevent MALT lymphomas. While the *H. pylori* infections are associated with this and other gastric disease, the eradication of *H. pylori* in asymptomatic individuals is not currently recommended for prevention of MALT lymphomas or gastric cancer.

Resources

BOOKS

Feldman, M, et al. *Sleisenger & Fordtran's Gastrointestinal and Liver Disease*. 8th ed. St. Louis: Mosby, 2005.

Goldman, Lee, and Andrew I. Schafer. *Goldman's Cecil Medicine*. 24th ed. Philadelphia: Saunders/Elsevier, 2012.

WEBSITES

Leukaemia Foundation. "Mucosa-Associated Lymphoid Tissue Lymphoma (MALT)." http://www.leukaemia.org.au/blood-cancers/lymphomas/non-hodgkin-lymphoma-nhl/mucosa-associated-lymphoid-tissue-lymphoma-malt (accessed October 31,2014).

ORGANIZATIONS

American Cancer Society, 250 Williams St. NW, Atlanta, GA 30303, (800) 227-2345, http://www.cancer.org.

Warren Maltzman, PhD

Mammography

Definition

Mammography is the study of the breast using **x-rays**. The actual test is called a mammogram. It is an x-ray of the breast that shows the fatty, fibrous, and glandular tissues. There are two types of mammograms: screening and diagnostic. A screening mammogram is ordered for women who have no problems with their

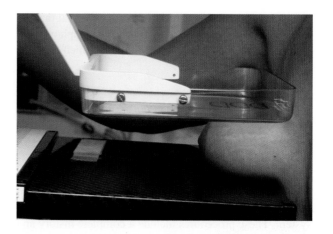

Breast compressed with a compression paddle during mammography. *(Southern Illinois University/Science Source)*

breasts. It consists of two x-ray views of each breast: a craniocaudal (from above) and a mediolateral oblique (from the sides). A diagnostic mammogram is for evaluation of abnormalities in either men or women. Additional x-rays from other angles, or special coned views of certain areas, are taken.

Purpose

The purpose of screening mammography is **breast cancer** detection. A **screening test** by definition is used for patients without any signs or symptoms in order to detect disease as early as possible. Many studies have shown that having regular mammograms increases a woman's chances of finding breast **cancer** in an early stage, when it is more likely to be curable. It has been estimated that a mammogram may find a cancer as much as two or three years before it can be felt. The American Cancer Society (ACS) guidelines recommend an annual screening mammogram for every woman of average risk beginning at age 40. Radiologists look specifically for the presence of microcalcifications and other abnormalities that can be associated with malignancy. New digital mammography and computer-aided reporting can automatically enhance and magnify the mammograms for easier identification of these tiny calcifications.

The highest risk factor for developing cancer is age. Some women are at an increased risk for developing breast cancer, such as those with a positive family history of the disease. Beginning screening mammography at a younger age may be recommended for these women.

Diagnostic mammography is used to evaluate an existing problem, such as a lump, discharge from the nipple, or unusual tenderness in one area. It is also done to evaluate further abnormalities that have been seen on screening mammograms. The radiologist normally views

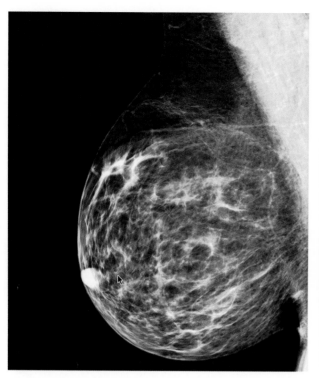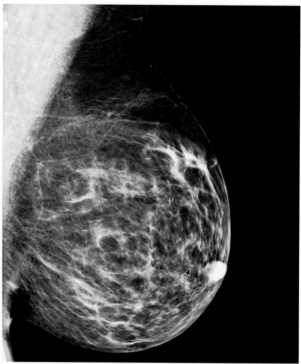

Mammogram of the breasts. *(Blue Planet Earth /Shutterstock.com)*

the films immediately and may ask for additional views, such as a magnification of one specific area. Additional studies such as an ultrasound of the breast may be performed as well to determine whether the lesion is cystic or solid. Breast-specific **positron emission tomography** (PET) and **magnetic resonance imaging** (MRI) scans may be ordered to further evaluate a tumor, but mammography is still the first choice in detecting small tumors on a screening basis.

Description

A mammogram may be offered in a variety of settings. Hospitals, outpatient clinics, physician's offices, or other facilities may have mammography equipment. In the United States, only places certified by the U.S. Food and Drug Administration (FDA) are legally permitted to perform, interpret, or develop mammograms. Mammograms are taken with dedicated machines using high frequency generators, low kVp (kilovolts peak), molybdenum targets, and specialized x-ray beam filtration. Sensitive high-contrast film and screen combinations along with prolonged developing enable the visualization of minute breast details.

In addition to the usual paperwork, a woman will be asked to fill out a questionnaire asking for information on her current medical history. Beyond her personal and family history of cancer, details about menstruation, previous breast surgeries, child bearing, birth control, and hormone replacement therapy are recorded. Information about breast self-examination (BSE) and other breast health issues are usually available at no charge.

At some centers, a technologist may perform a physical examination of the breasts before the mammogram. Whether or not this is done, it is essential for the technologist to record any lumps, nipple discharge, breast pain, or other concerns of the patient. All visible scars, tattoos, and nipple alterations must be carefully noted as well.

Clothing from the waist up is removed, along with necklaces and dangling earrings. A hospital gown or similar covering is put on. A small self-adhesive metal marker may be placed on each nipple by the x-ray technologist. This allows the nipple to be viewed as a reference point on the film for concise tumor location and easier centering for additional views. Large moles within the mammography field may be covered in the same way.

Patients are positioned for mammograms differently, depending on the type of mammogram being performed:

• For craniocaudal position (CC), the woman stands or sits facing the mammogram machine. One breast is exposed and raised to a level position while the height of the cassette holder is adjusted to the same level. The breast is placed mid-film with the nipple in profile and the head turned away from the side being x-rayed. The shoulder is relaxed and pulled slightly backward while the breast is pulled as far forward as possible. The technologist holds the breast in place and slowly lowers the compression with a foot pedal. The breast is compressed between the film holder and a rectangle of plastic (called a paddle). The breast is compressed until the skin is taut and the breast tissue firm when touched on the lateral side. The exposure is taken immediately and the compression released. Good compression can be uncomfortable, but it is necessary. Compression reduces the thickness of the breast, creates a uniform density, and separates overlying tissues. This allows for a detailed image with a lower exposure time and decreased radiation dose to the patient. The same view is repeated on the opposite breast.

• For mediolateral oblique position (MLO), the woman is positioned with her side toward the mammography unit. The film holder is angled parallel to the pectoral muscle, anywhere from 30 to 60 degrees depending on the size and height of the patient. The taller and thinner the patient, the higher the angle. The height of the machine is level with the axilla (armpit). The arm is placed at the top of the cassette holder with a corner touching the armpit. The breast is lifted forward and upward, and compression is applied until the breast is held firmly in place by the paddle. The nipple should be in profile and the opposite breast held away by the patient, if necessary. This procedure is repeated for the other breast. A total of four x-rays, two of each breast, are taken for a screening mammogram. Additional x-rays, using special paddles, different breast positions, or other techniques may be taken for a diagnostic mammogram.

The mammogram may be seen and interpreted by a radiologist right away, or it may not be reviewed until later. If there is any questionable area or abnormality, extra x-rays may be recommended. These may be taken during the same appointment. More commonly, especially for screening mammograms, the woman is called back on another day for these additional films.

A screening mammogram usually takes approximately 15 to 30 minutes. A woman having a diagnostic mammogram can expect to spend up to an hour for the procedure.

The cost of mammography varies widely. Many mammography facilities accept "self-referral." This means women can schedule themselves without a physician's referral; however, some insurance policies do require a doctor's prescription to ensure payment. Medicare covers annual screening mammograms for eligible women over age 40.

Preparation

The compression or squeezing of the breast necessary for a mammogram is a concern to many women. Mammograms should be scheduled when a woman's breasts are least likely to be tender. One to two weeks after the first day of the menstrual period is usually best, as the breasts may be tender during the menstrual period. Some women with sensitive breasts also find that stopping or decreasing caffeine intake from coffee, tea, colas, and chocolate for a week or two before the examination decreases any discomfort. Women receiving hormone therapy may also have sensitive breasts. Over-the-counter pain relievers are recommended an hour before the mammogram appointment when pain is a significant problem.

Women should not put deodorant, powder, or lotion on their upper body on the day the mammogram is performed. Particles from these products can get on the breast or film holder and may show up as abnormalities on the mammogram. Most facilities will have special wipes available for those patients who need to wash before the mammogram.

Aftercare

No special aftercare is required.

Risks

The risk of radiation exposure from a mammogram is considered minimal and not significant. Experts are unanimous that any negligible risk is by far outweighed by the potential benefits of mammography. Patients who have breast implants must be x-rayed with caution, and compression is minimally applied so that the sac is not ruptured. Special techniques and positioning skills must be learned before a technologist can x-ray a patient with breast implants.

Some breast cancers do not show up on mammograms, or "hide" in dense breast tissue. A normal (or negative) study is not a guarantee that a woman is cancer-free. The false-negative rate is estimated to be 15%–20%, and even higher in younger women and women with dense breasts.

False positive readings are also possible. Breast biopsies may be recommended on the basis of a mammogram and find no cancer. It is estimated that 75%–80% of all breast biopsies result in benign (no cancer present) findings. This is considered an acceptable rate, because recommending fewer biopsies would result in too many missed cancers.

Results

A mammography report describes details about the x-ray appearance of the breasts. It also rates the mammogram according to standardized categories, as part of the Breast Imaging Reporting and Data System (BI-RADS) created by the American College of Radiology (ACR):

- BI-RADS 0 means that the x-ray scan was incomplete and additional imaging scans are needed.
- BI-RADS 1 is considered normal or negative and means that no abnormalities were seen.
- BI-RADS 2 is also considered normal but refers to benign findings. One or more abnormalities were seen in the breast, but they were clearly benign (not cancerous) or variations of normal. Some kinds of calcifications, enlarged lymph nodes, or obvious cysts might generate a BI-RADS 2 rating.
- BI-RADS 3 means that either additional images are needed or that an abnormality was seen, but is probably (but not definitely) benign. A follow-up mammogram within a short interval of 6 to 12 months is suggested. This helps to ensure that the abnormality is not changing, or is "stable." Only the affected side will be x-rayed at this time. Some women are uncomfortable or anxious about waiting, and may want to consult with their doctor about having a biopsy.
- BI-RADS 4 means suspicious for cancer. A biopsy is usually recommended in this case.
- BI-RADS 5 means an abnormality is highly suggestive of cancer. A biopsy or other appropriate action should be taken.
- BI-RADS 6 refers to lesions that have been confirmed as malignant.

QUESTIONS TO ASK YOUR DOCTOR

- What do my results mean?
- What does my BI-RADS rating mean?
- Do I need a mammogram every year?

There are also ratings for breast density:

- BI-RADS 1 means that the breast is mostly fat (75% or more).
- BI-RADS 2 means that 25%–50% of the breast is fibrous and glandular tissue.
- BI-RADS 3 indicates that up to 75% of the breast is dense fibrous or glandular tissue, which can make it difficult to detect small masses.
- BI-RADS 4 means that more than 75% of the breast is fibrous or glandular tissue, which can potentially lead to a missed diagnosis.

Screening mammograms are not usually recommended for women under age 40 who have no special risk factors and normal physical breast examinations. A mammogram may be useful if a lump or other problem is discovered in a woman aged 30–40. Below age 30, breasts tend to be "radiographically dense," which means that the breasts contain a large amount of glandular tissue that is difficult to image in fine detail. Mammograms for this age group are controversial. An ultrasound of the breasts is usually done instead.

Health care team roles

The mammography technologist must be empathetic to the patient's modesty and anxiety. He or she must explain that compression is necessary to improve the quality of the image but does not harm the breasts. Patients may be very anxious when additional films are requested. Explaining that an extra view gives the radiologist more information will help to ease the patient's tension. According to the American Cancer Society, one in eight women will develop breast cancer at some point in her life, but educating the public on the importance of early diagnosis will help in achieving more positive outcomes.

Resources

BOOKS

Grant, Lee A., and Nyree Griffin. *Grainger & Allison's Diagnostic Radiology Essentials*. Philadelphia: Churchill Livingstone/Elsevier, 2013.

Ikeda, Debra. *Breast Imaging*. Philadelphia: Mosby/Elsevier, 2011.

Lentz, Gretchen, et al. *Comprehensive Gynecology.* 5th ed. St. Louis: Mosby/Elsevier, 2012.

Mettler, Fred A., Jr. *Essentials of Radiology.* 3rd ed. Philadelphia: Saunders/Elsevier, 2014.

PERIODICALS

Berg, Wendie A., et al. "Detection of Breast Cancer with Addition of Annual Screening Ultrasound or a Single Screening MRI to Mammography in Women with Elevated Breast Cancer Risk." *JAMA* 307, no. 13 (2012): 1394–1404. http://dx.doi.org/10.1001/jama.2012.388 (accessed October 3, 2014).

Bleyer, Archie, and H. Gilbert Welch. "Effect of Three Decades of Screening Mammography on Breast-Cancer Incidence." *New England Journal of Medicine* 367, no. 21 (2012): 1998–2005. http://dx.doi.org/10.1056/NEJMoa1206809 (accessed October 3, 2014).

Reis, Cláudia. "Quality Assurance and Quality Control in Mammography: A Review of Available Guidance Worldwide." *Insights into Imaging* (August 4, 2013): e-pub ahead of print. http://dx.doi.org/10.1007/s13244-013-0269-1 (accessed October 3, 2014).

OTHER

American College of Radiology. *The American College of Radiology BI-RADS® ATLAS and MQSA: Frequently Asked Questions.* August 2011. http://www.acr.org/~/media/ACR/Documents/PDF/QualitySafety/Resources/BIRADS/BIRADSFAQs.pdf (accessed October 3, 2014).

WEBSITES

American Cancer Society. "How Many Women Get Breast Cancer?" http://www.cancer.org/cancer/breastcancer/overviewguide/breast-cancer-overview-key-statistics (accessed October 3, 2014).

American Cancer Society. "Mammogram Reports—BI-RADS." http://www.cancer.org/treatment/understandingyourdiagnosis/examsandtestdescriptions/mammogramsandotherbreastimagingprocedures/mammograms-and-other-breast-imaging-procedures-mammo-report (accessed October 3, 2014).

Centers for Medicare & Medicaid Services. "Your Medicare Coverage: Mammograms." http://www.medicare.gov/coverage/mammograms.html (accessed October 3, 2014).

National Cancer Institute. "Mammograms." http://www.cancer.gov/cancertopics/factsheet/Detection/mammograms (accessed October 3, 2014).

ORGANIZATIONS

American Cancer Society, 250 Williams St. NW, Atlanta, GA 30303, (800) 227-2345, http://www.cancer.org.

National Cancer Institute, 6116 Executive Blvd., Ste. 300, Bethesda, MD 20892-8322, (800) 4-CANCER (422-6237), http://cancer.gov.

Lorraine K. Ehresman
Lee A. Shratter, MD
REVISED BY ROSALYN CARSON-DeWITT, MD

Mantle cell lymphoma

Definition

Mantle cell **lymphoma** (MCL) is a rare type of **non-Hodgkin lymphoma** (NHL) characterized under the microscope by expansion of the mantle zone area of the lymph node with a homogeneous (structurally similar) population of malignant small lymphoid cells. These cancerous cells have slightly irregular nuclei and very little cytoplasm, and are mixed with newly made normal lymphocytes (white blood cells) that travel from the bone marrow to the lymph nodes and spleen. Unlike normal lymphocytes, they do not mature properly and become cancerous instead.

Description

The body's immune system produces two types of lymphocytes or white blood cells: the B cells, which are made in the bone marrow, and the T cells, which are made in the thymus. Both types of cells are found in the lymph, the clear liquid that bathes tissues and circulates in the lymphatic system. Lymphomas are cancers that occur in this lymphatic system and B-Cell lymphomas—also called non-Hodgkin lymphomas—include follicular lymphomas, small non-cleaved cell lymphomas (Burkitt lymphomas), marginal zone lymphomas (MALT lymphomas), small lymphocytic lymphomas, large cell lymphomas, and also mantle cell lymphomas.

Mantle cell lymphoma accounts for 5% to 10% of all lymphomas diagnosed and 5% of B-cell lymphomas. There are three subsets of MCL cells: the mantle zone type, the nodular type, and the blastic or blastoid (immature) type. These various types often occur together to some degree, and approximately 30% to 40% of diagnoses are of mixed mantle and nodular type. As MCL develops further, the non-cancerous mantle centers also become invaded by cancerous cells. In about 20% of these cases, the cells become larger, and of the blastic type.

Extensive debates are ongoing concerning the grade of this cancer. European classification used to classify it as a low-grade cancer because it is initially slow-growing, while American classification considered it intermediate based on patients' shorter average survival rate. The combined European-American classification (REAL), is still discussing the status of mantle cell lymphoma. This is due to the mixed nature of MCL cells. Blastic type-MCL seems to be considered as a high-grade cancer because it spreads at about the rate of other lymphomas belonging to that category. The studies currently attempting to describe the precise nature of

KEY TERMS

Anemia—A condition caused by a reduction in the amount of red blood cells produced by the bone marrow. Its symptoms are general weakness and lack of energy, dizziness, shortness of breath, headaches, and irritability.

Antibody—A protein (immunoglobulin) produced by plasma cells (mature B cells) to fight infections in the body. They are released into the circulatory system in response to specific antigens and thus target those antigens that induced their production.

Antigen—An antigen is any substance which elicits an antibody response. As such, they are substances that stimulate a specific immune response of the body and are capable of reacting with the products of that response. Antigens may be foreign chemical substances or proteins located on the surface of viruses, bacteria, toxins, tumors and other infectious agents.

B-Cell lymphocyte—A type of lymphocyte (white blood cell). B cells react to the presence of antigens by dividing and maturing into plasma cells.

B-cell lymphomas—Non-Hodgkin lymphomas that arise from B cells.

Blood cell—Cellular component of blood. There are three general types: white blood cells, red blood cells, and platelets, all which are produced in the bone marrow.

Cytoplasm—The organized complex of organic and inorganic substances external to the nuclear membrane of a cell.

DNA—Deoxyribonucleic acid are nucleic acids that are the part of the cell nucleus that contains and controls all genetic information.

Edema—Swelling of a body part caused by an abnormal buildup of fluids.

Gene—The specific site on a chromosome, consisting of protein and DNA responsible for the transmittal and determination of hereditary characteristics.

Gene therapy—The use of genes to treat cancer and other diseases.

Immune system—The system within the body, consisting of many organs and cells, that recognizes and fights foreign cells and disease.

Lymph—A milky white liquid responsible for carrying the lymphocytes in the lymphatic vessels.

Lymphatic system—Tissues and organs such as the bone marrow, spleen, thymus and lymph nodes that produce and store cells to fight infection and disease. Also includes the lymphatic vessels that carry lymph.

Lymphocyte—A type of white blood cell that defends the body against infection and disease. Lymphocytes are found in the bloodstream, the lymphatic system, and lymphoid organs. The two main types of lymphocytes are the B cells (produced in the bone marrow) and the T cells (produced in the thymus).

Lymphoma—Cancers that starts in the lymphatic system. Lymphomas are classified into two categories: Hodgkin lymphoma and non-Hodgkin lymphoma.

Monoclonal antibody—An antibody raised against a specific antigen. Monoclonal antibodies are being used to target chemotherapy or radioactive substances directly to cancer cells.

Non-Hodgkin lymphomas—Lymphomas characterized by different types of cancerous lymphatic cells, excluding those characterized by Hodgkin lymphoma.

Remission—A complete or partial disappearance of the signs and symptoms of cancer, usually in response to treatment.

Stem cell—Primitive cell found in the bone marrow and in the blood stream. Stem cells become different types of mature blood cells, thus enabling them to rejuvenate the circulatory and immune systems.

Stem cell transplant—Treatment procedure by which young blood stem cells are collected from the patient (autologous) or another matched donor (allogeneic). High-dose chemotherapy and/or radiation is given, and the stem cells are reinserted into the patient to rebuild his or her immune system.

these cells will be key to any general agreement that is finally reached.

Demographics

Each year, mantle cell lymphoma cases are only about 6% of all NHL diagnoses. Mantle cell lymphoma is rare in persons under the age of 50. The average age of a Mantle cell lymphoma patient is 65. Most patients are men; out of 1,000 persons diagnosed with MCL, approximately 33% will be women. This **cancer** has the shortest average survival of all lymphoma types.

Causes and symptoms

The cause of MCL appears to be breakage in chromosome 11. A small piece of chromosome 11 is then transferred to chromosome 14. About 85% of all MCL patients display this chromosomal abnormality.

As a result of this chromosomal abnormality (deemed a reciprocal translocation), B cell lymphoma cells produce abnormally large quantities of a protein that encourages rapid cell growth.

Many of its symptoms are shared by other lymphomas as well and patients generally complain of **fatigue**, **anemia**, low grade fevers, **night sweats**, **weight loss**, rashes, digestive disturbances, chronic sinus irritation, recurrent infections, sore throat, shortness of breath, muscle and bone aches and edema.

More specific symptoms include spleen enlargement (in about 60%–80% of cases), particularly with nodular-type MCL. Swollen lymph nodes are an early-stage symptom, even though the general health of the patient is good. Mild anemia is also common. Some patients also report lower back pain, and burning pain in the legs and testicles. As MCL becomes more advanced, the lymph nodes increase in volume, and the general symptoms become more pronounced.

In the end stage of MCL, neurologic symptoms appear, indicating that the MCL has spread to the central nervous system.

Diagnosis

MCL is very similar to several other lymphoma types and special care must be taken with the diagnosis. It should not be made from blood or bone marrow specimens alone. It is believed that immunologic tests are required to make the correct diagnosis. Immunophenotyping is one such test, it is used to determine what kind of surface molecules are present on cells, and thus, the exact type of lymphoma from a tissue sample. The Lymphoma Research Foundation of America recommends that several opinions be sought from recognized mantle cell experts to confirm the accuracy of the diagnosis.

At the time of diagnosis, mantle cell lymphoma has usually spread into other tissues such as the lymph nodes, spleen, bone marrow (up to 90% of cases), or to Waldeyer's ring (the ring of adenoid, palatine and lingual tonsils at the back of the mouth) or to the gastrointestinal tract. MCL can also spread to the colon, in which case it is diagnosed as multiple lymphomatous polyposis.

Treatment

There is no formal staging system for mantle cell lymphoma and no standard treatment has yet been adopted for MCL patients. Patients have been treated with surgery, radiation, single drug or combination **chemotherapy**, and stem cell transplants. CHOP is one of the most common chemotherapy regimens for treating MCL. It derives its name from the combination of drugs used: **cyclophosphamide** (Cytoxan, Neosar), **doxorubicin** (Adriamycin), **vincristine** (Oncovin), and prednisone.

Alternative and complementary therapies

Because MCL is a cancer of the lymphatic system, immunologic therapies are often used, or combined with the more conventional radiation and chemotherapy treatments. Immunological therapies take advantage of the body's immune system. The immune system is a network of specialized cells and organs that defends the body against foreign invaders (antigens) by producing special "defense" proteins, an example of which are the antibodies. These substances recognize and attach to the antigens, usually found on the surface of cells and destroy them. There are reports of immunological therapies being used for MCL using interferon, one such natural substance produced by the body in response to a virus. Numerous studies show that **interferons** can stimulate the immune system to fight the growth of cancer, but there has not yet been enough evidence produced to see it emerge as a strong candidate for MCL treatment.

Other immunological therapies based on **monoclonal antibodies** (MABs or MOABs) have recently emerged, such as Rituxan (**rituximab**). MABs work on cancer cells in the same way natural antibodies work, by identifying and binding to the target cells, alerting other cells in the immune system to the presence of the cancer cells. MABs are very specific for a particular antigen, meaning that one designed for a B-cell lymphoma will not work on T-cell lymphomas. MABs used alone may enhance a patient's **immune response** to the cancer but they are thought to be more efficient when combined to another form of therapy, such as a chemotherapeutic drug. This way, the cancer is attacked on two fronts: chemical attack from the chemotherapy and immune response attack stimulated by the MAB.

Clinical trials

Clinical trials addressing the needs of MCL patients are very recent because the mantle cell lymphoma subtype has only recently been defined. There are now several trials being carried out in the United States specifically for mantle cell. Some other trials designed for patients with lymphomas may also accept mantle cell patients. Ongoing trials in this area

QUESTIONS TO ASK YOUR DOCTOR

- What kinds of diagnostic studies will be required to ascertain the type and spread of this tumor?
- Could there be a genetic component to this tumor? Should other family members be tested?
- What types of treatments are available?
- What types of side effects from treatments can I expect? What are your recommendations to help me deal with those side effects?
- Am I eligible for any clinical trials? Would these be helpful to consider?
- Are there any lifestyle changes that I should make?
- What type of diet should I follow? Are there foods I should avoid?
- Should I avoid any medications?
- How often should I be checked after treatment has ended?
- Is there a support group that I can join to hear about other people's experiences with this disease?

are chiefly concerned with investigating monoclonal antibodies. Information regarding clinical trials can be obtained through the Clinical Trials web site listed at the end of this entry.

The following clinical protocols are specifically designed for MCL patients:

- The MD Anderson Protocol (high-dose chemotherapy with or without stem cell transplant)
- Rituxan, by itself or with CHOP
- Bexxar
- Oncolym
- Flavopiridol
- Phenylacetate

Prognosis

There is no cure for mantle cell lymphoma. As with other slow-growing lymphomas, spontaneous remissions have been reported. Unfortunately, the median survival rate is only three to four years. All mantle cell lymphoma experts agree that the long-term prognosis of MCL

patients receiving conventional treatment is poor, and that there is an urgent need for new, improved therapies.

Prevention

Because the cause of MCL is unknown, no prevention measures can be recommended.

Coping with cancer treatment

It is important to have a caregiver system when receiving medical treatment for MCL, and it is just as important to have a network of support for coping with the non-medical aspects of the cancer. Friends, relatives, coworkers and health professionals all can provide help, as well as the national cancer associations, some specifically addressing the needs of lymphoma patients. Please refer to the Resources section at the end of this entry for contact information.

Because MCL is a cancer that usually involves chemotherapy and **radiation therapy**, it can be severely damaging to organ function and long-term resistance. In addition to the immediate side effects of these treatments, other effects appear after treatment is completed, one of which, called Post-Cancer Fatigue (PCF), is often seen with lymphoma patients. This is fatigue that persists after treatment and can sometimes be extreme. The medical team will be able to offer the best advice to deal with PCF.

See also Acute lymphocytic leukemia; Central nervous system lymphoma.

Resources

BOOKS

Hoffman R., et al. *Hematology: Basic Principles and Practice.* 4th ed. Philadelphia: Elsevier, 2005.

PERIODICALS

Rajguru S, Kahl., BS. "Emerging Therapy For The Treatment of Mantle Cell Lymphoma." *Journal of the National Comprehensive Cancer Network* 12, no. 9 (2014): 1311–18. http://www.ncbi.nlm.nih.gov/pubmed/25190697 (accessed October 31, 2014).

WEBSITES

"Mantle Cell Lymphoma." Lymphoma*Info*.net. http://www.lymphomainfo.net/nhl/types/mantle.html. (accessed October 15, 2014).

ORGANIZATIONS

American Cancer Society, 250 Williams St. NW, Atlanta, GA 30303, (800) 227-2345, http://www.cancer.org.

Monique Laberge, PhD

Marijuana *see* **Tetrahydrocannabinol**

Mastectomy

Definition

Mastectomy is the surgical removal of part or all of a breast—and sometimes additional tissue—for the treatment or prevention of **breast cancer**.

Purpose

More than 100,000 mastectomies are performed each year in the United States. Although the vast majority are performed to treat breast **cancer**, an increasing number of women are choosing prophylactic mastectomy.

Cancer treatment

Breast cancer is treated with mastectomy when:

• The cancer is advanced, and all of the breast tissue and possibly lymph nodes and muscles must be removed.
• The tumor is large and would be difficult to remove with good cosmetic results by breast-conserving surgery.
• The breast is small or shaped such that breast-conserving surgery would leave very little tissue.
• A sufficient amount of normal tissue surrounding the tumor—the margin of resection—cannot be removed along with the tumor.
• Radiation therapy following breast-conserving surgery is not appropriate or possible.

Many women with earlier-stage breast cancers choose to have a full mastectomy rather than a breast-conserving **lumpectomy** or segmental mastectomy, even though the latter are just as effective and survival rates are just as high as with a mastectomy. A 2013 study found that a majority of women under 40 opted for mastectomies rather than a more modest surgical procedure followed by radiation treatments. Some women fear radiation or are unable to undergo **radiation therapy** because of pregnancy, an underlying medical condition, or because of the time commitment, travel distance, or cost. Some women choose a mastectomy because they want **breast reconstruction** surgery. Other women are afraid that their cancer will recur and achieve greater peace of mind with a mastectomy. However, women in the United States are more likely to have mastectomies than women in other countries, and there is growing concern over the increase in unnecessary mastectomies.

Prophylactic mastectomy

Prophylactic or preventive mastectomy—removal of one or both breasts to prevent possible future breast cancer—is controversial. The rate of prophylactic mastectomies has increased by an estimated 50% in recent years. Some researchers worry that prophylactic mastectomies are reaching almost epidemic proportions with little medical justification. Fear generated by breast-cancer awareness campaigns, improvements in breast **reconstructive surgery**, and celebrity disclosures of prophylactic mastectomies all may be contributing to this trend. Nevertheless, undergoing a prophylactic mastectomy is no guarantee that breast cancer will not develop or recur.

About 5%–10% of breast cancers result from specific mutations in the breast cancer susceptibility genes BRCA1 and BRCA2. Women with these mutations have a very high likelihood of developing breast cancer, and the younger they are when the cancer develops, the more aggressive the disease. Many women with BRCA mutations choose to have prophylactic double (bilateral) mastectomies.

An increasing number of women are choosing double mastectomies after developing cancer in one breast, even though the risk of cancer in the healthy breast is only about 1% per year. By 2013, up to 15% of women with breast cancer were choosing double mastectomies, compared with less than 3% in the late 1990s. Studies have suggested that 70% of these double mastectomies may be unnecessary.

Bilateral prophylactic mastectomy is sometimes performed on high-risk women with lobular carcinoma-in-situ (LCIS), in which abnormal cells are found in the milk-producing glands. Although LCIS seldom becomes invasive, it increases the risk of breast cancer in either breast. While most surgeons consider prophylactic mastectomy for LCIS to be unnecessary, the number of such surgeries increased by 50% between 2000 and 2013.

Description

Mastectomies are typically performed under general anesthesia in a hospital and require at least an overnight stay. Immediate breast reconstruction requires a longer hospital stay; however, an increasing number of mastectomies are performed in specialized outpatient facilities. A mastectomy with lymph node dissection—the removal of axillary (underarm) lymph nodes—takes 90–120 minutes.

An oval-shaped incision is usually made around the nipple across the width of the breast. The type and location of the incision may vary according to breast reconstruction plans or other factors. The diseased and at-risk tissue is removed and sent to a pathology laboratory for analysis. If no immediate breast reconstruction is planned, surgical drains are left in place to prevent fluid

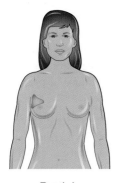
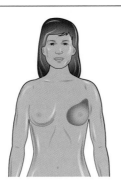
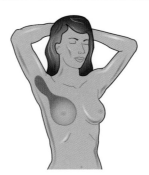
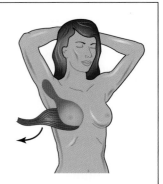

Partial mastectomy (quadrantectomy)   Simple mastectomy   Modified radical mastectomy with lymph nodes removed   Radical mastectomy with chest muscle removed

There are four types of mastectomies: partial mastectomy, or lumpectomy, in which the tumor and surrounding tissue is removed; simple mastectomy, where the entire breast and some axillary lymph nodes are removed; modified radical mastectomy, in which the entire breast and axillary lymph nodes are removed; and radical mastectomy, where the entire breast, axillary lymph nodes, and chest muscles are removed. *(Illustration by Electronic Illustrators Group. © Cengage Learning®.)*

accumulation. The skin is sutured and bandages or dressings are applied. The stitches later dissolve or surgical staples are removed at an office visit.

Types of mastectomies

With a total or **simple mastectomy**, the breast tissue is separated from the overlying skin and the underlying chest wall muscle. All the breast tissue—from the collarbone to the ribs and from the side of the body to the breastbone—is removed. One or more axillary lymph nodes may be removed through a separate incision to be checked for cancerous cells.

A **modified radical mastectomy** is the most common type. It removes the breast, nipple, an ellipse of skin, most of the underarm lymph nodes, and often the lining over the chest muscles, but usually leaves the chest muscles intact. The surgery leaves the woman with a more normal chest shape than a radical mastectomy and a less visible scar. It also allows for immediate or delayed breast reconstruction.

A radical or Halsted mastectomy removes the breast, all surrounding lymph nodes up to the collarbone, and the chest muscle. The procedure was developed in the late 1800s, when it was believed that extensive surgery was more likely to cure cancer. Radical mastectomies often left women disfigured and disabled, with a large defect in the chest wall requiring skin grafting and with significantly decreased sensation and motion in the arm. Radical mastectomies are now performed only for recurrent breast cancer or when the tumor has spread to the chest muscle.

Breast-conserving surgeries include lumpectomies, in which only the tumor and a small amount of surrounding normal tissue are removed, and partial or segmental mastectomies, in which the cancerous region, surrounding normal tissue, and possibly the lining over the chest muscles below the cancer are removed. **Lymph node dissection** may be performed at the same time, or later through a separate incision.

Skin-sparing mastectomy and breast reconstruction

If a woman is not going to have immediate breast reconstruction, the surgeon removes as much of the breast skin as is necessary to flatten the surface of the chest and scar. In contrast, a skin-sparing mastectomy removes the breast tissue through a small incision, leaving the breast skin to accommodate a soft-tissue reconstruction or breast implant. The nipple and areola may also be removed, although some studies have found little difference in recurrence rates after nipple-sparing mastectomy.

Breast reconstruction surgery may be performed at the time of the mastectomy or months or even years later, depending on the site and type of cancer and the woman's overall health. The reconstructive surgery is performed by a plastic surgeon. Mastectomy with reconstruction surgery can take up to five or six hours. Tissue-flap surgery reconstructs the breast with the patient's own muscle, fat, and skin taken from other parts of the body. Alternatively, reconstruction may use implants filled with saline or silicone gel. Surgery is sometimes performed on the other breast so that both breasts are approximately the same size and shape. A drain may be placed in the armpit after the surgery, which usually requires a hospital stay of three days or less. Insurance companies are required to cover breast reconstructions in conjunction with mastectomies.

Some women prefer not to have reconstructive surgery. Tissue flap is major surgery and may not be appropriate for women who are very thin or obese, who smoke, or who have other health conditions.

Precautions

A choice between a mastectomy and breast-conserving surgery should be considered carefully. Mastectomy results in a significant loss of sensation in the breast, which may affect self-image or sexual feelings. Furthermore, although studies have found that women who choose preventive mastectomy are generally satisfied with their choice, the women also report that they had inadequate prior information about the surgery, **genetic testing**, and breast reconstruction.

Preparation

Surgical treatment for breast cancer is often performed within a few weeks of diagnosis. Sometimes **chemotherapy** is used before surgery to shrink the tumor and reduce the amount of tissue that must be surgically removed. A recent study found that treatment with **aromatase inhibitors**, such as anastrozole, can shrink large, endocrine-rich tumors in postmenopausal women, allowing many of them to have breast-conserving surgery instead of a mastectomy.

Routine preoperative preparations, such as not eating or drinking the night before surgery, are typically required. The patient may be asked to donate blood in case a blood transfusion is necessary. Women should stop taking aspirin, **nonsteroidal anti-inflammatory drugs** such as ibuprofen, and possibly other medications several weeks before surgery.

Aftercare

Many mastectomy patients go home the same day or within a day or two; however, they may need to change bandages and/or care for the incision. Surgical drains must be properly attended to, including measuring and emptying the fluid. If a drain becomes blocked, fluid or blood may collect at the surgical site, which can cause infection and/or delay wound healing. Pain is usually controlled with prescribed medication. Severe pain may be a sign of complications. A return visit to the surgeon is usually scheduled seven to ten days after the procedure. Activities such as driving may be restricted.

Physical therapy is an integral part of mastectomy aftercare. Exercises to maintain shoulder and arm mobility may be prescribed as early as 24 hours after surgery; however, intense exercise should be avoided for a time. The affected area must be protected from infection, pressure, constriction, or injury, especially if axillary lymph nodes were removed.

Emotional care is an important aspect of recovery from a mastectomy. Women may experience anger, **depression**, negative self-image, and grief, as well as anxiety over possible cancer recurrence. Assistance in dealing with the psychological effects of a breast cancer diagnosis, as well as the surgery, can be invaluable.

Following a lumpectomy or mastectomy, a pathologist examines the removed tissue to confirm that the margins of resection are free of cancer cells. This ensures that all of the cancer has been removed. The size of the margins—the distance between the tumor and the edges of the tissue—helps determine the need for additional treatment. If cancer cells extend out to the edge, additional surgery called re-excision will be performed. Other breast cancer treatments following mastectomy may include chemotherapy, radiation therapy, hormone therapy, and/or targeted therapy. Radiation therapy almost always follows breast-conserving surgery.

Risks

Mastectomy risks include:

- risks associated with general anesthesia
- excessive bleeding during or after surgery, particularly with a double mastectomy or breast reconstruction
- numbness at the incision site and mild-to-moderate tenderness adjacent to the site due to severed nerves
- delayed wound healing from fluid or blood accumulation
- infection
- unexpected scarring
- phantom breast symptoms, such as itching or aching in a breast that has been removed
- scarring from lymph node removal, resulting in decreased arm mobility and requiring more intense physical therapy
- complications arising from breast reconstruction surgery

Approximately 10%–20% of patients develop lymphedema after axillary lymph node removal. This complication can arise at any time, even years after surgery. This mild-to-severe swelling of the arm caused by faulty lymph drainage is a chronic condition that requires continuing treatment. Severe cases can be disabling. A type of **biopsy** known as **sentinel lymph**

KEY TERMS

Areola—The pigmented ring around the nipple.

Aromatase inhibitor—A medication for preventing or treating breast cancer in postmenopausal women by inhibiting the body's production of estrogen.

Axillary lymph nodes—The glands of the lymphatic system located under the arms.

Biopsy—The removal of cells or tissue for examination by a pathologist.

BRCA1, BRCA2—Breast cancer susceptibility genes; specific mutations in these genes greatly increase the risk of breast and ovarian cancers.

Breast-conserving surgery—Breast cancer treatment, such as a lumpectomy or partial mastectomy, that removes only the cancerous tissue rather than the entire breast.

Lobular carcinoma-in-situ (LCIS)—Breast cancer that is confined to the milk-producing glands.

Lumpectomy—Excision of a breast tumor and a limited amount of surrounding tissue.

Lymph node dissection—The removal of underarm lymph nodes to check for the spread of cancer.

Lymphedema—Accumulation of lymphatic fluid in the soft tissues of the arms, hands, and sometimes the breast area following lymph node dissection.

Mammogram—A breast x-ray used to detect cancer.

Margin of resection—The area between the cancerous tumor and the edges of the removed tissue.

Modified radical mastectomy—Total mastectomy with axillary lymph node dissection, but with preservation of the chest muscles.

Partial mastectomy—Segmental mastectomy; removal of only the cancerous breast tissue and some of the surrounding normal tissue.

Prophylactic mastectomy—Removal of a healthy breast to prevent future breast cancer.

Radical mastectomy—Removal of the breast, chest muscles, axillary lymph nodes, and associated skin and subcutaneous tissue.

Skin-sparing mastectomy—Removal of the breast tissue, leaving the skin intact for breast reconstruction.

Tamoxifen—A drug that blocks the activity of estrogen; used to prevent or treat breast cancer.

Tissue-flap surgery—Breast reconstruction using tissues from elsewhere in the body.

Total mastectomy—Simple mastectomy; removal of only the breast tissue, nipple and a small portion of the overlying skin.

node mapping and biopsy often eliminates the need to remove lymph nodes.

Results

Women are usually cancer free following a mastectomy. For a single tumor of less than 1.6 in. (4 cm) that is removed with clear margins, a lumpectomy plus radiation is at least as effective as a mastectomy. For women with small invasive breast cancers, radiation therapy following lumpectomy reduces the likelihood of recurrence by two-thirds.

Prophylactic mastectomy in healthy women with BRCA mutations reduces their risk of breast cancer by 90%. However, it is not clear whether women undergoing this procedure are at lower risk of dying from breast cancer than high-risk women who use careful surveillance methods.

Abnormal results

Abnormal mastectomy results include incomplete removal of the cancer or chronic pain or impairment that

does not improve after several months of physical therapy. There is approximately a 9%–10% chance of recurrence following a lumpectomy plus radiation therapy, or recurrence of cancer on the chest wall following a mastectomy.

Morbidity and mortality rates

Morbidity rates are modest. The most common problems include postoperative infection, unwanted scarring, lymphedema, and issues related to emotional adjustment. Mortality is extremely uncommon, averaging fewer than ten deaths per year.

Alternatives

There is no alternative to a medically indicated mastectomy, although breast-conserving surgery is often an option. Alternatives to post-mastectomy reconstructive surgery include the use of pads or breast forms. There are alternatives to prophylactic mastectomy, including genetic testing for BRCA mutations. Women at high risk for breast cancer because of BRCA mutations can use careful surveillance with frequent mammograms. They may also be able to reduce their breast cancer risk by taking **tamoxifen** or an aromatase inhibitor. In the past, mastectomies were performed on young women with early breast cancer because of the risk of recurrence. However, a recent large-scale study found that there were no differences in recurrence or survival between young women who had mastectomies and those who had breast-conserving surgery.

Resources

BOOKS

Berger, Karen, John Bostwick, and Glyn E. Jones. *A Woman's Decision: Breast Care, Treatment & Reconstruction.* 4th ed. St. Louis, MO: Quality Medical, 2011.

Curran Baker, Amy, Linda Curran, and MaryBeth Curran Brown. *Now What? A Patient's Guide to Recovery After Mastectomy.* New York: Demos Health, 2012.

Delinsky, Barbara. *Uplift: Secrets from the Sisterhood of Breast Cancer Survivors.* 10th ed. New York: Atria, 2011.

Friedman, Sue, Rebecca Sutphen, and Kathy Steligo. *Confronting Hereditary Breast and Ovarian Cancer: Identify Your Risk, Understand Your Options, Change Your Destiny.* Baltimore: Johns Hopkins University, 2012.

Levy, Robyn Michele. *Most of Me: Surviving My Medical Meltdown.* Vancouver, BC: Greystone, 2012.

Love, Susan M., and Karen Lindsey. *Dr. Susan Love's Breast Book.* Cambridge, MA: Da Capo Press, 2010.

Patenaude, Andrea Farkas. *Prophylactic Mastectomy: Insights from Women Who Chose to Reduce Their Risk.* Santa Barbara, CA: Praeger, 2012.

Steligo, Kathy. *The Breast Reconstruction Guidebook: Issues and Answers from Research to Recovery.* Baltimore: Johns Hopkins University, 2012.

PERIODICALS

Fallbjörk, Ulrika, Pär Salander, and Birgit H. Rasmussen. "From 'No Big Deal' to 'Losing Oneself:' Different Meanings of Mastectomy." *Cancer Nursing* 35, no. 5 (September/October 2012): E41.

Hurley, Richard. "Jolie, Genes, and the Double Mastectomy." *British Medical Journal* 346, no. 7909 (May 25, 2013): 27.

Mallon, P., et al. "The Role of Nipple-Sparing Mastectomy in Breast Cancer: A Comprehensive Review of the Literature." *Plastic and Reconstructive Surgery* 131, no. 5 (2013): 969–84. http://dx.doi.org/10.1097/PRS.0b013e3182865a3c (accessed October 3, 2014).

Parker-Pope, Tara. "Facing Cancer, a Stark Choice." *New York Times*, January 22, 2013.

Stenger, Matthew. "Neoadjuvant Aromatase Inhibitor Therapy Converts Many Patients to Candidates for Breast-Conserving Surgery." *ASCO Post* 3, no. 6 (2012). http://www.ascopost.com/issues/april-15-2012/neoadjuvant-aromatase-inhibitor-therapy-converts-many-patients-to-candidates-for-breast-conserving-surgery.aspx (accessed February 5, 2015).

Zagouri, Flora, et al. "Prophylactic Mastectomy: An Appraisal." *American Surgeon* 79, no. 2 (February 2013): 205–12.

OTHER

American Cancer Society. "Breast Reconstruction After Mastectomy." http://www.cancer.org/acs/groups/cid/docu ments/webcontent/002992-pdf.pdf (accessed October 3, 2014).

National Cancer Institute. "Surgery Choices for Women with DCIS or Breast Cancer." http://www.cancer.gov/cancertopics/treatment/breast/surgerychoices.pdf (accessed October 3, 2014).

WEBSITES

BreastCancer.org. "Mastectomy." http://www.breastcancer.org/treatment/surgery/mastectomy (accessed October 3, 2014).

Fox, Maggie, and JoNel Aleccia. "More Women Opting for Preventive Mastectomy—But Should They Be?" NBC News, May 15, 2013. http://www.nbcnews.com/health/more-women-opting-preventive-mastectomy-should-they-be-1C9918752 (accessed October 3, 2014).

London, Susan. "Breast Cancer Does Not Mandate Mastectomy in Young." American College of Surgeons, *Surgery News UpDATE*, September 16, 2011. http://www.facs.org/surgerynews/update/mastectomy0911.html (accessed October 3, 2014).

National Cancer Institute. "Breast Cancer Treatment." http://www.cancer.gov/cancertopics/pdq/treatment/breast/Patient/page5 (accessed October 3, 2014).

ORGANIZATIONS

American Cancer Society, 250 Williams St. NW, Atlanta, GA 30303, (800) 227-2345, http://www.cancer.org.

American College of Surgeons, 633 N. Saint Clair St., Chicago, IL 60611-3211, (312) 202-5000, (800) 621-4111, Fax: (312) 202-5001, postmaster@facs.org, http://www.facs.org.

Breastcancer.org, 7 E. Lancaster Ave., 3rd Fl., Ardmore, PA 19003, http://www.breastcancer.org.

National Breast Cancer Coalition, 1101 17th St. NW, Ste. 1300, Washington, DC 20036, (202) 296-7477, (800) 622-2838, Fax: (202) 265-6854, http://www.breastcancerdeadline2020.org.

National Cancer Institute, 6116 Executive Blvd., Ste. 300, Bethesda, MD 20892-8322, (800) 4-CANCER (422-6237), http://cancer.gov.

REVISED BY L. FLEMING FALLON, JR., MD, DRPH
Margaret Alic, PhD

PERIODICALS

Zucker, Stanley, and Jian Cao, et al. "Selective Matrix Metalloproteinase (MMP) Inhibitors In Cancer Therapy." *Cancer Biology & Therapy* 8, no. 24 (2009): 2371–73. http://www.ncbi.nlm.nih.gov/pmc/articles/PMC2829367/ (accessed October 31, 2014).

Crystal Heather Kaczkowski, MSc.

Matulane *see* **Procarbazine**

Maxeran *see* **Metoclopramide**

Matrix metalloproteinase inhibitors

Definition

Matrix metalloproteinases are a class of enzymes that can break down proteins, such as collagen and gelatin. Since these enzymes require zinc or calcium atoms to function, they are referred to as metalloproteinases. Matrix metalloproteinases function in tumor cell invasion and **metastasis**, wound healing, and **angiogenesis** (supplying the tumor with blood). They are normally found in the spaces between cells (extracellular) in tissues and are involved in degrading extracellular matrix proteins like collagens and gelatins. The extracellular matrix compartments are the primary barriers to tumor growth and spread. Matrix metalloproteinase inhibitors are selective inhibitors of matrix metalloproteinases. These agents inhibit tumor metastasis and angiogenesis.

Description

Matrix metalloproteinases have been linked to cancers such as breast, ovarian, colorectal, and lung. Synthetic matrix metalloproteinase inhibitors are being explored for use in **cancer prevention** and treatment because of their demonstrated antimetastatic and antiangiogenic properties. Matrix metalloproteinase inhibitors include compounds such as: Marimastat (BB-2516), COL-3, BAY 12-9566, and KB-R7785. Marimastat (BB-2516) was the first orally bioavailable matrix metalloproteinase inhibitor to enter **clinical trials** in the field of oncology. Developing nontoxic, orally active, MMP inhibitors is important because these compounds will likely need chronic administration in combination with other therapies.

Resources

BOOKS

Chu, Edward, and Vincent T. DeVita Jr. *Physicians' Cancer Chemotherapy Drug Manual 2014.* Burlington, MA: Jones & Bartlett Learning, 2014.

Clendeninn, Neil J., and Krzysztof Appelt, eds. *Matrix Metalloproteinase Inhibitors In Cancer Therapy.* Totowa, N.J.: Humana Press, 2000.

Mechlorethamine

Definition

Mechlorethamine is a **chemotherapy** medicine used to treat **cancer** by destroying cancerous cells. Mechlorethamine is marketed as the brand name Mustargen. It is also commonly known as nitrogen mustard.

Purpose

Mechlorethamine is approved by the U.S. Food and Drug Administration (FDA) to treat **Hodgkin lymphoma** and non-Hodgkin **lymphoma**. It is also approved for certain types of leukemia, malignant lymphomas, and lung cancer. Mechlorethamine has been used to relieve symptoms caused by a build up of cancerous fluid in the lungs, abdomen, and around the heart.

Description

Mechlorethamine is one of the first chemotherapy drugs discovered to have an effect on cancer cells. **Clinical trials** with this agent began in the 1940s. Mechlorethamine is a member of the group of chemotherapy drugs known as alkylating agents. Alkylating agents interfere with the genetic material (DNA) inside the cancer cells, more specifically through cross-linking DNA strands, and prevent them from further dividing and growing more cancer cells. Mechlorethamine is commonly combined with other chemotherapy agents to treat cancer.

Recommended dosage

A mechlorethamine dose can be determined using a mathematical calculation that measures a person's body surface area (BSA). This number is dependent upon a patient's height and weight. The larger the person, the greater the body surface area. BSA is measured in the units known as square meter (m^2). The body surface area is calculated and then multiplied by the drug dosage in

KEY TERMS

Anemia—A red blood cell count that is lower than normal.

Antidote—A drug given to reverse the negative effects of another drug.

Chemotherapy—Specific drugs used to treat cancer.

Deoxynucleic acid (DNA)—Genetic material inside of cells that carries the information to make proteins that are necessary to run the cells and keep the body functioning smoothly.

Food and Drug Administration (FDA)—The government agency that oversees public safety in relation to drugs and medical devices, and gives the approval to pharmaceutical companies for commercial marketing of their products.

Intravenous—To enter the body through a vein.

Metastatic—Cancer that has spread to one or more parts of the body.

Neutropenia—A white blood cell count that is lower than normal.

milligrams per square meter (mg/m^2). This calculates the actual dose a patient is to receive.

Mechlorethamine is a yellowish liquid that is injected directly into a vein over a period of one to five minutes. It can also be applied onto the skin as an ointment for certain conditions.

Mechlorethamine is combined with other chemotherapeutic drugs **vincristine** (Oncovin), **procarbazine**, and prednisone for treatment of Hodgkin lymphoma. The dose of mechlorethamine used in this regimen is 6 mg per square meter on day 1 and day 8 of a treatment cycle. This regimen is referred to as MOPP, and was one the initial regimens that caused a breakthrough in the treatment of Hodgkin lymphoma.

Mechlorethamine can also be infused into certain compartments in the body where cancerous fluid has accumulated. The dose for this treatment is based on a patient's weight in kilograms (1 kilogram is 2.2 pounds). Mechlorethamine is given at a dose of 0.2 to 0.4 mg per kilogram of body weight, infused directly into the area where the fluid is building up.

Precautions

Patients should notify their doctors if they have had any previous allergic reactions to chemotherapy treatment or if they have received **radiation therapy**.

Blood counts should be monitored regularly while on mechlorethamine therapy. During a certain time period after receiving mechlorethamine, there may be an increased risk of getting infections. Caution should be taken to avoid unnecessary exposure to crowds and people with infections.

Patients who may be pregnant or are trying to become pregnant should tell their doctors before receiving mechlorethamine. Chemotherapy can cause men and women to become sterile, or unable to have children.

Patients should check with their doctors before receiving live virus vaccines while on chemotherapy.

Patients should increase their intake of fluids while on this medication.

Side effects

One of the most common side effects from receiving mechlorethamine is **nausea and vomiting**. The nausea and vomiting can begin within one hour from receiving the drug. Patients will be given **antiemetics** before and after receiving mechlorethamine to help prevent or decrease this side effect.

A common side effect from taking mechlorethamine is low blood cell counts (**myelosuppression**). When the white blood cell count is lower than normal (**neutropenia**), patients are at an increased risk of developing **fever** and infections. The platelet blood count can also be decreased. Platelets are blood cells in the body that cause clots to form to stop bleeding. When the platelet count is low, patients are at an increased risk for bruising and bleeding. Low red blood cell counts (**anemia**), make people feel tired, dizzy, and lacking in energy.

Less common side effects from mechlorethamine include **diarrhea**, loss of appetite (**anorexia**), mouth sores, liver problems, metallic taste in the mouth, fever, ringing in the ears or hearing loss, and inflammation at the injection site. Allergic reactions have been reported, some of them severe anaphylactic reactions.

Damage to nerves and nervous system tissues is uncommon with mechlorethamine therapy. However, some reports do exist of nerve damage that has resulted in numbness and tingling in the hands and feet.

Mechlorethamine can cause skin reactions. When applied on top of the skin, the area can become red, swollen, brown colored, itchy, and have a burning sensation.

Hair loss (**alopecia**), irritation, and change of color of the vein where the drug was injected can occur. If the drug is not given directly into the vein, or is accidentally injected into surrounding areas of tissue, an antidote must be administered to that area as soon as possible. The area will become painful, gray-colored, and the tissue will begin to die. This is considered a severe reaction, and medical personnel must be notified immediately.

Interactions

Radiation therapy along with mechlorethamine administration can cause severe damage to the bone marrow.

Resources

BOOKS

Chu, Edward, and Vincent T. DeVita Jr. *Physicians' Cancer Chemotherapy Drug Manual 2014*. Burlington, MA: Jones & Bartlett Learning, 2014.

WEBSITES

AHFS Consumer Medication Information. "Mechlorethamine." American Society of Health-System Pharmacists. Available from: http://www.nlm.nih.gov/medlineplus/druginfo/meds/a682223.html (accessed October 31, 2014).

American Cancer Society. "Mechlorethamine." http://www.cancer.org/treatment/treatmentsandsideeffects/guide tocancerdrugs/mechlorethamine (accessed November 3, 2014).

Nancy J. Beaulieu, R.Ph., B.C.O.P.

Meclizine

Definition

Meclizine is an antihistamine commonly used to control nausea, vomiting, and dizziness. It is known by the over-the-counter name Bonine. In the United States, the prescription brand name is Antivert.

Purpose

Meclizine may be given to help control **nausea and vomiting** that often occurs with **cancer** treatment, other medical conditions, or motion sickness. It is also used as part of palliative care for patients with terminal cancer.

More recently, meclizine has been reported to be effective in the treatment of panic disorder.

Description

Meclizine acts as a central nervous system depressant. It is believed its therapeutic actions occur due to the

KEY TERMS

Antihistamine—Agent that blocks or counteracts the action of histamine, which is released during an allergic reaction.

Palliative—Referring to treatments that are intended to relieve pain and other symptoms of disease but not to cure.

drug's drying effects and its ability to depress conduction of nerve messages in the inner ear. Meclizine begins working about one hour after ingestion. It continues being effective for eight to 24 hours.

Recommended dosage

The dosage to control nausea and vomiting associated with cancer treatment is 25–50 mg, every eight to 12 hours. When used to manage dizziness, patients generally take 25–100 mg daily in divided doses. Patients should not double up on this medication if a dose is missed.

Precautions

Patients with glaucoma, an enlarged prostate, bladder or bowel obstructions, or asthma or other breathing difficulties should discuss with the doctor the risks and benefits associated with this drug before taking it. Those who have experienced an allergic reaction to meclizine should not take it. The FDA recommends that youngsters under age 12 should not take this drug, except under the direction of a physician. Pregnant women and those trying to become pregnant should not take this medication. Animal reproductive studies have shown some deformities at elevated doses. Women who are breastfeeding should discuss this medication with their doctors prior to taking it.

Side effects

Meclizine may cause drowsiness and **fatigue**. Drowsiness is the most common adverse reaction. Alcohol and other central nervous system depressants, such as pain medication and tranquilizers, may increase this effect. Patients should refrain from drinking alcoholic beverages, and avoid driving or operating machinery or appliances when taking this drug. Less frequently, the drug also may produce the opposite effect. Excitability, nervousness, restlessness, mood enhancement and difficulty sleeping may develop. Rarely, it may cause a patient to see or hear things that are not present (hallucinations). Despite being used to treat nausea and vomiting, it may produce this effect. It may also cause constipation, **diarrhea**, an upset stomach or a poor appetite (**anorexia**). Other side effects include frequent or difficult urination, incomplete emptying of the bladder, low blood pressure, a rapid heart rate or palpitations. It may cause vision changes, a dry nose and throat, ringing in the ears, and a rash or hives. Some of the side effects may be more pronounced in older adults.

Side effects may decrease as the body adjusts to the medication. Ice chips or sugarless hard candy or gum may help relieve the dry mouth. If the feeling of a dry mouth persists for more than two weeks, the doctor should be notified.

Interactions

Central nervous system depressants, including alcohol, may increase drowsiness associated with meclizine. Pain medications, other antihistamines, seizure medications, sleeping pills and muscle relaxants can depress the central nervous system. Taking this drug with some medications used to treat **depression** may increase the risk of side effects. Patients should inform the doctor of all medications being taken. Patients should not start or stop any drugs without the approval of the doctor. The herbal supplement henbane may increase some of meclizine's side effects, including dry mouth and difficulty urinating.

Resources

BOOKS

Beers, Mark H., MD, and Robert Berkow, MD, editors. "Care of the Dying Patient." In *The Merck Manual of Diagnosis and Therapy*. Whitehouse Station, NJ: Merck Research Laboratories, 2007.

WEBSITES

Healthwise. "Meclizine." Norris Cotton Cancer Center, Dartmouth. http://cancer.dartmouth.edu/pf/health_encyclopedia/d00859a1 (accessed November 14, 2014).

Micromedex. "Meclizine, Buclizine, And Cyclizine (Oral Route, Parenteral Route)." Mayo Clinic. http://www.mayoclinic.org/drugs-supplements/meclizine-buclizine-and-cyclizine-oral-route-parenteral-route/description/drg-20069630 (accessed November 14, 2014).

ORGANIZATIONS

U.S. Food and Drug Administration, 10903 New Hampshire Ave., Silver Spring, MD 20993, (888) INFO-FDA (463-6332), http://www.fda.gov.

Debra Wood, R.N.
Rebecca J. Frey, PhD

Mediastinal tumors

Definition

A mediastinal tumor is a growth in the central chest cavity (mediastinum), which separates the lungs and contains the heart, aorta, esophagus, thymus, and trachea. Mediastinal tumors are also known as neoplasms of the mediastinum.

Description

Growths that originate in the mediastinum are called primary mediastinal tumors. Most of them are composed of reproductive (germ) cells or develop in thymic, neurogenic (nerve), lymphatic, or mesenchymal (soft) tissue.

Secondary (metastatic) mediastinal tumors originate in the lung, stomach, esophagus, and trachea, and spread through the lymphatic system to the chest cavity.

Although still relatively rare, malignant mediastinal tumors are becoming more common. Usually diagnosed in patients between 30 and 50 years old, they can develop at any age and arise from any tissue that exists in or passes through the chest cavity.

The mediastinum is traditionally divided into superior, anterior, middle, and posterior compartments, and is also described as having anterosuperior, middle, and posterior divisions. Boundaries of these divisions are not fixed, and they frequently overlap.

Mediastinal tumors

Cancer type	Occurs in
Thymomas	Anterior mediastinum, almost always form where heart and major vessels meet
Teratomas	Anterior mediastinum, along the center of the body between the skull and kidneys
Lymphomas	Anterior and middle mediastinum
Thyroid tumors	Thyroid (anterior mediastinum)
Mesenchymal tumors (soft tissue tumors)	Middle mediastinum
Carcinomas	Middle mediastinum
Neurogenic tumors (developing in nerve cells)	Posterior mediastinum
Malignant schwannomas	Posterior mediastinum
Neuroblastomas	Posterior mediastinum

Table listing types of mediastinal tumors. *(Table by GGS Creative Resources. © Cengage Learning®.)*

The anterosuperior compartment contains a vein and the thymus gland, superior vena cava, aortic arch, and thyroid gland. More than half (54%) of mediastinal tumors in adults and 43% of those in children occur in the anterosuperior compartment.

The middle mediastinum contains the pericardium, heart, nerves of the diaphragm (phrenic nerves), trachea, main bronchial stem, and lung hila. Twenty percent of adult mediastinal tumors and 18% of those in children occur in this division.

The posterior mediastinum contains the sympathetic chain, vagus nerve (which controls the heart, larynx, and gastrointestinal tract), thoracic duct (which drains lymph from the abdomen, legs, and left side of the head and chest), descending thoracic aorta, and the esophagus. Slightly more than one fourth (26%) of adult mediastinal tumors and 40% of those in children occur in the posterior mediastinum.

Each of these compartments also contains lymph nodes and fatty tissue.

Types of cancers

Anterior mediastinal tumors

The most common anterior mediastinal tumors are thymomas, teratomas, lymphomas, and thyroid tissue that has become enlarged or displaced (ectopic).

THYMOMAS. The cause of most adult mediastinal tumors and 15% of those in children, thymomas almost always form at the spot where the heart and great vessels meet. These tumors usually develop between the ages of 40 and 60.

About half of the people who have thymomas do not have any symptoms. Between 35% and 50% experience symptoms of **myasthenia gravis**, such as

• weakness of the eye muscles
• drooping of one or both eyelids (ptosis)
• fatigue

Early treatment of these slow-growing tumors is very effective. Most are benign, but thymomas can metastasize and should always be considered cancerous.

TERATOMAS. Most common in young adults, teratomas are made up of embryonic (germ) cells that did not develop normally and do not belong in the part of the body where the tumor is located. Found along the center of the body between the skull and kidneys, teratomas account for:

• 10%–15% of primary mediastinal tumors
• 70% of germ cell tumors in children
• 60% of germ cell tumors in adults

Teratomas may be solid or contain cysts. Malignant teratomas usually develop between the ages of 30 and 40, and almost all (90%) of them occur in men.

At least 90% of patients with these tumors experience:

• chest pain
• cough
• fever
• shortness of breath

These symptoms may not appear until the tumor has grown very large.

LYMPHOMAS. These tumors account for 10%–20% of anterior mediastinal tumors. Although lymphomas are the second most common mediastinal tumor in children, they are usually diagnosed between the ages of 30 and 40. Nonsclerosing **Hodgkin lymphoma** causes most adult mediastinal lymphomas.

Some patients with lymphomas do not have symptoms. Others cough or experience chest pain.

THYROID TUMORS. Most mediastinal thyroid tumors grow out of goiters and occur in women between the ages of 50 and 60. About 75% of these tumors extend to the windpipe (trachea). The rest extend behind it.

Mediastinal thyroid tumors are encapsulated and do not metastasize.

Middle mediastinal tumors

Tumors of the middle mediastinum include lymphomas, mesenchymal tumors, and carcinomas.

MESENCHYMAL TUMORS. Also called soft tissue tumors, mesenchymal tumors originate in connective tissue within the chest cavity. These tumors account for about 6% of primary mediastinal tumors. More than half (55%) of them are malignant.

The most common mesenchymal tumors are lipomas, liposarcomas, fibromas, and fibrosarcomas.

Posterior mediastinal tumors

Tumors of the posterior mediastinum include neurogenic tumors, mesenchymal tumors, and endocrine tumors.

NEUROGENIC TUMORS. Representing 19%–39% of mediastinal tumors, neurogenic tumors can develop at any age. They are most common in young adults.

Adult neurogenic tumors are usually benign. In children, they tend to be malignant and tend to metastasize before symptoms appear.

MALIGNANT SCHWANNOMAS. Also known as malignant sheath tumors, malignant sarcomas, and neurosarcomas, these tumors develop from the tube (sheath) enclosing the peripheral nerves that transmit impulses from the central nervous system (CNS) to muscles and organs.

Usually large and painful, these rare, aggressive tumors may invade the lungs, bones, and aorta.

NEUROBLASTOMAS. The most common malignant tumors of early childhood, neuroblastomas generally occur before the age of two. These tumors usually develop in the adrenal glands, neck, abdomen, or pelvis.

Neuroblastomas often spread to other organs. Most patients have symptoms that relate to the part of the body the tumor has invaded. Likelihood of survival is greatest in patients who are less than a year old and whose tumor has not spread.

Symptoms

About 40% of people who have mediastinal tumors do not have any symptoms. When symptoms exist, they usually result from pressure on an organ that the tumor has invaded, and indicate that the tumor is malignant.

The symptoms most commonly associated with mediastinal tumors are:

• chest pain
• cough
• shortness of breath

Other symptoms associated with mediastinal tumors include:

• hoarseness
• hemoptysis (coughing up blood)
• fatigue
• difficulty swallowing (dysphagia)
• night sweats
• systemic lupus erythematosus
• inflamed muscles (polymyositis)
• ulcerative colitis
• rheumatoid arthritis
• thyroid problems (thyroiditis, thyrotoxicosis,)
• fever
• glandular disorders (panhypopituitarism, adenopathy)
• high blood pressure
• low blood sugar (hypoglycemia)
• breast development in males (gynecomastia)
• wheezing
• vocal cord paralysis

• heart problems (superior vena cava syndrome, pericardial tamponade, arrhythmias)
• neurologic abnormalities
• weight loss
• other immune, autoimmune, and endocrine system disorders

Blood disorders associated with these tumors include abnormally high levels of calcium (**hypercalcemia**); abnormally low numbers of circulating blood cells (cytopenia), normal red blood cells (pernicious anemia), or antibodies (hypogammaglobulinemia); and an inability to produce red blood cells (red-cell aplasia).

Diagnosis

Imaging studies

Routine x-rays often detect mediastinal tumors. Doctors use **computed tomography** (CT) scans of the chest to determine tumor size and location, extent of disease, the tumor's relationship to nearby organs and tissues, and whether the tumor contains cysts or areas of calcification.

Magnetic resonance imaging (MRI) is more effective at clarifying the relationship between a tumor and nearby blood vessels, but is far more costly and time-consuming than CT scanning.

Other tests

Injecting radioactive substances into the patient's blood (radioimmunoassay) enables doctors to measure levels of hormones and other substances a tumor secretes and identify specific tumor types, evaluate the effectiveness of therapy, and monitor possible tumor recurrence.

Invasive procedures

Imaging studies play the most important role in initial diagnosis of mediastinal tumors, but before doctors can determine the most effective treatment for any tumor, they must know what kind of cells it contains.

Although invasive diagnostic procedures have been largely replaced by less invasive techniques (such as CT-guided percutaneous needle **biopsy**), some patients still require surgery.

MEDIASTINOSCOPY. Performed under general anesthesia, this relatively simple procedure enables doctors to accurately diagnose 80%–90% of mediastinal tumors, and 95%–100% of anterior mediastinal tumors.

Mediastinoscopy is especially useful in providing the large tissue specimens needed to diagnose lymphomas.

MEDIASTINOTOMY. Doctors perform mediastinotomy by using a lighted tube to:

- examine the center of the chest and nearby lymph nodes
- remove tissue for biopsy
- determine whether cancer has spread from the spot where it originated. Similar to mediastinoscopy, this procedure begins with a small incision next to the breastbone, rather than in the patient's neck.

Mediastinotomy also enables doctors to examine the lymph nodes closest to the heart and lungs. **Cancer** that originates in the left upper lobe of the lung often spreads to these nodes.

THORACOTOMY. Although some surgeons still perform this procedure to diagnose mediastinal tumors, **thoracoscopy** may be used instead in certain situations. In a **thoracotomy**, the physician gains access to the chest cavity by cutting through the chest wall. Thoracotomy allows for study, examination, treatment, or removal of any organs in the chest cavity. Tumors and metastatic growths can be removed, and a biopsy can be taken, through the incision. Thoracotomy also gives access to the heart, esophagus, diaphragm, and the portion of the aorta that passes through the chest cavity.

THORACOSCOPY. This 100% accurate, minimally invasive procedure is performed under general anesthesia. Enabling the surgeon to view the entire mediastinum, thoracoscopy may be used when a mediastinal tumor touches the mediastinal pleura; however, this procedure has limited applications.

Thoracoscopy cannot be performed on a patient who has thick scar tissue.

Treatment

Doctors use surgery, radiation, and single-agent or combination **chemotherapy** to treat mediastinal tumors.

Thymomas

A patient whose **thymoma** is surgically removed (resected) has the best chance of survival. To lessen the likelihood of new tumors developing (reseeding), surgeons do not recommend biopsy, and try to remove the tumor without puncturing the capsule that encloses it.

RADIATION. Thymomas respond well to radiation, which is used:

- to treat all stages of disease
- before or after surgical resection
- to treat recurrent disease

The course of treatment lasts three to six weeks. The most common complications of **radiation therapy** are formation of scar tissue in the lungs (pulmonary fibrosis), inflammation of the pericardium (pericarditis), and inflammation of the spinal cord (myelitis).

CHEMOTHERAPY. The use of chemotherapy to treat invasive thymomas is becoming more common. One or more drugs may be administered before or after surgery. Synthetic hormones (**corticosteroids**) can reverse the progression of tumors that do not respond to chemotherapy.

Teratomas

Teratomas are removed surgically. Chemotherapy and radiation are not used to treat these tumors. The prospect for long-term cure is excellent, and these tumors rarely recur.

Lymphomas

These tumors do not require surgery, except to make the diagnosis. Doctors treat them with chemotherapy and radiation.

Thyroid tumors

Doctors generally treat thyroid tumors with surgical resection, chemotherapy, and/or radiation.

Fibrosarcomas

Fibrosarcomas cannot usually be resected and do not respond well to chemotherapy.

Malignant schwannomas

Multiagent chemotherapy is used to treat these aggressive tumors, which tend to recur following surgery. The 5-year survival rate is 75%.

Neuroblastomas

Because these tumors sometimes regress spontaneously, doctors may postpone treatment if the patient has no symptoms or the tumor is not growing.

In other cases, doctors remove these tumors even before symptoms appear. Risks associated with removing these tumors from the spinal canal include:

- injury to the spinal cord or anterior spinal artery
- uncontrolled bleeding in the spinal canal
- decreased blood supply (ischemia) to tissues and organs.

See also CT-guided biopsy; Fibrosarcoma; Neuroblastoma; Thyroid cancer.

Resources

WEBSITES

A.D.A.M. Medical Encylopedia. "Mediastinal Tumor." MedlinePlus. http://www.nlm.nih.gov/medlineplus/ency/article/001086.htm (accessed November 19, 2014).

Boston Medical Center. "Mediastinal Tumor." http://www.bmc.org/thoraciconcology/diseases-conditions/mediastinal-tumor.htm (accessed November 19, 2014).

Maureen Haggerty

Mediastinoscopy

Definition

Mediastinoscopy is a surgical procedure that enables physicians to view areas of the mediastinum, the cavity behind the sternum (breastbone) that lies between the lungs. The organs in the mediastinum include the heart and its vessels; lymph nodes; and the trachea, esophagus, and thymus. Mediastinoscopy with **biopsy** is minor surgery for the removal of tissues from the mediastinum through very small incisions.

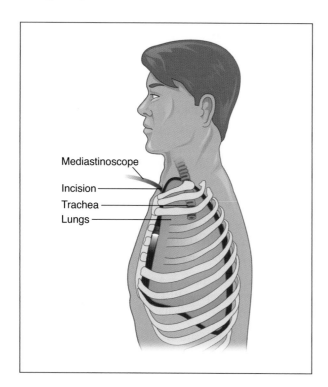

Mediastinoscope

Incision

Trachea

Lungs

A mediastinoscopy is a surgical procedure most commonly used to detect or stage cancer in the lungs and the surrounding areas. *(Illustration by Electronic Illustrators Group. © Cengage Learning®.)*

Purpose

Mediastinoscopy is most commonly used to detect or stage lung **cancer**, **mesothelioma**, or other cancers, such as **esophageal cancer**, and to determine whether the cancer has spread to the lymph nodes of the chest. It is also often the diagnostic method of choice for detecting **lymphoma** (cancer of lymphatic tissues), including **Hodgkin lymphoma**. Staging of lung and other cancers involves determining the level or progression of the cancer. Stages provide consistent definitions of cancer levels and may indicate the appropriate treatments. Staging also provides some guidance for prognosis. Mediastinoscopy and biopsy (tissue removal) from lymph nodes and other tissues or from abnormal growths in the front part of the mediastinum near the chest wall are likely to reveal whether a lung cancer has spread beyond the lungs. Mediastinoscopy is also useful for examining the outside surfaces of the airway tubes, such as the trachea, and for evaluating masses or tumors in the middle chest.

The lymph nodes between the lungs can also be biopsied during mediastinoscopy to check for infection. Mediastinoscopy is commonly performed on patients with enlarged lymph nodes to determine whether the enlargement is due to infection or a lung cancer that has spread to the nodes. Mediastinoscopy is used to detect infections such as tuberculosis, sarcoidosis (a chronic lung disease), and to confirm the diagnosis of certain other conditions and diseases of the respiratory organs, including autoimmune disorders.

Mediastinoscopy may be used to verify a diagnosis that was not confirmed by other methods, such as radiographic and laboratory studies. If a malignant tumor is confirmed during mediastinoscopy, the surgeon may immediately perform a surgical procedure to remove the tumor, combining the diagnostic and surgical procedures into one operation.

Description

Mediastinoscopy is usually performed in a hospital operating room under general anesthesia. Before the general anesthesia is administered, local anesthesia is applied to the throat for the insertion of an endotracheal tube through the nose or mouth into the trachea. This enables the patient to breathe under general anesthesia while the head is tilted far back for the procedure. The tube keeps the throat open with the neck bent backward. A very small incision of less than 1 in. (2.5 cm) is made, usually just below the neck or at the notch at the top of the sternum (breastbone) just above the clavicles. Carbon dioxide gas flows into the chest through this opening, and the lungs are allowed to collapse slightly, providing the

KEY TERMS

Biopsy—The removal of cells or tissue for examination by a pathologist.

Cauterize—To use heat or chemicals to stop bleeding, prevent the spread of infection, or destroy tissue.

Endotracheal tube—A tube placed down the trachea (windpipe).

Hodgkin lymphoma—A malignancy of lymphoid tissue in the lymph nodes, spleen, liver, or bone marrow.

Lymph nodes—Small round structures located throughout the body that contain immune system cells for fighting infection.

Mediastinoscope—A thin hollow tube for performing mediastinoscopy.

Mediastinotomy—Surgical incision into the mediastinum.

Mediastinum—The space in the chest between the lungs that contains the heart and its vessels, lymph nodes, the trachea, esophagus, and thymus.

Mesothelioma—A tumor derived from mesothelial tissue such as the lining of the lungs, thorax, or perineum.

Pleural space—The space between the layers of the pleura—the membrane lining the lungs and thorax.

Positron emission tomography (PET)—A method of medical imaging capable of displaying the metabolic activity of organs.

Sarcoidosis—A chronic disease characterized by nodules in the lungs, skin, lymph nodes, and bones, although any tissue or organ in the body may be affected.

Thymus—An organ in the mediastinal cavity that is important for the body's immune response.

Ultrasound—An imaging method in which high-frequency sound waves are used to outline an internal region of the body.

surgeon with space to work. The soft tissue of the neck is dissected down to the trachea. The surgeon may clear a path to first feel the lymph nodes for any abnormalities. The surgeon then inserts the mediastinoscope, a type of endoscope, through the incision along the side of the trachea. The mediastinoscope is a narrow, hollow tube with an attached light and a camera that projects images of the organs inside the mediastinum onto a video screen. Tools can be inserted through the hollow tube of the mediastinoscope for performing biopsies. A tissue sample from the lymph nodes or a mass along the trachea or major bronchial tubes can be removed and examined under a microscope or sent to a laboratory for further testing.

Mediastinotomy is the surgical opening of the mediastinum and is complementary to mediastinoscopy. Mediastinotomy provides direct access to lymph nodes that are inaccessible by mediastinoscopy and, like mediastinoscopy, is used to evaluate or excise diseased lymph nodes and stage cancers. One or two small incisions, usually next to the sternum and between the ribs, enable the surgeon to insert additional instruments to cut out and remove lymph nodes. Other instruments are used to cauterize bleeding blood vessels with a small electric current. A chest x-ray is usually taken after the procedure.

In some cases, if tissue sample analysis indicates a malignancy, surgery may be performed immediately, while the patient is already prepared and under anesthesia. In other cases, the surgeon will complete the visual study and biopsy, remove the instruments, reinflate the lungs, and stitch the small incisions closed. The patient will remain in the surgical recovery area until the effects of anesthesia have lessened, usually within a few minutes, and it is safe to leave the area. The entire procedure usually requires about 60–90 minutes, in addition to preparation and recovery time.

Mediastinoscopy is a safe, thorough, and cost-effective diagnostic tool that presents less risk than some other diagnostic procedures. However, **positron emission tomography** (PET) scanning has reduced the use of mediastinoscopy for staging cancers.

Demographics

Approximately 130,000 new pulmonary nodules are diagnosed each year in the United States, about half of which are malignant lung cancers. Many of these are diagnosed via mediastinoscopy.

Precautions

Because mediastinoscopy is a surgical procedure, it should only be performed when the potential benefits outweigh the risks of anesthesia and surgery. Patients who had mediastinoscopy previously should not have it again if there is scarring from the first procedure. Several other medical conditions, such as impaired cerebral circulation, obstruction or distortion of the upper airway, or thoracic aortic aneurysm (abnormal dilation of the thoracic aorta) may also preclude mediastinoscopy.

Certain structures in a person's anatomy that can be compressed by the mediastinoscope may complicate these pre-existing medical conditions. Mediastinal irradiation is also a contraindication for mediastinoscopy.

Preparation

Mediastinoscopy is generally performed after other imaging tests, such as **computed tomography** (CT) scans, have suggested that a cancer may have spread to the lymph nodes between the lungs. The specific procedures of the mediastinoscopy are discussed with the patient. Patients also meet with their anesthesiologist to discuss their medical history and the anesthesia to be used. Patients sign a consent form after reviewing the risks of the procedure and the known risks and reactions to anesthesia. The physician will normally instruct the patient not to eat or drink anything after midnight before the test, until after the procedure is completed. This helps prevent nausea from the anesthesia. Patients should inform their physician of all medications they are currently taking, including **vitamins**, supplements, and over-the-counter drugs, as it may be necessary to stop or adjust dosages of any substances that affect blood clotting before undergoing mediastinoscopy. The physician may prescribe a sedative the night before and again immediately before the procedure. A local anesthetic is usually applied to the throat to prevent discomfort during placement of the endotracheal tube.

Aftercare

Following mediastinoscopy, patients are carefully monitored for any changes in vital signs or symptoms of complications from the procedure or anesthesia. The patient may have a sore throat from the endotracheal tube, experience temporary chest pain, and/or have soreness or tenderness at the incision site. Discomfort at the incision site(s) may last for a few days. Patients usually go home the same day, but must be driven since the medications will leave them drowsy for several hours. They should not drink alcohol for the rest of the day and should notify the doctor if **fever**, shortness of breath, or shoulder or chest pain develop. The patient will be left with a small straight scar of less than 1 in. (2.5 cm).

Risks

Complications from mediastinoscopy are relatively rare, although the usual risks associated with general anesthesia also apply to this procedure. Major and minor complications from general anesthesia occur in 3%–10% of all surgical patients. These are primarily heart and lung problems or infections. Complications from mediastinoscopy occur in less than 1% of patients. There is a risk of puncturing the esophagus, trachea, or blood vessels, which can lead to bleeding. The following complications, in decreasing order of frequency, have also been reported:

- pneumothorax—air in the pleural space, which can cause lung collapse but may be treated by inserting a drainage tube in the chest between the ribs for a few days
- vocal cord weakening or paralysis, causing hoarseness, due to recurrent laryngeal nerve injury
- infection
- tumor implantation in the wound
- injury to a thoracic nerve
- esophageal injury
- chylothorax—milky lymphatic fluid in the pleural space—from injury to a lymphatic duct
- air embolism (an air bubble)
- transient hemiparesis (paralysis on one side of the body)

Results

Mediastinoscopy biopsy results are generally available in five to seven days. Normal results of lymph node biopsies will indicate small, smooth lymph nodes with no abnormal tissue, growths, or signs of cancer or infection. Abnormal findings may indicate lung cancer, tuberculosis, sarcoidosis, lymphoma, Hodgkin lymphoma, or spread of disease from elsewhere in the body. In the case of lung cancer staging, the results indicate the severity and progression of the cancer. Mediastinoscopy with **lymph node biopsy** can indicate whether a cancer is localized or has begun to spread, which may affect treatment options. Mediastinoscopy can also be useful for distinguishing between lung cancer and mesothelioma, since lung cancers often spread to the lymph nodes, whereas mesothelioma spreads less often.

Mediastinoscopy results in a diagnosis in 10%–75% of cases, depending on the histology, location, and size of the cancer. However, the rate of false positives—diagnosing disease that is not present—can be as high as 20% with mediastinoscopy.

Alternatives

Although mediastinoscopies continue to be performed, advancements in computed tomography (CT), **magnetic resonance imaging** (MRI), **ultrasonography** techniques, and PET scanning have led to a decline in its use. However, these less invasive techniques, especially ultrasound, are not as specific as mediastinoscopy and may not be as useful for diagnosis. Improved fine-needle aspiration (withdrawing fluid using suction) and core-

QUESTIONS TO ASK YOUR DOCTOR

- Why do I need mediastinoscopy?
- What information will the procedure provide?
- How long will the mediastinoscopy take?
- When will the results be available?
- What are the potential complications of mediastinoscopy?

needle biopsy (using a needle to obtain a small tissue sample) have reduced the need for mediastinoscopy and biopsy. New techniques in **thoracoscopy** (examination of the thoracic cavity with a lighted instrument called a thoracoscope) offer additional options for examining masses in the mediastinum. Mediastinoscopy may be required when other methods cannot be used or when the results from other methods are inconclusive.

Health care team roles

Mediastinoscopy is usually performed by a thoracic or general surgeon or a trained pulmonary specialist.

Resources

BOOKS

Karlet, Mary C. "Mediastinoscopy." In *Case Studies in Nurse Anesthesia*, edited by Sass Elisha. Sudbury, MA: Jones and Bartlett, 2011.

McKenna, Robert J., Ali Mahtabifard, and Scott J. Swanson. *Atlas of Minimally Invasive Thoracic Surgery (VATS)*. Philadelphia: Elsevier/Saunders, 2011.

Wetherall, Sharon, and Philip M. Hartigan. "Bronchoscopy and Mediastinoscopy." In *Essential Clinical Anesthesia*, edited by Charles A. Vacanti. New York: Cambridge University, 2011.

PERIODICALS

Waller, D., and K. M. Skwarski. "Is There Still a Role for Mediastinoscopy as the First Mediastinal Staging Procedure in Lung Cancer?" *Journal of the Royal College of Physicians of Edinburgh* 43, no. 2 (2013): 137–43. http://dx.doi.org/10.4997/JRCPE.2013.211 (accessed October 3, 2014).

WEBSITES

A.D.A.M. Medical Encyclopedia. "Mediastinoscopy with Biopsy." MedlinePlus. http://www.nlm.nih.gov/medlineplus/ency/article/003864.htm (accessed October 3, 2014).

Harvard Health Publications. "Mediastinoscopy." Harvard Medical School. http://www.health.harvard.edu/diagnostic-tests/mediastinoscopy.htm (accessed October 3, 2014).

Lechtzin, Noah. "Mediastinoscopy and Mediastinotomy." *The Merck Manual for Health Care Professionals*. http://www.merckmanuals.com/professional/pulmonary_disorders/diagnostic_pulmonary_procedures/mediastinoscopy_and_mediastinotomy.html (accessed October 3, 2014).

Marshall, M. Blair. "Lung/Thoracic Surgery." The Society of Thoracic Surgeons. http://www.sts.org/patient-information/lung/thoracic-surgery (accessed October 3, 2014).

ORGANIZATIONS

American Cancer Society, 250 Williams St. NW, Atlanta, GA 30303, (800) 227-2345, http://www.cancer.org.

American College of Surgeons, 633 N. Saint Clair St., Chicago, IL 60611-3211, (312) 202-5000, (800) 621-4111, Fax: (312) 202-5001, postmaster@facs.org, http://www.facs.org.

American Lung Association, 1301 Pennsylvania Ave. NW, Ste. 800, Washington, DC 20004, (202) 785-3355, (800) LUNG-USA (586-4872), http://www.lung.org.

The Society of Thoracic Surgeons, 633 N. Saint Clair St., Fl. 23, Chicago, IL 60611, (312) 202-5800, Fax: (312) 202-5801, http://sts.org.

L. Fleming Fallon, Jr., MD, DrPH
Margaret Alic, PhD

Medroxyprogesterone acetate

Definition

Medroxyprogesterone acetate (MPA) is used during **cancer** therapy to stop new cell growth in some cancers. It is also used outside of cancer treatment as a contraceptive. MPA is known by many different brand names in the United States including Amen, Depo-Provera, Provera, Prodasone, and Progeston.

Purpose

MPA is used to treat some advanced, hormone-responsive cancers of the breast, kidney, and lining of the uterus.

Description

MPA is a synthetic derivative of the female hormone progesterone. In healthy women, progesterone plays a major role in preparing the uterus for pregnancy. MPA has been approved by the Food and Drug Administration (FDA), and its use in cancer treatment is usually covered by insurance. Outside the area of cancer treatment, it is used to prevent pregnancy.

KEY TERMS

Endometrial cancer—Cancer of the uterus.

Food and Drug Administration (FDA)—The government agency that oversees public safety in relation to drugs and medical devices, and gives the approval to pharmaceutical companies for commercial marketing of their products.

Exactly why MPA stops tumor growth is unclear. Many cancerous tumors are sensitive to hormones. It appears that MPA, in some way, changes the hormonal climate of the tumor so that cells stop responding to other hormones and proteins that would normally stimulate their growth. This drug cannot tell the difference between normal cells and cancer cells, so some normal cells are also killed during treatment. But since cancer cells generally grow more rapidly than normal cells, more cancer cells are killed. MPA is considered very effective and relatively non-toxic.

MPA is usually given to women whose **breast cancer** has returned or whose cancer does not respond to **tamoxifen** or **toremifene**. Both drugs are **antiestrogens**, or agents that antagonize the actions of estrogen. For these women, it is an alternative to the new aromatase inhibiting drugs (anastrozole, letrozole, or aromasin). Aromatase is one of the enzymes involved in steroid biosynthesis. In **endometrial cancer** (cancer of the uterus), MPA is sometimes used when cancer has spread (metastasized) beyond the uterus or is inoperable.

Recommended dosage

MPA comes as tablets or as a liquid that is given as an intramuscular injection. For breast cancer, it is usually given as a tablet once a day at the same time each day. Occasionally, MPA is given in divided doses that are spaced evenly throughout the day. For kidney and uterine cancer, MPA is usually given as a shot once a week at first, then later once a month.

Precautions

People taking MPA daily should take it at the same time each day. The time of day is unimportant, but the regular spacing of the dose is important.

Women taking MPA should not get pregnant. It is believed that MPA causes birth defects in babies born to mothers who are taking this drug during the first four months of pregnancy.

Side effects

The number and severity of side effects vary widely among people. Not only is it dependent on each person's own unique body chemistry, side effects vary with the type of cancer, the health of the patient, and the other drugs being given. There is no way to predict who will experience side effects of MPA.

Among the more common side effects are:

- increased appetite and weight gain
- nausea
- swelling and fluid retention in the hands, legs, and breast
- breakthrough vaginal bleeding
- muscle cramps
- fatigue
- emotional or mood changes
- headaches

A less common, but serious, side effect is the development of blood clots that can lead to heart attack or stroke. People who have a history of clotting problems are not good candidates for using MPA.

Interactions

Aminoglutethimide (Cytadren: an inhibitor of steroid biosynthesis), when given with MPA, decreases the effectiveness of MPA.

Resources

BOOKS

Chu, Edward, and Vincent T. DeVita Jr. *Physicians' Cancer Chemotherapy Drug Manual 2014*. Burlington, MA: Jones & Bartlett Learning, 2014.

PERIODICALS

Li Cl, Beaber EF, Tang MT, Porter PL, Daling JR, and Malone KE. "Effect of Depo-Medroxyprogesterone Acetate On Breast Cancer Risk Among Women 20 To 44 Years of Age." *Cancer Research* 15, no. 72 (2012): 2028–35. http://www.ncbi.nlm.nih.gov/pubmed/22369929 (accessed November 3, 2014).

WEBSITES

American Cancer Society. "Hormone Therapy For Endometrial Cancer." http://www.cancer.org/cancer/endometrialcancer/detailedguide/endometrial-uterine-cancer-treating-horm one-therapy (accessed November 3, 2014).

Tish Davidson, A.M.

Medulloblastoma

Definition

Medulloblastoma is a solid cancerous tumor originating in the cerebellum of the brain, located at the back of the brain below the cerebral hemispheres. It is also known as a primitive neuroendocrine tumor or PNET. Medulloblastomas are classified as infratentorial tumors because they are found below the tentorium, the membrane that separates the cerebellum from the cerebral hemispheres.

Description

Medulloblastoma is the most common cancerous brain tumor of childhood, although it can also occur in adults. It accounts for 18%–30% of all childhood **brain tumors** but only 2% of all primary brain tumors overall. Medulloblastomas can occur soon after birth and into puberty, but most tumors occur either before age ten or at some point in the late teens or early twenties. Untreated tumors can spread to other areas of the brain and to the spine.

Medulloblastomas occur in the area of the brain known as the cerebellum. The cerebellum, located in the back of the brain above the neck, is the area of the brain responsible for controlling and integrating movement. A person could move his or her muscles without the aid of the cerebellum, but those movements would be clumsy

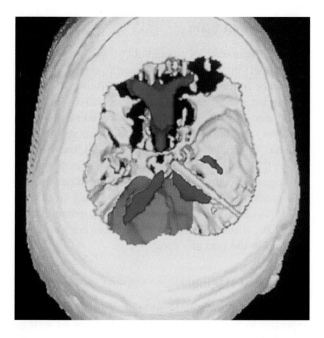

Colorized three-dimensional computed tomography brain scan showing a medulloblastoma tumor (red). *(CNRI/ Science Source)*

and disorganized. Medulloblastoma tumors in the cerebellum can result in loss of function of the cerebellum, leading to the uncoordinated movement called cerebellar ataxia.

There are five basic types of medulloblastoma, classified according to the appearance of the tumor cells:

- Classic medulloblastoma: the tumor appears as sheets of small, closely packed cells. Most medulloblastomas are of this type.
- Desmoplastic nodular medulloblastoma: the tumor cells appear as clumps or groups scattered within areas of less dense tissue. This form is more common in adults than in children and has a relatively favorable outcome.
- Anaplastic medulloblastoma: the tumor cells are large and rounded; it is also known as large-cell medulloblastoma and is associated with poorer outcomes.
- Medullomyoblastoma: the tumor includes striated and smooth muscle cells as well as nerve cells.
- Melanotic medulloblastoma: the tumor contains small undifferentiated cells containing the pigment melanin. These last two types are very rare.

If medulloblastomas are not detected early, they may spread **cancer** throughout the brain or spinal cord. If the cancer spreads to the spinal cord, a child may experience severe back pain, difficulty walking, and the inability to control bladder and bowel functions.

Demographics

Medulloblastoma is primarily a childhood cancer, occurring mainly in the first ten years of life. There are between 350 and 400 cases of medulloblastoma diagnosed in the United States each year; the incidence is similar worldwide. The median age of diagnosis is 7 years; and more than 70% of all pediatric medulloblastomas are diagnosed in children under age 10. Boys tend to develop the tumors more frequently than girls; the sex ratio is 1.7M:1F.

Medulloblastomas are rare in adults but do occur; about 33% of medulloblastomas diagnosed in the United States are found in adults between 20 and 44 years of age, The incidence drops off sharply in adults older than 45. Medulloblastomas are more common in men than in women but are equally common across different racial and ethnic groups.

Causes and symptoms

The cause of medulloblastoma is unknown as of 2014; however, researchers have identified alterations to chromosome 17 in about 50% of patients with medulloblastoma; similar changes on chromosomes 1, 7, 8, 9, 10q, 11, and 16 may also be involved. In addition, several tumor suppressor genes—most notably *RASSFTA*, *CASP8*, and *HICI*—are deactivated in about 30% of medulloblastoma patients.

This type of tumor can occur in association with three rare types of genetically-linked family cancer syndromes. Gorlin syndrome, **Li-Fraumeni syndrome**, and Turcot syndrome. Gorlin syndrome is caused by a defect in a gene known as *PTCH1* located on chromosome 9. This defect can result in medulloblastoma as well as cancers of the skin and ovary. Turcot syndrome is associated with mutations in the *MLH1*, *MSH2*, *MSH6*, and *PMS2* genes. Li-Fraumeni syndrome results from a mutation in the *TP53* tumor suppressor gene, and can present with cancer of the intestinal tract as well as medulloblastoma. However, these syndromes are quite rare and account for only a small fraction of reported cases of medulloblastoma.

Medulloblastoma can present in many ways. In infants, symptoms of the tumor may include an unusual increase in head size, vomiting, irritability, and lethargy. Since all infants generally have these symptoms at one time or another, it can be difficult for a parent or even a health care worker to recognize the initial presentation of medulloblastoma in babies and toddlers. The increase in head size results from the buildup of cerebrospinal fluid within the ventricles (internal hollow spaces) inside the brain, a condition known as hydrocephalus. Another telltale sign is the infant's inability to raise the eyes upward, sometimes called the sun-setting sign. In most cases, symptoms are present between 1 and 5 months before diagnosis.

In older children and teenagers, medulloblastoma can present the same as in infants or much differently. Such nonspecific symptoms as **nausea and vomiting**, morning headache, and vague visual disturbances may be the first sign of a tumor in the cerebellum. Other more striking signs may include double vision; stiff neck and head tilt; sudden difficulty writing; muscular weakness; and problems walking and moving that worsen over time.

Diagnosis

The diagnosis of medulloblastoma is made with both clinical observation and **imaging studies**. If a parent has noticed some of the signs and symptoms listed above, then a visit to a pediatrician is certainly warranted. In infants, the pediatrician may notice an increase in the circumference of the child's head or observe the sunsetting sign. During the office visit, various specialized neurological tests will be conducted to discern any sign of a problem in the cerebellum or surrounding brain structures. Examination of the patient's eyes may reveal

papilledema, or swelling of the optic disc caused by increased intracranial pressure. The physician may ask the patient to walk across the room to test for gait disturbances or head tilt.

There is no biochemical test that indicates the presence of a medulloblastoma. If the patient's history and office examination indicate the presence of a tumor, then imaging studies can be performed to detect the presence of a tumor. The two types of imaging studies conducted to detect medulloblastoma are **magnetic resonance imaging** (MRI) and **computed tomography** (CT) scan. The MRI uses a high-strength magnetic field to visualize the brain and is very useful for detecting medulloblastomas. The CT scan uses x-ray images reconstructed by computer. Like the MRI, a CT scan is also useful for detecting brain tumors as well as tumors that may have spread to the spine. CT scans to visualize the tumor may be performed with or without a contrast dye. Imaging modalities that may be used include **positron emission tomography** (PET), used most often to detect recurrent medulloblastomas; and magnetic resonance spectroscopy (MRS), used to distinguish between a growing malignant tumor and a benign static growth.

To confirm the diagnosis, a tissue sample will be obtained during surgery and sent to a pathologist to determine the specific type of medulloblastoma. In some cases a sample of cerebrospinal fluid (CSF from the tumor) will analyzed to assist in staging.

Treatment team

The treatment of medulloblastoma is optimally carried out in a specialized cancer center that has experience in treating this often difficult-to-treat cancer. A multidisciplinary team of cancer specialists, including a pediatric oncologist (a doctor specializing in the treatment of **childhood cancers**), a pediatric neurosurgeon (a doctor specializing in childhood brain surgery), as well as a pediatric neurologist and radiation oncologist (a doctor specializing in the use of radiation to treat cancer) usually work together to plan treatment. Child psychologists, physical therapists, rehabilitation specialists, dietitians, and social workers are also often involved in the patient's care.

Clinical staging

The staging of childhood brain tumors has become important to the selection of treatment plans, as well as providing information to make a more accurate prognosis. For medulloblastoma, there are four stages defined:

KEY TERMS

Ataxia—The inability to perform voluntary, coordinated muscular movements.

Cerebellum—The portion of the brain lying superior to the spinal cord, involved in coordinating voluntary muscular movements.

Chemotherapy—The application of certain medicinal chemicals to treat specific diseases, including cancer.

Gorlin syndrome—An inherited tendency to develop basal cell carcinoma and other conditions, including medulloblastoma, as the result of mutations in the *PTCH1* gene.

Hydrocephalus—The buildup of cerebrospinal fluid within the ventricles (cavities) in the brain.

Li-Fraumeni syndrome—A hereditary cancer syndrome caused by mutations in the *TP53* tumor suppressor gene. The syndrome increases a child's risk of medulloblastoma.

Papilledema—Swelling of the optic disc due to increased intracranial pressure.

Radiation therapy—The use of high-energy ionizing radiation in the treatment of cancerous tumors.

Shunt—A tube inserted beneath the skin to drain excess cerebrospinal fluid from the brain into the abdomen.

Tentorium—The membrane that separates the cerebrum from the cerebellum.

Turcot syndrome—A childhood cancer syndrome associated with mutations in the *MLH1*, *MSH2*, *MSH6*, and *PMS2* genes.

• T1: the tumor is less than 3 cm in diameter.

• T2: the tumor is greater than 3 cm in diameter and has invaded one other brain structure in addition to the cerebellum.

• T3: the tumor has invaded two other brain structures besides the cerebellum.

• T4: the tumor has spread down into the midbrain or upper spinal cord.

More recently, oncologists have moved away from this staging system for medulloblastoma to a simplified system in which patients are categorized as either low-risk or high-risk. Low-risk patients are those in which the tumor was completely removed during surgery; there is no evidence from imaging studies that the tumor has spread; and examination of a CSF sample shows no malignant cells. All other patients are in the high-risk category.

Treatment

Surgery

The treatment options for medulloblastoma have changed significantly over the past few decades. Surgery has been the first treatment option for medulloblastoma, and this is still the most common treatment. Surgery serves three purposes: to relieve pressure caused by the buildup of CSF in the brain; to obtain a tissue sample for analysis; and to remove as much of the tumor as possible. If the tumor cannot be removed completely, the surgeon may place a shunt, a long tube that passes from the brain into the abdomen, to divert excess cerebrospinal fluid.

After the surgery, further treatment depends upon whether the child has been placed in the low-risk or the high-risk group.

Chemotherapy and radiation therapy

Children with some tumor remaining after surgery will often have **radiation therapy** applied to the area in the brain where the medulloblastoma tumor was located. Radiation therapy is usually postponed in children younger than three, because the child's brain is still developing; radiotherapy in children below the age of three may result in growth retardation along with moderate to severe learning disabilities. For children at high risk, the current recommendation is to use both radiation and **chemotherapy**, since this combination improves overall survival rates for high-risk children.

Because of the possible side effect of radiation, especially in young children, chemotherapy is used more frequently for medulloblastoma. Researchers have found that medulloblastoma tumors are highly sensitive to chemotherapy, which spares the young brain from the side effects of radiation treatment. High-risk children are treated most often with a combination of **cyclophosphamide**, **vincristine**, and **cisplatin**, while children at average risk are treated with a combination of these three drugs and **lomustine**. Other chemotherapy drugs that may be used in children with medulloblastoma include **etoposide**, **methotrexate**, **carmustine**, **procarbazine**, **cytarabine**, or **hydroxyurea**. Delivering the chemotherapy drugs directly into the spinal column or the ventricles of the brain in order to reduce the risk of relapse is a newer technique.

Newer treatments for medulloblastoma under investigation include retinoids (Accutane), which appear to shrink tumors in animal models when combined with cisplatin; and drugs that target the WNT and NOTCH cell signaling pathways. These drugs include resveratrol and an investigational drug currently called MK-0752. As of 2014, a Phase I clinical trial of vismodegib, a drug developed to treat **basal cell carcinoma**, is being conducted for patients with medulloblastoma.

Alternative and complementary therapies

Alternative and complementary therapies are those that fall outside the scope of traditional, first-line therapies such as surgery, chemotherapy and radiation. Complementary therapies are intended to supplement traditional therapies with the objective of relieving symptoms. Alternative therapies are nontraditional, unproven attempts to cure the disease.

Common complementary therapies used in many types of cancer include aromatherapy, massage, meditation, music therapy, prayer, and certain forms of exercise. The objective of these therapies include reduction in anxiety and increase in sense of well-being.

Numerous alternative therapies exist in cancer treatment. Plant extracts, **vitamins**, protein therapies, and natural substances such as **mistletoe** and shark cartilage have all been touted as cancer-fighting remedies; however, some alternative therapies, such as Laetrile, can produce dangerous side effects and have shown no anticancer activity in **clinical trials**. Patients interested in alternative therapies should consult their doctors to ensure that they do not interfere with regular cancer treatment and that the products are safe, especially for children.

Prognosis

The prognosis for patients with medulloblastoma depends on five factors: age at diagnosis; the extent of CNS disease at the time of diagnosis; the amount of tumor remaining after surgery; the tissue type of the tumor; and the biological characteristics of the tumor cells. In 1930, the anticipated survival rate for a child with medulloblastoma after surgery was less than 2%. As of 2014, with the use of improved surgical techniques, radiation, and chemotherapy, the survival rates for older children with medulloblastoma range between 40% and 90%; the 20-year survival rate is 51%. Infants have a poorer prognosis, with five-year survival rates between 30% and 50%. In adults with medulloblastoma, the five-year survival rate is about 57% and the 10-year survival rate, 44%.

Coping with cancer treatment

During treatment, a child's health will be closely monitored by the team of physicians involved. Those physicians will be able to watch the child for any side effects from the treatments, especially if the child is receiving chemotherapy. The most frequent side effects of chemotherapy include nausea and vomiting, **diarrhea**, **fatigue**, and hair loss (**alopecia**); in some cases, radiation therapy combined with chemotherapy with cisplatin results in hearing loss. With medications, physicians can often treat some of the side effects, especially nausea, vomiting, and diarrhea.

Cancer treatment can be especially frightening for a young child. Family support is critical, and parents should consult their physician about organizations in the area to help their child cope with the effects of medulloblastoma and its treatment. The child should be referred to a neuropsychologist for learning and behavioral difficulties as he or she grows older, and to an endocrinologist for problems with growth or hormonal imbalances, particularly at puberty. Children recovering from medulloblastoma treatment frequently encounter learning difficulties when they return to school, and should be followed long-term for problems with memory or other cognitive disabilities. The risk of cognitive problems is greatest in children who were treated at younger ages and those who received more intense radiation therapy.

Clinical trials

There were many clinical trials underway as of 2014 to help improve treatment options for medulloblastoma. Some of the most promising were studies employing peripheral **stem cell transplantation**. This is a technique in which certain cells in the body, known as stem cells, replace the immune cells and blood cells that are destroyed in the process of chemotherapy. The hope is that stem cells will enable physicians to use higher doses of chemotherapy in order to destroy medulloblastomas.

Prevention

There are no known ways to prevent medulloblastoma, as this cancer is not associated with any environmental or lifestyle factors. Those who have the very rare genetic disorders which predispose them to medulloblastoma—Gorlin, Li-Fraumeni, and Turcot syndromes—should be especially aware of any signs or symptoms of medulloblastoma. Children of parents with these genetic disorders should undergo routine screening by a pediatrician for signs of a brain tumor.

See also Bone marrow transplantation.

Resources

BOOKS

Hayat, M.A. *Tumors of the Central Nervous System, volume 8: Astrocytoma, Medulloblastoma, Retinoblastoma,*

Chordoma, Craniopharyngioma, Oligodendroglioma, and Ependymoma. New York: Springer, 2012.

Kaye, Andrew H., and Edward R. Laws, Jr., eds. *Brain Tumors: An Encyclopedic Approach.* 3rd ed. New York: Saunders/Elsevier, 2012.

Niederhuber, J.E., et al. *Clinical Oncology.* 5th ed. Philadelphia: Elsevier, 2014.

Shiminski-Maher, Tania, Catherine Woodman, and Nancy Keene. *Childhood Brain and Spinal Cord Tumors: A Guide for Families, Friends and Caregivers*, 2nd ed. Bellingham, WA: Childhood Cancer Guides, 2014.

PERIODICALS

Aref, D., and S. Croul. "Medulloblastoma: Recurrence and Metastasis." *CNS Oncology* 2 (July 2013): 377–385.

Crawford, J. "Childhood Brain Tumors." *Pediatrics in Review* 34 (February 2013): 63–78.

Gerber, N.U., et al. "Recent Developments and Current Concepts in Medulloblastoma." *Cancer Treatment Reviews* 40 (April 2014): 356–365.

Hoang, D.H., et al. "Cognitive Disorders in Pediatric Medulloblastoma: What Neuroimaging Has to Offer." *Journal of Neurosurgery: Pediatrics* 14 (August 2014): 136–144.

Knight, S.J., et al. "Working Memory Abilities among Children Treated for Medulloblastoma: Parent Report and Child Performance." *Journal of Pediatric Psychology* 39 (June 2014): 501–511.

Kostaras, X., and J.C. Easaw. "Management of Recurrent Medulloblastoma in Adult Patients: A Systematic Review and Recommendations." *Journal of Neuro-Oncology* 115 (October 2013): 1–8.

Meiss, F., and R. Zeiser. "Vismodegib." *Recent Results in Cancer Research* 201 (2014): 405–417.

Ruggiero, A., et al. "Platinum Compounds in Children with Cancer: Toxicity and Clinical Management." *Anti-Cancer Drugs* 24 (November 2013): 1007–1019.

Schroeder, K., and S. Gururangan. "Molecular Variants and Mutations in Medulloblastoma." *Pharmacogenomics and Personalized Medicine* 7 (February 4, 2014): 43–51.

OTHER

American Brain Tumor Association (ABTA). "Medulloblastoma." http://www.abta.org/secure/medulloblastoma-brochure.pdf (accessed September 3, 2014).

American Cancer Society (ACS). "Brain and Spinal Cord Tumors in Children." http://www.cancer.org/acs/groups/cid/documents/webcontent/003089-pdf.pdf (accessed September 3, 2014).

WEBSITES

Jallo, George I. "Medulloblastoma." Medscape Reference. http://emedicine.medscape.com/article/1181219-overview (accessed September 3, 2014).

National Cancer Institute (NCI). "Childhood Central Nervous System Embryonal Tumors Treatment (PDQ)." http://www.cancer.gov/cancertopics/pdq/treatment/child-CNSembryonal/healthprofessional/page1/AllPages (accessed September 2, 2014).

ORGANIZATIONS

American Brain Tumor Association (ABTA), 855 West Bryn Mawr Avenue, Suite 550, Chicago, IL 60631, (773) 577-8750, (800) 886-2282, Fax: (773) 577-8738, info@abta.org, http://www.abta.org.

American Cancer Society (ACS), 250 Williams Street NW, Atlanta, GA 30303, (800) 227-2345, http://www.cancer.org/aboutus/howwehelpyou/app/contact-us.aspx, http://www.cancer.org/index.

Children's Oncology Group (COG), 222 E. Huntington Drive, Suite 100, Monrovia, CA 91016, (626) 447-0064, Fax: (626) 445-4334, HelpDesk@childrensoncologygroup.org, http://www.childrensoncologygroup.org/.

National Cancer Institute (NCI), BG 9609 MSC 9760, 9609 Medical Center Drive, Bethesda, MD 20892-9760, (800) 4-CANCER (422-6237), http://www.cancer.gov/global/contact/email-us, http://www.cancer.gov/.

Edward R. Rosick, D.O., M.P.H.
REVISED BY REBECCA J. FREY, PhD

Megace *see* Megestrol acetate

Megestrol acetate

Definition

Megestrol acetate is used to treat unexplained **weight loss** during **cancer** therapy and to stop new cell growth in some cancers. Megestrol acetate is also known by the brand name Megace.

Purpose

Megestrol acetate is used to treat some advanced hormone-responsive cancers of the breast, kidney, and uterus. It is also used in larger doses to help reverse weight loss for which there is no other treatable cause.

Description

Megestrol acetate is a synthetic derivative of the female hormone progesterone. In healthy women, progesterone plays a major role in preparing the uterus for pregnancy. It has been approved by the Food and Drug Administration (FDA), and its use is usually covered by insurance.

Exactly why megestrol acetate stops tumor growth is unclear. Many tumors are sensitive to hormones. It appears that megestrol acetate, in some way, changes the hormonal climate of the tumor so that cells stop responding to other hormones and proteins that would normally stimulate their growth. This drug cannot tell the difference between normal cells and cancer cells, so some

KEY TERMS

Food and Drug Administration (FDA)—The government agency that oversees public safety in relation to drugs and medical devices, and gives the approval to pharmaceutical companies for commercial marketing of their products in the United States.

Hormone—A chemical released by a gland that travels through the circulatory system and affects only the tissues at a distance from its release point that have receptors for the chemical.

Progesterone—A female hormone that prepares the uterus for pregnancy.

normal cells are also killed during treatment. But since cancer cells grow more rapidly than normal cells, more cancer cells are killed.

Megestrol acetate has another independent use in cancer treatment. In high doses, it is used to counteract weight loss that does not occur for any other treatable reason. Megestrol acetate appears to bring about weight gain through increased fat storage.

Recommended dosage

Megestrol acetate comes in both liquid and tablet form. To treat weight loss, the standard dosage is a single dose given in the morning with breakfast.

To reduce tumor growth, the dose of megestrol acetate is individualized, and depends on the type of cancer, the patient's body weight and general health, what other drugs are being given, and the way the cancer responds to hormones. A standard dose of Megace to treat **breast cancer** is 160 mg/day divided into four doses. A standard dose for **endometrial cancer** (cancer of the uterus) is 40–320 mg/day in divided doses. Treatment normally continues for about two months.

Precautions

Women taking megestrol acetate should not get pregnant. Megestrol acetate is believed to cause birth defects in babies born to mothers who are taking the drug.

Side effects

Megestrol acetate has several rare but serious side effects. Some people have been reported to develop **Cushing syndrome**. This is a hormonal imbalance in which people (usually women) develop fatty deposits in the face and neck, lose bone mass (osteoporosis), stop menstruating, develop diabetes, high blood pressure, and other signs of fluid and salt (electrolyte) imbalances.

Other common side effects of megestrol acetate include:

- worsening of diabetic symptoms
- pain in the chest or abdomen
- infection
- sarcoma (tumors of the skin or connective tissue)
- irregular heartbeat
- fluid retention
- breakthrough vaginal bleeding
- blood clots in legs or lungs
- nausea or constipation
- dry mouth or increased salivation
- abnormal white blood cell count
- confusion or abnormal thinking
- emotional and psychological changes
- rash, itching, abnormal sweating, or skin disorders
- cough, sore throat, lung disorders
- hair loss (alopecia)
- uncontrolled urination or urinary tract infection
- male impotence

Interactions

No specific interactions with other pharmaceuticals have been reported in people using megestrol acetate. However, many drugs interact with nonprescription (over-the-counter) drugs and herbal remedies as well as prescription drugs. Patients should always tell their health care providers about all remedies they are taking. Patients should also mention if they are on a special diet such as low salt or high protein.

Resources

BOOKS

Chu, Edward, and Vincent T. DeVita Jr. *Physicians' Cancer Chemotherapy Drug Manual 2014*. Burlington, MA: Jones & Bartlett Learning, 2014.

WEBSITES

AHFS Consumer Medication Information. "Megestrol." American Society of Health-System Pharmacists. Available from: http://www.nlm.nih.gov/medlineplus/druginfo/meds/a682003.html (accessed on November 3, 2014).
American Cancer Society. "Megestrol." http://www.cancer.org/treatment/treatmentsandsideeffects/guidetocancerdrugs/megestrol (accessed November 3, 2014).

Tish Davidson, A.M.

Mekinist *see* **Trametinib**

KEY TERMS

Adjuvant therapy—Treatment given to patients who are at risk of having microscopic untreated disease present but have no obvious symptoms.

Dysplastic nevus syndrome—A familial syndrome characterized by the presence of multiple atypical appearing moles, often at a young age.

Epidermis—The uppermost layer of skin cells.

Genome—The genetic makeup of a cell, composed of DNA.

Immunotherapy—A form of treatment that uses biologic agents to enhance or stimulate normal immune function.

Lymph node dissection—Surgical removal of a group of lymph nodes.

Lymphedema—Swelling of a limb (such as an arm or leg) following surgical removal of the lymph nodes that drain the limb.

Melanocytes—Skin cells derived from the neural crest that produce the protein pigment melanin.

Metastasis (plural, metastases)—A tumor growth or deposit that has spread via lymph or blood to an area of the body remote from the primary tumor.

Mohs surgery—A form of microscopically controlled surgery that allows for the precise removal of cancerous tissue. It is commonly used to treat various types of skin cancer, particularly in areas of the body where preserving as much tissue as possible is essential. Mohs surgery is also known as micrographic surgery.

Nevus (plural, nevi)—The medical term for mole.

Resection—The act of removing an organ or tissue surgically.

Targeted therapy—In cancer treatment, a type of drug therapy that blocks tumors by interfering with signaling pathways or specific molecules that the cancer cells need for growth. Also called biologic therapy, targeted therapy is less harmful to normal cells than traditional chemotherapy.

Xeroderma pigmentosum (XP)—A rare inherited skin disorder in which the skin cells lack an enzyme needed to repair damage to the cell's DNA caused by sunlight. People with XP are 1,000 times more likely to develop melanoma than people without the disorder.

Melanoma

Definition

Melanoma is a type of **skin cancer**; its name is derived from the Greek word for black. The **cancer** cells form in melanocytes, the pigmented cells that produce a brownish-black pigment known as melanin and are responsible for racial variations in skin color, the color of moles, and **tanning** in response to sun exposure. In malignant melanoma, melanocytes become cancerous and may spread throughout the body and invade other organs and tissues. Initially melanoma begins on the surface of the skin. If left untreated, melanoma can cause illness that may be fatal; however, if caught early, melanoma may be treatable with surgery, **chemotherapy**, **radiation therapy**, and **immunotherapy**.

Description

The epidermis, the outermost and upper layer of the skin, contains melanocytes, the skin cells that make melanin, the pigment that gives skin its hue. Melanin is responsible for the color of a person's skin, hair, and eyes. There are between 1,000 and 2,000 melanocytes in each square millimeter of human skin. The difference in skin color between fair-skinned and darker-skinned people does not depend on the number of melanocytes in the skin but on their level of activity. When skin is exposed to the sun, the melanocytes become more active, produce more melanin, and cause the skin to darken—that is, they cause a suntan. When a cancerous tumor develops in tissue containing melanocytes, a person has melanoma.

Most cases of melanoma occur in the skin (cutaneous melanoma), but sometimes melanoma can also occur in the iris, the colored part of the eye—a condition known as ocular melanoma.

Cutaneous melanoma

Sometimes melanoma arises out of normal skin, but it can also develop in a mole (also called a nevus). Moles are benign growths or collections of melanocytes on the skin. According to the American Academy of Dermatology, individuals usually have about 30 moles on their skin. The number and type of moles individuals have may increase the risk of developing melanoma. People with more than 50 moles or with moles that are unusual and irregular-looking (doctors call these dysplastic nevi or atypical moles) are at increased risk of developing melanoma.

There are four major types of cutaneous (skin-based) melanoma:

- Superficial spreading melanoma accounts for 70% of all cases of melanoma and typically occurs in younger people. This type of melanoma takes a long time to penetrate the top layer of skin, and the first sign of it is a flat or slightly raised skin lesion. The lesion may be discolored with irregular borders and may develop out of a previously benign mole. It is most likely to occur on the trunk in men, the legs in women, and the upper back in men and women.

- Lentigo maligna melanoma is another form of melanoma that is most often found in older adults. It begins as a flat or slightly raised tan, brown, or dark brown skin discoloration that remains close to the skin's surface. Once the malignancy spreads, it is referred to as lentigo maligna melanoma.

- Acral lentiginous melanoma is the most common type of melanoma in African Americans and Asians and is least common among Caucasians. The black or brown discoloration of acral letiginous melanoma first spreads on the surface of the skin, often under the nails or on the soles of the feet or palms of the hands.

- Nodular melanoma, which accounts for 10% to 15% of all melanoma cases, is the most aggressive form of melanoma, and by the time it is diagnosed, it may have spread to other areas of the body. This type of melanoma starts as a bump that is usually black. Nodular melanoma is found most frequently on the trunk, legs, and arms, and most often affects older people.

Superficial spreading melanoma, lentigo maligna melanoma, and acral lentiginous melanoma begin as in situ malignancies, which means they affect only the top layers of skin. Eventually, these forms of melanomas may become invasive and spread to other areas of the body. Nodular melanoma is often invasive by the time it is diagnosed.

Ocular melanoma

Ocular melanoma, or melanoma of the eye, is a cancer that develops in the parts of the eye that contain melanocytes—the iris and other nearby structures that belong to the middle pigmented layer of the eye. It affects about six persons per million per year in the United States and is most likely to develop in people with blue eyes and fair skin. Ocular melanoma is more common in Denmark and other Scandinavian countries than in the United States. It is slightly more common in men than in women. The average age of a person diagnosed with this type of melanoma is 55.

Ocular melanomas can grow slowly for years without producing any symptoms, although they eventually cause blurred vision, gradual loss of sight, and sometimes pain in the eye. This type of melanoma often spreads from the eye to the liver, lungs, or even the central nervous system before it is diagnosed. Most patients die from the spread of the cancer to these vital organs rather than from the effects of the cancer on the eye itself. About half of all patients diagnosed with ocular melanoma die within 10 years after diagnosis and treatment. The standard forms of treatment for this type of cancer are radiation therapy and surgical removal of the affected eye.

Risk factors

Malignant melanoma occurs in people of all ages and ethnicities. However, certain factors put people at greater risk for developing this disease, including the following:

- having fair skin
- having red or blond hair
- having blue or green eyes
- being older than 20 years; the rate rises sharply after age 50 and is highest among people in their 80s
- having excessive sun exposure, exposure to artificial ultraviolet light (such as in tanning beds), or a history of severe sunburns in childhood
- living in areas that get high levels of ultraviolet radiation, such as mountainous regions or countries closer to the equator
- having a previous personal history of melanoma or another type of skin cancer
- extensive scars or burns on the skin
- exposure to certain chemicals in the environment, including arsenic and some types of weed killers
- having a job that requires working outdoors during daylight hours
- having a close relative with melanoma
- having a high number of moles (50 or more)
- having moles that are unusual or irregular-looking

Because the development of melanoma is usually related to sun exposure, people with less melanin and lighter skin, hair, and eyes are at greater risk.

Having certain procedures or health conditions that weaken the immune system may also predispose a person to developing melanoma. Compared to people in the general population, those who have undergone organ transplants have a threefold risk of melanoma. Having human immunodeficiency virus (HIV) or acquired immunodeficiency syndrome (AIDS), other forms of cancer, or autoimmune diseases that require immunosuppressive treatments can also increase a person's risk of developing malignant melanoma.

A rare inherited condition known as xeroderma pigmentosum (XP) increases a person's risk of malignant melanoma. People with XP lack an enzyme that is needed to repair damage caused by sunlight to the DNA in skin cells. Without this protective enzyme, the DNA in individual skin cells can undergo mutations leading to melanoma and other types of skin cancer. Fewer than 40% of individuals with XP survive beyond the age of 20.

Demographics

Melanoma accounts for only 4% of skin cancers in the United States; however, it is responsible for 75% of deaths from skin cancer. Although melanoma is more common in women than men up to age 40, in adults over 40 it is more common in men. The average age of Americans at the time of diagnosis of melanoma is 61 years; however, it is the most common cancer in women between the ages of 25 and 29, and is second only to **breast cancer** in women between the ages of 30 and 34. In the United States, melanoma affects Caucasians 20 times more often than African Americans, and six times more often than Hispanics.

In the United States, 1 in 85 people is expected to develop melanoma during his or her lifetime. According to the **National Cancer Institute** (NCI), 76,100 new cases of melanoma will be diagnosed in the United States in 2014, about 43,890 in men and 32,210 in women; and 9,710 people will die from the disease, 6,470 men and 3,240 women. Melanoma was considered a rare form of cancer until the 1970s, but its rate among Caucasians in the United States has tripled since 1985. Unlike many cancers, which are declining in incidence as of 2014, the incidence of primary cutaneous malignant melanoma has been steadily increasing since 1980, possibly related to increased sun exposure. Currently, the risk is about 13 per 100,000 of the population. Melanoma affects all age groups but is most commonly seen in patients between 30 and 60 years of age; the average age at time of diagnosis is 61 as of 2014. Nonetheless, the rate of melanoma is rising faster among young people than

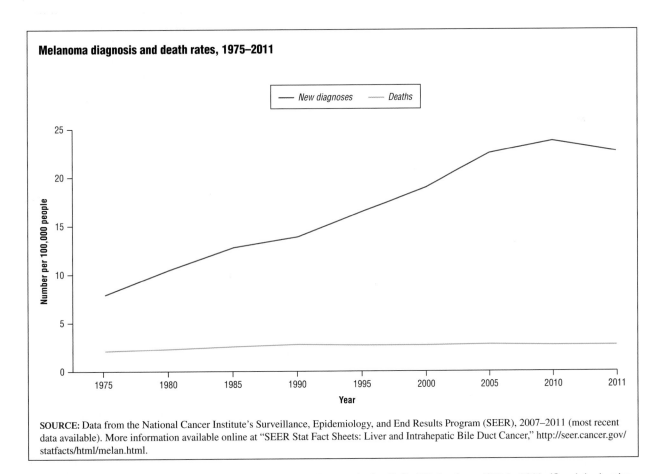

Melanoma diagnosis and death rates, 1975–2011

— New diagnoses ⸺ Deaths

Number per 100,000 people

Year

SOURCE: Data from the National Cancer Institute's Surveillance, Epidemiology, and End Results Program (SEER), 2007–2011 (most recent data available). More information available online at "SEER Stat Fact Sheets: Liver and Intrahepatic Bile Duct Cancer," http://seer.cancer.gov/statfacts/html/melan.html.

Line graph showing new diagnoses of and deaths from melanoma in the United States from 1975 to 2011. *(Graph by Lumina Datamatics Ltd. © 2015 Cengage Learning®.)*

among older adults; melanoma is now the most common cancer diagnosed in young adults between the ages of 25 and 29. The current overall lifetime risk of melanoma is about 28% (1 in 50) for Caucasians; 0.1% (1 in 1,000) for African Americans; and 0.5% (1 in 200) for Hispanics/Latinos. In Canada, doctors estimate that there are 10 to 13 cases of melanoma per 100,000 people.

The highest rates of melanoma in the world, however, are not found in the United States or Canada but in Australia, New Zealand, and Israel. There are approximately 57 cases of melanoma per 100,000 people per year in Australia and 40 cases per 100,000 people per year in Israel. The World Health Organization (WHO) reported that 232,000 cases of malignant melanoma were diagnosed worldwide in 2012 (the most recent year for which data are available), with 55,000 deaths.

One of the more unusual findings in the United States in recent years is the rapid increase of deaths from melanoma in older males. Although the death rate among younger men (44 years or younger) has dropped since the late 1990s, most likely as a result of public health education campaigns about the dangers of sun exposure, it has risen 66% in men between the ages of 45 and 64, and 157% in men over 65.

Causes and symptoms

Causes

ULTRAVIOLET RADIATION. The development of melanomas from normal skin is not completely understood. As of 2014, researchers think there may be two pathways to malignant melanoma, one involving exposure to sunlight and the other with melanocyte proliferation triggered by other factors. This hypothesis is based on the difference in distribution of moles on the body between patients who develop melanomas on the face and neck, and those who develop melanomas on the trunk or legs. A small percentage of melanomas arise within burn scar tissue. Researchers do not fully understand the relationship between deep burns and an increased risk of skin cancer. In general, however, melanoma is caused by the interaction of ultraviolet (UV) radiation from the sun and the melanin in melanocytes. UV radiation can damage the DNA in skin cells both directly and indirectly. Researchers have found that 92% of melanomas are caused by indirect damage to DNA and 8% by direct damage.

When the DNA in a skin cell is damaged by UV radiation, the cell can undergo a series of mutations that lead to abnormal multiplication of new cells. In some cases the changed DNA makes the cell more vulnerable

to the damaging effects of UV radiation. About 40% of melanomas begin in moles, with the remaining 60% starting in normal skin.

Melanomas grow in two stages or phases. The first is a phase of outward or radial growth. The second phase, which is much more dangerous, is a phase of vertical growth into deeper layers of tissue. It is during this second phase of growth that melanomas become harder to treat and able to spread to other parts of the body.

ENVIRONMENTAL CHANGES. Melanoma was a rare form of cancer until the twentieth century. The earliest known surgical removal of a melanoma was performed in 1787 by a British surgeon, but the disease was little studied until the 1840s and 1850s, when two other British doctors described the stages of melanoma and found that it runs in some families. The connection between melanoma and sun exposure was not made until 1956, when an Australian doctor named Henry Lancaster found that high intensity of sunlight is a risk factor for melanoma. In the 1970s, scientists began to notice that the ozone layer—a layer of the Earth's atmosphere consisting of ozone gas—was becoming thinner. The ozone layer helps to block a high-energy type of ultraviolet radiation known as UVB from reaching the surface of the earth, so doctors began to wonder whether a thinner ozone layer could contribute to an increase in the rate of melanoma and other skin cancers.

As of 2014, however, doctors do not think that the rise in cases of melanoma since the 1980s is due primarily to changes in the ozone layer. One reason is that depletion of the ozone layer is most severe over Antarctica, which is not a heavily populated continent. Another is that recent advances in genetics indicate that heredity plays a larger role in melanoma than was thought to be the case in the 1980s. Still another reason for skepticism about the role of the ozone layer in melanoma is that recent studies indicate that a lower-energy form of ultraviolet radiation called UVA triggers the development of melanoma rather than the UVB blocked by the ozone layer. If this finding is accurate, then the increased incidence of melanoma is not related to changes in the ozone layer. It is also likely that the increase in the number of reported cases of melanoma since the 1990s is due partly to better diagnostic tools and earlier diagnosis.

GENETIC FACTORS. The development of melanoma is also thought to have a strong genetic link, since many people who develop melanoma also have family members with the disease. Researchers have identified mutations in genes on chromosomes 1, 9, and 12 as linked to familial melanoma, including a gene called

BRAF that may play a role in the development of melanoma. A mutated form of *BRAF* is thought to switch on the malignant cells, allowing them to grow and divide. As of 2014, researchers think that mutations in the *BRAF* gene are responsible for 50%–60% of cases of melanoma. Another gene mutation called *p53* has also been associated with melanoma cases among families. A positive family history of one or two first-degree relatives having had melanoma substantially increases the risk on a genetic basis. A family tendency is observed in 8% to 12% of patients. There is a syndrome known as the dysplastic (atypical) nevus syndrome that is characterized by atypical moles with bothersome clinical features in children under age 10. Such individuals have to be observed closely for the development of malignant melanoma.

There are mutations in up to 50% of familial melanoma patients of the tumor-suppressing gene *CDKN2A* (also known as the *p16* gene) on chromosome 9. Mutations in another tumor suppressor gene known as *CDK4* have also been linked to melanoma.

Symptoms

The first sign of melanoma is a mole, sore, lump, or growth found on the skin. Melanomas can occur anywhere on the body, but they are most often found on the backs of men and the legs of women. Generally, melanomas are black or brown, but may be red, skin-colored, or white. Some may develop pinkish or bluish patches mixed in with darker areas.

Changes in a mole's appearance over time may also indicate malignant melanoma. Sometimes, a growth or mole may bleed, ooze, or itch, which indicates malignancy. Having satellite moles, new moles that grow near an existing mole, may also point to this form of skin cancer.

Early-stage melanomas may itch or shed small flakes of skin, while more advanced melanomas may bleed or ooze fluid as well as itch. Advanced melanomas may also become hard or lumpy in texture. Melanomas do not, however, usually cause pain.

People with moles, lumps, or growths that fit these criteria should be checked by a doctor.

Diagnosis

Diagnosis of melanoma begins with careful examination of the skin.

Examination

If a person finds an abnormal mark or mole on the skin, the first step should be to contact his or her healthcare provider for a skin examination. About 80% of all skin cancers are first noticed by the patient. The doctor or nurse

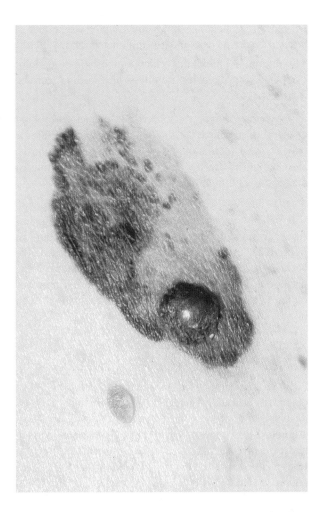

A close-up image of a malignant melanoma on a patient's back. *(Wellcome Image Library/Custom Medical Stock Photography)*

will carefully examine all moles, birthmarks, and pigmented areas over the person's entire body, including the back, legs, hands, feet, and scalp.

Doctors often use the ABCDE mnemonic when making a diagnosis of melanoma. The letters stand for the following signs:

- Asymmetry: Melanomas are usually asymmetrical. A normal mole is round, whereas a suspicious mole is unevenly shaped.

- Border: The edges of a melanoma may be ragged or blurred. A normal mole has a clear-cut border with the surrounding skin, whereas the edges of a suspect mole are often irregular or scalloped.

- Color: A malignant melanoma often has several colors or shades, whereas benign moles are typically one color. Normal moles are uniformly tan or brown, but cancerous moles may appear as mixtures of red, white, blue, brown, purple, or black.

• Diameter: Cancerous moles are usually larger than a pencil eraser or pea (about 6 millimeters or 1/4 inch).

• Evolution: A mole that changes over time in color or shape or develops itchiness or bleeding can be suspect.

A family doctor can often spot suspicious-looking changes in a patient's skin, but will usually refer the patient to a dermatologist for a definite diagnosis. Dermatologists are doctors with specialized training in diagnosing and treating skin disorders.

To diagnose cutaneous melanoma, a dermatologist will first use a dermatoscope, which is a special palm-sized instrument with a magnifying lens and built-in light. The use of dermatoscopes has increased the accuracy of diagnosing malignant melanoma by 20%, because a doctor can make digital images of suspicious moles or skin areas and save them for comparison with images from later checkups.

Tests

There are no blood or other laboratory tests as of 2014 that can be used to diagnose melanoma. The diagnosis is usually made by a combination of tissue analysis and (for advanced-stage disease) **imaging studies**. Most patients have an early-stage melanoma, and extensive testing is not usually warranted. Routine testing in this situation involves a complete blood count, a chest x-ray, and determinations of blood enzymes including lactic dehydrogenase and alkaline phosphatase.

If the patient has signs or symptoms of a more advanced disease, or if the lesion's depth of penetration is sizeable, imaging studies may be appropriate. These would involve **computed tomography** (CT) scans of the abdomen, the chest, or regional nodal areas, or a CT or **magnetic resonance imaging** (MRI) scan of the brain. A **positron emission tomography** (PET) scan may also be used to look for melanoma metastases. PET scans involve the use of radioactive glucose to look for cancer cells, as cancers take up sugar more rapidly than normal tissues.

Procedures

BIOPSIES. If the dermatoscope images suggest that the patient may have melanoma, the next step is to take a sample of the abnormal mole or area of skin to be sent to a laboratory for analysis under a microscope. This procedure is called a **biopsy**. In the case of melanoma, the doctor will remove the entire mole rather than just a portion of it, so as to obtain an accurate measurement of its depth. When dealing with an early malignant melanoma, it is very important to establish the exact thickness of penetration of the primary tumor. Any biopsy that does not remove the full vertical extent of the primary is inadequate. Therefore, if a skin lesion is suspicious, full-thickness excisional biopsy is the approach recommended. Shave biopsies and biopsies that remove only a portion of the suspect area are inappropriate. Often, in an early case, the excision involves just the suspicious lesion with minimal normal skin, but should be a full vertical excision of the skin. Early-stage melanomas can be excised by **Mohs surgery**, a technique that involves removal of the visible melanoma followed by removal of skin that may contain cancer cells one layer at a time. The surgeon examines each layer of skin under a microscope before proceeding to the next layer. When no more cancer cells are found, the Mohs surgery is complete. Biopsies are done under topical or local anesthesia.

To evaluate whether the melanoma may have spread beyond the skin, the doctor may perform a **sentinel lymph node biopsy**. A sentinel lymph node is the lymph node closest to the melanoma, the one to which it is most likely to spread.

STAGING. Malignant melanoma is curable if caught early. When a melanoma is not removed in its early stages, however, cancer cells will start to grow downward from the skin surface and invade healthy tissue. The disease can then spread to other parts of the body, where it is difficult to control. Measuring a cancer's size, thickness, and likelihood of spreading is called staging. Melanomas are graded in five stages from 0 to 4. The chief factor in determining a patient's chances of recovery is the thickness of the melanoma. This is measured in millimeters and is called Breslow's depth, after the doctor who first connected it to the patient's chances of survival in 1970.

The five stages of melanoma and a person's chances of five-year survival at each stage are as follows:

• Stage 0: The cancerous cells are found only in the outer layer of skin and have not invaded deeper tissues. At this stage the cancer is called melanoma in situ. The five-year survival rate is 99.9%.

• Stage I: The melanoma is no more than 1 millimeter (1/25 of an inch) thick and has not spread to nearby lymph nodes. Five-year survival rate is 92%–97%.

• Stage II: The tumor is between 1 and 2 millimeters (1/25 and 5/64 of an inch) thick but has not spread to nearby lymph nodes. Survival rate is 53%–81%.

• Stage III: The melanoma has spread to nearby lymph nodes or to skin just outside the original tumor. Survival rate after five years is 40%–60%.

• Stage IV: The melanoma cells have spread to other organs (often the lungs, liver, brain and bones); to lymph nodes; or to skin areas far away from the original tumor. The five-year survival rate is 10%–15%, with an average life expectancy of six to nine months.

Young children are an exception to the survival rates for adults. For some reason that is not yet known as of 2014, survival in children is more closely related to age than to the thickness of the cancer, with younger children being less likely to survive than older children or teenagers.

Treatment

Surgery

The only definite cure for malignant melanoma is surgical removal of the cancerous mole or patch of skin before the melanoma reaches a Breslow depth of 1 millimeter (1/25 of an inch). The surgeon will remove a margin of normal skin surrounding the melanoma as well as the tumor itself to make sure that no cancerous cells are left behind. A procedure known as microscopically controlled excision—also known as Mohs surgery after the physician who developed it in 1938—can be used to examine each layer of skin as it is removed to ensure that the proper amount is taken. Depending on the amount of skin removed, the cut is either closed with stitches or covered with a skin graft. When surgical excision is performed on such visible areas as the face, cosmetic surgery may also be performed to minimize the scar. Other techniques for removing skin tumors include burning, freezing with a probe containing liquid nitrogen (cryosurgery), or laser surgery. For skin cancer that is localized and has not spread to other areas of the body, excision may be the only treatment needed.

For advanced melanoma that has moved beyond the original tumor site, the local lymph nodes may be surgically removed.

Immunotherapy

Immunotherapy in the form of interferon or interleukin is being used more often with success for advanced melanoma. Interferon alpha 2a is an agent that stimulates the immune system. This adjuvant therapy may slightly increase the duration of a patient's disease-free state and lengthen overall survival. However, interferon alpha 2a has high toxicity and patients may not tolerate the side effects. Another drug used in immunotherapy for advanced-stage melanoma is ipilimumab, a synthetic version of an immune system antibody. Still another option is Bacille Calmette-Guérin (BCG) vaccine, which also stimulates the immune system.

Radiation therapy

Though radiation therapy has a minimal role in the primary treatment of malignant melanoma, for patients who have metastatic disease, radiation may be helpful in symptom relief. This is true in patients who have developed tumor deposits in such areas as the brain or bone. Therapy that is intended to relieve the symptoms of the disease rather than cure it is called palliative therapy.

Chemotherapy

Chemotherapy can be used to treat metastatic melanoma; however, it is not usually used as first-line therapy because melanomas are more resistant to chemotherapy than other cancers. The chemotherapeutic agent **dacarbazine**, or DTIC, seems to be the most active agent. Overall responses are noted in about 20% of patients. Combination chemotherapy may be an option. The regimen of DTIC+BCNU (**carmustine**) + **cisplatin** + **tamoxifen** delivers a response rate of 40%. Other chemotherapy drugs that may be used include **vinblastine**, **carboplatin**, and **temozolomide**. As of 2014, chemotherapy is more often given in combination with targeted therapy than used by itself.

Some very early-stage melanomas may be treated with imiquimod (Zyclara), a topical medication applied as a cream. It is used most often in areas where surgery would be disfiguring. It cannot be used for later-stage melanomas.

Targeted therapy

A newer treatment option for advanced-stage melanoma is targeted therapy. Targeted therapy is a type of drug therapy that blocks the growth of skin cancers by interfering with signaling pathways or specific molecules that the cancer cells need for growth. There are several types of targeted therapy drugs used for melanoma as of 2014. One group targets cells with mutations in the *BRAF* gene; it includes drugs like vemurafenib and **dabrafenib**, which attack the BRAF protein directly and shrink metastatic tumors, thus prolonging the patient's survival time. Some acral melanomas contain mutations in the *C-KIT* gene; they may respond to treatment with imatinib or **nilotinib**, drugs that are known to affect cells with *C-KIT* mutations.

Vaccines

Vaccines for melanoma are being studied in **clinical trials**, but have not been found helpful as of 2014.

Alternative and complementary therapies

There are no established alternative treatments for skin cancer. Preventive measures that can be helpful include minimizing exposure to the sun and sunburn, eating a diet high in **antioxidants**, and supplementation with antioxidant nutrients.

Patients diagnosed with melanoma may benefit from some complementary therapies such as prayer, meditation, humor therapy, art therapy, pet therapy, and aromatherapy. While these approaches should not be used as replacements for conventional treatments, they can help to lift the patient's spirits following surgery.

"Look Good...Feel Better" is a free public service program approved by the American Cancer Society; it helps patients with any kind of cancer cope with changes in their looks related to cancer treatment. It began in 1987 when a doctor asked the president of the Personal Care Products Council to help a patient who was so depressed by her appearance during chemotherapy that she refused to leave her hospital room. The president sent a makeup artist to visit the patient, who was so delighted with her makeover that she began to respond better to her cancer treatment. Look Good...Feel Better has expanded to include programs for teens, men, and Spanish-speaking patients; groups are available in all 50 states, the District of Columbia, and Puerto Rico.

Prognosis

Whether the melanoma has spread to the body's organs and the thickness of the lesion at the time of diagnosis have significant impact on the prognosis. Patients diagnosed and treated before their melanoma spreads to the lymph nodes have a five-year survival rate of 91% however, those whose melanoma has spread to the lungs or liver have a five-year survival rate of only 10%–15%, with an average life expectancy of six to nine months.

Other factors may also influence survival rates. For example, although melanoma among African Americans is rare, it is more lethal. Melanomas also tend to be thinner in females, so women have more favorable survival rates. In addition, older adults generally have shorter periods of survival after melanoma diagnosis.

Prevention

Skin protection

People cannot change their skin type, but they can lower their risk of melanoma by taking the following precautions against sun exposure:

- Avoid using tanning booths and sun lamps. Legislation has been proposed in several states as of 2014 to prohibit minors from visiting tanning salons. In addition, the U.S. Food and Drug Administration (FDA) issued a formal warning on May 29, 2014, about the use of sunlamps and similar indoor tanning

QUESTIONS TO ASK YOUR DOCTOR

- How does my sun/ultraviolet light exposure history affect my risk of melanoma?
- How often do I need skin examinations for melanoma?
- Do I have any moles or lesions that I should watch carefully?
- How far has my melanoma spread beneath the skin?
- What is my prognosis, based on the stage of melanoma I have?
- Are there risks and side effects associated with cancer treatment?
- How should I care for my skin after melanoma treatment?
- What steps should I take to avoid sun exposure now that I have been treated for melanoma?

devices, stating that they must carry warning labels regarding the increased risk of skin cancer associated with their use, and that they should not be used by persons under the age of 18.

- Stay out of the sun between 10 A.M. and 4 P.M.

- Use a sunscreen with a sun protection factor (SPF) of 15 or higher every day. People with very fair skin should use a product with an SPF of 30 or higher. Sunscreens as high as 100 SPF are now available. SPF 15 sunscreens filter out about 93% of UVB rays; SPF 30 sunscreens filter out about 97%; SPF 50 sunscreens about 98%; and SPF 100 sunscreens about 99%. Always check the expiration date on sunscreen products; most are good for two to three years.

- Apply sunscreen over the entire body 30 minutes before going outside, and reapplying the product every two hours.

- Use a lip balm that contains sunscreen.

- Wear clothing that covers as much of the body as possible, including a broad-brimmed hat and sunglasses to protect the eyes. Some companies now make clothing that is more tightly woven and is coated with special products to block out UV radiation.

- Keep in mind that UV rays can be reflected from the surface of the ocean, sandy beaches, or snow-covered ski slopes. It is a good idea to check the local weather forecast for the UV index for the day before heading outdoors.

- Remember that children need special protection against the sun as their skin burns more easily, they spend more time outdoors than most adults, and they are less knowledgeable about the dangers of too much sun. Parents should keep infants under six months out of the sun altogether, and use sunscreen on infants older than six months.

Although melanoma has been linked to mutations in several specific genes as of 2014, **genetic testing** is not presently recommended as a preventive strategy, even when several members of a family have been diagnosed with the disease. Regular skin examinations by a dermatologist and periodic self-examination are more useful in detecting early-stage melanoma.

Because slightly more than half of melanomas do not start in moles, doctors do not think that removing normal moles in teenagers or young adults is a useful way to prevent melanoma.

Self-examination

Another important form of preventive care is regular self-examination of one's skin. The American Academy of Dermatology (AAD) outlines the steps:

- A person should first become familiar with his or her birthmarks, moles, freckles, and other skin blemishes in order to spot new growths or suspicious changes.

- Use a well-lit private room with a full-length mirror; take along a handheld mirror in order to see the back, buttocks, and other parts of the body that require a second mirror.

- It is important to check all parts of the body, not just those exposed to sunlight. Begin with the upper body, front and back; then the arms. Women should look underneath their breasts.

- Sitting in front of the mirror, examine the legs, genitals, soles of the feet, and the skin between the toes.

- Examine the back of the neck and scalp using the handheld mirror. Part the hair at intervals to check the entire scalp.

Nutrition

Some research suggests that eating a diet rich in antioxidants, **folic acid**, fats, and proteins and whole, unprocessed foods may aid in the prevention of skin cancer such as melanoma. Specific plant flavonoids have also been studied for their skin-protective properties, including apigenin (found in vegetables, fruits, tea, and wine), curcumin (found in the spice turmeric), resveratrol (found in grape skins, red wine, and peanuts), and quercetin (found in apples and onions).

Health care team roles

A physician makes an initial diagnosis that the patient has a problematic mole, but in most cases refers the patient to a dermatologist for a specialized examination. The dermatologist and a pathologist may confirm the diagnosis. A surgeon removes most lesions. A plastic and reconstructive surgeon may repair or minimize surgical scars. Nurses and nurse practitioners will participate in prevention education with patients.

Resources

BOOKS

Baldi, Alfonso, Paola Pasquali, and Enrico P. Spugnini, eds. *Skin Cancer: A Practical Approach.* New York: Humana Press, 2014.

Barnhill, Raymond L., ed. *Pathology of Melanocytic Nevi and Melanoma.* New York: Springer, 2013.

Crowson, A. Neil, Cynthia M. Magro, and Martin C. Mihm. *The Melanocytic Proliferations: A Comprehensive Textbook of Pigmented Lesions,* 2nd ed. Hoboken, NJ: John Wiley and Sons, 2013.

Jones, Alexander C., ed. *Melanoma: Molecular Biology, Risk Factors and Treatment Options.* Hauppauge, NY: Nova Science Publishers, 2013.

Handbook of Cutaneous Melanoma. New York: Springer, 2013.

PERIODICALS

Abbas, O., D.D. Miller, and J. Bhawan. "Cutaneous Malignant Melanoma: Update on Diagnostic and Prognostic Biomarkers." *American Journal of Dermatopathology* 36 (May 2014): 363–379.

Abello-Poblete, M.V., et al. "Histologic Outcomes of Excised Moderate and Severe Dysplastic Nevi." *Dermatologic Surgery* 40 (January 2014): 40–45.

Damian, D.L., R.P. Saw, and J.F. Thompson. "Topical Immunotherapy with Diphencyprone for In-transit and Cutaneously Metastatic Melanoma." *Journal of Surgical Oncology* 109 (March 2014): 308–313.

Hallemeier, C.L., et al. "Adjuvant Hypofractionated Intensity Modulated Radiation Therapy after Resection of Regional Lymph Node Metastases in Patients with Cutaneous Malignant Melanoma of the Head and Neck." *Practical Radiation Oncology* 3 (April-June 2013): e71–e77.

Hawryluk, E.B., and M.G. Liang. "Pediatric Melanoma, Moles, and Sun Safety." *Pediatric Clinics of North America* 61 (April 2014): 279–291.

Holman, D.M., et al. "Strategies to Reduce Indoor Tanning: Current Research Gaps and Future Opportunities for Prevention." *American Journal of Preventive Medicine* 44 (June 2013): 672–681.

O'Leary, R.E., J. Diehl, and P.C. Levins. "Update on Tanning: More Risks, Fewer Benefits." *Journal of the American Academy of Dermatology* 70 (March 2014): 562–568.

Olszanski, A.J. "Current and Future Roles of Targeted Therapy and Immunotherapy in Advanced Melanoma." *journal of Managed Care Pharmacy* 20 (April 2014): 346–356.

Saranga-Perry, V., et al. "Recent Developments in the Medical and Surgical Treatment of Melanoma." *CA: A Cancer Journal for Clinicians* 64 (May 2014): 171–185.

Shackelford, R., et al. "Malignant Melanoma with Concurrent BRAF E586K and NRAS Q81K Mutations." *Case Reports in Oncology* 7 (May 6, 2014): 297–300.

Sondak, V.K., and G.T. Gibney. "Surgical Management of Melanoma." *Hematology/Oncology clinics of North America* 28 (June 2014): 455–470.

OTHER

American Cancer Society (ACS). "Melanoma Skin Cancer." http://www.cancer.org/acs/groups/cid/documents/webcontent/003120-pdf.pdf (accessed June 29, 2014).

WEBSITES

American Academy of Dermatology (AAD). "Melanoma." http://www.aad.org/dermatology-a-to-z/diseases-and-treatments/m—p/melanoma (accessed June 29, 2014).

American College of Mohs Surgery (ACMS). "The Mohs Step-by-Step Process." http://www.skincancermohssurgery.org/mohs-surgery/step-by-step-process.php (accessed July 6, 2014).

Food and Drug Administration (FDA). "FDA to Require Warnings on Sunlamp Products." http://www.fda.gov/newsevents/newsroom/pressannouncements/ucm399222.htm (accessed June 30, 2014).

Heistein, Jonathan B. "Melanoma." Medscape Reference. http://emedicine.medscape.com/article/1295718-overview (accessed June 29, 2014).

Melanoma Research Foundation. "Understand Melanoma." http://www.melanoma.org/understand-melanoma (accessed June 29, 2014).

National Cancer Institute (NCI). "What Does a Mole Look Like?" http://www.cancer.gov/cancertopics/prevention/skin/molephotos (accessed June 23, 2014).

National Cancer Institute (NCI). "What You Need to Know about Melanoma and Other Skin Cancers." http://www.cancer.gov/cancertopics/wyntk/skin/page1/AllPages (accessed June 23, 2014).

National Human Genome Research Institute (NHGRI). "Learning about Skin Cancer." http://www.genome.gov/10000184 (accessed July 4, 2014).

Skin Cancer Foundation. "Melanoma." http://www.skincancer.org/skin-cancer-information/melanoma (accessed July 4, 2014).

ORGANIZATIONS

American Academy of Dermatology (AAD), P.O. Box 4014, Schaumburg, IL 60168, (847) 240-1280, (866) 503-SKIN (7546), Fax: (847) 240-1859, http://www.aad.org/Forms/ContactUs/Default.aspx, http://www.aad.org/.

American Cancer Society (ACS), 250 Williams Street NW, Atlanta, GA 30303, (800) 227-2345, http://www.cancer.org/aboutus/howwehelpyou/app/contact-us.aspx, http://www.cancer.org/index.

American College of Mohs Surgery (ACMS), 555 East Wells Street, Suite 1100, Milwaukee, WI 53202, (414) 347-1103, (800) 500-7224, http://www.

skincancermohssurgery.org/contact.php, http://www.skincancermohssurgery.org/.

American Society of Clinical Oncology (ASCO), 2318 Mill Road, Suite 800, Alexandria, VA 22314 , (571) 483-1300, (888) 651-3038, contactus@cancer.net, http://www.asco.org/.

Look Good . . . Feel Better (LGFB),(800) 395-LOOK (5665), http://lookgoodfeelbetter.org/contact, http://lookgoodfeelbetter.org/.

Melanoma Research Foundation, 1411 K Street, NW, Suite 800, Washington, DC 20005, (202) 347-9675, (800) 673-1290, Fax: (202) 347-9678, info@melanoma.org, http://www.melanoma.org/.

National Cancer Institute (NCI), BG 9609 MSC 9760, 9609 Medical Center Drive, Bethesda, MD 20892-9760, (800) 4-CANCER (422-6237), http://www.cancer.gov/global/contact/email-us, http://www.cancer.gov/.

Office of Cancer Complementary and Alternative Medicine (OCCAM), 9609 Medical Center Dr., Room 5-W-136, Rockville, MD 20850, (240) 276-6595, Fax: (240) 276-7888, ncioccam1-r@mail.nih.gov, http://cam.cancer.gov/.

Skin Cancer Foundation, 149 Madison Avenue, Suite 901, New York, NY 10016, (212) 725-5176, http://www.skincancer.org/contact-us, http://www.skincancer.org/.

Amy Sutton
Rebecca J. Frey, PhD

Melphalan

Definition

Melphalan is an anticancer (antineoplastic) agent. It also acts as a suppressor of the immune system. It is available under the brand name Alkeran.

Purpose

Melphalan is primarily used to treat **ovarian cancer** and **multiple myeloma**, which is a type of **cancer** of the bone marrow. It is also used to treat cancers that have metastasized to the liver.

Although not specifically labeled for use in the treatment of these cancers, melphalan is also used in some patients with:

- breast cancer
- cancers of the blood and lymph system
- endometrial cancer
- malignant melanoma
- Waldenström macroglobulinemia

KEY TERMS

Antineoplastic—A drug that prevents the growth of a neoplasm by interfering with the maturation or proliferation of the cells of the neoplasm.

Neoplasm—New abnormal growth of tissue.

More recently, melphalan has been used to prevent rejection of transplanted stem cells in the treatment of metastatic **breast cancer** and renal cell **carcinoma**.

Description

Melphalan is a nitrogen mustard derivative and belongs to the group of alkylating anticancer agents. It chemically interferes with the synthesis of genetic material (DNA and RNA) of cancer cells, which prevents these cells from being able to reproduce and continue the growth of the cancer.

Recommended dosage

Melphalan may be taken either orally in pill form or as an injection in liquid form. The dosage prescribed may vary widely depending on the patient, the cancer being treated, and whether or not other medications are also being taken.

A typical dosage for multiple **myeloma** is 6 mg per day for two to three weeks. After this initial dose, the drug is halted for up to 4 weeks, then resumed at a dose of 2 mg per day, depending on blood counts of the drug in the patient's blood test.

A typical dosage for ovarian cancer is 0.2 mg per kilogram (2.2 pounds) of body weight once per day for five days.

Precautions

Melphalan should be taken with food to minimize stomach upset. Melphalan should always be taken with plenty of fluids.

Melphalan can cause an allergic reaction in some people. Patients with a prior allergic reaction to melphalan should not take the drug.

Melphalan can cause serious birth defects if either the man or the woman is taking this drug at the time of conception, or if the woman is taking this drug during pregnancy. Also, male sterility is a possible side effect of melphalan. This sterility may either be temporary or permanent.

Because melphalan is easily passed from mother to child through breast milk, breastfeeding is not recommended while melphalan is being taken.

Melphalan suppresses the immune system and interferes with the normal functioning of certain organs and tissues. For these reasons, it is important that the prescribing physician is aware of any of the following pre-existing medical conditions:

• a current case of, or recent exposure to, chicken pox
• herpes zoster (shingles)
• a current case, or history of, gout or kidney stones
• all current infections
• kidney disease

Because melphalan is such a potent immunosuppressant, patients taking this drug must exercise extreme caution to avoid contracting any new infections. They should do their best to:

• avoid any person with any type of infection
• avoid any person who has received a polio vaccine in the last two months
• avoid bleeding injuries, including those caused by brushing or flossing the teeth
• avoid contact of the hands with the eyes or nasal passages unless the hands have just been washed and have not touched anything else since this washing
• avoid contact sports or any other activity that could cause a bruising or bleeding injury

Side effects

There are no common side effects of melphalan. Side effects that may occur, however, include:

• increased susceptibility to infection
• nausea and vomiting
• diarrhea
• mouth sores
• skin rash, itching, or hives
• swelling in the feet or lower legs

A doctor should be consulted immediately if the patient experiences black, tarry, or bloody stools, blood in the urine, persistent cough, **fever** and chills, pain in the lower back or sides, painful or difficult urination, or unusual bleeding or bruising.

Interactions

Melphalan should not be taken in combination with any prescription drug, over-the-counter drug, or herbal remedy without prior consultation with a physician. It is particularly important that the prescribing physician be aware of the use of any of the following drugs:

• amphotericin B
• antithyroid agents

- azathioprine
- chloramphenicol
- colchicine
- flucytosine
- ganciclovir
- interferons
- plicamycin
- probenecid
- sulfinpyrazone
- zidovudine
- any radiation therapy or chemotherapy medicines

Resources

WEBSITES

AHFS Consumer Medication Information. "Melphalan." American Society of Health-System Pharmacists. Available from: http://www.nlm.nih.gov/medlineplus/druginfo/meds/a682220.html (accessed November 3, 2014).

American Cancer Society. "Melphalan." http://www.cancer.org/treatment/treatmentsandsideeffects/guidetocancerdrugs/melphalan (accessed November 3, 2014).

Cancer Research UK. "Melphalan (Alkeran)." http://www.cancerresearchuk.org/about-cancer/cancers-in-general/treatment/cancer-drugs/melphalan (accessed November 3, 2014).

ORGANIZATIONS

U.S. Food and Drug Administration, 10903 New Hampshire Ave., Silver Spring, MD 20993, (888) INFO-FDA (463-6332), http://www.fda.gov.

Paul A. Johnson, EdM
Rebecca J. Frey, PhD

Memory change

Description

Many people with **cancer** experience memory changes—such as mild forgetfulness, an inability to concentrate on more than one task, or more severe memory loss—after undergoing **chemotherapy** or radiation treatments. In other cases, as in a person with a brain tumor, the cancer itself may cause memory changes. Surgical interventions, particularly for brain cancer, may also lead to memory loss.

Causes and symptoms

Studies show that patients experience trouble with memory and language skills after chemotherapy. Scientists are searching for the exact cause, but they believe the chemotherapy agents may be associated with this side effect. The drugs are designed to attack cancer cells, but often kill healthy cells in the process. Researchers are studying whether chemotherapy agents may be damaging healthy brain cells. Others believe the cancer itself may be responsible for the memory changes.

Similarly, **radiation therapy** also may cause people with cancer to lose some mental abilities, including memory. Physicians use radiation waves to penetrate cancer cells and stop them from growing. During the process, the rays may damage some healthy tissue. The severity of damage depends on the dose and duration of the radiation treatments. In some cases, cells killed by radiation can form a tumor-like mass in the brain, which can lead to memory loss. Children who undergo radiation treatments for a brain tumor may have developmental delays later in life.

Other side effects of cancer, such as **fatigue**, pain, and **depression**, may lead to memory impairment as a person struggles to cope with cancer. Living with constant pain, for example, takes a great deal of energy and can cause a person to become more distracted than usual. Sometimes, especially in elderly patients, it can be difficult to tell if the memory changes are caused by an existing dementia or the cancer treatment.

Treatment

Depending on the type and intensity of cancer treatment, memory difficulties may fade over time. Some people, however, will experience a permanent loss. Families can help by offering useful strategies, such as making lists of daily tasks, using a calendar or daily organizer, reducing stress, and encouraging the person to ask for help if disoriented.

Patients scheduled for radiation therapy should discuss their concerns about memory loss with their physician before the treatment begins. The radiologists may be able to control the dosage to minimize damage to healthy cells. For instance, many hospitals use a gamma knife for brain cancer treatment. The device allows radiation therapists to simultaneously attack a tumor with high-energy rays from several different angles. The gamma knife sends a concentrated dose to the tumor without damaging surrounding brain tissue.

Occupational therapists can assist people who find that cancer-related memory changes are interfering with their ability to work or perform normal activities. Many people learn helpful coping strategies from other cancer survivors by joining a support group. Since more damage occurs in younger patients, children who go through radiation therapy for **brain tumors** may need extra tutoring, or special education programs when they go to school.

Alternative and complementary therapies

Often, when physicians prescribe medication to ease a person's pain or depression, the patient's memory may improve as well. Researchers also are studying the ability of the herb *ginkgo biloba* to increase mental sharpness. Although it has not yet been proven to be completely effective, some people with memory loss find it helpful. Since ginkgo can cause circulatory problems, it is important to check with a doctor before taking it.

Resources

PERIODICALS

Kanaskie ML, and Loeb SJ. "The Experience of Cognitive Change in Women With Breast Cancer Following Chemotherapy." *Journal of Cancer Survivorship: Research and Practice* Published electronically ahead of print October 25, 2014. http://www.ncbi.nlm.nih.gov/pubmed/25343970 (accessed November 3, 2014).

Zheng Y, Luo J, Bao P, Cai H, Hong Z, Ding D, Jackson JC, Shu XO, and Dai Q. "Long-term Cognitive Function Change Among Breast Cancer Survivors." *Breast Cancer Research and Treatment* 146, no. 3 (2014): 599–609. http://www.ncbi.nlm.nih.gov/pubmed/25005574 (accessed November 3, 2014).

WEBSITES

American Cancer Society. "Chemo Brain." http://www.cancer.org/treatment/treatmentsandsideeffects/physicalsideeffects/chemotherapyeffects/chemo-brain (accessed November 3, 2014).

Melissa Knopper, M.S.

Memory loss *see* **Memory change**

MEN syndrome *see* **Multiple endocrine neoplasia**

Meningioma

Definition

A meningioma is a benign tumor of the central nervous system that develops from cells of the meninges, the membranes that cover and protect the brain and spinal cord.

Description

The meninges

The delicate tissues of the brain and spinal cord are protected by a layer of bone and an inner covering called the meninges. The meninges are composed of three layers:

• dura mater

• arachnoid

• pia mater

The tough, thick dura mater forms the outer layer of the meninges and is attached to the bone of the skull and spinal cord. The arachnoid and pia mater layers are thinner and more delicate than the dura mater. The innermost pia mater layer is attached directly to the brain and spinal cord. Meningiomas arise from the middle arachnoid layer, and most remain attached to the dura mater by a dural tail.

Types of meningiomas

Meningiomas account for 15%–20% of all **brain tumors**, and 25% of all spinal cord tumors. The World Health Organization (WHO) classifies meningiomas into 11 different categories according to their cell type. However, because there are so many different cell types and so much overlap between types, meningiomas are most often placed into three general categories, including benign, atypical, and malignant.

Benign meningiomas are by far the most common, accounting for more than 90% of all meningiomas. These tumors grow slowly and produce symptoms only if they become large enough to compress nearby brain tissue. In some patients, meningiomas can grow very large with almost no symptoms. This happens because the tumor has grown very slowly and has gradually compressed the brain over time. Meningiomas can also cause fluid to build up in the brain, and can sometimes block veins. They may also grow into nearby bone, causing the bone to become thicker.

Up to 7% of meningiomas are classified as atypical. These tumors grow more quickly than benign meningiomas and are more likely to be symptomatic. Malignant meningiomas are fast-growing aggressive tumors and are the most rare, accounting for only about 2% of all meningiomas. It is extremely unusual for meningiomas to metastasize to other organs. When they do, the lungs are the most common site.

Only about one tenth of meningiomas are found in the spine. These slow-growing tumors cause symptoms when they begin to compress the spinal cord. Spinal meningiomas usually grow in the spinal canal between the neck and the abdomen, and are almost always benign.

Demographics

Only one person in every 50,000 is diagnosed with a symptomatic meningioma annually. Most of these patients are women. Women develop brain meningiomas almost twice as often as men and spinal meningiomas four to five times more often than men. The disease usually strikes middle-aged and elderly patients. Men are most affected between the ages of 50 and 60 years, while women are most affected between the ages of 60 and 70 years. Atypical and malignant meningiomas are more common in men. Meningiomas do not occur very often in children.

Causes and symptoms

Causes

Although no single factor has been found that causes meningiomas, several risk factors are known. Some patients have developed a meningioma after being exposed to radiation. These patients tend to be younger than typical meningioma patients, and their tumors often grow more quickly. According to one study, the average age of patients with radiation-induced meningiomas is 38 years.

There is also a genetic component to meningioma. Patients who suffer from neurofibromatosis, a rare genetic disease, often develop multiple meningiomas.

Since meningioma cells recognize the female sex hormone progesterone, some researchers believe that female sex hormones may play a role in the development of meningiomas. This possible link is still being investigated.

A group of researchers at the **National Cancer Institute** reported in 2004 that people in certain occupations have a higher than normal risk of developing meningiomas. These higher-risk occupations include auto body painting, industrial production supervision, teaching, business management, interior decorating and design, and career military service. Further research is needed to determine whether there is a common causal factor linking these different fields of work.

Symptoms

Up to 75% of meningiomas produce no symptoms because they grow slowly and remain small. Often, tumors are discovered only when patients are being investigated for an unrelated illness. When symptoms do appear, it results that the tumor has grown large enough to compress part of the brain or spinal cord.

Patients experience different symptoms depending on the location of the tumor. Most brain meningiomas are located either just below the top of the skull, or between

---

---

the two hemispheres of the brain. If the tumor is located in these areas, symptoms include:

- headaches
- seizures
- dizziness
- problems with memory
- behavior changes
- protrusion of one or both eyeballs (exophthalmos)

More rarely, tumors are near sensory areas of the brain such as the optic nerve or close to the ears. Patients with these tumors experience vision or hearing losses.

Spinal meningiomas are usually found in the spinal column between the neck and the abdomen. The most common symptoms are:

- pain
- weakness and stiffness of the arms and legs
- episodes of partial paralysis

Diagnosis

Meningiomas are diagnosed using a painless noninvasive technique called **magnetic resonance imaging** (MRI). MRI works by exposing the patient to harmless radio waves and a magnetic field, which produce clear images of the brain and the spine that show the size and location of tumors. No special preparation is required for the test.

Diagnosis can also be made by **computed tomography** (CT) scan. The CT scan uses low-dose x-rays to generate a picture of the inside of the body. Sometimes a dye is injected into the patient's vein to improve the visibility of tissues. If the meningioma has grown into nearby bone, a CT scan will show the extent of bone

---

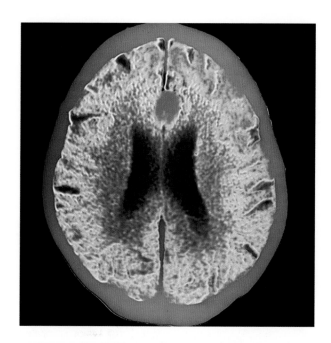

Colored computed tomography (CT) scan of the brain showing a meningioma. At upper center is the tumor (red). The cerebrum is colored yellow and light purple. *(DPT CLINICAL RADIOLOGY SALSBURY HOSPITAL/Science Source)*

invasion better than MRI. Women who are pregnant, or who think they might be pregnant, should tell their doctors before having a CT scan.

Treatment team

The treatment team for a patient with a symptomatic meningioma may include a radiologist, a neurologist (specialist of the nervous system), and a neurosurgeon.

If surgery is necessary, a neurosurgeon will perform the procedure with the help of a surgical team. The team includes two or three nurses, and an anesthesiologist.

A small number of patients receive radiotherapy for their meningioma either because the tumor is too difficult to remove surgically, or because the surgeon had to leave some tumor behind. These patients will be referred to a radiation oncologist (specialist in giving radiation to **cancer** patients).

Clinical staging

Meningiomas are classified into three different grades depending upon the likelihood of recurrence and aggressive growth:

• Grade I: Low risk of recurrence and slow growth

• Grade II: Greater likelihood of recurrence and/or aggressive growth

• Grade III: High recurrence rates and aggressive growth.

The vast majority of meningiomas are grade I. Atypical tumors are grade II, and malignant tumors are grade III.

Treatment

Medical treatment for meningiomas is necessary when tumors cause symptoms. Fortunately, only about a quarter of meningiomas become symptomatic. Most patients are cured by surgery.

The objective of surgery is to remove not only the entire meningioma, but also the tail that attaches the tumor to the meninges. If the tumor has grown into bone, the bone is removed, too. If the tumor is in a difficult location in the brain, the surgeon may leave some tumor behind in order to preserve brain tissue.

Spinal meningioma is the most successfully treated meningioma, and the most successfully treated of all spinal tumors. Most of these tumors are removed completely, and they rarely recur. Even patients with quite severe symptoms fully recover after surgery.

For the few patients who are inoperable (usually because of tumor location), **radiation therapy** can stop the growth of tumors. Recently, stereotactic radiosurgery has been successfully used. This procedure uses images of the patient's skull to construct a frame that allows precise aiming of radiation, thus minimizing harm to nearby healthy tissue. Another option is fractionated radiotherapy, which also delivers precise doses of radiation to very small areas of tissue.

Not every patient with a meningioma receives surgery or radiation. Asymptomatic patients with small or slow-growing tumors can receive periodic MRI tests to check tumor growth. Treatment may also not be necessary for patients with mild or minimal symptoms.

Alternative and complementary therapies

Unlike many other cancers, conventional medical treatment of meningioma has very high success rates. As a result, alternative therapies are not commonly used for these tumors.

Prognosis

The prognosis following brain meningioma treatment is very good. For the few patients who are not cured, prognosis depends on how completely the tumor is removed. If some tumor is left behind, recurrence is more likely, particularly for patients with grade II or grade III meningiomas. Ten years after surgery, 7%–20% of patients with benign grade I tumors have a recurrence. For patients with malignant grade III tumors, up to 78%

have a recurrence. A second surgery is sometimes necessary for patients with recurrent tumors.

Coping with cancer treatment

When first diagnosed with a meningioma, many patients experience anxiety, resulting in nervousness, sleepless nights, and even nausea. Patients can often relieve many of their fears by learning more about the disease and its course of treatment. Nevertheless, about 21% of patients with meningiomas develop psychiatric disorders, most commonly **depression** or an anxiety disorder.

The majority of meningioma patients are treated with surgery alone. Surgery will involve a hospital stay of at least a week. Before going home, patients are usually given medications to help prevent pain and swelling. Once home, patients can expect to feel some headache pain, and will become tired easily. If headaches and weakness become worse, a doctor should be contacted. Patients should make sure they get plenty of rest and eat a balanced, nutritious diet. Most patients can begin to resume their normal activities in about six to eight weeks.

Clinical trials

Chemotherapy is seldom given to meningioma patients because surgery (and/or radiotherapy) is usually successful. For patients with tumors that do not respond to these treatments, however, chemotherapy is available within a clinical trial.

Clinical trials have investigated several drugs to treat patients whose meningioma recurs following failure of both surgery and radiotherapy. **Hydroxyurea**, a drug used to treat some other cancers, has been shown to slow the growth of meningioma cells. Studies of hydroxyurea continue. Some trials have explored the link between meningioma and female sex hormones. **Tamoxifen**, an anti-estrogen drug used to fight **breast cancer**, has produced disappointing results. Trials using RU-486, an anti-progesterone agent, are underway. Information on these and other open clinical trials is available on the Internet from the National Cancer Institute at http://www. nci.nih.gov.

Prevention

The most avoidable risk factor for the development of meningioma is exposure to radiation. Children exposed to small amounts of radiation in the 1950s to treat tinea captis, a fungal infection of the scalp, developed meningiomas at an unusually high rate. There is also a clear relationship between radiation dose and

---

QUESTIONS TO ASK YOUR DOCTOR

- Will I need to have surgery?
- Can I expect a full recovery after surgery?
- Will I need radiotherapy?
- How often will I need to return for an MRI or CT scan?
- How soon can I return to work after surgery?

---

meningioma: the higher the radiation dose, the greater the probability of developing a meningioma.

Special concerns

Geriatric

In very elderly people, the symptoms of a meningioma can be very similar to normal aging. These patients typically experience difficulty with learning and remembering things as a result of the tumor. Headaches, a classic symptom of a meningioma, are not usually reported. Treatment of very elderly patients may be difficult if the patient is too frail for surgery.

Pediatric

On the rare occasions that meningiomas are diagnosed in children, they tend to be large, fast growing, and located in unusual positions. Treatment for children is the same as for adults: complete **tumor removal** with surgery and/or radiotherapy.

Neurofibromatosis

Neurofibromatosis (NF) is actually two different genetic diseases: NF Type 1 and NF Type 2. NF Type 2 is the more rare of the two diseases, affecting only one in 40,000 individuals. These patients often develop multiple brain meningiomas. Although there is no cure for NF, meningioma tumors can be removed with surgery.

Resources

BOOKS

Beers, Mark H., MD, and Robert Berkow, MD, editors. "Exophthalmos." In *The Merck Manual of Diagnosis and Therapy*. Whitehouse Station, NJ: Merck Research Laboratories, 2007.

WEBSITES

Johns Hopkins Medicine. "What is a Meningioam?" http:// www.hopkinsmedicine.org/neurology_neurosurgery/

centers_clinics/brain_tumor/center/meningioma/meningi oma-brain-tumor.html (accessed on November 3, 2014).

Mayo Clinic. "Meningioma." http://www.mayoclinic.org/dis eases-conditions/meningioma/basics/definition/CON-20026098?p=1 (accessed on November 3, 2014).

ORGANIZATIONS

American Brain Tumor Association, 8550 W. Bryn Mawr Ave., Ste. 550, Chicago, IL 60631, (773) 577-8750, (800) 886-2282, Fax: (773) 577-8738, info@abta.org, http://www.abta.org.

International Meningioma Society,info@meningiomasociety.org, http://meningiomasociety.org.

National Brain Tumor Society, 55 Chapel St., Ste. 200, Newton, MA 02458, (617) 924-9997, http://www.brain tumor.org.

National Cancer Institute, 9609 Medical Center Dr., BG 9609 MSC 9760, Bethesda, MD 20892-9760, (800) 4-CANCER (422-6237), http://www.cancer.gov.

Alison McTavish, M.Sc.
Rebecca J. Frey, PhD

KEY TERMS

Agonist—A drug that binds to cell receptors and stimulates activities normally stimulated by naturally occurring substances.

Endorphin—Short for endogenous morphine, it is a naturally occurring substance that binds to opioid receptors in the brain.

Narcotic analgesic—A classification of medications that relieves pain by temporarily depressing the central nervous system.

Opioid—A drug that possesses some properties characteristic of opiate narcotics but not derived from opium.

Patient controlled analgesic (PCA)—A device resembling an intravenous pump that allows patients to self-medicate within pre-established dosage parameters for pain control.

Meperidine

Definition

Meperidine, available as hydrochloride salt, is a narcotic analgesic, a classification term used to describe medications capable of producing a reversible depression of the central nervous system for pain control. Because of its potential for physical and psychological dependence, meperidine is a carefully controlled substance. It is commonly referred to by one of its brand names, Demerol.

Purpose

There are several possible indications for the administration of meperidine. It is commonly used for the relief of moderate to severe pain, particularly in obstetrics. Meperidine is also widely used preoperatively, and as an adjunct to anesthesia during surgery. Meperidine is not recommended for long-term management of chronic pain, such as pain caused by **cancer**, because of its potential for psychological and physical dependence.

Description

Meperidine is a synthetic compound that acts as an agonist—meaning it attaches to opioid receptors in the central nervous system and stimulates physiologic activity normally stimulated by naturally occurring substances such as endorphins (short for endogenous morphine). Meperidine acts much like morphine, although constipation, suppression of the cough reflex, and smooth muscle spasm are all reduced with meperidine.

Meperidine is available in a banana-flavored syrup, in a tablet, and in a liquid form for injection. Oral meperidine tends to be less effective than the injectable form. When taking the syrup, patients should dilute it with approximately one half glass of water to reduce temporary anesthesia to the mouth and tongue.

Recommended dosage

The recommended dosage of meperidine depends on the purpose for which it is prescribed, as well as the population in whom it is administered. For example, elderly patients, or patients with underlying medical problems that increase side effects or decrease drug metabolism, should generally be given reduced dosages. Meperidine can be taken orally, in tablet or syrup form, intravenously (directly into a vein), or by injection into the muscle (intramuscularly) or connective tissue (subcutaneously).

Generally, repeated doses administered to manage pain should be given by injection intramuscularly. The subcutaneous route is acceptable for occasional administration. When given intravenously, meperidine should be diluted and administered very slowly. When taken in conjunction with phenothiazine or other tranquilizers, the dose should be decreased by as much as a half. Specific dosages are as follows.

FOR RELIEF OF MODERATE TO SEVERE PAIN. The recommended dosage for adults for pain relief is 50–150 mg every three to four hours by oral or intramuscular route. When given intravenously through a patient-controlled analgesia (PCA) device, an initial dose of 10 mg should be administered. The PCA should be programmed to administer between 1–5 mg every 6–10 minutes. If meperidine is given continuously through an intravenous line, the dose should be adjusted based on patient response to a range of 15–35 mg an hour. Children should be given 1–1.8 mg per kg (2.2 pounds) intramuscularly or subcutaneously.

FOR PREOPERATIVE MEDICATION. Adults may be given 50–100 mg of meperidine intramuscularly, or subcutaneously 30–90 minutes prior to surgery. Children's dosages should be reduced to 1–2 mg per kg through the same routes.

For obstetric pain control. The recommended dosage for control of regular (not sporadic) pain in this setting is 50–100 mg every 1–3 hours intramuscularly or subcutaneously.

Precautions

Other patients who should avoid meperidine use include those with previous hypersensitivity to narcotics, or those with underlying respiratory problems. Meperidine, even in recommended therapeutic doses, can decrease the respiratory drive. Conditions such as asthma or chronic obstructive pulmonary disease may increase the likelihood of respiratory difficulty. Meperidine can also impair judgment, and should not be used in individuals engaging in activities that require alertness, such as driving.

Because its effects on a fetus are unknown, meperidine is not recommended in pre-labor stage pregnant women. Even in labor, when it may be indicated for pain control, meperidine may cause respiratory depression of the mother and her baby, particularly premature babies. Meperidine is excreted in breast milk, and, if needed, should be administered several hours before breastfeeding to minimize ingestion by the infant.

Side effects

The most common adverse effects of meperidine are lightheadedness, dizziness, sedation, nausea and/or vomiting, and sweating. Less common, but more severe, side effects include respiratory depression and abnormally low blood pressure.

Interactions

Individuals who are taking or have recently taken drugs called monoamine oxidase (MAO) inhibitors (a class of antidepressants) should not be given meperidine. Reactions have been reported in this population that are characterized by a variety of signs and symptoms including respiratory distress, coma, abnormally low or abnormally high blood pressure, hyperexcitability, and even death. If administration of a narcotic is required, it should be given in small, gradually increasing test doses under careful supervision.

Adverse effects such as respiratory depression and decreased blood pressure are more common when meperidine is administered in conjunction with other narcotic analgesics, anesthetics, phenothiazines, sedatives, or any other type of drug that suppresses the central nervous system. Alcohol should also be avoided.

Resources
BOOKS
Chu, Edward, and Vincent T. DeVita Jr. *Physicians' Cancer Chemotherapy Drug Manual 2014*. Burlington, MA: Jones & Bartlett Learning, 2014.

WEBSITES
AHFS Consumer Medication Information "Meperidine." American Society of Health-System Pharmacists. Available from: http://www.nlm.nih.gov/medlineplus/druginfo/meds/a682117.html (accessed November 4, 2014).
American Cancer Society. "Meperidine." http://www.cancer.org/treatment/treatmentsandsideeffects/guidetocancerdrugs/meperidine (accessed November 4, 2014).

Tamara Brown, R.N.

Mercaptopurine
Definition

Mercaptopurine is a medicine used to prevent the formation and spread of **cancer** cells. Mercaptopurine is also called 6-mercaptopurine or 6-MP, and is available under the brand name Purinethol.

Purpose

Mercaptopurine is used as part of the consolidation and maintenance treatment for **acute lymphocytic leukemia** (ALL) and acute myelocytic leukemia (AML).

Description

Mercaptopurine is an analog of purine, a component of DNA/RNA, and belongs to antimetabolites that prevent the biosynthesis, or utilization, of normal cellular metabolites. It has been used for several decades in combination with other **chemotherapy** drugs for the treatment of different types of acute adult and childhood leukemias (ALL and AML). It has also been shown to be effective for the treatment of inflammatory bowel disease (IBD), which includes Crohn's disease and ulcerative colitis; certain types of arthritis; and polycythemia vera, which is an above normal increase in red cells in the blood. Mercaptopurine helps to decrease the dose of steroids in patients with IBD, and to reduce their dependence on steroids to control symptoms of their disease. The medicine is taken up by red cells in the blood and works by decreasing the formation of certain genetic material (DNA and RNA) in patients with cancer and by altering the activity of the immune system in patients with IBD.

Recommended dosage

Doses vary between different chemotherapy protocols. The usual dose is 2.5 mg per kg (2.2 pounds) per day in adults and children—50 mg daily in an average 5-year old child or 100–200 mg daily in adults. The total daily dose is calculated to the nearest multiple of 25 mg and is given all at one time. Another way of dosing 6-MP is based on body surface area (BSA), and is usually 75 mg per square meter in children and 80–100 mg per square meter in adults.

Doses of 1.5–2.5 mg per kg per day is recommended for leukemia patients. For those patients with inflammatory bowel disease, doses of 1.5 mg per kg per day have been used in research studies.

Administration

This medicine is usually taken by mouth and should be given at the same time every day, preferably on an empty stomach, one hour before meals or two hours after meals. Children with leukemia should be taking this medicine at bedtime for maximum effectiveness. All patients should drink plenty of fluids—at least eight glasses of water per day—while taking this medication, unless otherwise directed by a physician.

Precautions

The use of 6-MP in pregnant women should be avoided whenever possible, especially during the first three months of pregnancy, as 6-MP can cause birth defects and spontaneous abortions.

As 6-MP can lower the body's ability to fight infections, patients are advised to avoid contact with people who have a cold, flu, or other infections.

Mercaptopurine should be used with caution in the following populations:

- people who had an allergic reaction to 6-MP in the past
- people at risk for pancreatitis (inflammation of the pancreas)
- breastfeeding mothers (it is not known if 6-MP crosses in to breast milk)
- people with liver or kidney disease
- people with gout (6-MP can exacerbate the symptoms of gout)
- people taking allopurinol for gout
- people with suppressed bone marrow (tissue filling the empty spaces inside the bone)

Patients are encouraged to stop taking 6-MP, and contact a physician immediately, if any of the following symptoms develop:

- fever, chills, or sore throat
- yellowing of the skin or eyes
- blood in the urine or stools
- black stools

• unusual bleeding or bruising

• stomach pain with nausea, vomiting, or loss of appetite

Patients taking 6-MP must see a physician before starting medication therapy, and also occasionally during therapy, to have blood tests for the monitoring of a complete blood count and kidney and liver functions.

Side effects

This is a very potent medicine that can cause serious side effects. These side effects include skin rash, nausea, vomiting, **diarrhea**, mouth sores, yellowing of the eyes or skin, clay-colored stools, dark urine, decreased ability to fight infections, pinpoint red dots on the skin, and darkening of the skin. **Nausea and vomiting**, diarrhea, and stomach pain are less common in children than in adults.

Interactions

Mercaptopurine can decrease the effectiveness of blood thinners such as **warfarin** (Coumadin).

The drug can exacerbate the symptoms of gout. The anti-gout medication, **allopurinol**, can increase blood levels of 6-MP and increase the risk of its side effects. The dose of 6-MP needs to be decreased—or its use should be avoided—in patients taking allopurinol, which interferes with the degradation of 6-MP.

Risk of liver disease may be increased in patients taking both **doxorubicin** (a cancer chemotherapy drug) and 6-MP. Other medicines that decrease the function of the liver can cause increased toxicity with 6-MP. Patients should inform their doctor or pharmacist about all the prescription drugs and over-the-counter medications that they are taking.

Resources

BOOKS

Chu, Edward, and Vincent T. DeVita Jr. *Physicians' Cancer Chemotherapy Drug Manual 2014*. Burlington, MA: Jones & Bartlett Learning, 2014.

WEBSITES

American Cancer Society. "Mercaptopurine." http://www. cancer.org/treatment/treatmentsandsideeffects/guidetocan cerdrugs/mercaptopurine (accessed November 4, 2014).

The Scott Hamilton CARES Initiative. "Mercaptopurine."-Chemocare.com http://chemocare.com/chemotherapy/ drug-info/Mercaptopurine.aspx (accessed November 4, 2014).

Olga Bessmertny, Pharm.D.

Merkel cell carcinoma

Definition

Merkel cell **carcinoma** (MCC) is a rare form of **cancer** that develops on, or just beneath, the skin and in hair follicles. It is also known as neuroendocrine cancer of the skin or trabecular cancer.

Description

Merkel cells are cells that lie in the middle layers of the skin. They are named for their discoverer, a German professor of anatomy named Friedrich Sigmund Merkel (1845–1919). These cells are organized around hair follicles and are believed to act as some type of touch receptors. MCC begins in these cells.

MCC usually appears as firm shiny skin lumps, or tumors. These tumors are painless and can range in size from less than a quarter of an inch (0.6 cm) to over two inches (5.1 cm) in diameter. They may be red, pink, or blue. Tumors first appear on the head and neck in about 48% of cases, and less frequently on other sun-exposed parts of the body.

MCC is very aggressive, it spreads very rapidly, and it often invades other tissues and organs (metastasizes). The most common sites of **metastasis** of MCC are the lymph nodes, liver, bones, lungs, and brain. Metastasis to the lymph nodes generally occurs within seven to eight months after the first skin tumors appear. Nearly half of all people affected with MCC will develop systemic metastases within 24 months, and 67%–74% of these people will die within five years.

Local recurrence of MCC after the removal of the primary tumor occurs in approximately one-third of all patients and is usually apparent within four months.

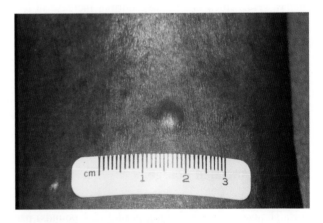

A Merkel cell tumor on a patient's leg. *(Caliendo, RBP FBPA/ Custom Medical Stock Photo)*

Several other names have been used to describe MCC, among these are: anaplastic carcinoma of the skin, apudoma, endocrine carcinoma of the skin, neuroendocrine carcinoma of the skin (NEC), primary small-cell carcinoma of the skin, primary undifferentiated carcinoma of the skin, and trabecular cell carcinoma. The two most commonly used names are MCC and NEC.

Demographics

The American Cancer Society estimates that approximately 1,500 cases of MCC are diagnosed each year in the United States. It is seen almost exclusively (94% of known cases) in Caucasians. It affects males more often than females. Seventy-six percent of cases reported in the United States have been diagnosed in people older than 65, but MCC has also been seen in a child as young as seven and a woman as old as 97.

Causes and symptoms

The cause of MCC has not been positively identified. It is believed to be caused by the skin damage associated with exposure to ultraviolet light from the sun.

Some researchers believe that Merkel cell carcinoma may also be associated with immunodeficiency syndromes, as six of the 1043 patients recorded in the United States developed MCC after being diagnosed with **chronic lymphocytic leukemia**.

The only symptom of primary MCC is the appearance of the characteristic tumors in the skin. Lymph node metastases show enlarged, firm, lymph nodes in the region of the primary tumor. Other systemic metastases show as masses in the affected organs. The location of the primary tumor is not related to the location of these systemic metastases.

Diagnosis

The diagnosis of MCC is performed by examining and testing a **biopsy** of the tumor. MCC is difficult to differentiate from several other forms of abnormal tissue growth (neoplasms). This diagnosis cannot be made just by examining the tumor cells under a microscope. It is done by performing a variety of chemical tests on these cells. Testing must be performed to make sure this is not metastatic oat-cell (lung) cancer.

Treatment team

MCC is generally first identified by a microbiologist who examines a biopsy sample. Most MCC tumor removals are performed by dermatologists. Post-operative radiation treatments are generally ordered by the dermatologist and performed by a radiation therapist under the direction of a radiologist and/or a radiation physicist.

Because of the rapid and possibly invasive nature of MCC, patients are generally referred to a physician specializing in cancer (oncologist) to ensure that the disease has not spread to other parts of the body. **Chemotherapy** for MCC is considered investigational.

Clinical staging

MCC is classified into three clinical stages. Stage I MCC is defined as a disease that is localized to the skin. Stage II MCC is characterized by a spreading of the disease to the lymph nodes that are near the primary skin tumor or tumors. Stage III MCC is characterized by systemic metastases.

Treatment

Treatment of stage I MCC involves wide local excision and follow-up **radiation therapy**. Wide local excision is a procedure in which the tumor and a small area of the surrounding healthy tissue are surgically removed. Since MCC is so aggressive, all patients are considered to be at high risk for recurrence and metastasis. For this reason, all patients will undergo radiation therapy of the lymph nodes near the site of the primary tumor that was removed. A technique called lymphoscintigraphy is used to determine the precise location of the lymph nodes that are most likely to be affected.

Treatment of stage II MCC is the same as for stage I MCC with the additional removal of the affected lymph nodes.

Treatment of stage III MCC is generally chemotherapy. But, because the number of known cases of MCC is relatively small, there is no generally prescribed chemotherapy regimen. It has been treated with **etoposide**, **cisplatin**, and **fluorouracil** with varying degrees of success.

Alternative and complementary therapies

Naturopathic remedies believed by some to be beneficial in the prevention of skin cancers include regular cleansing by fasting, enema, or herbal supplements. Many naturopaths also recommend a daily scrubbing of the skin with a sauna brush prior to bathing to increase circulation. **Vitamins** A, C, and E, as well as zinc, are believed by some to be essential supplements to a high fiber diet in the prevention of skin damage. However, these remedies have not been proven effective in treating Merkel cell tumors. Traditional medical treatments that have succeeded include surgery, radiation therapy, and chemotherapy, as well as rare success with stem cell transplant.

Prognosis

The prognosis for patients affected with MCC is generally poor. Half will have a recurrence within two years and one-third will develop systemic involvement (stage III). The average time span from diagnosis of stage III MCC to death is eight months. The two-year survival rate for people affected with MCC is approximately 50%. Factors that improve the patient's length of survival include location of the tumor on the limbs rather than the face; localization of the disease; and female sex.

Coping with cancer treatment

The radiation therapy necessary for follow-up treatment after MCC **tumor removal** can become stressful for some patients. Additionally, most of these cancers occur in the head and neck region, and their removal can be very disfiguring. It is important that all patients receive adequate counseling and other psychological support prior to and during such treatments.

Clinical trials

In late 2014, there were six active trials for Merkel cell carcinoma listed on the National Cancer Institute website. Information on **clinical trials** can be found by conducting a search at: http://www.cancer.gov/clinical-trials/search.

Prevention

Because MCC is believed, at least in some cases, to be caused by long-term exposure to ultraviolet light, it may possibly be prevented by avoiding sun exposure when possible and by wearing a PABA containing sunscreen daily.

QUESTIONS TO ASK YOUR DOCTOR

- What stage is my cancer in?
- How long will my radiation therapy treatments last after the tumor is removed?
- What are the possible side effects of the particular radiation or chemotherapy treatments that I will receive?
- How often should I continue to be checked for possible recurrence of MCC?

Special concerns

MCC is very aggressive and can metastasize quickly. For these reasons, medical treatment needs to be sought quickly when MCC is suspected. Recurrence of MCC, either on the skin or in the lymph nodes or other bodily organs, is quite common. It is extremely important that all MCC patients—even if they believe that they have no symptoms—have follow-up examinations monthly for at least two years after they have finished their initial radiation treatments.

Resources

PERIODICALS

Hughes, M.P., Hardee, M.E., Cornelius, L.A., Hutchins, L.F., Becker, J.C., and Gao, L. "Merkel Cell Carcinoma: Epidemiology, Target, and Therapy." *Current Dermatology Reports* 22, no. 3 (2014): 46–53. http://www.ncbi.nlm.nih.gov/pmc/articles/PMC3931972/ (accessed November 4, 2014).

Rabinowits, G. "Systemic Therapy for Merkel Cell Carcinoma: What's on the Horizon?" *Cancers* 6, no. 2 (2014): 1180–94. http://www.ncbi.nlm.nih.gov/pubmed/24840048 (accessed November 4, 2014).

WEBSITES

National Cancer Institute. "General Information About Merkel Cell Carcinoma." http://www.cancer.gov/cancertopics/pdq/treatment/merkelcell/Patient/page1 (accessed November 4, 2014).

ORGANIZATIONS

American Academy of Dermatology, PO Box 4014, Schaumburg, IL 60168, (847) 240-1280, (866) 503-SKIN (7546), Fax: (847) 240-1859, http://www.aad.org.

American Cancer Society, 250 Williams St. NW, Atlanta, GA 30303, (800) 227-2345, http://www.cancer.org.

Skin Cancer Foundation, 149 Madison Ave., Ste. 901, New York, NY 10016, (212) 725-5176, http://www.skincancer.org.

Paul A. Johnson, EdM
Rebecca J. Frey, PhD

Mesna

Definition

Mesna is a medicine that helps protect the inside lining of the bladder from damage due to certain **chemotherapy** drugs. Mesna may also be referred to as 2-mercaptoethane sulfonate, sodium salt, or Mesnex (its brand name).

Purpose

Mesna is a medicine that is approved by the Food and Drug Administration (FDA) for use in combination with the chemotherapy drug **ifosfamide** to protect the bladder lining from irritation due to the chemotherapy. It has also been shown useful in protecting the bladder lining when used in combination with large doses of the chemotherapy drug **cyclophosphamide**. Irritation to the bladder lining can cause bleeding and this is referred to as hemorrhagic cystitis. Mesna is not administered to treat **cancer**.

Description

Mesna is a clear, colorless solution with a foul odor. It is usually administered intravenously through a vein to prevent bleeding of the inside lining of the bladder. Sometimes it can be given to a patient to mix in a beverage and drink. When ifosfamide and cyclophosphamide are given, they break down in the body and form a poisonous substance called acrolein. Acrolein concentrates in the bladder and causes irritation that can lead to severe bleeding from the bladder into the urine. When mesna is administered it also concentrates in the bladder and combines with the toxic acrolein to form a nontoxic substance that is removed from the body by urinating.

Recommended dosage

Mesna is usually administered through a vein over at least five minutes. This same drug can also be mixed with a beverage and taken by mouth—flavored drinks like grape juice, cola, and chocolate milk are good choices to hide the taste of the mesna.

The mesna dose depends on the amount of chemotherapy drugs, ifosfamide or cyclophosphamide, that a patient receives. The mesna dose can vary with the time frame the chemotherapy drugs are being administered. The standard mesna dose is equal to 20% of the total ifosfamide dose given at three separate time intervals through a vein infused over at least five minutes. The first dose is right before the ifosfamide, often referred to as hour 0. The second dose is four hours

KEY TERMS

Acrolein—A breakdown product of the chemotherapy drugs ifosfamide and cyclophosphamide that concentrates in the bladder and irritates the bladder lining and causes bleeding.

Bladder—Organ in the body that collects urine from the kidneys.

Chemotherapy—Specific drugs used to treat cancer.

Food and Drug Administration—A government agency that oversees public safety in relation to drugs and medical devices. The FDA gives the approval to pharmaceutical companies for commercial marketing of their products.

Hemorrhagic cystitis—Irritation of the bladder lining that causes bleeding.

Nontoxic—Does not cause harm.

after the start of the infusion and the third dose is eight hours after the start of the infusion. Mesna is given in this way each day the ifosfamide is administered.

Mesna can be given at a dose of 100% of the ifosfamide. This mesna would be mixed directly with the ifosfamide in the same intravenous infusion bag. This type of dosing may or may not have the patient receive a small dose of mesna right before or after the ifosfamide infusion.

Precautions

Mesna can cause allergic reactions that range from a mild rash to severe life-threatening, full-body allergic reactions. Patients with a known previous allergic reaction to mesna or thiol-like medicines should tell their doctor before receiving mesna.

Mesna that contains the preservative benzyl alcohol must not be used in premature babies or infants and must be used with caution in older children.

Mesna should prevent most bleeding from the bladder, however patients may be asked to check their urine for traces of blood with a chemical strip that is dipped into the urine sample.

Side effects

Side effects due only to the mesna are uncommon and difficult to determine since the drug is not given alone. However in clinical studies mesna has been known to cause **nausea and vomiting**, **diarrhea**, abdominal pain, and a bad taste in the mouth. Other reported side effects include; headache, **fatigue**, pain in arms and legs, drop in blood pressure, and allergic reactions.

All side effects a patient experiences should be reported to his or her doctor.

Interactions

Mesna can cause a false positive test of the urine for ketone bodies. This may be most important in diabetic patients who routinely check their urine for ketones.

Resources

BOOKS

Chu, Edward, and Vincent T. DeVita Jr. *Physicians' Cancer Chemotherapy Drug Manual 2014*. Burlington, MA: Jones & Bartlett Learning, 2014.

WEBSITES

AHFS Consumer Medication Information. "Mesna." American Society of Health-System Pharmacists. Available from: http://www.nlm.nih.gov/medlineplus/druginfo/meds/a613013.html (accessed November 4, 2014).
American Cancer Society. "Mesna." http://www.cancer.org/treatment/treatmentsandsideeffects/guidetocancerdrugs/mesna (accessed November 4, 2014).

Nancy J. Beaulieu, RPh, BCOP

Mesnex *see* **Mesna**

Mesothelioma

Definition

Malignant mesothelioma is a rare form of **cancer**. In mesothelioma, malignant cells are found in the sac lining of the chest (the pleura) or the abdomen (the peritoneum). The majority of people with mesothelioma have a job history that exposed them to asbestos, an insulation material. Twenty to fifty years may pass between exposure and diagnosis.

Description

A layer of specialized cells called mesothelial cells are found in the chest and abdominal cavities, the cavity around the heart (pericardial sac), and around the outer surface of most internal organs. These cells form tissue called mesothelium.

Mesothelium performs a protective function for the internal organs by producing a lubricating fluid that permits the organs to move around. For example, this

---

KEY TERMS

Asbestos—A group of naturally occurring fibrous minerals called silicates (e.g., magnesium and silicon) that are found in soil and rocks around the world. These silicates are heat resistant and have an ideal structure for use in building materials and textiles. Accordingly, asbestos has been used as an insulating material since ancient times. Exposure to asbestos dust is the primary risk factor for developing malignant mesothelioma.

Mediastinoscopy—Mediastinoscopy is a minimally invasive procedure in which a lighted fiberoptic instrument with a tiny video camera is passed through a small incision in the mediastinum, about 1 inch above the breast bone. It is performed to assess the lymph nodes in the pleural cavity and obtain a biopsy of mediastinal tissue.

Pleurodesis—Pleurodesis is a procedure that attaches the outside of the lung to the inside of the chest wall to help prevent the lung from collapsing. This may be a surgical procedure or it can be accomplished by instilling a chemical irritant such as talc into the lung, which causes the pleura to adhere to the chest wall.

---

fluid makes it easier for the lungs to move inside the chest while people breathe. The mesothelium of the abdomen is known as the peritoneum, and the mesothelium of the chest is called the pleura. Pericardium refers to the mesothelium of the pericardial cavity.

Malignant mesotheliomas are classified into three distinct types based on the specific cancer cell type:

- Epithelial mesothelioma is characterized by well defined, elongated epithelial cells that are easily identified microscopically. It accounts for about 50%–75% of mesotheliomas and has the highest survival rate.

- Sarcomatoid mesothelioma is characterized by a less common cell that comes from supportive structures in the body such as muscle and bone. It represents from 7% to 20% of mesotheliomas.

- Biphasic mesotheliomas are those characterized by a mix of epithelial and sarcomatoid cells. It is the second most common type of mesothelioma and accounts for 20%–40% of cases.

Benign or non-malignant forms of mesothelioma can also develop. Symptoms of this benign type are similar but appear many years sooner in people exposed to asbestos. Treatment is usually successful. Individuals diagnosed with a non-malignant mesothelioma are advised to have regular check-ups to watch for any signs of more serious asbestos-related diseases.

Approximately 90% of all mesotheliomas begin in the chest cavity and are known as pleural mesotheliomas, which is one type of environmental pulmonary disease. The remaining 10% include peritoneal mesothelioma, which appears in the cavity around the heart. Pericardial mesothelioma occurs less often.

Demographics

Mesothelioma is a relatively rare form of cancer. According to the American Cancer Society, about 3,000 new cases are diagnosed each year in the United States. Although asbestos use has declined since the 1980s, the reported cases of mesothelioma are related to the widespread use of asbestos from the 1940s to the end of the 1970s. Rates have leveled off in the United States and are expected to decrease due to the decrease in workplace exposure; however, mesothelioma is still on the rise in some countries.

The average age at diagnosis of malignant mesothelioma is between 50 and 70, reflecting the long time period between exposure and presentation of symptoms. The disease affects men three to five times more frequently than women and is more common among whites and Hispanics/Latinos than among African Americans or Asian Americans.

Causes and symptoms

Asbestos exposure is the primary risk factor for mesothelioma. Asbestos workers have a 10% risk of developing the disease at some point in their lives. In the past, asbestos was used as an effective type of insulation. The use of this material, however, has declined since its link with mesothelioma has become evident. It is believed that when the fibers of asbestos are inhaled, some reach the ends of the small airways and penetrate the pleural lining. Once that occurs, the fibers may directly harm mesothelial cells, eventually causing mesothelioma. If the fibers are swallowed, they can reach the abdominal cavity, where they contribute to the development of peritoneal mesothelioma.

Exposure to certain types of radiation as well as to a chemical related to asbestos known as zeolite has also been associated with the development of mesothelioma.

The early symptoms of mesothelioma are subtle and often mistaken for more common ailments. The typical symptoms include:

• pain in the lower back or at the side of the chest
• shortness of breath
• difficulty swallowing
• persistent cough
• fever
• fatigue
• abdominal pain, weight loss, and nausea and vomiting (peritoneal mesothelioma)

As the disease progresses, other symptoms may be develop, including **anemia** and blood clotting disorders, bowel obstruction, fluid build-up (peritoneal effusion) in the pleura or pericardium, and the coughing up of blood (**hemoptysis**). Peritoneal effusion may affect the functioning of other abdominal organs. Pleural mesothelioma can spread either locally into lymph nodes of the chest or into the pericardium, diaphragm, peritoneum of the abdomen, the liver, adrenal glands, and rarely, the testicles.

Diagnosis

Individuals who experience shortness of breath, chest pain, or pain or swelling in the abdomen are advised to see a doctor. The doctor will perform a complete physical examination, take a thorough medical history, and may also order abdominal and/or chest **x-rays**. One or more of the following methods may be used to determine whether mesothelioma is present.

• Imaging tests such as x-rays, computed tomography (CT scans), or magnetic resonance imaging (MRI) to visualize the area in question. CT and MRI also will help determine staging based on the location, size, and extent of the cancer, including the involvement of lymph nodes and other organ systems.
• Pleural biopsy. Diagnosing mesothelioma requires an adequate biopsy specimen. However, because

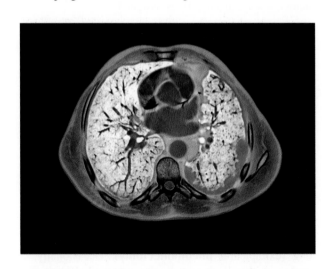

Computed tomography (CT) scan revealing mesothelioma in the left lung of a 69-year-old patient. The tumor is shown in orange in the lower right corner. (DU Cane Medical Imaging Ltd./Science Source)

mesothelioma usually arises from the lower part of the diaphragmatic and/or parietal pleura, it is sometimes difficult to obtain enough tissue. A simple, or closed, pleural biopsy involves inserting a needle into the chest cavity to obtain tissue and pleural fluid from the pleural membrane for analysis. This technique is minimally invasive and normally requires only local anesthesia. However, the needle biopsy may not provide sufficient material to identify cell types and confirm a diagnosis of mesothelioma. Also, since the biopsy is not performed under direct vision, the needle might not take tissue from the exact area of the tumor. If the diagnosis cannot be made with the less invasive needle biopsy, an open pleural biopsy may be necessary. With this approach, a surgeon makes an incision on the patient's side and goes into the pleural space to remove an adequate tumor sample. This method has the advantage of allowing maximum exploration of the pleural membranes, but it does require general anesthesia.

- Thoracoscopy. A thoracoscopy allows the doctor to see directly into the chest (pleural) cavity at the tumor site and surrounding area and to obtain a tissue sample for analysis of cells (histopathologic analysis). The thoracoscopy is performed by making a tiny incision in the chest while the patient is under anesthesia. A lighted fiber optic instrument (endoscope) with a tiny video camera attached is passed through the incision to examine the area. Forceps are then used to obtain a tissue biopsy of the tumor or chest wall. Biopsy of a peritoneal tumor may be obtained using a similar approach called a laparoscopy to view the inside of the abdomen and obtain a sample of the affected peritoneum.

- Bronchoscopy. A bronchoscopy, which examines the airways, or a mediastinoscopy, which looks at the lymph nodes in the chest, allows the doctor to view the target area using a lighted fiber optic instrument with a camera attached. Samples may be taken with a needle and sent to the pathology laboratory to determine the presence of cancer cells. However, bronchoscopy and mediastinoscopy are not often used to diagnose mesothelioma, as the disease is seldom found within the airways or the lymph nodes.

- Surgery. This allows the doctor to obtain a larger tumor sample or, on occasion, remove the entire tumor.

Diagnosing mesothelioma is often difficult, even with tissue biopsies. Microscopically, the tissue and cells that characterize mesothelioma are hard to distinguish from several other forms of cancer. For this reason, certain laboratory tests are important for accurate diagnosis. Some lab tests involve the use of specific antibodies to distinguish lung cancer from mesothelioma. Sometimes an accurate diagnosis involves the use of a highly sensitive electron microscope to view the tissue samples.

Treatment team

A person with symptoms of mesothelioma is likely to seek help from a primary physician initially. In the diagnostic phase, radiologic technicians will perform various **imaging studies**. A specially-trained physician—a thoracic surgeon or, rarely, a pulmonologist—performs other diagnostic tests such as **pleural biopsy** and **thoracoscopy**. A pathologist then views the tissue samples to determine the cell type involved and confirm the diagnosis of mesothelioma. Following diagnosis, the patient treatment may entail surgery, **radiation therapy**, **chemotherapy**, or a combination of these. The patient may receive care from a thoracic surgeon, an anesthesiologist, medical and radiation oncologists, and specially-trained nurses who administer chemotherapy.

Clinical staging

The treatment and outlook for people with mesothelioma depends a great deal on the stage of the cancer and whether it is local or has spread to lymph nodes or other body organs. Staging is done with results of chest CT, **mediastinoscopy**, and MRI. A staging system is used only with pleural mesothelioma, which represents the majority of cases. Pleural mesothelioma was once staged with the Butchart system, but has since been replaced with the TNM system, now used as the standard.

TNM first assesses the size of the tumor (T), whether or not the cancer has spread to nearby lymph nodes (N), and if the cancer has metastasized (M). Based on these factors, a stage from I–IV is assigned.

Treatment

Treatment for mesothelioma is primarily supportive care, which may include surgery (pleurectomy) to relieve shortness of breath (dyspnea) and remove **pleural effusion**, **pleurodesis** to prevent lung collapse, and chemotherapy to shrink tumors and relieve symptoms. Surgery is an option only when the cancer is limited to one place and the patient is able to withstand surgery. During surgery, the physician may remove the cancerous portion of the lining of the chest (pleurectomy) or abdomen (peritonectomy) and some of the tissue or lymph nodes that surround it. Depending on the extent of disease spread, it may become necessary to remove a lung (extrapleural **pneumonectomy**). Occasionally, a portion of the diaphragm is also removed. If it is not possible to treat the cancer, less invasive measures may be used for symptom relief. These palliative measures are intended only to improve symptoms.

Radiation therapy is not considered appropriate for pleural mesothelioma since the disease itself is not usually limited to one precise area, but may be used to relieve symptoms such as local pain and difficulty swallowing in patients for whom surgery is not an option.

Chemotherapy involves the use of drugs to kill cancer cells. The most commonly used drugs for this cancer are **doxorubicin**, **cisplatin**, and **methotrexate**. The medicines are injected into a vein or taken by mouth. In the treatment of mesothelioma, they may also be injected directly into the chest or abdominal cavity. Chemotherapy is primarily applied to shrink the tumor and may be given in addition to surgery, depending on the type and stage of the cancer.

Pain is controlled with analgesic medicines, either orally or by injection. Opioid drugs are commonly used. Some patients, particularly in the latter stages of the disease, may need to have an in-dwelling catheter, which delivers the pain medications consistently.

Intraoperative **photodynamic therapy** may be applied for the treatment of pleural mesothelioma that is confined to the lung. This treatment uses special photosensitive drugs that make cancer cells easier to kill with laser light treatment. The drugs are administered intravenously 24 to 48 hours before surgery. Normal cells will have released the drug at the time of surgery but the cancer cells will retain the drug and die when the pleura is exposed to laser beams.

Alternative and complementary therapies

Few alternative therapies are appropriate for treatment of mesothelioma. Nevertheless, many well-studied complementary treatments may increase a patient's comfort and sense of well-being. Integrative oncology includes all of the conventional treatments described above and adds complementary approaches such as acupuncture, massage, and reflexology to help manage pain, anxiety, restlessness, and symptoms related to chemotherapy treatments. Other approaches may include meditation to aid in relaxation and guided imagery to help prevent nausea. Because the prognosis for mesothelioma is often poor, many patients may opt to try other avenues of treatment. Patients should always consult with their physicians before attempting non-standard treatment.

Prognosis

Mesothelioma, whether pleural or peritoneal, is an incurable cancer and survival rates are low. By the time symptoms appear and mesothelioma is diagnosed, the disease is often advanced. The average survival period after diagnosis is 9 to 12 months. If the cancer is

---

QUESTIONS TO ASK YOUR DOCTOR

- What type of mesothelioma do I have?
- Has my cancer spread beyond the primary site?
- What stage is my cancer in? What are the treatment options?
- What is my prognosis?
- Are any experimental therapies available that I may benefit from? Where are they being performed?

---

discovered before it has spread and is treated aggressively, about half of the patients may live two years after diagnosis, and up to 20%, usually younger patients with a shorter duration of symptoms, may survive up to five years. Long-term survival is uncommon.

Coping with cancer treatment

Coping with cancer treatment can be difficult and exhausting. Patients receiving therapy for mesothelioma will benefit from finding a group of family and friends to help with household responsibilities, provide transportation, and offer psychological support. Patients should avoid rushing back to normal activities after treatment is completed.

Clinical trials

A great deal of research is being conducted in the area of mesothelioma. Much of the research is focused on understanding the process whereby asbestos changes mesothelial cells to malignant mesothelioma. In addition, new surgical procedures and new combinations of **anticancer drugs** are being investigated in **clinical trials**. **Gene therapy** and **immunotherapy** using interleukins and **interferons** to activate the immune system are also being investigated. National professional organizations focused on cancer or lung disease will often help patients and their families find a suitable clinical trial offering experimental therapies.

Prevention

The only preventive measure for mesothelioma is to avoid or limit exposure to asbestos. People who might experience asbestos exposure at work include miners, insulation manufacturers, construction workers, ship builders, and factory workers. Use of asbestos has declined markedly since the 1980s but sources of asbestos are not always known and exposure still occurs.

Resources

BOOKS

Fishman, Alfred P., Jack A. Elias, Jay A. Fishman, Michael A. Grippi, editors. " Asbestos-Related Lung Disease." In *Fishman's Pulmonary Diseases and Disorders*. 4th edition. New York, NY: McGraw-Hill, 2008.

Porter, Robert S., MD, and Justin L. Kaplan, MD, editors. "Mesothelioma, Section 14: Pulmonary Disorders." In *The Merck Manual of Diagnosis and Therapy*. 19th edition. Whitehouse Station, NJ: Merck Research Laboratories, 2011.

PERIODICALS

Ismail-Khan, Roohi, Lary A. Robinson. "Malignant Pleural Mesothelioma: A Comprehensive Review." *Cancer Control: Journal of the Moffit Cancer Center* 13 (April 2006) 255–263.

WEBSITES

American Cancer Society. "How is Malignant Mesothelioma Staged?"http://www.cancer.org/cancer/malignantmesothelioma/detailedguide/malignant-mesothelioma-staging (accessed July 29, 2014).

Mesothelioma Alliance. "Pleural Mesothelioma." http://www.mesothelioma.com/mesothelioma/types/pleural.htm (accessed July 3, 2014).

ORGANIZATIONS

American Cancer Society, 250 Williams St. NW, Atlanta, GA 30303, (800) 227-2345, http://www.cancer.org.

American Lung Association, 55 W. Wacker Dr., Ste. 1150, Chicago, IL 60601, (800) LUNG-USA (586-4872), Fax: (202) 452-1805, http://www.lung.org.

National Cancer Institute, 9609 Medical Center Dr., BG 9609 MSC 9760, Bethesda, MD 20892-9760, (800) 4-CANCER (422-6237), http://www.cancer.gov.

L. Lee Culvert
Deanna Swartout-Corbeil, R.N.

Metastasis

Definition

Metastasis is the spread of **cancer** cells from the **primary site** in the body where the cancer originated to other tissues and organs. Distant metastasis is the spread of cancer farther from the primary site. The tumors produced by metastasis are sometimes called secondary tumors. Metastasis is responsible for 90% of cancer deaths.

Description

Metastasis occurs when cancer cells break away from a primary tumor and travel through the bloodstream or lymph vessels to other parts of the body. Most of these breakaway cells die, but some settle in new areas, grow, and form new tumors. If only a single secondary tumor develops, it is called a metastasis or a metastatic tumor. "Metastases" refers to two or more such tumors.

The ability to invade and metastasize are defining characteristics of many cancers. Invasion is the ability of cancer cells to penetrate the membranes that separate them from healthy tissues and blood vessels. The English word "metastasis" comes from a Greek word meaning "a change." Metastatic cancer cells are generally of the same type as the primary cancer from which they originated, and the metastatic cancer is named according to the primary cancer. Metastatic cancer cells usually share many features with the original cancer cells, such as the production of specific proteins or certain changes to chromosomes. Once a cancer manages to spread through the body, patients do not usually survive more than a few months.

The first step in cancer development—carcinogenesis—is a change or mutation of the DNA in the chromosomes of a cell. Mutations can be triggered by many different factors, including environmental **carcinogens** (such as tobacco smoke or ultraviolet radiation), viruses, and chronic irritation and inflammation. Mutations can inactivate tumor suppressor genes that prevent uncontrolled cell growth and division. Mutations in oncogenes can cause cells to multiply uncontrollably. Most cancers are the end result of multiple genetic alterations in both oncogenes and tumor suppressor genes. Mutations also prevent apoptosis or programmed self-destruction that normally occurs when a cell recognizes damage to its DNA. The protein produced by the p53 gene ordinarily encourages apoptosis in cells with defective DNA, and these cells are more likely to survive and replicate if the p53 gene has been altered or deactivated. Many cancers also involve rearrangement or loss of parts of whole chromosomes.

Most cancer cells originate within the epithelium—the layer of tissue that covers body surfaces and lines the inner surfaces of body cavities and blood vessels. Cancer cells in epithelial tissue are genetically unstable and have a high mutation rate. Following genetic alterations, the cell replicates—copies itself—at a fast rate.

Steps in metastasis

For cancer cells to metastasize, they must evolve the ability to:

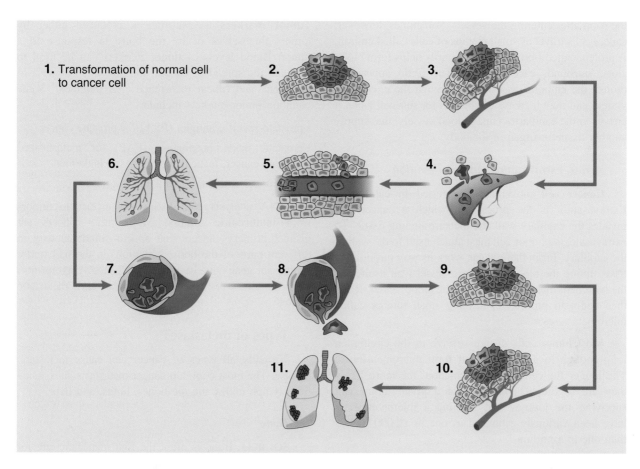

1. Transformation of normal cell to cancer cell

2.

3.

4.

5.

6.

7.

8.

9.

10.

11.

Illustration depicting the transformation of a normal cell to a cancerous cell. (1) A cell is transformed. (2) Cancerous cell proliferates and cells pile up to form a malignant tumor. (3) Angiogenesis: the tumor acquires a blood supply, which also allows (4) the cancer cells access into the circulatory system. (5) Cancer cells travel through the blood stream. (6) The cells stop in a capillary bed and (7) adhere to the layer of cells that line the blood vessel. (8) The cells invade the essential, functional tissue of the organ surrounding the blood vessel. (9) In this new organ, cancer cells pile up to form secondary tumors, which (10) induce angiogenesis. (11) Metastases (secondary tumors) are now evident. *(Illustration by Argosy Publishing. © Cengage Learning®.)*

- separate from the primary tumor
- survive independently
- break through the blood or lymph vessel wall
- evade the immune system
- anchor and grow in a new location

Studies indicate that cells from the same tumor vary in their metastatic potential; those that eventually form metastases are said to have a higher degree of malignancy. Some researchers believe that cancer cells gain metastatic potential by "macromutations,"or major rearrangements of their genetic material.

Local invasion

The first stage in the development of metastasis is the tumor's penetration of the basement membrane, which separates epithelial tissue from underlying connective tissue. The basement membrane is a specialized layer of extracellular matrix—a mass of tissue fibers and proteins that support and nourish the connective tissues. Normally, the extracellular matrix is a barrier that keeps cells from moving away from their sites of origin. Cancer cells secrete several different enzymes that digest the proteins in the basement membrane. When the membrane has been sufficiently weakened, the tumor can push through, causing local invasion of nearby normal tissue.

Intravasation and embolization

Individual cancer cells break off from the tumor and invade and move through the walls of nearby blood or lymph vessels in a process called intravasation. Even a small tumor can shed as many as a million cancer cells into blood or lymph vessels each day. Most of these cells die soon after entering the vessels. Sometimes, however, cancer cells travel as small clumps of cells called emboli. A protein called fibrin, which ordinarily helps form blood clots, surrounds each embolus. The fibrin appears to protect the embolus as it moves through the circulatory system and may increase its chances for survival when it arrives in the capillaries (small blood vessels) that supply another tissue or organ of the body.

Arrest, extravasation, and proliferation

Cancer cell movement is arrested in capillaries. Extravasation is the process in which a cancer cell invades the capillary wall and the surrounding tissue. To extravasate, the tumor cell must attach itself to the wall of the capillary. From there, it can work its way through the tissue lining the blood vessel, the vessel wall itself, and the basement membrane covering the blood vessel. It can then begin to proliferate, forming small tumors called micrometastases.

Most tumor cells do not survive in the circulation long enough to extravasate and form micrometastases. The longer the cells are in circulation, the more likely they are to die. The chances of a given tumor cell surviving the journey and forming a micrometastasis have been variously estimated as one in 10,000 to less than one in a million.

Angiogenesis

Angiogenesis is the process in which a tumor creates its own blood supply by releasing growth factors—especially vascular endothelial growth factor (VEGF)—that attract vascular cells to form new blood vessels within the tumor. Angiogenesis is sometimes called vascularization, which means blood vessel formation. Angiogenesis is a significant step in the development of metastasis for two reasons: the formation of new blood vessels supplies the tumor with nutrients that speed up its growth, and these vessels provide pathways for cancer cells to travel from the primary tumor to other organs. Micrometastases stimulate angiogenesis to supply oxygen and nutrients for the growth of secondary tumors in the new locations. A similar process of vessel formation can involve the lymph system. The secondary tumor can eventually release its own cancer cells into the circulation and produce further metastases.

Diagnosis and monitoring

Some primary cancers, such as lung and ovarian cancers, begin to shed tumor cells that metastasize before the primary cancer is large enough to be detected by standard diagnostic techniques. However, some marker molecules of circulating cancer cells can be detected.

Tumor markers are substances produced either by tumors themselves or by the body in response to a tumor. Blood levels of tumor markers can be used to evaluate the spread of cancer, the patient's response to treatment, and cancer recurrence after treatment. Some common tumor markers include:

- prostate-specific antigen (PSA) for prostate cancer
- prostatic acid phosphatase (PAP) for metastasized prostate cancer, testicular cancer, and leukemia
- CA (cancer antigen) 125 for many cancers

DNA analysis can distinguish metastatic tumors from multicentric tumors. Multicentric cancers are distinct primary cancers that appear simultaneously in different parts of the body. Mutations in the p53 tumor suppressor gene have been used as "genetic fingerprints" to differentiate between multicentric and metastatic tumors.

Types of metastases

Virtually all types of cancer can cause metastatic disease. The most common cancer metastasis sites, aside from lymph nodes, are the bones, lungs, and liver.

Bone

SOURCES. Bone is often the first metastatic site for breast and prostate cancers. More than two-thirds of metastatic breast and prostate cancers spread to the bone, and about one-third of metastatic lung, thyroid, and kidney cancers spread to the bone. Breast, prostate, and lung cancers are responsible for about 80% of bone metastases, and more than half of patients with these three types of primary cancers will develop bone metastases. Other common sources of bone metastases are bladder and uterine cancers and **melanoma**. Primary bone cancers are less common than bone metastases.

Bone metastases usually are caused by tumor cells carried through the bloodstream and are typically multiple. About 70% of bone metastases occur in the ribs, spine, sacrum (lowest portion of spine, attached to pelvis), or head; most of the remainder occur in the long bones of the body. Patients with lung cancer that has metastasized to bone survive, on average, for less than six months, but breast and **prostate cancer** patients may have lengthy periods of survival with bone metastases.

Breast cancer is the leading cause of cancer death in women worldwide, but death is usually caused by distant metastasis and/or local cancer recurrence. This appears to be due to a small proportion of aggressive cancer cells called cancer stem cells, cancer metastasis-initiating cells, or tumor-initiating cells. Breast cancer stem cells have unique characteristics including self-renewal, the ability to differentiate into other types of cells, and resistance to most **chemotherapy** agents and radiation treatment.

SYMPTOMS. Bone metastasis is a common cause of pain in patients with late-stage cancer. Metastases in the spine can compress the spinal cord and damage the nervous system. Bone metastases also make bones prone to fracture.

DIAGNOSIS. Bone metastases may be detected with bone scans, **computed tomography** (CT) scans, **magnetic resonance imaging** (MRI), or **positron emission tomography** (PET) scans. Bone metastasis is confirmed by a **biopsy**. Bone metastases may also be detected by simple tests for substances released into the blood or urine:

- Bone metastases can dissolve bones, leading to high blood calcium levels.

- Alkaline phosphatase levels can increase as bones dissolve.

- N-telopeptide may be released into urine when bone is damaged.

TREATMENT. Treatment can often slow the growth of or shrink bone metastases and relieve pain and other symptoms. Treatment options for bone metastases depend on a variety of factors; for example, localized treatments are used for just one or a few bone metastases. Bone metastases treatments may include:

- systemic (full-body) chemotherapy

- removal of the ovaries to lower estrogen levels or the testicles to lower testosterone, which may promote the growth of some breast and uterine cancers and prostate cancers, respectively; may also administer drugs that block hormone production or interfere with hormonal action on cancer cells

- external radiation therapy

- injection of radioactive elements that settle in the bone and kill cancer cells, particularly for blastic metastases that often occur with prostate cancer, in which the cancer stimulates bone cells called osteoblasts to form new bone

- use of drugs—bisphosphonates and denosumab—to slow the action of bone cells called osteoclasts that dissolve bone, a condition known as lytic metastasis

- surgery to stabilize a weakened bone

- surgical removal of part of the vertebrae (laminectomy) of the spine, followed by radiation treatment, to prevent compression of the spinal cord

- ablation, which inserts a needle or probe directly into the tumor and destroys it with heat, cold, or a chemical agent

- injection of a quick-setting bone cement or glue to strengthen and stabilize a bone and relieve pain

- pain medications

Lung

SOURCES. Metastatic tumors in the lungs can result from a primary lung cancer or from malignancies elsewhere in the body that spread to the lungs through the circulatory system or by direct extension. Almost any type of cancer can metastasize to the lung, but the most common tumors that spread to the lung are breast cancer, sarcomas, **non-Hodgkin lymphoma**, **neuroblastoma**, and **Wilms tumor**. Other primary tumors that often metastasize to the lung are bladder, colorectal, kidney, ovarian, pancreatic, prostate, stomach, thyroid, and uterine cancers and melanoma. Between 20% and 54% of fatal cancers have lung metastasis.

DIAGNOSIS. Diagnosis is usually the appearance of masses on a chest x-ray. Evaluation of lung metastases is initially directed at diagnosing/locating the primary tumor.

TREATMENT. The treatment for secondary lung cancers is usually appropriate systemic therapy for the primary tumor. Surgery for secondary lung tumors may be beneficial if there are four or less metastases. Surgery is usually only performed if the primary tumor is treatable, all metastases can be removed, chemotherapy or other nonsurgical approaches cannot be used, and there are no metastases elsewhere in the body. The five-year survival rate for surgical treatment of secondary lung tumors is 20%–35%.

Liver

SOURCES. The most common form of **liver cancer** is metastatic, and liver metastases are often the first evidence of a primary cancer elsewhere in the body. This is because the central role of the liver in circulation makes it a common arrest point for tumor emboli. The most common sites of primary tumors that metastasize to the liver are the lungs, breasts, colon, pancreas, and stomach. Other cancers that commonly metastasize to the liver include ovarian, bladder, thyroid, prostate, colorectal, kidney, and uterine cancers and melanoma.

DIAGNOSIS. Diagnosis of liver metastasis is usually difficult unless the cancer is well advanced. Ultrasound, CT scans, and liver function tests are used to screen patients with primary cancer for metastases in the liver, but the results are not totally reliable. A definitive diagnosis depends on a **liver biopsy**.

TREATMENT. Metastatic cancer to the liver is considered incurable. Systemic chemotherapy may temporarily shrink tumors and extend life but does not cure the cancer. Radiation treatment may relieve pain.

KEY TERMS

Angiogenesis—The formation of new blood vessels to supply a tumor with nutrients and help carry tumor emboli into the larger vessels of the circulatory system.

Apoptosis—The programmed self-destruction of a cell when DNA damage is detected.

Basement membrane—A specialized layer of extracellular matrix that separates epithelial tissue from underlying connective tissue; cancer cells must break through the basement membrane to migrate to other parts of the body and form metastases.

Carcinoma of unknown primary origin (CUP)—Metastatic cancer in which the type of cancer or site of origin is unknown.

Computed tomography (CT)—A diagnostic and screening technique that uses x-rays to obtain cross-sectional images of tissues.

Embolus (plural, emboli)—A clump of tumor cells that breaks off from a primary tumor to travel through the circulatory system and lodge in a capillary in another part of the body; embolization is the process of emboli formation.

Epithelium—The layer of tissue that covers body surfaces and lines the internal surfaces of body cavities, blood vessels, and hollow organs. Most cancer cells arise within epithelial tissue.

Extracellular matrix—A collection of connective-tissue proteins and fibers that supports and nourishes body tissues. The extracellular matrix forms a physical barrier to the movement of tumor cells.

Extravasation—The process of reverse invasion by which tumor cells that have invaded vessels and traveled to other organs force their way back out of the vessels and into the tissues surrounding their new site.

Intravasation—The entrance of cancer cells from a tumor into a vessel.

Magnetic resonance imaging (MRI)—A diagnostic technique that provides cross-sectional images of body structures.

Micrometastasis (plural, micrometastases)—Small tumors formed by cancer cells that have broken off from a primary tumor and traveled through blood or lymph vessels to different sites in the body where they have begun to grow and multiply.

Multicentric—Primary cancers that develop at two or more sites simultaneously.

Oncogene—A gene that has the potential to turn a cell cancerous; mutated forms of proto-oncogenes that promote normal cell growth and division.

RAS—A member of a family of genes that can mutate to oncogenes that are linked to common human cancers.

Tumor markers—Substances produced by a tumor or an immune response to a tumor that can be detected in the blood, urine, or tissues of patients with certain types of cancer.

Tumor necrosis factor (TNF)—A protein that destroys cells showing abnormally rapid growth; used in immunotherapy to shrink tumors.

Tumor suppressor genes—Genes that encode proteins such as p53 that inhibit cell division and replication; tumor suppressor genes are damaged or inactive in many types of cancer cells.

Vascular endothelial growth factor (VEGF)—A factor released by tumor cells that attracts vascular (blood vessel) cells to the tumor to form new blood vessels.

Surgery is sometimes used, particularly if the primary tumor is in the colon and there is a solitary metastasis.

Brain

SOURCES. The most common source of brain metastasis is primary cancer of the lung. Other sources include malignant melanomas and cancers of the breast, kidney, or digestive tract.

SYMPTOMS. Symptoms of metastatic tumors to the brain are similar to those of primary brain tumors—increased pressure inside the head and disturbances in brain function, including headaches, seizures, loss of sensation or balance, or personality changes.

DIAGNOSIS. Secondary **brain tumors** are usually detected with CT scans or MRI.

TREATMENT. A single secondary brain tumor can sometimes be surgically removed, followed by radiation treatment. Otherwise, radiation is used alone. Steroids may reduce brain swelling and treat headaches and other symptoms. Because most chemotherapy drugs cannot

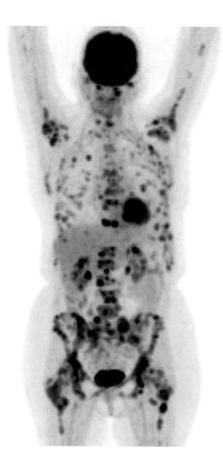

Positron emission tomography (PET) scan revealing metastasis; the black areas indicate the spread of cancer throughout the body. *(Living Art Enterprises/Science Source)*

cross the blood-brain barrier, systemic chemotherapy is of little use; however, **intrathecal chemotherapy** injects drugs directly into the spinal fluid to treat brain metastases. Patients with multiple metastases in the brain or widespread cancer elsewhere in the body have a poor prognosis.

Metastatic cancers of unknown primary origin

Between 0.5% and 7% of all cancers are carcinomas of unknown primary origin (CUPs). The patient's history and a physical examination are used for signs of breast, prostate, pelvic, rectal, and **gastrointestinal cancers**. The pattern of CUP metastasis may indicate whether the primary tumor is above or below the diaphragm. Lung metastases are twice as common from primary tumors located above the diaphragm, whereas liver metastases are more common if the primary site is below the diaphragm.

CUP metastases are usually treated by chemotherapy. They generally have a poor prognosis, with an average survival of three to four months. Fewer than 10% of patients survive five years. Male gender and liver involvement are negative prognostic factors.

Other metastatic sites

Other metastatic sites include:

• the peritoneum (lining of the abdominal cavity) with colorectal, ovarian, pancreatic, stomach, and uterine cancers
• the adrenal gland with kidney, lung, and prostate cancers
• the uterus from vaginal cancer
• skin or muscle with melanoma
• rarely, the lung, heart, central nervous system, or other tissues for blood and lymphatic system cancers (leukemia, multiple myeloma, lymphoma)

Treatment

Most metastatic cancers are incurable. Therefore, the primary goal of treatment is to control cancer growth and/or relieve symptoms. Although some treatments can prolong life, most patients die from metastatic cancer.

Surgery

Surgery is of limited use. It is sometimes used to remove large secondary tumors that are causing pain or interfering with body functions. In some cases, such as limited metastases to the lung or liver, it offers a survival advantage.

Chemotherapy

Systemic chemotherapy is frequently used to treat micrometastases. Because of side effects and risks—such as **nausea and vomiting** or the possibility of some chemotherapy drugs causing other cancers—the likelihood of tumor responsiveness must be balanced against the patient's quality of life.

Isolated perfusion is the delivery of high doses of chemotherapy drugs directly into a blood vessel. It is used in the treatment of metastatic melanoma and **sarcoma** to the extremities and certain other cancers. It allows for the regional delivery of drugs that would be very toxic or lethal if delivered systemically.

Radiation

Radiation therapy can be especially effective for metastases to the bones or brain, although it can only treat a limited area. It is also associated with an increased rate of secondary cancers in patients who have been previously treated for malignancies. The risk is particularly high in patients who were treated with a combination of radiation and chemotherapy.

Immunotherapy

Immunotherapy is systemic therapy that mobilizes the patient's own immune system to fight cancer or uses synthetic versions of immune system proteins to destroy cancer cells. Major categories of immunotherapy include:

- interferons—proteins produced by immune system cells that limit viral replication and stimulate resistance to infection
- interleukins—small proteins that promote the growth and activation of immune system cells, including interleukin-2 (IL-2 or aldesleukin) used to treat metastatic melanoma and renal cell carcinoma
- tumor necrosis factor (TNF)—a protein that stimulates the production of interleukins and destroys cells that are growing unusually rapidly
- monoclonal antibodies produced in laboratory-grown cell clones that recognize specific tumor markers and help the immune system destroy the cells
- vaccines that stimulate immune-system killer T cells to attack tumor cells

Hyperthermia

Hyperthermia is the use of therapeutic heat to shrink or destroy cancers on and inside the body. The treatment can be delivered directly to the tumor, to an area of the body, or to the whole body. Some forms of radiation therapy and chemotherapy are enhanced when combined with hyperthermia.

Newer therapies

Research into treatments for metastatic cancer has increased dramatically in recent years, and **clinical trials** of new treatments are ongoing. Some newer experimental treatments include:

- gene therapy to replace mutant p53 tumor suppressor genes
- inhibition of activated *ras* oncogenes
- angiogenesis inhibitors
- anti-VEGF antibodies
- substances that trigger apoptosis in defective cells
- substances that inhibit uncontrolled replication of tumor cells

Alternative and complementary therapies

Clinical trials have not shown alternative cancer treatments to be safe or effective, and they pose the risk of delaying or interrupting medical treatments that may be beneficial. Complementary therapies are used in addition to standard treatments to relieve pain or treat side effects, or reduce stress and improve quality of life.

See also Cancer biology; Cancer genetics; Carcinogenesis; Hepatic arterial infusion.

QUESTIONS TO ASK YOUR DOCTOR

- Is my cancer likely to metastasize?
- Where would it likely spread?
- Can metastasis be prevented?
- How is metastasis diagnosed?
- Can metastasis be treated?

Resources

BOOKS

Pecorino, Lauren. *Molecular Biology of Cancer: Mechanisms, Targets, and Therapeutics*. 3rd ed. Oxford: Oxford University, 2012.

Seyfried, Thomas N. *Cancer as a Metabolic Disease: On the Origin, Management, and Prevention of Cancer*. Hoboken, NJ: John Wiley & Sons, 2012.

Shockney, Lillie, and Gary R. Shapiro. *100 Questions & Answers About Advanced and Metastatic Breast Cancer*. Sudbury, MA: Jones & Bartlett Learning, 2012.

PERIODICALS

Brabletz, Thomas, et al. "Roadblocks to Translational Advances in Metastasis Research." *Nature Medicine* 19, no. 9 (September 2013): 1104–9.

Damsky, W. E., N. Theodosakis, and M. Bosenberg. "Melanoma Metastasis: New Concepts and Evolving Paradigms." *Oncogene* 33, no. 19 (May 8, 2014): 2413–22.

Geng, Shao-Qing, Aris T. Alexandrou, and Jian Jian Li. "Breast Cancer Stem Cells: Multiple Capacities in Tumor Metastasis." *Cancer Letters* 349, no. 1 (July 10, 2014): 1–7.

McGowan, Kat. "MicroRNA Halts Breast Cancer Protein." *Discover* 35, no. 1 (January/February 2014): 70.

Slezak, Michael. "The Making of a Monster." *New Scientist* 221, no. 2953 (January 25–31): 8.

Wan, Liling, Klaus Pantel, and Yibin Kang. "Tumor Metastasis: Moving New Biological Insights into the Clinic." *Nature Medicine* 19, no. 11 (November 2013): 1450–64.

OTHER

American Cancer Society. "Bone Metastasis." http://www.cancer.org/acs/groups/cid/documents/webcontent/003087-pdf.pdf (accessed August 17, 2014).

Bone and Cancer Foundation. "Questions and Answers About Breast Cancer, Bone Metastases, & Treatment-Related Bone Loss." http://www.boneandcancerfoundation.org/pdfs/Breast_Cancer_Q+A.pdf (accessed August 17, 2014).

WEBSITES

National Cancer Institute. "Metastatic Cancer." http://www.cancer.gov/cancertopics/factsheet/Sites-Types/metastatic (accessed August 16, 2014).

Sol Goldman Pancreatic Cancer Research Center. "Metastasis." Johns Hopkins Medicine. http://pathology.jhu.edu/pan creas/DiagMetastasis.php?area=di (accessed August 17, 2014).

ORGANIZATIONS

American Cancer Society, 250 Williams Street NW, Atlanta, GA 30303, (800) 227-2345, http://www.cancer.org.

Bone and Cancer Foundation, PO Box 287452, New York, NY 10128-0025. bcfdn@aol.com, http://www.boneandcancer foundation.org.

National Cancer Institute, 6116 Executive Boulevard, Suite 300, Bethesda, MD 20892-8322, (800) 4-CANCER (422-6237), http://www.cancer.gov.

Rebecca J. Frey, PhD
REVISED BY MARGARET ALIC, PhD
REVIEWED BY MELINDA GRANGER OBERLEITNER, RN, DNS, APRN, CNS

Methadone *see* **Opioids**

Methotrexate

Definition

Methotrexate is a **folic acid** derivative that interferes with folic acid metabolism (folate antagonist). It is a cytotoxic agent (a chemical that is directly toxic to cells) with multiple characteristics and may be described as an antimetabolite, antineoplastic, and immunosuppressant. In the United States, methotrexate is also recognized by the trade names Folex and Mexate, or the generic name amethopterin.

Purpose

Methotrexate is administered to **cancer** patients diagnosed with various malignancies. These conditions may include **breast cancer**, lung cancer, non-metastatic bone cancer, cancers associated with the head and neck, **acute lymphocytic leukemia**, meningeal leukemia, advanced non-Hodgkin lymphomas, and uterine tumors. Certain other cancers may be treated with methotrexate as prescribed by the oncologist.

Description

Methotrexate was granted FDA approval in 1986. Methotrexate is a highly effective chemical compound that targets a specific enzyme required by cells for normal function. When this enzyme activity is blocked by methotrexate, certain processes within the cell are shut down and cell death results. The growth of some normal cells may be affected by methotrexate; however, because

---

KEY TERMS

Antimetabolite—Anti-cancer drugs which prevent cells from growing and dividing by blocking the chemical reactions required in the cell to produce DNA.

Antineoplastic—Agents that inhibit or prevent the development of cancers by stopping the maturation and proliferation of malignant cells.

BCD—The combined chemotherapy treatment of bleomycin, cyclophosphamide, and dactinomycin.

Cytotoxic—Chemicals that are toxic to cells, and prevent their reproduction or growth.

Hodgkin lymphoma—A human malignant disorder of lymph tissue that appears to originate in a particular lymph node and later spreads to the spleen, liver, and bone marrow.

Immunosuppressant—Any chemotherapeutic agent which also has the effect of suppressing the immune system.

Leucovorin—The antidote for high dose treatments of methotrexate.

Lymphocytic leukemia—An acute form of childhood leukemia characterized by the development of abnormal cells in the bone marrow and lymph cells found in blood-forming tissues.

Metastatic—Refers to the spread of a cancer from its place of origin to another site in the body.

Oncologist—A physician who specializes in the diagnosis and treatment of patients with cancer.

---

this is a process associated with actively dividing cells, the accelerated rate at which cancer cells grow and divide make them more susceptible to the effects of methotrexate. Methotrexate may be given as a single agent, often followed by **leucovorin** rescue. Methotrexate may also be administered in a combination regimen with steroids to produce and maintain rapid remission of certain cancers or as part of an adjuvant therapy regimen with **doxorubicin**, **cisplatin**, or the BCD combination of **bleomycin**, **cyclophosphamide**, and **dactinomycin**.

Recommended dosage

Methotrexate is available is both injectable and tablet form. The injectable form may be given intravenously (IV), intramuscularly (IM), or intrathecal (directly into the spinal fluid). The dose amount varies over a wide range for patients receiving methotrexate. The final dose and treatment cycle will be determined by the oncologist based on what the medication is being used for, what cancer type is being treated, whether methotrexate is being used as a single agent or in concert with other **anticancer drugs**, and the method by which the medication is being administered. It is extremely important to take methotrexate in the correct timetable prescribed by the oncologist. If a dose is missed, the patient should not take the missed dose at a later time, or double the next prescribed dose. Rather, the patient should maintain the schedule prescribed and notify the oncologist about the missed dose.

Precautions

To maximize treatment effects, patients receiving methotrexate should observe certain guidelines. Including any modifications given by the oncologist, these guidelines should include regular visits with the oncologist and laboratory testing for white blood cell count, kidney, liver, and bone marrow function. Avoid any immunizations not approved or prescribed by the oncologist. Avoid contact with individuals taking or that have recently taken oral polio vaccine, or individuals that have an active infection. When necessary wear a protective facemask. Avoid prolonged or direct exposure to sunlight, as some patients experience an increased sensitivity. Ask for specific instructions on oral hygiene procedures to reduce the risk of gum abrasion, and avoid touching the eye and nasal areas unless hands have been properly washed immediately prior to contact. To reduce bleeding and bruising complications, patients should exercise extreme caution when handling sharp instruments and decline participation in contact sports. Prior to treatment, the patient's medical history should be thoroughly reviewed to avoid complications that might arise from previous conditions such as gout, kidney stones or kidney disease, liver disease, chickenpox, shingles, intestinal blockage, colitis, immunosuppression, stomach ulcers, mouth sores, or a history of allergic reactions to various drugs. The oncologist should also be made aware if the patient is pregnant or if there is the possibility the patient might be pregnant, or if the patient is a breast-feeding mother. Only prescribed medications or over the counter (OTC) drugs approved by the oncologist should be taken by a patient receiving methotrexate.

Side effects

The beneficial effects of methotrexate are usually accompanied by less desirable side effects. Side effects correlate in severity with dose amount and length of treatment. It is important to encourage the patient to discuss any presenting side effects. Some side effects do not require medical attention, but still cause the patient concern. Side effects that fall into this category may include loss of hair (**alopecia**) and appetite (**anorexia**), nausea or vomiting, skin rash with **itching**, pale skin tone, and the appearance of boils or acne. These side effects tend to diminish as the body adjusts to the therapy, or if they become bothersome, the oncologist may prescribe interventions. Side effects that should be reported immediately to the oncologist include mouth sores; back, lower side, joint or stomach pain; **fever** or chills; headaches; bloody or dark urine; drowsiness; dizziness; black tarry stools; bloody stools or vomit; **diarrhea**; redness or pinpoint red spots on the skin; swelling of the feet or lower legs; the development of a cough or hoarseness; and shortness of breath.

Interactions

Anti-inflammatory medications should be avoided while the patient is receiving methotrexate. These drugs elevate the effects of methotrexate to potentially harmful levels. Vaccines should be avoided due to the immunosuppression action of methotrexate, and alcohol should be avoided to reduce the risk of liver complications.

Resources

BOOKS

Chu, Edward, and Vincent T. DeVita Jr. *Physicians' Cancer Chemotherapy Drug Manual 2014*. Burlington, MA: Jones & Bartlett Learning, 2014.

WEBSITES

American Cancer Society. "Methotrexate." http://www.cancer.org/treatment/treatmentsandsideeffects/guidetocancerdrugs/methotrexate (accessed November 4, 2014).

The Scott Hamilton CARES Initiative. "Methotrexate." Chemocare.com. http://chemocare.com/chemotherapy/drug-info/Methotrexate.aspx (accessed November 4, 2014).

Jane Taylor-Jones, Research Associate, M.S.

Methylphenidate

Definition

Methylphenidate is a mild central nervous system stimulant. It is the most commonly prescribed medication for treating children with attention-deficit/hyperactivity disorder (ADHD) and is also used to treat narcolepsy and certain other conditions.

Purpose

The primary use of methylphenidate, first developed in 1956, is in the treatment of ADHD in children and adults. ADHD is the most common childhood neurobehavioral disorder. Every year more than 2.5 million children are medicated for ADHD. Methylphenidate increases the release of the neurotransmitters norepinephrine and dopamine. Although the drug can cause restlessness in normal individuals, it generally calms children with ADHD, improving their ability to focus and helping to control motor restlessness, inattention, and impulsivity. Hyperactive children who take methylphenidate have improved self-control, make fewer errors in their schoolwork, and get along better with their peers. Children with ADHD often take methylphenidate only during the school year.

Methylphenidate is also used to prevent daytime sleep episodes in patients with severe narcolepsy. On occasion it is used to decrease sedation and lethargy from opioid pain medications and to help relieve **depression** in terminally ill patients. It is sometimes used to increase appetite and energy levels in **cancer** patients.

Description

Methylphenidate comes in a variety of strengths and forms:

- 5-, 10-, and 20-milligram (mg) tablets
- chewable tablets
- immediate-release tablets
- intermediate-acting (extended-release) 20 mg tablets
- long-acting (extended-release) capsules and tablets
- solutions
- skin patches for children aged 6–12

U.S. brand names

- Ritalin, Ritalin LA, Ritalin-SR
- Metadate CD, Metadate ER
- Methylin, Methylin ER
- Concerta (long-acting tablets)
- Daytrana (patch) p

Canadian brand names

- Ritalin, Ritalin SR
- PMS-Methylphenidate
- Riphenidate
- Concerta

International brand names

- Ritalin
- Ritalina
- Rubifen
- Concerta

Recommended dosage

Methylphenidate dosages depend on the form of the drug, body weight, and individual responses. For treating ADHD, regular tablet and solution forms are usually introduced with two low daily doses—preferably 35–45 minutes before breakfast and lunch—of 0.3 mg/kilogram (kg) of body weight or 2.5–5 mg per dose. The dosage is increased at weekly intervals by 0.1 mg/kg/dose or 5–10 mg/day, to a maximum of 2 mg/kg/day or 90 mg/day. The usual therapeutic dose is 0.5–1 mg/kg/day or 20–30 mg per day.

The recommended dosage for treating narcolepsy in adults is 5–20 mg two to three times a day, 30–45 minutes before meals.

The usual adult dose to counteract opiate side effects is 2.5–15 mg once or twice per day.

Methylphenidate should be taken exactly as directed. The last dose of the day should be short-acting and taken before 6 P.M. because it can interfere with sleep. Tablets should be swallowed whole: crushing or breaking them changes the absorption time. A missed dose should be taken as soon as possible, but two tablets should not be taken at the same time.

Precautions

It is relatively easy to become physically and/or psychologically dependent on methylphenidate, particularly if it is taken at higher dosages or for longer than necessary. Signs of physical dependency include:

- having to increase the dosage to achieve the same effect
- mental depression
- unusual behavior
- fatigue or weakness

Methylphenidate should be tapered off gradually before discontinuing. Halting the drug abruptly can cause withdrawal symptoms including:

- headache
- irritability
- nausea
- abnormal chewing and tongue movements
- anxiety
- agitation
- sleep disturbance
- depression
- paranoia
- suicidal thoughts

Patients should not drive or operate machinery or appliances until they understand how methylphenidate affects them, since it makes some people lightheaded or dizzy.

Methylphenidate may cause changes in the composition of the blood and in liver function. Patients should receive regular blood tests and blood pressure and pulse checks while taking this drug.

Pediatric

Methylphenidate has undergone more testing than any other drug prescribed for children. Although it is generally considered safe and effective for the treatment of ADHD, the increasing frequency with which it is prescribed for younger and younger children has caused a great deal of controversy. Some medical professionals believe that methylphenidate is over-prescribed. They call for better diagnostic procedures conducted by trained personnel, rather than relying on subjective observations by parents and teachers for diagnosing ADHD. Children should have a drug-free period ("drug holiday") for at least several weeks every year. Methylphenidate should not be prescribed for children under age six.

Methylphenidate can cause sudden death in children, teenagers, and adults, especially those with heart defects or other serious heart problems. The American Heart Association recommends that children be monitored for heart problems before administration of methylphenidate.

Pregnant or breastfeeding

Methylphenidate is in pregnancy category C, meaning that there have been no adequate studies in pregnant women. It is not usually prescribed for women in their childbearing years, unless the physician determines that the benefits outweigh the risks. It is not known whether methylphenidate passes into breast milk; however breastfeeding is not recommended while taking this drug.

Other conditions and allergies

Methylphenidate can cause sudden death, heart attack, or stroke, especially in those with heart defects or other serious heart problems. It should be used with caution in patients with high blood pressure or a history of seizures. Methylphenidate is contraindicated for patients with:

- severe anxiety, tension, or agitation
- severe depression
- mental or emotional instability
- certain other mental-health conditions
- a history of alcohol or drug abuse

- epilepsy
- Tourette's syndrome
- tic disorders
- glaucoma

Side effects

The most common side effects of methylphenidate are nervousness, sleep disturbances, rapid heartbeat, and increased blood pressure. Reducing the dose, changing the time of day the drug is taken, or having regular drug-free periods may reduce some side effects.

Other side effects of methylphenidate may include:

- agitation
- dizziness
- irritability
- vision changes
- drowsiness
- nausea
- vomiting
- loss of appetite
- stomach pain
- diarrhea
- heartburn
- dry mouth
- headache
- muscle tightness
- restlessness
- numbness, burning, or tingling in the hands or feet
- decreased sexual desire
- painful menstruation

Less common side effects of methylphenidate include:

- chest pain
- heart palpitations
- joint pain
- skin rash
- uncontrolled speech or movements
- blood in the urine or stool
- muscle cramps
- red dots on the skin
- bruising

At higher dosages or with long-term use, side effects of methylphenidate may include **weight loss** or mental changes such as confusion, false beliefs, mood changes, hallucinations, or dissociative symptoms.

QUESTIONS TO ASK YOUR DOCTOR

- How should I give this medication to my child?
- What if my child misses a dose?
- What side effects are to be expected?
- Can I take my child off this drug whenever I want?
- Should my child have drug-free periods?

Symptoms of methylphenidate overdose include:

- inappropriate happiness
- sweating
- flushing
- headache
- fever
- fast, pounding, or irregular heartbeat
- widening of pupils
- dry mouth or nose
- vomiting
- agitation
- muscle twitching
- uncontrollable shaking of a part of the body
- confusion
- hallucinations
- loss of consciousness

Pediatric

The most serious pediatric side effect of methylphenidate is growth suppression. It may slow a child's rate of growth or weight gain. Other common side effects in children include insomnia, appetite loss, and stomach pains.

Interactions

Methylphenidate may have adverse interactions with many drugs including:

- amphetamines
- appetite suppressants
- caffeine
- cocaine
- asthma medications
- cold, sinus, and hay fever medications
- nabilone
- pemoline

- monoamine oxidase inhibitors (MAOIs) and other antidepressants
- pimozide
- anticoagulants (blood thinners)
- anti-seizure drugs
- high blood pressure medications

Methylphenidate should not be taken within two weeks of having taken an MAOI.

Resources

BOOKS

Diller, Lawrence H. *The Last Normal Child: Essays on the Intersection of Kids, Culture, and Psychiatric Drugs.* Westport, CT: Praeger, 2006.

Iversen, Leslie L. *Speed, Ecstasy, Ritalin: The Science of Amphetamines.* New York: Oxford University Press, 2006.

Tone, Andrea, and Elizabeth Siegel Watkins. *Medicating Modern America: Prescription Drugs in History.* New York: New York University Press, 2007.

PERIODICALS

Ahuja, Anjana. "Ritalin? Does It Work?" *The Times* (London) (November 16, 2007): 6.

Godfrey, J. "The Prevalence and Correlates of Adult ADHD in the United States: Results from the National Comorbidity Survey Replication." *American Journal of Psychiatry* 163 (2006): 716–723.

Kessler, R. C., et al. "Safety of Therapeutic Methylphenidate in Adults: A Systematic Review of the Evidence." *Journal of Psychopharmacology* 23, no. 2 (March 2009): 194.

Rubin, Rita. "Sudden Death in Kids, ADHD Drugs Linked." *Miami Times* 86, no. 43 (June 24–30, 2009): 11B.

WEBSITES

American Society of Health-System Pharmacists. "Methylphenidate." *MedlinePlus.* http://www.nlm.nih.gov/medlineplus/druginfo/meds/a682188.html (accessed October 15, 2014).

National Institute on Drug Abuse. "NIDA InfoFacts: Stimulant ADHD Medications—Methylphenidate and Amphetamines." http://www.drugabuse.gov/infofacts/ADHD.html (accessed October 15, 2014).

Vetter, Victoria L., et al. "Cardiovascular Monitoring of Children and Adolescents With Heart Disease Receiving Medications for Attention Deficit/Hyperactivity Disorder: A Scientific Statement From the American Heart Association Council on Cardiovascular Disease in the Young, Congenital Cardiac Defects Committee, and the Council on Cardiovascular Nursing." *Circulation.* http://circ.ahajournals.org/cgi/content/full/117/18/2407 (October 14, 2014).

ORGANIZATIONS

American Academy of Pediatrics, 141 Northwest Point Blvd., Elk Grove Village, IL 60007-1098, (847) 434-4000, (800) 433-9016, Fax: (847) 434-8000, http://www.aap.org.

American Heart Association, 7272 Greenville Ave., Dallas, TX 75231, (800) AHA-USA-1 (242-8721), http://www.heart.org.

National Institute on Drug Abuse (NIDA), Office of Science Policy and Communications, Public Information and Liaison Branch, 6001 Executive Blvd., Rm. 5213, MSC 9561, Bethesda, MD 20892-9561, (301) 443-1124, http://www.drugabuse.gov.

U.S. Food and Drug Administration, 10903 New Hampshire Ave., Silver Spring, MD 20993, (888) INFO-FDA (463-6332), http://www.fda.gov.

Debra Wood, RN
L. Fleming Fallon, Jr, MD, DrPH.
Margaret Alic, PhD

Methylprednisolone *see* **Corticosteroids**

Metoclopramide

Definition

Metoclopramide (Reglan, Octamide, Maxeran) is a drug used to prevent the **nausea and vomiting** caused by **cancer chemotherapy**, diabetic **neuropathy**, gastro-esophageal reflux, and similar conditions. It has also been approved by the Food and Drug Administration (FDA) to treat the small bowel prior to intubation. Metoclopramide is one of the drugs most frequently used in palliative care for cancer patients.

Purpose

Nausea and vomiting are among the most common side effects of cancer chemotherapy. They are also among the most unpleasant and upsetting side effects for patients. If left untreated, persistent nausea and vomiting can lead to dehydration, dental decay, digestive abnormalities, and nutritional deficiencies. In addition, persistent vomiting may force some patients to stop taking their chemotherapy and risk a recurrence of their cancer. It is therefore very important that these symptoms be adequately treated.

The nausea and vomiting that occurs with chemotherapy is often divided into three types: anticipatory, acute, and delayed. Anticipatory nausea and vomiting usually occurs before or during chemotherapy. These symptoms are thought to be caused by anxiety, and often occur in patients who have been previously treated with very toxic chemotherapy. Acute nausea and vomiting occurs within a few minutes to several hours after drug administration and usually stops within 24 hours.

Delayed nausea and vomiting occurs several hours after chemotherapy, and can last several days.

Description

For the majority of patients, nausea and vomiting can be successfully treated with antiemetic medication. Metoclopramide is one of the most widely used and effective **antiemetics** for treating the delayed nausea and vomiting caused by chemotherapy. It has been used since the 1980s, and works in two ways. It affects a part of the brain known to trigger vomiting, and also affects the speed of intestinal motion. As a result, the stomach empties into the intestines more quickly, and the contents of the intestines move more quickly in the correct direction.

Metoclopramide is most often used in patients taking **cisplatin** (Platinol) chemotherapy. Cisplatin is used to treat a wide range of cancers including **bladder cancer**, **ovarian cancer** and **non-small cell lung cancer**. Compared with other cancer chemotherapy, cisplatin is often considered to cause the most severe nausea and vomiting. For 60%–70% of patients taking cisplatin, however, metoclopramide provides adequate control of nausea and vomiting.

Recommended dosage

Although metoclopramide can be taken either orally or intravenously, cancer patients on chemotherapy usually receive the drug intravenously. Metoclopramide is usually given 30 minutes before chemotherapy, and then two more times after chemotherapy at two hour intervals.

The recommended dose varies from patient to patient, and depends on both the severity of nausea and vomiting, and on the toxicity of the drug. A higher dose will be given to patients with severe symptoms. Higher doses will also be given to patients receiving drugs such as cisplatin that are known to cause severe nausea and vomiting. Some patients receiving cisplatin may be given a combination of three different drugs to help combat their nausea: metoclopramide, **dexamethasone** (Dexone), and **lorazepam** (Ativan). The three work on different areas of the body and produce a greater effect together than they do when given separately.

Precautions

Metoclopramide can cause sleepiness and lack of concentration. Patients should avoid tasks that require mental alertness such as driving or operating machinery. Patients should also be aware that metoclopramide may enhance their response to alcohol and drugs that depress the central nervous system. Because metoclopramide can cause **depression**, patients with a history of serious clinical depression should take this drug only if absolutely necessary.

Metoclopramide can make the symptoms of Parkinson's disease worse, and patients with a history of seizures should not take metoclopramide, because the frequency and severity of the seizures may increase. The drug should also not be used in patients with intestinal problems such as bleeding, tears, or blockages. The safety of metoclopramide for pregnant women or children is unknown. The drug is found in the breast milk of lactating mothers.

Side effects

The most frequent side effects of metoclopramide are restlessness, drowsiness, and **fatigue**. These occur in about 10% of patients. Less common side effects include insomnia, headache, and dizziness. These occur in only 5% of patients. Feelings of anxiety or agitation may also occur, especially after a rapid intravenous injection of the drug. Some women may experience menstrual irregularities.

Metoclopramide therapy can cause some patients to make abnormal involuntary movements, a condition known as dyskinesia. These reactions are most common in young adults of 18–30 years of age, and often disappear about a day after the patient stops taking the drug. Among geriatric patients, particularly women, dyskinesia sometimes develops when patients stop taking metoclopramide after long term treatment.

Interactions

Patients who are also taking cabergoline (Dostinex), a drug used to treat hormonal problems and Parkinson's disease, should not take metoclopramide. Because metoclopramide affects the functioning of the intestines, it can interfere with the absorption of certain drugs. The effect of digoxin (Lanoxin), for example, may be reduced, whereas the effects of other drugs like aspirin, **cyclosporine** (Neoral, Sandimmune, SangCya) and tetracycline (Minocin, Vibramycin) may be enhanced.

Resources

BOOKS

Karch, A. M. *Lippincott's Nursing Drug Guide.* Springhouse, PA: Lippincott Williams & Wilkins, 2003.

PERIODICALS

Duby, J. J., R. K. Campbell, S. M. Setter, et al. "Diabetic Neuropathy: An Intensive Review." *American Journal of Health-System Pharmacy* 61 (January 15, 2004): 160–173.

Nauck, F., C. Ostgathe, E. Klaschik, et al. "Drugs in Palliative Care: Results from a Representative Survey in Germany." *Palliative Medicine* 18 (March 2004): 100–107.

Steely, R. L., D. R. Collins Jr., B. E. Cohen, and K. Bass. "Postoperative Nausea and Vomiting in the Plastic Surgery Patient." *Aesthetic Plastic Surgery* 28 (January-February 2004): 29–32.

ORGANIZATIONS

ASHP (formerly the American Society of Health-System Pharmacists), 7272 Wisconsin Ave., Bethesda, MD 20814, (301) 664-8700, (866) 279-0681, custserv@ashp.org, http://www.ashp.org.

U.S. Food and Drug Administration, 10903 New Hampshire Ave., Silver Spring, MD 20993, (888) INFO-FDA (463-6332), http://www.fda.gov.

Alison McTavish, M.Sc.
Rebecca J. Frey, PhD

Metronidazole *see* **Antibiotics**

Mexate *see* **Methotrexate**

Miacalcin *see* **Calcitonin**

Micronutrients and cancer prevention

Definition

Micronutrients include all of the essential **vitamins** and minerals that are required in very small amounts for normal growth, development, and health. Micronutrients also include the thousands of phytonutrients or phytochemicals present in plant foods, the majority of which have not yet been identified. Although potential roles for micronutrients in **cancer prevention** have been studied for decades, the contributions of specific micronutrients remain unclear.

Description

Vitamins and minerals

There are 13 essential vitamins and a similar number of essential minerals. Most of these micronutrients must be obtained from foods, although vitamins D and K are also produced by the body. Vitamins A, C, D, and E (in the form of alpha-tocopherol), the B-complex vitamins folate or **folic acid** and niacin, and the mineral selenium have been studied for their cancer-preventing potential.

Naturally occurring and synthetic vitamin A and closely related compounds are called retinoids. Vitamin A is obtained directly from animal products such as egg yolks, dairy, liver, and fish oil. Provitamin A carotenoids, including alpha- and beta-carotenes, are retinoids that are converted to retinol—a form of vitamin A—in the small intestine.

Selenium is a trace element that is an essential component of selenoenzymes and selenoproteins. Plants incorporate selenium from the soil into various sulfur-containing micronutrients such as selenomethionine.

Phytonutrients

In addition to vitamins, provitamin A carotenoids, and minerals from plant foods, many other phytonutrients are of interest for potentially reducing the risk of some cancers. More than 40 different carotenoids are present in red, orange, yellow, and green fruits and vegetables, of which lycopene, lutein, zeaxanthin, and beta-cryptoxanthin are of particular interest.

Polyphenols of interest include:

- flavonoids found in a wide range of fruits, vegetables, and grains, including colorful anthocyanins, and quercetin in apples, onions, teas, and red wine
- isoflavones in supplements and foods such as soy, red clover, garbanzo beans, and licorice
- lignans in whole grains and flaxseed
- ellagic acid in berries and walnuts
- resveratrol in grapes and red wine
- curcumin that gives the spice turmeric its yellow color
- phenolic compounds in coffee

Sulfur-containing phytochemicals are of particular interest. Glucosinolates in cruciferous vegetables—including broccoli, kale, watercress, arugula, and collard greens—are converted to compounds such as isothiocyanates and indole-3-carbinol (I3C) when the vegetables are chopped or chewed. Allyl sulfides are present in garlic and onions. Cabbage and kale are good sources of sulforaphane.

Other phytochemicals that have been suggested to protect against some cancers include:

- lunasin in soy
- capsaicin in hot peppers
- chlorophylls and chlorophyllin—a semi-synthetic mixture derived from chlorophyll
- inositol hexaphosphate (IP6 or phytic acid) from legumes, cereals, nuts, and soybeans

Function

The majority of known micronutrients that are potentially involved in **cancer** prevention are **antioxidants**. Antioxidants are substances that block or reverse the activity of free radicals and other oxidants. Free radicals are highly reactive molecules formed during normal metabolism. Free radicals and other oxidants are also present in environmental toxins, such as tobacco smoke. They can cause various types of oxidative damage to cells, including DNA damage that can lead to cancer. Dietary antioxidants—especially those in fruits, vegetables, and whole grains—may help prevent cancer-promoting free-radical damage. However, there is no conclusive evidence that any specific antioxidant, either in foods or dietary supplements, can reduce cancer risk, and some may even increase the risk of certain cancers.

Some micronutrients have anti-inflammatory activities that may play a role in cancer prevention. Inflammation is the immune system's protective response to infection or injury, but chronic inflammation is associated with some cancers. Inflammation can inhibit cell death and cause cells to multiply (proliferate) and grow new blood vessels (angiogenesis)—characteristics of cancer cells.

In addition to antioxidant and anti-inflammatory activities, some micronutrients may prevent or delay the development of cancers by:

- directly detoxifying or deactivating carcinogens
- activating enzyme systems that detoxify carcinogens
- repairing DNA damage
- promoting cancer cell death

Specific functions

Although only some carotenoids are retinoids that are converted to vitamin A, most carotenoids have antioxidant activity. They also help stimulate communication between cells, which is important for maintaining cells in their differentiated state. Cancer cells often revert to an undifferentiated (immature) state.

Numerous anticancer activities have been attributed to selenium:

- improving immune system function
- directly causing cancer cell death
- increasing selenium-containing metabolites that inhibit tumor cell growth
- maximizing the activity of antioxidant selenoproteins
- affecting the metabolism of carcinogens
- influencing DNA repair
- inhibiting blood vessel formation required by growing tumors
- incorporation into the protein Sep15, which has been implicated in cancer prevention

It has been suggested that resveratrol:

- inhibits the expression and activity of enzymes that metabolize compounds into carcinogens
- increases the expression and activity of an enzyme that promotes excretion of carcinogens
- inhibits the activities of some inflammatory enzymes
- inhibits the activity of at least one enzyme that helps cancer cells invade normal tissue
- inhibits angiogenesis required by invasive tumors
- may inhibit cancer cell proliferation and induce cancer cell death

Glucosinolates are antioxidants. Their metabolic products have been suggested to:

- help eliminate carcinogens from the body
- alter cell-signaling pathways to prevent normal cells from becoming cancerous
- alter the metabolism or activity of hormones such as estrogen or stimulate enzymes that lower estrogen activity, thereby possibly inhibiting the development of hormone-sensitive cancers, such as some breast cancers

Chlorophylls and chlorophyllin can form tight complexes with some **carcinogens** in tobacco smoke and cooked meat and with aflatoxin-B1. Aflatoxin is a potent fungal carcinogen in moldy grains and legumes that causes severe outbreaks of **liver cancer** in parts of Africa and Asia. Binding of chlorophyll or chlorophyllin may interfere with absorption of these carcinogens by the gastrointestinal tract. Chlorophyllin is also an antioxidant.

Specific cancer-preventing functions have been attributed to some other micronutrients:

- Alpha-tocopherol (vitamin E) can neutralize free radicals that cause oxidative damage to DNA.
- Folate is required both for DNA synthesis and repair and for synthesis of the amino acid methionine, which

is necessary for DNA methylation, a biochemical process that regulates gene expression. Cancers can arise from DNA damage that outpaces DNA repair and from the inappropriate expression of certain genes.

- Some polyphenols, including some flavonoids such as anthocyanins and quercetin, are antioxidants.
- Isoflavones and lignans are phytoestrogens that may have activities similar to the female hormone estrogen.
- Ellagic acid is an antioxidant.
- Allyl sulfides may strengthen the immune system and stimulate enzymes that help rid the body of carcinogens.
- Sulforaphane stimulates carcinogen-detoxifying enzymes.
- Lunasin may suppress the proliferation of tumor cells and increase expression of genes that monitor DNA damage.
- Capsaicin is thought to protect DNA from carcinogens.
- IP6 in whole grains has antioxidant activity.
- Saponins are phytonutrients that can interfere with DNA replication, thereby preventing cancer-cell proliferation.

Benefits

Although no single micronutrient has been proven to help prevent cancer in humans, a large body of evidence indicates that diets that are low in fat and include a variety of fruits, vegetables, legumes, and whole grains reduce the risk of at least some cancers. At least five daily servings of fruits and vegetables have been consistently associated with lower cancer incidence. Some studies have associated diets high in cruciferous vegetables with a lower risk for several cancers. Consumption of whole grains is associated with reduced risk for colon and certain other cancers. Phytonutrients in the bran and germ of whole grains may help protect against certain cancers, but only when consumed in whole foods. This may be because their effects are additive, synergistic with each other or with fiber and minerals in whole grains, and/or complementary to micronutrients in fruits and vegetables when consumed together.

Traditional Asian diets include foods that are high in vitamins, minerals, antioxidants, and other micronutrients. Asians following traditional diets are among the healthiest and longest-lived people, with lower rates of cancer and many other chronic diseases. Asian and other high-fiber diets that are rich in IP6 appear to suppress the growth and progression of early-stage **prostate cancer**. As more Asians adopt Western diets, their cancer rates

Allyl sulfides—Phytochemicals in garlic and onions that may have a role in cancer prevention.

Angiogenesis—The formation and differentiation of blood vessels.

Anthocyanins—Plant pigments with antioxidant activities.

Antioxidant—Substances, including many micronutrients, that prevent or reduce oxidative damage.

Capsaicin—An active ingredient from hot chili peppers that may have cancer-preventive activity.

Carcinogen—A substance or agent that promotes cancer, either directly or following activation in the body.

Carotenes—Pro-vitamin A carotene; orange or red carotenoids such as beta-carotene that can be converted to vitamin A.

Carotenoids—Red or yellow plant pigments and phytonutrients with various biological activities in the human body.

Chlorophyllin—A semi-synthetic chlorophyll derivative that may help protect against the fungal carcinogen aflatoxin.

Differentiated—Refers to cancer cells that multiply slowly and are closer in structure to normal cells.

Undifferentiated cancer cells spread quickly and do not reach the matured state of normal cells.

Ellagic acid—A phenolic antioxidant in many fruits and vegetables.

Flavonoids—A large group of aromatic compounds, including many plant pigments and antioxidants.

Folate—Folic acid; vitamin B9; a micronutrient required for normal fetal development and possibly involved in cancer prevention.

Free radical—A reactive atom or group of atoms that damage cells, proteins, and DNA.

Glucosinolates—Sulfur-containing phytonutrients in cruciferous plants that are metabolized to bioactive compounds such as isothiocyanates and indoles that may be anticarcinogenic.

Indole-3-carbinol (I3C)—A metabolite of glucosinolates that may have cancer-preventing activity.

Inflammation—A response to irritation, infection, or injury; chronic inflammation is associated with some cancers.

Inositol hexaphosphate (IP6)—Phytic acid; a phytochemical in high-fiber foods that may have cancer-preventing properties.

---

increase. Mediterranean diets are also being studied in relation to cancer prevention.

There are numerous claims of cancer prevention by specific micronutrients:

• Low levels of folate cause birth defects and have been associated with colorectal and certain other cancers, although it is unclear whether higher amounts of folate from foods or supplements help prevent cancer.

• Selenium may help prevent the development and progression of cancer, although this remains unclear.

• Isoflavones and lignans are of interest with regard to hormone-dependent cancers such as breast and prostate cancers.

• Intestinal microflora help convert plant lignans into mammalian lignans—enterolactone and enterodiol—which may help protect against hormone-related cancers by helping fat cells remove excess estrogen.

• Phytoestrogens in soybeans may lower the risk of breast cancer.

• Resveratrol and phenolic compounds in coffee have been suggested to protect against certain cancers.

• Glucosinolates may help fight prostate cancer.

• Isothiocyanates may lower the risk of lung and colon cancers, although protective effects may depend on an individual's genetic makeup.

• Sulforaphane may help prevent colon cancer in genetically susceptible people.

• Lunasin may reduce the risk of several cancers, including prostate cancer.

• IP6, saponins, phenolic acids, and protease inhibitors in whole grains lower the risk of colon and breast cancers.

• Withanolides include a large group of antioxidant steroids that may help prevent colon cancer.

Isoflavones—Common phytonutrients with antioxidant and estrogenic activities.

Lignans—A class of plant phenolic compounds with antioxidant and estrogenic activities.

Lunasin—A peptide in soy and some cereal grains that may have anticancer properties.

Lycopene—A red plant pigment with antioxidant properties.

Niacin—Nicotinic acid; vitamin B3.

Oxidants—Molecules such as free radicals that can cause oxidative damage to cellular components including DNA.

Phenolic acids—Common plant metabolites that can function as phytonutrients.

Phytochemicals—Phytonutrients; micronutrients in plants that may have physiological activities.

Phytoestrogens—Plant compounds that have activities of the human hormone estrogen.

Polyphenols—Antioxidant phytochemicals that prevent or neutralize the effects of free radicals.

Quercetin—A yellow plant pigment with antioxidant activity.

Recommended dietary allowance (RDA)—Recommended daily allowance; the approximate amount of a nutrient that should be ingested daily.

Resveratrol—A phytonutrient found especially in grapes and red wine, which may reduce the risk of cancer.

Retinoids—Various naturally occurring and synthetic analogs of vitamin A.

Saponins—Mostly toxic plant glucosides that produce a soapy lather.

Selenium—An essential trace element in meat and grains that may reduce the risk of cancer.

Selenoprotein—Enzymes and other proteins containing the element selenium.

Sulforaphane—An anticarcinogenic isothiocyanate in cruciferous vegetables that is thought to stimulate the production of enzymes that detoxify carcinogens.

Vitamin A—Any of several fat-soluble vitamins with antioxidant activities.

Vitamin D—A fat-soluble steroid vitamin produced by the body through exposure to sunlight and with multiple activities in the human body.

Vitamin E—Alpha-tocopherol; an essential fat-soluble vitamin with antioxidant activity.

Precautions

Attributing any effects on cancer prevention to specific micronutrients is extremely difficult for several reasons. Micronutrients interact with and may function synergistically with each other and with other components in foods, so their activities may depend on other dietary constituents. Food preparation and cooking can also affect the availability and physiological activity of micronutrients. Micronutrient supplements, therefore, are not equivalent to micronutrients in foods and may be less likely to help prevent cancer. In addition, the vast majority of micronutrients in whole grains and other foods remain unidentified, so their contributions to cancer prevention are unknown. Genetic differences between individuals clearly influence at least some of the cancer-preventative effects of micronutrients. Microorganisms in the gut have very important roles in the digestion and metabolism of micronutrients and the compositions of gut microflora (microbiomes) differ significantly between individuals. Finally, micronutrient studies utilizing laboratory animals or cell cultures are not necessarily of relevance to humans.

Most people do not get the recommended dietary allowances (RDAs) of one or more essential vitamins and minerals. RDAs for other micronutrients have not been determined. Nevertheless, there is little or no evidence that any micronutrient dietary supplements—including multivitamins/minerals—reduce the risk of cancer for most people. Rather, there is near-unanimous agreement among experts that the best way for healthy, well-nourished people to obtain micronutrients that may help prevent cancer is to follow a diet that is high in a variety of fruits, vegetables, whole grains, and fiber. Although an estimated 40% of American adults take a daily multivitamin—often to compensate for poor dietary habits—the evidence is clear that supplements cannot substitute for micronutrients obtained from a healthy diet. The U.S. Preventive Services Task Force has found inadequate evidence either for or against vitamin/mineral supplements for cancer prevention in healthy adults without nutrient deficiencies. However, they do advise against vitamin E and beta-carotene supplements.

Pediatric

Children should never be given micronutrient supplements except under medical supervision.

Geriatric

Many physicians suggest that older adults take multivitamin/mineral supplements. Because they may absorb and metabolize micronutrients less efficiently, older adults are more likely to be deficient in one or more essential micronutrients.

Pregnant or breastfeeding

Pregnant and breastfeeding women should use micronutrient supplements only under medical supervision.

Other conditions and allergies

Little is known about the estrogenic activities of phytoestrogens and resveratrol. Women with a history of estrogen-sensitive breast, ovarian, or uterine cancer are specifically advised against taking resveratrol or phytoestrogen supplements.

Risks

Dietary supplements are not required to prove that they are either safe or effective, and their manufacture is not well regulated. They may contain varying amounts of active ingredients or dangerous contaminants. Interactions with foods, medications, and other supplements are usually unknown and may be potentially dangerous. Some supplements, especially in large amounts, may cause side effects.

Some micronutrient supplements carry specific risks.

- High doses of vitamin A are toxic.
- Long-term use of high-dose beta-carotene supplements may increase lung cancer risk in current and former smokers and former asbestos workers.
- Two trials found an association between folate supplementation and increased risk of prostate cancer, although results of other studies have been mixed. High doses of supplemental folate may accelerate tumor growth in cancer patients.
- Both low and very high selenium levels have been associated with increased cancer risk.
- Large amounts of supplemental selenium can be toxic.

- One clinical trial found that selenium supplements increased the likelihood of developing type 2 diabetes.
- There is no evidence to support claims that potassium can prevent cancer, and excess potassium can be toxic.
- Experts advise against the use of supplements containing I3C or diindoylmethane (DIM) (a breakdown product of I3C with antioxidant properties), because their potential risks and benefits are unknown, and animal studies have yielded contradictory results.

Research and general acceptance

There is clear consensus that diets high in a variety of fruits, vegetables, and whole grains reduce the overall risk of cancer and other chronic diseases. Epidemiological studies indicate that foods high in vitamin A and carotene and diets high in carotenoid-rich fruits and vegetables reduce the risk of certain cancers. Laboratory and animal studies indicate that antioxidants in foods and supplements prevent free-radical damage associated with the development of cancer. Resveratrol arrests cell growth, inhibits proliferation, and induces cell death in various cancer cell lines, and chlorophyllin supplementation may reduce the risk of liver cancer in populations at high risk for aflatoxin exposure. Beyond this, there is very little definitive evidence for cancer-preventive effects of specific micronutrients.

- Studies of vitamin and mineral supplements have shown no clear cancer-prevention benefit.
- Human studies of antioxidant supplements for reducing cancer risk have yielded mixed results, although randomized, controlled, clinical trials—the research gold standard—have generally showed no significant effect on cancer risk from various combinations of supplements.
- Large, controlled studies have indicated that high-dose beta-carotene supplements do not lower cancer risk.
- Laboratory and animal studies have found that vitamin D may slow or prevent cancer development. Higher intake or high blood levels of vitamin D in humans have been associated with reduced risk for colorectal cancer, but results have been inconclusive for all other cancers.
- Studies of alpha-tocopherol levels or intake and cancer risk have reported no association, mixed results, or increased risk.
- Although adequate folate intake prevents neural tube and other birth defects, studies on folate and cancer prevention have been inconclusive.
- Some laboratory and animal studies have suggested a role for niacin in cancer prevention, but there have been few large studies with humans.

QUESTIONS TO ASK YOUR DOCTOR

- Am I likely to be deficient in any micronutrients?
- What changes should I make in my diet to ensure that I am getting required micronutrients?
- Do you recommend that I take a multivitamin/mineral supplement?
- Do you recommend any phytonutrient supplements?
- Will micronutrient supplements help prevent cancer?

• Death rates from cancer have been shown to be significantly lower in regions with high soil selenium levels compared with populations with low soil selenium and relatively low selenium intake. However, results of studies on selenium supplements in humans have been mixed.

Vitamin supplements

Although the available evidence indicates that cancer-preventive benefits come from micronutrients in foods rather than supplements, some experts continue to recommend multivitamin/mineral and other supplements for lowering cancer risk. Nutritional supplements constitute a multibillion-dollar industry and are very heavily marketed by some alternative practitioners as well as by manufacturers.

Resources

BOOKS

Meyskens, Frank L., Jr., and Kedar N. Prasad, editors. *Vitamins and Cancer: Human Cancer Prevention by Vitamins and Micronutrients*. New York: Humana, 2013.

Shankar, Sharmila, and Rakesh Srivastava, editors. *Nutrition, Diet, and Cancer*. New York: Springer, 2012.

PERIODICALS

"Are You Really Benefiting from Your Multivitamins?" *Tufts University Health & Nutrition Letter* 32, no. 1 (March 2014): 4–5.

Holzapfel, Nina Pauline, et al. "The Potential Role of Lycopene for the Prevention and Therapy of Prostate Cancer: From Molecular Mechanisms to Clinical Evidence." *International Journal of Molecular Sciences* 14, no. 7 (2013): 14620–46.

Hossein-nezhad, Arash, and Michael F. Holick. "Vitamin D for Health: A Global Perspective." *Mayo Clinic Proceedings* 88, no. 7 (July 2013): 720–55.

Major, Jacqueline M., et al. "Genetic Variants Reflecting Higher Vitamin E Status in Men Are Associated with Reduced Risk of Prostate Cancer." *American Journal of Nutrition* 144, no. 5 (May 2014): 729–33.

Nile, Shivraj Hariram, and Se Won Park. "Edible Berries: Bioactive Components and Their Effect on Human Health." *Nutrition* 30, no. 2 (February 2014): 134–44.

Tio, Martin, Juliana Andrici, and Guy D. Eslick. "Folate Intake and the Risk of Breast Cancer: A Systematic Review and Meta-Analysis." *Breast Cancer Research and Treatment* 145, no. 2 (June 2014): 513–24.

Wang, Lian, et al. "Specific Carotenoid Intake is Inversely Associated with the Risk of Breast Cancer Among Chinese Women." *British Journal of Nutrition* 111, no. 9 (May 14, 2014): 1686–95.

WEBSITES

American Cancer Society. "Folic Acid." http://www.cancer.org/treatment/treatmentsandsideeffects/complementaryandalternativemedicine/herbsvitaminsandminerals/folic-acid (accessed July 2, 2014).

American Cancer Society. "Phytochemicals." http://www.cancer.org/treatment/treatmentsandsideeffects/complementaryandalternativemedicine/herbsvitaminsandminerals/phytochemicals (accessed July 2, 2014).

American Cancer Society. "Selenium." http://www.cancer.org/treatment/treatmentsandsideeffects/complementaryandalternativemedicine/herbsvitaminsandminerals/selenium (accessed July 2, 2014).

American Cancer Society. "Vitamin A, Retinoids, and Provitamin A Carotenoids." http://www.cancer.org/treatment/treatmentsandsideeffects/complementaryandalternativemedicine/herbsvitaminsandminerals/vitamin-a-and-beta-carotene (accessed July 2, 2014).

Higdon, Jane. "Niacin." Micronutrient Information Center, Linus Pauling Institute, Oregon State University. http://lpi.oregonstate.edu/infocenter/vitamins/niacin (accessed July 2, 2014).

National Cancer Institute. "Antioxidants and Cancer Prevention." http://www.cancer.gov/cancertopics/factsheet/prevention/antioxidants (accessed July 1, 2014).

Scudellari, Megan. "Mutagens and Multivitamins." *Scientist*, June 1, 2014. http://www.the-scientist.com//?articles.view/articleNo/40054/title/Mutagens-and-Multivitamins (accessed July 4, 2014).

ORGANIZATIONS

American Cancer Society, 250 Williams Street NW, Atlanta, GA 30303, (800) 227-2345, http://www.cancer.org.

Linus Pauling Institute, Oregon State University, 307 Linus Pauling Science Center, Corvallis, OR 97331, (541) 737-5075, Fax: (541) 737-5077, lpi@oregonstate.edu, http://lpi.oregonstate.edu/infocenter.

National Cancer Institute, 6116 Executive Boulevard, Suite 300, Bethesda, MD 20892-8322, (800) 4-CANCER (422-6237), http://www.cancer.gov.

Margaret Alic, PhD

Mistletoe

Description

Mistletoe is a parasitic evergreen plant that lives on trees such as oak, elm, fir, and apple. The parasitic plant has yellowish flowers, small yellowish green leaves, and waxy white berries. There are many species of this plant in the Viscacea and Loranthacea plant families. European mistletoe (*Viscum album*) and American mistletoe (*Phoradendron leucarpum*) are used as medical remedies. In addition to Europe and North America, mistletoe is also found in Australia and Korea.

Mistletoe berries are poisonous to cats and other small animals. There is, however, some debate about how toxic the berries are to humans, and there is controversy about whether it is safe to use mistletoe as a remedy. Mistletoe is also known as mystyldene, all-heal, bird lime, golden bough, and devil's fuge.

General use

Mistletoe is known popularly as the plant sprig that people kiss beneath during the Christmas season. That custom dates back to pagan times when, according to legend, the plant was thought to inspire passion and increase fertility.

Over the centuries, mistletoe has acquired a reputation as an all-purpose herbal remedy. In the seventeenth century, French herbalists prescribed mistletoe for nervous disorders, epilepsy, and the spasms known as the St. Vitus dance.

Mistletoe has also been used in folk medicine as a digestive aid, heart tonic, and sedative. It was used to treat arthritis, hysteria and other mental disturbances, **amenorrhea**, wounds, asthma, bed wetting, infection, and to stimulate glands.

For centuries, mistletoe also served as a folk medicine treatment for **cancer**. Iscador, an extract of the European mistletoe plant, is said to stimulate the immune system and kill cancer cells. It reportedly reduces the size of tumors and improves the quality of life. Iscador is one brand name of the mistletoe extract in Europe, and other brand names include Helixor and Eurixor.

Although in alternative medicine mistletoe is viewed as a multipurpose remedy, there is disagreement among medical experts about the safety and effectiveness of this herb. The number of possible interactions with other medications described below indicates that mistletoe should be used with caution.

Preparations

In alternative medicine, the leaves, twigs, and sometimes the berries of mistletoe are used. In Europe, mistletoe remedies range from tea made from mistletoe leaves to injections of Iscador; however, the berries may be poisonous and the herb may cause liver damage.

Since 2005 mistletoe has not been tested by the United States Food and Drug Administration (FDA), many experts urge caution until more research is completed.

Home remedies

Mistletoe tea may be an alternative treatment for conditions that include high blood pressure, asthma, epilepsy, nervousness, **diarrhea**, and amenorrhea. The tea is prepared by adding 1 tsp. (5 g) of finely cut mistletoe to 1 cup (250 mL) of cold water. The solution is steeped at room temperature for 12 hours and then strained.

Mistletoe wine is prepared by mixing 8 tsp. (40 g) of the herb into 34 oz. (1 L) of wine. After three days, the wine can be consumed. Three to four glasses of medicinal wine may be consumed each day.

Mistletoe must be stored away from light and kept above a drying agent.

Cancer treatment

Iscador, the European extract, may be injected before surgery for cancers of the cervix, ovary, breast, stomach, colon, and lung. Cancer treatments can take several months to several years. The treatment is given by subcutaneous injection, preferably near the tumor. Iscador may be injected into the tumor, especially tumors of the liver, cervix, or esophagus.

The dosage of Iscador varies according to the patient's age, sex, physical condition, and type of cancer. The treatment usually is given in the morning three to seven days per week. As treatment continues, the dosage may be increased or adjusted.

Advocates of Iscador believe it can stimulate the immune system, kill cancer cells, inhibit the formation of tumors, and extend the survival time of cancer patients. They maintain that mistletoe can help prevent cancer and be complementary to standard medical cancer treatments. They also think that mistletoe could possibly repair the DNA that is decreased by **chemotherapy** and radiation.

Precautions

Opinions are sharply divided on how safe and effective the herb is as a home remedy and in the treatment of conditions such as cancer. There is controversy about which parts of the plants are poisonous. Although the berries are classified as poisonous in the United States, some sources say that eating berries is only dangerous for babies, and only if handfuls are consumed. Pregnant or breast-feeding women, however, should not use the plant.

According to a report from the Hepatitis Foundation International, mistletoe is toxic to the liver; however, the *PDR for Herbal Medicines* advises that there are no health hazards when mistletoe is taken properly and in designated therapeutic dosages.

People considering mistletoe should consult with their doctors or practitioners. Until there is definitive proof otherwise, there is a risk that the herbal remedies will conflict with conventional treatment.

Side effects

Mistletoe may be toxic to the liver. For people diagnosed with hepatitis, use of an herb such as mistletoe may cause additional liver damage; however, advocates of mistletoe maintain it is safe, at least under certain circumstances.

Commercial mistletoe extracts may produce fewer side effects. The body temperature may rise and there may be flu-like symptoms. The patient may experience nausea, abdominal pain, and—if given the extract injection—inflammation around the injection sight. Allergy symptoms may result.

Interactions

Mistletoe should not be used by people who take monoamine oxidase (MAO) inhibitor antidepressants such as Nardil. Potential reactions include a dangerous rise in blood pressure and a lowering of blood potassium levels (hypokalemia). In addition, mistletoe may interfere with the action of antidiabetic medications, to increase the activity of diuretics, and to increase the risk of a toxic reaction to aspirin or NSAIDs. Cancer patients considering mistletoe treatment should first consult with their doctors or practitioners.

Resources

PERIODICALS

Marvibaigi, M., Supriyanto, E., Amini, N., Abdul Majid, F.A., Jaqanathan, S.K. "Preclinical and Clinical Effects of Mistletoe Against Breast Cancer." *Biomed Research International* http://www.ncbi.nlm.nih.gov/pubmed/25136622 (accessed November 4, 2014).

WEBSITES

American Cancer Society. "Mistletoe." http://www.cancer.org/treatment/treatmentsandsideeffects/

complementaryandalternativemedicine/herbsvitaminsandminerals/mistletoe (accessed November 8, 2014).

National Cancer Institute. "Mistletoe Extracts (PDQ®)." http://www.cancer.gov/cancertopics/pdq/cam/mistletoe/patient/page1 (accessed November 8, 2014).

ORGANIZATIONS

National Center for Complementary and Alternative Medicine, 9000 Rockville Pike, Bethesda, MD 20892, (888) 644-6226, TTY: (866) 464-3615, http://nccam.nih.gov.

Office of Cancer Complementary and Alternative Medicine (OCCAM), 9609 Medical Center Dr., Rockville, MD 20850, (240) 276-6595, ncioccam1-r@mail.nih.gov, http://cam.cancer.gov.

Liz Swain
Rebecca J. Frey, PhD

Mithramycin *see* **Plicamycin**

Mitomycin-C

Definition

Mitomycin-C is also known as mitomycin and MMC. It is an antineoplastic, or medicine that kills **cancer** cells. It is sold under the trade name Mutamycin.

Purpose

Mitomycin-C may be used to fight a number of different cancers, including cancer of the stomach, colon, rectum, pancreas, breast, lung, uterus, cervix, bladder, head, neck, eye, and esophagus.

It is impossible to provide a detailed description of how mitomycin-C may be combined with other medications in the treatment of each of these cancers, but some examples can be presented. In the treatment of **non-small cell lung cancer** (NSCLC), one therapeutic regimen that may be used is known as MT, which consists of mitomycin-C, **vindesine**, and **cisplatin**.

Mitomycin-C is sometimes used in patients with colorectal cancer metastatic to the liver. However, the side effects of mitomycin-C, especially those involving the bone marrow and **fatigue**, are so great that other medications may be tried first. In treating **breast cancer** metastatic to the liver, mitomycin is regarded as salvage therapy.

For advanced **stomach cancer**, the FAM regimen may be used, which consists of **fluorouracil**, **doxorubicin** (Adriamycin), and mitomycin-C. Mitomycin-C may also be used for colorectal cancer metastatic to the liver in combination with other medicines.

More recently, mitomycin has been found effective in treating malignant **melanoma** of the eye.

In addition to cancer treatment, mitomycin is sometimes used as a topical application in eye surgery to prevent visual haze after operations on the cornea (the transparent exterior coat that covers the front of the eye where light enters). It is also used topically by some doctors to keep incisions in the ear drum open in children with recurrent ear infections without the need to place ventilation tubes in the incisions. This use of mitomycin is considered experiental.

Description

Mitomycin-C is an antitumor antibiotic. Mechanistically however, it belongs to DNA covalent binding (alkylating) agents. Mitomycin-C, upon bioactivation, kills cancer cells by disrupting the activity of DNA within the cells. DNA is an acid that contains genetic material.

Recommended dosage

Twenty milligrams per square meter should be given intravenously every six to eight weeks when this medication is used alone. Alternately, five to ten milligrams per square meter may be given every six weeks when the drug is used in combination with other drugs. Mitomycin-C, **leucovorin**, and fluorouracil may be used to treat metastatic **rectal cancer**; this regimen includes an injection of 10 milligrams per square meter of mitomycin-C. When mitomycin-C is combined with vindesine and cisplatin in the treatment of non-small cell lung cancer, eight milligrams per square inch are administered intravenously on days one and twenty-nine of a six-week cycle.

Precautions

Because of the side effects associated with mitomycin-C, some physicians perform blood tests and order chest x-rays (of the lungs) for patients receiving this therapy. The likelihood that lung problems will appear in patients receiving mitomycin-C increases if oxygen therapy and/or x-ray therapy are administered.

Patients receiving less than 60 mg of mitomycin-C are at reduced risk of developing a complex medical condition called cancer-associated hemolytic uremia syndrome (HUS). HUS is characterized by **anemia**, other blood defects, and kidney problems. Doctors should carefully observe patients receiving mitomycin-C, as cancer-related HUS is best treated early. However, HUS is not likely to develop until four or more months after the patient received the final dose of mitomycin-C. To achieve early diagnosis of HUS, the doctor may carefully monitor kidney function and blood levels. In addition, transfusions may be avoided as well as certain other procedures involving the blood, as these may increase the risk HUS will develop.

Side effects

The ability of the bone marrow to produce blood cells may be affected. This side effect can be serious. If it occurs, the doctor may decide to reduce the dose of medicine administered. However, mitomycin-C may cause delayed, rather than immediate, bone marrow suppression. Once such suppression does occur it may last for as many as eight weeks.

Major lung problems may occur. Such lung deficits may start as no more than cough, fatigue, and breathing problems. Doctors may conduct lung function tests and obtain x-rays to observe whether lung problems are developing. If these lung problems do occur, **corticosteroids** may provide effective therapy. Stopping mitomycin-C therapy may also be recommended.

Mitomycin-C may also cause cancer-associated HUS.

In addition, there may be **nausea and vomiting**, loss of appetite (**anorexia**), stomach problems, fatigue, **fever**, hair loss (**alopecia**), and lung problems. If bleeding does occur, there may be damage to the surrounding skin.

Resources

WEBSITES

Cancer Research UK. "Mitomycin C." http://www.cancerre searchuk.org/about-cancer/cancers-in-general/treatment/cancer-drugs/mitomycin-c (accessed November 8, 2014).

National Cancer Institute. "Mitomycin." http://www.cancer.gov/cancertopics/druginfo/mitomycinc (accessed November 8, 2014).

The Scott Hamilton CARES Initiatve. "Mitomycin-C." Chemocare.com. http://chemocare.com/chemotherapy/drug-info/MitomycinC.aspx (accessed November 8, 2014).

ORGANIZATIONS

ASHP (formerly the American Society of Health-System Pharmacists), 7272 Wisconsin Ave., Bethesda, MD 20814, (301) 664-8700, (866) 279-0681, custserv@ashp.org, http://www.ashp.org.

U.S. Food and Drug Administration, 10903 New Hampshire Ave., Silver Spring, MD 20993, (888) INFO-FDA (463-6332), http://www.fda.gov.

Bob Kirsch
Rebecca J. Frey, PhD

KEY TERMS

Adrenocortex—The outer part of adrenal gland that sits on top of the kidneys.

Anorexia—A condition of uncontrolled lack or loss of desire for food.

Mitotane

Definition

Mitotane, also known by the brand name Lysodren, is a medicine that has been proven to be effective in the treatment of **adrenocortical carcinoma**.

Purpose

Mitotane destroys cells of the adrenocortex. The adrenocortex, also called the adrenal cortex, is a section of adrenal gland that sits on top of the kidneys. Mitotane is usually used for patients whose **cancer** cannot be treated surgically and for patients whose cancer has metastasized.

Description

As a chemical, mitotane resembles the insecticides DDD and DDT, although mitotane does not harm people as these do. Scientists do not understand why, but the drug causes damage to the adrenocortex in such a way as to be helpful for some patients with adrenocortical tumors. In addition, mitotane restricts the ability of the gland to produce chemicals.

Recommended dosage

The dose of mitotane given to patients varies, although between four and eight grams (0.12–0.25 oz.) per day is a typical dose. Patients vary in how much mitotane they tolerate, some patients tolerating two grams (0.1 oz.) per day while others tolerate sixteen grams (0.5 oz.) per day. The doses are given orally. At the beginning of the therapy, the patient may receive 500 milligrams of mitotane twice a day. At any one time a

third or a quarter of an entire day's dose is taken. If the patient has difficulty tolerating a certain dose, the doctors may adjust this and use a somewhat smaller dose. Mitotane should be given for at least three months. If the medicine is effective, it may be continued indefinitely. However, most patients respond to the x-ray treatment of the pituitary gland and so do not need mitotane treatment to continue indefinitely.

Many doctors use mitotane in conjunction with **radiation therapy** directed to the pituitary gland, but other approaches to this medicine may also be taken.

Precautions

Many patients on mitotane should receive adrenocorticosteroids.

Side effects

Four out of five patients receiving mitotane experience **anorexia** and nausea. About one-third of patients experience lethargy and sleepiness. Roughly one in five develop skin problems with the medicine. However, patients who experience these side effects do not have to stop taking the medication, although the doctor may lower the dose the person is receiving.

Interactions

Mitotane should not be given with spironolactone (a diuretic/water pill).

Resources

BOOKS

Chu, Edward, and Vincent T. DeVita Jr. *Physicians' Cancer Chemotherapy Drug Manual 2014*. Burlington, MA: Jones & Bartlett Learning, 2014.

WEBSITES

AHFS Consumer Medication Information. "Mitotane." American Society of Health-System Pharmicists. Available from: http://www.cancer.org/treatment/treatmentsandsideeffects/guidetocancerdrugs/mitotane (accessed November 8, 2014).

American Cancer Society. "Mitotane." http://www.cancer.org/
treatment/treatmentsandsideeffects/guidetocancerdrugs/
mitotane (accessed November 8, 2014).

Bob Kirsch

Mitoxantrone

Definition

Mitoxantrone, also known by its trade name Novantrone, is an anticancer agent effective against certain kinds of leukemias. It is also used in Multiple Sclerosis (MS), and was approved by the Federal Drug Administration in 1987.

Purpose

Mitoxantrone is used with other drugs to treat acute non-lymphocytic leukemia (ANLL), a category that includes myelogenous, promyelocytic, monocytic and erythroid acute leukemia. In adults, ANLL accounts for up to 85% of all adult leukemia cases. Mitoxantrone may also be used in the treatment of **acute lymphocytic leukemia**, **chronic myelocytic leukemia**, **ovarian cancer**, advanced or recurrent **breast cancer**, **prostate cancer**, and MS.

Description

Mitoxantrone is classified as an anthracycline antitumor antibiotic, and closely resembles another drug in this category, **daunorubicin**. Although its precise mechanism is not clear, mitoxantrone is cell cycle non-specific, meaning that it is toxic to cells that are dividing, as well as those that are not.

Recommended dosage

Mitoxantrone is given intravenously over a thirty-minute time period. **Chemotherapy** dosages are based on a person's body surface area (BSA), which is calculated in square meters using height and weight measurements. Drug dosages are ordered in milligrams per square meter (mg/m^2).

In patients with **cancer**, the recommended dosage for induction therapy is 12 mg/m^2 administered on the first three days of treatment. After that time, another chemotherapy drug is usually infused. This course of treatment is often adequate to induce remission, but may be repeated if it does not. In the second induction course, the dosage remains the same, but mitoxantrone is given

KEY TERMS

Body surface area (BSA)—A measurement, based on a patient's height and weight, that helps determine appropriate chemotherapy dosages.

Mucositis—A severe, painful inflammation of the mucous membranes.

Myelosuppression—A condition in which bone marrow activity is diminished, resulting in decreased platelet, red blood cell, and white blood cell counts.

Remission—The time period during which symptoms of a disease are absent.

for two days, rather than three, followed by other chemotherapy agents. Dosages may be altered, depending on the level of bone marrow toxicity the patient develops.

For patients with solid tumors, such as advanced hormone-refractory prostate cancer, a single dose of 12 mg/m^2 is administered, and repeated every three to four weeks. Recent studies show that mitoxantrone used with glucocorticoids has resulted in improved pain control and quality of life in men with prostate cancer.

Precautions

Mitoxantrone's use in children has not been studied sufficiently to determine whether its use is safe and effective. It should not be used in individuals who have experienced a previous reaction to it.

Mitoxantrone is excreted by the liver and kidneys. It may alter the appearance of urine, causing it to be a blue-green color for approximately 24 hours. The sclera, or whites of the eyes, may temporarily be blue-tinged. Patients should not be alarmed by this change, but should alert their doctors if it is prolonged or is accompanied by other symptoms.

Mitoxantrone should not be administered to pregnant women, as damage to the fetus may occur. Throughout treatment, women should use methods to prevent pregnancy. It is excreted in breast-milk, so breast-feeding should be avoided during treatment.

Side effects

Mitoxantrone can cause severe and sometimes rapid **myelosuppression** leading to decreased white blood cell, red blood cell, and platelet counts. Blood counts should be monitored frequently throughout treatment. The white blood cells tend to nadir, or drop to their lowest point, within ten to fourteen days after mitoxantrone is administered. Patients should also be examined for symptoms of low white blood cell count, which typically resemble those of an infection: sore throat, burning with urination, increased temperature, or swelling. Patients should also be carefully monitored for indications that platelet count is low. Symptoms may include unexplained bruises, bleeding or increased bleeding with menstruation, and headache.

Mitoxantrone can damage the heart, possibly causing changes that lead to congestive heart failure (CHF). Patients especially at risk are those previously treated with anthracyclines or radiation to the chest area, or those with an already existing heart condition. Symptoms to watch for include swelling of the hands and ankles, difficulty breathing, or heart palpitations.

Mitoxantrone can cause a severe, painful inflammation of the mucous membranes called **mucositis**. The condition may develop within a week of treatment. A patient may experience a burning sensation in his or her throat, as well as mouth pain. Mucositis typically resolves in a few weeks on its own, but there are measures one can take to hasten the process and provide comfort during healing. Hydration is very important to keep the mouth moist. Good oral hygiene is important—the teeth should be brushed with a very soft toothbrush, and flossed gently with unwaxed dental floss. If bleeding occurs, using a toothbrush may not be safe. Patients should talk to their health care providers should this occur. Your doctor or nurse may recommend a special mouthwash that helps relieve pain.

Patients undergoing treatment with mitoxantrone may be at risk for **tumor lysis syndrome**, a potentially life-threatening condition that develops when large numbers of cells rupture and release their contents into the blood stream. Preventative measures should be implemented to prevent adverse effects.

Interactions

Because mitoxantrone can alter normal blood counts, medications that contain aspirin should be avoided. Aspirin acts as a blood-thinner, and can predispose a person to bleeding. Patients should discuss all medications, whether they are prescribed or over-the-counter drugs, with their doctor to ensure there are no potential interactions. **Cytarabine**, another drug used to treat cancer, may increase the toxicity of mitoxantrone if the drugs are used together.

Resources

BOOKS

Chu, Edward, and Vincent T. DeVita Jr. *Physicians' Cancer Chemotherapy Drug Manual 2014*. Burlington, MA: Jones & Bartlett Learning, 2014.

WEBSITES

American Cancer Society. "Mitoxantrone." http://www.cancer.org/treatment/treatmentsandsideeffects/guidetocancerdrugs/mitoxantrone (accessed November 8, 2014).

Cancer Research UK. "Mitoxantrone (Onkontrone)." http://www.cancerresearchuk.org/about-cancer/cancers-in-general/treatment/cancer-drugs/mitoxantrone (accessed November 8, 2014).

Tamara Brown, R.N.

MMPIs *see* **Matrix metalloproteinase inhibitors**

Modified radical mastectomy

Definition

A modified radical **mastectomy** is a surgical procedure that removes the breast, surrounding tissue, and nearby lymph nodes affected by **cancer**.

Purpose

The purpose of modified radical mastectomy is the removal of **breast cancer** (abnormal cells in the breast that grow rapidly and replace normal healthy tissue). Modified radical mastectomy is the most widely used surgical procedure to treat operable breast cancer. This procedure leaves a chest muscle called the pectoralis major intact. Leaving this muscle in place will provide a soft tissue covering over the chest wall and a normal-appearing junction of the shoulder with the anterior (front) chest wall. This sparing of the pectoralis major will avoid a disfiguring hollow defect below the clavicle. Additionally, the purpose of modified radical mastectomy is to allow for the option of **breast reconstruction**, a procedure that is possible, if desired, due to intact muscles around the shoulder of the affected side. The modified radical mastectomy procedure involves removal of large multiple tumor growths located underneath the nipple, as well as cancer cells on the breast margins.

Description

The surgeon's goals during this procedure are to minimize any chance of local/regional recurrence, avoid

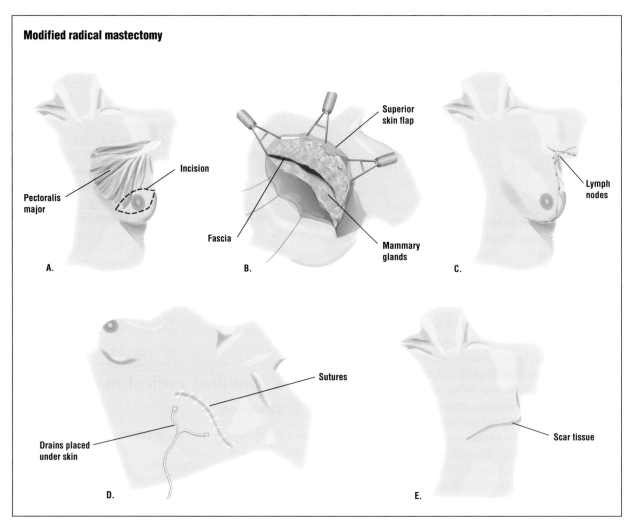

Modified radical mastectomy

A.

Pectoralis major

Incision

B.

Superior skin flap

Fascia

Mammary glands

C.

Lymph nodes

D.

Drains placed under skin

Sutures

E.

Scar tissue

In a modified radical mastectomy, the skin on the breast is cut open (A). The skin is pulled back, and the tumor, lymph nodes, and breast tissue are removed (B and C). The incision is then closed (D). *(Illustration by GGS Information Services. © Cengage Learning®.)*

any loss of function, and maximize options for breast reconstruction. Incisions are made to avoid visibility in a low-neckline dress or bathing suit. An incision in the shape of an ellipse is made. The surgeon removes the minimum amount of skin and tissue so that the remaining healthy tissue can be used for possible reconstruction. Skin flaps are made carefully and as thinly as possible to maximize removal of diseased breast tissues. The skin over a neighboring muscle (pectoralis major fascia) is removed, after which the surgeon focuses in the armpit (axillary) region. In this region, the surgeon carefully identifies vital anatomical structures such as blood vessels (veins, arteries) and nerves. Accidental injury to specific nerves like the medial pectoral neurovascular bundle will result in destruction of the muscles that this surgery attempts to preserve, such as the pectoralis major. In the armpit region, the surgeon carefully protects the vital structures while removing cancerous tissues. After

axillary surgery, breast reconstruction can be performed if desired by the patient.

Demographics

When all ages are taken into account, white women are more likely to contract breast cancer than other ethnicities, although in women under age 45, African American women have a higher risk of developing the disease. Additionally, African American women are more likely to die of the disease. The lowest risk of breast cancer development or death is in women of Asian, Hispanic, or Native American backgrounds.

While considerably less common, men can also have breast cancer. According to the American Cancer Society, in 2013 there were approximately 2,240 new breast cancer diagnoses in men, with 410 deaths.

Known risk factors in women include a strong genetic correlation, with greatly increased risk among women with a close relative (mother, sister, maternal aunt, or maternal grandmother) who has had breast cancer. Increased susceptibility for development of breast cancer can occur in females who never breastfed a baby, had a child after age 30, started menstrual periods very early, or experienced menopause very late.

Breast cancer is the most common cancer in women, other than **skin cancer**. The American Cancer Society estimated that in 2013, 296,980 new cases of breast cancer were diagnosed in the United States, with 39,620 women dying as a result of the disease. Approximately one in eight women will develop breast cancer at some point in her life. The risk of developing breast cancer increases with age. Without even considering genetic and environmental factors, women aged 30 to 40 have a 1 in 252 chance of developing breast cancer, women aged 40 to 50 have a 1 in 68 chance, women aged 50 to 60 have a 1 in 35 chance, and women aged 60 to 70 have a 1 in 27 chance.

Diagnosis

Modified radical mastectomy is a surgical procedure to treat breast cancer. In order for this procedure to be an option, a definitive diagnosis of breast cancer must be established. The first clinical sign for approximately 80% of women with breast cancer is a mass (lump) located in the breast. A lump can be discovered by monthly self-examination or by a health professional who can find the 10%–25% of breast cancers that are missed by yearly mammograms (a low-radiation x-ray of the breasts). A **biopsy** can be performed to examine the cells from a lump that is suspicious for cancer. The diagnosis of the extent of the cancer and whether it has spread to regional lymph nodes determines the treatment course—i.e., whether to combat the cancer with surgery, **chemotherapy**, or **radiation therapy**, either singly or in combination. Staging the cancer can estimate the amount of tumor, which is important not only for diagnosis but for prognosis (statistical outcome of the disease process). Patients with a type of breast cancer called ductal **carcinoma** in situ (DCIS), which is a stage 0 cancer,

have the best outcome—nearly all these patients are cured of breast cancer. Persons whose cancer has spread to other places within the body (metastases) have stage IV cancer and the worst prognosis (potential for survival). At present, people affected with stage IV breast cancer have essentially no chance of cure.

Persons affected with breast cancer must undergo the staging of the cancer to determine the extent of cancerous growth and possible spread (**metastasis**) to distant organs. Patients with stage 0 disease have noninvasive cancer with a very good outcome. Stages I and II are early breast cancer without lymph node involvement (stage I) and with node-positive results (stage II). Persons with stage III cancer have locally advanced disease and about a 50% chance for five-year survival. Stage IV disease is the most severe, since the breast cancer cells have spread through lymph nodes to distant areas and/or other organs in the body. It is very unlikely that persons with stage IV metastatic breast cancer will survive 10 years after diagnosis.

It is also imperative to assess the degree of cancerous spread to lymph nodes within the armpit region. Of primary importance to stage determination and regional lymph node involvement is identification and analysis of the sentinel lymph node. The sentinel lymph node is the first lymph node to which any cancer would spread. The procedure for sentinel node biopsy involves injecting a radioactively labeled tracer (technetium 99) or a blue dye (isosulfan blue) into the tumor site. The tracer or dye will spread through the lymphatic system to the sentinel node, which should be surgically removed and examined for the presence of cancer cells. If the sentinel node and one or two other neighboring lymph nodes are negative, it is very likely that the remaining lymph nodes will not contain cancerous cells, and further surgery may not be necessary.

Once a breast lump (mass) has been identified by **mammography** or physical examination, the patient should undergo further evaluation to histologically (studying the cells) identify or rule out the presence of cancer cells. A procedure called fine-needle aspiration allows the clinician to extract cells directly from the lump for further evaluation. If a diagnosis cannot be established by fine-needle biopsy, the surgeon should perform an open biopsy (surgical removal of the suspicious mass).

Preparation

Preparation for surgery is imperative. The patient should plan for both direct care and recovery time after modified radical mastectomy. Preparation immediately prior to surgery should include no food or drink after midnight before the procedure. Postsurgical preparation should include caregivers to help with daily tasks for several days.

Aftercare

After breast cancer surgery, women should undergo frequent testing to ensure early detection of cancer recurrence. It is recommended that mammograms, physical examinations, or additional tests (biopsies) be performed annually. Aftercare can also include psychotherapy, since mastectomy is emotionally traumatic. Affected women may be worried or have concerns about appearance, the relationship with their sexual partner, and possible physical limitations. Community-centered support groups usually made up of former breast cancer surgery patients can be a source of emotional support after surgery. Patients may stay in the hospital for one to two days. For about five to seven days after surgery, there will be one or two drains left inside the body to remove any extra fluid from the area after surgery. Usually, the surgeon will prescribe medication to prevent pain. Restrictions on movement should be specifically discussed with the surgeon.

Risks

There are several risks associated with modified radical mastectomy. The procedure is performed under general anesthesia, which itself carries risk. Women may have short-term pain and tenderness. The most frequent risk of breast cancer surgery—with extensive lymph node removal—is edema, or swelling of the arm. This effect is usually mild, but the presence of fluid can increase the risk of infection. Leaving some lymph nodes intact instead of removing all of them may help lessen the likelihood of swelling. Nerves in the area may be damaged. There may be numbness in the arm or difficulty moving shoulder muscles. There is also the risk of developing a lumpy scar (keloid) after surgery. Another risk is that the surgery did not remove all the cancer cells and that further treatment may be necessary with chemotherapy and/or radiotherapy. By far, the worst risk is recurrence of cancer; however, immediate signs of risk following surgery include **fever**, redness in the incision area, unusual drainage from the incision, and increasing pain. If any of these signs develop, it is imperative to call the surgeon immediately.

Results

If no complications develop, the surgical area should completely heal within three to four weeks. After mastectomy, some women may undergo breast reconstruction, which can also be done during mastectomy.

QUESTIONS TO ASK YOUR DOCTOR

- What is the prognosis for the stage (0, I, II, III, IV) of my type of cancer?
- Will my movement be restricted after surgery?
- What care will I need on a daily basis following surgery?
- When should we set up a follow-up consultation/examination?
- Will I require other treatment (chemotherapy and/or radiation therapy) following surgery?
- What kind of mental health treatment should I pursue (psychotherapy, community-centered support groups, etc.) following surgery?
- What options do I have for breast reconstruction? When would that treatment begin?

Recent studies have indicated that women who undergo cosmetic **reconstructive surgery** have a higher quality of life and a better sense of well-being than those who do not utilize this option.

Morbidity and mortality rates

The outcome of breast cancer is very dependent on the stage at the time of diagnosis. The five-year survival rates for the various stages are:

- Stage 0, 93%
- Stage I (early/lymph node–negative), 88%
- Stage II (early/lymph node–positive), 74%–81%
- Stage III disease (locally advanced), 41%–67%
- Stage IV (metastatic), 15%

Approximately 17% of patients develop lymphedema after axillary **lymph node dissection**, while only 3% of patients develop lymphedema after sentinel node biopsy. Five percent of women are unhappy with the cosmetic effects of the surgery.

Alternatives

There are no effective alternatives to mastectomy. A mastectomy is recommended for tumors with dimensions over 2 in. (5 cm). Additional treatment (adjuvant) is typically recommended, with chemotherapy and/or radiation therapy administered to destroy any remaining cancer. Modified radical mastectomy is one of the standard treatment recommendations for stage III breast cancer.

Health care team roles

The procedure is typically performed by a surgeon who has received five years of general surgery training and additional training in the specialty of **surgical oncology**. A surgeon who specializes in this field has expertise in removing cancerous tissues or areas. The procedure is performed in a hospital and requires that the hospital have a surgical care unit. In the surgical care unit, the patient will be treated by a team of professionals that includes, but is not limited to, physicians, nurses, physician assistants, and medical assistants.

Resources

BOOKS

Lentz, Gretchen, et al. *Comprehensive Gynecology.* 5th ed. St. Louis: Mosby/Elsevier, 2012.

Niederhuber, John E., et al. *Abeloff's Clinical Oncology.* 5th ed. Philadelphia: Saunders/Elsevier, 2013.

Townsend, Courtney M., et al. *Sabiston Textbook of Surgery.* 19th ed. Philadelphia: Saunders/Elsevier, 2012.

PERIODICALS

Ribeiro, G. H., et al. "Modified Radical Mastectomy: A Pilot Clinical Trial Comparing the Use of Conventional Electric Scalpel and Harmonic Scalpel." *International Journal of Surgery* 11, no. 6 (2013): 496–500. http://dx.doi.org/10.1016/j.ijsu.2013.03.013 (accessed October 3, 2014).

Sun, M. Q., et al. "Comparison of Psychological Influence on Breast Cancer Patients between Breast-Conserving Surgery and Modified Radical Mastectomy." *Asian Pacific Journal of Cancer Prevention* 14, no. 1 (2013): 149–52.

WEBSITES

A.D.A.M. Medical Encyclopedia. "Mastectomy." MedlinePlus. http://www.nlm.nih.gov/medlineplus/ency/article/002919.htm (accessed October 3, 2014).

Breastcancer.org. "What Is Mastectomy?" http://www.breastcancer.org/treatment/surgery/mastectomy/what_is (accessed October 3, 2014).

ORGANIZATIONS

ABCD (After Breast Cancer Diagnosis), 5775 N. Glen Park Rd., Ste. 201, Glendale, WI 53209, (414) 977-1780, (800) 977-4121, abcdinc@abcdmentor.orghelpline@abcdmentor.org, http://www.abcdbreastcancersupport.org.

American Cancer Society, 250 Williams St. NW, Atlanta, GA 30303, (800) 227-2345, http://www.cancer.org.

National Breast Cancer Coalition, 1101 17th St. NW, Ste. 1300, Washington, DC 20036, (202) 296-7477, (800) 622-2838, Fax: (202) 265-6854, http://www.breastcancerdeadline2020.org.

National Cancer Institute, 6116 Executive Blvd., Ste. 300, Bethesda, MD 20892-8322, (800) 4-CANCER (422-6237), http://cancer.gov.

Laith Farid Gulli, MD
Nicole Mallory, MS, PA-C

REVISED BY ROSALYN CARSON-DEWITT, MD

Mohs surgery

Definition

Mohs surgery—also called Mohs micrographic surgery or microscopically controlled surgery—is a precise, highly specialized technique that removes **skin cancer** by progressively removing individual layers of tissue and examining each layer under a microscope for **cancer** cells. This enables the removal of all of the cancer while preserving healthy tissue.

Purpose

Malignant skin tumors may appear as asymmetrical shapes with long, finger-like projections that extend laterally across the skin or deep down into the skin. These extensions may be composed of only a few cells that cannot be seen or felt. It is possible to miss these cancerous cells with standard surgical removal (excision), which might lead to recurrence of the tumor. In some cases, the cancer requires removal of a large piece of skin. If the cancer is on the face, many patients find this prospect cosmetically unacceptable. Mohs surgery enables the surgeon to excise precisely the entire tumor without removing excessive amounts of surrounding healthy tissue. It is used to remove complicated skin cancers or those in sensitive areas, since it usually spares more healthy tissue for functional or cosmetic purposes and leaves less of a scar than other procedures, while ensuring that the cancer is entirely removed.

The most common uses of Mohs surgery are for:

• cancer recurrences following other treatments, especially local recurrences of basal-cell carcinoma (BCC)

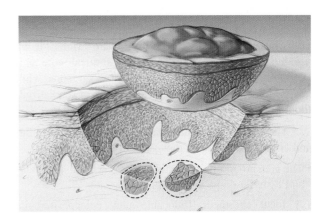

Mohs surgery is used to remove skin cancer tumors of many types, including melanoma. Here, the main portion of the tumor is excised (debulked) using a spoon-shaped tool (curette). Further layers of tissue will be removed as necessary. *(Art & Science, Inc/Custom Medical Stock Photo)*

- cancers that have a high risk of recurrence
- squamous-cell carcinomas larger than 2 cm (0.8 in.) across or with poorly defined edges
- cancers that are spreading along nerves under the skin
- cancers on certain areas of the genitals or face, such as on or near the eyes, eyelids, lips, nose, ears, forehead, or hairline

Although Mohs surgery is not usually the surgical choice for melanomas, which require more extensive excision, this surgery may be used for acral lentiginous melanoma—an aggressive cancer usually affecting dark-skinned people—because Mohs surgery can often avoid **amputation** of fingers or toes. Mohs surgery is sometimes used for:

- large tumors
- tumors without well-defined edges
- cancers whose extent is unknown
- cancers on the fingers, hands, feet, or scalp
- primary treatment of BCC or squamous-cell carcinomas of the skin
- the rare skin cancers microcystic adnexal carcinoma and Merkel cell carcinoma
- Bowen's disease (a precancerous lesion of the skin or mucous membranes)
- extramammary Paget disease (a rare breast cancer)
- leiomyosarcoma (a cancer partially composed of smooth muscle cells)
- laryngeal cancer
- malignant fibrous histiocytoma (a bone cancer)
- mucoepidermoid carcinoma (a salivary gland tumor)

Description

The Mohs procedure was developed in the 1930s by the American surgeon Frederic Edward Mohs. It is usually performed in an office with a surgical suite and laboratory for examining the tissue by surgeons who have generally undergone at least one year of specialized training in the procedure.

The surgery is usually started in the early morning and completed the same day.

- The area around the tumor is cleansed with disinfectant and a sterile drape is placed over the site.
- A local anesthetic (lidocaine plus epinephrine) is injected into the area.
- To define the area to be excised and enable accurate mapping of the tumor, identifying marks are made with a surgical marking pen, dye, stitches, staples, fine scalpel cuts, or temporary tattoos.

- The visible tumor and a thin layer of surrounding tissue are excised (debulked) using a spoon-shaped curette (first Mohs excision).
- The tissue is taken to the laboratory for processing and analysis while the patient waits.
- The excised tissue is divided into sections, stained, and color-coded with marks corresponding to those on the skin to indicate the source of each section and make a Mohs map of the surgical site.
- A technician freezes the tissue sections, removes very thin slices from the entire edge and undersurface of the tumor, and prepares microscopic slides for examination by the surgeon. This process may take an hour or more.
- If there is evidence of cancer in any sections, the surgeon removes a deeper layer of skin from that section (second Mohs excision).
- These steps are repeated until all excised sections are cancer-free, which generally requires three or fewer excisions. However, depending on the extent of the cancerous roots, more excisions may be required, and the procedure may take as long as an entire day.
- The surgical site is repaired.

Precautions

Mohs surgery is significantly more complex and time-consuming—and much more expensive—than other skin cancer treatments, although the outcomes are often better, with a generally higher cure rate that avoids the need for a second procedure. Many additional doctors are being trained in Mohs surgery, and as of 2014, its use in the United States had increased more than 400% in just over a decade. It is used far less often in other countries. In 2013, Medicare placed it at the top of its list of overused or overpriced procedures. The American Academy of Dermatology has stated that it is sometimes used inappropriately and together with Mohs surgeons' associations developed guidelines for recommending its use based, in part, on the size and type of skin cancer and locations such as the nose or eyelids.

Preparation

Patients should provide the physician with a complete list of all prescription and over-the-counter medications, **vitamins**, and supplements. Use of anticoagulants such as aspirin, **warfarin**, or **heparin** might need to be temporarily suspended to reduce the risk of bleeding. Depending on the location of the tumor and the patient's health status, prophylactic **antibiotics** might be prescribed prior to the procedure. Patients might be asked to stop smoking and not consume certain foods or beverages some hours before the procedure. However, patients are encouraged to eat prior to the surgery and to bring snacks in case of a lengthy procedure. Since it is difficult to predict how long a Mohs surgery will take, patients should be prepared to spend the entire day. Surgery on some locations of the body might require that the patient be driven home.

Aftercare

Following the procedure, the surgeon assesses the wound and discusses options for functional and/or cosmetic repair or reconstruction. Most often, the surgeon performs reconstruction on the same day.

• Small, simple wounds might be allowed to heal naturally.

• Somewhat larger wounds might be stitched together.

• Large or complicated wounds might require a skin graft taken from elsewhere in the body or closure with a flap of skin adjacent to the wound.

• Rarely, repair requires a plastic surgeon or reconstructive surgical specialist.

Patients will receive specific wound-care instructions for changing bandages and cleaning the surgical site. Wounds that were repaired with absorbable stitches or skin grafts are generally covered with a bandage for one week. Wounds that were repaired using nonabsorbable stitches are covered with a bandage, which should be replaced daily until the stitches are removed one–two weeks later. Prescription or over-the-counter medications or topical ointments may be prescribed. There is not usually any significant pain, but discomfort can be treated

---

QUESTIONS TO ASK YOUR DOCTOR

• Why is Mohs surgery preferable for my condition?

• How long have you been performing Mohs surgeries?

• What will the procedure entail?

• Will I need to alter my current medication use?

• What happens if you do not locate the border of the cancerous lesion?

• How will the wound be repaired?

• What is the cure rate with Mohs surgery for this type of cancer?

• What are the chances that the tumor will recur?

• How often will I need follow-up appointments?

---

with acetaminophen. Bruising, swelling, or small amounts of bleeding around the wound may occur. Patients will be told when they can return to activities such as showering, exercise, or applying makeup and how to treat the surgery scar to ensure healing and quick fading. Signs of infection—such as redness, pain, or drainage—should be reported to the physician immediately.

Post-surgical checkups monitor recovery and check for any cancer recurrence. The checkups may continue for years, since about 40% of patients with skin cancer will develop a second skin cancer within five years. Patients are also told how to recognize symptoms of skin cancer.

Risks

• Fresh-tissue Mohs surgery on a large tumor requires high amounts of local anesthetic, which can be toxic.

• Infection, bleeding, scarring, or nerve damage can occur.

• Tiny nerve endings that are cut during the surgery can cause temporary or permanent numbness in and around the surgical site.

• The area may remain tender for weeks or months after the surgery.

• Large tumors or extensive surgery can result in temporary or permanent weakness in the area, but this is unusual.

• Rarely, there is intermittent itching or shooting pain in the area.

• Skin grafts or flaps might require additional repair.

Results

Mohs surgery has the highest cure rates for malignant skin tumors. BCC recurrence following Mohs surgery is less than 5%, compared with up to 15% or higher for some other procedures, although this varies with the size of the tumor.

Abnormal results

Tumors spread in unpredictable patterns. Sometimes a seemingly small tumor is found to be quite large and widespread, resulting in a much larger excision than was anticipated. In addition, technical errors, such as those occurring during processing or interpretation of the tissue sections, may lead to local recurrence of the cancer.

Resources

BOOKS

Nouri, Keyvan. *Mohs Micrographic Surgery.* London, UK: Springer, 2012.

PERIODICALS

Ad Hoc Task Force. "Appropriate Use Criteria for Mohs Micrographic Surgery: A Report of the American Academy of Dermatology, American College of Mohs Surgery, American Society for Dermatologic Surgery Association, and the American Society for Mohs Surgery." *Journal of the American Academy of Dermatology* 67 (2012): 531–50.

Cimons, Marlene. "Not Safe From the Sun." *Washington Post* (August 5, 2014): E1.

Rosenthal, Elisabeth. "Patients' Costs Skyrocket; Specialists' Incomes Soar." *New York Times* (January 19, 2014): A1.

Turner, John Brad, and Brian Rinker. "Melanoma of the Hand: Current Practice and New Frontiers." *Healthcare* 2, no. 1 (2014): 125–38.

OTHER

"Patient Information: Mohs Micrographic Surgery in the Treatment of Skin Cancer." American Society for Mohs Surgery. http://www.mohssurgery.org/files/public/patient_information_brochure.pdf (accessed August 18, 2014).

WEBSITES

American College of Mohs Surgery. "About Mohs Surgery." Mohs Surgery Patient Education. http://www.skincancer mohssurgery.org/mohs-surgery (accessed August 18, 2014).

Goldman, Glenn. "Mohs Surgery Comes Under the Micro-scope." American Academy of Dermatology. November 8, 2013. http://www.aad.org/members/publications/member-to-member/2013-archive/november-8-2013/mohs-surgery-comes-under-the-microscope (accessed August 18, 2014).

ORGANIZATIONS

American Academy of Dermatology, PO Box 4014, Schaumburg, IL 60168, (847) 240-1280, Fax: (847) 240-1859, (866) 503-SKIN (7546), http://www.aad.org.

American College of Mohs Surgery, 555 East Wells Street, Suite 1100, Milwaukee, WI 53202-3823, (414) 347-1103, (800) 500-7224, http://www.skincancermohssurgery.org.

American Society for Dermatologic Surgery, 5550 Meadow-brook Drive, Suite 120, Rolling Meadows, IL 60008, (847) 956-0900, http://www.asds.net.

American Society for Mohs Surgery, 5901 Warner Avenue, Box 391, Huntington Beach, CA 92649-4659, (714) 379-6262, Fax: (714) 379-6272, (800) 616-ASMS (2767), info@mohssurgery.org, http://www.mohssurgery.org.

Belinda Rowland, PhD
Rebecca J. Frey, PhD
Margaret Alic, PhD

Monoclonal antibodies

Definition

Monoclonal antibodies (mAbs) are proteins produced in the laboratory from a single clone of a B cell, the cells of the immune system that make antibodies.

Description

Antibodies, also known as immunoglobulins (Igs), are proteins that help identify foreign substances to the immune system, such as bacteria or viruses. Antibodies bind to the foreign substance to mark it as foreign. The substance that the antibody binds to is called an antigen. All monoclonal antibodies of a particular type bind to the same antigen.

The structure of most antibodies can be divided into two parts: the section that binds the antigen and the section that identifies the type of antibody. The latter is referred to as a constant region, because it is essentially the same within the same type of antibody. The most common type of antibody is IgG (immunoglobulin gamma), which is found in blood and other bodily fluids. For **cancer** treatments, monoclonal antibodies are often humanized, which involves using human sequences for the constant regions and using mouse or other animal-derived sequences for the binding region. Humanization reduces the immune reaction of a patient to the antibody itself.

When used as a treatment for cancer, there are three general strategies with monoclonal antibodies. One uses the ability of the antibodies to bind to the cancer cells that have the tumor antigens on their surface. The immune system will see the cancer cells marked with bound antibodies as foreign and destroy them. A second strategy is to use the antibodies to block the binding of cytokines or other proteins that are needed by the cancerous cells to maintain their growth. These types of monoclonal antibodies bind to the receptors for the cytokine that are on the tumor cell surface.

A final strategy involves special antibodies that are linked (conjugated) to a substance that is deadly to the cancer cells. Radioactive isotopes, like yttrium 90, and toxins produced by bacteria, like pseudomonas exotoxin, have both been successfully conjugated to antibodies. The antibodies are then used to destroy the tumor cells with the radioactivity or toxic substance.

The first two strategies utilize naked mAbs, which are so-called because they are not joined with any other material. Examples include **alemtuzumab** (Campath) and **trastuzumab** (Herceptin). The third method uses conjugated mAbs such as **ibritumomab** tiuxetan (Zevalin), brentuximab vedotin (Adcetris), and **ado-trastuzumab emtansine** (Kadcyla).

Side effects

Side effects vary depending upon the drug being used, but some general side effects of mAbs include:

• chills

• diarrhea

• drop in blood pressure

• fever

• general weakness

• headache

• nausea and vomiting

• skin rashes

Resources

WEBSITES

American Cancer Society. "Monoclonal Antibodies to Treat Cancer." http://www.cancer.org/treatment/treatmentsand sideeffects/treatmenttypes/immunotherapy/immunother apy-monoclonal-antibodies (accessed October 3, 2014).

Mayo Clinic staff. "Monoclonal Antibody Drugs for Cancer: How They Work." Mayo Clinic. http://www.mayoclinic. org/diseases-conditions/cancer/in-depth/monoclonal-anti body/ART-20047808 (accessed October 3, 2014).

Michelle Johnson, MS, JD

Monoclonal gammopathy of undetermined significance see **Multiple myeloma**

Morphine see **Opioids**

Mouth dryness see **Xerostomia**

Mozobil *see* **Plerixafor**

MRI *see* **Magnetic resonance imaging**

▌Mucositis

Definition

Mucositis is an inflammatory condition involving the lining of the mouth and digestive tract.

Description

Mucositis frequently occurs in **cancer** patients after **chemotherapy** and **radiation therapy**. The cheek, gums, soft plate, oropharynx, top and sides of tongue, and floor of the mouth may be affected, as well as the esophagus and rectal areas. Along with redness and swelling, patients typically experience a strong, burning pain.

Risk factors

Although there are factors that increase the likelihood and severity of mucositis, there is no reliable manner to predict who will be affected. Not only is mucositis more common in elderly patients, the degree of breakdown is often more debilitating. The severity of mucositis tends to be increased if a patient exercises poor oral hygiene or has a compromised nutritional status. A preexisting infection or irritation to the mucous membrane may also result in a more severe case of mucositis.

Causes and symptoms

The precise mechanism by which cancer treatment induces mucositis is not clear, but it is believed to damage the rapidly dividing epithelial cells in the mucous membranes. This damage leads to inflammation and swelling, and then actual breakdown of the mucosa, the lining of the mouth and digestive tract. Another theory is that the body's natural defenses are weakened. For example, the immunoglobulin IgA is normally found in saliva. In patients who developed mucositis after undergoing cancer treatment with **methotrexate**, IgA levels in saliva were decreased.

The types of drug used to treat cancer and the schedule by which they are given influence the risk of developing mucositis. **Doxorubicin** and methotrexate, for example, frequently cause mucositis. The chemotherapy agent **fluorouracil** does not usually severely affect the mucous membranes when administered in small doses over continuous intravenous (IV) infusion. When the schedule is adjusted so that a higher dose is given over a shorter period of time (typically over five days), fluorouracil can cause very severe, painful, dose-limiting cases of mucositis. Patients undergoing treatment with high-dose chemotherapy and bone marrow rescue usually develop mucositis.

In addition, mucositis also tends to develop in radiation therapy administered to the oral cavity, or in dosages that exceed 180 cGy per day over a five-day period. Combination therapy, either multiple chemotherapy agents or chemotherapy and radiation therapy to the oral cavity, can increase the incidence of mucositis.

Treatment

Because there is no real cure for mucositis, treatment is aimed at prevention and management of symptoms. Mucositis typically resolves a few weeks after treatment as the cells regenerate, and treatment cessation is only occasionally required. In some cases, drug therapy will be altered so that a less toxic agent is given.

Patients at risk for mucositis should be meticulous about their oral hygiene, brushing frequently with a soft toothbrush and flossing carefully with unwaxed dental floss. If bleeding of the gums develops, patients should replace their toothbrushes with soft toothettes or gauze. Dentures should also be cleaned regularly. Patients should be well-hydrated, drinking fluids frequently and rinsing the mouth several times a day. Mouthwashes that contain alcohol or hydrogen peroxide should be avoided as they may dry out the mouth and increase pain. Lips should also be kept moist. Physical irritation to the mouth should be avoided. If time permits, dental problems, such as cavities or ill-fitting dentures, should be resolved with a dentist prior to beginning cancer treatment. Patients are generally more comfortable eating mild, medium-temperature foods. Spicy, acidic, very hot or very cold foods can irritate the mucosa. Tobacco and alcohol should also be avoided.

Hospital personnel and the patients themselves should inspect the mouth frequently to look for signs and symptoms of mucositis. Evidence of mucositis—inflammation, white or yellow shiny mucous membranes developing into red, raw, painful membranes—may be present as early as four days after chemotherapy administration.

Sodium bicarbonate mouth rinses are sometimes used to decrease the amount of oral flora and promote comfort, though there is no scientific evidence that this is beneficial. Typically, patients will rinse every few hours with a solution containing 1/2 teaspoon (tsp) salt and 1/2 tsp baking soda in one cup of water.

Pain relief is often required in patients with mucositis. In some cases, rinsing with a mixture of maalox, xylocaine, and **diphenhydramine** hydrochloride relieves pain. However, because of xylocaine's numbing effects, taste sensation may be altered. Worse, it may reduce the body's natural gag reflex, possibly causing problems with swallowing. Coating agents such as kaopectate and aluminum hydroxide gel may also help relieve symptoms. Rinsing with benzydamine has also shown promise, not only in managing pain, but also in preventing the development of mucositis. More severe pain may require liquid tylenol with codeine, or even intravenous opioid drugs. Patients with severe pain may not be able to eat, and may also require nutritional supplements through an IV (intravenous line).

Alternative and complementary therapies

A treatment called **cryotherapy** has shown promise in patients being treated with fluorouracil administered in the aforementioned five-day, high-dose schedule. Patients continuously swish ice chips in their mouth during the thirty-minute infusion of the drug, causing the blood vessels to constrict, thereby reducing the drug's ability to affect the oral mucosa.

Chamomile and **allopurinol** mouthwashes have been tried in the past to manage mucositis, but studies have found them to be ineffective. Biologic response modifiers are being evaluated to determine their possible role in managing mucositis. Recent studies using topical antimicrobial lozenges have shown promise as well, but more research is needed.

Resources

BOOKS

Berger, Ann M., Shuster, Jr., John L., Von Roenn, Jamie, eds. *Principles and Practice of Palliative Care and Supportive Oncology*. 4th ed. Philadelphia: Wolters Kluwer Health, and Lippincott Williams & Wilkins, 2013.

Fawcett, Josephine N., and McQueen, Anne, eds. *Perspectives on Cancer Care*. Chichester, West Sussex, UK: Wiley-Blackwell, 2011.

WEBSITES

National Cancer Institute. "Oral Mucositis." http://www.cancer.gov/cancertopics/pdq/supportivecare/oralcomplications/HealthProfessional/page5 (accessed November 8, 2014).

Tamara Brown, R.N.

Multiple endocrine neoplasia

Definition

The multiple endocrine neoplasia (MEN) is a group of three related disorders in which two or more

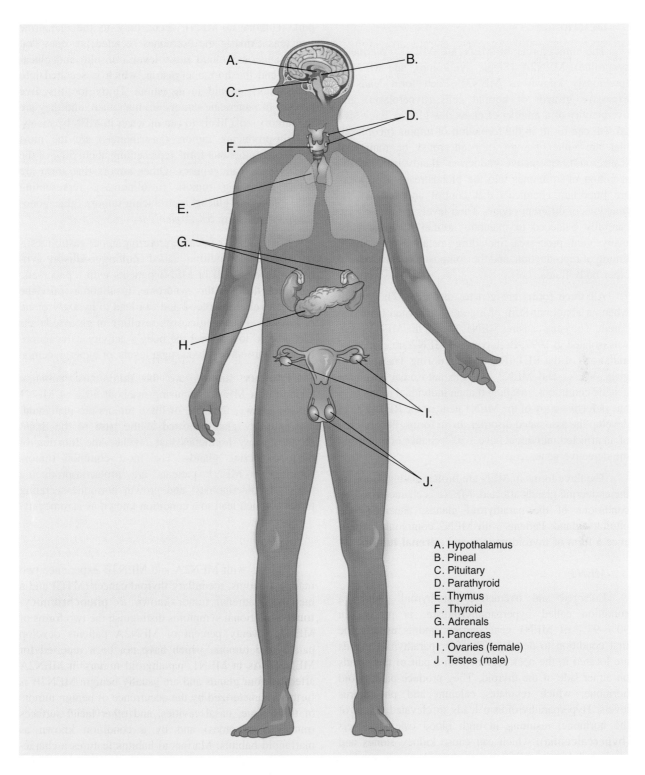

A. Hypothalamus
B. Pineal
C. Pituitary
D. Parathyroid
E. Thymus
F. Thyroid
G. Adrenals
H. Pancreas
I . Ovaries (female)
J . Testes (male)

The human endocrine system: A. Hypothalamus. B. Pineal gland. C. Pituitary gland. D. Parathyroid glands. E. Thymus. F. Thyroid. G. Adrenals. H. Pancreas. I. Ovaries (female). J. Testes (male). *(Illustration by Electronic Illustrators Group. © 2015 Cengage Learning®.)*

of the hormone-secreting (endocrine) glands of the body develop tumors. Commonly affected glands are the thyroid, parathyroids, pituitary, adrenals, and pancreas. Two common cancers are medullary **thyroid cancer** and gastrinomas. MEN is sometimes called familial multiple endocrine neoplasia (FMEN) and previously has been known as familial endocrine adenomatosis.

Description

The three forms of MEN are MEN1 (Wermer's syndrome), MEN2A (Sipple syndrome), and MEN2B (previously known as MEN3). Each form leads to excessive growth of normal cells (hyperplasia) and overactivity of a number of endocrine glands. Excessive growth can result in the formation of tumors (neoplasia) that are either benign (noncancerous) or malignant (cancerous). Overactive endocrine glands increase the secretion of hormones into the bloodstream. Hormones are important chemicals that control and instruct the functions of different organs. Their levels in the body are carefully balanced to maintain normal functioning of many vital processes, including metabolism, growth, timing of reproduction, and the composition of blood and other body fluids.

All three forms are genetic disorders. They result when an abnormal form of a gene is inherited from one parent. The gene causing MEN1, named the MEN1 gene, was isolated in 1997. Both types of MEN2 are caused by mutations of the RET (REarranged during Transfection) gene. MEN1 and MEN2 are both autosomal dominant genetic conditions, meaning that an individual needs only one defective copy of the MEN1 gene or the RET gene to develop the associated disorder. In all forms, the children of an affected individual have a 50% chance of inheriting the defective gene.

The three forms of MEN are further distinguished by the endocrine glands affected. MEN1 is characterized by conditions of the parathyroid glands, pancreas, and pituitary gland. Patients with MEN2 commonly experience a form of thyroid **cancer** and **adrenal tumors**.

MEN1

Enlarged and overactive parathyroid glands, a condition called hyperparathyroidism, is present in 90%–97% of MEN1 gene carriers and is usually the first condition to develop. The four parathyroid glands are located in the neck region, with a pair of the glands on either side of the thyroid. They produce parathyroid hormone, which regulates calcium and phosphorus levels. Hyperparathyroidism leads to elevated levels of the hormone, resulting in high blood calcium levels (**hypercalcemia**), which can cause kidney stones and weakened bones. All four parathyroid glands tend to develop tumors, but most tumors are benign and **parathyroid cancer** is rare. Hyperparathyroidism may be present during the teenage years, but most individuals are affected by age 40.

Pancreatic tumors occur in 40%–75% of individuals with the MEN1 gene. The pancreas, which sits behind the stomach, has two parts, an endocrine part and an exocrine part. Tumors in MEN1 occur only in the endocrine pancreas. Among the hormones secreted are ones that lower and raise blood sugar levels—insulin and glucagons—and the hormone gastrin, which is secreted into the stomach to aid in digestion. Thirty to thirty-five percent of pancreatic tumors are malignant, and they are the tumors most likely to cause cancer in MEN1 patients. Gastrin-producing tumors (gastrinomas) are the most common tumors that form, representing about 50% of the MEN1 pancreatic tumors. Other tumors that form are insulin-producing tumors (insulinomas), representing 25%–30%, and glucagon-producing tumors (glucagonomas), representing 5%–10%.

Gastrinomas can cause recurring upper gastrointestinal ulcers, a condition called **Zollinger-Ellison syndrome**. About half of MEN1 patients with a pancreatic condition develop this syndrome. Insulinomas raise the insulin level in the blood and can lead to hypoglycemia, or low blood sugar (glucose), resulting in glucose levels that are too low to fuel the body's activity. Glucagonomas can cause high blood sugar levels, or hyperglycemia.

Pituitary tumors are the third most common condition in MEN1, occurring in about 50% of MEN1 patients. Fewer than 5% of these tumors are malignant. The pituitary gland, located at the base of the brain, secretes many hormones that regulate the function of other endocrine glands. The most common tumors forming in MEN1 patients are prolactin-producing tumors (prolactinomas) and growth hormone–secreting tumors, which lead to a condition known as acromegaly.

MEN2

Patients with MEN2A and MEN2B experience two main symptoms, medullary thyroid cancer (MTC) and a medullary adrenal tumor known as **pheochromocytoma**. Additional symptoms distinguish the two forms of MEN2. Twenty percent of MEN2A patients develop parathyroid tumors, which have not been reported for MEN2B. As in MEN1, parathyroid tumors in MEN2A affect all four glands and are usually benign. MEN2B is further characterized by the occurrence of benign tumors of the tongue, nasal cavities, and other facial surfaces (mucosal neuromas) and by a condition known as marfanoid habitus. Marfanoid habitus features a characteristic appearance resulting from severe wasting of the proximal muscles. A distinct facial appearance—an elongated face with a thick forehead, wide-eyed look, and broad nose—is often noted at birth. Gastrointestinal, skeletal, and pigmentation abnormalities may also occur. Mucosal neuromas occur in all MEN2B patients, and marfanoid habitus occurs in 65%. About 5% of MEN2 cases are MEN2B.

Association of multiple endocrine neoplasias with other conditions

Form	Associated diseases/conditions
MEN 1 (Wermer's syndrome)	Parathyroid hyperplasia
	Pancreatic islet cell carcinomas, Pituitary hyperplasia
	Thymus, adrenal, carcinoid tumors (less common)
MEN 2A (Sipple syndrome)	Medullary thyroid carcinoma, Pheochromocytoma
	Parathyroid hyperplasia
MEN 2B	Medullary thyroid carcinoma, Pheochromocytoma
	Parathyroid hyperplasia
	Swollen lips
	Tumors of mucous membranes (eyes, mouth, tongue, nasal cavities)
	Enlarged colon
	Skeletal problems such as spinal curving
Familial medullary thyroid carcinoma	Medullary thyroid carcinoma

Table listing diseases and conditions associated with multiple endocrine neoplasias. *(Table by GGS Creative Resources. © Cengage Learning®.)*

Ninety-five percent of MEN2A patients and 90% of MEN2B patients develop medullary thyroid **carcinoma** (MTC). Medullary thyroid carcinoma forms from the C-cells of the thyroid. C-cells make the hormone **calcitonin**, which is involved in regulating the calcium levels in the blood and calcium absorption by the bones. The thyroid, which is located in the front of the neck between the Adam's apple and the collarbone, also secretes hormones that are essential for the regulation of body temperature, heart rate, and metabolism.

Medullary thyroid carcinoma causes high blood levels of calcitonin. In MEN2B, MTC develops earlier and is more aggressive than in MEN2A. It has been described in MEN2B patients younger than one year, whereas in MEN2A patients it is likely to occur between the ages of 20 and 40.

Pheochromocytoma is found in 50% of MEN2A patients and 45% of MEN2B patients. A tumor of the medulla portion of the adrenal gland, it is usually a slow-growing and benign adrenal tumor. The two flat adrenal glands, one situated above each kidney, secrete the hormones epinephrine and norepinephrine to increase heart rate and blood pressure, along with other effects. Excessive secretion of these adrenal hormones can cause life-threatening hypertension and cardiac arrhythmia. Tumors form on both adrenal glands in 50% of MEN2 patients diagnosed with a pheochromocytoma. Tumor malignancy is very rare.

Demographics

MEN syndromes are rare. MEN1 occurs in about three to twenty persons out of 100,000, and MEN2 occurs in about three out of 100,000 people. Both MEN1 and MEN2 show no geographic, racial, or ethnic trend, and men and women have an equal chance of acquiring the MEN syndromes.

Ninety-eight percent of MEN1 gene carriers will develop varying combinations of tumors by age 30, but cancer has not been reported in patients younger than 18. Seventy percent of MEN2A gene carriers will have symptoms by age 70, with most diagnoses occurring between the ages of 30 and 50. MEN2B can occur before one year of age, but most symptoms appear anytime between the ages of 20 and 70.

Causes and symptoms

MEN1

MEN1 is caused by mutations of the MEN1 gene. The MEN1 gene encodes for a previously unknown protein named menin. The role of menin in tumor formation in endocrine glands is not known. But the MEN1 gene is thought to be one of a group of genes known as a tumor suppressor gene. A patient who inherits one defective copy of a tumor suppressor gene from either parent has a strong predisposition to the disease because of the high probability of incurring a second mutation in at least one dividing cell. That cell no longer possesses even one normal copy of the gene. When both copies are defective, tumor suppression fails and tumors develop.

A number of different mutations have been discovered in the MEN1 gene, but people having the same mutation do not always develop the same endocrine conditions. Members within a single family can show different sets of conditions. The symptoms of MEN1 depend on the endocrine condition present:

• Hyperparathyroidism: weakness, fatigue, constipation, kidney stones, loss of appetite (anorexia), and bone and joint pain.

• Gastrinoma: peptic ulcers of the stomach and small intestine, diarrhea, and weight loss.

• Insulinoma: hypoglycemia characterized by weakness, shakiness, fast heartbeat, and difficulty concentrating.

• Glucagonoma: hyperglycemia characterized by inflammation of the tongue or stomach, anemia, weight loss, diarrhea, and blood clots.

• Prolactinoma: secretion of milk in women who are not nursing, headaches, sweating, fatigue, weight gain,

KEY TERMS

Endocrine—A term used to describe the glands that produce hormones in the body.

Exocrine—A term used to describe organs that secrete substances outward through a duct.

Hyperplasia—An overgrowth of normal cells within an organ or tissue.

Medullary thyroid cancer (MTC)—A slow-growing tumor of which about 20% are associated with MEN2.

Neoplasm—An abnormal formation of tissue; for example, a tumor.

Oncogene—A gene with a mutation that causes cell growth and division, leading to the formation of cancerous tumors.

Pheochromocytoma—A tumor of the medullary of the adrenal gland.

RET (REarranged during Transfection) gene—Located on chromosome 10q11.2, mutations in this gene are associated with two very different disorders, the multiple endocrine neoplasia (MEN) syndromes and Hirschsprung disease.

Tumor suppressor gene—A type of gene that instructs cells on the appropriate time to die. A mutation can turn off the gene, resulting in cell growth and tumor formation.

fertility problems in men and women, and visual problems.

• Acromegaly: enlarged hands and feet, enlarged face, thickened oily skin, fatigue, sweating, bone and joint pain, weight gain, and high blood sugar.

MEN2

Both types of MEN2 are caused by mutations of the RET gene. The RET gene is a cancer-causing gene, or an oncogene. A number of different mutations lead to MEN2A, but only one specific genetic alteration leads to MEN2B.

Unlike for MEN1, the likelihood of developing different conditions in MEN2A is associated with specific mutations of the RET gene. Family history can indicate which conditions current family members are likely to develop. The symptoms of MEN2 are those that accompany hyperparathyroidism, MTC, and pheochromocytoma:

• Medullary thyroid cancer: enlargement of thyroid or neck swelling; lumps or nodules in the neck, pain in the neck region going to the ears, persistent cough unrelated to a cold, cough with bleeding, diarrhea or constipation, hoarseness, and difficulty swallowing or breathing.

• Pheochromocytoma: headaches, sweating, chest pains, feelings of anxiety.

The conditions of MEN2B patients show a variety of additional symptoms, including the occurrence of mucosal neuromas and marfanoid habitus, which is characterized by an elongated face, a thick forehead, and poor muscle development.

Diagnosis

The occurrence of one endocrine condition does not immediately lead to a suspicion of MEN syndromes. Diagnoses is based on the occurrence of one or more endocrine conditions and a family history of MEN1 or MEN2.

Since 1994, **genetic testing** using DNA technology has been available for both MEN1 and MEN2. The identification of the MEN1 gene in 1997 has made genetic screening for this gene more accurate.

A blood sample is usually analyzed for DNA testing, although other tissue can be used. The sample is sent to a laboratory that specializes in DNA diagnosis. There a geneticist will perform several tests on the DNA collected from the cells in blood sample. The exact tests performed will depend on whether MEN1 or MEN2 is suspected. Because different regions of the RET gene are associated with different endocrine conditions in MEN2A, several regions of the gene are examined. A positive result means the defective gene is present, and a negative result means the defective gene is not present.

The test results for the RET gene mutations are more reliable than for the MEN1 gene because detection techniques for identifying MEN1 are still being developed. A clinical diagnosis of MEN2 is confirmed with genetic testing 90%–95% of the time. Even when a genetic test is negative, family medical records will be carefully reviewed to confirm the presence of MEN2, and periodic screening of related conditions will likely continue until age 30 or 40. The time required to obtain the test results for MEN2 is about 2–4 weeks, but MEN1 results will likely take longer because there are fewer diagnostic labs set up for MEN1 analysis.

Those considered at risk for MEN1 or MEN2 based on genetic tests or family history are offered preventative surgery, regular screening for associated endocrine conditions, or a combination of these treatment options.

Conditions are screened following the accepted procedure for each condition. Diagnosis is based on clinical features and on testing for elevated hormone levels.

MEN1

Hyperparathyroidism is diagnosed when high levels of calcium and intact parathyroid hormone are measured in a blood sample. Normal values of calcium for adults is 4.4–5.3 mg/dL (milligrams per deciliter), and normal values of parathyroid hormone are 10–55 pg/mL (picograms per milliliter). Prior to the parathyroid test, no food should be eaten for at least six hours. An x-ray of bones may be taken and then examined by a radiologist for signs of low bone density. An x-ray of the abdominal region can reveal kidney stones. Patients should be screened yearly.

Diagnosis of a gastrinoma follows established procedures and includes measuring the levels of gastrin in the blood and the level of stomach gastric acid production. Hypoglycemia associated with insulinomas is diagnosed by measuring blood glucose levels. This test may be administered while a patient is experiencing symptoms related to low insulin levels or during a supervised period of fasting. Depending on the type of test given, no food should be eaten from 6–12 hours prior to the test. Normal glucose levels range between 64–128 mg/dL. Blood glucagon levels above the normal range of 50–100 pg/mL can indicate hyperglycemia, which is associated with glucagonomas. Large pancreatic tumors are identified using **computed tomography** (CT scans) or radionuclide imaging, but **ultrasonography** conducted during surgery is the best method for detecting small tumors. There is no accepted system for staging the pancreatic tumors associated with MEN1.

Prolactinomas, the pituitary tumors most often associated with MEN1, are diagnosed when prolactin levels are greater than 20 ng/l (nanograms per liter). A tumor is identified using **magnetic resonance imaging** (MRI). Tumors secreting excess growth hormone are diagnosed when hormone levels are above the upper normal range of 3 ng/l and from observable changes in physical appearance.

MEN2

Medullary thyroid carcinoma is diagnosed by measuring calcitonin levels in blood and urine samples and from a **biopsy** of any thyroid nodules. Levels of calcitonin above 50 pg/mL can indicate the presence of MTC. Patients showing normal calcitonin levels may require a different test, in which calcitonin is measured at regular intervals after an injection of pentagastrin, a synthetic hormone.

Fine needle aspiration is the biopsy procedure used to diagnose MTC and other forms of thyroid cancer. A sample of cells is removed from a nodule, and the cells are then examined under a microscope by a pathologist to determine if cancer cells are present. MTC has four stages, based on the size of the tumor and where the cancer has spread. **Tumor staging** follows the system established for other forms of thyroid cancer.

A high level of epinephrine relative to norepinephrine indicates a pheochromocytoma on one or both adrenal glands. A CT scan, an MRI, or radionuclide imaging will be performed to locate the tumor.

Diagnosis of hyperparathyroidism in MEN2A patients is identical to its diagnosis for MEN1 patients, but with screening recommended every two to three years.

Treatment team

Conditions of MEN syndromes are first diagnosed by a pathologist who interprets blood and urine samples collected at a doctor's office or a clinic. Depending on the specific condition, a doctor specializing in conditions of the endocrine gland (an endocrinologist) may be consulted. When MEN syndromes are suspected, a genetic counselor will help prepare a patient for the genetic testing procedures and results. A geneticist will perform and interpret genetic tests. Since MEN syndromes often require surgery, the surgical team will likely consist of a surgeon experienced in operating on endocrine glands.

Treatment

No comprehensive treatment is available for genetic disorders such as MEN, but the symptoms of many conditions are treatable. Surgical removal of tumors is the recommended treatment for most conditions, and most MEN patients will require more than one endocrine gland surgery during a lifetime.

An important distinction between an endocrine condition in MEN patients and the same condition in patients not diagnosed with MEN is that endocrine tumors for MEN patients are likely to arise in many locations of a single gland or on multiple glands. Treatment options that work for patients with a single endocrine condition may not be effective in MEN patients. Surgery is often more extensive for MEN patients.

Genetic testing can exclude family members who do not have mutations of the RET or MEN1 gene. The advantage of testing is the early treatment and improved outcomes for those who carry the defective gene and relief from unnecessary anxiety and clinical testing for those not having the defective gene.

MEN1

A common approach to treating MEN1 is with regular screening. Surgical procedures may be delayed until a patient has developed clinical symptoms caused by excess hormone or an easily identifiable tumor.

There are two surgical options for MEN1 patients showing multiple symptoms of hyperparathyroidism or for patients having high blood calcium levels (hypercalcemia), even when no symptoms of the condition are present. All parathyroid tissue is identified and removed and parathyroid tissue is implanted in the forearm, or the surgeon removes three parathyroids and one half of the fourth. After surgery, blood calcium levels are regularly tested to ensure that the remaining parathyroid tissue has not enlarged and caused the condition to return. If hyperparathyroidism recurs, a portion of the remaining tissue is removed until calcium levels return to normal or all the remaining tissue is removed. For MEN1 patients, recurrence is likely within 15 years of the first surgery. Patients with no parathyroid tissue must take daily calcium and vitamin D supplements to prevent hypercalcemia.

There are two views on the best screening strategy for pancreatic tumors in MEN1 patients. One approach is yearly screening, particularly for gastrinomas. This strategy emphasizes the earliest possible detection and surgical removal of tumors. The other approach is screening every 2–3 years, with the reasoning that although tumors are detected at a later stage, they can be better managed with drugs and, if necessary, with surgery.

Surgical removal of insulinomas and glucagonomas, as well as of other less commonly occurring pancreatic tumors in MEN1 patients, is generally the recommended treatment because these tumors are difficult to treat with medication.

The best treatment option for gastrinomas is complex because in MEN1 patients there can be multiple gastrinomas of varying sizes on the pancreas and upper portion of the small intestine (duodenum), and they have a tendency to recur. Most doctors support the use of medication to control the condition and do not recommend surgical intervention. Common treatment of symptoms is the use of drugs that block acid production, called acid pump inhibitors. Others recommend surgery that includes removal of the duodenum and a section of the pancreas and cutting nerves to the section of the stomach involved in acid secretion. Surgery is supported as a way to reduce the risk for **metastasis**. In some cases,

gastrin levels and gastric acid levels returned to normal, and MEN1 patients experienced no symptoms after the surgery. A treatment no longer recommended is removal of the entire stomach. Malignant gastrinomas cause death in 10%–20% of MEN1 patients with this condition, and 30%–50% will eventually spread to the liver.

Treatment of pituitary tumors in MEN1 patients rarely involves surgery. For prolactinomas, medications are effective in returning prolactin levels to normal and preventing tumor growth.

MEN2

Medullary thyroid carcinoma is the primary concern for those testing positive for the RET gene mutations. Since genetic testing became available for MEN2, two approaches have emerged to manage this cancer. Some recommend removing the entire thyroid gland (thyroidectomy) before any symptoms occur, although doctors disagree at what age to perform this surgery. This strategy emerged owing to a number of cases in which thyroids removed from identified MEN2 patients showing no clinical signs of MTC were found to be cancerous. Preventative thyroid surgery is offered to those with RET gene mutations beginning at age 5. Some recommend surgery after age 10, unless calcitonin tests are positive earlier. They contend that surgery before age 10 may increase the chance of damaging the larynx or the parathyroids.

The second approach is yearly blood calcitonin testing beginning in early childhood. A thyroidectomy is performed after the first abnormal calcitonin test. There is only a 10% chance of recurrence 15–20 years after surgery for those identified using this method. The advantage of this method is to delay surgery until it is necessary. The disadvantages are the cost and discomfort of yearly testing. Also, the first detection of elevated levels of calcitonin in the blood may occur after the cancer has already reached an advanced stage.

A thyroidectomy is the standard treatment for all stages of MTC. If MTC is diagnosed in an advanced stage, the spread of the cancer may have already occurred. Metastasis is very serious in MTC because **chemotherapy** and **radiation therapy** are not effective in controlling metastasis. Further tests are likely to include a CT scan and an MRI.

All MTC patients must take thyroid hormone medication for the rest of their lives in order to maintain normal body functions. Follow-up treatment to assure that the cancer has not recurred includes monitoring the levels of calcitonin in the blood. The survival rate ten years after the initial diagnosis is 46%. If the cancer is detected using genetic screening before the patient shows signs of having the disease, surgical removal of the thyroid gland can cure MTC.

Pheochromocytoma may occur after the MTC diagnosis by as much as 20 years. Pheochromocytoma in MEN2 can be cured by surgical removal of the affected adrenal gland. If a pheochromocytoma occurs on only one gland, there is some debate on whether to remove both adrenal glands or only the affected gland. Fifty percent of MEN2 patients who underwent removal of one adrenal gland developed a pheochromocytoma in the other gland within ten years. Because malignancy is rare, most doctors recommend removing the affected glands first and then monitoring hormone levels to see if a second tumor occurs. If both glands are removed, hormone replacement therapy is required.

Alternative and complementary therapies

There are no alternative treatments specifically targeted for people with MEN syndromes, although cow and shark cartilage treatments are being investigated as a way to decrease tumor growth in some cancers. These treatments are administered orally, by injection, or as an enema, but studies of the effectiveness of this treatment for humans are inconclusive.

Coping with cancer treatment

The surgery that most MEN syndromes patients will face can cause anxiety and fear. Patients should discuss their concerns about an operation with their personal physician, the surgeon, nurses, and other medical personnel. Getting specific answers to questions can provide a clear idea of what to expect immediately after the surgery as well as any long-term changes in quality of life.

Clinical trials

Clinical studies of MEN syndromes focus on understanding the genes involved in the inheritance of MEN1 and MEN2 and on the unique treatment needs for the endocrine gland conditions occurring in MEN patients. Information on clinical trials is available online at http://www.clinicaltrials.gov.

Prevention

There is no preventive measure to block the occurrence of the genetic mutations that cause MEN syndromes. Medullary thyroid carcinoma, one of the most serious conditions of MEN2, can be prevented by thyroidectomy.

QUESTIONS TO ASK YOUR DOCTOR

- Are the tumors associated with this condition cancerous?
- Can one endocrine tumor spread to other endocrine glands?
- What are the long-lasting effects of this disorder?
- What are the long-lasting effects of treatment?
- After treatment, what are the chances that a condition will recur?
- Are there alternative treatments to surgery?
- Will I need to take hormone supplements, if so, for how long?
- Will this disorder affect my ability to have children?
- What is the current status of predictive gene testing?
- Who in my family should be tested for this disorder?

Special concerns

It is important to seek professional genetic counseling before proceeding with genetic testing, particularly for children. Adults may have to make treatment decisions for children.

Genetic tests are often expensive. Whether or not **health insurance** will cover the costs of counseling and testing will depend on individual policies. Some insurance companies cover the costs only when a patient shows symptoms of a condition. Genetic tests raise issues of privacy. Most states in the United States have legislation that restricts the use of genetic test results by insurance companies and employers.

See also Cancer genetics; Familial cancer syndromes; Pancreatic cancer, endocrine; Thyroid cancer.

Resources

BOOKS

Sperling, Mark A., ed. *Pediatric Endocrinology*. 3rd ed. Philadelphia: Saunders/Elsevier, 2008.

PERIODICALS

Callender, GG., Rich, TA., Perrier, ND. "Multiple Endocrine Neoplasia Syndromes." *The Surgical Clinics of North America* 88, no. 4 (2008): 863–95. http://www.ncbi.nlm. nih.gov/pubmed/18672144 (accessed November 8, 2014).

WEBSITES

U.S. National Library of Medicine. "Multiple Endocrine Neoplasia." Genetics Home Reference. http://ghr.nlm.nih.gov/condition/multiple-endocrine-neoplasia (accessed November 8, 2014).

ORGANIZATIONS

Genetic Alliance, Inc., 4301 Connecticut Ave. NW, Ste. 404, Washington, DC 20008-2369, (202) 966-5557, info@geneticalliance.org, http://www.geneticalliance.org.

G. Victor Leipzig
Monica McGee, M.S.

Multiple myeloma

Definition

Multiple **myeloma** is a type of **cancer** caused by uncontrolled growth of abnormal plasma cells that form tumors. Plasma cells normally make antibodies that help the body fight infection.

Description

Multiple myeloma is an uncommon cancer of the blood, accounting for approximately 1% of all cancers. Multiple myeloma is a disease in which malignant plasma cells spread through the bone marrow and the hard outer portions of the large bones of the body. These myeloma cells may form tumors called plasmacytomas. Eventually, multiple soft spots called osteolytic lesions form in the bones.

Bone marrow is the spongy tissue within the bones. The breastbone, spine, ribs, skull, pelvic bones, and the long bone of the thigh all are particularly rich in marrow. Bone marrow is a very active tissue that is responsible for producing the cells that circulate in the blood. These include the red blood cells that carry oxygen, the white blood cells that develop into immune system cells, and platelets, which cause blood to clot.

Plasma cells and immunoglobulins

Plasma cells develop from B lymphocytes or B cells, a type of white blood cell. B cells, like all blood cells, develop from stem cells in the bone marrow. Each B cell carries a specific antibody that recognizes a specific foreign substance called an antigen. Antibodies are large proteins called immunoglobulins (Igs), which recognize and destroy foreign substances and organisms such as bacteria. When a B cell encounters its antigen, it begins

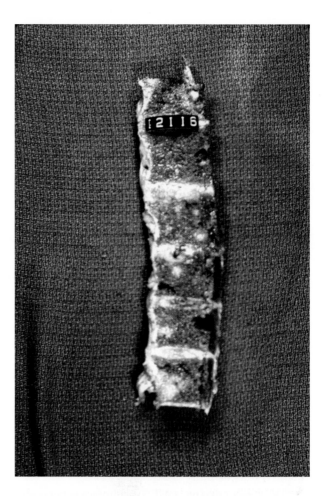

Portion of spine from patient with multiple myeloma. In this disease, malignant plasma cells spread through the bone marrow and hard outer portions of the body's large bones. As malignant plasma cells increase in the bone marrow and replace normal marrow, they exert pressure on the bone. Bones become soft and may fracture; spinal bones may collapse. *(O.J. Staats MD/Custom Medical Stock Photo)*

to divide rapidly to form mature plasma cells. These plasma cells are all identical (monoclonal). They produce large amounts of identical antibody that are specific for the antigen.

Malignant plasma cells

Multiple myeloma begins when the genetic material (DNA) is damaged during the development of a stem cell into a B cell in the bone marrow. This causes the cell to develop into an abnormal or malignant plasmablast, an early form of plasma cell. Plasmablasts produce adhesive molecules that allow them to bond to the inside of the bone marrow. A growth factor, called interleukin–6, promotes uncontrolled growth of these myeloma cells in the bone marrow and prevents their natural death. Whereas normal bone marrow contains less than 5%

Amyloidosis—A complication of multiple myeloma in which amyloid protein accumulates in the kidneys and other organs, tissues, and blood vessels.

Anemia—Any condition in which the red blood cell count is below normal.

Antibody—Immunoglobulin produced by immune system cells that recognizes and binds to a specific foreign substance (antigen).

Antigen—Foreign substance that is recognized by a specific antibody.

B cell (B lymphocyte)—Type of white blood cell that produces antibodies.

Bence-Jones protein—Light chain of an immunoglobulin that is overproduced in multiple myeloma and is excreted in the urine.

Beta 2-microglobulin—Protein produced by B cells; high concentrations in the blood are indicative of multiple myeloma.

Cryoglobulinemia—Condition triggered by low temperatures in which protein in the blood forms particles, blocking blood vessels and leading to pain and numbness of the extremities.

Electrophoresis—Use of an electrical field to separate proteins in a mixture (such as blood or urine), on the basis of the size and electrical charge of the proteins.

Hemoglobin—Protein in red blood cells that carries oxygen.

Hypercalcemia—Abnormally high levels of calcium in the blood.

Hyperviscosity—Thick, viscous blood, caused by the accumulation of large proteins, such as immunoglobulins, in the serum.

Immunoglobulin (Ig)—Antibody; large protein produced by B cells that recognizes and binds to a specific antigen.

M-protein—Monoclonal or myeloma protein; paraprotein; abnormal antibody found in large amounts in the blood and urine of individuals with multiple myeloma.

Malignant—A characteristic of cancer cells that grow uncontrollably and invade other tissues.

Monoclonal—Identical cells or proteins; cells (clones) derived from a single, genetically distinct cell, or proteins produced by these cells.

Monoclonal gammopathy of undetermined significance (MGUS)—Common condition in which M-protein is present, but there are no tumors or other symptoms of disease.

Neoplasm—Tumor made up of cells with no function, usually cancerous cells.

Osteoblast—Bone-forming cell.

Osteoclast—Cell that absorbs bone.

Osteolytic lesion—Soft spot or hole in bone caused by cancer cells.

Osteoporosis—Condition in which the bones become weak and porous, due to loss of calcium and destruction of cells.

Paraprotein—M-protein; abnormal immunoglobulin produced in multiple myeloma.

Plasma—The liquid part of blood.

Plasma cell—A type of white blood cell developed from B lymphocytes that produces antibodies.

Platelet—Blood cell that is involved in blood clotting.

Stem cell—Undifferentiated cell that retains the ability to develop into any one of numerous cell types.

---

plasma cells, bone marrow of a person with multiple myeloma contains more than 10% plasma cells.

In most cases of multiple myeloma, the malignant plasma cells all make an identical Ig. Immunoglobulins are made up of four protein chains that are bonded together. Two of the chains are light and two are heavy. There are five classes of heavy chains, corresponding to five types of Igs with different immune system functions. The Igs from myeloma cells are nonfunctional and are called paraproteins. All of the paraproteins from any one individual are monoclonal (identical) because the myeloma cells are identical clones of a single plasma cell. Thus, the paraprotein is a monoclonal protein or M-protein. The M-proteins crowd out the functional Igs and other components of the immune system. They also cause functional antibodies, which are produced by normal plasma cells, to rapidly break down. Thus, multiple myeloma depresses the immune system.

In about 75% of multiple myeloma cases, the malignant plasma cells also produce monoclonal light chains, or incomplete Igs. These are called Bence–Jones proteins and are secreted in the urine. About 1% of multiple myelomas are called nonsecretors because they do not produce any abnormal Ig.

Osteolytic lesions

About 70% of people who have multiple myeloma have soft spots or lesions in their bones. These lesions can vary from quite small to grapefruit size. In part, these lesions occur because the malignant plasma cells rapidly outgrow the normal bone–forming cells. In addition, malignant myeloma cells produce factors that affect cells called osteoclasts. These are the cells that normally destroy old bone, so that new bone can be produced by cells called osteoblasts. The myeloma cell factors increase both the activation and the growth of osteoclasts. As the osteoclasts multiply and migrate, they destroy healthy bone and create lesions. Osteoporosis, or widespread bone weakness, may develop.

Demographics

The American Cancer Society predicted that 24,000 new cases of multiple myeloma would be diagnosed by the end of 2014, with 11,000 deaths. The disease occurs slightly more in men than in women.

In Western industrialized countries, approximately four people in 100,000 develop multiple myeloma. The incidence of multiple myeloma among African Americans is 9.5 per 100,000, about twice that of Caucasians. Asians have a much lower incidence of the disease. In China, for example, the incidence of multiple myeloma is only one in 100,000. The offspring and siblings of individuals with multiple myeloma are at a slightly increased risk for the disease.

At diagnosis, the average age of a multiple myeloma patient is 68 to 70. Although the average age at onset is decreasing, most multiple myelomas still occur in people over 40.

Causes and symptoms

Causes

The cause of multiple myeloma has not been determined, but researchers have learned more about how changes in a person's DNA can lead to plasma cell cancer. Certain oncogenes, which are genes that can cause a cell to become cancerous, have been identified that may be associated with multiple myeloma. When these oncogenes have abnormalities, they can cause myeloma cells to form. Researchers have also identified changes in certain tumor suppressor genes that might lead to multiple myeloma. Tumor suppressor genes normally slow or stop cancerous cell division, but if the gene has an abnormality, it fails to stop cancer cell growth. Ongoing research continues to examine what parts of a missing chromosome might make myeloma more aggressive in some patients, and what role a process called translocation—which involves switching of chromosomes in the body—might play in the development of myeloma.

RELATED DISORDERS. Monoclonal gammopathy of undetermined significance (MGUS) is a common condition in which a monoclonal Ig is detectable. However, there are no tumors or other symptoms of multiple myeloma. MGUS occurs in about 1% of the general population and in about 3% of those over age 70. Over a period of years, about 16%–20% of those with MGUS will develop multiple myeloma or a related cancer called malignant **lymphoma**.

Occasionally, only a single plasmacytoma develops, either in the bone marrow (isolated plasmacytoma of the bone) or other tissues or organs (extramedullary plasmacytoma). Some individuals with solitary plasmacytoma may develop multiple myeloma.

Symptoms

The accumulation of malignant plasma cells can result in tiny cracks or fractures in bones. Malignant plasma cells in the bone marrow can suppress the formation of red and white blood cells and platelets. About 80% of people who have multiple myeloma are anemic due to low red blood cell formation. Low white blood cell formation results in increased susceptibility to infection, since new, functional antibodies are not produced. In addition, normal circulating antibodies are rapidly destroyed. Low platelet formation can result in poor blood clotting. It is rare, however, that people go to their doctors with these symptoms as indicators of multiple myeloma.

EARLY SYMPTOMS. The following are early symptoms of multiple myeloma:

- pain in the lower back or ribs
- fatigue and paleness due to anemia (low red blood cell count)
- frequent and recurring infections, including bacterial pneumonia, urinary–tract and kidney infections, and shingles (herpes zoster)
- excessive bleeding

BONE DESTRUCTION. Bone pain, particularly in the backbone, hips, and skull, is often the first symptom of multiple myeloma. As malignant plasma cells increase in the bone marrow, replacing normal marrow, they exert pressure on the bone. As overly active osteoclasts (large cells responsible for the breakdown of bone) remove bone tissue, the bone becomes soft. Fracture and **spinal cord compression** can occur.

Plasmacytomas (malignant tumors of plasma cells) may weaken bones, causing fractures. Fractured bones or weak or collapsed spinal bones, in turn, can place unusual pressure on nearby nerves, resulting in nerve pain, burning, or numbness and muscle weakness. Proteins produced by myeloma cells also may damage nerves.

Calcium from the destroyed bone enters the blood and urine, causing **hypercalcemia**, a medical condition in which abnormally high concentrations of calcium compounds exist in the bloodstream. High calcium affects nerve cell and kidney function. The symptoms of hypercalcemia include:

• weakness and fatigue
• depression
• mental confusion
• constipation
• increased thirst
• increased urination
• nausea and vomiting
• kidney pain
• kidney failure

Hypercalcemia affects about one-third of multiple myeloma patients.

SERUM PROTEINS. The accumulation of M-proteins in the serum (the liquid portion of the blood minus certain proteins) may cause additional complications such as hyperviscosity syndrome, or thickening of the blood, though it is rare in multiple myeloma patients. Symptoms of hyperviscosity include:

• fatigue
• headaches
• shortness of breath
• mental confusion
• chest pain
• kidney damage and failure
• vision problems
• Raynaud's disease

Raynaud's phenomenon can affect any part of the body, but particularly the fingers, toes, nose, and ears.

Cryoglobulinemia occurs when the protein in the blood forms particles under cold conditions. These particles can block small blood vessels and cause pain and numbness in the toes, fingers, and other extremities during cold weather.

Amyloidosis is a rare complication of multiple myeloma. It usually occurs in individuals whose plasma cells produce only Ig light chains. These Bence–Jones proteins combine with other serum proteins to form amyloid protein. This starchy substance can invade tissues, organs, and blood vessels. In particular, amyloid proteins can accumulate in the kidneys, where they block the tiny tubules that are the kidney's filtering system. Indicators of amyloidosis include:

• carpal tunnel syndrome
• kidney failure
• liver failure
• heart failure

Diagnosis

Blood and urine tests

Often, the initial diagnosis of multiple myeloma is made from routine blood tests that are performed for other reasons. Blood tests may indicate:

• anemia
• abnormal red blood cells
• high serum protein levels
• high levels of beta-2 microglobulin
• low levels of normal antibody
• high calcium levels
• high blood urea nitrogen (BUN) levels
• high creatinine levels

Urea and creatinine normally are excreted in the urine. High levels of urea and creatinine in the blood indicate that the kidneys are not functioning properly to eliminate these substances.

Protein electrophoresis is a laboratory technique that uses an electrical current to separate the different proteins in the blood and urine based on size and charge. Since all of the multiple myeloma M–proteins in the blood and urine are identical, electrophoresis of blood and urine from a patient with multiple myeloma shows a large M–protein spike, corresponding to the high concentration of monoclonal Ig. Electrophoresis of the urine also can detect Bence–Jones proteins.

Bones

In a **bone marrow aspiration**, a doctor uses a very thin, long needle to remove a sample of marrow from the hip bone. Alternatively, a **bone marrow biopsy** with a larger needle removes solid marrow tissue. The marrow is examined under a microscope for plasma cells and tumors. If 10%–30% of the cells are plasma cells, multiple myeloma is the usual diagnosis.

X-rays are used to detect osteoporosis, osteolytic lesions, and fractures. **Computed tomography** (CAT

International staging system for multiple myeloma

Stage	Criteria	Median length of patient survival, in months
I	Beta-2-microglobulin levels < 3.5 mg/L and albumin levels ≥ 3.5 g/dL	62
II	Beta-2-microglobulin levels < 3.5 mg/L and albumin levels < 3.5 g/dL OR Beta-2-microglobulin levels 3.5–5.5 mg/L	44
III	Beta-2-microglobulin levels ≥ 5.5 mg/L	29

dL = deciliter
g = grams
L = liter
mg = milligrams

SOURCE: National Cancer Institute, "Table 2. The International Staging System for Multiple Myeloma," *Plasma Cell Neoplasms (Including Multiple Myeloma) Treatment (PDQ®)*. Available online at: http://www.cancer.gov/cancertopics/pdq/treatment/myeloma/HealthProfessional/Table2.

The international staging system for multiple myeloma.
(Table by Lumina Datamatics Ltd. © 2015 Cengage Learning®.)

or CT) scans can detect lesions in both bone and soft tissue. **Magnetic resonance imaging** (MRI) may give a more detailed image of a certain bone or a region of the body.

Cell testing

New tests can examine the cells obtained during a **biopsy** to look for signs of cancer and identify specific types of cancer cells. For example, **flow cytometry** analyzes the surface of sample cells to identify the type of cell and specific materials on the cells by passing them under a laser beam after treating them with an antibody. Other techniques check for abnormalities in a patient's chromosomes. These include cytogenetic testing and fluorescent in situ hybridization (FISH).

Treatment team

After the initial diagnosis, the treatment team for multiple myeloma can include a hematologist (a specialist in diseases of the blood) and an oncologist (cancer specialist), although often these may be the same person. If radiation is used in treatment, a radiation oncologist may join the team. The treatment of multiple myeloma involves complex decisions, and obtaining second opinions from additional specialists may be important.

Clinical staging

Staging of cancer is a method used by doctors to classify the extent of the cancer so that doctors can plan treatment and help predict the outlook, or prognosis, for a patient. By using uniform staging, doctors can also better compare treatment success and conduct **clinical trials** to improve treatment for patients with various cancers.

Multiple myeloma staging is based on the levels of beta–2 microglobulin and albumin in a patient's blood. Beta– 2 microglobulin is a protein in plasma cells, and albumin is a substance that makes up a large part of plasma. Patients who have multiple myeloma usually have more beta–2 microglobulin than normal and less albumin than normal. There are three stages of multiple myeloma. As the stage number gets higher, measured beta–2 microglobulin levels increase and albumin levels decrease.

Treatment

Since multiple myeloma often progresses slowly, and since the treatments can be toxic, the disease is sometimes not treated until patients have symptoms and laboratory tests indicate a need to address the disease. In particular, MGUS might be followed closely but not treated. Solitary plasmacytomas are treated with radiation and/or surgery and followed closely with examinations and laboratory tests.

Patients often receive treatment in three phases. The first phase is induction therapy, which is used to reduce the disease. **Chemotherapy**, steroid therapy, and targeted therapy are part of the induction treatment. The second phase is called consolidation therapy, which is meant to kill remaining cancer cells. Patients usually receive high doses of chemotherapy and a stem cell transplant. In the maintenance therapy phase, treatment is designed to keep multiple myeloma in remission.

Chemotherapy

Chemotherapy, or treatment with anti-cancer drugs, is used for multiple myeloma. A combination of drugs works better than any single drug. **Melphalan** and prednisone, the combination of an anticancer drug and a steroid, has been a standard treatment for many years. Several other drugs are used for patients who have multiple myeloma, depending on their specific stage and health.

Multiple myeloma can recur, or come back, after the end of chemotherapy. Although the chemotherapy can be repeated after each recurrence, the disease is progressively less responsive to treatment.

Side effects of chemotherapy may include:

- anemia
- hair loss (alopecia)
- nausea and vomiting
- diarrhea
- mood swings
- swelling
- acne

These side effects disappear after treatment is discontinued.

Biologic therapy

Biologic therapy, also called **immunotherapy**, uses substances made from living organisms. For multiple myeloma, this often means the use of interferon, which is a substance similar to hormones. Interferon can keep some patients in remission longer.

Targeted therapy

As researchers and doctors learn more about the cells and chromosomes responsible for cancers like multiple myeloma, they can design treatments targeted to destroy certain cancer cells in a patient's body. Chemotherapy usually destroys all rapidly dividing cells, but targeted therapy can destroy only particular cells, causing fewer side effects. Targeted therapy often is given in clinical trials.

Other drug treatments

Bisphosphonates are drugs that inhibit the activity of osteoclasts. These drugs can slow the progression of bone disease, reduce pain, and help prevent bone fractures. Different types of bisphosphonates inhibit osteoclasts in different ways. They also reduce the production of interleukin–6 by bone marrow cells. Laboratory studies suggest that bisphosphonates may kill or inhibit the growth of multiple myeloma cells. Pamidronate is the most common bisphosphonate for treating multiple myeloma.

Bone and peripheral blood stem cell transplantation

Bone marrow or peripheral blood stem cell transplantations (PBSCT) are used to replace the stem cells of the bone marrow following high–dose chemotherapy. Chemotherapy destroys the bone marrow stem cells that are necessary to produce new blood cells. In an autologous transplant, the patient's bone marrow stem cells or peripheral blood stem cells (immature bone marrow cells found in the blood) are collected, treated with drugs to kill any myeloma cells, and frozen prior to chemotherapy. Growth factors are used to increase the number of peripheral stem cells prior to collection. A procedure called apheresis is used to collect the peripheral stem cells. Following high–dose chemotherapy, the stem cells are reinserted into the individual. In an allogeneic transplant, the donor stem cells come from a genetically related individual such as a sibling.

Other treatments

Blood transfusions may be required to treat severe **anemia**.

Plasmapheresis, or plasma exchange transfusion, may be used to thin the blood to treat hyperviscosity syndrome. In this treatment, blood is removed and passed through a machine that separates the plasma, containing the M-protein, from the red and white blood cells and platelets. The blood cells are transfused back into the patient, along with a plasma substitute or donated plasma.

Multiple myeloma may be treated with high–energy x-rays directed at a specific region of the body. **Radiation therapy** is used for treating bone pain.

Once multiple myeloma is in remission, calcium and vitamin D supplements can improve bone density. It is important not to take these supplements when the myeloma is active. Individuals with multiple myeloma must drink large amounts of fluid to counter the effects of hyperviscous blood.

Prognosis

The prognosis for individuals with MGUS or solitary plasmacytoma is very good. Most do not develop multiple myeloma; however, approximately 15% of all patients with multiple myeloma die within three months of diagnosis. About 60% respond to treatment and live for an average of two and a half to three years following diagnosis. Approximately 23% of patients die of other illnesses associated with advanced age.

The prognosis for a given individual may be based on the prognostic indicators described above. Doctors track survival by stage, and survival improves with lower stages of multiple myeloma. In general, survival with treatment has improved in recent decades and ranges from nearly three years to slightly more than five years.

With treatment, multiple myeloma may go into complete remission. This is defined as:

- M–protein absent from the blood and urine
- myeloma cells not detectable in the bone marrow
- no clinical symptoms
- negative laboratory tests

With very sensitive testing, a few myeloma cells are usually detectable and eventually lead to a recurrence of the disease, in the bone or elsewhere in the body. One reason for recurrence is **drug resistance**, or the ability of cancer cells to ignore and survive the toxic effects of chemotherapy drugs. In 2013 a group of researchers identified a gene in multiple myeloma patients that was associated with drug resistance and poor outcome in multiple myeloma. They found that by blocking the gene, called NEK2, patients survived longer.

Coping with cancer treatment

Techniques such as biofeedback, guided imagery, and meditation may be helpful for reducing stress and relieving pain. Pain medication is usually prescribed for multiple myeloma. Back or neck braces may help relieve bone pain. Exercise, if possible, is important for retaining calcium in the bones.

Clinical trials

There are hundreds of ongoing clinical trials for the treatment of multiple myeloma. These take place throughout the United States and are sponsored by both government and industry. Clinical trials of treatments for multiple myeloma include:

- use of lenalidomide or observation for patients who have no symptoms and have high–risk smoldering multiple myeloma
- skeletal targeted radiotherapy (STP), in which a radioactive element is attached to a drug that binds to bone
- new anti–cancer drugs
- new combinations of drugs
- preventing graft–versus–host disease in patients who have peripheral blood stem cell transplants
- drugs for relapsed or refractory multiple myeloma

Prevention

There are no clearly established risk factors for multiple myeloma that people can control. It is possible that a combination of factors interact to cause the disease. Thus, there is no method for preventing multiple myeloma.

Special concerns

Since there is a high probability that multiple myeloma will recur after treatment, patients are followed carefully. Blood tests, x-rays, and other **imaging studies** may be used to check for a recurrence.

See also Bone marrow transplantation; Immuno-electrophoresis; Pheresis.

Resources

BOOKS

Holland, Jimmie C., and Sheldon Lewis. *The Human Side of Cancer: Living with Hope, Coping with Uncertainty.* New York: HarperCollins, 2000.

WEBSITES

American Cancer Society "Multiple Myeloma." http://www.cancer.org/cancer/multiplemyeloma/detailedguide/index (accessed August 4, 2014).

Brown, Jennifer. "Team Finds Gene that Promotes Drug Resistance in Cancer." Iowa*Now*, The University of Iowa, January 14, 2013. http://now.uiowa.edu/2013/01/team-finds-gene-promotes-drug-resistance-cancer (accessed October 23, 2014).

Leukemia & Lymphoma Society. "Myeloma." http://www.lls.org/#/diseaseinformation/myeloma/ (accessed October 23, 2014).

Multiple Myeloma Research Foundation. "About Multiple Myeloma." http://www.themmrf.org/multiple-myeloma/ (accessed October 23, 2014).

National Cancer Institute. "Plasma Cell Neoplasms (Including Multiple Myeloma) Treatment (PDQ®)." http://www.cancer.gov/cancertopics/pdq/treatment/myeloma/Patient (accessed October 23, 2014).

ORGANIZATIONS

International Myeloma Foundation, 12650 Riverside Dr., Ste. 206, North Hollywood, CA 91607, (818) 487-7455, (800) 452-CURE (2873), TheIMF@myeloma.org, http://myeloma.org.

Leukemia & Lymphoma Society, 1311 Mamaroneck Ave., Ste. 310, White Plains, NY 10605, (914) 949-5213, Fax: (914) 949-6691, infocenter@lls.org, http://www.lls.org.

Multiple Myeloma Research Foundation, 383 Main Ave., 5th Fl., Norwalk, CT 06851, (203) 229-0464, info@themmrf.org, http://www.themmrf.org.

Margaret Alic, PhD
REVISED BY TERESA G. ODLE

Mustargen *see* **Mechlorethamine**

Mutamycin *see* **Mitomycin-C**

Myasthenia gravis

Definition

Myasthenia gravis (MG) is an autoimmune disease that causes muscle weakness.

Description

MG affects the neuromuscular junction, interrupting the communication between nerve and muscle, and thereby causing weakness. People with MG may have difficulty moving their eyes, walking, speaking clearly, swallowing, and even breathing, depending on the severity and distribution of weakness. Increased weakness with exertion, and improvement with rest, is a characteristic feature of MG.

MG has been associated with malignant **thymoma**, a disease in which **cancer** cells are found in the tissues of the thymus.

Demographics

About 30,000 people in the United States are affected by MG. It can occur at any age, but is most common in women who are in their late teens and early twenties, and in men in their sixties and seventies.

Causes and symptoms

Myasthenia gravis is an autoimmune disease, meaning that it is caused by the body's own immune system. In MG, the immune system attacks a receptor on the surface of muscle cells. This prevents the muscle from receiving the nerve impulses that normally make it respond. MG affects "voluntary" muscles, which are those muscles under conscious control responsible for movement. It does not affect heart muscle or the "smooth" muscle found in the digestive system and other internal organs.

A muscle is stimulated to contract when the nerve cell controlling it releases acetylcholine molecules onto its surface. The acetylcholine lands on a muscle protein called the acetylcholine receptor. This leads to rapid chemical changes in the muscle which cause it to contract. Acetylcholine is then broken down by acetylcholinesterase enzyme, to prevent further stimulation.

In MG, immune cells create antibodies against the acetylcholine receptor. Antibodies are proteins normally involved in fighting infection. When these antibodies attach to the receptor, they prevent it from receiving acetylcholine, decreasing the ability of the muscle to respond to stimulation.

Why the immune system creates these self-reactive "autoantibodies" is unknown, although there are several hypotheses:

- During fetal development, the immune system generates many B cells that can make autoantibodies, but B cells that could harm the body's own tissues are screened out and destroyed before birth. It is possible that the stage is set for MG when some of these cells escape detection.

- Genes controlling other parts of the immune system, called MHC genes, appear to influence how susceptible a person is to developing autoimmune disease.

- Infection may trigger some cases of MG. When activated, the immune system may mistake portions of the acetylcholine receptor for portions of an invading virus, though no candidate virus has yet been identified conclusively.

- About 10% of those with MG also have thymomas, or tumors of the thymus gland. The thymus is a principal organ of the immune system, and researchers speculate that thymic irregularities are involved in the progression of MG. A definite relationship exists between MG and thymoma: of patients with MG, 15% also have thymoma, and of patients with thymoma, 50% have MG.

Treatment

While there is no cure for myasthenia gravis, there are a number of treatments that effectively control symptoms in most people. Even though no rigorously tested treatment trials have been reported and no clear consensus exists on treatment strategies, MG is one of the most treatable immune disorders. Several factors require consideration before initiating treatment, such as the severity, distribution, and rapidity of the MG progression.

Edrophonium (Tensilon) is a drug used to block the action of acetylcholinesterase, prolonging the effect of acetylcholine and increasing strength. An injection of edrophonium rapidly leads to a marked improvement in most people with MG. An alternate drug, neostigmine, may also be used.

Pyridostigmine (Mestinon) is usually the first drug tried. Like edrophonium, pyridostigmine blocks acetylcholinesterase. It is longer-acting, taken by mouth, and well-tolerated. Loss of responsiveness and disease progression combine to eventually make pyridostigmine ineffective in tolerable doses in many patients.

Thymectomy, or removal of the thymus gland, has increasingly become a standard form of treatment for MG. Up to 85% of people with MG improve after thymectomy, with complete remission eventually seen in about 30%. The improvement may take months or even several years to fully develop. Thymectomy is not usually recommended for children with MG, since the thymus continues to play an important immune role throughout childhood.

Immune-suppressing drugs are used to treat MG if patient response to pyridostigmine and thymectomy is not adequate. These drugs include **corticosteroids** such as prednisone, and the non-steroids **azathioprine** (Imuran) and **cyclosporine** (Sandimmune).

Plasma exchange may also be performed to treat the condition or to strengthen very weak patients before thymectomy. In this procedure, blood plasma is removed and replaced with purified plasma free of autoantibodies. It can produce a temporary improvement in symptoms, but is too expensive for long-term treatment. Another blood treatment, intravenous immunoglobulin therapy, is also used. In this procedure, large quantities of purified immune proteins (immunoglobulins) are injected. For unknown reasons, this leads to symptomatic improvement in up to 85% of patients. It is also too expensive for long-term treatment. There are indications that IVIg is an effective immunoglobulin for some categories of MG patients.

People with weakness of the bulbar muscles may need to eat softer foods that are easier to chew and swallow. In more severe cases, it may be necessary to obtain nutrition through a feeding tube placed into the stomach (gastrostomy tube).

Alternative and complementary therapies

No alternative therapies have been shown to be effective for the treatment of MG. Reports claiming that herbal remedies or alternative treatments alleviate or cure MG have not been corroborated by properly controlled **clinical trials**, which are required to evaluate the benefit of such treatments.

Among complementary MG therapies, prescription of low dose atropine can help relieve the cramping and **diarrhea** often caused by the drug Mestinon. Propantheline bromide (ProBanthine) is a drug similar to atropine, and it may also be prescribed to treat gastrointestinal discomfort. Caution must be taken not to take too much atropine because it cancels the beneficial effects of the anticholinesterase drugs. Ephedrine is sometimes also used with anticholinesterase therapy to strengthen the muscle tissue of MG patients.

Resources

BOOKS

Lisak, Robert P., ed. *Handbook of Myasthenia Gravis and Myasthenic Syndromes*. New York: M. Dekker, 1994.

WEBSITES

A.D.A.M. Medical Encyclopedia. "Myasthenia Gravis." MedlinePlus. http://www.nlm.nih.gov/medlineplus/ency/article/000712.htm (accessed November 8, 2014).

Mayo Clinic. "Myasthenia Gravis." http://www.mayoclinic.org/diseases-conditions/myasthenia-gravis/basics/definition/CON-20027124 (accessed November 8, 2014).

Richard Robinson
Monique Laberge, PhD

Myasthenic syndrome of Lambert-Eaton *see* **Lambert-Eaton myasthenic syndrome**

Mycophenolate mofetil

Definition

Mycophenolate mofetil (brand name CellCept) is a drug that has been shown to inhibit tumor growth in rodents, and that may prove useful in treating tumors in humans.

Purpose

The U.S. Food and Drug Administration (FDA) approved the use of mycophenolate mofetil in August 2000 for use in patients undergoing liver transplants, and the drug is used primarily to ease the acceptance of a transplanted organ by a recipient. The drug makes acceptance of the transplanted organ more likely because it prevents the recipient from mounting an **immune response** to the organ, or treating it like a foreign invader. The drug also seems to have the ability to inhibit tumor growth, and may prove effective in treating certain kinds of **cancer**.

In laboratory studies, mycophenolate mofetil has inhibited tumor growth in cancers of the pancreas, colon, lung, and blood. The value of the drug for anticancer therapy is still being evaluated.

In addition to its use in treating cancer, mycophenolate mofetil has been used by dermatologists to treat pyoderma gangrenosum, a rare skin disorder of unknown origin characterized by ulcerated areas on the legs. Pyoderma gangrenosum is associated with systemic diseases in about half the patients diagnosed with it, and mycophenolate mofetil has been found to be effective in treating these patients either alone or in combination with prednisone.

Mycophenolate mofetil is reported to be effective in relieving pain in patients with cluster headache; however, this use of the drug is considered investigational.

KEY TERMS

B cell—A type of cell in the lymphatic system that contributes to immunity by releasing compounds that attack foreign bodies, such as bacteria and viruses.

Clearance—A measure of the rate at which a drug or other substance is removed from the blood.

Intravenous line—A tube that is inserted directly into a vein to carry medicine directly to the blood stream, bypassing the stomach and other digestive organs that might alter the medicine.

Kilogram—Metric measure that equals 2.2 pounds.

Lymphatic system—The system that collects and returns fluid in tissues to the blood vessels and produces defensive agents for fighting infection and invasion by foreign bodies.

Milligram—One-thousandth of a gram, and there are one thousand grams in a kilogram. A gram is the metric measure that equals about 0.035 ounces.

Mutant—Altered, not normal.

T cell—A cell in the lymphatic system that contributes to immunity by attacking foreign bodies, such as bacteria and viruses, directly.

Description

Mycophenolate mofetil suppresses, or prevents activity of, cells in the lymphatic system, both T cells and B cells. Under normal circumstances, T cells mount an immune response by reacting directly with foreign materials in the body and B cells release compounds that attack foreign materials. But during a transplant, T cells and B cells can cause a reaction that leads to the rejection of a donor organ.

Recommended dosage

The drug is given orally and by intravenous line. Dosages given for cancer therapy are experimental. To prevent immune response during organ transplants, the drug is dispensed in capsules of 250 mg, tablets of 500 mg, and by intravenous line in doses of 500 mg. Time intervals between dosages are determined according to the rate of the drug's breakdown in the patient's body.

Precautions

Mycophenolate mofetil is known to cause or may cause lymphomas and **skin cancer**. The benefit of taking

the drug must be weighed against the increased risk of the cancers it causes.

It is critical for the patient's doctor to monitor blood levels carefully when using this drug, as patients vary widely in their rate of clearance of mycophenolate mofetil, particularly when it is given in combination with other immunosuppressants.

Side effects

In addition to increasing the risk of lymphomas and skin cancer, mycophenolate mofetil may cause a number of other unwanted reactions. They include dizziness, headache, trembling, as well as pain in the chest, swelling (edema), and high blood pressure (hypertension). Many digestive tract upsets from constipation to **diarrhea** to vomiting are also possible side effects. There is also a chance of hemorrhage, or uncontrolled bleeding in the digestive tract.

Interactions

Taking the drug is likely to make oral contraceptives ineffective and another form of birth control should be used. Stomach medications that contain magnesium and aluminum hydroxides, such as antacids, can block the uptake of mycophenolate mofetil across the gut. They should be avoided. As always, the physician in charge of the care plan should be told of every drug a patient is taking so that the potential for interactions can be avoided. The drug is considered superior to some others used as a suppressant of the immune response in transplants because it does not show as many drug interactions as other drugs do. But the short list of interactions might be in part related to its limited time on the market, and interactions that are yet unidentified.

Resources
WEBSITES
AHFS Consumer Medication Information. "Mycophenolate." American Soceity of Health-System Pharmicists. Available from: http://www.nlm.nih.gov/medlineplus/druginfo/meds/a601081.html (accessed November 8, 2014).

Healthwise. "Mycophenolate Mofetil." Norris Cotton Cancer Center, Dartmouth. http://cancer.dartmouth.edu/pf/health_encyclopedia/d03839a1 (accessed November 8, 2014).

Micromedex. "Mycophenolate Mofetil (Oral Route)." Mayo Clinic. http://www.mayoclinic.org/drugs-supplements/mycophenolate-mofetil-oral-route/description/drg-20073191 (accessed November 8, 2014).

ORGANIZATIONS
ASHP (formerly the American Society of Health-System Pharmacists), 7272 Wisconsin Ave., Bethesda, MD 20814,

(301) 664-8700, (866) 279-0681, custserv@ashp.org, http://www.ashp.org.

U.S. Food and Drug Administration, 10903 New Hampshire Ave., Silver Spring, MD 20993, (888) INFO-FDA (463-6332), http://www.fda.gov.

Diane M. Calabrese
Rebecca J. Frey, PhD

Mycosis fungoides

Definition

Mycosis fungoides is a **skin cancer** characterized by patches, plaques, and tumors where cancerous T lymphocytes have invaded the skin.

Description

Mycosis fungoides, the most common type of **cutaneous T-cell lymphoma**, originates from a type of white blood cell called a T lymphocyte or T cell. In mycosis fungoides, cancerous T cells accumulate in the skin. These cells and the skin irritation they create become visible as growths or changes in the skin's color or texture.

Mycosis fungoides usually develops and progresses slowly. It often begins as an unexplained rash that can wax and wane for years. Whether this stage represents early mycosis fungoides or a precancerous stage is controversial. The classic symptoms of mycosis fungoides are red, scaly skin patches that develop into raised plaques, then into large, mushroom-shaped tumors. The patches often originate on parts of the body that are covered by clothing and sometimes improve when they are exposed to sunlight. **Itching** can be intense.

As the **cancer** progresses, the cancer cells lose their affinity for the skin and spread to nearby lymph nodes and other internal organs. The normal T cells also start to disappear. Because T cells are very important in immunity, this leaves the patient susceptible to infections. Treatment at an earlier stage of the disease can often stop or slow this progression.

Sézary syndrome is a variant of mycosis fungoides. Sézary syndrome is characterized by red, thickened skin and large numbers of cancer cells in the blood.

Demographics

Mycosis fungoides is usually diagnosed after the age of 50, but has been seen as early as childhood. Mycosis fungoides develops twice as often in men as in women and is more common in people of African than of European origin.

Causes and symptoms

Environmental chemicals, virus infections, allergies, and genes have all been suggested as possible causes of this cancer.

The symptoms of mycosis fungoides include:

- Patches: patches are red or brown, sometimes scaly, flat areas. There may be one patch or many. Patches may itch and can resemble psoriasis, eczema, allergies, or other skin diseases. Some patients do not have a patch stage.

- Plaques: plaques are red or brown, sometimes scaly, raised areas. Itching is usually more intense than during the patch stage. The hair sometimes falls out in the affected skin. If the face is involved, the facial features can change.

- Tumors: tumors can originate from plaques, red skin, or normal skin. They are usually reddish brown or purple. The itching can diminish, but the tumors may develop painful open sores or become infected. Some tumors can become very large. Patches, plaques, and tumors can co-exist.

- Erythrodermic form: in the erythrodermic form, the skin becomes red, thickened, and sometimes peels and flakes. The palms and soles thicken and may crack. Itching is usually intense. More than 90% of the time, the erythrodermic form is associated with Sézary syndrome.

- Other, more rare symptoms are also seen, including itching alone.

Diagnosis

A physical examination, history of the symptoms, blood tests, and **skin biopsy** are usually the key to diagnosing this cancer. The blood tests examine the health of the internal organs and look for cancer cells in the blood. The skin **biopsy** checks for the typical microscopic changes seen in this disease. This biopsy is a brief, simple procedure often done in the doctor's office. After numbing the skin with an injection of local anesthetic, the doctor snips out one or more tiny pieces of abnormal skin. The skin samples are sent to a trained pathologist for examination, and results may take up to a week to come back.

During its early stages, mycosis fungoides can be very difficult to diagnose. The symptoms resemble other skin diseases and numerous biopsies may be needed before the typical features are found. Special stains and DNA tests on the skin sample may find the cancer a little earlier.

Acyclovir—A drug used to kill viruses.

Antibody—A protein made by the immune system. Antibodies attach to target molecules and can be useful as drugs.

Biopsy—A sample of an organ taken to look for abnormalities. Also, the technique used to take such samples.

Computed tomography (CT)—A special x-ray technique that produces a cross-sectional image of the body.

Cutaneous T-cell lymphoma—A type of skin cancer originating from T lymphocytes.

Electron beam—A type of radiation composed of electrons. Electrons are tiny, negatively charged particles found in atoms.

Hypericin—A chemical derived from plants that kills cells after being activated by visible light.

Interferon alpha—A chemical made naturally by the immune system and also manufactured as a drug.

Local anesthetic—A liquid used to numb a small area of the skin.

Lymph node—A small organ full of immune cells that are found in clusters throughout the body. Lymph nodes are where reactions to infections usually begin.

Myelosuppression—A decrease in blood cell production from the bone marrow. This can result in anemia, an increased risk of infections, or bleeding tendencies.

Oncologist—A doctor who specializes in the treatment of cancer.

Pancreatitis—Inflammation of the pancreas. This disease is potentially serious and life-threatening.

Pathologist—A doctor who specializes in examining cells and other parts of the body for abnormalities.

Precancerous—Abnormal and with a high probability of turning into cancer, but not yet a cancer.

Remission—A decrease in the symptoms of the cancer. In a complete remission, there is no longer any evidence of the cancer, although it may still be there.

Retinoids—Drugs related to vitamin A.

T lymphocyte or T cell—A type of white blood cell. Some T cells, known as helper T cells, aid other cells of the immune system. Other T cells, called cytotoxic T cells, fight viruses and cancer.

Ultraviolet light—Light waves that have a shorter wavelength than visible light, but longer wavelength than x-rays. UVA light is closer to visible light than UVB.

White blood cells—The cells in the blood that fight infections. There are several types of white blood cells. Also called immune cells.

To stage this cancer, the lymph nodes are checked for abnormal size or texture and, if necessary, biopsied. The doctor may also recommend x-ray studies of the chest, **computed tomography**, or biopsies of the internal organs to look for cancer cells.

Treatment team

Patients diagnosed with mycosis fungoides are often referred to an oncologist. A dermatologist may also become involved. Depending on the treatment chosen, the team may include other specialists, such as a radiation oncologist, specially trained nurses, a dietitian, or a social worker.

Clinical staging

In stage I, the lymph nodes look normal and cancer cells cannot be found in the internal organs. In stage IA,

patches or plaques cover less than 10% of the skin. In stage IB, they are present on more than 10%.

In stage IIA, some of the lymph nodes look swollen or abnormal. Patches or plaques may cover any amount of skin. In stage IIB, the lymph nodes may or may not look abnormal, but there is at least one tumor on the skin. Neither the lymph nodes nor the internal organs contain detectable cancer cells in stage IIA or IIB.

In stage III, the skin looks thickened, red and sometimes scaly. The lymph nodes sometimes look abnormal, but no cancer cells can be detected in them or within internal organs.

In stage IVA and IVB, the skin may have patches, plaques, tumors, or widespread reddening. In stage IVA, cancer cells have been found in the lymph nodes but not in other internal organs. In stage IVB, cancer cells have been found in internal organs and sometimes the lymph nodes.

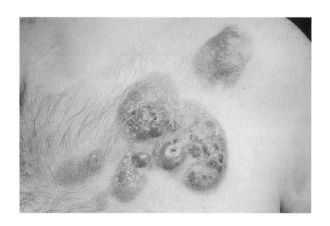

Red, scaly plaque on skin of patient with mycosis fungoides. *(Wellcome Image Library/Custom Medical Stock Photography)*

Treatment

Mycosis fungoides is rarely cured. Instead, most treatments are aimed at controlling the symptoms, improving the quality of life, and preventing the disease from progressing into later stages. This cancer responds well to a variety of therapies and frequently goes into remission, particularly if it is caught early. Even in stage IV, treatment can significantly improve the symptoms in the skin.

In stages III and IV, treatments directed against the cancer cells in the skin may be combined with **chemotherapy** or other therapies against metastatic cells. Experimental treatments are sometimes offered, especially in stage III or stage IV. If the cancer relapses, re-treatment may be possible or other therapies can be tried.

One treatment option for early cancers is ultraviolet B (UVB) light. UVB light can treat mycosis fungoides patches, but not plaques or tumors. About 70% of patients go into complete remission and 15% into partial remission. The side effects can include itching, sunburn, aging of the skin, and a risk of developing other skin cancers. The eyes must be protected from UVB light.

Psoralen and ultraviolet A (PUVA) photochemotherapy is an option for all stages, although earlier stages usually have a better response. In PUVA, the drug methoxypsoralen is taken before exposure to ultraviolet A (UVA) light. The drug sensitizes the cancer cells to the light. The complete remission rate with this treatment is 62%–90%. The side effects may include itching, dry skin, sunburn, nausea, nail discoloration, and a risk of developing other skin cancers. The eyes must be protected to prevent damage to the retina and possibly cataracts.

Total skin electron-beam irradiation (TSEB) is also effective for all stages. TSEB is a type of radiation treatment that uses beams of electrons to irradiate the skin. The electrons stop at the skin and do not penetrate deeper tissues. Up to 80% of patients in stages II and III will respond. The side effects can include flaking of the skin, **alopecia** or hair loss (usually temporary), loss of sweat glands, skin irritation, blisters, dryness, temporary loss of the nails, and a risk of developing other skin cancers. These side effects limit the number of times this treatment can be given. TSEB is not available everywhere.

Other types of radiation—for instance, focused electron beam irradiation or x-rays—can shrink or destroy some tumors or plaques.

Mechlorethamine (nitrogen mustard) is a drug that can be painted onto the skin to suppress the cancer. A thin layer is applied to the whole skin at bedtime, then washed off in the morning. The side effects can include dryness, skin irritation, darkening of the skin, allergies to the ingredients, and possibly a risk of other skin cancers. Half to 80% of mycosis fungoides patients in stage IA and 25%–75% of patients in stage IB or IIA go into complete remission. In stage IIB, the complete remission rate is up to 50%. In stage III, it is 20%–40% and, in stage IV, up to 35%. In stages III and IV, this treatment is used to decrease the skin symptoms and is often combined with other treatments.

Carmustine (BCNU) is an alternative drug. Its effectiveness is similar to mechlorethamine. In addition to side effects in the skin, this drug may cause **myelosuppression**.

Bexarotene is a drug used for cases that do not respond to other treatments. About 40% of patients have a complete or partial remission. The side effects may include dryness of the mucous membranes, aching joints or muscles, headaches, **fatigue**, and increased fragility of the skin. One of the most serious side effects is an increase in the fats in the blood, which can lead to pancreatitis.

Aldesleukin fusion toxin contains a poison that damages cells, attached to a molecule that directs that poison to T cells. About 10% of patients have complete remissions and 40% respond to some extent. The side effects can include chills, nausea, fluid retention, and allergic reactions to the drug.

Chemotherapy is sometimes combined with other therapies for stages III and IV. In stage IV, chemotherapy is directed against the metastatic cells in the lymph nodes or internal organs. Approximately 60% of mycosis fungoides patients in stage IV respond to single drugs, but the remission usually lasts less than six months.

No cures have been reported, and it is not certain whether chemotherapy lengthens survival.

Corticosteroids are sometimes added to other treatments. These drugs decrease skin irritation and can destroy T cells. Fifty percent of patients have complete remissions on corticosteroids and 40% have partial remissions.

Supportive therapies can also help. Antihistamines or other drugs can decrease the itching. Mild moisturizing soaps and moisturizers can also combat the dryness and itching. If infection sets in, **antibiotics** may be necessary.

Alternative and complementary therapies

Complementary treatments can decrease stress, reduce the side effects of cancer treatment, and help patients feel more in control. For instance, some people find activities such as biofeedback, hypnosis, pet therapy, yoga, massage, pleasant distractions, meditation and prayer, mild physical exercise, or visualization helpful. Patients should check with their doctors before starting any complementary or alternative treatment. This is particularly important for alternative treatments that attempt to cure the cancer, boost the immune system, or reduce the side effects of conventional treatments. Some alternative treatments may interfere with the standard medical treatments or be dangerous when they are combined.

Prognosis

If mycosis fungoides is caught early, the prognosis is very good. If treatment begins during stage IA, most patients can expect to live as long as someone of the same age and gender who does not have this cancer. Median survival in stage IA is at least 20 years and most people die of diseases unrelated to the cancer. The overall 5-year survival in stage I is 80%–90%. In stage II, five-year survival is 60%–70%. As tumors develop and the cancer cells spread internally, the prognosis becomes worse. Five-year survival drops to 30% in stage IIB, 40%–50% in stage III, and 25%–35% in stage IV. Cancer cells can spread into almost any organ in the later stages of mycosis fungoides. Once this happens, many patients die of cancer complications, particularly skin infections that spread into the blood. Overall, half of mycosis fungoides patients live for at least ten years after their cancer is diagnosed.

Coping with cancer treatment

Many of the treatments used for mycosis fungoides can dry and irritate the skin. Some ways to help are:

QUESTIONS TO ASK YOUR DOCTOR

- What stage is my cancer?
- If it is treated, is my cancer likely to progress?
- Which treatment(s) do you recommend?
- What are the side effects of these treatments?
- Can you recommend anything to help with those side effects?
- How should I prepare for the treatment?
- Are there any other treatments which might work as well?
- Do you expect me to go into remission and, if so, how long can I expect it to last?
- How often should I return for check-ups?

- Wear soft, loose clothing over the affected areas.
- Protect the skin from the sun.
- Don't scratch or rub the affected areas.
- Check with a doctor or nurse before using lotions, moisturizers, sunscreens, or cosmetics on the area.
- If allowed, use moisturizer and a moisturizing soap.

Clinical trials

Because mycosis fungoides is unlikely to be cured with the standard treatments, all patients with this disease are candidates for **clinical trials**. Patients should check with their medical insurers before enrolling in a clinical trial. Insurers may not pay for some treatments; however, this varies with the insurer and each individual case.

Some clinical trials are testing new drugs, including some retinoids, acyclovir, and hypericin.

In extracorporeal photochemotherapy, the white blood cells are exposed to a chemical called a psoralen, temporarily separated from the rest of the blood and treated with UVA light, then returned to the body. This treatment may stimulate the immune system to destroy the cancer cells.

Interferon alpha is a drug that is injected into plaques and tumors. About 55% of patients have some response and 17% go into complete remission. The side effects may include fevers, fatigue, loss of appetite (**anorexia**), decreases in the number of white blood cells, or irregular heartbeats.

Antibodies can block important molecules on the cancer cells or carry poisons or radioactive molecules to the cancer.

Some clinical trials are testing whether **bone marrow transplantation** can produce lasting remissions.

Prevention

The risk factors for mycosis fungoides are unknown and there is no known means of prevention.

Special concerns

Because mycosis fungoides is rarely cured, patients must usually return periodically for check-ups or treatments to maintain the remission. Between visits, patients should also be alert for skin infections. These infections can spread into the blood and become serious if they are not controlled. Because mycosis fungoides can affect the appearance, patients may wish to discuss cosmetic concerns with a doctor, other professional, or support group. Mycosis fungoides increases the risk of developing other types of lymphocyte cancers.

See also Body image; Lymph node biopsy.

Resources

PERIODICALS

Humme, D., Nast, A., Erdmann, R., Vandersee, S., Beyer, M. "Systematic Review of Combination Therapies for Mycosis Fungoides." *Cancer Treatment Reviews* 40, no. 8 (2014): 927–33. http://www.ncbi.nlm.nih.gov/pubmed/24997678 (accessed November 8, 2014).

WEBSITES

National Cancer Institute. "General Information About Mycosis Fungoides and the Sézary Syndrome." http://www.cancer.gov/cancertopics/pdq/treatment/mycosisfungoides/Patient/page1 (accessed November 8, 2014).

U.S. National Library of Medicine. "Mycosis Fungoides." http://ghr.nlm.nih.gov/condition/mycosis-fungoides (accessed November 8, 2014).

ORGANIZATIONS

Cutaneous Lymphoma Foundation, PO Box 374, Birmingham, MI 48012-0374, (248) 644-9014, http://www.clfoundation.org.

Anna Rovid Spickler, D.V.M., PhD

Myelodysplastic syndromes

Definition

Myelodysplastic syndromes (MDS) are a group of similar bone marrow cancers also known as hematopoietic neoplasms. In each of these syndromes, the bone marrow does not produce enough blood cells, which leads to reduced numbers of mature cells in the blood. Normally the bone marrow produces healthy stem cells that become mature cells as time progresses. However, the blood cells of people with MDS do not mature normally and abnormal numbers of immature cells called blast cells are found in the blood and bone marrow. The bone marrow produces three major types of blood cells—red blood cells, white blood cells, and platelets. Patients with MDS may have decreased production of one, two, or all three types of blood cells. Different types of myelodysplastic syndromes occur based on specific changes that take place in both the bone marrow and the blood cells produced. The outcomes may vary for each disease.

Description

Blood cells perform many essential functions in the body. Red blood cells contain the iron-bearing protein hemoglobin that carries oxygen to all tissues and organ systems. Different types of white blood cells seek out and destroy invading pathogens that cause infection, such as bacteria, viruses, and fungi, and special white cells target and kill **cancer** cells. Platelets are an essential component of the body's coagulation system and are active in forming clots to control bleeding. Blood cells are formed and stored in the bone marrow, which is the spongy tissue inside most bones, especially the large bones. The bone marrow makes myeloid stem cells that mature to become red blood cells and platelets, and other stem cells that become myeloblasts and mature into certain types of white blood cells. The marrow also makes lymphoid stem cells that first become lymphoblasts and then mature into lymphocytes, the powerful cell-killing white cells that help fight cancer.

Normally, when the body needs a specific type of blood cell, the bone marrow uses its stockpile of stem cells to produce the type of mature cells needed for that particular situation. In patients who have MDS, the stem cells fail to develop and mature normally. The bone marrow is unable to develop a normal number of mature blood cells and is also not able to increase blood cell production when mature cells are needed in the bloodstream. Instead, the marrow eventually becomes filled with immature blast cells and the functions normally performed by blood cells are unfulfilled.

MDS subtypes

MDS comprises eight different syndromes or subtypes classified based on the number of blast cells in the bone marrow, changes in the type and numbers of blood cells in the blood, and the risk of developing acute myeloid leukemia. Diagnosis of the specific subtypes is important, because each subtype affects patients differently and requires specific treatment. The World Health Organization (WHO) developed a classification system to help standardize the different subtypes. The subtypes based on the WHO classification system are as follows:

- Refractory anemia (RA). Bone marrow with less than 5% blast cells and too few red blood cells in the blood (anemia) while the number of immature red cell blasts is abnormally high. White cell and platelet counts are normal.

- Refractory anemia with ring sideroblasts (RARS). The bone marrow has 5% red blood cell blasts and not enough red blood cells in the blood. The red cells that are present contain too much iron. White cells and platelets remain normal.

- Refractory anemia with excess blasts (RAEB). The bone marrow has 5%–19% blasts and too few red blood cells in the blood, a condition that can lead to acute myeloid leukemia. White cells and platelets may also be abnormal.

- Refractory cytopenia with multilineage dysplasia (RCMD). The bone marrow has less than 5% of blasts and there are fewer than 1% of blasts in the blood. The blood contains reduced numbers of at least two types of blood cells (cytopenia). In some forms of RCMD, the red blood cells may have too much (more than 15%) iron; this is called refractory cytopenia with multilineage dysplasia and ringed sideroblasts (RCMD-RS). These diseases may progress to acute myeloid leukemia.

- Refractory cytopenia with unilineage dysplasia (RCUD). The bone marrow has less than 5% of blasts and the blood has less than 1% of blasts. The blood has too few of one type of blood cell and at least 10% of the other two types of blood cells will have changes.

- Myelodysplastic syndrome associated with chromosome abnormality. The bone marrow and the blood have less than 5% of blasts. Red blood cells are reduced in the blood and the patient is anemic. A lack of genetic material is found in the del (5q) chromosome.

- Chronic myelomonocytic leukemia (CMML) and juvenile myelomonocytic leukemia (JMML). The bone marrow has 5%–20% blasts and an abnormal number of monocytes (a specific type of white blood cell) that have undergone mutations are found in the blood. The white blood cell count is higher than in other MDS subtypes.

- Unclassified myelodysplastic syndrome (MDS-U). A normal number of blasts are found in the bone marrow and the blood, but there are too few mature cells in the blood of any or all blood cell types. The disease does not precisely fit any of the other MDS subtypes.

Demographics

The incidence of MDS increases significantly with age and is most prevalent among white males. Approximately 10,000 new cases of MDS, regardless of subtype, are diagnosed annually in the United States, and 60,000 people are being treated for the disease at any given time. The average age at diagnosis is 70. The most common types are refractory **anemia** and refractory anemia with ring sideroblasts. CMML occurs most often in people aged 65 to 75, while JMML is found in children younger than age 6. However, a diagnosis of MDS is rare before age 50.

Causes and symptoms

Causes and risk factors

No clear cause is identified in the majority of MDS cases, which are referred to as primary or *de novo* myelodysplastic syndromes. Previous cancer treatments such as radiation and/or **chemotherapy** are responsible for most other cases of MDS. This type of MDS is called secondary or treatment-related MDS and it typically develops from three to seven years after the patient's exposure to radiation or chemotherapy drugs. It is found more often in younger people while primary MDS is found more often in older adults.

Other possible causative agents for secondary MDS include exposure to radiation, cigarette smoke, or toxic chemicals such as certain **pesticides**, fertilizers, and the solvent **benzene**. Exposure to heavy metals such as mercury or lead may also cause MDS. Children with pre-existing chromosomal abnormalities such as Down syndrome have a higher risk of developing MDS. MDS does not appear to run in families, nor can it be spread to other individuals.

Symptoms

MDS symptoms are related to the type of blood cells that the body lacks. The earliest symptoms usually arise from anemia, which results from a shortage of mature red blood cells. Anemia causes patients to feel tired and out of breath because of the reduction in red cells that transport oxygen throughout the body. MDS may also lead to a shortage of white blood cells, resulting in an increased likelihood of developing bacterial or viral infections. Another symptom of MDS may be a tendency to bleed due to decreased numbers of platelets; this may be indicated by blood in the stool, nose bleeds, increased bruises, or bleeding gums. These symptoms can occur in any combination, depending on a given patient's specific subtype of MDS.

Diagnosis

Blood tests

MDS is usually discovered when patients report to their primary care physicians with symptoms of anemia such as **fatigue** and shortness of breath. After preliminary blood tests, the patients are usually referred to a hematologist (a physician who specializes in blood diseases). The diagnosis of MDS requires a complete analysis of the patient's blood and bone marrow, which is performed in the hematology laboratory and reviewed by the hematologist. A complete blood count (CBC) is done to determine the number of each blood cell type within the sample. Low numbers of red blood cells, white blood cells, and or platelets are signs of MDS, but other blood diseases must be ruled out. Low blood counts (cytopenias) can also be the result of other conditions, including bleeding, nutritional deficiencies, or adverse reactions to certain medications. Therefore, the hematologist will investigate other possible causes for low blood counts before assigning a diagnosis of MDS. Staining the blood cells and examining them under a microscope may reveal abnormal white cells and a large number of blast cells, which can help to identify the type of MDS or may suggest another disease. Immunocytochemistry tests may be performed to identify substances on the surfaces of bone marrow cells (antigens) that helps to differentiate MDS from leukemia or other blood diseases. Immunophenotyping also helps to diagnose specific types of leukemia by comparing antigens on the cancer cells to those on normal immune system cells. The number, size, and shape of cells along with the percentage of live cells and the possible presence of **tumor markers** on the cell surfaces can be determined by **flow cytometry**, a technology that uses laser to analyze the reactions of stained cells to the light. Chromosome abnormalities may also be identified by a technique called fluorescence in situ hybridization (FISH), which uses fluorescent dyes and light to examine genes and chromosomes in cells and tissues.

Bone marrow biopsy

A **bone marrow biopsy** is required to confirm the diagnosis of MDS and determine the correct MDS subtype. This procedure involves a needle to aspirate a sample of marrow from inside the bone. Marrow samples are usually taken from the back of the hip bone (iliac crest). The area of the skin where the needle is inserted is numbed and sometimes the patient is also sedated. Patients may experience some discomfort but the procedure is safe and quick. A sample of the marrow, known as an aspirate, and a small piece of bone are both removed with the needle.

A hematologist or a pathologist (a specialist in diagnosing diseases through the examination of cells, tissue, and body fluids) will carefully examine the bone marrow sample under a microscope. Microscopic examination allows the doctor to determine the number and type of blast cells within the marrow in order to identify the specific MDS subtype. The chromosomes of the marrow cells are analyzed (cytogenetic testing). Abnormal bone marrow chromosomes are found in 40% to 70% of patients with MDS. The pattern of these abnormalities helps to predict response to a particular treatment. Thus, the full set of information provided by a bone marrow **biopsy**, CBC, and other laboratory tests will usually confirm the diagnosis and allow the doctor to recommend the most effective treatment plan.

Clinical staging

International Prognostic Scoring System (IPSS) for MDS

Because MDS is a bone marrow cancer, it is not staged in the conventional way. Instead, once a diagnosis of MDS is established, the likely longterm outcome or prognosis for each patient is calculated using the International Prognostic Scoring System (IPSS) for MDS, which helps to determine treatment. Using the IPSS calculator, the patient's score is calculated by adding the separate scores for bone marrow blast percentage, chromosomal abnormalities (karyotype), and number of different blood cells that are reduced (number of cytopenias). Scores range from 0 to 3.5 for each patient. Patients with lower scores have a better prognosis, including longer survival, and treatment will focus on improving blood cell production (hematopoiesis) and reducing iron overload. Patients with a higher score have more aggressive disease and may therefore undergo more aggressive treatment to delay transformation to acute leukemia and increase survival time.

Treatment

Supportive care

Treatment for MDS is tailored to the patient's age, general health, specific MDS subtype, and IPSS score. Treatment varies for each patient, but most treatment strategies are designed to control the symptoms of MDS. This approach is called supportive care and aims to correct certain disease symptoms to improve the patient's quality of life.

Supportive care for the MDS patients commonly includes red blood cell transfusions to relieve symptoms related to anemia. Red cell transfusions are relatively safe and the physician will review the risks and benefits of this approach. Platelet transfusions can also control excessive bleeding. However, transfused cells of any type are short-lived; therefore, patients require repeat transfusions at defined intervals. Based on results of regular blood tests, the doctor determines the timing for transfusions. **Antibiotics** often help combat infections that occur more frequently in patients with low white blood cell counts.

Certain drugs function to increase the number of mature red blood cells produced in the bone marrow and to reduce the symptoms of anemia. Erythropoietin-stimulating agents and recombinant human erythropoietin (rHuEPO) are sometimes used to treat anemia in MDS. Human erythropoietin (procrit) is a growth factor produced naturally in the body to support production of healthy blood cells. Administered only by injection, it has been shown to safely and effectively increase red blood cell counts with few side effects.

Lenalidomide is a drug that may be given to MDS patients who are known to have an abnormality of the del (5q) chromosome and who also require frequent red blood cell transfusions. This drug has been shown to reduce the need for transfusions. Immunosuppressive therapy with antithymocyte globulin (ATG) has also been shown to reduce the need for red blood cell transfusions by weakening immune system activity.

Growth factors—natural proteins the body normally uses to control blood production—may be given to increase white blood cell counts. These substances stimulate the patient's bone marrow to produce healthy blood cells. Growth factors that stimulate white cell production are G-CSF (neupogen, **filgrastim**) and GMCSF (leukine, **sargramostim**).

Frequent transfusions sometimes result in iron overload in some types of MDS. Excess iron in the blood has been associated with poor survival among some low risk patients. Therefore, treatment to reduce iron overload may be advised if a patient has a history of 20 or more blood transfusions. Iron chelation is one such treatment. Deferoxamine and deferasirox are FDA-approved iron chelation drugs that reduce iron overload in patients in the United States. These drugs have been shown to be effective but studies are still underway to investigate adverse effects and the effects of these drugs on overall survival.

Chemotherapy

Chemotherapy with drugs such as **azacitidine** and decitabine has been used to treat MDS by killing rapidly dividing cells. The use of such cell-killing drugs may also damage healthy cells and are associated with certain side effects. For these reasons, chemotherapy is generally not indicated until the disease becomes more aggressive or the patient has a high IPSS score. In acute myeloid leukemia—which has a high number of blasts in the bone marrow—reducing the risk of progression to acute leukemia may require chemotherapy. Chemotherapy is also used with **stem cell transplantation**.

Stem cell/bone marrow transplantation

Stem cells are extremely versatile and have the ability to divide and develop into other cell types. Stem cells in the bone marrow that make blood cells (hematopoietic stem cells) produce red blood cells, white blood cells, and platelets, any of which may be called for in MDS treatment, depending on the MDS subtype. Transplantation of stem cells from the bone marrow (sometimes called **bone marrow transplantation** or BMT) or stem cells obtained from the blood stream (peripheral blood stem cell transplant or PBSCT) is considered the only curative treatment for MDS. Stem cell transplantation is performed in combination with chemotherapy. Abnormal stem cells are first killed with chemotherapy, and then the blood-forming cells that will replace abnormal cells with healthy stem cells are transplanted. This treatment strategy depends on the otherwise good health of the patient, since the procedure is rigorous; therefore, it is more likely used in younger patients but is considered for patients older than age 60 based on their health status.

Two different types of transplantation include autologous transplant, which uses the patient's own stem cells, or allogeneic transplant, which uses bone marrow or peripheral blood stem cells from a sibling or other family member or an unrelated matching donor (found through a donor services program). Allogeneic transplants are considered the best source of stem cells because they come from healthy donors, whereas an autologous transplant runs the risk of reinfusing cancer cells from the patient's own body. The transplantation procedure follows a course of high-dose chemotherapy called "conditioning." Some patients may also undergo total body irradiation. A mini-transplantation procedure with less intense conditioning is sometimes used to reduce the risk of side effects in certain patients, such as older patients with a rapidly progressing form of MDS.

In autologous stem cell transplantation, the patient is first treated with white blood cell growth factors to increase the level of white blood cells, and in a week or so, stem cells are removed from the patient's blood (autologous hematopoietic stem cells) through a transplant catheter and are frozen for storage. After the conditioning chemotherapy and/or **radiation therapy**, the stem cells are thawed and infused back into the patient. The entire procedure takes one or two weeks. Many patients are able to complete the procedure on an outpatient basis, but others are hospitalized, depending on their condition. The stem cells will remain in the bloodstream for about 24 hours and then migrate to the bone marrow to become mature cells, restoring the type of blood cells needed. The treatment is not as effective in patients who have had previous chemotherapy. The growth of new blood cells takes about two to four weeks, sometimes longer, and patients may be hospitalized in order to monitor their progress.

In allogeneic stem cell transplant, a type of protein on the surface of the patient's white blood cells (human leukocyte antigens commonly referred to as HLA) must match or be compatible with the donor stem cells that will be infused into the patient. The donor cells usually come from the bone marrow or blood of a sibling or other family member with matching HLA. Siblings are considered the best match. This can be a problem for older adult patients who may not have a living sibling or one who is healthy enough to donate blood or bone marrow. Stem cells can also come from the bone marrow or blood of a donor who is HLA compatible. Donors are located through donor services in the hospital or cancer center where the patient is being treated or through the national donor registry. After the donor is treated with white blood cell growth factors to increase the level of white blood cells, stem cells will be obtained either from the donor's blood or bone marrow and reserved for transplantation. The same procedure is used to collect stem cells from the bone marrow for transplantation as is used for bone marrow biopsy. As with autologous stem cell transplantation, the whole process takes several weeks. One advantage of allogeneic transplant is that the immune system is regenerated once the immune system cells are destroyed by chemotherapy; in effect, the new cells resume the body's fight against the cancer. One disadvantage of an allogeneic stem cell transplant is increased risk of tissue rejection. Research is ongoing to determine effective combinations of treatment that employ stem cell transplantation. Researchers are also exploring techniques to improve the safety and effectiveness of treatment for older adult MDS patients.

Compatible umbilical cord blood that is rich with stem cells is another possible source for patients who have not found a compatible donor. Umbilical cord blood is being used in cancer centers worldwide and the results in children are especially promising. However, more research is needed before this technology is widely used in adults.

Prognosis

The prognosis for MDS patients depends on their risk of developing leukemia, which is indicated by the subtype of MDS and the individual's IPSS score. For low-risk patients with few blasts, normal karyotype (chromosomes) and 0-1 reduced cell counts, the median survival is 5-6 years; for patients with higher risk, survival ranges from 4 to 14 months. The 5-year survival rate for low risk patients (leukemia risk 15%) is 55%, for intermediate risk-1 patients (leukemia risk 30%) 35%, for intermediate risk-2 patients (leukemia risk 65%) 7% and for high-risk patients (leukemia risk 100%) 0%. Patients with refractory anemias only rarely develop leukemia and may respond to treatment and live with disease for some years. Higher-risk subtypes such as RCMD, RCMD-RS, or CMML progress more rapidly, and aggressive therapy will usually be applied to manage the disease.

Managing MDS requires frequent appointments with a physician to monitor disease progression and to evaluate the response to treatment. Advances in therapy have significantly enhanced patients' ability to cope with MDS, and new therapies are in development. Along with increased awareness of MDS, the development of new, experimental drugs, and a better understanding of the disease may help to reduce the significant morbidity and high mortality associated with high-risk MDS subtypes.

Clinical trials

MDS is the subject of extensive research. New combination treatments are under development, including lenalidomide with epoetin alfa; **busulfan, fludarabine**, and total-body irradiation for MDS patients undergoing stem cell transplantation; chemotherapy and unrelated donor stem cell transplantation; chemotherapy drugs (fludarabine phosphate, cyclophosphamide), total body irradiation, and bone marrow transplant followed by donor natural killer cell therapy; and many other ongoing trials. In addition to treatment by their local hematologist or oncologist, motivated patients can join a clinical trial and undergo experimental treatments at major medical centers. Many **clinical trials** are underway to test novel drug therapies or procedures for patients with MDS. Although these treatments have not yet been determined to be effective for MDS, initial studies indicate that the treatments have certain benefits. Patients can consult their physicians or cancer organizations about finding appropriate clinical trials. The **National Cancer Institute** (NCI) has a list on its website of thousands of clinical trials that are underway.

Prevention

There is no definite prevention for MDS, although tobacco smoke and toxic chemicals that increase risk (e.g., pesticides, fertilizers, benzene) can be avoided. MDS patients must carefully monitor daily activities and avoid the use of aspirin-like products that reduce platelet counts in the blood; this may help prevent secondary complications of MDS such as bruising and bleeding. Good hygiene and avoiding crowds or people with infections can help to prevent infections. A well-balanced diet is recommended to increase overall energy.

Resources

BOOKS

Aguayo, Alvaro, Jorge Cortes, and Hagop Kantarjian. "Mye lodysplastic Syndromes," In *Cancer Management: A Multidisciplinary Approach*, edited by Richard Pazdur, et al. 13th ed. PRR, Inc, 2012.

PERIODICALS

Duong, V. H., R. S. Komrokji, and A. F.List. "Update on the Pharmacotherapy for Myelodysplastic Syndromes." *Expert Opinion in Pharmacotherapy* 15 (Sept 2014): 1811–25.

Greenberg, P., et al. "International Scoring System for Evaluating Prognosis in Myelodysplastic Syndromes." *Blood* 89 (March 1997) 2079–88.

Ma, X. "Epidemiology of Myelodysplastic Syndrome." *American Journal of Medicine* 125, suppl. (July 2012): S2–S5.

Troy, J. D., E. Atallah, J. T. Geyer, and W. Saber. "Myelodysplastic Syndromes in the United States: An Update for Clinicians." *Annals of Medicine* 46 (Aug 2014): 283–289.

ORGANIZATIONS

Aplastic Anemia and MDS International Foundation, 100 Park Avenue, Suite 108, Rockville, MD 20850, (301) 279-7202, (800) 747-2820, help@aamds.org, http://www.aamds.org.

Leukemia & Lymphoma Society, 1311 Mamaroneck Ave., Ste. 310, White Plains, NY 10605, (914) 949-5213, Fax: (914) 949-6691, infocenter@lls.org, http://www.lls.org.

MDS Foundation, 4573 South Broad St., Suite 150, Yardville, NJ 08620, (800) MDS-0839, http://www.mds-foundation.org.

National Cancer Institute, 9609 Medical Center Dr., BG 9609 MSC 9760, Bethesda, MD 20892-9760, (800) 4-CANCER (422-6237), http://www.cancer.gov.

L. Lee Culvert
Andrea Ruskin, M.D.

Myelofibrosis

Definition

Myelofibrosis is a rare disease of the bone marrow in which collagen builds up fibrous scar tissue inside the

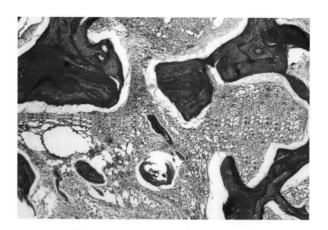

Magnified photomicrograph of myelofibrosis. Fibrosis occurs when scar tissue replaces normal bone marrow tissue, which impacts the production of blood cells. *(Ida Wyman/Phototake)*

marrow cavity. This is caused by the uncontrolled growth of a blood cell precursor, which results in the accumulation of scar tissue in bone marrow. Myelofibrosis goes by many names including idiopathic myelofibrosis, agnogenic myeloid metaplasia, chronic myelosclerosis, aleukemic megakaryocytic myelosis, and leukoerythroblastosis.

Description

Myelofibrosis can be associated with many other conditions including **breast cancer**, **prostate cancer**, **Hodgkin lymphoma**, non-Hodgkin lymphomas, acute myelocytic leukemia, **acute lymphocytic leukemia**, **hairy cell leukemia**, **multiple myeloma**, **myeloproliferative diseases**, tuberculosis, Gaucher disease, and Paget disease of bone. Myelofibrosis typically becomes progressively worse and can cause death.

In myelofibrosis, abnormal cells (hematopoietic stem cells) grow out of control and begin to produce both immature blood cells and excess scar (fibrous) tissue. The fibrous tissue builds up (fibrosis) primarily in the bone marrow, the place where blood cells are produced. The fibrous tissue interferes with the production of normal blood cells. The outcome of this is that the blood made by the bone marrow is of poor quality. To compensate for this, blood cell production occurs in other parts of the body (extramedullary hematopoiesis), but most notably in the spleen and liver. This causes enlargement of the spleen (splenomegaly) and the liver (hepatomegaly). Extramedullary hematopoiesis is not effective and, combined with the reduced production of blood cells by the bone marrow, a condition called **anemia** results.

The abnormal stem cells can spread throughout the body, settle in other organs, and form tumors that produce more abnormal blood cells and fibrous tissue. These tumors are most commonly found in the adrenals, kidneys, lymph nodes, breast, lungs, skin, bowel, thymus, thyroid, prostate, and urinary tract.

Demographics

Most patients with myelofibrosis are over 50 years old. The average age at diagnosis is 65 years; however, myelofibrosis can occur at any age. Myelofibrosis occurs with equal frequency in women and men, but in children it affects girls twice as often as it does boys.

Causes and symptoms

Myelofibrosis is caused by an abnormality in a single stem cell, which causes it to grow out of control. Myelofibrosis tumors that have originated from a single cell are called monoclonal. The cause of the stem cell abnormality is unknown. Persons who were exposed to **benzene** or high doses of radiation have developed myelofibrosis. There may be an association between myelofibrosis and autoimmune diseases, such as systemic lupus erythematosus and scleroderma, in which the immune system treats certain molecules of the body as foreign invaders.

Symptoms usually appear slowly over a long period of time. About one quarter of all patients with myelofibrosis have no symptoms (asymptomatic). An enlarged spleen discovered at an annual medical examination may be the first clue. Symptoms of myelofibrosis include:

- fatigue
- weight loss
- paleness
- fever
- sweating
- weakness
- heart palpitations
- shortness of breath
- itching
- feeling full after eating a small amount of food
- stomach pain or discomfort
- pain in the left shoulder or upper left portion of the body
- unexpected bleeding
- bone pain, especially in the legs

Diagnosis

Because symptoms are similar to other diseases (mostly leukemias), myelofibrosis is not easy to diagnose. The doctor would use his or her hands to feel (palpate) for enlargement of the spleen and liver. Blood tests and urine tests would be performed. **Bone marrow aspiration and biopsy** can help make a diagnosis, but they often fail because of the fibrosis. X-ray imaging and **magnetic resonance imaging** (MRI) may be performed.

Treatment

Many asymptomatic patients, if stable, do not require treatment. There is no cure for myelofibrosis, although **bone marrow transplantation** is curative in some cases. Treatment is aimed at reducing symptoms and improving quality of life.

Medications

Male hormones (androgens) can be used to treat anemia but, in women, these drugs can cause the development of male characteristics (e.g., hair growth on the face and body). Glucocorticoid therapy is also an effective treatment of anemia and can improve myelofibrosis in children. Nutrients that stimulate blood formation (hematinics), such as iron, **folic acid**, and vitamin B$_{12}$, may reduce anemia. Cancer chemotherapy (usually **hydroxyurea**) can decrease splenomegaly and hepatomegaly, reduce symptoms of myelofibrosis, lessen anemia, and sometimes reduce bone marrow fibrosis. The bone marrow of myelofibrosis patients is often not strong enough to withstand the harsh **chemotherapy** drugs, so this treatment is not always an option. Interferon-alpha has been shown to reduce spleen size, reduce **bone pain**, and, in some cases, increase the number of blood platelets (structures involved in blood clotting).

Other treatments

In certain cases, the enlarged spleen may be removed (**splenectomy**). Conditions that warrant splenectomy include spleen pain, the need for frequent blood transfusion, very low levels of platelets (**thrombocyto-penia**), and extreme pressure in the blood vessels of the liver (portal hypertension).

Radiation therapy is used to treat splenomegaly, spleen pain, bone pain, tumors in certain places such as next to the spinal cord, and fluid accumulation inside the abdomen (**ascites**). Patients who are not strong enough to undergo splenectomy are often treated with radiation therapy.

Bone marrow transplantation may be used to treat some patients with myelofibrosis. This procedure may be performed on patients who are less than 50 years old, have a poor life expectancy, and have a brother or sister with blood-type similarities.

Patients with severe anemia may require blood transfusions.

Prognosis

Similar to leukemias, myelofibrosis is progressive and often requires therapy to control the disease. Myelofibrosis can progress to acute lymphocytic leukemia or **lymphoma**. Although a number of factors to predict the survival time have been proposed, advanced age or severe anemia are consistently associated with a poor prognosis. The average survival rate of patients diagnosed with myelofibrosis is five years. Death is usually caused by infection, bleeding, complications of splenectomy, heart failure, or progression to leukemia. Spontaneous remission is rare.

Prevention

Persons who have been exposed to radiation, benzene, or radioactive thorium dioxide (a chemical used during certain diagnostic radiological procedures) are at risk for myelofibrosis.

Resources

PERIODICALS

Tefferi, A. "Primary Myelofibrosis: 2014 Update on Diagnosis, Risk-Stratification, and Management." *American Journal of Hematology* 89, no. 9 (2014): 915–25. http://www.ncbi. nlm.nih.gov/pubmed/25124313 (accessed November 8, 2014).

WEBSITES

A.D.A.M. Medical Encyclopedia. "Myelofibrosis." Medline Plus. http://www.nlm.nih.gov/medlineplus/ency/article/000531.htm (accessed November 8, 2014).
National Cancer Institute. "Primary Myelofibrosis." http://www.cancer.gov/cancertopics/pdq/treatment/myeloproliferative/Patient/page4 (accessed November 8, 2014).

Belinda Rowland, PhD
J. Ricker Polsdorfer, M.D.

Myeloma
Definition

Cancer that arises in the bone marrow and involves plasma cells, a type of white blood cell that produces proteins called immunoglobulins.

Resources

WEBSITES

American Cancer Society. "Multiple Myeloma." http://www.cancer.org/cancer/multiplemyeloma/ (accessed November 8, 2014).
Leukemia & Lymphoma Society. "Myeloma." http://www.lls.org/diseaseinformation/myeloma/ (accessed November 8, 2014).
Micromedex. "Multiple Myeloma." Mayo Clinic. http://www.mayoclinic.org/diseases-conditions/multiple-myeloma/basics/definition/con-20026607 (accessed November 8, 2014).

Kate Kretschmann

Myeloproliferative diseases
Definition

The myeloproliferative diseases, which are called myeloproliferative neoplasms (MPN), comprise six bone marrow cancers in which the bone marrow produces too many of certain types of blood cells. These diseases are all characterized by an excess of the specific stem cells in the bone marrow and related expansion of the same cells in the bloodstream. Essential thrombocythemia (ET) is the overproduction of platelets, polycythemia vera (PV) is the

KEY TERMS

Androgen—Androgens are male sex hormones. A drug related to the male sex hormones may be referred to as an androgen.

Autoimmune disease—A disease that develops when white blood cells of the immune system attack normal cells of different organ systems as though they were foreign cells.

Biopsy—A sample of tissue taken and stained to examine under the microscope for cellular abnormalities. The technique used to obtain such samples is also called biopsy.

Bone marrow—A group of cells and molecules found in the centers of most bones.

Computed tomography (CT)—A special x-ray technique that produces a cross-sectional image of the organs inside the body.

Corticosteroids—A class of drugs, related to hormones produced by glands in the body, that suppress the immune system. Prednisone (Deltasone) and cortisone are examples of corticosteroids.

Erythromelalgia—A condition characterized by warmth, redness, and pain in the hands and especially the feet.

Erythropoietin—A drug that stimulates the bone marrow to make more red blood cells. It is also known as epoetin alfa.

Extracorporeal photochemotherapy—A treatment procedure in which the white blood cells are exposed to a chemical called psoralen, which is removed from the blood and treated with UVA light, then reinfused into the body.

Gout—A painful swelling of the joints, especially the feet, that results from an accumulation of uric acid crystals. This disease often affects the big toe.

Granulocyte—Any of three types of white blood cells (neutrophils, eosinophils, and basophils) that contain visible granules.

Lymph node—A small, bean-shaped organ of the immune system that contains white blood cells and lymphatic fluid. Lymph nodes are found singly and in clusters throughout the body. Reactions to infections usually begin in the lymph nodes, which may swell in response.

Median—A type of middle or average value. The median is the number in the middle of a sequence of numbers.

Myeloid progenitor cell—A stem cell normally found in the bone marrow that is responsible for making red blood cells, platelets, and some white blood cells (granulocytes and monocytes).

Phlebotomy—The removal of blood, usually through a vein.

Platelets—Tiny cells that are an essential component of the body's coagulation system, which act to begin the blood clotting process.

Red blood cells—The cells in the blood that carry iron-bearing hemoglobin, which delivers oxygen to tissues throughout the body.

Spleen—An organ in the abdomen near the stomach. The spleen makes white blood cells, stores red blood cells, and removes old blood cells from circulating blood.

Transfusion—An infusion of blood or blood products from a donor to another person.

Ultrasound—A diagnostic imaging technique that uses sound waves to form images of organs and blood vessels inside the body.

White blood cells—A group of cells in the blood, also known as immune cells, that fight infection.

overproduction of red blood cells, and **chronic myelocytic leukemia** (CML) is the overproduction of white cells called granulocytes. In two other MPNs, chronic neutrophilic leukemia and chronic eosinophilic leukemia, specific types of white cells are overproduced. The sixth disease, primary **myelofibrosis** (PMF)—also called idiopathic myelofibrosis or agnogenic myeloid metaplasia—is somewhat different. Initially, the bone marrow overproduces normal cells as in the other myeloproliferative diseases. However, in myelofibrosis, the bone marrow is replaced by fibrous tissue and the liver and spleen take over the production of blood cells, which leads to most of the associated symptoms. Some of these chronic MPNs can become acute leukemia, characterized by the production of too many abnormal white blood cells. Unclassifiable MPNs are also found, in which the characteristics do not fit into any of the other MPNs.

Description

The prefix "myelo-" refers to marrow. Bone marrow, a reddish or yellowish spongy substance in the middle of most bones, produces blood cells. In the myeloproliferative diseases, the bone marrow makes too many blood cells of a specific kind. Blood contains red blood cells to carry oxygen, white blood cells to fight infections, and platelets to begin blood clotting. Myeloproliferative diseases develop when a myeloid progenitor cell, a type of stem cell responsible for making either red blood cells, platelets, or certain types of white blood cells, becomes overactive. The abnormal progenitor cell continues to make normal blood cells, but makes too many of them. The excess of blood cells results in varying symptoms, depending on the progenitor cell involved.

Other problems develop when some of the abnormal myeloid progenitor cells travel to the spleen, liver, or lymph nodes and begin making blood cells there, as in primary myelofibrosis or advanced stages of the other chronic myeloproliferative diseases. Most often, they migrate to the spleen. An enlarged spleen can crowd other organs in the abdomen and cause discomfort or digestive troubles. Massively swollen spleens can use large amounts of energy and cause muscle wasting and **weight loss**. They may also travel to the liver, which becomes enlarged and subsequently has its functions compromised.

In the later stages of myeloproliferative diseases, the bone marrow can become scarred and fibrous, as in primary myelofibrosis. This may leave no space for progenitor cells. As a result, blood cell production can drop to dangerously low levels. The abnormal progenitor cells may also mutate and develop into acute leukemia. These two serious complications are rare in some myeloproliferative diseases but common in others.

Types of myeloproliferative disease

The six main myeloproliferative diseases include: essential thrombocythemia, polycythemia vera, primary myelofibrosis, chronic myelocytic leukemia, chronic neutrophilic leukemia, and chronic eosinophilic leukemia.

In essential thrombocythemia (primary thrombocythemia), the myeloid progenitor cell makes too many platelets, the tiny blood cells that are involved in blood clotting. Blood containing too many platelets may either clot too easily or too slowly. Blood that clots too easily can lead to a variety of health problems, including strokes or heart attacks. Blood that clots too slowly can cause symptoms such as easy bruising, frequent nosebleeds, bleeding from the gums, or life-threatening hemorrhages. Excessive numbers of platelets can also cause headaches or erythromelalgia, an unusual condition characterized by warmth, redness, and pain in the hands or feet. Typically, patients with this disease have long periods without symptoms, interspersed with clotting or bleeding episodes. Some patients may have no symptoms at all. Rarely, this disease ends in scarring of the bone marrow or leukemia. Patients with bone marrow scarring have symptoms identical to primary myelofibrosis.

In polycythemia vera (primary polycythemia, Vaquez disease), the bone marrow makes too many red blood cells. Large numbers of red blood cells can make the blood too thick. Viscous blood flows sluggishly, pools in the veins, and delivers oxygen poorly. Patients may experience headaches, dizziness, **fatigue**, chest pains, or weakness and cramping in the calves while walking. The abnormal blood flow can also result in bleeding tendencies or blood clotting inside the veins. Many patients also have increased numbers of white blood cells or platelets, but most symptoms are caused by the sluggish blood flow. The spleen often enlarges. Polycythemia rarely leads to leukemia, but occasionally ends in bone marrow scarring. Patients with polycythemia vera will usually have a reddish, ruddy complexion.

In chronic myelocytic leukemia (chronic myelogenous leukemia), the myeloid progenitor cell makes too many of the type of white blood cells called granulocytes, as their microscopic appearance is granular. The number of platelets can also increase in this disease. In the early stages of the disease, the white blood cells have a normal appearance, but in 90%–95% of patients, two chromosomes—number 9 and number 22— inside the progenitor cell have exchanged locations (chromosomal translocation). This chromosome rearrangement is known as the Philadelphia chromosome, and this genetic abnormality destabilizes these cells and inevitably they become cancerous. Two variations of this disease include chronic neutrophilic leukemia (in which white cells known as neutrophils are overproduced) and chronic eosinophilic leukemia (in which white cells called eosinophils are overproduced).

Primary myelofibrosis (idiopathic myelofibrosis, myelofibrosis with myeloid metaplasia, or agnogenic myeloid metaplasia) begins like other myeloproliferative diseases, with overproduction of blood cells. However, bone marrow scarring develops very quickly and the marrow is replaced by fibrous tissue. The production of blood cells shifts to the liver and spleen, which causes most of the symptoms. Without progenitor cells in the bone marrow, blood cell numbers drop, causing fatigue and weakness from **anemia**. Many of the cells found in the blood are also immature cells called blasts or are oddly shaped. Although myeloid progenitor cells in the spleen and liver can compensate to some degree, the enlargement of these organs creates additional problems. Occasionally, this disease also progresses to acute leukemia.

Demographics

Essential **thrombocytopenia**, polycythemia vera, and primary myelofibrosis are usually diagnosed in the sixth and seventh decades of life, at a median age of 67.

Essential thrombocythemia is found in 2.5 people in 100,000, which is the lowest of all chronic MPNs. It is slightly more common in younger women and the median age is 60 years, slightly younger than that of the other MPNs.

Polycythemia vera occurs in about 5 people in one million, more often in men. It has been shown to develop more often in people of Eastern European Jewish ancestry, but not all studies confirm this.

Primary myelofibrosis is found in 0.5 to 1.5 people per 100,000. It is more common in Caucasians, with men and women affected equally.

Causes and symptoms

No consistent chromosomal abnormalities have been discovered in essential thrombocythemia, polycythemia vera, or primary myelofibrosis. CML is the only MPN with a chromosomal translocation, although the JAK2 mutation is present in more than 90% of patients with PV and in about 50% of patients with the other MPNs. Activation of the JAK-STAT pathway is associated with uncontrolled cell growth. The presence of the JAK2 mutation may indicate a higher risk of developing cardiovascular complications. Risk of developing PV is greater in people exposed to the solvent **benzene**, or radiation such as that from atomic bombs. The cause of the abnormal mutation in stem cells (progenitor cells) that leads to these diseases is unknown, but research continues to investigate genetic origins.

Myeloproliferative diseases share many features, such as enlargement of the spleen and abnormalities in blood clotting. Symptoms that can be seen in any of these diseases include:

- fatigue
- poor appetite (anorexia)
- weight loss
- night sweats
- fullness in the stomach after eating only a small amount
- abdominal pain or discomfort, especially in the upper left side
- nosebleeds, bleeding from the gums, easy bruising, or intestinal bleeding
- symptoms of blood clots including strokes, heart attacks, pain and swelling in the legs, or difficulty breathing
- disturbances in vision

Other symptoms of essential thrombocythemia can include:

- weakness
- dizziness
- headaches
- prickling or tingling in the skin
- erythromelalgia (warmth, redness, and pain in the extremities)

Other symptoms of polycythemia vera can include:

- headaches
- dizziness
- ringing in the ears
- pain in the chest (angina)
- weakness or cramping pains in the legs that disappears during rest
- redness of the face
- a blue tinge to the skin and other body surfaces (cyanosis)
- high blood pressure
- itching, especially after a warm bath or shower
- tingling or prickling of the skin
- erythromelalgia
- ulcers
- kidney stones
- gout

Other symptoms of primary myelofibrosis can include:

- fever
- gout
- bone pain

Diagnosis

The diagnosis of a myeloproliferative disease relies mainly on a physical examination, diagnostic laboratory tests on blood samples, and sometimes a **bone marrow biopsy**. In a complete blood count and differential examination of a stained blood sample, the doctor will find excessive numbers of the cells characteristic of each disease and the number and kinds of white blood cells. The appearance of the cells on a peripheral blood smear may also help confirm the diagnosis. Chromosome studies (**cytogenetic analysis**) of blood and bone marrow can often distinguish chronic myelocytic leukemia from the other three diseases based on chromosomal changes. A JAK2 gene mutation test may also be done on blood or bone marrow to determine if this particular mutation is present; it is often found in essential thrombocythemia, polycythemia vera, or primary myelofibrosis. Bone marrow samples reveal increased cell production of specific cell types and sometimes scarring of bone marrow tissue. An enlarged spleen and/or enlarged liver can often be detected during palpation of the abdomen during a physical examination, but occasionally ultrasound or **computed tomography** scans may be necessary.

Myeloproliferative diseases can resemble normal reactions to infections and other diseases. Various diagnostic tests may be done to rule out such diseases.

Clinical staging

Although the World Health Organization has classified MPNs, there is no defined staging system for essential thrombocythemia or polycythemia vera. The Dynamic International Prognostic Scoring System (DIPSS) is used for staging primary myelofibrosis. It includes eight risk factors associated with survival, including: being over 65 years old, hemoglobin less than 8 g/dL, white blood cell count over 25×10^9/L, increased immature (blast) cells in the blood, weight loss or **fever** for more than one month, presence of the Philadelphia chromosome and/or JAK-2 gene mutation, low platelet count, and dependence on red blood cell transfusions. Each risk factor is one point and high risk is three points or more, with higher scores indicating greater risk of developing leukemia and poor survival.

Treatment

No curative treatments are available for the myeloproliferative diseases other than stem cell/bone marrow transplantation, which is not an appropriate procedure for all patients. Therefore, treatment will primarily involve the management of symptoms for each different disease unless the patient is a candidate for **stem cell transplantation**.

Essential thrombocythemia

Treatments for essential thrombocythemia lower the risk of bleeding or blood clots. Many patients only require careful watching with regular platelet counts. Higher-risk patients require cell reducing (cytoreductive) therapies. **Hydroxyurea** (Hydrea), a drug that suppresses platelet production, is often given to reduce risk of developing blood clots. Hydroxyurea has few side effects but can occasionally cause a rash, intestinal upsets, sores on the skin, or a fever. This drug may also slightly increase the risk of leukemia. Another drug, **anagrelide** (Agrylin), is effective in more than 90% of patients. It does not promote leukemia, but can cause dizziness, headaches, **diarrhea**, fluid retention, rapid heartbeat, and rare cases of heart failure. Hydroxyurea and anagrelide

both increase the risk of miscarriages during the first trimester in pregnant women. Interferon alfa is another option for patients with ET, but it is reserved mainly for high-risk women of childbearing age.

A patient under age 60 who has never had a blood clot has a 3% chance of developing one in the future. Some doctors recommend treatment for these patients only during high-risk situations such as surgery. Low-dose aspirin (81 mg) is sometimes given to reduce the risk of developing blood clots and to control symptoms such as erythromelalgia.

Polycythemia vera

Treatment of PV focuses on reducing hemoglobin levels and maintaining an acceptable balance between red cells and serum (hematocrit) in the blood. Periodically removing about a pint of blood, a process called phlebotomy, is a safe and effective way to treat polycythemia vera. Phlebotomy may increase the risk of blood clotting in the arm used to remove blood, but this is not likely to occur when the hematocrit (the percentage of red blood cells in the blood) is kept below 45% in men and 42% in women. Phlebotomy can result in symptoms of iron deficiency such as abnormal food cravings (particularly a craving for ice).

Patients who are unlikely to develop blood clots may not need any other treatments, although radioactive phosphorus and myelosuppressive drugs may be given to reduce the red blood cell production. Higher risk patients are sometimes given hydroxyurea, a cell reducing therapy, in addition to phlebotomy. This drug has relatively few side effects, but it may increase the chance of developing leukemia. In some studies, 3%–5% of patients taking hydroxyurea eventually developed leukemia, compared to 1.5%–2% treated with phlebotomy alone. Alternatives to hydroxyurea include interferon alpha and anagrelide. These drugs do not increase the risk of leukemia, but they tend to have more side effects. Interferon alpha may be particularly difficult to tolerate. Its side effects include flu-like symptoms (fever, chills, postnasal drip, and poor appetite), fatigue, weight loss, **depression**, insomnia, memory loss, and nausea.

Radioactive phosphorus is used mainly in elderly patients who do not expect to need many years of treatment. In 80%–90% of patients, this treatment can suppress the disease symptoms for six months to several years; however, up to 17% of patients develop leukemia within 15 years.

Other symptoms of polycythemia vera are treated with a variety of drugs. **Itching** is sometimes suppressed by phlebotomy, but antihistamines are often needed as well. Other options include extracorporeal photochemotherapy, hydroxyurea, or interferon alpha. **Allopurinol** (Zyloprim) prevents kidney stones and gout. Aspirin can suppress the symptoms of erythromelalgia.

One of the most difficult complications to treat is enlargement of the spleen. In the early stages of the disease, this enlargement can often be controlled by phlebotomy. Later, interferon alpha, hydroxyurea, or surgical removal may be necessary. Surgery to remove a very large spleen is difficult and can be fatal in up to 10% of patients. Complications can include infections, bleeding, serious blood clotting, or increased numbers of white blood cells and platelets. Radiation treatments directed at the spleen may be another option, but they can suppress the bone marrow.

Primary myelofibrosis

Primary myelofibrosis may sometimes be cured by a stem cell transplant from a healthy donor, obtaining stem cells from either the donor's blood or bone marrow. Stem cell transplantation successfully replaces the abnormal stem cells with healthy stem cells in about one-third of patients who are eligible for this treatment. It may not be feasible for older patients or those in poor health since the procedure can have serious or fatal complications, including infections, organ damage, and bleeding. In addition, compatible donors are not available for all patients and older patients are less likely to have healthy siblings as stem cell donors. Stem cell transplantation is reserved for patients aged 45 to 60, while patients older than 60 are considered for **investigational drugs**.

Other treatments for this disease are not curative and are mainly intended to improve the patient's quality of life. Anemia is often treated with regular transfusions of red blood cells. Adverse effects can include heart failure or damage to the liver from excess iron. Drugs can sometimes make red blood cells last longer. **Corticosteroids** (prednisone) combined with an androgen (**fluoxymesterone**) are effective in about a third of all patients. **Danazol**, another androgen, works in about 20% of patients. These drugs may damage the liver and can produce masculine traits in women. Injections of erythropoietin, a hormone that stimulates red blood cell production, also work in a few patients. Granulocyte-colony stimulating factor is given for decreased white blood cell counts (**neutropenia**). Immunomodulatory drugs such as **thalidomide**, lenalidomide, and **pomalidomide** are all being investigated for PMF treatment.

About half of all patients with anemia improve after surgical removal of the spleen (**splenectomy**). This surgery can also help patients who have abdominal discomfort, weight loss, muscle wasting, or high blood pressure in the liver. However, the surgery itself is dangerous and can sometimes be fatal. In some cases, removal of the spleen may make the disease progress more quickly.

A painfully enlarged spleen can also be treated with hydroxyurea, interferon alpha, or radiation treatments. Hydroxyurea has few side effects, but it may increase the risk of leukemia. Interferon alpha shrinks the spleen in 30%–50% of patients, but has many side effects. Radiation treatments can decrease the symptoms for three to six months, but sometimes fatally suppress the blood-producing cells.

Alternative and complementary therapies

In traditional Chinese and Japanese medicine, herbal preparations are used to treat symptoms of chronic illnesses such as fatigue, loss of appetite, and **night sweats**, or to decrease red blood cell formation in polycythemia vera. Patients who are interested in complementary remedies are advised to discuss them with their doctors. Some may have dangerous side effects or be harmful when combined with conventional treatment.

Prognosis

Patients with essential thrombocythemia can expect a near normal life-span. The average (median) survival is 12 to 15 years. The chance of developing leukemia is less than 10%, and less than 5% for developing myelofibrosis of the bone marrow. Most patients with ET die from complications associated with blood clots (thrombosis). The 5-year survival rate is 74% to 93%.

Patients with polycythemia vera can usually be managed with therapeutic phlebotomies to maintain relatively normal red blood cell counts. With treatment, the average survival rate is about 10 years in older patients and more than 15 years in younger patients. Many patients can reach their normal life expectancy if they do not develop myelofibrosis of the bone marrow or leukemia. The risk of bone marrow scarring (myelofibrosis) after 10 years is approximately 15%–20%. If polycythemia vera is treated with phlebotomy alone, the risk of developing leukemia is 2%. Without treatment, patients with polycythemia vera usually die from bleeding (hemorrhage) or blood clotting (thrombosis) within months.

Patients with primary myelofibrosis may have a few years of relatively good health status, but overall, PMF has the worst prognosis. Unless PMF patients are able to receive a successful stem cell transplant, the disease will become progressively worse. The anemia becomes more severe and the liver and spleen remain enlarged, resulting in discomfort and digestive disturbances. The average survival time for this disease is 3.5 to 5.5 years, but survival is often unpredictable and may be much longer or much shorter. Acute leukemia develops in about 10%–25% of patients. In other patients, death occurs from heart failure, infections, bleeding (hemorrhage) or blood clots (thrombosis).

If patients with any of the MNPs develop fibrosis in the bone marrow, the risk of developing acute myeloid leukemia is much greater and patients typically die within three years.

Coping with cancer treatment

Acetaminophen and antidepressant drugs can help reduce some of the side effects of interferon alpha. Taking this drug at night may also make it easier to tolerate.

Clinical trials

The following therapies are being tested in **clinical trials**. Patients are advised to check with their medical insurers before enrolling in a clinical trial. Insurers may not pay for some treatments, but this varies with the insurer and each individual case.

Interferon alpha injections are being tested in essential thrombocythemia. This drug can lower platelet numbers and decrease the size of the spleen in about 80% of patients.

Several new drugs are in clinical trials. Thalidomide and SU5416 are being tested in patients with primary myelofibrosis. R115777 and 12-O-tetradecanoylphorbol-13-acetate (TPA) are in clinical trials open to patients with various myeloproliferative diseases.

Another possible treatment for primary myelofibrosis is to extract and purify normal progenitor cells and return them to the body after destroying the abnormal progenitor cells with **chemotherapy**.

Prevention

The following environmental factors have been linked to myeloproliferative diseases:

- working as an electrician or in a petroleum manufacturing plant
- prolonged use of dark hair dyes
- exposure to nuclear bomb blasts or thorium dioxide

Special concerns

Whether polycythemia vera, essential thrombocythemia, and primary myelofibrosis progress to leukemia is influenced by the specific treatment strategies. Some treatments, particularly radioactive phosphorus, can substantially increase the risk of disease progression to acute myeloid leukemia.

See also Acute myelocytic leukemia; Bone marrow aspiration and biopsy; Chromosome rearrangements; Cytology; Hypercoagulation disorders; Leukemias, chronic; Myelosuppression; Radiation therapy; Ultrasonography.

Resources

BOOKS

Duggan, Peter. "Polycythemia Vera." In *Conn's Current Therapy 2014; Expert Consult*, 55th ed. Philadelphia: W. B. Saunders, 2014, 856–863.

PERIODICALS

Passamonti, F., F. Cervantes, and A. M. Vannucchi, et al. "A Dynamic Prognostic Model to Predict Survival in Primary Myelofibrosis: a Study by the IWG-MRT (International Working Group for Myeloproliferative Neoplasms Research and Treatment)." *Blood* 115 (Jan 2010): 1703–1708.

Tefferi, A., and W. Vainchenker. "Myeloproliferative Neoplasms: Molecular Pathophysiology, Essential Clinical Understanding, and Treatment Strategies." *Journal of Clinical Oncology* 29 (May 2011): 573–582.

Tefferi, A., J. Thiele, and A. Orazi, et al. "Proposals and Rationale for Revision of the World Health Organization Diagnostic Criteria for Polycythemia Vera, Essential Thrombocythemia, and Primary Myelofibrosis." *Blood* 110 (May 2007): 1092–1097.

Tonkin, J., Y. Francis, A. Pattinson, et al. "Myeloproliferative Neoplasms: Diagnosis, Management and Treatment." *Nursing Standards* 26 (Aug 2012): 44–51.

WEBSITES

Keng, Michael, Anjali Advani, and Karl Theil. "The Myeloproliferative Neoplasms." Cleveland Clinic Medical Education. http://www.clevelandclinicmeded.com/medical pubs/diseasemanagement/hematology-oncology/chronic-myelproliferative-disorders/ (accessed October 2, 2014).

National Cancer Institute "General Information About Chronic Myeloproliferative Neoplasms." http://www.cancer.gov/cancertopics/pdq/treatment/myeloproliferative/Patient/page1 (accessed October 2, 2014).

ORGANIZATIONS

MPD-Net Online Support Group from Myeloproliferative Diseases Research Center, Inc., 115 East 72nd Street, New York, NY 10021, http://inform.acor.org/mpd/index.htm.

The National Organization for Rare Disorders, PO Box 8923, New Fairfield, CT 06812-8923, (800) 999-6673, http://www.rarediseases.org.

L. Lee Culvert
Anna Rovid Spickler, DVM, PhD

Myelosuppression

Definition

Myelosuppression is a decrease in the production of blood cells by the bone marrow.

Description

Normally, the blood contains large numbers of cells, including red blood cells to carry oxygen, white blood cells to fight infection, and platelets to begin the clotting process when needed. These cells are all made in the bone marrow, a reddish or yellowish substance found in the centers of most bones. Healthy bone marrow makes large numbers of stem cells each day that will mature into red blood cells, white blood cells, and platelets, replacing those that wear out and die off and ensuring that the functions of each cell type will continue. In myelosuppression, the bone marrow's production of stem cells is suppressed and too few mature cells are found in the blood. The functions performed by each cell type will be diminished, which will lead to the development of symptoms. Myelosuppression can occur as a result of a disease process such as **cancer**, induced by cell-killing (cytotoxic) drugs and radiation used in cancer treatment, or exposure to other toxic substances.

A decrease in the number of red blood cells, called **anemia**, occurs in about 70% to 90% of cancer patients whose cells are being exposed to **chemotherapy** or radiation. A drop in numbers of white blood cells often creates complications during chemotherapy. A type of white blood cell called neutrophils are affected most severely. A decrease in these cells is called **neutropenia**. Because neutrophils are responsible for defending the body against bacteria and other invading pathogens, neutropenia increases the chance of an infection. **Thrombocytopenia**, a drop in the number of platelets in the blood, is more rare; a reduction in the number of platelets that is low enough to cause problems occurs in fewer than 10% of cancer patients.

Myelosuppression is a painless condition, but the decreases in important blood cells can result in **fatigue** and shortness of breath if red cells are reduced, an increased risk of infection if white cells are reduced, and bruising and excessive bleeding if platelets are reduced. The consequences vary from mild to life-threatening, depending on which cells are affected and how low the blood cell numbers fall.

Causes and symptoms

The most common cause of myelosuppression is cancer treatment, including both radiation and chemotherapy. Although chemotherapy and radiation are targeted at killing cancer cells, their effects also destroy normal cells. Many of the drugs used in chemotherapy temporarily suppress the bone marrow. **Radiation therapy** that reaches the bone marrow is also destructive and may suppress cell production. Cancer cells themselves may also cause myelosuppression. Some cancers invade the bone marrow and crowd out the cells normally found there. Others can suppress the bone marrow without invasion. Nutritional deficiencies, common in cancer patients, also slow blood cell production, as do viruses and certain non-chemotherapy drugs.

Myelosuppression usually starts seven to ten days after an injury to the bone marrow. However, the bone marrow generally returns to normal within the next few weeks. Less often, cumulative damage can be caused. Occasionally, irreversible damage causes permanent myelosuppression. High-dose chemotherapy or intensive radiation therapy can destroy all of the cells in the bone marrow.

The symptoms of myelosuppression depend on the type of blood cell that is depleted, and the severity of the depletion. Low red blood cells result in anemia, which can cause severe fatigue, shortness of breath, and decreased functional capacity. Low white blood cells result in an increased risk of serious infection, which may

KEY TERMS

Anemia—Too few red blood cells in the blood.

Blood cells—The red blood cells, white blood cells, and platelets produced in the bone marrow and released into the blood.

Bone marrow—A spongy tissue in the center of most bones that makes all of the cells found in the blood.

Erythropoietin—A growth factor that stimulates the bone marrow to make more red blood cells. It is also known as epoetin alfa.

Febrile neutropenia—A reduced neutrophil count (less than 0.5×10^9/l) accompanied by fever (an elevated oral temperature greater than 101.3°F [38.5°C]).

Granulocyte colony-stimulating factor (G-CSF)—A protein and a type of hormone called a growth factor that stimulates the bone marrow to make neutrophils and some other types of white blood cells. Pharmaceutical granulocyte colony-stimulating factors are filgrastim (Neupogen) and lenograstim (Granisetron).

Granulocyte-macrophage colony-stimulating factor (GM-CSF)—A growth factor that stimulates the bone marrow to make neutrophils and some other types of white blood cells. Pharmaceutical GM-CSFs are sargramostim and molgramostim.

Growth factor—A hormone that can stimulate body cells to grow or stimulate the bone marrow to make more cells. Growth factors are found naturally in the body, but synthetic versions can also be manufactured as drugs.

Interleukin 11 (IL-11)—A growth factor that stimulates the bone marrow to make platelets. Its pharmaceutical counterpart is oprelvekin.

Neutropenia—Too few of the white cells called neutrophils in the blood.

Neutrophil—A type of white blood cell that seeks out and attacks pathogens such as bacteria, viruses, and fungi.

Packed red blood cells—Blood obtained from a donor that has had the fluid portion (plasma) removed so that only red cells are transfused.

Platelets—Tiny cells in the blood that are an essential component of the body's coagulation system. Platelets begin the blood clotting process.

Red blood cells—The cells in the blood that deliver oxygen to all tissues throughout the body.

Thrombocytopenia—Too few platelets in the blood.

Transfusion—A transfer of blood or blood products donated by one person to be given to another.

Transfusion reaction—An allergic reaction of the recipient of donated blood to some of the cells or proteins in donor blood.

White blood cells—The cells in the blood that fight infection, including different types called neutrophils, lymphocytes, monocytes, and eosinophils, among others.

---

manifest in **fever** and symptoms specific to the area of the infection. If fever is present, the patient may have a condition called febrile neutropenia, which can result in serious complications. A low platelet count may result in an increased risk of bruising and bleeding, including the possibility of severe hemorrhage.

Treatment

Myelosuppression is not always treated, especially if it is mild. Blood cell counts are monitored closely and treatments are primarily focused on stimulating the bone marrow to resume the growth of cells. If myelosuppression is a result of chemotherapy or radiation therapy, the cancer treatments may be stopped, delayed, or reduced to give the bone marrow a chance to recover. This may mean that the full dose of the treatment is not received.

Antibiotic therapy

Careful monitoring of possible neutropenia in cancer patients is important. If a cancer patient has a fever and other signs of possible infection, the physician may treat the patient with intravenous **antibiotics**, possibly for several days.

Transfusion therapy

Restoring red blood cell counts and platelet counts may require replacing them with transfusions of packed red blood cells or concentrated platelets. These treatments can be very effective in the short term; however, the transfused cells are short-lived and the treatment may need to be repeated. The possibility of a transfusion reaction must also be considered, although the risk is low.

Growth factors

Injections of growth factors may be used to stimulate production of cells by the bone marrow. Hematopoietic growth factors are hormones produced naturally in the body. Synthetic hematopoietic growth factors are given to stimulate the bone marrow to make stem cells that will mature into specific blood cells. The pharmaceutical growth factors in common use include erythropoietin (EPO), granulocyte colony-stimulating factor (G-CSF, or **filgrastim**), granulocyte-macrophage colony-stimulating factor (GM-CSF, or **sargramostim**), and interleukin II (**oprelvekin**). Erythropoietin injections can stimulate red blood cell production, decrease the need for transfusions, and generally improve patients' quality of life. This drug has few side effects if the kidneys are healthy, but it may not be effective if the body is already making enough natural erythropoietin. G-CSF and GM-CSF products can speed the growth and return of healthy neutrophils. A form of filgrastim called pegfilgrastim is given as a single dose by cutaneous injection once in each chemotherapy cycle. **Clinical trials** have shown that this treatment simply, safely, and effectively maintains neutrophil counts in patients undergoing myelosuppressive chemotherapy. G-CSF has also been shown to ameliorate the effects of ionizing radiation. The side effects of this type of growth factor therapy may include **bone pain**, fevers, rashes, muscle pains, and nausea, which are easily treated with appropriate medications. Interleukin II is given to increase platelet counts. Its side effects may include fluid retention, a rapid heartbeat, red eyes, and difficulty breathing. Growth factors are expensive and several injections are usually needed.

Other treatments

Chemotherapy- or radiation-induced myelosuppression may lead to complete destruction of the bone marrow, called residual bone marrow injury, which is incompatible with life. If the bone marrow is severely damaged, a bone marrow transplant may be necessary to provide new, healthy stem cells that will grow into mature red and white blood cells and platelets if the bone marrow responds.

Supportive therapy can help to minimize the effects of myelosuppression. If nutrition is a contributing factor, iron or vitamin supplements may be beneficial. Antibiotics may be used prophylactically to aid in preventing infections. Some patients find that mild exercise and enjoyable distractions help with fatigue.

Prognosis

The prognosis of myelosuppression depends on the underlying cause, the ability to reverse it, and the level

---

QUESTIONS TO ASK YOUR DOCTOR

- What is causing my reduced cell counts?
- Should treatment that may be causing the myelosuppression be stopped or postponed?
- What types of additional treatment would you recommend to increase my blood cell counts?
- What types of side effects can I expect from treatment?
- What are your recommendations to help me deal with those side effects?
- Am I eligible for any clinical trials? Would these be helpful to consider?

---

of severity. Severe myelosuppression can result in life-threatening anemia, infections, and massive bleeding. The risk of death and shortened survival time is increased by 65% in patients with anemia from myelosuppressive chemotherapy and radiation compared to cancer patients without anemia. The death rate in febrile neutropenia is 5% in patients with solid tumors, 11% in patients with blood cancers, and 18% in patients with bacterial infections that lead to sepsis. In addition, dose reduction and delays in chemotherapy or radiation can compromise treatment outcomes and decrease patients' overall survival. Frequently, however, the prognosis can be improved through timely treatments that address the underlying deficiency and help to encourage cell growth.

Prevention

Prevention of chemotherapy- and radiation-induced myelosuppression is limited. However, the use of simultaneous treatments such as growth factor administration may at least minimize the effects of chemotherapy on cell growth and keep myelosuppression from becoming severe. In time, certain aspects of myelosuppression may be preventable. The administration of stem cell factor (SCF) constantly during chemotherapy has been shown to proactively prevent chemotherapy-induced anemia and thrombocytopenia in mice, leading researchers to believe that this strategy may become part of supportive therapy for cancer patients. Gene therapies that increase tolerance to chemotherapy are also being explored in clinical trials.

See also Bone marrow transplantation; Immunosuppression; Transfusion therapy.

Resources

BOOKS

Hoffman, Ronald, Edward J. Benz, Leslie E. Silberstein, et al, eds. *Hematology: Basic Principles and Practice*. 6th ed. Philadelphia: Saunders Elsevier, 2013.

Niederhuber, John E., James O. Armitage, James H. Doroshow, and Michael B. Kastan, eds. *Abeloff's Clinical Oncology*. 5th ed. Philadelphia: Elsevier, 2014.

PERIODICALS

Bartucci, M., R. Dattilo, and D. Martinetti, et al. "Prevention of Chemotherapy-induced Anemia and Thrombocytopenia by Constant Administration of Stem Cell Factor." *Clinical Cancer Research* 17 (Oct 2011): 6185–6191.

De Naurois, J., I. Novitzky-Basso, and M. J. Gill, et al. "Management of Febrile Neutropenia: ESMO Clinical Practice Guidelines." *Annals of Oncology* 21 (2010) Suppl 5: 252–256.

Gilreath, J. A., D. D. Stenehjem, and G. M. Rodgers. "Diagnosis and Treatment of Cancer-related Anemia." *American Journal of Hematology* 89 (Feb 2014): 203–212.

Li, D., Y. Wang, and H. Wu, et al. "Mitigation of Ionizing Radiation-induced Bone Marrow Suppression by p38 Inhibition and G-CSF Administration." *Journal of Radiation Research* 52 (Oct 2011): 712–716.

Strati, P., W. Wierda, and J. Burger, et al. "Myelosuppression After Frontline Fludaravine, Cyclophosphamide, and Rituximab in Patients With Chronic Lymphocytic Leukemia: Analysis of Persistent and New-onset Cytopenia." *Cancer* 119 (Nov 2013): 3805–3811.

Teuffel, O., and L. Sung. "Advances in Management of Low-risk Febrile Neutropenia." *Current Opinion in Pediatrics* 24 (Feb 2013): 40–45.

ORGANIZATIONS

National Cancer Institute, Building 31 Room 10A31 31 Center Drive MSC 2580, Bethesda MD 20892-2580, (800) 4-CANCER (422-6237), http://cancernet.nci.nih.gov.

L. Lee Culvert
Anna Rovid Spickler, DVM, PhD

Myleran *see* **Busulfan**

Nasal cancer

Definition

Nasal **cancer** includes any cancer that occurs within the nose, either in the nasal vestibule (the immediate interior of the nose, just beyond the nostrils), or the nasal cavity (the deep interior of the nose). Many different types of cancer can occur within the nose, and the type of treatment and the chance of cure will vary according to the type of cancer that occurs.

Description

Nasal cancers are very rare, making up less than 2% of all tumors of the respiratory tract in the United States. Fewer than 50 cases a year are diagnosed in the United States. Although squamous cell **carcinoma** is the most common type of cancer that occurs within the nose, many other types can also occur, including: **adenocarcinoma**, **melanoma**, different kinds of sarcomas, inverted papilloma, **lymphoma**, and esthesioneuroblastoma.

Squamous cell carcinomas arise from skin tissue. They are the most common type and are often the result of either cigarette smoking or occupational exposure to dusts or chemical fumes. Adenocarcinomas are malignancies that resemble glandular tissue. Nasal adenocarcinomas are also often associated with occupational exposure to dusts or chemical fumes. T-cell lymphomas (non-Hodgkin) in the nasal area are strongly associated with a virus (**Epstein-Barr virus**, EBV). Although nasal T-cell lymphomas are fairly common in some parts of the world, they are very rare in the United States.

Inverted papillomas are associated with another virus (**human papillomavirus**, HPV) and arise from benign but locally invasive nasal polyps. They are rare, comprising only about 0.5% of all nasal tumors. Although a definite association with HPV has been shown, a tumor may require interaction of the virus with chemicals or other factors, which appear to cause transformation of the inverted papilloma into squamous cell carcinoma in the nose. Esthesioneuroblastoma is a very rare nasal tumor, with fewer than 200 cases reported in the last 25 years. They are tumors that arise in the nerves in the nose, and have occurred most commonly in teenagers and older adults.

Demographics

Although the overall risk of nasal cancer is quite low (because this type of cancer is very rare), relative risks for some specific groups are fairly high. For example, nasal T-cell lymphomas are virus-associated and occur in high incidence in Asia and South America. Nasal squamous cell carcinomas occur much more frequently in cigarette smokers and individuals who have occupational exposures to dusts or chemical fumes, especially in Europe. Consumption of salted and pickled foods creates an increased relative risk of nasal cancer in Asia. Nasal cancers are also more frequent in some African populations that use mahogany wood in cooking fires.

In the United States, nasal cancers are rare; about 2,000 are diagnosed in an average year. Recent evidence indicates that Caucasians are slightly more likely than members of other races or ethnic groups to develop nasal cancers. Males experience all types of nasal cancer in significantly greater numbers than women, probably due to greater occupational exposure to agents that can cause these types of cancer. About 80% of nasal cancers occur in people aged 55 or over, although the rare esthesioneuroblastoma has occurred in relatively high percentages in adolescents. Nasal cancers are very rare in children; fewer than 300 have been recorded in the United States from 1973 through 2010, with children below the age of 4 and adolescents between 15 and 19 having the lowest survival rates.

Causes and symptoms

All cancers are caused when a genetic mutation is made in a gene that is involved in the control of cell

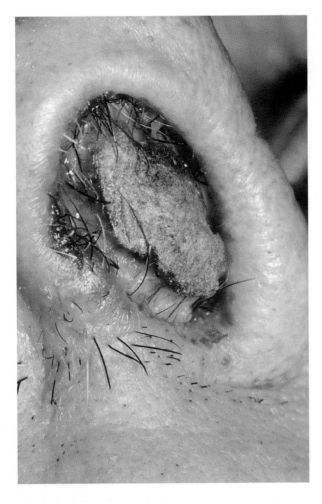

Cancerous tumor in the nose. *(J. Barabe/Custom Medical Stock Photo)*

usually metastasize, but which may turn malignant. These are also thought to be caused by a virus, although a different one: human papillomavirus (HPV). Some nasal cancers have a strong hereditary component: people with genetic alterations that cause hereditary **retinoblastoma** (a type of eye cancer usually found in children) have a much higher incidence of nasal cancers than average, which indicates that the genetic change that caused their original disease may also contribute to nasal cancer.

People with nasal cancer may think that they have a cold or chronic sinus infections. They may experience a feeling of stuffiness or blockage in the nose, persistent nasal drainage, or frequent nose bleeds. Other symptoms can occur if the tumor has invaded other tissues around the nose, particularly the orbit of the eye or the base of the skull. Other symptoms may include:

• double vision

• pain above or below the eye

• pus draining from the nose

• numbness or pain in parts of the face

• pain or pressure in one of the ears

• decreased sense of smell

• bulging of the eye

• a lump on the face or around the eye

• loose teeth

• frequent headaches

In advanced stages, patients with nasal cancers may suffer from **fatigue**, **weight loss**, lack of appetite (**anorexia**), and **fever**.

Diagnosis

There were no screening tests for nasal cancer as of 2014, partly because the disease is rare, and partly because of the complex structure of the mouth, throat, and nasal cavity. When otherwise unexplainable symptoms lead a doctor or dentist to suspect that a patient may have nasal cancer, often he or she will arrange for an endoscopic examination of the nasal cavity (and possibly the sinuses) in order to see if there is a tumor. In most cases, the patient will be referred to an otolaryngologist, a doctor who specializes in diagnosing and treating disorders of the head and neck.

Definite diagnosis requires a **biopsy**, in which a small piece of the tumor is cut out and examined to see what types of cells it contains. After a nasal cancer is diagnosed (depending on the type of cancer), many doctors will ask the patient to have an x-ray, **computed tomography** scanning (CT scan), or **magnetic resonance imaging** (MRI). These techniques visualize the tumor and show the doctor how much the tumor has

division. This mistake can arise naturally, can be inherited, or it can be caused by a virus, by sunlight or other radiation, or by some chemical that a person is exposed to, usually through eating, drinking, or breathing. For nasal cancers, all of these factors have been shown to play a part. There are, however, no known (as of 2014) inherited tendencies for nasal cancer.

The use of tobacco products has been strongly associated with the occurrence of nasal adenocarcinomas and squamous cell carcinomas. Chronic occupational exposures to baking flour, leather, wool, wood dust, chemical mixtures (particularly nickel, dioxane, nitrosamine, and chromium used in dye manufacturing), mustard gas, rubbing alcohol, or formaldehyde have a demonstrated association with nasal adenocarcinomas and squamous cell carcinomas as well. Some rare nasal T-cell lymphomas have been shown to be very strongly associated with the Epstein-Barr virus (EBV). Some nasal malignancies (about 5%) begin as inverted papillomas, a locally aggressive tumor which does not

KEY TERMS

Brachytherapy—A form of radiation therapy in which small pellets of radioactive material are placed inside or near the area to be treated. It is also known as internal radiation therapy or sealed-source radiotherapy.

Carcinoma—Any malignant tumor.

Endoscopy—A diagnostic procedure in which a miniature videocamera on the end of a flexible tube is inserted into internal body cavities so that the physician can view the internal structures.

Lymphoma—A type of cancer that arises in the lymph nodes.

Nasal polyp—A noncancerous teardrop-shaped mass that grows out from the inner lining of the nasal cavity.

Palliative care—Care intended to relieve pain and other symptoms rather than cure the disease.

Papilloma—A wart-like growth with a bumpy surface that can grow inside the nasal cavity and destroy healthy tissue. Papillomas are not themselves cancerous, but can give rise to squamous cell carcinomas.

Prosthesis—An artificial device used to replace a missing body part.

Retinoblastoma—A type of eye cancer that usually develops in children. There is some evidence that retinoblastoma is a risk factor for nasal cancer.

Sarcoma—A tumor that arises from bone or connective tissue.

Squamous cell carcinoma—A malignancy that arises from outer skin cells.

Targeted therapy—In cancer treatment, a type of drug therapy that blocks tumors by interfering with specific molecules that the cancer cells need for growth. Also called biologic therapy, targeted therapy is less harmful to normal cells than traditional chemotherapy.

invaded surrounding tissues. Because treatment for nasal cancer, as well as **paranasal sinus cancer**, involves surgery in a small, complex space that requires the surgeon to set very precise surgical boundaries, and because most nasal cancers are advanced by the time a patient sees a doctor, it is very important that the doctor evaluate the tumor thoroughly before planning treatment. If the tumor appears to have invaded other tissues, often a

doctor will schedule a surgical exploration of the tumor in order to better evaluate the cancer, with the goal of constructing the best possible treatment plan. In addition, sometimes surgical exploration is necessary to determine whether the position and invasion of the tumor into surrounding tissue make surgical removal of the tumor impossible.

Treatment team

As the understanding of cancer grows and new treatment approaches are developed, the complexity of cancer treatment also increases. Today, a multidisciplinary approach to cancer treatment is considered necessary for effective patient care. People involved in the treatment of a nasal cancer will typically include the referring physician, an otolaryngologist, an anesthesiologist, a medical oncologist, a pathologist, and a nurse. If **radiation therapy** is pursued, a radiation oncologist, radiation therapist, radiation nurse, radiation physicist, and a dosimetrist will also be involved. Treatment can also include a psychologist, nutritionist, dentist, social worker, or religious advisor. For nasal cancers, a reconstructive or plastic surgeon may be necessary for optimum cosmetic results after removal of a nasal tumor. If surgical removal of the eye is necessary, specialists in prosthetic eye replacement will be necessary as well.

Clinical staging

When a cancer develops, the original tumor can spread, usually through the blood or lymph system, to other parts of the body. Since the cancer spreads through the lymph system, often the lymph nodes in the area of the original tumor are the first other sites where cancerous cells can be found. Other common places that metastatic disease may appear are the lungs, the liver, and the bones.

One of the foremost goals of a doctor's assessment of a cancer patient is to determine how far the cancer has already spread and how likely it is to spread further, both of which are key factors in the likelihood that the patient will be cured. The assessment of the tumor's spread is termed staging, and the assessment of how aggressive the cancer cells are is termed grading.

Staging of nasal cancers is performed by visual inspection of tumors (perhaps through endoscopy) or visualization of tumors by imaging techniques like **x-rays**, MRIs, or CT scans. The doctor may also attempt to feel for tumors manually. This information will be used to create an official stage for the tumor that is a standardized expression of how much the tumor has already spread.

Because tumors of the nasal vestibule and cavity are rare, and because they are comprised of so many different types, no single staging system has been defined for use with these cancers. Cancers of the paranasal sinuses have a defined staging system based on the TNM system, and this system is often used for describing nasal cancers. The T in the TNM system represents the growth of the local tumor, N describes the spread of the tumor to the lymph nodes, and M describes the spread, or **metastasis**, of the cancer to distant body sites. The cancer is given various numbered ratings in each letter category, and these are used to create a standardized stage. Generally, tumors that are limited to the upper surface of the nasal mucosa with no invasion of local tissues are described as stage I, while tumors with minimal invasion of local tissues are identified as stage II. Tumors that have extensive local invasion or that have spread to the lymph nodes but not metastasized are described as stage III or early stage IV (A and B). Stage IVC tumors are any tumors that have metastasized to other body organs.

Most nasal cancers (up to 80%) have already spread to other body sites by the time the symptoms prompt patients to see their doctor. This fact, combined with the fact that the area is anatomically complex and tightly constructed, makes it very important that the first attempt at treatment is well planned, with input from a multidisciplinary team and thorough evaluation of the cancer before treatment is begun.

Treatment

Because cancers of the nasal cavity and vestibule include many different types of cancers, treatment will vary depending on the type of cancer involved, where it is located, and the extent to which it has already spread. Because of this, and because of the complexity of the anatomy in the area and the multitude of other important structures that may be involved in later stages, treatment of nasal cancers is highly individualized, with no firm standard practice guidelines.

For most nasal cancers, treatment will involve surgical removal of the tumor, plus an area of normal skin surrounding it. This procedure is called a wide local excision and is followed by four to five weeks of radiation therapy. If the cancer has reached the skin or has deeply invaded the structure of the nose itself, part or all of the nose may need to be removed. In such cases, the nose can be reconstructed from tissues taken from the face or other parts of the body, or a prosthetic (artificial) nose may be used.

In advanced cancers, preoperative radiation therapy may also be employed. However, since radiation therapy has proven very effective for nasal cancers and because radiation has better cosmetic results than surgical removal of a tumor, for many nasal cancers (especially T-cell lymphomas and esthesioneuroblastomas), radiation will be the initial treatment option. If the doctor decides to remove as much of the tumor as possible surgically, radiation therapy (external) will usually be used for four to five weeks after surgery in order to destroy any remaining cancerous tissue. One exception is the case of inverted papillomas, for which surgical excision alone is usually employed. Surgery, because of the tight anatomical area in which a surgeon must work, may also involve more recent techniques like cryosurgery (freezing tissue) or laser surgery.

Tumors initially treated by either radiation or surgery alone may, if they come back, be treated by the untried option or by employing both. External radiation may be supplemented, especially in advanced nasal vestibule cancer, by internal radioactive implants; this type of radiation therapy is known as brachytherapy. In addition, nasal cancer may be treated by **chemotherapy**, usually involving a combination of drugs. Chemotherapy was previously reserved for only advanced or recurrent nasal cancers, but is being used more frequently as a first-line or concurrent treatment. Drugs are used in combination in most chemotherapy because combinations of different drugs (with different side effects) deliver the highest cancer-destroying effect, while minimizing the chance for a serious adverse reaction to the therapy. The drug combinations used in nasal cancer vary depending on the type of cancer and may include: **cisplatin, fluorouracil, bleomycin, carboplatin, vinblastine,** or **methotrexate**. A newer form of pharmacotherapy is targeted therapy (sometimes called biologic therapy), which uses drugs that block the growth of cancer cells by targeting specific molecules that the cancer cells need for growth and reproduction. The targeted drug used most often to treat advanced nasal cancer is **cetuximab**, which may be combined with radiation therapy. In addition, nasal cancers described as stage III or IV will probably be treated with preventive radiation therapy of the neck area, in order to destroy cancerous cells that may have traveled to the lymph nodes.

Alternative and complementary therapies

Alternative and complementary therapies are treatments that are not traditional, first-line therapies like surgery, chemotherapy, and radiation. Complementary therapies are those that are meant to supplement traditional therapies and usually have the objective of relieving symptoms or helping cancer patients cope with the disease or traditional treatments. Alternative therapies are nontraditional treatments that are chosen instead of traditional treatments in an attempt to cure the disease. Alternative therapies have typically not been proven to be effective in the same way that traditional drugs are evaluated; that is, through **clinical trials**.

Common complementary therapies that may be employed by patients with nasal cancer are art therapy, massage, meditation, visualization, music therapy, prayer, t'ai chi, and yoga or other forms of exercise, which reduce anxiety and can increase a patient's feeling of well-being.

Prognosis

Although nasal cancers are made up of many different types of cancer, all types of nasal cancers are considered aggressive. The majority of nasal cancers are already in advanced stages when a patient seeks medical help, because symptoms mimic upper respiratory illnesses and often do not occur until the cancer has already filled the nasal cavity and invaded surrounding tissues. For this reason, and because treatment is difficult because of the complexity of the anatomical area, five-year survival rates are low. According to the American Cancer Society, only 63% of patients with stage I nasal cancer are alive five years later. The five-year figures for later stages are as follows: stage II, 61%; stage III, 50%; and stage IV, 35%. If the first treatment attempt is successful and a patient is cancer-free at two years, however, chances of longer-term survival improve greatly.

Nasal cancer is unusual in that, although many patients have metastasis to the lymph nodes or beyond (usually to the lungs), metastasis is not usually the reason for a patient's death. Most nasal cancer patients who succumb to the disease die from invasion of the tumor into vital areas of the brain.

Coping with cancer treatment

Treatment of nasal cancers commonly includes surgery, radiation therapy, and chemotherapy. Although the use of chemotherapy and radiation therapy in addition to surgery has improved the chance of survival for nasal cancer patients, both of these treatments unavoidably result in damage to some healthy tissues and other undesirable side effects.

Fatigue is a very common side effect of both radiation therapy and chemotherapy. Side effects of the actual treatments combine with the natural depletion of the body's resources as it fights off the disease. This makes coping with fatigue a very significant aspect of dealing with cancer treatment. In addition, there are the normal psychological consequences of the disease, such as stress and **depression**. The best way to deal with these symptoms is to cut back on stressful activities and take plenty of time to allow the body to heal. It is also important to try to maintain a well-balanced, nutritious diet, and to exercise. Patients should avoid as much extra stress as possible and should limit visitors, if needed, to avoid being overtired. At the same time, it is also important for the psychological health of patients to pursue their interests as much as possible and to avoid becoming isolated.

The biggest problem for those undergoing radiation therapy is the development of dry, sore, "burned" skin in the area being treated. (Radiation does not hurt during treatment and does not make the person radioactive.) Skin in the treatment area will become red, get itchy and sore, and may blister and peel, becoming painful. Patients with fair skin or those who have undergone previous chemotherapy have a greater risk of more serious reactions. Dry, itchy, or sore skin is temporary, but affected skin may be more sensitive to sun exposure for the rest of the patient's lifetime, so a good sunscreen and a hat should be used whenever affected skin is exposed to sunlight.

Other effects, specific to the nasal area, may also occur. Sometimes very thick mucus is produced that may be difficult to cough up. Some patients become hoarse and find it difficult to eat. It is important for patients to keep well-hydrated by drinking plenty of fluids and to eat as much protein as possible. If patients cannot eat enough to maintain a high-protein diet, liquid high-protein drinks should be consumed. Patients may be more susceptible to upper respiratory infections after treatment, so some physicians will prescribe preventative **antibiotics**. If eating is extremely painful, acetaminophen can be consumed in milk about 30 minutes before a meal for pain relief. Patients should be prepared for the fact that symptoms of radiation treatment can persist for up to a month after the last treatment.

Some of the more common side effects of chemotherapy include hair loss, nausea, and vomiting. Hair loss (**alopecia**) is a difficult part of dealing with cancer treatment for most patients, especially women. Hair may thin out gradually, or it may fall out in big clumps. To slow down the rate of hair loss, the patient should avoid any unnecessary sources of damage to the hair, like curling, blow-drying, or chemical treatments.

Different patients choose different ways of coping with the loss of their hair. Some patients may find they are more comfortable hiding hair loss with a wig. It is a good idea to cut off a lock of hair before hair loss begins in case a wig is later desired. Some patients may choose to remain bald, or may want to choose hats or scarves instead of wigs. In any case, it is important to remember that the loss of hair is a sign that the medication is doing its job, and that hair loss is temporary. Hair usually begins regrowth within a few months of the end of intensive chemotherapy, although it may return in a different color or texture from the original hair.

Nausea and vomiting are other fairly common side effects of many chemotherapy drugs. (Radiation to the brain or the GI tract can also cause nausea and vomiting.) After a few courses of chemotherapy drugs, some patients will become nauseated just from thinking about an upcoming treatment or from smelling certain odors. Drugs that combat nausea and vomiting can be prescribed, but are often not effective for anticipatory nausea. If nausea and vomiting are a problem, heavy, regular meals should be avoided in favor of small, frequent snacks made up of light but nourishing foods like soup. Avoiding food smells and other strong odors may help.

Desensitization, hypnosis, guided imagery, and relaxation techniques may be used if nausea and vomiting are severe. These techniques help to identify the triggers for the nausea and vomiting, decrease patient anxiety, and distract the patient from thinking about getting sick. Acupressure bands (commonly used for seasickness) and acupuncture may also provide some relief for some patients.

Both radiation therapy and chemotherapy treatments require a substantial level of commitment from the patient in terms of time and emotional energy. Fear and anxiety are major factors in coping with cancer and cancer treatments. The feelings are completely normal. Some patients find that concentrating on restful, pleasurable activities like hobbies, prayer, or meditation is helpful in decreasing negative emotions. It is also very important that patients have people to whom they can express their fears and other negative emotions. Support groups may help to provide an environment where fears can be freely expressed and understood. Patients for whom all treatments have failed often benefit from palliative care, which is care intended to control pain and relieve other symptoms rather than bring about a cure. At the end of life, patients may wish to consider **hospice care**, which can be given at home as well as in a separate hospice facility.

Clinical trials

Clinical trials are studies in which new treatments for disease are evaluated in patients. There were 104 open clinical trials for nasal cancer in the United States as of mid-2014. Many of these are trials of new targeted therapies for nasal cancer, either as stand-alone treatments or in addition to chemotherapy. Others are trials of various forms of radiation therapy.

Prevention

Although mutations in genetic material happen frequently, most of these do not result in cancer. This is because a healthy body repairs most mistakes before a cancer develops and because, if a cancer does develop, the immune system of a healthy body will usually destroy it. In general, therefore, a healthy lifestyle that includes exercise, plenty of sleep, a diet rich in fruits and vegetables, regular health screenings, and the avoidance of stress, excessive sun exposure, tobacco use, or excessive alcohol consumption will help to prevent most cancers.

Since nasal cancers in particular are often caused by chemical exposure, many of these cancers are preventable by avoiding excessive inhalation of wood dust or chemical mixtures and by avoiding use of all tobacco products. (Nasal cancers resulting from wood dust appear to require high-dose, long-term exposure, especially to hardwoods.)

One type of nasal cancer appears to be virus-associated and is more prevalent in people with a history of nasal polyps. People who are diagnosed with nasal polyps should discuss their removal with their physicians and have existing polyps checked regularly in order to detect a malignant polyp as quickly as possible.

Patients with nasal cancer can increase their chances of a cure by making sure that they see their doctors for all scheduled follow-up appointments. This is especially important for the first two years (when most recurrences of nasal cancer occur), but it is also important to maintain follow-up beyond that. Many nasal cancer patients experience a second tumor somewhere else in the upper respiratory tract.

Special concerns

One of the unique aspects of dealing with nasal cancer is the fact that surgical removal of a nasal tumor can result in substantial facial disfigurement. Patients who are dealing with this aspect of nasal cancer are forced to cope with the substantial emotional burden of disfigurement, in addition to the other emotional ramifications of the disease. People with facial disfigurement may be forced to cope with negative reactions from other people in public places, including staring, whispering, rude remarks or averted eyes, and other avoidance of interpersonal interaction.

In addition, the loss of the accustomed appearance will be experienced much like a bereavement. Patients will probably initially feel numb, then experience intense, overwhelming feelings of sadness, fear, and anger. The period characterized by intense, almost unbearable emotions is usually followed by a period of time when the patient feels completely empty, fatigued, and apathetic. Given time, most patients will come to an acceptance of their new reality and begin to enjoy old

QUESTIONS TO ASK YOUR DOCTOR

- Can you explain what kind of cancer I have?
- Can you explain the grade and stage of my cancer? What are the chances that it will come back?
- How was this cancer diagnosed?
- What is my prognosis?
- How much will the surgery alter my facial appearance?
- What treatments are we going to pursue? What happens if these don't work?
- Do you have experience in treating this type of cancer?
- Is there anything I can do to optimize treatment? Are there any particular side effects I should expect?
- Are there complementary therapies that you would recommend? Are there any other things that would help me cope with the diagnosis or treatment?
- How often will I need further check-ups? Is there anything I can do to keep this cancer from coming back?

friends and activities again. It is important not to expect patients in such circumstances to immediately accept their situation or to suppress the natural emotions that accompany the change in their appearance. Patients can ease the process by trying to focus on one day at a time and by finding people who can help them work through the process by listening and accepting their emotions. It is very important that a patient dealing with these changes have friends or family members to whom they can express their feelings of grief and anger. A support group might also be helpful.

See also Cryotherapy; Tumor grading; Tumor staging.

Resources

BOOKS

Harrison, Louis B., et al, eds. *Head and Neck Cancer: A Multidisciplinary Approach.* 4th ed. Philadelphia, PA: Wolters Kluwer Health/Lippincott Williams and Wilkins, 2014.

Medeiros, Aloisio, and Carlitos Veloso, eds. *Nose and Viral Cancer: Etiology, Pathogenesis and Treatment.* New York: Nova Science Publishers, 2010.

PERIODICALS

Bruschweiler, E. D., et al. "Workers Exposed to Wood Dust Have an Increased Micronucleus Frequency in Nasal and Buccal Cells: Results from a Pilot Study." *Mutagenesis* 29 (May 2014): 201–207.

D'Aguillo, C. M., et al. "Demographics and Survival Trends of Sinonasal Adenocarcinoma from 1973 to 2009." *International Forum of Allergy and Rhinology* 4, no. 9 (2014): 771–76.

Gerth, D. J., J. Tashiro, and S. R. Thailer. "Pediatric Sinonasal Tumors in the United States: Incidence and Outcomes." *Journal of Surgical Research* 190 (July 2014): 214–220.

Neto, R., et al. "An Engineering-Based Approach for Design and Fabrication of a Customized Nasal Prosthesis." *Prosthetics and Orthotics International* (June 4, 2014): e-pub ahead of print. http://dx.doi.org/10.1177/0309364614535232 (accessed November 18, 2014).

OTHER

American Cancer Society (ACS). "Nasal Cavity and Paranasal Sinus Cancers." http://www.cancer.org/acs/groups/cid/documents/webcontent/003123-pdf.pdf (accessed September 2, 2014).

WEBSITES

American Society of Clinical Oncology (ASCO). "Nasal Cavity and Paranasal Sinus Cancer." http://www.cancer.net/cancer-types/nasal-cavity-and-paranasal-sinus-cancer (accessed September 2, 2014).

Mayo Clinic. "Nasal and Paranasal Tumors." http://www.mayoclinic.org/diseases-conditions/nasal-paranasal-tumors/basics/definition/CON-20036284 (accessed September 2, 2014).

National Cancer Institute (NCI). "Paranasal Sinus and Nasal Cavity Cancer Treatment (PDQ®)" http://www.cancer.gov/cancertopics/pdq/treatment/paranasalsinus/HealthProfessional/page1/AllPages (accessed September 2, 2014).

ORGANIZATIONS

American Academy of Otolaryngology—Head and Neck Surgery, 1650 Diagonal Road, Alexandria, VA 22314-2857, (703) 836-4444, http://entnet.org/content/contact_us, http://entnet.org/.

American Cancer Society (ACS), 250 Williams Street NW, Atlanta, GA 30303, (800) 227-2345, http://www.cancer.org/aboutus/howwehelpyou/app/contact-us.aspx, http://www.cancer.org/index.

American Society of Clinical Oncology (ASCO), 2318 Mill Road, Suite 800, Alexandria, VA 22314, (571) 483-1300, (888) 651-3038, contactus@cancer.net, http://www.asco.org/.

National Cancer Institute (NCI), BG 9609 MSC 9760, 9609 Medical Center Drive, Bethesda, MD 20892-9760, (800) 4-CANCER (422-6237), http://www.cancer.gov/global/contact/email-us, http://www.cancer.gov/.

Office of Cancer Complementary and Alternative Medicine (OCCAM), 9609 Medical Center Dr., Room 5-W-136, Rockville, MD 20850, (240) 276-6595, Fax: (240) 276-7888, ncioccam1-r@mail.nih.gov, http://cam.cancer.gov/.

Wendy Wippel, MSc
REVISED BY REBECCA J. FREY, PhD

Nasopharyngeal cancer

Definition

Nasopharyngeal **cancer** is an uncontrolled growth of cells that begins in the nasopharynx, the passageway at the back of the nose.

Description

The nasopharynx connects the nose (hence, naso) to the pharynx, the shared passageway for air and food at the back of the nose and mouth. Air moves through the pharynx on its way into and out of the trachea, the tube that carries air to the lungs. Food passes through the pharynx on its way to the esophagus, the muscular tube that carries food to the stomach.

Although it is possible for people to breathe through the mouth, breathing through the nose is better. The nose warms and moistens air, and the interior of the nose has hairs to filter particles from the air. Thus, any blockage, such as a tumor or cancer in the nasopharynx, interferes with normal breathing.

Not all tumors that grow in the nasopharynx are malignant (cancerous). Many are benign (noncancerous), but the tumors still cause problems because they often grow into the vessels that supply blood to the nose. Malignant cancers in the nasopharynx grow from squamous, or flat, epithelial cells. Epithelial cells form body coverings, such as skin. Cancers that originate in epithelial cells are known as carcinomas.

Demographics

Nasopharyngeal cancer is rare in most parts of the world including the United States, where, according to the American Cancer Society, about 2,900 new cases were diagnosed in 2013. The exception is in Southeast Asia, where there are as many as 40 new cases each year for every 100,000 people. Men have twice the risk of developing nasopharyngeal cancer as compared to women. Although all age groups can be affected by this cancer, like many other cancers, people over the age of 40 tend to be more susceptible.

Causes and symptoms

Several factors put people at risk for nasopharyngeal cancer. One appears to be an infection with a type of herpes virus called **Epstein-Barr virus** (EBV). However, EBV infection is so common worldwide that other factors must also play a role. Genetic makeup, or inherited DNA, also appears to be a factor. Other factors that may promote the development of nasopharyngeal cancer include a diet very heavy in salted meats and salted fish, exposure to

certain workplace chemicals such as formaldehyde, and exposure to radioactivity.

In certain parts of China, the soil has a high concentration of uranium and thorium, which break down into radioactive elements such as radium and radon. The elements are taken up by trees, which are burned for wood and become airborne. They also dissolve in water, and fish and plants draw them up. The fish are eaten, and some of the plants are used for tea. This scenario seems to increase the risk of nasopharyngeal cancer, since white children growing up in China have a much higher risk of developing this cancer than white children growing up in the United States.

Symptoms of nasopharyngeal cancer include:

- lump or swelling in the nose or neck
- headaches
- ear pain
- numbness on the side of the face

KEY TERMS

Biopsy—A diagnostic procedure in which a tissue sample is removed from the body for examination.

Computed tomography (CT)—A radiographic technique in which multiple x-ray images assembled by a computer give a three-dimensional image of a structure.

Epstein-Barr virus (EBV)—A herpes virus that causes infectious mononucleosis.

Lymph—Clear, slightly yellow fluid carried by a network of thin tubes to every part of the body. Cells that fight infection are carried in the lymph.

Lymphatic system—Primary defense against infection in the body. The lymphatic system consists of tissues, organs, and channels (similar to veins) that produce, store, and transport lymph and white blood cells to fight infection.

Lymph nodes—Small, bean-shaped collections of tissue found in a lymph vessel. They produce cells and proteins that fight infection, and also filter lymph. Nodes are sometimes called lymph glands.

Magnetic resonance imaging (MRI)—Magnetic fields and radio frequency waves are used to image internal structures of the body.

Nasoscope—A type of endoscope designed specifically to be inserted through the nose and used for examination of the nasal cavity.

- difficulty breathing
- difficulty speaking

Diagnosis

Most nasopharyngeal cancer is diagnosed because the individual visits the doctor for relief of symptoms associated with the cancer. Early detection is uncommon. A physician examines the nasopharynx in various ways, usually starting with an instrument such as a nasoscope. The nasoscope allows a look at the inside of the nasal cavity. Palpating, or touching, lymph nodes in the neck to check for enlarged nodes is also part of the examination.

If suspicious growths are found, a **biopsy** is done to take a tissue sample. Different types of biopsy can be used. An incision may be made to obtain tissue, or a needle with a small diameter may be inserted into a suspicious mass (fine needle biopsy) to obtain cells, especially if there is a lump in the neck.

Computed tomography (CT) and **magnetic resonance imaging** (MRI) scans are also used. They help determine whether the cancer has spread from the walls of the nasopharynx. MRI offers a good way to examine the tonsils and the back of the tongue, which are soft tissues. CT is used as a way of studying the jaw, which is bone.

Treatment team

Generally, physicians with special training in the organs of the nose and throat take initial responsibility for the care of a patient with nasopharyngeal cancer. They are called otolaryngologists, or occasionally, otorhinolaryngologists. Otolaryngologists are usually labeled ENT (for ear, nose, and throat) specialists. An ENT specializing in cancer will probably lead the team, accompanied by radiation therapists and oncologists.

Clinical staging

Staging cancer involves determining how large the tumor is and how far the cancer has spread. Stage I nasopharyngeal cancer describes a cancer that has not spread or has only minimally spread. It is not in the lymph nodes and is localized in the nasopharynx. Stage II describes a larger cancer, one that affects more than half the area of the nasopharynx, but that is not in the lymph nodes. Stage III nasopharyngeal cancer has spread beyond the nasopharynx; it might affect the oropharynx, the cavity at the back of the mouth, or part of the throat. It may also have spread to the lymph nodes. Stage IV involves one or more of the following indications:

- spread of cancer to a site near the original site, such as the bones and nerves of the head

- more than one lymph node with cancer
- spread to other parts of the body, such as the larynx, the trachea, the bronchi, the esophagus, or more distant points, such as the lungs

Treatment

Treatment for nasopharyngeal cancer depends on the stage in which the cancer is diagnosed. For stage I and stage II, radiation or **chemotherapy** treatment of the affected area is sometimes all that is required to halt the cell growth. Decisions about which method to use depend on many factors, but the tolerance a patient has for radiation or chemotherapy and the size of the tumor are important.

Alternative and complementary therapies

Any technique, such as yoga, meditation, or biofeedback, that helps a patient cope with anxiety over the condition and discomfort from treatment is useful and should be explored as an option. Many herbal remedies are available to ease the symptoms of nausea that accompany treatment. The patient's physician, however, should be notified of any supplements or remedies, herbal or otherwise, that are taken, because these complementary therapies may interfere with the action of chemotherapy drugs being given.

Prognosis

The outlook for early-stage diagnoses of nasopharyngeal cancer is good. The five-year survival rate is about 72% for stage I cancers and 64% for stage II cancers. The five-year survival rate for stage III cancers is 63%, but drops dramatically to 38% for stage IV cancers. Unfortunately, about half of all people diagnosed with nasopharyngeal cancer are not diagnosed until the cancer is far advanced, which leads to a poorer prognosis.

Clinical trials

Participating in a clinical trial is often an option for cancer patients in advanced stages of the disease. **Clinical trials** are government-regulated studies of new treatments and techniques that may prove beneficial in diagnosing or treating a disease. Participation is always voluntary and at no cost to the participant. Clinical trials are conducted in three phases. Phase 1 tests the safety of the treatment and looks for harmful side effects. Phase 2 tests the effectiveness of the treatment. Phase 3 compares the treatment to other treatments available for the same condition.

The selection of clinical trials underway changes frequently. Patients and their families can search for new trials on the **National Cancer Institute** website at http://www.cancer.gov/clinicaltrials/search.

Coping with cancer treatment

The patient should be an active member of the treatment team, listening to information and making decisions about which course of treatment to take. Premier cancer centers encourage such a role.

Appetite might be affected before, during, and after treatment. Before treatment, the presence of a tumor can interfere with chewing and swallowing food, and food might not seem as appealing as it once did. During treatment, particularly radiation treatment, the treated nasopharynx will be sore, and eating and breathing may be difficult.

Patients should also seek out a support network to help them cope with the psychological implications of cancer. In addition to family and friends, local support organizations can offer guidance, answer questions, and link newly diagnosed patients with others who have survived a similar experience.

Prevention

There is no known way to prevent nasopharyngeal cancer; however, avoiding heavy alcohol and tobacco use is recommended, as is avoiding heavy consumption of salted meats and fish. Workplaces should be well ventilated. The EBV virus is so common that infection prevention is unrealistic.

Special concerns

Additional cancers that begin in the nasopharynx can start in the lymph cells found there. Because of their origin, these cancers are called lymphomas.

See also Oral cancer; Oropharyngeal cancer.

Resources

WEBSITES

American Cancer Society. "Nasopharyngeal Cancer." http://www.cancer.org/cancer/nasopharyngealcancer/detailed-guide/index (accessed August 22, 2014).

National Cancer Institute. http://www.cancer.gov/clinicaltrials/search (accessed August 22, 2014).

Paulino, Arnold. "Nasopharyngeal Cancer." Medscape Reference. http://emedicine.medscape.com/article/988165-overview (accessed August 22, 2014).

"Throat Cancer." MedlinePlus. http://www.nlm.nih.gov/medlineplus/throatcancer.html (accessed August 22, 2014).

ORGANIZATIONS

American Academy of Otolaryngology—Head and Neck Surgery, 1650 Diagonal Road, Alexandria, VA 22314-2857, (703) 836-4444.

American Cancer Society, 1599 Clifton Rd., NE, Atlanta, GA 30329, (404) 320-3333, (800) ACS-2345, http://www.cancer.org.

National Cancer Institute, BG 9609 MSC 9760, 9609 Medical Center Drive, Bethesda, MD 20892-9760, (800) 4-CANCER, TTY: (800) 332-8615, http://www.cancer.gov.

Diane M. Calabrese
REVISED BY TISH DAVIDSON, AM

National Cancer Institute

Description

The National Cancer Institute (NCI) is the institute within the U.S. National Institutes of Health (NIH) responsible for all aspects of **cancer research**. The NCI coordinates the National Cancer Program, which supports and conducts research, training, and dissemination of information on the causes, diagnosis, prevention, and treatment of cancer, as well as the rehabilitation and ongoing care of cancer patients and their families. The NCI Center for Cancer Research and the Division of Cancer Epidemiology and Genetics support scientists working in NCI laboratories and at the NIH Clinical Center in Bethesda, Maryland. The NCI also funds about 5,000 investigator-initiated research grants at institutions across the country.

NCI-supported research focuses on the mechanisms common to different types of cancer and also on the differences in molecular mechanisms, clinical manifestations, and epidemiology among various cancers. NCI considers the public health impact of cancer and recognizes that scientific breakthroughs are difficult to predict; breakthroughs sometimes come from unexpected lines of research.

The NCI has been at the forefront of the molecular biology revolution, which has dramatically increased knowledge about cancer genomes—changes in genes that lead to the development of cancer. Knowledge about signaling pathways in cells that control normal cell and cancer cell growth and the origin, development, behaviors, and microenvironments of various types of cancer cells has increased exponentially in recent years. This growth in knowledge has resulted in more precise and targeted treatments, especially immunological therapies, as well as new and improved classification of cancer types. Understanding about how to prevent and screen for some cancers has also advanced significantly in recent years. Currently, the NCI promotes screening for lung cancer, which is predicted to reduce deaths from that disease.

Provocative questions initiative

The NCI has actively solicited research proposals for its provocative questions initiative. This is a list of 20 important but somewhat neglected issues in laboratory, clinical, and population cancer sciences. The questions are grouped into five categories:

- cancer prevention and risk
- mechanisms of tumor development and recurrence
- tumor detection, diagnosis, and prognosis
- cancer therapy and outcomes
- clinical effectiveness

Examples of provocative questions include:

- Why are people reluctant to alter behaviors, such as smoking, known to increase cancer risk?
- How does physical activity affect cancer risk and prognosis?
- How does obesity increase cancer risk?
- What mechanisms affect susceptibility to cancer risk factors at various life stages?
- What properties of precancerous cells and their microenvironments predict progression to cancer?
- Why are some cancers so responsive to conventional chemotherapy?
- How can cancer treatments that meet guidelines be initiated and maintained in community settings?
- Can survival be prolonged by halting the further growth of treatment-resistant cancers?
- What causes cancer recurrences?

Overdiagnosis/overtreatment

One of the more controversial recent NCI initiatives has been its focus on overdiagnosis and overtreatment.

In 2013, an NCI working group recommended redefining cancer to eliminate the term from some common diagnoses. The intent was to delay potentially harmful treatments for some precancerous conditions that might never develop into cancer at all. Improvement in cancer screening techniques has resulted in the identification of many more precancerous, or *in situ*, breast, prostate, thyroid, and lung lesions. As an example, many physicians do not regard ductal **carcinoma** in situ of the breast as cancer, but upon hearing the word "carcinoma," patients may immediately decide to undergo **mastectomy** (breast removal) and other aggressive treatments that may not be necessary or advisable. The group suggested reclassifying these from cancers to "indolent lesions of epithelial origin" (IDLE), a change in terminology that may be less frightening to patients and might affect their treatment decisions. A similar situation occurred when the terms used for common cervical conditions found in Pap tests were changed; new terminology greatly reduced the number of unnecessary procedures performed for conditions that often disappear on their own.

Recent recommendations that heavy smokers undergo annual **computed tomography** (CT) scans have increased concerns about overdiagnosis for smoking-related diseases. Although potentially saving 20,000 lives a year, the scans would significantly increase both radiation exposure and the number of risky—and potentially unnecessary—invasive medical procedures. Recommendations for "watchful waiting" rather than immediate treatment include:

- 50%–60% of prostate cancer cases
- 33% of breast cancer cases
- 20%–30% of thyroid cancer cases
- 10% of lung cancer cases

Cancer experts debate the NCI group's recommendations. For example, physicians cannot say with certainty which precancerous conditions are too slow-growing to ever cause a problem and which ones will progress to potentially fatal cancers. Others point out that the incidence of invasive cancers has not decreased, despite years of aggressive treatment of precancerous conditions, suggesting that overdiagnosis and overtreatment are problematic. The NCI working group called for more research to establish guidelines to help distinguish between benign or slow-growing and aggressive tumors. This recommendation was added to the NCI's list of provocative questions.

Other initiatives

In 2013, the NCI launched a new initiative to target therapies for mutations in the RAS oncogene family.

RAS genes produce signaling proteins that ultimately determine whether a cell proliferates (multiplies) or dies. About 30% of human cancers have RAS mutations that lead to uncontrolled cell proliferation. Although RAS oncogenes have been known for more than three decades, no drugs have been developed that target their signaling pathways. This research is centered at the NCI's contract lab in Frederick, Maryland.

Other new and priority NCI initiatives include:

• the Cancer Genome Atlas—a collaboration with the National Human Genome Research Institute that is analyzing major mutations in 10,000 tumor samples from about 20 cancer types

• at the Center for Cancer Genomics: managing the massive amounts of genomic data; standardizing cancer tissue collection, DNA sequencing, and analysis; and encouraging patient tissue donations

• an unconventional clinical trial that is mapping the gene variations in approximately 1,000 patients whose cancers do not respond to conventional treatments and matching them with one of about 30 experimental drugs aimed at specific mutations

• analyzing the genes of exceptional responders whose cancers shrink or disappear in response to drugs that are typically ineffective

• encouraging oncologists to utilize tumor genetics in their treatment plans

• studying how obesity, heart disease, and diabetes complicate cancer treatment

• studying circulating tumor cells and the mechanisms of cancer metastasis

• reducing cancer health disparities among racial and ethnic groups

• controlling cancer in developing countries; for example, through expanding vaccinations against the human papillomavirus (HPV) that causes cervical cancer

Budget

The NCI is supported primarily by the public through the U.S. Congress. Its budget is about $5 billion per year, the largest share of the total NIH budget. This is supplemented by charitable donations through the National Cancer Institute Gift Fund and purchases of Breast Cancer Research Stamps, but the NCI does not solicit funds or conduct fundraising campaigns. Over the years, the NCI budget increased steadily, especially after passage of the National Cancer Act of 1971—President Richard Nixon's "War on Cancer." The resulting growth of the NCI led to the identification of numerous genes involved in cancer and the establishment of the molecular basis of oncogenesis—research that is now transforming the diagnosis and treatment of cancer. A subsequent five-year doubling of the NIH budget, beginning in 1998, resulted in a second period of rapid growth for the NCI, which helped speed completion of the Human Genome Project. Between 2003 and 2014, however, the NCI and total NIH budgets increased only minimally, with an overall loss of about 20% due to inflation. The NCI was forced to close about 130 of its 300 in-house laboratories, eventually reopening only about half of them.

About 40% of the NCI budget is dedicated to outside Research Project Grants. As of 2014, the NCI funded research grant proposals that ranked in approximately the top 9%. Applications with scores in the top 9%–25% were further reviewed for novelty, current investigator funding, and NCI priorities.

History

The NCI was established by the National Cancer Institute Act of 1937, making it the first dedicated institute within the NIH. As of 2014, the NIH included 27 institutes and centers. The National Cancer Act of 1971 broadened the NCI's scope and responsibilities and created the National Cancer Program, with the NCI director as its leader. It also established the Frederick National Laboratory for Cancer Research. Since 1971, legislative amendments have added NCI mandates for disseminating information and assessing clinical incorporation of new treatments.

Harold Varmus, MD, became NCI director in 2010, 45 years after he first joined an NIH laboratory as a research trainee. A 1989 Nobel Laureate for his work on the use of retroviruses to identify cancer genes, Varmus returned to the NIH in 1993 as its director, remaining there until 1999. Then, after ten years as president of the Memorial Sloan Kettering Cancer Center, he agreed to become director of the NCI, at a salary cut of almost 90%.

Membership

Divisions and centers

The NCI includes the:

• Division of Cancer Biology
• Division of Cancer Control and Population Sciences
• Division of Cancer Epidemiology and Genetics
• Division of Cancer Prevention
• Division of Cancer Treatment and Diagnosis
• Division of Extramural Activities
• Center for Cancer Research
• Center for Strategic Scientific Initiatives
• Center to Reduce Cancer Health Disparities

- Office of Cancer Centers
- Office of Cancer Complementary and Alternative Medicine

The Center for Global Health was established in 2011. Its goals include assisting low- and middle-income countries in establishing cancer registries and national cancer plans, and examining the high incidence of certain cancers in some countries, such as **gallbladder cancer** in Chile.

The newly established Center for Cancer Genomics is applying genome science to the diagnosis and treatment of cancer. Its research focuses on:

- identifying the genetic causes and drivers of cancer
- advancing precise diagnosis and treatment of tumors
- educating patients and doctors in genome-influenced cancer care
- protecting patient privacy while furthering treatment and research

External members

External advisory boards and working groups include the:

- President's Cancer Panel
- National Cancer Advisory Board
- Director's Consumer Liaison Group
- Board of Scientific Advisors
- Clinical Trials and Translational Research Advisory Committee
- Provocative Questions workshops for soliciting important but neglected areas of research
- National Frederick Advisory Committee for oversight of the Frederick National Laboratory for Cancer Research

Members of boards and working groups are drawn from:

- private pharmaceutical and biotechnology companies
- medical and scientific societies
- disease advocacy and volunteer organizations
- state research programs
- research institutions, universities, and medical schools
- 67 NCI-designated cancer centers, located in every region of the country

Mission

The NCI's mission is to:

- reduce the incidence of and morbidity and mortality from cancer
- extend survival

- increase the quality of life of cancer patients

Its mission includes:

- financial support and coordination of cancer research projects carried out by universities, hospitals, research foundations, and businesses nationwide and abroad, through research grants and cooperative agreements
- research conducted in NCI laboratories and clinics
- financial support for basic and clinical science education and training of pre-professionals and professionals in cancer research and treatment programs, through career awards, training grants, and fellowships
- financial support for research projects on cancer control
- financial support for a network of nationwide cancer centers
- collaborations with national and foreign institutions and voluntary organizations involved in cancer research and training
- encouragement and coordination of cancer research by industry
- collection and dissemination of information on cancer
- construction grants for laboratories, clinics, and other facilities involved in cancer research

Publications

The NCI makes available a great many free publications in various formats, including fact sheets, collections, e-books, and lists of **clinical trials**. Some materials are available in Spanish as well as English. These publications cover various cancer topics and cancer types and are geared to specific audiences. The NCI also publishes a newsletter, *CCR Connections*, and the *Journal of the National Cancer Institute*.

Services

Services of the NCI include:

- extensive web-based information on cancer topics and statistics, including frequently asked questions, a dictionary of cancer terms, and a drug dictionary
- the Cancer Information Service, which answers cancer-related questions from patients, family members and friends, healthcare providers, and researchers, by telephone in English and Spanish and by live online chat, e-mail, and regular mail
- clinical trials
- funding of research for university-, hospital-, and organization-based scientists nationwide
- in-house research support at NCI campuses and centers in Maryland
- announcements of funding opportunities

National Comprehensive Cancer Network

KEY TERMS

Clinical trial—A scientifically controlled study of the safety and effectiveness of a treatment that uses consenting human subjects.

Computed tomography (CT) scan—A diagnostic and screening technique that uses x-rays to obtain cross-sectional images of tissues.

Genome—The DNA sequences of all of the genes in a cell; cancer cell genomes differ in various ways from normal cell genomes.

Genomics—The science of mapping genes and sequencing the DNA of an organism, collecting the results in a database, and analyzing and applying those results.

Human Genome Project—An international project begun in 1990 and completed in 2003 that sequenced the three billion bases of DNA in the human genome.

Metastasis—The spread of cancer from its initial site to another part of the body.

Oncogene—A gene that has the potential to turn a normal cell into one that is cancerous.

Oncology—The study of cancer.

Pap test—A screening test for cervical cancer.

RAS—A member of a family of genes that can mutate to oncogenes that are linked to common human cancers.

- information about preparing research grant applications and the grant review process

- funding for cancer training and career development at NCI and at universities and institutions nationwide

- funding for small business development and biotechnology collaborations and partnerships

- online research tools, services, and resources for cancer researchers

- research directories

Resources

BOOKS

Division of Cancer Control and Population Sciences, National Cancer Institute. *Understanding and Influencing Multilevel Factors Across the Cancer Care Continuum.* Bethesda, MD: Oxford University, 2012.

Health Communication and Informatics Research Branch. *Cancer Prevention and Control in the Changing Communication Landscape: Behavioral Research Program*

(National Cancer Institute, Division of Cancer Control and Population Sciences). Cary, NC: Oxford University, 2013.

National Cancer Institute. *Coping with Advanced Cancer.* Bethesda, MD: National Cancer Institute, 2012.

Nordstrom, Robert J. *Translational Research in Biophotonics: Four National Cancer Institute Case Studies.* Bellingham, WA: SPIE, 2014.

PERIODICALS

Manrow, Richard E., Margaret Beckwith, and Lenora E. Johnson. "NCI's Physician Data Query (PDQ) Cancer Information Summaries: History, Editorial Processes, Influence, and Reach." *Journal of Cancer Education* 29, no. 1 (March 2014): 198–205.

Parker-Pope, Tara. "Scientists Urge Narrower Rules to Define Cancer." *New York Times* (July 30, 2013): A1.

OTHER

Vanchieri, Cori, and Sarah C.P. Williams. "The National Cancer Program: Managing the Nation's Research Portfolio: An Annual Plan and Budget Proposal for Fiscal Year 2013." National Cancer Institute. November 2012. http://www.cancer.gov/aboutnci/budget_planning_leg/plan-archives/NCI_Plan_2013.pdf (accessed July 6, 2014).

WEBSITES

Kaiser, Jocelyn. "Varmus's Second Act." *Science* 342 (October 25, 2013): 416–19. http://www.cancer.gov/aboutnci/director/speeches/science_interview_2013 (accessed July 6, 2014).

"Provocative Questions: Identifying Perplexing Problems to Drive Progress Against Cancer." National Cancer Institute. http://provocativequestions.nci.nih.gov (accessed July 9, 2014).

ORGANIZATIONS

National Cancer Institute, 6116 Executive Boulevard, Suite 300, Bethesda, MD 20892-8322, (800) 4-CANCER (422-6237), http://www.cancer.gov.

National Institutes of Health, 9000 Rockville Pike, Bethesda, MD 20892, (301) 496-4000, NIHinfo@od.nih.gov, http://www.nih.gov.

Margaret Alic, PhD

National Comprehensive Cancer Network

Description

The National Comprehensive Cancer Network (NCCN) is a nonprofit alliance of 25 major cancer centers. The NCCN develops resources for **cancer research**, education, and healthcare delivery to improve patient care.

Its most important function is the development and maintenance of clinical practice guidelines for use by clinicians, patients, and other decision-makers within the healthcare delivery system. The guidelines are developed in cooperation with clinicians at its member institutions. These clinicians are experts in the diagnosis and treatment of a broad range of cancers, including those that are particularly complex, aggressive, and/or rare.

The NCCN Board of Directors comprises leaders from each of the member institutions. As of 2014, Samuel M. Silver, MD, PhD, of the University of Michigan Comprehensive Cancer Center, was Chairman of the Board of Directors. Robert W. Carlson, MD, served as chief executive officer. The NCCN Corporate Council is an independent advisory body of pharmaceutical and biotechnology companies that supports the work of the NCCN.

The NCCN Foundation is the charitable NCCN affiliate. As of 2014, Ellen O. Tauscher served as Chair of the Foundation Board of Directors. She is a former congresswoman from California and former Undersecretary of State for Arms Control and International Security.

History

The NCCN was formally incorporated in 1993. In 1995, it announced the creation of a national alliance of 13 member institutions; its goals include the development and dissemination of cancer treatment standards, research on treatment outcomes, and delivery of high-quality, cost-effective cancer services nationwide. Its first annual conference in 1996 included 500 attendees.

In 1996, the NCCN released its first seven Clinical Practice Guidelines in Oncology, covering breast, ovarian, colon, rectal, prostate, lung, and pediatric cancers. Its first database, the NCCN Oncology Outcomes Database for Breast Cancer, was launched at five member institutions in 1997. In 1998, the NCCN launched its clinicians' website, as well as its Treatment Guidelines for Patients. Its Oncology Research Program was established the following year. The first complete library of NCCN Guidelines became available in 2001. The first issue of *JNCCN—Journal of the National Comprehensive Cancer Network* was published in January of 2003. The first chapter of the NCCN Drugs & Biologics Compendium became available the following year. The NCCN 1st Annual Congress: Hematologic Malignancies was held in September of 2006. **Chemotherapy** order templates for bladder, kidney, and prostate cancers and for chronic myelogenous leukemia became available in 2008. The NCCN website for patients was launched in 2009. Its first live webinar program—on case management for non-small cell lung cancer—attracted more than 230 attendees in that year. The NCCN Foundation was created in 2010, and the NCCN Guidelines for Patients also became available that year. Its Biomarkers Compendium launched in 2012. In 2013, the NCCN introduced its International Educational Activities Program and Patient and Caregiver Resources.

Membership

The 25 NCCN member institutions are the:

- City of Hope Comprehensive Cancer Center in Los Angeles, California
- Dana-Farber/Brigham and Women's Cancer Center and Massachusetts General Hospital Cancer Center in Boston
- Duke Cancer Institute in Durham, North Carolina
- Fox Chase Cancer Center in Philadelphia, Pennsylvania
- Fred & Pamela Buffett Cancer Center at the Nebraska Medical Center in Omaha
- Fred Hutchinson Cancer Research Center/Seattle Cancer Care Alliance, which includes Seattle Children's and University of Washington (UW) Medicine
- Huntsman Cancer Institute at the University of Utah in Salt Lake City
- Mayo Clinic Cancer Centers in Phoenix/Scottsdale, Arizona; Jacksonville, Florida; and Rochester, Minnesota
- Memorial Sloan Kettering Cancer Center in New York City
- Moffitt Cancer Center in Tampa, Florida
- Ohio State University Comprehensive Cancer Center at the James Cancer Hospital and Solove Research Institute in Columbus, Ohio
- Robert H. Lurie Comprehensive Cancer Center of Northwestern University in Chicago, Illinois
- Roswell Park Cancer Institute in Buffalo, New York
- Sidney Kimmel Comprehensive Cancer Center at Johns Hopkins in Baltimore, Maryland
- Siteman Cancer Center at Barnes-Jewish Hospital and Washington University School of Medicine in St. Louis, Missouri
- St. Jude Children's Research Hospital/University of Tennessee Health Science Center in Memphis
- Stanford Cancer Institute in Stanford, California
- University of Alabama at Birmingham Comprehensive Cancer Center
- University of California San Diego Moores Cancer Center in La Jolla
- University of California San Francisco Helen Diller Family Comprehensive Cancer Center

- University of Colorado Cancer Center in Aurora, Colorado
- University of Michigan Comprehensive Cancer Center in Ann Arbor
- University of Texas MD Anderson Cancer Center in Houston
- Vanderbilt-Ingram Cancer Center in Nashville, Tennessee
- Yale Cancer Center/Smilow Cancer Hospital in New Haven, Connecticut

NCCN members are widely regarded as the nation's best hospitals for cancer care, and they all utilize multidisciplinary teams for both patient care and research. Together, the member institutions represent more than 1,000 physicians and cancer researchers. However, the majority of these centers are not included in most of the healthcare plans available under the individual state **health insurance** exchanges established by the Patient Protection and Affordable Care Act.

Mission

The mission of the NCCN "is to improve the quality, effectiveness, and efficiency of cancer care so that patients can live better lives." Its vision is: "To be the world's leader in defining and advancing high-quality, high-value cancer care."

Publications

The *NCCN eBulletin* is an electronic newsletter sent on alternate Mondays to all registered users. The newsletter covers news, clinical and operational trends in cancer care, oncology health policy, notifications of guideline updates, and links to important advances in treatment and research at member institutions. Its international edition is delivered monthly to registered users outside of the United States. It also publishes a member institution edition, as well as the *JNCCN— Journal of the National Comprehensive Cancer Network*.

The NCCN publishes compendiums, surveys and data, video modules, and flash updates. Insurance companies and other payers refer to the compendiums for coverage decision; they are updated on a continuous basis along with the NCCN guidelines. The NCCN Drug & Biologics Compendium is designed to aid decisions about appropriate cancer drugs and biologics for specific conditions, based on evaluation of the scientific literature and expert advice. The types of evidence and degree of consensus for each drug recommendation are explained. The compendium includes both drug uses approved by the U.S. Food and Drug Administration (FDA) and medically appropriate uses beyond the FDA-approved label. It also includes uses that are no longer recommended, as well as information about licensing and permissions. The compendium is organized by chapters according to: detection, prevention, and risk reduction; treatment site; and supportive care. It can be browsed by generic drug name. The NCCN Biomarkers Compendium provides information on biomarker testing for cancer as recommended by the NCCN guidelines. These biomarkers are tests for changes in genes or gene products that can be used for screening, diagnosis, monitoring and surveillance, and prognosis.

Services

Guidelines

The NCCN Clinical Practice Guidelines in Oncology, commonly called the NCCN Guidelines, are at the core of the organization's mission. These guidelines represent the recognized standards for clinical cancer care and the most comprehensive and frequently updated clinical practice standards in any field of medicine. They cover 97% of all cancer patients. The guidelines are designed as decision-making tools to enable physicians to determine the best treatment plan based on diagnosis, cancer stage, and other factors such as patient age. They include pros and cons for each treatment option. The guidelines are continuously updated, based on current treatment protocols, reviews of the evidence from **clinical trials**, and other information, as well as judgments of experts and recommendations by panels of representatives from member institutions. Each panel focuses on a specific area: tumor type, prevention, detection, risk reduction, and supportive care.

As of 2014, there were 58 clinical guidelines, available free-of-charge from the NCCN website with free registration. The information is also available for tablet computers and smart phones. Specific guidelines for each type of cancer are organized by treatment; detection, prevention, and risk reduction; and supportive care. Age-related recommendations are also available. As of December 2013, there were more than 4.9 million downloads of NCCN guidelines.

The NCCN Guidelines for Patients are layperson translations of the clinical guidelines, designed to help patients discuss treatment options with their physicians. As of 2014, 13 patient guidelines were available:

- breast cancer
- chronic myelogenous leukemia
- colon cancer
- esophageal cancer
- malignant pleural mesothelioma
- melanoma

- multiple myeloma
- non-small cell lung cancer
- lung cancer screening
- ovarian cancer
- pancreatic cancer
- prostate cancer
- caring for adolescents and young adults (AAYA)—including recommendations that teen and young adult cancer patients be referred to centers with specific expertise in caring for patients in these age groups and utilizing holistic approaches to physical and psychosocial issues

Other patient resources

The NCCN makes available other resources for patients and caregivers, including:

- understanding a diagnosis
- explanations of guideline updates
- lists of support and advocacy organizations
- clinical trials and enrollment information
- life with cancer
- life after cancer
- patient and payment assistance resources for clinicians and others working with cancer patients
- a dictionary of terms

In conjunction with the National Business Group on Health, the NCCN publishes a Cancer Resource Guide that includes three sections: cancer risk and how to reduce the risk, information for cancer patients, and information for family members and other caregivers of cancer patients. It also includes five fact sheets:

- "Advance Care Planning"
- "Cancer Risk and Genetic Testing"
- "End-of-Life Care: Making Your Preferences Known"
- "Palliative Care: Is it Right for You?"
- "Cancer Survivorship"

The NCCN recently introduced its first patient information webinar, which focused on **non-small cell lung cancer**. Planned future live patient-information webinars include overviews of cancer types, treatment options, and resources for obtaining more information about treatment options and making informed decisions about those options. The webinars enable patients and their caregivers to listen to expert discussions and will include live question-and-answer sessions with an expert from an NCCN cancer center. The Guidelines for Patients library and patient information webinars are major initiatives of the NCCN Foundation.

KEY TERMS

Biologics—Natural compounds in the human body, usually proteins, which are used to treat disease.

Biomarker—A biological indicator, such as a metabolite in the blood, of a disease such as a specific type of cancer.

Clinical trial—A scientifically controlled study of the safety and effectiveness of a treatment using consenting human subjects.

Other professional resources

The NCCN sponsors professional webinars, online learning, and an International Educational Activities Program. Its professional meetings include:

- an annual conference (Advancing the Standard of Cancer Care)
- an annual congress (Hematologic Malignancies)
- oncology policy programs
- state oncology society forums
- a congress series

The NCCN Oncology Research Program obtains funding for clinical trials at member institutions. It has garnered millions of dollars in research grants from major pharmaceutical companies for investigator-initiated clinical trials, including evaluations of drug combinations and regimens, mechanisms of drug action, **drug resistance**, and extended uses for specific treatment agents.

The NCCN foundation funds Young Investigator Awards for young researchers at NCCN cancer centers. One goal of these awards is to emphasize research into better utilization of the NCCN guidelines for improving quality of care, extending coverage of quality care, and patient education.

Resources

PERIODICALS

Atlas, Scott W. "The Coming Two-Tier Health System." *Wall Street Journal* (May 1, 2014): A15.

Jenks, Susan. "Cancer Experts Issue First Guidelines for Survivors, Rare Cancer." *Journal of the National Cancer Institute* 105, no. 14 (July 17, 2013): 995.

Landro, Laura. "The Informed Patient: Cancer's Overlooked Patients—More Hospitals Tailor Care for the 'No Man's Land' of Teens and Young Adults." *Wall Street Journal* (April 29, 2014): D1.

Wood, Douglas E., and Ella A. Kazerooni. "Medicare's Puzzling Refusal to Cover Lung-Cancer Screening." *Wall Street Journal* (June 18, 2014): A13.

WEBSITES

"About NCCN." National Comprehensive Cancer Network. 2014. http://www.nccn.org/about/default.aspx (accessed July 8, 2014).

ORGANIZATIONS

National Comprehensive Cancer Network, 275 Commerce Drive, Suite 300, Fort Washington, PA 19034, (215) 690-0300, Fax: (215) 690-0280, http://www.nccn.org.

U.S. Food and Drug Administration, 10903 New Hampshire Avenue, Silver Spring, MD 20993-0002, (888) INFO-FDA (463-6332), http://www.fda.gov.

Margaret Alic, PhD

Nausea and vomiting

Definition

Nausea and vomiting are recognized as two separate and distinct conditions. Nausea is the subjective, unpleasant feeling or urge to vomit, which may or may not result in vomiting. Vomiting, also called emesis, is the forceful expelling of the contents of the stomach and intestines through the mouth. To some, nausea is a more distressing symptom than vomiting.

Description

Nausea and vomiting are major problems for patients being treated for **cancer**, with approximately 50% of patients experiencing nausea and vomiting as a result of cancer treatments, even when **antiemetics** (antiemesis medications) are used. In addition, more than 50% of cancer patients experience nausea and vomiting as a result of disease progression, or as a result of exposure to other therapies used to treat the cancer.

Not all patients diagnosed with cancer will experience nausea and vomiting. However, nausea and vomiting remain two of the most-feared side effects associated with cancer and cancer treatment. The negative aspects of nausea and vomiting can influence all facets of a patient's life. If nausea and vomiting are not controlled in the patient with cancer, the result can be serious metabolic problems such as disturbances in fluid and electrolyte balance and nutritional status. Psychological problems associated with nausea and vomiting

KEY TERMS

Antiemetic—Antiemetic drugs are drugs used to alleviate treatment-related nausea and vomiting.

Asthenia—A feeling of extreme weakness and fatigue.

Emesis—The expelling of stomach contents, also called vomiting, associated with cancer treatments or other causes.

Emetogenic—The relative tendency or likelihood of a drug to produce vomiting in patients receiving it as cancer therapy.

Nausea—The subjective feeling of abdominal discomfort associated with the urge to vomit.

include anxiety and **depression**. Uncontrolled nausea and vomiting can also lead to a patient's decision to stop potentially curative cancer therapy.

Causes and symptoms

The most common causes of nausea and vomiting in cancer patients include treatment with **chemotherapy** and **radiation therapy**; tumor spread to the gastrointestinal tract, liver, and brain; digestive disturbances and constipation; infection; and use of certain **opioids**, which are drugs that work on the central nervous system to treat cancer pain. The mechanisms that control nausea and vomiting are not fully understood, but both are controlled by the central nervous system. Nausea is thought to arise from stimulation of the autonomic nervous system. It is theorized that chemotherapy causes vomiting by stimulating areas in the gastrointestinal tract and the brain. The areas in the brain that are stimulated are the chemoreceptor trigger zone (CTZ) and the emetic or vomiting center (VC). When the VC is stimulated, muscular contractions of the abdomen, chest wall, and diaphragm occur, which result in the expulsion of stomach and intestinal contents.

Chemotherapy-induced nausea and vomiting

Not all chemotherapeutic agents cause nausea and vomiting. Chemotherapy drugs vary in their ability or potential to cause nausea and vomiting. This variation is known as the "emetogenic potential" of the drug, or the potential of the drug to cause emesis. Chemotherapy drugs are classified as having high (greater than 90% of patients exposed to this drug will experience nausea and vomiting), moderate (30% to 90% experience nausea and vomiting), low (10% to 30% experience nausea and vomiting), and minimal (less than 10% experience nausea and vomiting) emetogenic potential.

The incidence and severity of chemotherapy-induced nausea and vomiting varies and is related to the emetogenic potential of the drug, the drug dosage, the schedule of administration of the drug, and the route of the drug. For example, even a drug with a low emetogenic potential may cause nausea and vomiting if given at higher doses. Factors associated with increased nausea and vomiting after chemotherapy include female gender, age over six in children, age under 50 in adults, history of motion sickness, and history of vomiting in pregnancy.

The nausea and vomiting that can result with chemotherapy is classified as anticipatory, acute, or delayed. Anticipatory nausea and vomiting occur prior to the actual chemotherapy treatment in patients who have previously experienced significant nausea and vomiting episodes during treatment. That is, smelling the odor alone may be enough to induce or trigger nausea and vomiting in the sensitized patient. Acute nausea and vomiting occur shortly after administration of the chemotherapeutic agent, usually within 1–2 hours and peaking at 4–6 hours. Delayed nausea and vomiting occur more than 24 hours after chemotherapy administration.

Radiation therapy-induced nausea and vomiting

Although not all patients receiving radiation therapy will experience nausea and vomiting, patients receiving radiation therapy to the gastrointestinal tract and brain are most likely to experience those side effects. Radiation therapy to the brain is believed to stimulate the CTZ, the VC, or both. The higher the radiation therapy dose and the larger the amount of gastrointestinal tract tissue exposed to radiation, the higher the potential for nausea and vomiting. In other words, the potential for nausea and vomiting increases as the dosage increases. Nausea and vomiting associated with radiation therapy usually occurs a half hour to several hours after a treatment and usually does not occur on the days when the patient is not undergoing treatment.

Treatment

Pharmacologic management

The most commonly used intervention to manage nausea and vomiting in cancer patients is the use of antiemetic drugs. Many of these drugs work by inhibiting stimulation of the CTZ and perhaps the VC. The three most commonly used drug categories used to treat nausea and vomiting associated with cancer treatment are 5-HT$_3$ receptor antagonists, also called serotonin receptor antagonists; neurokinin (NK-1) receptor antagonists, also called substance P neurokinin receptor antagonists; and **corticosteroids**, specifically glucocorticoids. Cannabinoids may be recommended for some patients. Other

antiemetic drugs are available such as dopaminergic antagonists and dopamine 2 (D2) antagonists, but these are antipsychotic drugs that produce sedation and have a higher incidence of reactions affecting patients' ability to move (pyramidal reactions), so they are not widely used for alleviating treatment-related nausea and vomiting. Antiemetics may be given as single agents or a combination of drugs may be prescribed.

5-HT$_3$ RECEPTOR ANTAGONISTS. Drugs known as 5-HT$_3$ receptor antagonists, also called serotonin receptor antagonists because of their mechanism of action, are considered as first-line therapy for treatment-related nausea and vomiting. These drugs are thought to prevent nausea and vomiting by preventing serotonin produced in the gastrointestinal tract from initiating a central nervous system response that results in vomiting. Four first-generation serotonin receptor antagonists are FDA approved for use as antiemetics, including granisetron (Kytril), dolasetron (Anzemet), ondansetron (Zofran), and tropisetron (Navoban). These drugs are used for nausea and vomiting associated with chemotherapy and with anesthesia used during surgery. They are often used in combination with a corticosteroid drug such as **dexamethasone**. Ondansetron is approved for nausea and vomiting associated with radiation therapy as well as chemotherapy. An orally disintegrating ondansetron formulation that dissolves rapidly under the tongue and does not have to be taken with water is also available. A transdermal formulation of granisetron can be worn as a patch. These drugs are reported to be safe for children over age 4 and adults, including adults over age 65 and those with impaired kidney function (renal insufficiency). No major differences are found between dolasetron, granisetron, and ondansetron in terms of efficacy and toxicity. Palonosetron (Aloxi) is a second generation 5-HT$_3$ receptor antagonist approved for treating delayed emesis associated with chemotherapeutic drugs that produce mild to moderate nausea and vomiting.

A common adverse effect of the 5-HT$_3$ serotonin antagonists is asthenia, a state of unusual **fatigue** and weakness. Asthenia usually occurs two to three days after treatment with serotonin antagonists and may last one to four days.

NEUROKININ RECEPTOR ANTAGONISTS. The neurokinin receptor antagonists are used in combination with other antiemetics and corticosteroids for relief of acute and delayed nausea and vomiting caused by high-dose chemotherapy, most often caused by the drug **cisplatin**. These drugs are most often combined with 5-HT$_3$ antagonists and corticosteroids (dexamethasone). Aprepitant (Emend) and fosaprepitant dimeglumine (Emend Injection) are the most commonly used NK-1 receptor antagonists. Fosaprepitant is an intravenous prodrug of aprepitant and is given by injection into a vein. These drugs inhibit emesis-related chemotherapy actions in the brain. They are often given as part of a regimen including ondansetron and dexamethasone, which has been shown to effectively prevent chemotherapy-induced nausea and vomiting.

CORTICOSTEROIDS. Steroid hormone drugs (corticosteroids) are sometimes used alone to treat mild to moderately emetogenic chemotherapy. Glucocorticoids, a specific type of corticosteroid, bind to glucocorticoid receptors in most cells in the body. They are used both to reduce swelling and inflammation associated with cancer pain and to control and prevent nausea and vomiting associated with chemotherapy. The glucocorticoid dexamethasone is commonly used in combination with a 5-HT_3 serotonin antagonist (ondansetron) and a neurokinin-1 antagonist (aprepitant) to treat moderate to highly emetogenic chemotherapy. Corticosteroid use is limited to short-term use because of the multiple adverse effects associated with long-term use.

CANNABINOIDS. Cannabinoids are synthetic versions of cannabis that may be effective in selected patients who have not responded to the more commonly used antiemetic drugs. They are usually not prescribed as first-line therapy due to generally low rates of effectiveness. Synthetic cannabinoids produce an antiemetic effect by acting on the cannabinoid receptor system found in nerve tissues. Dronabinol (Marinol) and nabilone (Cesamet) are the main synthetic cannabinoid drugs used. Dronabinol has been found to work synergistically with prochlorperazine to enhance the antiemetic effect and these two drugs are sometimes used in combination to treat chemotherapy-induced nausea and vomiting. Controversy still exists related to the use of cannabinoids, which may not be an accepted cultural or societal practice for some patients. Side effects of synthetic cannabinoids include physical and psychogenic effects such as fatigue, weakness, abdominal pain, nausea, vomiting, heart palpitations, fast heart rate, facial flushing, dry mouth, amnesia, anxiety, depression or other abnormal mental state, depersonalization, confusion, dizziness, and euphoria.

Alternative and complementary therapies

The use of antiemetics is considered the cornerstone of therapy to treat chemotherapy-induced vomiting. Non-pharmacologic therapies may be used in conjunction with pharmacologic agents to enhance the effects of the drugs. Non-pharmacologic strategies include behavioral interventions such as guided imagery, hypnosis, systematic desensitization, and attentional distraction. Dietary interventions such as eating cold or room temperature foods and foods with minimal odors while avoiding spicy,

---

QUESTIONS TO ASK YOUR DOCTOR

- Should I expect to experience nausea and vomiting during or after chemotherapy?
- Do the specific chemotherapy drugs I will be taking produce nausea and vomiting? Is it usually mild, moderate or severe?
- What medications can I take to relieve treatment side effects such as nausea and vomiting?
- How are these medications given?
- Are these drugs taken only when I am receiving chemotherapy or during the whole treatment period?
- Are there any risks and side effects associated with these medications?
- What alternative or complementary treatments are available to help relieve nausea and vomiting from chemotherapy or radiation?

---

salty, sweet, or high-fat foods may be beneficial to some patients while undergoing chemotherapy treatments. Another dietary recommendation is the use of ginger or ginger capsules to decrease episodes of nausea and vomiting. Acupressure, specifically stimulation of the Nei Guan point (P6) of the dominant arm or stimulation of the Inner Gate and ST36 or Three Mile point (below the knee and lateral—outside area—to the tibia) has proven helpful to some patients. Music therapy interventions have also been effective as diversional interventions to reduce incidence and severity of chemotherapy-induced nausea and vomiting.

See also Antiemetics.

Resources

PERIODICALS

Barbour, S. Y. "Corticosteroids in the Treatment of Chemotherapy-Induced Nausea and Vomiting." *Journal of the National Comprehensive Cancer Network* 10 (April 2012): 493–99.

Celio, L. F. Ricchini, and F. DeBraud. "Safety, Efficacy, and Patient Acceptability of Single-Dose Fosaprepitant Regimen for Chemotherapy-Induced Nausea and Vomiting." *Patient Preference and Adherence* 7 (May 2013): 391–400.

Lorenzen, S., S. Spori, and F. Lordick. "Incidence and Treatment of Chemotherapy-Induced Nausea and Emesis in Gastrointestinal Cancer." *Z Gastroentrology* 52 (August 2014): 821–30.

Roila, F., et al. "Guideline Update for MASCC and ESMO in the Prevention of Chemotherapy- and Radiotherapy-Induced Nausea and Vomiting: Results of the Perugia

Consensus Conference." *Annals of Oncology* 21, suppl. 5 (2010): 232.

WEBSITES

American Society of Clinical Oncology. "Antiemetics: ASCO Clinical Practice Guideline Update." http://www.asco.org/quality-guidelines/antiemetics-asco-clinical-practice-guideline-update (accessed September 16, 2014).

Hesketh, Paul J. "Prevention and Treatment of Chemotherapy-Induced Nausea and Vomiting." UpToDate®. http://www.uptodate.com/contents/prevention-and-treatment-of-chemotherapy-induced-nausea-and-vomiting (accessed September 16, 2014).

National Cancer Institute. "Nausea and Vomiting (PDQ®)." http://www.cancer.gov/cancertopics/pdq/supportivecare/nausea/Patient (accessed September 16, 2014).

ORGANIZATIONS

American Cancer Society, 1599 Clifton Rd. NE, Atlanta, GA 30329, (800) ACS-2345 (227-2345), http://www.cancer.org.

National Cancer Institute, 9609 Medical Center Dr., BG 9609 MSC 9760, Bethesda, MD 20892-9760, (800) 4-CANCER (422-6237), http://www.cancer.gov.

L. Lee Culvert
Melinda Granger Oberleitner, RN, DNS
Teresa G. Odle

Navelbine *see* **Vinorelbine**

Neck cancers *see* **Head and neck cancers**

Neoral *see* **Cyclosporine**

Neosar *see* **Cyclophosphamide**

Nephrectomy

Definition

A nephrectomy is a surgical procedure for the removal of a kidney (radical nephrectomy) or a section of a kidney (partial nephrectomy, also known as nephron-sparing surgery).

Purpose

Nephrectomy, or kidney removal, is performed on patients with severe kidney damage from disease, injury, or congenital conditions. These include **cancer** of the kidney (renal cell **carcinoma**), polycystic kidney disease, hydronephrosis (kidney swelling), and serious kidney infections. It is also used to remove a healthy kidney from a donor for the purposes of kidney transplantation.

KEY TERMS

Hemostasis—Slowing down or stopping bleeding.

Hydronephrosis—Severe swelling of the kidney due to backup of urine. It may occur because of an obstruction, calculi, tumor, or other pathological conditions.

Morcellation—The division of tissue or tumors into smaller pieces.

Pneumoperitoneum—The presence of air or gas in a cavity.

Polycystic kidney disease—A hereditary kidney disease that causes fluid- or blood-filled pouches of tissue called cysts to form on the tubules of the kidneys. These cysts impair normal kidney function.

Renal cell carcinoma—Cancer of the kidney.

Trocar—A small sharp instrument used to puncture the abdomen at the beginning of the laparoscopic procedure.

Description

Nephrectomy may involve removing a small portion of the kidney or the entire organ and surrounding tissues. In partial nephrectomy, only the diseased or infected portion of the kidney is removed. Radical nephrectomy involves removing the entire kidney, a section of the tube leading to the bladder (ureter), the gland that sits atop the kidney (adrenal gland), lymph nodes, and the fatty tissue surrounding the kidney. A simple nephrectomy performed for living donor transplant purposes requires removal of the kidney and a section of the attached ureter. A nephrectomy may be performed as an open procedure or in some situations may be performed laparoscopically.

Open nephrectomy

In a traditional, open nephrectomy, the kidney donor is administered general anesthesia and a 6–10 in. (15.2–25.4 cm) incision is made through several layers of muscle on the side or front of the abdomen. A rib resection may be necessary for access to the kidney and other structures. The blood vessels connecting the kidney to the donor are cut and clamped, and the ureter is also cut between the bladder and kidney and clamped. Depending on the type of nephrectomy procedure being performed, the ureter, adrenal gland, and/or surrounding tissue may also be dissected. The kidney is removed and the vessels and ureter are then tied off or sutured to achieve hemostasis. The incision is approximated and sutured (sewn up). The surgical procedure can take up to three hours, depending on the type of nephrectomy being performed.

Laparoscopic nephrectomy

Laparoscopic nephrectomy is a form of minimally invasive surgery that utilizes specialized instruments and endoscopic components to access, dissect, and remove the kidney. The surgeon views the kidney and surrounding tissue with a flexible endoscope. A trocar port is inserted into the abdomen to gain access. Pneumoperitoneum is established by inserting carbon dioxide into the abdominal cavity to inflate the cavity and improve visualization of the kidney and surrounding tissue. Additional trocar ports are inserted into the abdominal cavity for insertion of the instrumentation and camera components. The kidney and tissue are identified and dissected free. Hemostasis is achieved and the kidney is isolated. The kidney may be removed by morcellation or by securing it in a bag and pulling it through a trocar port. Although laparoscopic nephrectomy takes slightly longer than a traditional nephrectomy, it promotes a faster recovery time, shorter hospital stays, and reduced postoperative pain.

A modified laparoscopic technique called hand-assisted laparoscopic nephrectomy may also be used to remove the kidney. In the hand-assisted surgery, a small incision of 3–5 in. (7.6–12.7 cm) is made in the patient's abdomen. The incision allows the surgeon to place his or her hand in the abdominal cavity using a special surgical glove that also maintains a seal for the inflation of the abdominal cavity with carbon dioxide. This technique gives the surgeon the benefit of using his or her hands to feel the kidney and related structures. The kidney is then removed by hand through the incision instead of with a bag.

Demographics

The HCUP Nationwide Inpatient Sample from the Agency for Healthcare Research and Quality (AHRQ) reports that 61,905 patients underwent partial or radical nephrectomy surgery for non-transplant-related indications in the United States in 2010. Patients with **kidney cancer** accounted for more than half of those procedures. About 65,150 new cases of renal cell carcinoma were expected to be diagnosed in 2013, per the American Cancer Society, as well as 13,680 kidney cancer-related deaths.

According to the United Network for Organ Sharing (UNOS), 5,622 people underwent nephrectomy to become living kidney donors in 2012. Of these, 2,107 were male and 3,515 were female. Related donors were more common than non-related donors, with full siblings being the most common relationship between living donor and kidney recipients, and child to parent being the next most common relationship between living donor and kidney recipients. Nearly 3,000 new patients are added to the kidney waiting list each month.

Preparation

Prior to surgery, blood samples will be taken from the patient to type and crossmatch in case a transfusion is required during surgery. A catheter will also be inserted into the patient's bladder. The surgical procedure will be described to the patient, along with the possible risks.

Aftercare

Nephrectomy patients may experience considerable discomfort in the area of the incision. Patients may also experience numbness, caused by severed nerves, near or on the incision. Pain relievers are administered following the surgical procedure and during the recovery period on an as-needed basis. Although deep breathing and coughing may be painful due to the proximity of the incision to the diaphragm, breathing exercises are encouraged to prevent **pneumonia**. Patients should not drive an automobile for a minimum of two weeks.

Risks

Possible complications of the nephrectomy procedure include infection, bleeding (hemorrhage), and postoperative pneumonia. There is also the risk of kidney failure in a patient with impaired function or disease in the remaining kidney.

Results

Normal results of a nephrectomy are dependent on the purpose of the procedure and the type of nephrectomy performed. Immediately following the procedure, it is normal for patients to experience pain near the incision site, particularly when coughing or breathing deeply. Renal function of the patient is monitored carefully after surgery. If the remaining kidney is healthy, it will increase its functioning over time to compensate for the loss of the removed kidney.

Length of hospitalization depends on the type of nephrectomy procedure. Patients who have undergone laparoscopic radical nephrectomy may be discharged two to four days after surgery. Traditional open nephrectomy patients are typically hospitalized for about a week. Recovery time will also vary, from three to six weeks on average.

Morbidity and mortality rates

Survival rates for living kidney donors undergoing nephrectomy are excellent; mortality rates are only 0.03% or three deaths for every 10,000 donors. Many

QUESTIONS TO ASK YOUR DOCTOR

- How many procedures of this type have you performed, and what are your success rates?
- Will my nephrectomy surgery be performed with a laparoscopic or an open technique?
- Will my nephrectomy be partial or radical, and what are the risks involved with my particular surgery?
- What will my recovery time be after the procedure?
- What are the chances that the transplant will be successful (if donating a kidney)?
- Will I require adjunctive treatment such as chemotherapy or immunotherapy?

of the risks involved are the same as for any surgical procedure—infection, hemorrhage, blood clot, or allergic reaction to anesthesia.

For patients undergoing nephrectomy as a treatment for renal cell carcinoma, survival rates depend on several factors, including the stage of the cancer and the patient's overall health and medical history. According to the American Cancer Society, the five-year survival rate for patients with stage I renal cell carcinoma is 81%, while the five-year survival rate for stage II kidney cancer is 74%. Stage III and IV cancers have metastasized, or spread, beyond the kidney and have a lower survival rate: 53% for stage III and about 8% for stage IV. **Chemotherapy**, radiation, and/or **immunotherapy** may also be required for these patients.

Alternatives

Because the kidney is responsible for filtering wastes and fluid from the bloodstream, kidney function is critical to life. Nephrectomy candidates diagnosed with serious kidney disease, cancer, or infection usually have few treatment choices aside from this procedure. However, if kidney function is lost in the remaining kidney, the patient will require chronic dialysis treatments or transplantation of a healthy kidney to sustain life.

Health care team roles

If nephrectomy is required for the purpose of kidney donation, it will be performed by a transplant surgeon in one of over 200 UNOS-approved hospitals nationwide. For patients with renal cell carcinoma, nephrectomy

surgery is typically performed in a hospital setting by a surgeon specializing in urologic oncology.

Resources

BOOKS

Brenner, B. M., and F. C. Rector, eds. *Brenner & Rector's The Kidney.* 9th ed. Philadelphia: Saunders/Elsevier, 2012.

Wein, Alan J., et al. *Campbell-Walsh Urology.* 10th ed. Philadelphia: Saunders/Elsevier, 2012.

PERIODICALS

Alberts, Victor, et al. "Transplant Nephrectomy: What Are the Surgical Risks?" *Annals of Transplantation* 18 (April 16, 2013): 174–81. http://dx.doi.org/10.12659/AOT.883887 (accessed October 3, 2014).

Alyami, Fahad A., and Ricardo A. Rendon. "Laparoscopic Partial Nephrectomy for >4 cm Renal Masses." *Canadian Urological Association Journal* 7, nos. 5–6 (2013): E281–86. http://dx.doi.org/10.5489/cuaj.1003 (accessed October 3, 2014).

Cohen, Jason, et al. "Do Hemostatic Agents Impact Negative Outcomes following Robotic Partial Nephrectomy?" *Journal of Endourology* (July 24, 2013): e-pub ahead of print. http://dx.doi.org/10.1089/end.2013.0136 (accessed October 3, 2014).

Hwan Kang, Su, Hyun Yul Rhew, and Taek Sang Kim. "Changes in Renal Function After Laparoscopic Partial Nephrectomy: Comparison with Laparoscopic Radical Nephrectomy." *Korean Journal of Urology* 54, no. 1 (2013): 22–25. http://dx.doi.org/10.4111/kju.2013.54.1.22 (accessed October 3, 2014).

Lavallée, Luke T., et al. "The Association between Renal Tumour Scoring Systems and Ischemia Time during Open Partial Nephrectomy." *Canadian Urological Association Journal* 7, nos. 3–4 (2013): E207–14. http://dx.doi.org/10.5489/cuaj.11202 (accessed October 3, 2014).

Patel, Nilay, et al. "Renal Function and Cardiovascular Outcomes after Living Donor Nephrectomy in the UK: Quality and Safety Revisited." *BJUI International* 112, no. 2 (2013): E134–42. http://dx.doi.org/10.1111/bju.12213 (accessed October 3, 2014).

WEBSITES

American Cancer Society. "Surgery for Kidney Cancer." http://www.cancer.org/cancer/kidneycancer/detailedguide/kidney-cancer-adult-treating-surgery (accessed October 3, 2014).

American Cancer Society. "What Are the Key Statistics about Kidney Cancer?" http://www.cancer.org/cancer/kidney-cancer/detailedguide/kidney-cancer-adult-key-statistics (accessed October 3, 2014).

Weill Cornell Medical College. "Open Donor Nephrectomy." New York-Presbyterian Hospital. http://cornellsurgery.org/patients/services/livingdonor/surgery-recovery-donor health.html (accessed October 3, 2014).

ORGANIZATIONS

American Cancer Society, 250 Williams St. NW, Atlanta, GA 30303, (800) 227-2345, http://www.cancer.org.

International Association of Living Organ Donors, http://www.livingdonorsonline.org.

National Kidney Foundation, 30 E. 33rd St., New York, NY 10016, (212) 889-2210, (800) 622-9010, Fax: (212) 689-9261, http://www.kidney.org.

United Network for Organ Sharing (UNOS), 700 N. 4th St., Richmond, VA 23219, (804) 782-4800, http://www.unos.org.

Paula Anne Ford-Martin
REVISED BY TAMMY ALLHOFF, CST/CSFA, AAS

Nephrostomy

Definition

A nephrostomy is a surgical procedure by which a tube, stent, or catheter is inserted through the skin and into the kidney.

Purpose

The ureter is the fibromuscular tube that carries urine from the kidney to the bladder. When this tube is blocked, urine backs up into the kidney. Serious, irreversible kidney damage can occur because of this backflow of urine. Infection is also a common consequence of this stagnant urine.

Nephrostomy is performed in several different circumstances:

- The ureter is blocked by a kidney stone.
- The ureter is blocked by a tumor, abscess, or fluid collection.
- There is a hole in the ureter or bladder and urine is leaking into the body. This may occur after trauma or accidental injury during surgery (iatrogenic injury), or severe hemorrhagic cystitis.
- The ureter is obstructed during pregnancy.
- Access is needed in order to infuse materials/medications directly into the kidney, such as antibiotics, antifungal agents, chemotherapeutic agents, or chemicals that will dissolve stones.
- As a diagnostic procedure to assess kidney anatomy.
- As a diagnostic procedure to assess kidney function.

Description

To begin the procedure, the patient is given an anesthetic to numb the area where the catheter will be inserted. The doctor then inserts a needle into the kidney. There are several imaging technologies such as ultrasound

and **computed tomography** (CT) that are used to help the doctor guide the needle into the correct place.

Next, a fine guide wire follows the needle. The catheter, which is about the same diameter as intravenous (IV) tubing, follows the guide wire to its proper location. The catheter is then connected to a bag outside the body that collects the urine. The catheter and bag are secured so that the catheter will not pull out. The procedure usually takes one to two hours.

Demographics

For unknown reasons, the number of people in the United States with kidney and ureter stones has been increasing over the past 20 years. White Americans are more prone to develop kidney stones than African Americans. Stones occur more frequently in men. The condition strikes most typically between the ages of 20 and 40. Once a person gets more than one stone, others are likely to develop.

Upper tract tumors develop in the renal pelvis (tissue in the kidneys that collects urine) and in the ureters. These cancers account for less than 1% of cancers of the reproductive and urinary systems. Upper tract tumors are often associated with **bladder cancer**.

Precautions

People preparing for a nephrostomy should review with their doctors all the medications they are taking.

People taking anticoagulants (blood thinners such as Coumadin) may need to stop medication. People taking metformin (Glucophage) may need to stop taking the medication for several days before and after nephrostomy. Diabetics should discuss modifying their insulin doses because fasting is required before the procedure.

Preparation

Either the day before or the day of the nephrostomy, blood samples are taken. Other diagnostic tests done before the procedure may vary, depending on why the nephrostomy is being done, but the patient may have a CT scan or ultrasound to help the treating physician locate the blockage.

Patients should not eat for eight hours before a nephrostomy. On the day of the procedure, the patient will have an IV line placed in a vein in the arm. Through this line, the patient will receive **antibiotics** to prevent infection, medication for pain, and fluids. The IV line will remain in place after the procedure for at least several hours, and often longer.

Aftercare

Outpatients are usually expected to stay in the clinic or hospital for 8 to 12 hours after the procedure to make sure the nephrostomy tube is functioning properly. They should plan to have someone drive them home and stay with them for at least the first 24 hours after the procedure. Inpatients may stay in the hospital several days. Generally, people feel sore where the catheter is inserted for about a week to ten days.

Care of the nephrostomy tube is important. It is located on the patient's back, so it may be necessary to have someone help with its care. The nephrostomy tube should be kept dry and protected from water when taking showers. The skin around it should be kept clean, and the dressing over the area changed frequently. It is the main part of the urine drainage system, and it should be treated very carefully to prevent bacteria and other germs from entering the system. If any germs get into the tubing, they can easily cause a kidney infection. The drainage bag should not be allowed to drag on the floor. If the bag should accidentally be cut or begin to leak, it must be changed immediately. It is not recommended to place the drainage bag in a plastic bag if it leaks.

Risks

A nephrostomy is an established and generally safe procedure. As with all operations, there is always a risk of allergic reaction to anesthesia, bleeding, and infection.

QUESTIONS TO ASK YOUR DOCTOR

- Why am I having a nephrostomy?
- How do I prepare for surgery?
- How long will I have to stay in the hospital?
- How long do you expect the nephrostomy tube to stay in?
- How much help will I need in caring for the nephrostomy tube?

Bruising at the catheter insertion site occurs in about half of people who have a nephrostomy. This is a minor complication. Major complications include the following:

- injury to surrounding organs, including bowel perforation, splenic injury, and liver injury
- infection, leading to septicemia
- significant loss of functioning kidney tissue (<1%)
- delayed bleeding, or hemorrhage (<0.5%)
- blocking of a kidney artery (<0.5%)

Results

In a successful nephrostomy, the catheter is inserted, and urine drains into the collection bag. How long the catheter stays in place depends on the reason for its insertion. In people with pelvic **cancer** or bladder cancer where the ureter is blocked by a tumor, the catheter will stay in place until the tumor is surgically removed. If the cancer is inoperable, the catheter may have to stay in place for the rest of the patient's life.

Health care team roles

A nephrostomy is performed by an interventional radiologist or urologist with special training in the procedure. It can be done either on an inpatient or outpatient basis, depending on why it is required. For most cancer patients, nephrostomy is an inpatient procedure. Specially trained nurses called wound, ostomy, and continence nurses (WOCN) are commonly available for consultation in most major medical centers to assist patients.

Resources

BOOKS

Brenner, B. M., and F. C. Rector, eds. *Brenner & Rector's The Kidney.* 9th ed. Philadelphia: Saunders/Elsevier, 2012.

Townsend, Courtney M., et al. *Sabiston Textbook of Surgery*. 19th ed. Philadelphia: Saunders/Elsevier, 2012.

Wein, Alan J., et al. *Campbell-Walsh Urology*. 10th ed. Philadelphia: Saunders/Elsevier, 2012.

PERIODICALS

Ali, S. M., et al. "Frequency of Complications in Image Guided Percutaneous Nephrostomy." *Journal of the Pakistani Medical Association* 63, no. 7 (2013): 816–20.

Li, Albert C., and Sidney P. Regalado. "Emergent Percutaneous Nephrostomy for the Diagnosis and Management of Pyonephrosis." *Seminars in Interventional Radiology* 29, no. 3 (2012): 218–25. http://dx.doi.org/10.1055/s-0032-1326932 (accessed October 3, 2014).

OTHER

National Institutes of Health Clinical Center. *Caring for Your Percutaneous Nephrostomy Tube*. http://www.cc.nih.gov/ccc/patient_education/pepubs/percneph.pdf (accessed October 3, 2014).

WEBSITES

Cardiovascular and Interventional Radiological Society of Europe. "Nephrostomy." http://www.cirse.org/index.php?pid=152 (accessed October 3, 2014).

Macmillan Cancer Support. "Nephrostomy." http://www.macmillan.org.uk/Cancerinformation/Cancertreatment/Treatmenttypes/Supportivetherapies/Nephrostomy.aspx (accessed October 3, 2014).

ORGANIZATIONS

American Cancer Society, 250 Williams St. NW, Atlanta, GA 30303, (800) 227-2345, http://www.cancer.org.

American College of Radiology, 1891 Preston White Dr., Reston, VA 20191, (703) 648-8900, info@acr.org, http://www.acr.org.

Cardiovascular and Interventional Radiological Society of Europe (CIRSE), Neutorgasse 9/6, 1010 Vienna, Austria, +43 1 904 2003, Fax: +43 1 904 2003 30, info@cirse.org, http://www.cirse.org.

United Ostomy Associations of America, Inc. (UOAA), PO Box 512, Northfield, MN 55057-0512, (800) 826-0826, info@ostomy.org, http://www.ostomy.org.

Urology Care Foundation, 1000 Corporate Blvd., Linthicum, MD 21090, (410) 689-3700, (800) 828-7866, Fax: (410) 689-3998, info@urologycarefoundation.org, http://auafoundation.org.

Tish Davidson, AM
Monique Laberge, PhD

Neumega *see* **Oprelvekin**

Neupogen *see* **Filgrastim**

Neuroblastoma

Definition

Neuroblastoma is a type of **cancer** that begins in nerve cells outside the brain. Tumors usually develop in the nerve tissue of the adrenal glands, neck, chest, abdomen, pelvis, or spinal cord.

Description

Neuroblastoma usually occurs when children are young, and sometimes before they are born, although it may not be noticed until later. If the cancer is not found until later, it has often spread to the lymph nodes, liver, lungs, bones, or bone marrow. Approximately two-thirds of neuroblastomas start in the adrenal glands, glands above each kidney that produce hormones.

Demographics

Neuroblastoma is the most common cancer that occurs in infants, and approximately 7% of **childhood cancers** are neuroblastomas. Most cases are diagnosed when children are between one and two years old, and the cancer is rarely diagnosed in a child older than age ten. According to some reports, African American children develop the disease at a slightly higher rate than Caucasian children.

Causes and symptoms

Neuroblastoma can be inherited, or passed in the genes from parent to child. When this is the case, it is found at an earlier age than in children who have not inherited the gene mutation that causes the cancer. Most

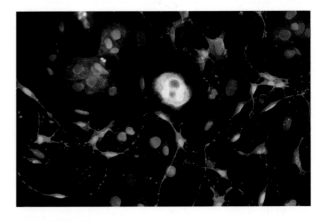

Immunofluorescent light micrograph of human neuroblastoma cancer cells. The normal epithelial cells appear green, the cytoplasm of neuroblastoma is red, and the nuclei are blue. (*NANCY KEDERSHA/Science Source*)

KEY TERMS

Adjuvant chemotherapy—Treatment of a cancer with drugs after surgery to kill as many of the remaining cancer cells as possible.

Adrenal gland—Gland located above each kidney consisting of an outer wall (cortex) that produces steroid hormones and an inner section (medulla) that produces other important hormones, such as adrenaline and noradrenaline.

Alternative therapy—A therapy is generally called alternative when it is used instead of conventional cancer treatments.

Biopsy—A small sample of tissue removed from the site of the tumor to be examined under a microscope.

Complementary therapy—A therapy is called complementary when it is used in addition to conventional cancer treatments.

Conventional therapy—Treatments that are widely accepted and practiced by the mainstream medical community.

Disseminated—Spread to other tissues.

Hormone—A substance produced by specialized cells that affects the way the body carries out the biochemical and energy-producing processes required to maintain health (metabolism).

Localized—Confined to a small area.

Monoclonal antibody—A protein substance which is produced in the laboratory by a single population of cells and can be used to target cancer treatment.

Neoadjuvant chemotherapy—Treatment of the tumor with drugs before surgery to reduce the size of the tumor.

Neuroblast cells—Cells produced by the fetus that mature into nerve cells and adrenal medulla cells.

Resectable cancer—A tumor that can be surgically removed.

Salvage therapy—Treatment measures taken late in the course of a disease after other therapies have failed. It is also known as rescue therapy.

Staging system—A system that describes cancer based on how far the cancer has spread from its original site, developed to help the physician determine how to best treat the disease.

Unresectable cancer—A tumor that cannot be completely removed by surgery.

---

causes of neuroblastoma are still unknown, although doctors know that neuroblastomas develop when cells produced by the fetus (neuroblast cells) fail to mature into normal nerve or adrenal cells and keep growing and proliferating.

The first symptom of a neuroblastoma is usually an unusual growth or lump, found in most cases in the abdomen of the child, causing discomfort or a sensation of fullness and pain. Other symptoms such as numbness and **fatigue** arise because of pressure caused by the tumor. **Bone pain** also occurs if the cancer has spread to the bone. The cancer may cause protruding eyes and dark circles around the eyes. Some children have weakness or paralysis from compression of the spinal cord. **Fever** is also reported in one case out of four. High blood pressure, persistent **diarrhea**, rapid heartbeat, reddening of the skin, and sweating occur occasionally. Some children may also have uncoordinated or jerky muscle movements, or uncontrollable eye movements, but these symptoms are rare. If the disease spreads to the skin, blue or purple patches are observed.

Diagnosis

A diagnosis of neuroblastoma usually requires blood and urine tests to investigate the nature and quantity of chemicals (neurotransmitters) released by the nerve cells. These are broken down by the body and released in urine. Additionally, scanning techniques are used to identify neuroblastoma tumors. These techniques produce images or pictures of the inside of the body and include **computed tomography** scan (CT scan) and **magnetic resonance imaging** (MRI). To confirm the diagnosis, the physician will surgically remove some of the tissue from the tumor or bone marrow (**biopsy**). The biopsy sample is examined under a microscope, often using one or more advanced techniques to look for changes in cells. For example, **immunohistochemistry** uses antibodies and a special dye to cause the tissue to light up under a microscope.

Treatment team

The treatment team usually consists of an pediatric oncologist who is experienced in the treatment of neuroblastoma, a surgeon to perform biopsies and possibly attempt surgical removal of the tumor, a **radiation therapy** team and, if indicated, a **bone marrow transplantation** team.

Clinical staging

Once neuroblastoma has been diagnosed, the physician will perform more tests to determine if the cancer has spread to other tissues in the body. This process, called staging, is important for the physician to determine how to treat the cancer and also check liver and kidney function. The staging system for neuroblastoma is based on how far the disease has spread from its original site to other tissues in the body. Doctors often place stages into categories of risk to help determine a patient's risk and the best treatment choices. The common staging system for neuroblastoma is:

- Stage 1 neuroblastoma is confined to the site of origin, with no evidence that it has spread to other tissues, and the cancer can be surgically removed.
- Stage 2 is divided into A and B. Stage 2A is neuroblastoma located only where it began, but unable to be removed completely using surgery. Stage 2B is in the original area, may or may not be completely removed by surgery, and nearby lymph nodes have signs of cancer.
- Stage 3 neuroblastoma is a tumor that cannot be completely removed by surgery that has spread to the other side of the body and to nearby lymph nodes; or remains on one side of the body, but has spread to lymph nodes on the other side of the body; or a tumor in the center of the body that has spread to lymph nodes or tissues on both sides and cannot be removed by surgery.
- Stage 4 neuroblastoma has spread to lymph nodes further from the tumor. In stage 4S, the cancer has spread to the skin, liver, or bone marrow, and the tumor cannot be completely removed during surgery. In addition, cancer cells may be in lymph nodes near the tumor. Stage 4S is also used to describe children with neuroblastoma who are younger than one year old.

Treatment

Treatments are available for children with all stages of neuroblastoma. More than one of these treatments may be used, depending on the stage of the disease. The four types of treatment used are:

- Surgery (removing the tumor in an operation)
- Radiation therapy (using high-energy x-rays to kill cancer cells)
- Chemotherapy (using drugs to kill cancer cells)

- High-dose chemotherapy and radiation therapy with stem cell rescue (removing the patient's stem cells, or immature bone marrow cells, and giving high doses of therapy, then returning the stem cells through an infusion).

Surgery is used whenever possible to remove as much of the cancer as possible, and can generally cure the disease if the cancer has not spread to other areas of the body. Before surgery, **chemotherapy** may be used to shrink the tumor so that it can be more easily removed; this is called neoadjuvant chemotherapy. New chemotherapy drugs are tested often, and some studies have shown promising results in children who have intermediate-risk neuroblastoma without using chemotherapy, so that side effects are less severe. Radiation therapy is often used after surgery; high-energy rays (radiation) are used to kill as many of the remaining cancer cells as possible. Chemotherapy (called **adjuvant chemotherapy**) can also be used after surgery to kill remaining cancer cells. Bone marrow transplantation is used to replace bone marrow cells killed by radiation or chemotherapy. In some cases, the patient's own bone marrow is removed prior to treatment and saved for transplantation later. Other times the bone marrow comes from a matched donor, such as a sibling.

New therapies are tested in **clinical trials**. These trials have led to advances such as targeted therapy, which uses drugs or other materials to find and attack neuroblastoma cells or changes in a certain gene without harming a patient's normal cells. An example is tyrosine kinase inhibitor, which blocks the signals that neuroblastoma tumors need so they can grow. Another novel therapy is vaccine therapy. Vaccines are a type of biologic therapy, also called **immunotherapy**, which uses a patient's own immune system to fight cancer. Doctors are also using a drug that prevents new blood vessels from providing blood to neuroblastoma tumors, which stops their growth. Sometimes, a clinical trial offers the best treatment choice, especially for a rare cancer. Participation in clinical trials is voluntary.

Alternative and complementary therapies

No alternative therapy has been reported to substitute for conventional neuroblastoma treatment.

Prognosis

The chances of recovery from neuroblastoma depend on the stage of the cancer, the age of the child at diagnosis, the location of the tumor, and the state and nature of the tumor cells evaluated under the

QUESTIONS TO ASK YOUR DOCTOR

- What treatment choices do we have?
- Has the neuroblastoma spread to other parts of the body?
- What is the stage of the cancer?
- Based on your experience in treating neuroblastoma, how long do you think my child will survive if there is no response to treatment or the cancer comes back?
- How long will it take to recover from treatment?
- Will my child develop any long-term risks or complications from the cancer or its treatment?
- Can you recommend a support group for people who are coping with neuroblastoma?

microscope. Infants have a higher rate of cure than do children over one year of age, even when the disease has spread. In general, the prognosis for a young child with neuroblastoma is good: the predicted five-year survival rate is approximately 87% for children who had the onset of the disease in infancy, and up to 65% for those whose disease developed later. In general, survival rates for the disease have been improving. Doctors continue to use DNA and genetic information to help determine a child's risk for a poor outcome or a return of the cancer so they can plan more aggressive treatment if necessary. Studies of 13-cis-retinoic acid, a drug related to vitamin A, have shown promise when this agent is given to high-risk children after stem cell transplant or chemotherapy.

Coping with cancer treatment

Neuroblastoma is a childhood cancer and it must be recognized that children, adolescents, and their families have very special needs. These are best met at cancer centers for children that maintain communication between the treatment team and the primary care physician. These centers have experience in recognizing the unique needs of children having to cope with cancer, and they are staffed by pediatric support professionals other than the oncology treatment team while being associated with a children's hospital.

Clinical trials

In 2014, the **National Cancer Institute** was supporting at least 37 clinical trials involving neuroblastoma. These trials were evaluating a variety of anticancer drug combinations or other treatments. Some studies also involved **stem cell transplantation** and the rejection of transplanted cells from a donor. Other clinical trials were aimed specifically at treatments for neuroblastoma that resists typical treatment or returns.

Prevention

Because an increased risk for development of neuroblastoma can be passed down from parents, anyone with a history of this cancer in his or her family should consider genetic counseling regarding the risk of neuroblastoma occurring in their children. Otherwise, there are no known steps to take for preventing neuroblastoma. Detecting the disease as early as possible can improve a child's prognosis.

Special concerns

After completion of a course of treatment for neuroblastoma, children need regular follow-up care. The follow-up visits can include lab tests and imaging examinations to check for signs of the cancer remaining or returning. Parents should be sure to keep all follow-up appointments to catch any return of the cancer as early as possible in their child.

See also Bone marrow aspiration and biopsy.

Resources

BOOKS

Beers, Mark H., and Robert Berkow, eds. "Neuroblastoma." In *The Merck Manual of Diagnosis and Therapy.* Whitehouse Station, NJ: Merck Research Laboratories, 2007.

PERIODICALS

Brodeur, G. M., and R. Bagatell. "Mechanisms of Neuroblastoma Regression." *Nature Reviews: Clinical Oncology* 11, no. 12 (2014): 704–13. http://dx.doi.org/10.1038/nrclinonc.2014.168 (accessed December 22, 2014).

Liu, Y. L., J. S. Miser, and W. M. Hsu. "Risk-Directed Therapy and Research in Neuroblastoma." *Journal of the Formosan Medical Association* 113, no. 12 (2014): 887–89. http://dx.doi.org/10.1016/j.jfma.2014.11.001 (accessed December 22, 2014).

OTHER

American Cancer Society. "Neuroblastoma." http://www.cancer.org/acs/groups/cid/documents/webcontent/003125-pdf.pdf (accessed October 4, 2014).

WEBSITES

American Society of Clinical Oncology. "Neuroblastoma, Childhood Overview." Cancer.Net. http://www.cancer.net/cancer-types/neuroblastoma-childhood/overview (accessed October 4, 2014).

MD Anderson Cancer Center. "Neuroblastoma Basics." http://www.mdanderson.org/patient-and-cancer-information/cancer-information/cancer-types/neuroblastoma/index.html (accessed October 4, 2014).

National Cancer Institute. "General Information about Neuroblastoma." http://www.cancer.gov/cancertopics/pdq/treatment/neuroblastoma/Patient/page1 (accessed October 4, 2014).

ORGANIZATIONS

American Cancer Society, 250 Williams Street NW, Atlanta, GA 30303, (800) 227-2345, http://www.cancer.org.

National Cancer Institute, 9609 Medical Center Drive, Bethesda, MD 20892, (800) 422-6237, http://www.cancer.gov.

Lisa Christenson
Monique Laberge, PhD
Rebecca J. Frey, PhD
REVISED BY TERESA G. ODLE

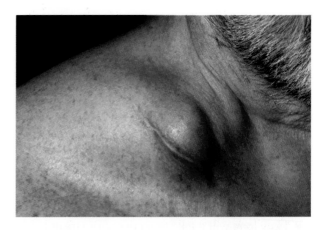

Neuroendocrine tumor located on the shoulder. Neuroendocrine tumors are rare; this tumor was caused by the spread of a primary cancer located elsewhere in the body. (*Dr. P. Marazzi/Science Source*)

Neuroendocrine tumors

Definition

Neuroendocrine tumors are tumors that develop from the cells in the body that release hormones into the blood when they receive signals from the body's nervous system. These tumors can occur in many different areas of the body.

Description

The endocrine system is a network of glands made up of endocrine cells that produce hormones in the body. The neuroendocrine system cells are specialized endocrine cells of the nervous system that produce neurohormones. Neuroendocrine cells do not form a specific gland; instead, they are found throughout several of the body's organs, where they help regulate body function. An example of a function is controlling how quickly or slowly food moves through a person's gastrointestinal tract once swallowed.

Neuroendocrine tumors represent a large class of cancers that can occur wherever neuroendocrine cells are found in the body. They are sometimes called carcinoid tumors, but it is more accurate to consider carcinoid tumors as a type within the larger family of neuroendocrine tumors. GI carcinoid tumors are most often found in the digestive system and the lung. Statistically, 38% occur in the appendix, 23% in the ileum, 13% in the rectum, and 11.5% in the bronchi. About 8,000 GI carcinoid cancers are diagnosed in the United States each year.

Neuroendocrine pancreatic tumors are rare cancers. Only about 1,000 cases are diagnosed each year in the United States. They occur with the same frequency in men and women and the average age at diagnosis is 53 years. Neuroendocrine pancreatic tumors are also known as islet cell tumors. Islet cells are the hormone-producing cells in the pancreas that form the tumors. It is possible that some neuroendocrine tumors are not reported.

Because they can occur wherever neuroendocrine cells are found, neuroendocrine tumors come in a wide variety of types and have been classified according to their site of origin, which can become confusing. For example, some forms of **thyroid cancer** begin in the thyroid's neuroendocrine cells.

Neuroendocrine carcinoma

There are many different types of malignant, or cancerous, tumors. One of these is **carcinoma**. A carcinoma is a **cancer** that begins in epithelial cells, the cells that usually line or cover an organ. Though most neuroendocrine cancers cannot be described as a certain type, neuroendocrine carcinomas can be found in several areas of the body, including the brain, lungs, and GI tract.

Pancreatic neuroendocrine tumors

Most neuroendocrine pancreatic tumors produce multiple hormones, but usually there is excessive production of only one hormone. This is why neuroendocrine pancreatic tumors are often classified according to the predominant hormone secreted or resulting symptoms observed. For example, insulinomas produce excessive amounts of insulin, and gastrinomas produce

KEY TERMS

Apudoma—A tumor capable of Amine Precursor Uptake and Decarboxylation (APUD).

Bronchi—Air passages to the lungs.

Diffuse neuroendocrine system—Concept developed by Feyrter, a German pathologist, more than 60 years ago, to unify tumors that occur in various parts of the body and possess secretory activity as well as similar properties when examined under a microscope.

Epithelial cells—Cells that cover the surface of the body and line its cavities.

Gastrointestinal tract—The GI tract, also called the digestive tract, starts from the oral cavity (mouth) and proceeds to the esophagus, the stomach, the duodenum, the small intestine, the large intestine (colon), the rectum, and the anus. It processes all the food we eat. Along its way, food is digested, nutrients are extracted, and waste is eliminated from the body in the form of stool and urine.

Gland—An organ that produces and releases substances for use in the body, such as fluids or hormones.

Hormone—Chemical substances produced by endocrine glands and transported by the bloodstream to the organs that require them to regulate their function.

Ileum—The last portion of the small intestine.

Metastasis—The transfer of cancer from one location or organ to another one not directly related to it.

Nervous system—The network of nerve tissue of the body. It includes the brain, the spinal cord and the ganglia (group of nerve cells).

Neurohormone—A hormone produced by specialized neurons or neuroendocrine cells.

Neuron—Specialized cell of the nervous system that transmits nervous system signals. It consists of a cell body linked to a long branch (axon) and to several short ones (dendrites).

Syndrome—A series of symptoms or medical events occurring together and pointing to a single disease as the cause.

---

excessive amounts of the peptide gastrin. Glucagonomas are associated with skin lesions and irritation around the eyes, and somatostatinomas are associated with gallstones, mild diabetes, and **diarrhea** or constipation.

Pheochromocytomas

These rare tumors develop in cells of the adrenal glands called chromaffin cells. One adrenal gland is located just above each kidney. Chromaffin cells release hormones during stress. Pheochromocytomas often are benign, or noncancerous, but must be treated because they release excessive amounts of hormones into the bloodstream that increase heart rate and blood pressure.

Merkel cell cancer

This rare type of neuroendocrine tumor grows rapidly. It begins in cells just beneath the skin that make hormones, and it is usually diagnosed near the head and neck.

Diagnosis

The diagnosis of neuroendocrine tumors is based on a doctor's physical examination and patient's medical history, along with a combination of laboratory and imaging examinations. Diagnosis varies depending on the site of the neuroendocrine tumor and the hormones, organs, and body functions affected.

Lab tests

Blood and urine tests can measure substances such as hormones in a patient's body to indicate an imbalance caused by a neuroendocrine tumor. A 24-hour urine test requires a patient to collect urine for 24 hours so that the lab can measure amounts of hormones released in the urine. **Tumor markers**, certain substances in the body that might indicate neuroendocrine cancer, can also be found in blood or urine samples.

Medical imaging exams

Using imaging exams helps doctors identify and stage neuroendocrine tumors throughout the body. A doctor may use **computed tomography** (CT) scans, **magnetic resonance imaging** (MRI), or **positron emission tomography** (PET) for these purposes. **Nuclear medicine scans**, which use a small amount of injected radioactive dye and a special camera to highlight cancerous tumors, are useful for detecting small tumors around the body. **Ultrasonography** uses sound waves instead of **x-rays** to image inside a patient's body, and a doctor might place the ultrasonography probe at the end of a long thin tube called an endoscope to see inside a patient's GI tract.

Biopsy

A **biopsy**, or sample of cells or tissue from a tumor, is the only way to confirm whether a tumor is cancerous. Doctors may gather the tissue or cells using a needle or during surgery to remove a neuroendocrine tumor. They also can gather samples during **colonoscopy** or endoscopy, which are procedures that use a thin, lighted tube with a camera on the end to examine the inside of the body.

Clinical staging

A recent classification from the World Health Organization groups neuroendocrine tumors into types according to where the tumor developed, how aggressively the tumor is growing, and characteristics of the tumor's cells. The system also takes into account whether the tumor is functional or nonfunctional, meaning whether it causes clinical problems for a patient because of its effect on hormones and body functions. Doctors use this and other information to plan treatment. There is no staging system specific to neuroendocrine tumors; most are staged along with the body organ or location in which they develop. For example, pancreatic neuroendocrine tumors are staged with other pancreatic cancers. Merkel cell cancer has its own staging system.

Treatment

Surgery

The only truly effective treatment for neuroendocrine tumors is to remove the tumor using surgery. Doctors can remove the tumor one of several ways, depending on where the tumor is located and its size. The doctor may have to remove all or part of the organ in which the tumor originated. Sometimes, doctors can use special techniques such as cryosurgery, which freezes and destroys the cancer cells, or **radiofrequency ablation**, which uses high-energy radio waves to destroy the cells. These techniques result in shorter recovery times than invasive surgery.

Chemotherapy

Although **chemotherapy** is sometimes used when **metastasis** has occurred, it is rarely effective. The treatment for carcinoid syndrome is typically meant to decrease the severity of symptoms. Patients should try to avoid stress and any foods that produce symptoms. Some medications can be given for symptomatic relief; for example, tumors of the gastrointestinal tract may be treated with octreotide (Sandostatin) or lanreotide (Somatuline) to relieve such symptoms as diarrhea and flushing. These drugs are known as somatostatin analogs. Some patients may receive regional chemotherapy, which delivers the drugs directly to the area where the neuroendocrine tumor is located.

Other therapies

Radiation therapy usually delivers a targeted beam of x-rays from outside the patient's body to destroy cancer cells. Doctors treat some neuroendocrine tumors with a radioactive substance that is infused or delivered directly to the cancerous cells.

Hormone therapy is often used to treat neuroendocrine tumors. Special hormone therapy drugs can block, add, or remove hormones to stop production of hormones that are causing illness in the patient and the growth of tumors.

Targeted and novel therapies

Targeted therapies are new approaches to treating neuroendocrine and other cancers. The therapy uses drugs and other materials to identify and attack only specific cancer cells and spare normal, healthy cells. Several substances are used or being tested for use in metastatic or recurrent (returning) neuroendocrine cancers. Some patients participate in **clinical trials** where new therapies are being investigated.

Prognosis

The prognosis for patients with neuroendocrine tumors is related to the specific growth patterns of the tumor, the tumor's location, and how far the cancer has advanced. Doctors look at indicators of how the tumor is affecting the patient's health, as well. Researchers continue to look for ways to measure certain proteins and markers in a patient's blood to better predict prognosis.

Prevention

Neuroendocrine tumors such as carcinoid tumors are rare, and there is little that can be done to prevent them. Some medical conditions place people at higher risk for certain types of GI carcinoid tumors, which people should discuss with their doctors. A hereditary condition called **multiple endocrine neoplasia** type 1 increases risk of neuroendocrine tumors, so patients who have the condition in their family should discuss their history with their doctor. Smoking tobacco may also increase risk of neuroendocrine tumors.

See also Adenoma; Carcinoid tumors, gastrointestinal; Carcinoid tumors, lung; Cushing syndrome; Endocrine system tumors; Lung cancer, small cell; Merkel cell carcinoma; Pancreatic cancer, endocrine; Parathyroid cancer; Pituitary tumors; Zollinger-Ellison syndrome.

Resources

BOOKS

Beers, Mark H., and Robert Berkow, eds. "Carcinoid Tumors." In *The Merck Manual of Diagnosis and Therapy*. Whitehouse Station, NJ: Merck Research Laboratories, 2007.

PERIODICALS

Grat, M., et al. "Outcomes following Liver Transplantation for Metastatic Neuroendocrine Tumors." *Transplant Proceedings* 46, no. 8 (2014): 2766–69.

Hallet, J., et al. "Exploring the Rising Incidence of Neuroendocrine Tumors: A Population-Based Analysis of Epidemiology, Metastatic Presentation, and Outcomes." *Cancer* (October 13, 2014): e-pub ahead of print. http://dx.doi.org/10.1002/cncr.29099 (accessed November 11, 2014).

Raj, N., and D. Reidy-Lagunes. "Current Clinical Trials of Targeted Agents for Well-Differentiated Neuroendocrine Tumors." *Pancreas* 43, no. 8 (2014): 1185–89.

OTHER

American Cancer Society. "Gastrointestinal Carcinoid Tumors." http://www.cancer.org/acs/groups/cid/docu ments/web-content/003102-pdf.pdf (accessed August 28, 2014).

WEBSITES

American Society of Clinical Oncology. "Neuroendocrine Tumor: Overview." Cancer.Net. http://www.cancer.net/cancer-types/neuroendocrine-tumor/overview (accessed August 28, 2014).

MD Anderson Cancer Center. "Carcinoid Tumor Prevention and Screening." http://www.mdanderson.org/patient-and-cancer-information/cancer-information/cancer-types/carcinoid-tumors/prevention/index.html (accessed August 28, 2014).

National Cancer Institute. "General Information about Gastrointestinal Carcinoid Tumors." http://www.cancer.gov/cancertopics/pdq/treatment/gastrointestinalcarcinoid/Patient (accessed August 28, 2014).

National Cancer Institute. "General Information about Pancreatic Neuroendocrine Tumors (Islet Cell Tumors)." http://www.cancer.gov/cancertopics/pdq/treatment/isletcell/Patient (accessed August 28, 2014).

ORGANIZATIONS

American Cancer Society, 250 Williams Street NW, Atlanta, GA 30303, (800) 227-2345, http://www.cancer.org.

The Carcinoid Cancer Foundation, 9333 Mamaroneck Avenue, No. 492, White Plains, NY 10605, (888) 722-3132, http://www.carcinoid.org.

National Cancer Institute, 9609 Medical Center Drive, Bethesda, MD 20892, (800) 422-6237, http://www.cancer.gov.

Monique Laberge, PhD
Rebecca J. Frey, PhD
REVISED BY TERESA G. ODLE
REVIEWED BY MELINDA GRANGER OBERLEITNER, RN, DNS, APRN, CNS

Neurofibromatosis *see* **von Recklinghausen neurofibromatosis**

Neurontin *see* **Gabapentin**

Neuropathy

Definition

Neuropathy is a condition of nerves that causes tingling, pain, numbness, or weak muscles in areas of the body. People who have **cancer** may have neuropathy because of **chemotherapy** treatment, infection, or another cause.

Description

Neuropathy is also called peripheral neuropathy for the nerves (known as the peripheral nerves) that help the muscles to contract (motor nerves) and allow a range of sensations to be felt (sensory nerves). Peripheral nerves carry messages to and from the brain and between the spinal cord and the rest of the body. They help control some of the involuntary functions of the autonomic nerves, which regulate the sweat glands, blood pressure, and internal organs. Peripheral nerves are fragile and easily damaged. The symptoms of neuropathy depend on the cause and on which nerve, or nerves, are involved.

Cancer patients may develop neuropathy because of effects from certain chemotherapy drugs, tumors formed by cancer, or other diseases and medications. If the sensory nerves are involved, the symptoms may include pain, numbness and tingling, burning, or a loss of feeling. If the motor nerves are affected, the patient may have weakness or paralysis of the muscles that the nerves help control. These symptoms may begin gradually.

Chemotherapy drugs associated with peripheral neuropathy

Name of drug
5-azacytidine
5-fluorouracil
Bortezomib (Velcade)
Cytarabine (in high doses)
Epothilones, such as ixabepilone (Ixempra)
Gemcitabine
Hexamethylmelamine
Ifosfamide
Lenalidomide (Revlimid)
Misonidazole
Plant alkaloids, such as vinblastine, vincristine, vinorelbine, and etoposide
Platinum drugs, such as cisplatin, carboplatin, and oxaliplatin
Suramin
Taxanes, including paclitaxel (Taxol) and docetaxel (Taxotere)
Teniposide (VM-26)
Thalidomide (Thalomid)

Table listing chemotherapy drugs known to cause peripheral neuropathy. (*Table by Lumina Datamatics Ltd. © 2015 Cengage Learning®.*)

Depending on the specific nerves involved, symptoms can range from mild tingling or numbness in the fingers or toes to severe pain in the hands or feet. Patients may also describe these symptoms as burning, prickling, or pinching. Some patients report that the skin is so sensitive that the slightest touch is painful. They may also experience heaviness or weakness in the arms and legs. As neuropathy increases in severity, patients might have an unsteady gait and can have difficulty feeling the floor beneath them. Patients who have autonomic neuropathy might experience dizziness, constipation, difficulty urinating, impotence, vision changes, and hearing loss.

Causes and symptoms

Neuropathy occurs in cancer patients for a number of reasons. A cancerous tumor can press on nerves, causing pain or problems with nerve function. Patients sometimes have other diseases such as diabetes, nutritional imbalances, alcoholism, and kidney failure, which can also cause neuropathy. The doctor will look carefully at a patient's medical history, physical condition, and diagnostic tests to determine the cause. The most common cause in cancer patients, however, is chemotherapy drugs. Neuropathy occurs in approximately 10%–20% of cancer patients receiving chemotherapy. The most common chemotherapy drugs that cause neuropathy include:

- platinum compounds (e.g., cisplatin and carboplatin)
- taxanes (e.g., docetaxel and paclitaxel)
- vincristine

The following chemotherapy agents can also cause neuropathy, but the incidence is relatively small compared to the prior ones listed. These include:

- procarbazine
- cytosine arabinoside (Ara C or cytarabine)

Treatment

Patients may undergo physical or occupational therapy to help keep their muscles strong and to work on improving balance and coordination. Exercising regularly can help lessen the pain from neuropathy.

In addition, a variety of medications are available that can ease symptoms for those suffering from neuropathy. These medications include:

- Pain relievers. Pain medicines available over-the-counter, such as acetaminophen (Tylenol), and nonsteroidal anti-inflammatory drugs (NSAIDs) such as aspirin and ibuprofen (Advil, Motrin IB, Nuprin), can help to alleviate mild symptoms. For more severe symptoms, the physician may recommend a prescription NSAID.
- Tricyclic antidepressants. Certain antidepressant medications have been used to help relieve peripheral neuropathy.
- Duloxetine (Cymbalta), a newer antidepressant known as an SNRI, has been recommended by the American Society of Clinical Oncology as the most effective antidepressant medication.
- Certain drugs intended to treat epilepsy can be effective in treating jabbing, shooting pain.
- Some topical treatments (applied to the skin), such as pain patches, may offer some relief.

The physician or pharmacist should be consulted regarding potential side effects or interactions with other medications.

Alternative and complementary therapies

Several other drug-free techniques can be helpful in providing pain relief. These are frequently used in conjunction with medication. These include:

- Biofeedback. This therapy uses a special machine to teach the patient how to control certain responses that can reduce pain.
- Transcutaneous electronic nerve stimulation (TENS). The physician may prescribe this treatment to try to prevent pain signals from reaching the brain. It is generally more effective for acute pain than chronic pain.
- Acupuncture. This may be effective for chronic pain, including the pain of neuropathy.
- Hypnosis. The patient under hypnosis typically receives suggestions intended to decrease the perception of pain.
- Relaxation techniques. These techniques can help decrease the muscle tension that aggravates pain. They may include deep-breathing exercises, visualization, and meditation.

If a patient has severe and chronic, or ongoing, neuropathy, doctors might perform surgery to repair injuries or destroy the nerves causing the pain and other symptoms. **Clinical trials** continue to explore better methods for treating peripheral neuropathy in patients who have cancer and chemotherapy. A trial testing the effectiveness of a drug called **amifostine** was ongoing during the summer of 2014.

Resources

BOOKS

Yarbo, Connie, Debra Wujcik, and Barbara Holmes Gobel. *Cancer Symptom Management.* 4th ed. Burlington, MA: Jones & Bartlett Learning, 2014.

PERIODICALS

Ezendam, Nicole P. M., et al. "Chemotherapy-Induced Peripheral Neuropathy and Its Impact on Health-Related Quality of Life among Ovarian Cancer Survivors: Results from the Population-Based PROFILES Registry." *Gynecologic Oncology* (September 30, 2014): e-publication ahead of print. http://dx.doi.org/10.1016/j.ygyno.2014.09.016 (accessed October 24, 2014).

Park, Ranhee, and Chaisoon Park. "Comparison of Foot Bathing and Foot Massage in Chemotherapy-Induced Peripheral Neuropathy." *Cancer Nursing* (October 1, 2014): e-publication ahead of print. http://dx.doi.org/10.1097/NCC.0000000000000181 (accessed October 24, 2014).

Seretny, Marta, et al. "Incidence, Prevalence, and Predictors of Chemotherapy-Induced Peripheral Neuropathy: A Systematic Review and Meta-Analysis." *Pain* (September 25, 2014): e-publication ahead of print. http://dx.doi.org/10.1016/j.pain.2014.09.020 (accessed October 24, 2014).

OTHER

American Cancer Society. "Peripheral Neuropathy Caused by Chemotherapy." http://www.cancer.org/acs/groups/cid/documents/webcontent/002908-pdf.pdf (accessed September 30, 2014).

WEBSITES

American Society of Clinical Oncology. "Peripheral Neuropathy." Cancer.Net. http://www.cancer.net/navigating-cancer-care/side-effects/peripheral-neuropathy (accessed September 30, 2014).

Johns Hopkins Medicine. "Peripheral Neuropathy." http://www.hopkinsmedicine.org/healthlibrary/conditions/nervous_system_disorders/peripheral_neuropathy_134,51/ (accessed September 30, 2014).

National Cancer Institute. "Managing Chemotherapy Side Effects: Nerve Changes." http://www.cancer.gov/cancer-topics/coping/chemo-side-effects/nerve.pdf (accessed September 30, 2014).

Deanna Swartout-Corbeil, RN

REVISED BY TERESA G. ODLE

Neurotoxicity

Definition

Neurotoxicity is damage or nerve cell destruction in the brain or other parts of the nervous system. Radiation and a number of naturally occurring and artificial substances can cause this damage. These substances are called neurotoxins. **Radiation therapy** and **chemotherapy** for treating **cancer** are common causes of neurotoxicity.

Description

Neurotoxicity occurs when a person is exposed to a toxic substance that causes the nervous system to work differently. Eventually, this disrupts or destroys the brain's neurons, which send and process signals in the brain and throughout the nervous system. Chemotherapy and radiation therapy, along with several types of heavy metals, **pesticides**, and industrial solvents, are types of neurotoxins.

Neurotoxicity can lead to conditions called neuropathies. Peripheral neuropathies involve damage to the motor, sensory, or vasomotor nerves of the peripheral nervous system (the extremities). Cranial neuropathies involve damage to the brain. Polyneuropathies are degenerative nerve diseases that are usually caused by toxins such as lead, but that involve many peripheral nerves at once. Most neurotoxicity involves the degeneration or "dying back" of the axons of nerve cells, especially the longest peripheral nerves. However, some neurotoxins cause demyelination of nerve cells or target specific types of nerve cells, such as Schwann cells, spinal ganglia, or autonomic neurons.

Neurotoxicity of the peripheral nervous system has some general features:

- The extent and severity of the neurotoxicity is related to the degree of exposure to the toxin.
- All individuals exposed to a given neurotoxin exhibit similar signs and symptoms.
- Neurotoxic illness usually occurs upon or shortly after exposure, with the common exceptions of organophosphates, which have a two- to four-week latency period, and cisplatin, which sometimes has a two-month latency period.
- Improvement of symptoms usually begins as soon as the patient is no longer exposed to the toxin.

Occupational and/or environmental toxins may play a role in some progressive neurodegenerative disorders, including:

- Parkinson's disease
- amyotrophic lateral sclerosis (Lou Gehrig's disease)
- multiple sclerosis
- dementia

Chemotherapy-induced (chemo-induced) peripheral **neuropathy** (CIPN) is a collection of neurotoxic symptoms caused by peripheral nerve damage from chemotherapy. Neurotoxicity is the dose-limiting factor for three common chemotherapy drugs—cisplatin, **vincristine**, and paclitaxel.

Central neurotoxicity from chemotherapy is the result of chemotherapy's effects on the brain. Depending on which part of the brain is affected, central neurotoxicity can lead to memory loss, seizures, or problems with cognitive (thinking) skills. Patients may experience symptoms such as: loss of balance, problems with movement, confusion, and memory issues. Effects of central neurotoxicity may occur soon after the patient receives drugs, or the effects may be delayed.

Radiation-induced neurotoxicity can involve both the central and peripheral nervous systems. Although peripheral nerves are relatively resistant to radiation-induced damage, the brachial and lumbosacral plexuses are susceptible. Radiation damage can be acute, sub-acute, and transient, or progressive, permanent, and disabling. Radiation-induced damage may not become fully apparent until months or years after treatment.

Radiation-induced nerve damage depends on:

- the total radiation dose
- its duration
- the method of administration
- the volume of irradiated nerve tissue
- the amount of irradiated healthy tissue
- individual susceptibility

The most important determinant of radiation-induced neurotoxicity is the amount of healthy tissue that is irradiated:

- One-session radiosurgery targets little or no healthy tissue.
- Fractionated radiation therapy targets more healthy tissue, but the intervals between treatments may allow for more healing.
- Whole brain radiation therapy targets large areas of the brain and is more neurotoxic.
- Radiation-induced brachial plexopathy occurs when radiation therapy is directed at the chest, axillary (armpit) region, thorax, or neck.
- Radiation-induced lumbosacral plexopathy occurs when radiation therapy is directed at cancers in the abdominal and pelvic regions.

Risk factors

Radiation therapy or chemotherapy for cancer treatment are major risk factors for neurotoxicity. Occupations involving toxic chemicals are also major risk factors.

Certain disorders can make a person more or less susceptible to neurotoxins:

- Some patients are more vulnerable to neurotoxic drugs because of an underlying genetic or acquired neuropathy, such as neuropathies caused by cancer or HIV/AIDS.

- Some brain disorders in children may develop through interactions between genes and neurotoxic environmental triggers.
- Genetic impairments in metabolism sometimes either increase or decrease the neurotoxicity of certain drugs.
- Certain forms of genes that promote nerve cell survival can counter neurotoxicity.

Demographics

Unlike many cancers and diseases, researchers do not track every diagnosis of neurotoxicity that occurs as a side effect or complication of the use of certain drugs or treatments. However, various reports and studies have tracked neurotoxicity in some cancer patients. For example, a 2010 report said that 4%–11% of patients who have stem cell transplants have neurotoxicity as a complication of the treatment.

Some statistics are available on the incidence of radiation-induced neurotoxicity in the United States:

- Brachial plexopathy (injury to the brachial plexus—the nerve bundles located on each side of the neck that give rise to the individual nerves controlling the muscles of the shoulders, arms, and hands) has been estimated to occur in 1.8%–4.9% of patients treated with radiation, most often for breast or lung cancer.
- Lumbosacral plexopathy (injury to the lumbosacral plexus—the network of nerves in the lower back region) occurs in 0.3%–1.3% of patients receiving radiation therapy.
- The incidence of severe radiation-induced dementia from whole brain radiation therapy (WBRT) ranges from 11% in one-year survivors to 50% in those surviving for two years.

Causes and symptoms

In as many as 25% of neuropathies the source of the neurotoxicity cannot be identified. Drugs are among the most common causes of neurotoxicity and a large number of drugs are associated with or suspected of being neurotoxic. Chemotherapy drugs most often associated with central neuropathy include:

- methotrexate
- ifosfamide
- cytarabine

Chemotherapy drugs associated with peripheral neuropathy include:

- 5-azacytidine
- 5-fluorouracil
- bortezomib (Velcade)

- cytarabine (in high doses)
- epothilones such as ixabepilone (Ixempra)
- gemcitabine
- hexamethylmelamine
- ifosfamide
- lenalidomide (Revlimid)
- misonidazole
- plant alkaloids such as vinblastine, vincristine, vinorelbine, and etoposide
- platinum drugs such as cisplatin, carboplatin, and oxaliplatin
- suramin
- taxanes including paclitaxel (Taxol) and docetaxel (Taxotere)
- teniposide (VM-26)
- thalidomide (Thalomid)

Antibiotics associated with peripheral neuropathy include:

- chloroquine
- chloramphenicol
- clioquinol
- dapsone
- ethambutol
- fluoroquinolones
- griseofulvin
- isoniazid (INH)
- mefloquine
- metronidazole
- nitrofurantoin
- nucleoside analogs
- podophyllin resin
- sulfonamides
- streptomycin

Other drugs associated with peripheral neuropathy include:

- allopurinol
- almitrine
- botulinum toxin
- cimetidine
- clofibrate
- colchicine
- cyclosporin A
- dichloroacetate
- disulfiram
- etretinate
- gold salts

- immunosuppressants
- interferons alpha-2A and 2B
- penicillamine
- pyridoxine (if abused)
- sulfasalazine
- tacrolimus (FK506, ProGraf)
- zimelidine

Symptoms of neurotoxicity can appear immediately upon exposure to the toxin or they can develop later. The most common symptoms of neurotoxicity are pain, tingling, or numbness in the feet. Other symptoms may include:

- weakness, numbness in the limbs, possibly accompanied by restless leg syndrome
- difficulty walking
- sensory loss
- impaired reflexes
- vision loss
- headache
- memory loss
- cognitive or behavioral problems
- sexual dysfunction

CIPN can begin at any time during or after chemotherapy and sometimes worsens over the course of chemotherapy. It often affects both sides of the body in similar ways; for example, the toes of both feet may be affected. The neuropathy often starts in the feet and later appears in the hands, which is called a "stocking/glove distribution." CIPN can cause severe pain and affect daily movements, including walking or writing. Symptoms of CIPN depend on which nerves are affected. Common symptoms include:

- pain
- numbness
- tingling or burning sensations
- weakness
- muscle shrinkage
- balance problems, tripping, or stumbling
- loss of reflexes
- increased sensitivity to temperature (usually cold) or pressure
- constipation
- difficulty urinating
- blood pressure changes
- difficulty swallowing

Severe problems from CIPN include:

- changes in heart rate
- breathing difficulties

• paralysis

• organ failure

Acute reactions to radiation normally occur during or immediately following therapy and are usually caused by swelling. Acute toxicity lessens with subsequent treatments. Symptoms of acute radiation neurotoxicity include:

• headache

• nausea

• vomiting

• drowsiness

Neurotoxicity from localized radiation therapy often involves specific neurologic deficits. Following radiation therapy to the neck or upper thorax, early-delayed neurotoxicity can result in a myelopathy characterized by an electric shock-like sensation radiating down the back and into the legs when the neck is flexed. This myelopathy resolves spontaneously. Radiation therapy for extraspinal tumors, such as **Hodgkin lymphoma**, can cause late-delayed symptoms such as progressive paralysis and sensory loss.

Symptoms of acute neurotoxicity from WBRT include hair loss (**alopecia**), nausea, vomiting, lethargy, middle-ear inflammation, and severe cerebral swelling. Some of these effects are transient, but others can last for months following radiation therapy. Late-delayed neurotoxicity reactions are usually permanent and may be progressive. They can vary from moderate to severe and can include:

• memory impairment

• confusion

• personality changes

• progressive dementia

• cerebral atrophy

• rarely, the development of new cancers

Diagnosis

Examination

Neurotoxicity is often diagnosed based solely on exposure to known neurotoxins. For patients who have undergone radiation therapy or chemotherapy, a diagnosis of neurotoxicity is usually obvious on physical examination. In other cases diagnosis may be much more difficult. The physician will conduct a complete physical examination and a medical history focusing on drug use, medications, and occupational and environmental exposures. A neurological exam will be performed to check a patient's motor and sensory functions. When a potential source of the neurotoxicity can be identified, the dose, duration of exposure, and level of protection are estimated.

Tests

Tests for neurotoxicity may include:

• facial nerve testing

• blink reflex testing

• blood and urine tests for the presence of known neurotoxins

• a variety of laboratory tests, depending on the suspected source of the neurotoxicity

Procedures

Diagnostic procedures may include:

• electromyography (EMG), which measures electrical activity associated with functioning skeletal muscle

• studies of nerve conduction, such as nerve conduction velocity (NVC) measurements

• nerve and/or muscle biopsies to obtain tissue for examination by a pathologist

• MRI or CT scans to visualize damage from neurotoxicity or rule out tumors

Treatment

Treatment for neurotoxicity depends on the cause. The most important treatment is to eliminate or reduce exposure to the neurotoxin. In cases of CIPN, treatment may be postponed, the doses of chemotherapy drugs lowered, or the drug that is causing the CIPN may be eliminated.

Drugs

Acute neurotoxicity from radiation therapy and pain from CIPN may be treated with:

• corticosteroids

• tricyclic antidepressants in smaller doses than are used to treat depression

• anticonvulsants

• numbing patches or topical creams, such as lidocaine patches or capsaicin cream, applied to the painful area

• opioids or narcotics for severe pain

Alternative

Alternative medicines for neurotoxicity include:

• alpha-lipoic acid

• evening primrose, which contains the omega-6 essential fatty acids linoleic acid and gamma-linoleic acid (GLA)

• vitamin E

Alternative treatments for neuropathic pain include:

• physical therapy

• acupuncture

- massage
- biofeedback
- relaxation therapy
- occupational therapy

Home remedies

Home remedies for neuropathy include:

- maintaining a balanced diet
- vitamin B supplements
- soaking in cool water
- applications of heat
- elevating or lowering limbs
- remaining seated as much as possible if the neuropathy is in the feet
- caring for the feet—checking often for open sores or using special shoes or inserts
- exercise
- avoiding anything that worsens the neuropathy, such as heat or cold or tight clothes or shoes
- avoiding alcohol, which can damage nerves and make the neuropathy worse
- controlling blood sugar, since high blood sugar can damage nerves

Prognosis

The prognosis for neurotoxicity varies tremendously depending on the neurotoxin, the degree and duration of exposure, and the severity of the damage to the nervous system. Depending on the circumstances, patients can fully recover following treatment, survive without full recovery, or have lasting effects. In severe cases, neurotoxicity can cause death.

CIPN may be short-term and disappear after treatment stops, may take up to two years to completely resolve, or may develop into a chronic disorder requiring long-term treatment. Some cases may be both severe and permanent. The prognosis for CIPN depends on:

- the chemotherapy drug(s)
- the drug dose
- the total chemotherapy dose over time
- the patient's age
- a personal or family history of neuropathy
- the existence of other medical conditions that can cause neuropathy, such as diabetes or HIV infection

Prevention

Doctors can use several techniques for chemotherapy or radiation therapy to lessen the risk of neurotoxicity, including:

- smaller chemotherapy doses over a longer period of time (two or three times per week, instead of one large dose)
- the same dose administered over six hours instead of over one hour
- the same dose as a continuous, very slow infusion over a few days
- use of stereotactic radiosurgery instead of whole brain radiation therapy to target a tumor more precisely and spare healthy brain tissue

Bortezomib administered subcutaneously (into the skin) instead of intravenously (into a vein) is associated with a lower risk of CIPN.

Possible preventions for CIPN that are being studied include:

- vitamin E, an antioxidant that may help protect against nerve damage caused by cisplatin and paclitaxel
- calcium and magnesium infusions before and after oxaliplatin
- the anticonvulsant drug carbamazepine, which may help treat as well as prevent CIPN
- various supplements, including amino acids and proteins, given before and after chemotherapy

Resources

BOOKS

Davidson, Philip William, Gary J. Myers, and Bernard Weiss, eds. *Neurotoxicity and Developmental Disabilities.* London: Elsevier, 2006.

DeAngelis, Lisa M., and Jerome B. Posner. *Neurological Complications of Cancer,* 2nd ed. New York: Oxford University Press, 2009.

Dobbs, Michael R. *Clinical Neurotoxicity.* Philadelphia: Saunders/Elsevier, 2009.

PERIODICALS

Visovsky C., et al. "Putting Evidence into Practice: Evidence-Based Interventions for Chemotherapy-Induced Peripheral Neuropathy." *Clinical Journal of Oncology Nursing* 11 (2007): 901-913.

Wickham, R. "Chemotherapy-Induced Peripheral Neuropathy: A Review and Implications for Oncology Nursing Practice." *Clinical Journal of Oncology Nursing* 11 (2007): 361-376.

OTHER

"Peripheral Neuropathy Caused by Chemotherapy." American Cancer Society. http://www.cancer.org/acs/groups/cid/documents/webcontent/002908-pdf.pdf (accessed December 22, 2014).

Weimer, Louis H. "Medication-Induced Neuropathies." The Neuropathy Association. http://www.neuropathy.org/site/DocServer/Medication-Induced_Neuropathies.pdf?docID=1604 (accessed October 4, 2014).

WEBSITES

"Central Neurotoxicity, Memory Loss, and Their Relationship to Chemotherapy." eMedicine. http://emedicine.medscape.com/article/316497-overview (accessed October 4, 2014).

Kaplan, Robert J. "Radiation-Induced Brachial Plexopathy." The Scott Hamilton CARES Initiative. http://chemocare.com/chemotherapy/side-effects/central-neurotoxicity-memory-loss.aspx#.U_4ad_mwLjs (accessed October 4, 2014).

"NINDS Neurotoxicity Information Page." National Institute of Neurological Disorders and Stroke. http://www.ninds.nih.gov/disorders/neurotoxicity/neurotoxicity.htm (accessed October 4, 2014).

"Radiation Injury to the Brain." International RadioSurgery Association. http://www.irsa.org/radiation_injury.html (accessed October 4, 2014).

Rutchik, Jonathan S. "Toxic Neuropathy." eMedicine. http://emedicine.medscape.com/article/1175276-overview (accessed October 4, 2014).

ORGANIZATIONS

American Cancer Society, 250 Williams Street NW, Atlanta, GA 30303, (800) 227-2345, http://www.cancer.org.

National Cancer Institute, 9609 Medical Center Drive, Bethesda, MD 20892, (800) 422-6237, http://www.cancer.gov.

Margaret Alic, PhD
REVISED BY TERESA G. ODLE

Neutrexin *see* **Trimetrexate**

Neutropenia

Description

Neutropenia is an abnormally low level of neutrophils in the blood. Neutrophils are white blood cells (WBCs) produced in the bone marrow, and they comprise about 60% of the blood. These cells are critically important to an **immune response** and migrate from the blood to tissues during an infection. They ingest and destroy particles and germs. Germs are microorganisms such as bacteria, protozoa, viruses, and fungi that cause disease.

People who have **cancer** can have low white cell counts, or neutropenia, because of the cancer's effects on blood cells or because of cancer treatment. Neutropenia is an especially serious disorder for cancer patients who may have reduced immune functions, because it makes the body vulnerable to bacterial and fungal infections. White blood cells are especially sensitive to **chemotherapy**. The number of cells killed during **radiation therapy** depends upon the dose and frequency of radiation, and how much of the body is irradiated.

Neutrophils can be segmented (segs, polys, or polymorphonuclear cells, called PMNs) or banded (bands). Bands are newly developed, immature neutrophils. If there is an increase in new neutrophils (bands), this may indicate that an infection is present and the body is attempting a defense. Neutropenia is sometimes called agranulocytosis or granulocytopenia because neutrophils display characteristic multi-lobed structures and granules in stained blood smears.

The normal level of neutrophils in human blood varies slightly by age and race. Infants have lower counts than older children and adults. African Americans have lower counts than Caucasians or Asians. The average adult level is 1,500 cells/mm^3 of blood. Neutrophil counts (in cells/mm^3) are interpreted as follows:

• Greater than 1,000. Normal protection against infection.

• 500–1,000. Some increased risk of infection.

• 200–500. Great risk of severe infection.

• Lower than 200. Risk of overwhelming infection; requires hospital treatment with antibiotics.

Neutropenia has no specific symptoms except the severity of the patient's current infection. In severe neutropenia, the patient is likely to develop periodontal disease, oral and rectal ulcers, **fever**, and bacterial **pneumonia**. Fever recurring every 19–30 days suggests cyclical neutropenia.

Causes and symptoms

Neutropenia may result from three processes.

Decreased WBC production

Lowered production of white blood cells is the most common cause of neutropenia. It can result from:

• cancer, including certain types of leukemia

• radiation therapy

- medications that affect the bone marrow, including cancer drugs (chemotherapy), chloramphenicol (Chloromycetin), anticonvulsant medications, and antipsychotic drugs (Thorazine, Prolixin, and other phenothiazines) (In hematopoietic stem cell transplantation [HSCT], high levels of total body irradiation or chemotherapy are used to kill cancer cells, or these treatments may be combined. Two types of HSCT treatments are bone marrow transplantation and peripheral blood stem cell transplantation. During the treatment process, the patient's normal bone marrow stem cells are killed along with the cancer cells. The stem cells are not able to mature into immune cells such as neutrophils, causing neutropenia. To reduce neutropenia, the normal stem cells from the patient may be removed before treatment and given back at a later time. Cells can also be supplied from another donor.)
- hereditary and congenital disorders that affect the bone marrow, including familial neutropenia, cyclic neutropenia, and infantile agranulocytosis
- exposure to pesticides
- vitamin B_{12} and folate (folic acid) deficiency

Destruction of white blood cells

WBCs are used and die at a faster rate due to:

- acute bacterial infections in adults
- infections in newborns
- certain autoimmune disorders, including systemic lupus erythematosus (SLE)
- penicillin, phenytoin (Dilantin), and sulfonamide medications (Benemid, Bactrim, Gantanol)

Sequestration and margination of WBCs

Sequestration and margination are processes in which neutrophils are removed from the general blood circulation and redistributed within the body. These processes can occur because of:

- hemodialysis
- Felty syndrome or malaria—the neutrophils accumulate in the spleen
- bacterial infections—the neutrophils remain in the infected tissues without returning to the bloodstream

Symptoms

It is important to detect infections early. Some signs that indicate infection include:

- coughing, difficulty breathing, and congestion
- an oral temperature greater than 105° with typical fever symptoms of chills and sweating
- problems in the mouth such as white patches, sores, and swollen gums
- sore throat
- changes in urination or in stools
- abdominal pain
- anal sores
- drainage and pain from any cuts or tubes used in the cancer treatments such as catheters and feeding tubes
- vaginal redness or discharge
- an overall feeling of illness

Diagnosis

Diagnosis is based on a white blood cell count and differential. The cause of neutropenia can be difficult to establish and depends on a combination of the patient's medical history, genetic evaluation, **bone marrow biopsy**, and repeated measurements of the WBC. However, in cancer patients it is usually an expected side effect of chemotherapy or radiation. The overall risk of infection depends on the type of cancer an individual has as well as the treatment received. Patients at greater risk include those with blood and bone marrow cancers (leukemias and **lymphomas**) and those who receive bone marrow transplants.

Treatment

Treatment of neutropenia depends on the underlying cause.

Medications

Patients with fever and other signs of infection are treated with **antibiotics**. Some antibiotics used in the treatment of cancer patients include imipenem, meropenem, aminoglycoside, antipseudomonal penicillin, rifampin, and vancomycin. Combination therapy that uses several types of antibiotics to stop the infection can be utilized, but some of the drugs may be toxic or costly. As of 2014, Spectrum Pharmaceuticals was about to begin phase 3 **clinical trials** on a new biologic therapy granulocyte-stimulating factor called SPI-2012.

Patients receiving chemotherapy for cancer may be given drugs even while healthy to help restore the WBC to normal. A blood growth factor called **sargramostim** (Leukine, Prokine) stimulates WBC production. Another drug class commonly used to reduce neutropenia in cancer patients is granulocyte colony-stimulating factors, which include **filgrastim** (Neupogen) or pegfilgrastim (Neulasta). This substance is normally produced in the body at low levels. G-CSF helps the body produce more neutrophils to fight infection. This is especially useful in that many bacteria cannot be killed by antibiotics due to antibiotic resistance.

Throughout the course of treatment it is important that the patient be monitored closely. This requires hospitalization for some patients, while others may be adequately treated at home. Blood cell counts tend to drop to their lowest levels about one to two weeks following chemotherapy administration. This is the time when neutropenia and resulting infection are most likely to occur. Doctors withhold the next round of chemotherapy until a patient's blood cell counts return to an acceptable level.

Alternative and complementary therapies

A healthy lifestyle should be adopted that includes good nutrition, plenty of sleep, and appropriate levels of exercise. Avoid uncooked foods that may contain harmful bacteria. A nutritionist should be consulted to determine an appropriate, healthy diet.

Psychological stress can also weaken the immune system, making a person more susceptible to illness. It is important to find emotional support through family, friends, support groups, or spiritual means.

Special concerns

Often the infections that develop in a cancer patient are opportunistic infections. That is, the organisms responsible for the infection normally would not cause disease in a healthy person, but do so in a cancer patient because the immune system is weak. Several steps can be taken on a daily basis to reduce the risk of developing an infection:

- Care should be taken to keep the body clean. Hands should be washed after using the bathroom and before eating.

- Stagnant or still water in the environment that might contain bacteria should be avoided. This might include flower vases and birdbaths, or containers that may hold items such as dentures.

- Use non-alcoholic antiseptic mouthwashes to cleanse the mouth.

- Use deodorant instead of antiperspirant. Antiperspirants will not allow the body to sweat, trapping bacteria within the body that may increase the risk of infection.

- Women with neutropenia should consider using sanitary napkins instead of tampons during their menstruation to help prevent possible infections such as toxic shock syndrome.

- Avoid others who are ill and large crowded areas where one might encounter illness.

- Avoid activities that may increase the chance of physical injury and protect the body by wearing gloves, shoes, and other items. Tend to all injuries as soon as possible.

- Avoid foods that may cause illness in an immunosuppressed patient, such as raw or undercooked meats or eggs; unpasteurized juice, beer, and dairy products; aged cheese in any product; and unwashed raw fruits and vegetables (all foods should be cooked).

- Do not garden or be around fresh flowers.

- Avoid being around pets and do not clean any litter boxes or aquariums.

- Use a soft toothbrush and use an electric shaver (if necessary) to prevent small cuts in the gum and skin that could result in infection.

- Avoid constipation.

- Consult with the treating physician before receiving any vaccinations.

See also Immunologic therapies; Infection and sepsis; Chronic myelocytic leukemia.

Resources

BOOKS

Abeloff, Martin D., et al. *Clinical Oncology*. 5th ed. New York: Churchill Livingstone, 2014.

Ferri, Fred. *Ferri's Best Test*. 3rd ed. Philadelphia: Saunders, 2015.

Hoffman R., et al. *Hematology: Basic Principles and Practice*. 6th ed. Philadelphia: Elsevier, 2012.

McPherson, R. A., et al. *Henry's Clinical Diagnosis and Management By Laboratory Methods*. 22nd ed. Philadelphia: Saunders, 2011.

Niederhuber, J. E., et al. *Clinical Oncology*. 5th ed. Philadelphia: Elsevier, 2014.

OTHER

American Cancer Society. "Infections in People with Cancer." http://www.cancer.org/acs/groups/cid/documents/webcontent/002871-pdf.pdf (accessed October 21, 2014).

WEBSITES

American Society of Clinical Oncology. "Neutropenia." http://www.cancer.net/navigating-cancer-care/side-effects/neutropenia (accessed October 21, 2014).

MedlinePlus. "Low White Blood Cell Count and Cancer." U.S. National Library of Medicine. http://www.nlm.nih.gov/medlineplus/ency/patientinstructions/000675.htm (accessed October 21, 2014).

National Cancer Institute. "Side Effects and Ways to Manage Them." http://www.cancer.gov/cancertopics/coping/chemotherapy-and-you/page7#SE8 (accessed October 21, 2014).

University of Pennsylvania Oncolink. http://www.oncolink.upenn.edu (accessed October 21, 2014).

Rebecca Frey, PhD
Jill Granger, MS
REVISED BY TERESA G. ODLE

Nexavar *see* **Sorafenib**

Night sweats

Description

Night sweats can be a side effect of **cancer** treatment or a symptom of certain cancers. Night sweats are part of a variety of symptoms referred to as vasomotor. Vasomotor symptoms stem from the body's thermoregulatory center, which is affected by circulating hormones.

Women may undergo **oophorectomy** (the surgical removal of one or both ovaries), either for **ovarian cancer** or when accompanied by hysterectomy for **endometrial cancer** or uterine **sarcoma**, as part of their cancer treatment. Pelvic radiation may also damage the ovaries. Removal or permanent damage to the ovaries results in immediate menopause. Many women with ovarian cancer have already gone through menopause, as a function of their age. However, when ovarian or reproductive tract cancer strikes a pre-menopausal woman, the immediate, versus gradual, loss of circulating hormones is dramatic, and is a concern in the immediate post-operative period. In an *American Cancer Society News Today* on January 29, 2001, the ACS reported on a study that found women undergoing systemic treatment for **breast cancer**, especially those on **tamoxifen**, reported a higher frequency and intensity of menopausal symptoms such as night sweats, hot flashes, and **fatigue**. Men may also experience vasomotor symptoms with metastatic **adenocarcinoma** of the prostate, or following removal of the prostate for **prostate cancer**.

Vasomotor symptoms such as night sweats add to the existing stress for individuals undergoing cancer treatment, as they can reduce the quality of sleep, make daily life very uncomfortable, and decrease the quality of life.

Night sweats can be a sign of infection in the immuno-compromised cancer patient, as well as a symptom of undiagnosed cancer and early AIDS. Drenching night sweats may be a sign of Hodgkin or **non-Hodgkin lymphoma**, both in children as well as in adults. Night sweats may also be present with liver hemangioma tumors. Generalized symptoms such as night sweats, **fever**, chills, and sweating are sometimes referred to as B symptoms. Night sweats have also been associated with malignant **melanoma** and with metastatic compression of the optic nerve. Children who are ultimately diagnosed with a malignancy may present to a rheumatologist with a variety of symptoms, including night sweats. Night sweats in the absence of explained fever or perimenopause should be brought to the attention of one's healthcare provider for evaluation.

Causes and symptoms

The ovary produces the hormone estrogen. When the ovary is removed, there is a dramatic termination of circulating estrogen, with symptoms such as night sweats, hot flashes, and vaginal dryness. Estrogen replacement therapy (ERT) can relieve these symptoms. However, the use of ERT is controversial with some cancers, because of the association with estrogen-receptor positive cancers. Women who are approaching menopause at the time of **chemotherapy** may lose ovarian function as a result of treatment, thus undergoing significant menopausal symptoms. The use of tamoxifen in postmenopausal women has been associated with an increase in vasomotor symptoms.

Hodgkin and non-Hodgkin lymphomas are cancers of the lymphatic system. Symptoms include night sweats; painless swelling in the lymph nodes, especially in the neck, underarm, or groin; unexplained **weight loss**; recurrent fevers; and itchy skin. The night sweats in **Hodgkin lymphoma** appear to be related to an instability in the thermoregulatory center of the hypothalamus. Risk factors for Hodgkin and non-Hodgkin lymphomas include reduced immune function, transplant surgery, occupational exposure to herbicides and other toxic chemicals, Sjögren's syndrome, and **Epstein-Barr virus**.

Treatment

Some research has been conducted using estrogen-androgen replacement therapy. The concerns about ERT and estrogen-sensitive cancers remain the same. The androgen component assists in the healing process, as well as in a sense of well-being, sexual desire and arousal, and increased energy level. The use of androgens can result in hirsutism (growth of male-pattern hair), which may be dose-dependent.

Successful diagnosis of the cause of the night sweats can lead to proper treatment for the condition. Successful treatment of Hodgkin or non-Hodgkin **lymphoma** resolves the night sweats.

Alternative and complementary therapies

Acupuncture has been effective for both men and women. Individuals considering herbal remedies or supplements for reproductive-related night sweats associated with cancer treatment should seek the counsel of a knowledgeable practitioner. Substances that function through mimicking estrogenic properties could have an adverse effect in estrogen-sensitive tumors.

Resources

WEBSITES

Mayo Clinic staff. "Night Sweats." Mayo Clinic. http://www.mayoclinic.org/symptoms/night-sweats/basics/definition/sym-20050768 (accessed November 14, 2014).
National Cancer Institute Cancer Trials. http://www.cancer.gov/clinicaltrials (accessed November 19, 2014).

ORGANIZATIONS

American Cancer Society, 250 Williams St. NW, Atlanta, GA 30303, (800) 227-2345, http://www.cancer.org.

National Cancer Institute, 9609 Medical Center Dr., BG 9609 MSC 9760, Bethesda, MD 20892-9760, (800) 4-CANCER (422-6237), http://www.cancer.gov.
National Center for Complementary and Alternative Medicine, 9000 Rockville Pike, Bethesda, MD 20892, (888) 644-6226, TTY: (866) 464-3615, http://nccam.nih.gov.

Esther Csapo Rastegari, RN, BSN, EdM

Nilotinib

Definition

Nilotinib (Tasigna) is a second generation BCR-ABL inhibitor drug manufactured by Novartis Pharmaceuticals. It is used for the treatment of Philadelphia positive chronic myeloid leukemia (Ph+ CML).

Purpose

Nilotinib is used to treat chronic myeloid leukemia (CML), also called chronic myelogenous leukemia, in people who carry a specific genetic abnormality called the Philadelphia chromosome. CML is **cancer** that develops in myeloid cells in the bone marrow and results in the production of abnormal blood cells. These blood cells mature incorrectly or incompletely and live longer than normal so that they build up in the blood, causing symptoms of CML.

CML accounts for 10%–15% of all leukemias, and almost all CML is associated with a specific non-inherited genetic defect called the Philadelphia chromosome. When cells divide, their chromosomes double and also divide in order for each cell to have a complete set of genetic information. Sometimes during this doubling and division process material from one chromosome incorrectly gets attached to or exchanged with material from another chromosome. This process is called translocation. CML starts when part of chromosome 9 is exchanged with part of chromosome 22. The resulting abnormal chromosome 22 is known as the Philadelphia chromosome. People who have it are said to be Philadelphia chromosome positive or Ph+. Although it is not clear what factors cause this translocation, almost everyone with CML is Ph+.

As the result of the formation of the translocation between chromosomes 9 and 22, a new gene called bcr-abl is formed on the Philadelphia chromosome. This gene produces a tyrosine kinase protein called BCR-ABL. BCR-ABL causes myeloid cells to become cancer (malignant) cells. These malignant cells grow and reproduce abnormally. Nilotinib is a tyrosine kinase inhibitor. It interferes with the activities of the BCR-ABL protein and stops the production of cancerous myeloid cells while allowing the production of normal blood cells to continue.

Nilotinib is approved for use during the chronic (early) phase of CML and in the accelerated (second) stage of CML. It normally is used only after another tyrosine kinase inhibitor drug, **imatinib mesylate** (Gleevec), has been tried. Imatinib mesylate successfully treats CML in many people. Those people whose cancer does not respond to the drug or who cannot tolerate the side effects of imatinib mesylate may be treated with nilotinib.

Description

Nilotinib is sold in the United States and the European Union under the brand name of Tasigna. The drug was first approved by the U.S. Food and Drug Administration (FDA) on October 27, 2007 and by the European Union on November 17, 2007. The drug is also approved in the European Union to treat gastrointestinal stroma tumors, a type of digestive system cancer.

Nilotinib is a light yellow hard gel capsule with red printing. Each capsule has a strength of 200 mg. Capsules should be stored at controlled room temperature. Nilotinib continues to be tested in **clinical trials** in the United States for use against other cancers and in combination with other therapies. A list of clinical trials currently enrolling volunteers can be found at http://www.clinicaltrials.gov.

Recommended dosage

Nilotinib must be taken *exactly* as prescribed, and the dosage should not be changed or the drug discontinued except on order of a physician. The usual recommended dosage in patients with CML Ph+ is 400 mg taken twice daily 12 hours apart. Nilotinib capsules must be taken whole; they should never be crushed or divided. They may not be taken with food; nothing should be eaten for at least two hours before and one hour after the dose is taken. Grapefruit juice or dietary supplements containing extracts from grapefruit juice should not be used while taking this drug. Patients who forget to take a dose should not take a make-up dose. Instead they should skip the dose and then take the next dose at their regularly scheduled time.

There are special dosage recommendations and restrictions for use of nilotinib in some individuals including those with certain heart conditions, liver function abnormalities, or suppression of normal production of blood cells in the bone marrow (**myelosuppression**), or those taking certain drugs. See Precautions and Drug Interactions for additional information.

The safety and effectiveness of this drug have not been established in children.

No information is available on overdosage.

Precautions

Nilotinib can cause serious and life-threatening side effects. Sudden deaths have occurred with the administration of nilotinib. The drug carries a black-box warning concerning administration of the drug. An electrocardiogram (ECG) and various blood tests must be done before the drug can safely be started.

The following black box warnings must be observed:

• Nilotinib can prolong a phase of the heart contraction cycle called the QT interval. This drug should not be used in patients with long QT interval. Heart monitoring (ECG) should be done before the drug is started, one week after starting the drug, when dosage is changed, and at regular intervals during treatment to check for long QT interval. Other drugs known to prolong the QT interval should be avoided. If long QT interval occurs, dosage must be substantially reduced or the drug must be discontinued.

• Nilotinib should not be given to individuals with low blood potassium levels (hypokalemia) and low blood magnesium levels (hypomagnesemia). Blood electrolyte levels should be checked regularly and corrected when possible.

• Nilotinib should be used with caution in patients with liver (hepatic) impairment.

The following precautions also should be observed:

• Severe decrease in the number of normal blood cells (myelosuppression) may occur. Decrease in the number of blood platelets (thrombocytopenia) may reduce the ability of the blood to clot and increase the risk of bleeding episodes. Decrease in the number of neutrophils (neutropenia) may decrease the ability of the body to fight infection. Decrease in the number of red blood cells (anemia) may reduce the ability of the blood to supply oxygen. Blood count should be monitored frequently; dosage may need to be reduced.

• Patients with a history of pancreatitis may have elevated serum lipase levels. Serum lipase should be monitored.

• Patients with impaired liver function may have a variety of abnormally elevated measures of liver function (e.g., bilirubin, alkaline phosphatase). Liver function should be monitored.

• Nilotinib can cause abnormal blood levels of phosphate, potassium, calcium, and sodium. Electrolytes should be monitored and corrected.

• Food increases the amount of nilotinib in the blood. All food should be avoided for two hours before and one hour after each dose.

Pregnant or breastfeeding

Nilotinib is a pregnancy category D drug. Woman who are pregnant or who might become pregnant should not use nilotinib. It is not known whether the drug is excreted in breast milk. Women taking this drug should not breastfeed, as there is the potential for this drug to cause serious adverse effects on nursing infants.

Side effects

Nilotinib has many side effects, the most serious of which is sudden death. The two most common serious side effects reported during clinical trials were **thrombocytopenia** and **neutropenia** (see Precautions). Other common serious side effects included **pneumonia**, **fever**, elevated serum lipase levels, and intracranial hemorrhage (bleeding in the brain). Additional serious side effects included fluid retention around the heart (**pericardial effusion**) and lungs (**pleural effusion**), inflammation of the pancreas, and liver damage.

Common but less serious side effects reported in more than 10% of patients during clinical trials included rash, nausea, vomiting, constipation, **diarrhea**, and headache.

Interactions

Nilotinib is known to interact with many drugs and all food. If these drugs cannot be avoided, the dosage of nilotinib may need to be adjusted. All interactions are not known. Patients should provide their doctor and pharmacist with a complete list of all prescription and nonprescription drugs, herbs, and dietary supplements that they are taking.

When taken with nilotinib, these drugs are likely to increase the amount of nilotinib circulating in the blood.

• ketoconazole (Nizoral)

• itraconazole (Sporanox)

• ritonavir (Norvir)

• atazanavir sulfate (Reyataz)

• indinavir (Crixivan)

• nelfinavir (Viracept)

• saquinavir (Invirase)

• telithromycin (Ketek)

• erythromycin (E-mycin)

• clarithromycin (Biaxin)

QUESTIONS TO ASK YOUR DOCTOR

• How long will I need to take this drug before you can tell if it is helping?

• How often do I have to have blood work and other laboratory tests done to check the effect the drug is having?

• Is this drug safe to take with the other drugs that I am currently taking?

• What side effects should I watch for? When should I call the doctor about them?

• Are there any clinical trials of this drug combined with other therapies that might benefit me?

When taken with nilotinib, these drugs are likely to decrease the amount of nilotinib circulating in the blood.

• dexamethasone (Decadron)

• phenytoin (Dilantin)

• carbamazepine (Tegretol)

• rifampin (Rimactane)

• phenobarbital (Luminal)

Taking nilotinib with food increases the amount of drug in the blood.

Nilotinib contains a small amount of lactose as an inactive ingredient. Individuals who are lactose-intolerant should discuss this with their physician.

Resources

PERIODICALS

Usküdar Teke, H. "Pleural Effusion: A Rare Side Effect of Nilotinib—A Case Report." *Case Reports in Medicine* (September 9, 2014). http://dx.doi.org/10.1155/2014/203939 (accessed November 17, 2014).

WEBSITES

American Cancer Society. "Detailed Guided Leukemia, Chronic Myeloid (CML)." http://www.cancer.org/docroot/CRI/CRI_2_3x.asp?rnav=cridg&dt=83 (accessed October 15, 2014).

MedlinePlus. "Leukemia, Adult Chronic." http://www.nlm.nih.gov/medlineplus/leukemiaadultchronic.html (accessed October 14, 2014).

National Cancer Institute. "FDA Approval for Nilotinib." http://www.cancer.gov/cancertopics/druginfo/fda-nilotinib (accessed October 14, 2014).

ORGANIZATIONS

American Cancer Society, 250 Williams St. NW, Atlanta, GA 30303, (800) 227-2345, http://www.cancer.org.

Leukemia & Lymphoma Society, 1311 Mamaroneck Ave., Ste. 310, White Plains, NY 10605, (914) 949-5213, Fax: (914) 949-6691, infocenter@lls.org, http://www.lls.org.

National Cancer Institute, 9609 Medical Center Dr., BG 9609 MSC 9760, Bethesda, MD 20892-9760, (800) 4-CANCER (422-6237), http://www.cancer.gov.

Tish Davidson, AM

Nilutamide *see* **Antiandrogens**

Nipent *see* **Pentostatin**

Nitrogen mustard *see* **Mechlorethamine**

Nolvadex *see* **Tamoxifen**

Cancer Research UK. "Non-Hodgkin Lymphoma (NHL)." http://www.cancerresearchuk.org/about-cancer/type/non-hodgkins-lymphoma/ (accessed November 8, 2014).

National Cancer Institute. "Non-Hodgkin Lymphoma." http://www.cancer.gov/cancertopics/types/non-hodgkin (accessed November 8, 2014).

Kate Kretschmann

Non-melanoma skin cancer *see* **Skin cancer, non-melanoma**

Non-small cell lung cancer *see* **Lung cancer, non-small cell**

Non-Hodgkin lymphoma

Definition

Non-Hodgkin lymphoma is one of two general types of lymphomas (cancers that begin in lymphatic tissues and can invade other organs) differing from **Hodgkin lymphoma** by a lack of Hodgkin-specific Reed-Sternberg cells.

Description

Non-Hodgkin **lymphoma** (NHL) is a **cancer** of lymphocytes, a type of white blood cell that moves around the body as part of its role in the immune system. NHL is much less predictable than HD and is more likely to spread to areas beyond the lymph nodes.

NHL is comprised of approximately 10 subtypes and 20 different disease entities. Division is based on whether the lymphoma is low-grade (progressing slowly) or high-grade (progressing rapidly). NHL is also grouped according to cell type—B cells or T cells. Physicians can diagnose the type of lymphoma by performing a **biopsy**, in which a lymph node is removed and examined in the laboratory. Some of the non-Hodgkin lymphoma types include **Burkitt lymphoma**, diffuse large B-cell lymphoma, follicular center lymphoma, and **mantle cell lymphoma**.

Resources

WEBSITES

American Cancer Society. "Non-Hodgkin Lymphoma." http://www.cancer.org/cancer/non-hodgkinlymphoma/detailed-guide/non-hodgkin-lymphoma-what-is-non-hodgkin-lymphoma (accessed November 8, 2014).

Nonsteroidal anti-inflammatory drugs

Definition

Nonsteroidal anti-inflammatory drugs (NSAIDs) are a type of drug that reduces pain and inflammation.

Purpose

NSAIDs often are used to relieve mild to moderate pain for all types of **cancer**, as well as the pain of arthritis, menstrual cramps, sore muscles following exercise, and tension headaches. Most NSAIDs are available in over-the-counter formulations.

Ibuprofen and naproxen are two NSAIDs that are also used to bring down **fever** and treat the side effects of **radiation therapy**.

Description

This class of drugs eases discomfort by blocking the pathway of an enzyme that forms prostaglandins (hormones that cause pain and swelling). By doing so, the drugs lessen the pain in different parts of the body.

Some of the NSAIDs used in cancer treatment include: ibuprofen (Motrin, Advil, Rufen, Nuprin), naproxen (Naprosyn, Naprelan, Anaprox, Aleve), nabumetone (Relafen), ketorolac, sulindac, and diclofenac (Cataflam, Voltaren). The class of drugs known as cyclooxygenase-2 inhibitors that emerged in the late 1990s for dealing with arthritis pain, such as the brand names Celebrex and Vioxx, is also considered part of the group of NSAIDS.

If NSAIDs are not strong enough to keep a cancer patient comfortable, physicians often will combine them with such **opioids** (narcotics) as codeine. In later stages, doctors also may combine NSAIDs with stronger opioids like morphine, to treat very severe pain.

NSAIDs have been studied for their potential effectiveness in lowering the risk of certain types of cancer, particularly colon, prostate, and ovarian cancers. More research needs to be done, however, to confirm the drugs' ability to protect against cancer.

Recommended dosage

Patients typically take NSAIDs on an as-needed basis. Doses vary depending on the type of NSAID being used. For example, the most common type, ibuprofen, is available over the counter in 200 milligram (mg) caplets, which can be taken at regular intervals throughout the day. The maximum daily dose for ibuprofen is 1,200 mg.

Precautions

Most doctors recommend taking NSAIDs with a full glass of water. Avoid taking these drugs on an empty stomach. Smoking **cigarettes** and drinking alcohol while taking NSAIDs may irritate the stomach.

People who take NSAIDs should notify their doctors before having surgery or dental work, because these drugs can prevent wounds from healing properly.

Women who are pregnant or breastfeeding should check with their doctors before taking NSAIDs, because they may be harmful to a developing fetus or a newborn.

People with diabetes or who take aspirin, blood thinners, blood pressure medications, or steroids should also check with their doctors before taking NSAIDs.

Side effects

Many NSAID users experience mild side effects, such as an upset stomach. In 4%–7% of cases, more serious complications develop, such as stomach ulcers. Typically, elderly people experience the most serious complications.

Common side effects include stomach upset, constipation, dizziness, and headaches.

More severe side effects include stomach ulcers and bleeding ulcers. If a person has black, tarry stools or starts vomiting blood, it may be caused by a bleeding ulcer.

Kidney dysfunction is another severe complication of long-term NSAID use. Signs of kidney problems include dark yellow, brown, or bloody urine. NSAID use also may cause liver function problems over longer periods of time.

To guard against ulcers, physicians may ask patients to take NSAIDs with such anti-ulcer medications as omeprazole or misoprostol. Another option is to take the NSAID in a different, non-oral form. Often topical creams or suppositories are available. Finally, doctors may decide to switch to a different type of pain killer, such as a cyclooxygenase-2 (COX-2) inhibitor like Celebrex, which may be easier on the stomach. Some studies indicate that the use of COX-2 inhibitors may postpone the need to prescribe narcotic medications for severe pain.

Some patients who have had problems with side effects from NSAIDs may benefit from acupuncture as an adjunctive treatment in **pain management**. A study done in New York found that older patients with lower back pain related to cancer reported that their pain was relieved by acupuncture with fewer side effects than those caused by NSAIDs.

Interactions

NSAIDs can be taken with most other prescription and over-the-counter drugs without any harmful interactions. Certain drug combinations, however, should be avoided. For instance, when ibuprofen is combined with **methotrexate** (used for **chemotherapy** and arthritis treatment) or certain diabetic medicines and antidepressants, it can amplify negative side effects. Patients should check with a pharmacist before taking NSAIDs with other drugs.

NSAIDs may also interact with certain herbal preparations sold as dietary supplements. Among the herbs known to interact with NSAIDs are bearberry (*Arctostaphylos uva-ursi*), feverfew (*Tanacetum parthenium*), evening primrose (*Oenothera biennis*), and gossypol, a pigment obtained from cottonseed oil and used as a male contraceptive. In most cases, the herb increases the tendency of NSAIDs to irritate the digestive tract. It is just as important for patients to inform their doctors of herbal remedies that they take on a regular basis as it is to give the doctors lists of their other prescription medications.

Resources

BOOKS

Wilkes, Gail M., and Margaret Barton-Burke. *2013 Oncology Nursing Drug Handbook*. Burlington, MA: Jones & Bartlett Learning, 2013.

PERIODICALS

Brasky, Theodore M., et al. "Non-Steroidal Anti-Inflammatory Drugs (NSAIDs) and Breast Cancer Risk: Differences by Molecular Subtype." *Cancer Causes Control* 22, no. 7 (2011): 965–75.

Wang, X., et al. "Meta-Analysis of Nonsteroidal Anti-Inflammatory Drug Intake and Prostate Cancer Risk." *World Journal of Surgical Oncology* 12 (October 5, 2014): 304.

WEBSITES

American Cancer Society. "Non-Steroidal Anti-Inflammatory Drugs." http://www.cancer.org/treatment/treatmentsandsideeffects/physicalsideeffects/pain/paindiary/pain-control-non-steroid-anti-inflammatory-drugs (accessed November 6, 2014).

Harvard Medical School. "12 Things You Should Know about Pain Relievers." http://www.health.harvard.edu/fhg/updates/12-things-you-should-know-about-pain-relievers.shtml (accessed November 6, 2014).

ORGANIZATIONS

U.S. Food and Drug Administration, 10903 New Hampshire Ave., Silver Spring, MD 20993, (888) INFO-FDA (463-6332), http://www.fda.gov.

Melissa Knopper, MS
Rebecca J. Frey, PhD

Novantrone *see* **Mitoxantrone**

NSAIDs *see* **Nonsteroidal anti-inflammatory drugs**

Nuclear medicine scans

Definition

A nuclear medicine scan is a test in which radioactive material is taken into the body and is used to create an image of a specific organ or bone.

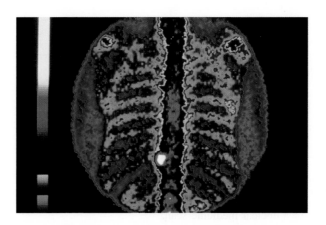

False-color bone scintigram (nuclear bone scan) of a person suffering from a secondary (metastatic) bone cancer (white area) affecting the dorsal spine. (CNRI/ Science Source)

Purpose

The purpose of a nuclear medicine scan is to locate areas of impaired function in the organ or bone being scanned. Nuclear medicine scans are widely used for diagnosis and monitoring of many different conditions. In the diagnosis and treatment of **cancer**, nuclear medicine scans are used to identify cancerous sites, for tumor localization and staging, and to judge response to therapy.

Description

A nuclear medicine scan is an extremely sensitive test that can provide information about the structure and function of specific parts of the body. Types of nuclear scans include bone scans, heart scans, lung scans, kidney and bladder scans, thyroid scans, liver and spleen scans, and gallbladder scans. Brain scans are done to detect malignancy.

In a nuclear medicine scan, a small amount of radioactive material, or tracer, is injected or taken orally by the patient. After a period of time during which the radioactive material accumulates in one area of the body, a scan is taken by a special radiation detector, called a radionuclide scanner. This machine produces an image of the area for analysis by the medical team.

This test is performed in a radiology facility, either in a hospital department or an outpatient x-ray center. During the scan, the patient lies on his or her back on a table, but may be repositioned to the stomach or side during the study. The radionuclide scanner is positioned against the body part to be examined. Either the camera, the table, or both may change position during the study. Depending on the type of scan, the procedure may take anywhere from 15 to 60 minutes. It is important for the patient not to move except when directed to do so by the technologist.

Precautions

Women who are pregnant or breast-feeding should not undergo this test. A patient who is unable to remain still for an extended period of time may require sedation for a nuclear medicine scan.

Preparation

The required preparation for nuclear medicine scans ranges from slight to none. The doctor may advise that certain prescription medications be discontinued before the test or that the patient not eat for three to four hours before the test. Depending on the type of test, a reference scan or specialized blood studies may be done before the scan is taken. Jewelry or metallic objects should be removed.

The patient should advise the doctor of any previously administered nuclear medicine scans; recent surgeries; sensitivities to drugs, allergies, or prescription medications; and if there is a chance of pregnancy.

Aftercare

No special care is required after the test. Fluids are encouraged after the scan to aid in the excretion of the radioactive material. It should be almost completely eliminated from the body within 24 hours.

Risks

The risks of nuclear medicine scans are very low. Most scans use the same or a lesser amount of radiation as a conventional x-ray and the radioactive material is quickly passed through the body. Side effects or negative reactions to the test are very rare.

Results

A normal result is a scan that shows the expected distribution of the tracer and no unusual shape, size, or function of the scanned organ.

Abnormal results

Depending on the tracer and technique used, the scan can identify and image particular types of tumors or certain cancers. Too much tracer in the spleen and bones, compared to the liver, can indicate potential hypertension or cirrhosis. Liver diseases such as hepatitis may also

cause an abnormal scan, but are rarely diagnosed from the information revealed by this study alone.

In a bone scan, a high concentration of tracer occurs in areas of increased bone activity. These regions appear brighter and may be referred to as "hot spots." They may indicate healing fractures, tumors, infections, or other processes that trigger new bone formation. Lower concentrations of tracer may be called "cold spots." Poor blood flow to an area of bone, or bone destruction from a tumor, may produce a cold spot.

See also Imaging studies; Magnetic resonance imaging.

Resources

WEBSITES

American Cancer Society. "Nuclear Scans." http://www.cancer.org/treatment/understandingyourdiagnosis/examsandtest-descriptions/imagingradiologytests/imaging-radiology-tests-nuc-scan (accessed November 8, 2014).

National Cancer Institute. "Uses of Imaging." http://imaging.cancer.gov/patientsandproviders/cancerimaging/usesofimaging (accessed November 8, 2014).

U.S. National Library of Medicine. "Nuclear Scans." MedlinePlus. http://www.nlm.nih.gov/medlineplus/nuclearscans.html (accessed November 8, 2014).

ORGANIZATIONS

Society of Nuclear Medicine and Molecular Imaging, 1850 Samuel Morse Dr., Reston, VA 20190, (703) 708-9000, Fax: (703) 708-9015, http://www.snmmi.org.

Ellen S. Weber, MSN
Paul A. Johnson, EdM

Nutritional support

Description

Achieving adequate nutritional support is difficult during **cancer** treatment. However, it is important for cancer patients to preserve body composition and proper nutrition. This means not gaining or losing too much weight and maintaining strength. Doing so can improve daily function and the ability to cope with cancer therapies. Adequate nutrition may help a cancer patient feel better and stronger and will help to fight off infection.

Malnutrition is a primary concern and is a primary cause of illness in cancer patients who often have difficulty consuming enough calories and nutrients. Protein-energy malnutrition (or protein-calorie malnutrition) is a particular problem. It is the most common secondary illness in cancer patients and occurs when not enough protein and energy (calories) are consumed to sustain the body's composition, causing **weight loss**. When body stores are severely compromised, a patient's body cannot function as it should, which may lead to illness and even death. Exhaustion, weakness, decreased resistance to infection, muscle wasting, and difficulties tolerating cancer therapies may result from inadequate nutrition.

People who have cancer commonly experience **anorexia**, or loss of appetite. Anorexia is the most common cause of malnutrition and deterioration in patients who have cancer. Another common problem in cancer is weight loss and cachexia. Cachexia, also known as wasting syndrome, is a condition where a person's body weight wastes away, characterized by a constant loss of weight, muscle, and fat. Cachexia can occur in people who consume enough food, but because of disease complications, cannot absorb enough nutrients. Malnutrition, anorexia, and cachexia are serious concerns in cancer patients.

Causes and symptoms

There are many reasons for malnutrition in cancer patients, including the effect of the tumor, side effects of treatment, or psychological issues such as **depression**. The growth of tumors in a patient's digestive system may cause blockage, lead to **nausea and vomiting**, or cause poor digestion or poor absorption of nutrients.

Cancer therapies and their side effects may also lead to nutrition difficulties. For example, following some intestinal surgeries, malabsorption of protein and fat may occur. In addition, there may be an increased requirement for energy due to infection or **fever**.

Treatment

Nutritional problems related to side effects should be addressed to make sure cancer patients have adequate nutrition and do not lose too much weight. The following suggestions help patients deal with side effects such as loss of appetite, nausea, vomiting, **fatigue**, and **taste**

alteration. To deal with appetite loss and weight loss, patients can:

- Eat more when feeling the hungriest.
- Eat foods that are enjoyed the most.
- Eat several small meals and snacks instead of three large meals.
- Have ready-to-eat snacks on hand such as cheese and crackers, granola bars, muffins, nuts and seeds, canned puddings, ice cream, yogurt, and hard-boiled eggs.
- Eat high-calorie foods and high-protein foods.
- Begin with small portions during a meal to enjoy the satisfaction of finishing a meal, and have additional servings if still hungry.
- Eat in a pleasant atmosphere with family and friends if desired.
- Make sure to consume at least 8–10 glasses of water per day to maintain fluid balance.
- Consider commercial liquid meal replacements.
- Discuss with a physician the possibility of using appetite-increasing medications.

Nausea is a common side effect of several cancer treatments including surgery, **chemotherapy**, biological therapy, and radiation. If nausea is a problem, the following methods may provide relief:

- Avoid fatty, fried, spicy, greasy, or hot foods with a strong odor.
- Eat small meals frequently but slowly.
- Consume dry toast or crackers before getting out of bed for nausea that is worse in the morning.
- Consume such foods as clear liquids, toast, crackers, yogurt, sherbet, pretzels, oatmeal, skinned chicken (baked or broiled), angel food cake, and fruits and vegetables that are soft or bland.
- Drink cold beverages.
- Avoid hot foods that may add to nausea and consume foods at room temperature or cooler.
- Drink or sip liquids (using a straw if necessary) throughout the day, but not during meals, or suck on ice chips.
- Discuss with a physician the possibility of using antinausea medications (also called antiemetics).

Vomiting may occur because of the cancer, the treatment, or emotional upset. If vomiting occurs, the following guidelines may help:

- Avoid drinking or eating until vomiting has subsided, then consume small amounts of clear liquids.
- Consume a fully liquid diet (including dairy products unless they are difficult to digest).

• Once able to tolerate liquids, begin with small quantities and gradually return to a regular diet once nausea and vomiting improve.

If fatigue is preventing the patient from receiving adequate nutrition, the following strategies may help:

• Buy frozen, canned, or ready-to-use foods.

• Eat high-calorie foods.

• Have ready-to-eat snacks on hand such as cheese and crackers, granola bars, muffins, nuts and seeds, canned puddings, ice cream, yogurt, and hard-boiled eggs.

• Use a service such as Meals on Wheels or another delivery or home-care service.

• Invite friends or family over to assist with meal preparation.

• Use commercial liquid meal replacements.

Taste changes can give foods a metallic or off flavor. The following strategies can alleviate taste changes.

• If meats have a metallic taste, other sources of protein such as dairy products, poultry, fish, seafood, peanut butter, eggs, seeds, nuts, tofu, and legumes can be substituted.

• Use of plastic utensils can decrease metallic flavor.

• Tart foods such as citrus juices, lemonade, cranberry juice, and pickles can help alleviate a metallic taste. However, these foods can irritate a sore mouth and throat.

• Consume a variety of foods and try different seasonings, herbs, and sauces.

• Patients can choose foods that look and smell appealing.

• Drinks that are too strong or sweet can be diluted with water.

• Rinsing the mouth often with baking soda and water helps clear the metallic taste.

Alternative and complementary therapies

There is no alternative or complementary nutritional therapy that has proved effective for **cancer prevention** or cancer treatment. It has been shown, however, that nutrition can play a role in cancer prevention. Eating a plant-based diet that is low in fat and salt, avoiding tobacco, and keeping alcohol use to a minimum can contribute to lower risk of many cancers. Maintaining a healthy weight and remaining physically active can also lower cancer risks. In addition, several foods and nutraceuticals such as garlic, plant sterols, green and black tea polyphenols, and soybean products (soy isoflavones) have shown promise in previous research for anticarcinogenic properties. Many of these products are actively being tested in **clinical trials** to elucidate anticarcinogenic properties. It is important to check with

---

QUESTIONS TO ASK YOUR DOCTOR

• What effect will the treatment or disease have on my body nutritionally, and my ability to eat, digest food, and absorb nutrients?

• How long will the negative side effects last?

• Is there a risk of malnutrition or weight loss with this type of cancer or treatment?

• What nutrients are most important to obtain during treatment?

• Are there any nutritional supplements that may be required?

---

a dietitian or doctor before taking nutritional supplements or alternative therapies because they may interfere with cancer medications or treatments.

Special concerns

Cancer patients should maintain an adequate intake of fluids, energy, and protein. The patient's nutrient requirements should be calculated by a dietitian or doctor because requirements vary considerably from patient to patient.

Enteral nutrition may be administered through a nose tube (or surgically placed tubes) for patients with eating difficulties, such as difficulty swallowing, esophageal narrowing, blockage caused by a tumor, stomach weakness, paralysis, or other conditions that affect normal food intake. If a patient's gastrointestinal tract is working and is not affected by the cancer treatments, then enteral support is preferable. Parenteral nutrition (most often an infusion into a vein) can be used if the patient's gut is not functioning properly or for other reasons that prevent enteral feeding.

Resources

BOOKS

Quillin, Patrick, and Noreen Quillin. *Beating Cancer with Nutrition—Revised.* Sun Lakes, AZ: Bookworld Services, 2001.

PERIODICALS

Alberts, D. S., et al. "Lack of Effect of a High-Fiber Cereal Supplement on the Recurrence of Colorectal Adenomas." *New England Journal of Medicine* 2000: 1156–62.

Schatzkin, A., et al. "Lack of Effect of a Low-Fat, High-Fiber Diet on the Recurrence of Colorectal Adenomas." *New England Journal of Medicine* 2000: 1149–55.

Singletary, Keith. "Diet, Natural Products and Cancer Chemoprevention." *The Journal of Nutrition* 2000: 465S–466S.

WEBSITES

American Cancer Society. "Nutrition for People with Cancer." http://www.cancer.org/treatment/survivorshipduringandaftertreatment/nutritionforpeoplewithcancer/index (accessed December 22, 2014).

National Cancer Institute. "Overview of Nutrition in Cancer Care." http://www.cancer.gov/cancertopics/pdq/supportivecare/nutrition/Patient/page1 (accessed August 4, 2014).

ORGANIZATIONS

The National Cancer Institute (NCI). Public Inquiries Office, Building 31, Room 10A31, 31 Center Drive, MSC 2580, Bethesda, MD 20892-2580, (301) 435-3848, (800) 422-6237, http://www.cancer.gov.

National Center for Complementary and Alternative Medicine (NCCAM), 31 Center Dr., Room #5B–58, Bethesda, MD 20892, (301) 495-4957, (800) 422-6237, http://nccam.nih.gov/.

Crystal Heather Kaczkowski, MSc

REVISED BY TERESA G. ODLE

Nystatin *see* **Antifungal therapy**

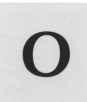

Obesity and cancer risk

Definition

Obesity increases the risk for certain cancers, for reasons that are not well understood. Obesity may also worsen **cancer** prognosis.

Description

Obesity is caused by consuming more calories than the body uses for basic metabolism and physical activity. The extra calories are stored in fat cells. This excess fat increases the risk of many serious diseases, including high blood pressure, heart disease, stroke, type 2 diabetes, liver and gallbladder disease, sleep apnea and respiratory problems, arthritis, infertility in women, and various cancers. People who are overweight or obese, on average, have shorter life spans than people who maintain a healthy weight throughout their lives.

Associations between overweight/obesity and cancer development are complicated. Although overweight and obesity are usually determined by body mass index (BMI)—a measure of body fat based on weight and height—cancer is sometimes associated with fat distribution in the body. Abdominal fat, as measured by waist circumference, is associated with increased risk for colorectal cancer, regardless of body weight, and is probably linked to higher risks for endometrial (uterine lining), colorectal, and pancreatic cancers, as well as **breast cancer** in postmenopausal women.

Higher BMI and obesity are significantly associated with poorer prognoses for many cancers. They reduce survival rates and appear to increase the risk of cancer recurring after treatment.

Association studies

The American Cancer Society's Cancer Prevention Study II found significant increases in cancer among people who were the most overweight. Overweight/ obesity was an important risk factor for endometrial and esophageal cancers; breast cancer in postmenopausal women; and colorectal, kidney, and pancreatic cancers. Overweight and obesity probably increased the risk of thyroid, gallbladder, and liver cancers; **non-Hodgkin lymphoma; multiple myeloma**; cervical and ovarian cancers; aggressive forms of **prostate cancer**; and possibly some others.

A large Finnish study published in 2014 reported correlations between increasing BMI in men and increasing incidence of colon, kidney, liver, and bladder cancers and of all cancers combined. Increasing BMI correlated with increasing incidence of colon, gallbladder, stomach, and ovarian cancers in women. However, increasing BMI was associated with decreasing incidence of lung cancer in men and lung and breast cancers in women. High BMI was associated with increased overall cancer risk in people who had never smoked but with reduced risk in smokers.

Endometrial and esophageal cancers

Endometrial cancer and esophageal adenocarcinoma are the cancers most strongly associated with obesity. Both premenopausal and postmenopausal overweight and obese women have two to four times the risk of endometrial cancer as normal-weight women. The risk appears to increase with weight gain during adulthood, especially among women who have never had menopausal hormone therapy (MHT). This increased risk from obesity may be associated with diabetes and possibly with physical inactivity. People who are overweight or obese have twice the risk of esophageal adenocarcinoma as healthy-weight people. Obesity does not increase the risk—and may even reduce the risk—of squamous cell cancer, the other major type of **esophageal cancer**.

Breast cancer

Overweight/obesity has consistently been associated with a modest increase in the risk of breast cancer in postmenopausal women, primarily in women who have

Cancers associated with excess body fat

Colorectal
Endometrial
Esophageal
Gallbladder
Kidney
Ovarian
Pancreatic
Postmenopausal breast cancer

SOURCE: World Cancer Research Fund International, "Cancers Linked with Greater Body Fatness." Available online at: http://www.wcrf.org/int/cancer-facts-figures/link-between-lifestyle-cancer-risk/cancers-linked-greater-body-fatness.

Table listing cancers known to be associated with excess body fat. *(Table by Lumina Datamatics Ltd. © 2015 Cengage Learning®.)*

never had MHT and who have hormone receptor-positive breast cancers that grow in response to the female hormones estrogen and/or progesterone. The strongest association appears to be in women who gained weight as adults, usually between the ages of 18 and 50–60. One study found a 6% increase in risk for every 11 lb. (5 kg) gained since age 20. Increased exercise is associated with decreased risk, especially in premenopausal women. High BMI is independently associated with poor prognosis for receptor-positive breast cancer. Obesity may also be a risk factor for **male breast cancer**.

A 2013 study reported that obesity had no overall association with breast cancer in African American women and was associated with reduced risk for receptor-negative breast cancer. However, larger waist and hip circumferences were associated with increased risk for premenopausal breast cancer. Obese Hispanic American women may also be at lower risk than obese white women.

Colorectal cancer

Higher BMI is strongly associated with increased risk for colorectal cancer in men, with abdominal fat presenting the greatest risk. BMI and waist circumference are associated with **colon cancer** in women, but the link is less strong and may be affected by MHT in postmenopausal women. High BMI is associated with a modestly increased risk for **rectal cancer**.

Other cancers

• Obesity has been consistently associated with renal cell cancer—the most common type of kidney cancer. Although high blood pressure is a risk factor for renal cell cancer, obesity is an independent risk factor.

• Overweight/obesity, especially waist circumference, is associated with a slightly increased risk of pancreatic cancer.

• Increasing weight is associated with increased risk for thyroid cancer.

• Gallbladder cancer risk increases with increasing BMI, possibly because of the high incidence of gallstones—a strong risk factor for gallbladder cancer—in obese people.

• There may be a very slight increase in overall risk for prostate cancer associated with obesity. Several studies have shown a higher risk for aggressive prostate cancer in obese men.

• Obesity may be associated with increased risk for cholangiocarcinoma, a bile duct tumor.

• Population studies have shown strong links between obesity and liver cancer.

• Studies of BMI and ovarian cancer risk have reported conflicting results.

Risk factors

In addition to abdominal fat, the timing of weight gain may be important for some cancers. In general, excess weight during childhood and young adulthood may present a greater risk. Some research suggests that overweight teenagers, but not women who gain weight as adults, may be at greater risk for premenopausal **ovarian cancer**.

Demographics

About one-third of adults in the United States are obese, and another one-third are overweight. Furthermore, about 17% of children and teens—12.5 million—are obese, and most overweight children and teens grow up to be overweight or obese adults. Overweight/obesity rates for children and teens have increased by 300% since 1980. Overweight and obesity rates for adults in the developed world have also increased dramatically in recent decades. Obesity is now considered a global epidemic. Overweight/obesity puts a very large segment of the population at risk for serious chronic diseases and cancers.

It is estimated that one out of every three cancer deaths in the United States is associated with overweight or obesity, poor nutrition, and/or physical inactivity. Although these factors are interrelated, the strongest link is between body weight and cancer risk. It has been estimated that overweight/obesity alone contributes to as many as one in five cancer deaths. In 2007, it was estimated that about 34,000 new cancers in men in the United States (4% of male cancers) and 50,500 new cancers in women (7%) were caused by obesity. The percentages of specific cancers resulting from obesity vary greatly, with a high of about 40% for **endometrial cancer** and esophageal **adenocarcinoma**. If these trends continue, it is projected that obesity will cause an additional 500,000 cancers in the United States by 2030.

Causes and symptoms

The mechanisms by which obesity increases cancer risk are not well understood. This is one of the "provocative questions" being addressed by the **National Cancer Institute**.

Inflammation and cytokines

Excess fat can cause inflammation and impaired immune system function. Obesity often causes chronic low-level or subacute inflammation, and chronic inflammation has been associated with increased risk for various cancers, including breast cancer. Obesity may alter immune responses, increase oxidative stress, or affect the nuclear-factor kappa-beta system, which regulates immune responses and has been linked to inflammation and cancer. Fat (adipose) tissues produce immune system and cell-signaling proteins called cytokines that promote inflammation. Chronic inflammatory microenvironments caused by cytokines in fat tissue may promote cancer spread (**metastasis**). High cytokine levels in tumors and blood are associated with poorer breast cancer outcomes.

Fat cells produce cytokines, growth factors, and other proteins called adipokines that may inhibit or stimulate cell growth. Obese people have higher levels of leptin, an adipokine that appears to promote cell proliferation—a characteristic of cancer cells—and lower levels of adiponectin, an adipokine that may help prevent cell proliferation. Fat cells also may directly or indirectly affect tumor growth regulators, such as mammalian target of rapamycin (mTOR) and AMP-activated protein kinase.

Although the cause of increased esophageal cancer risk from obesity is unknown, overweight and obese people are more likely to have a history of **Barrett's esophagus** or gastroesophageal reflux, which increase the risk for esophageal adenocarcinoma. Obesity may increase esophageal inflammation associated with these conditions.

Hormones

Excess fat may affect levels of hormones, especially insulin and estrogen, or proteins that influence the utilization of certain hormones, such as sex hormone–binding globulins. Body fat may affect factors that

KEY TERMS

Adipokines—Cytokines and growth factors secreted by adipose (fat) cells.

Adiponectin—A hormone secreted by fat cells that regulates glucose and lipid metabolism.

Adipose tissue—Fat tissue.

Androgens—Male sex hormones.

Bariatric surgery—Weight-loss surgery.

Body mass index (BMI)—A measure of body fat: the ratio of weight in kilograms to the square of height in meters.

Cytokines—Proteins that regulate immune responses and mediate intercellular communication.

Inflammation—An immune response to irritation, infection, or injury; chronic inflammation is associated with increased cancer risk.

Insulin—A hormone required for the metabolism of carbohydrates, lipids, and proteins and the regulation of blood sugar levels; lack of insulin or insulin insensitivity results in high blood sugar levels and diabetes.

Insulin-like growth factor-1 (IGF-1)—An insulin-like growth factor that normally declines after puberty, but that is produced by fat cells and may be associated with increased cancer risk.

Leptin—A peptide hormone produced by fat cells that acts on the hypothalamus to suppress appetite and burn stored fat.

Menopausal hormone therapy (MHT)—Treatment of menopausal symptoms with estrogen or estrogen and progesterone.

Nonsteroidal anti-inflammatory drugs (NSAIDs)—Over-the-counter and prescription medications for reducing pain and inflammation that may have a role in cancer prevention.

control cell division, such as insulin-like growth factor-1 (IGF-1). Obese people often have increased blood levels of both insulin and IGF-1, which may promote the growth of some tumors. High levels of insulin or IGF-1 are among proposed mechanisms for increased colon cancer risk. High insulin levels may also play a role in **kidney cancer**. IGF-1 levels, as well as levels of certain other hormones and growth factors, have been associated with prostate cancer risk.

Fat tissues produce excess estrogen, which is associated with risk for endometrial, breast, and certain other cancers. In particular, increased estrogen levels are believed to be responsible for the increased risk of postmenopausal estrogen-responsive breast cancer in obese women. High estrogen levels from fat tissue probably also have a role in endometrial cancer risk. In men, fat cells convert male androgens to estrogen, which may increase the risk of male breast cancer.

Diagnosis

BMI is the most common screening for overweight/obesity. BMI is weight in kilograms divided by the square of height in meters (or weight in pounds divided by the square of height in inches) and multiplied by 703. For adults aged 20 and over, BMI ranges are:

- less than 18.5—underweight
- 18.5–24.9—normal weight
- 25–29.9—overweight
- 30 or above—obese

For children and teens, overweight/obesity is based on the Centers for Disease Control and Prevention's sex-specific BMI-for-age growth charts: overweight is classified as being within the 85th to less than the 95th percentile, and obesity is at or above the 95th percentile.

However, BMI does not necessarily accurately reflect body fat associated with cancer risk. Heavily muscled athletes may have high BMIs but significantly less body fat. Chronic dieters who have lost significant muscle mass may have low BMIs but elevated body fat. Direct caliper measurements of body fat determine skin-fold thickness at the back of the upper arm and other sites. Waist circumference as a measure of abdominal fat is also a better predictor than BMI for the risk of some cancers.

Treatment

Treating obesity to reduce cancer risk usually requires lifelong management of diet and exercise or bariatric (weight-loss) surgery. A realistic weight-loss goal is 10% of body weight over a six-month period, although without permanent changes in eating habits and exercise patterns, lost weight is often quickly regained. Typical recommendations include a medically approved commercial weight-loss program or:

- a balanced diet of 1,000–1,600 daily calories
- replacing fats and sugar with fruits, vegetables, and whole grains
- no more than 30% of calories from fat; no more than one-third of those from saturated fats
- 60–90 minutes of daily physical activity

QUESTIONS TO ASK YOUR DOCTOR

- Is my excess weight increasing my cancer risk?
- Will losing weight reduce my cancer risk?
- Do you recommend bariatric surgery for reducing my cancer risk?
- Does my obesity affect my cancer prognosis?
- Does my obesity increase the risk that my cancer will recur?

- behavior modification, including monitoring food intake, portion control, and recognition of responses to foods and overeating triggers

Overweight/obese cancer patients may attempt to lose moderate amounts of weight during and after treatment through a well-balanced diet and increased physical activity and under close medical monitoring.

Prognosis

Bariatric surgery for obesity lowers the risk for obesity-associated cancers. The effects on cancer risk of **weight loss** through dieting and increased physical activity are less clear. Weight-loss surgery combined with lifestyle changes results in an average loss of about 30% of body weight, compared with about 7%–10% by conventional methods, and it is not yet clear whether this more moderate weight loss reduces cancer risk. However, intentional weight loss by overweight/obese people reduces insulin, estrogen, and androgen levels, and some evidence indicates that even moderate weight loss may reduce the risk of postmenopausal breast cancer, more aggressive types of prostate cancer, and possibly other cancers. Numerous studies addressing whether weight loss reduces cancer risk are underway.

Prevention

It has been estimated that if every adult in the United States reduced their BMI by 1%—a loss of 2.2 lb. (1 kg) for an average-weight adult—about 100,000 new cancer cases would be avoided. Evidence also suggests that regular physical activity can improve survival for people with breast, prostate, and colon cancers.

A 2014 study found that regular use of **nonsteroidal anti-inflammatory drugs** (NSAIDs) reduced breast cancer risk, especially in overweight women. Although combination MHT with both estrogen and progestin appears to lower the risk of endometrial cancer in overweight/obese women, this is not generally recommended because of other adverse health effects from MHT.

Resources

BOOKS

Surh, Young-Joon. *Nutrition and Physical Activity in Aging, Obesity, and Cancer: The Third International Conference.* Boston: Blackwell, 2012.

Sutton, Amy L. *Breast Cancer Sourcebook.* Detroit: Omnigraphics, 2012.

PERIODICALS

Alzahrani, Badr, Tristan J. Iseli, and Lionel W. Hebbard. "Non-Viral Causes of Liver Cancer: Does Obesity Led Inflammation Play a Role?" *Cancer Letters* 345, no. 2 (April 10, 2014): 223–29.

Banderal, Elisa V., et al. "Body Fatness and Breast Cancer Risk in Women of African Ancestry." *BMC Cancer* 13 (October 14, 2013): 475.

Catsburg, Chelsea, et al. "Associations between Anthropometric Characteristics, Physical Activity, and Breast Cancer Risk in a Canadian Cohort." *Breast Cancer Research and Treatment* 145, no. 2 (June 2014): 545–52.

Cui, Yong, et al. "Use of Nonsteroidal Anti-Inflammatory Drugs and Reduced Breast Cancer Risk among Overweight Women." *Breast Cancer Research and Treatment* 146, no. 2 (July 2014): 439–46.

Gilbert, Candace A., and Joyce M. Slingerland. "Cytokines, Obesity, and Cancer: New Insights on Mechanisms Linking Obesity to Cancer Risk and Progression." *Annual Review of Medicine* 64 (2013): 45.

Lashinger, Laura M., Nikki A. Ford, and Stephen D. Hursting. "Interacting Inflammatory and Growth Factor Signals Underlie the Obesity-Cancer Link." *Journal of Nutrition* 144, no. 2 (February 2014): 109–13.

Riboli, Elio. "The Cancer-Obesity Connection: What Do We Know and What Can We Do?" *BMC Biology* 12 (2014): 9.

Song, Xin, et al. "Body Mass Index and Cancer Incidence: The FINRISK Study." *European Journal of Epidemiology* 29, no. 7 (July 2014): 477–87.

OTHER

American Cancer Society. "Body Weight and Cancer Risk." http://www.cancer.org/acs/groups/cid/documents/webcon tent/002578-pdf.pdf (accessed August 4, 2014).

WEBSITES

American Society of Clinical Oncology (ASCO). "Obesity and Cancer." http://www.asco.org/practice-research/obesity-and-cancer (accessed November 11, 2014).

Cancer Research UK. "Obesity, Body Weight and Cancer." http://www.cancerresearchuk.org/cancer-info/healthyliv ing/obesity-bodyweight-and-cancer/obesity-body-weight-and-cancer (accessed November 11, 2014).

Foxhall, Lewis E. "The Obesity-Cancer Connection, and What We Can Do about It." American Cancer Society. http://www.cancer.org/cancer/news/expertvoices/post/2013/02/28/the-obesity-cancer-connection-and-what-we-can-do-about-it.aspx (accessed August 4, 2014).

National Cancer Institute. "Obesity and Cancer Risk." http://www.cancer.gov/cancertopics/factsheet/Risk/obesity (accessed August 4, 2014).

ORGANIZATIONS

American Cancer Society, 250 Williams Street NW, Atlanta, GA 30303, (800) 227-2345, http://www.cancer.org.

Centers for Disease Control and Prevention (CDC), 1600 Clifton Rd., Atlanta, GA 30333, (800) CDC-INFO (232-4636), http://www.cdc.gov.

National Cancer Institute, 6116 Executive Boulevard, Suite 300, Bethesda, MD 20892-8322, (800) 4-CANCER (422-6237), http://www.cancer.gov.

Margaret Alic, PhD

REVIEWED BY MELINDA GRANGER OBERLEITNER, RN, DNS, APRN, CNS

Obinutuzumab

Definition

Obinutuzumab (Gazyva) is a type of targeted **immunotherapy** drug called a monoclonal antibody. It is used to treat **chronic lymphocytic leukemia** (CLL), a **cancer** of immune-system white blood cells, primarily B lymphocytes (B cells).

Purpose

Obinutuzumab injection was approved by the U.S. Food and Drug Administration (FDA) in 2013 for treatment, in combination with **chlorambucil** (Clb), of CLL patients who have not been previously treated for the disease. The approval was based on a clinical trial that demonstrated improved progression-free survival (PFS) with combination Gazyva/chlorambucil (GClb) treatment compared with Clb treatment alone for CD20-positive CLL. The trial also compared **rituximab** in combination with Clb (RClb) with GClb; as of 2014, the full results were not yet available. However, in a trial of previously untreated elderly CLL patients with multiple debilitating coexisting conditions, the GClb group had a median PFS of 26.7 months compared with 15.2 months for the RClb group and 11.1 months for the Clb group. In addition to significantly prolonging PFS, GClb was associated with an increased rate of complete remission. GClb also resulted in significantly increased overall survival compared with Clb alone. In the past, the treatment goal for elderly patients with CLL and coexisting conditions has been to control symptoms.

KEY TERMS

Apoptosis—Programmed self-destruction by a cell.

B cell—A type of white blood cell or lymphocyte derived from bone marrow that secretes antibodies, has other complex functions in the immune system, and is overproduced in chronic lymphocytic leukemia; the target of obinutuzumab.

CD20—A surface protein on B cells that is the target of obinutuzumab.

Chlorambucil (Clb)—A chemotherapy drug used to treat chronic lymphocytic leukemia.

Chronic lymphocytic leukemia (CLL)—A cancer characterized by an abnormal increase in mature lymphocytes, especially B cells, that primarily affects older adults.

Gazyva/chlorambucil (GClb)—Combined treatment with obinutuzumab and chlorambucil.

Glycoengineering—The production of drugs, such as monoclonal antibodies, with specific sugar molecules attached to enhance their activity.

Hepatitis B virus (HBV)—A virus that attacks the liver and that can be reactivated by obinutuzumab treatment.

Monoclonal antibodies—Identical antibodies that recognize and bind to specific proteins; commonly used for targeted drug therapies.

Ofatumumab—A monoclonal antibody used to treat chronic lymphocytic leukemia.

Progression-free survival (PFS)—The length of time patients survive without their cancer progressing; used in clinical trials to measure the effectiveness of a drug.

Progressive multifocal leukoencephalopathy (PML)—A life-threatening brain infection that is a rare side effect of obinutuzumab.

Receptor—A molecule, usually a protein such as CD20, inside or on the surface of a cell, that binds a specific chemical group or molecule to initiate a sequence of events.

Rituximab/chlorambucil (RClb)—A combination monoclonal antibody/chlorambucil treatment for chronic lymphocytic leukemia.

Targeted immunotherapy—An immunological drug, such as a monoclonal antibody, that interferes with specific molecules involved in cancer cell growth and/or survival.

Tumor lysis syndrome—Excess uric acid, potassium, and phosphate in the blood due to the rapid destruction of large numbers of cancer cells.

These clinical-trial results suggest that long-term disease control may be possible. Obinutuzumab is also being studied for the treatment of other types of cancer.

Description

CLL is a chronic, debilitating disease that can lead to severe infections. Previously available treatments usually induced remission but did not cure the disease. Obinutuzumab is a monoclonal antibody produced in the laboratory that seeks out and binds strongly to a specific protein receptor called CD20 on the surfaces of B cells—some normal B cells as well as CLL B cells. Obinutuzumab is known as a third-generation type 2 anti-CD20 glycoengineered fully humanized IgG1 monoclonal antibody. "Glycoengineered" means that special carbohydrate (sugar) molecules have been added to a portion of the antibody to strengthen its binding to CD20 receptors. "Fully humanized" means that the human immune system will not recognize and destroy the drug as "foreign." By binding to CD20, obinutuzumab both tags the B cells for destruction by the immune system and induces apoptosis—B cell self-destruction. The type 2

CD20 binding of obinutuzumab differentiates it from the type 1 binding of the **monoclonal antibodies** rituximab and **ofatumumab**, which are also used to treat CLL. Obinutuzumab binding activates a different signaling pathway within B cells than the signaling pathway activated by rituximab and ofatumumab and increases direct cell killing. The binding also decreases the internalization into the cell of the obinutuzumab-CD20 complex, which means that the drug remains active for longer.

Brand names

Obinutuzumab is made by Genentech, Inc., and marketed under the brand name Gazyva in the United States, Canada, and Australia. It was approved in Europe in 2014, where it is marketed by Roche under the brand name Gazyvaro. It is also known as GA101, afutuzumab, and anti-CD20 monoclonal antibody R7159.

Recommended dosage

Obinutuzumab is a liquid that is added to fluid and administered by infusion into a vein (IV) by a doctor or nurse in a medical office or hospital. It is usually injected in six cycles of 28 days each.

- On Day 1 of Cycle 1, a small dose of 100 milligrams (mg) is infused slowly over four hours to monitor for infusion reactions.
- The next day (Day 2), 900 mg is injected over at least three hours.
- If no problems arise, the third infusion of 1,000 mg is six days later (Day 8).
- The fourth infusion of 1,000 is a week later (Day 15). The third and fourth infusions are over at least two hours each.
- Cycles 2–6 are 1,000 mg infused over at least two hours once a month for five months.

The day before the first infusion, the patient may be given medications and plenty of fluids to reduce the risk of a serious side effect called **tumor lysis syndrome**, which can occur when large numbers of cancer cells are killed simultaneously, releasing their contents and overwhelming the bloodstream. Between 30 minutes and two hours before each infusion, the patient is given medications, including acetaminophen (Tylenol), to reduce the risk of reactions. For at least the first two treatments, an oral or IV antihistamine, such as **diphenhydramine** (Benadryl), and an IV corticosteroid are also administered.

Precautions

Obinutuzumab comes with a "black box warning" concerning the possibility of potentially fatal reactivation of hepatitis B virus (HBV) or progressive multifocal **leukoencephalopathy** (PML). The patient is given a blood test for HBV before the first treatment, and blood tests for hepatitis may be administered during treatment. PML is a rare brain infection that cannot be prevented, treated, or cured and that usually results in severe disability or death.

Some people have infusion reactions during or within 24 hours of obinutuzumab administration, particularly with the first two treatments. Mild reactions are usually **fever** and chills. Less common, more serious reactions can be dangerous and may include:

- low blood pressure causing lightheadedness or dizziness
- fainting
- headache
- flushing or feeling warm
- itching or hives
- cough or shortness of breath
- changes in heart rate

- back or abdominal pain
- swelling of the face, tongue, or throat

Some adverse reactions may necessitate interrupting or halting obinutuzumab treatment.

- Tumor lysis syndrome can occur within a day of the first transfusion in patients with large numbers of leukemia cells. Tumor lysis syndrome can lead to kidney failure and may affect the heart and nervous system.
- Blood cell counts and tests for effects on other organs are performed throughout the treatment to determine whether other medications are needed or whether the treatment should be reduced, delayed, or halted.
- Obinutuzumab can lower white blood cell counts and have other effects on the immune system that can increase the risk of infection.
- Patients should not receive vaccines during and for some time after treatment without consulting their doctor, since obinutuzumab could make the vaccine less effective or lead to serious infection.
- Patients should avoid contact with people who have recently received a live virus vaccine, such as oral polio or nasal-spray flu vaccines.
- Obinutuzumab can lower platelet counts, increasing the risk of bleeding. Patients should consult their doctors before taking drugs or supplements that increase bleeding risk, including aspirin, warfarin (Coumadin), or vitamin E.

Pediatric

The safety and effectiveness of obinutuzumab have not been established in pediatric patients.

Geriatric

Since CLL typically affects the elderly, the median age in **clinical trials** was 73, and many of the patients had multiple coexisting conditions.

Pregnant or breastfeeding

It is not known whether obinutuzumab affects fertility. The effects of obinutuzumab on a fetus are unknown, so women should avoid becoming pregnant during treatment and for at least 12 months after treatment ends. Women should not breastfeed while receiving obinutuzumab.

Other conditions and allergies

Patients should inform their doctors if they:

- are allergic to anything, including medicines, dyes, additives, or foods

- have ever tested positive for HBV
- have any type of infection or have ever had a long-term or intermittent infection
- have any type of heart disease
- are taking medicine for high blood pressure
- have any other medical conditions, such as kidney or liver disease, congestive heart failure, diabetes, or gout
- have ever had heart or lung disease
- are planning to have surgery, including dental surgery

Side effects

The most common side effects of obinutuzumab are infusion reactions, especially with the first two infusions, and lowered white blood cell counts that increase the risk of infection. Less common side effects are:

- lowered platelet count with increased risk of bleeding
- lowered red blood cell count (anemia)
- fever
- cough
- muscle or bone pain

Rare side effects of obinutuzumab are reactivation of HBV infection, tumor lysis syndrome, PML, and death from heart problems. Patients should immediately contact their doctor or seek emergency medical treatment if they have:

- symptoms of HBV infection or hepatitis, including jaundice
- symptoms of a brain infection, including confusion or dizziness
- severe or long-lasting muscle or joint pain
- fever, chills, cough, sore throat, or other signs of infection
- unusual bleeding or bruising
- nausea, vomiting, diarrhea, and fatigue within 12–24 hours of an infusion
- reduced need to urinate or production of less than usual amounts of urine

Interactions

Patients should inform their physicians of all prescription and over-the-counter medicines, **vitamins**, nutritional supplements, and herbs that they are taking, especially blood pressure medications. They should inform their doctors if they drink alcohol. Since obinutuzumab can lower blood platelets, patients may need to avoid drugs or supplements that interfere with blood clotting and may increase the risk of bleeding. These include:

QUESTIONS TO ASK YOUR DOCTOR

- Will any of my drugs or over-the-counter remedies interact with obinutuzumab?
- What side effects can I expect from obinutuzumab?
- What reactions require emergency medical attention?

- nonsteroidal anti-inflammatory drugs (NSAIDs), such as aspirin, ibuprofen (Advil, Motrin), naproxen (Aleve), and many others, including many cold, flu, fever, and headache remedies that contain aspirin or ibuprofen
- warfarin (Coumadin), dabigatran (Pradaxa), rivaroxaban (Xarelto), apixaban (Eliquis), or other blood thinners, including any type of heparin injections
- anti-platelet drugs, such as clopidogrel (Plavix) or prasugrel (Effient)
- vitamin E

Resources

PERIODICALS

Goede, Valentin, et al. "Obinutuzumab plus Chlorambucil in Patients with CLL and Coexisting Conditions." *New England Journal of Medicine* 370, no. 12 (March 20, 2014): 1101–10.

Rai, Kanti R., and Jacqueline C. Barrientos. "Movement Toward Optimization of CLL Therapy." *New England Journal of Medicine* 370, no. 12 (March 20, 2014): 1160–2.

OTHER

Genentech. "Full Prescribing Information." Food and Drug Administration. November 2013. http://www.accessdata. fda.gov/drugsatfda_docs/label/2013/125486s000lbl.pdf (accessed September 29, 2014).

WEBSITES

"Obinutuzumab." American Cancer Society. November 4, 2013. http://www.cancer.org/treatment/treatmentsandsi deeffects/guidetocancerdrugs/obinutuzumab (accessed September 27, 2014).

"Obinutuzumab." DrugBank. January 23, 2014. http://www. drugbank.ca/drugs/DB08935 (accessed September 29, 2014).

"Obinutuzumab." National Cancer Institute. September 18, 2014. http://www.cancer.gov/cancertopics/druginfo/obi nutuzumab (accessed September 27, 2014).

"Obinutuzumab Injection." MedlinePlus. March 15, 2014. http://www.nlm.nih.gov/medlineplus/druginfo/meds/ a614012.html (accessed September 27, 2014).

ORGANIZATIONS

American Cancer Society, 250 Williams Street NW, Atlanta, GA 30303, (800) 227-2345, http://www.cancer.org.

National Cancer Institute, 6116 Executive Boulevard, Suite 300, Bethesda, MD 20892-8322, (800) 4-CANCER (422-6237), http://www.cancer.gov.

U.S. Food and Drug Administration, 10903 New Hampshire Avenue, Silver Spring, MD 20993-0002, (888) INFO-FDA (463-6332), http://www.fda.gov.

Margaret Alic, PhD

Occupational exposures and cancer

Definition

Occupational exposures to various substances that may increase the risk of specific cancers can occur at indoor workplaces including factories, restaurants, or medical facilities, or outdoors in mines or on construction sites or farms. Although many such exposures have been documented, because cancers can take years to develop and new occupational chemicals and hazards are continually being introduced, additional occupational exposures may be identified in the future.

Description

Occupational exposures to known or suspected carcinogens do not mean that a worker will develop cancer. Occupational exposures are just one of many factors that may increase the risk of developing particular cancers. As well as the degree of occupational exposure to carcinogens, cancer risk depends on many other factors that may or may not interact with occupational exposures in cancer development. These factors include:

- personal characteristics such as age and sex
- genetic susceptibilities and family history
- diet and lifestyle habits, including lack of exercise, cigarette smoking, alcohol consumption, and obesity
- exposure to environmental carcinogens such as secondhand smoke or radon gas

In identifying occupational exposures, researchers often examine cancer clusters—unusual concentrations of particular cancers occurring in a group of workers, especially primary cancers (not metastases) that are uncommon in the general population. However, cancers from occupational exposures are usually not discovered

until many years after the initial exposure. Some cancers—such as cancers of the lung, bladder, nasal cavity and sinuses, and larynx—can be caused by a wide variety of occupational exposures. Other common cancers associated with occupational exposures include skin cancers, leukemia, **lymphoma**, soft-tissue sarcomas, and throat and liver cancers.

Specific cancers

LUNG CANCERS AND MESOTHELIOMA. Although smoking is the greatest risk factor for lung cancer, lung cancer is also associated with occupational exposures.

- Exposure to secondhand smoke that can cause lung cancer affects employees in smoke-filled environments such as bars, restaurants, casinos, bingo halls, and bowling alleys. Although indoor smoking has been extensively banned in the United States, cancers resulting from years of occupational exposure to secondhand smoke will continue to develop long into the future.

- Workers exposed to asbestos are seven times more likely than others to die from lung cancer. Asbestos workers who smoke are 50–90 times more likely to develop lung cancer. Asbestos also causes malignant mesothelioma, an incurable and fatal cancer of the lining of the lungs, chest, and abdomen. Mesothelioma may not be detected until as long as 45 years after exposure. Asbestos in insulation exists in schools, offices, factory buildings, and homes. Workers who remove asbestos from buildings must take special precautionary measures to avoid inhalation of asbestos fibers and wear special clothing to avoid bringing asbestos dust home on their clothing. Other occupational exposures to asbestos occur among construction workers, railroad workers, shipbuilders, and factory workers. Asbestos exposure can also lead to cancers of the larynx, esophagus, pancreas, kidney, and colon.

- Workers exposed to diesel fumes—such as railroad crews and truck drivers—may have a 40% greater risk of lung cancer. Diesel fumes contain carcinogens such as benzene, formaldehyde, and dioxins. Formaldehyde used as a disinfectant in hospitals, in carpet and furniture glues, and in embalming can also cause respiratory cancers.

- Exposure to fine silica particles increases risk for lung cancer. Silica occurs in sand, rock, and mineral ores and is used in sandblasting, masonry, tunnel construction, ceramics, laying of railroad track, soap and glass manufacturing, shipbuilding, and agriculture. It is estimated that 2.2 million workers in the United States are exposed to silica. This includes workers in the construction industry and those involved in the cutting, grinding, crushing, or drilling of concrete, masonry, tile, or rock. About 320,000 workers are exposed in industries such as brick, concrete, and pottery manufacturing and in foundries that use sand and sandblasting. Many more workers are being exposed to silica with the dramatic increase in hydraulic fracturing (fracking) of gas and oil wells.

- Metal workers and electroplaters are exposed to chromium, a risk factor for lung cancer.

- Painters, printers, and chemists are at increased risk for lung cancer from occupational exposures to various chemicals.

- Uranium and talc miners have increased lung cancer risk.

- Miners and workers who manufacture and apply pesticides are at risk for lung, skin, and liver cancers from arsenic exposure.

- Radon gas is a lung cancer risk factor among underground miners and workers in buildings with radon leaking from the underlying soil.

- Workers in shoe manufacturing may be at increased risk of lung cancer death from repeated exposure to low levels of organic solvents such as toluene.

- Petroleum workers and others exposed to soots, tars, and oils from coal and gas are at increased risk for lung, liver, and skin cancers.

- Occupational exposures to vinyl chloride, nickel chromates, mustard gas, chloromethyl ethers, beryllium, and various other materials increase the risk of lung cancer.

BLADDER CANCER. Bladder cancer from occupational exposures is most common in people who work with radiation or with dyes involving aromatic amines such as benzidine and naphthylamine, including factory workers and hair colorists. Chemical, dye, and rubber workers risk exposure to naphthylamine. More than 5,000 different chemicals are used in hair dyes, and some of these chemicals have been reported to be carcinogenic in animals. Epidemiologic studies have reported increased risk of bladder cancer among hairdressers and barbers. A working group of the International Agency for Research on Cancer reported in 2008 that some hair dye chemicals are likely human carcinogens. Exposure to leather dust in shoe manufacturing is a risk factor for bladder and nasal cancers. The risk of bladder cancer rises with age, and smoking further increases the risk significantly.

SKIN CANCER. Skin cancer is commonly caused by exposure to ultraviolet (UV) radiation from sunlight. Outdoor workers in occupations such as road and building construction, landscaping, and painting, and beach and boat workers are at greater risk, with the risk proportional to the degree of UV exposure. Exposures to coal tars, pitch, paraffin, certain oils, creosote, arsenic, and radium can also cause skin cancer.

LARYNGEAL CANCER. Cancer of the larynx can be caused by heavy exposure to wood dust, paint fumes, and asbestos. Exposure to certain chemicals in metalworking, petroleum, plastic, and textile industries increases the risk for laryngeal and hypopharyngeal cancers. Tobacco and heavy alcohol use can further increase risk for these cancers by as much as 100-fold.

LYMPHATIC AND HEMATOPOIETIC (BLOOD) CANCERS. Long-term exposure to herbicides and insecticides increases risk for leukemias and lymphomas in farmers and other agricultural workers as well as those involved in herbicide and insecticide production. Lymphatic and hematopoietic cancers can also be caused by occupational exposures to **benzene** and radiation. Petroleum, rubber, and chemical workers are at risk for benzene exposure. A study examining a possible association between perchloroethylene exposure in dry-cleaning workers and higher cancer death rates found instead a possible link between formaldehyde exposure and death from myeloid leukemia. Studies have also found a significantly increased risk of leukemia among oncology nurses.

OTHER CANCERS. Other cancers associated with occupational exposures include:

• Salivary gland cancer may be linked to exposure to nickel alloys, silica dust, and radioactive substances.

• Exposure to sawdust in furniture manufacturing can cause nasal cancer.

• Chemicals used in leather, pesticides, and some industrial solvents may increase the risk of a type of salivary gland cancer that occurs in the nose and sinuses.

• Pancreatic cancer appears to be associated with significant exposures to pesticides, certain dyes, and chemicals found in gasoline.

• Exposure to asbestos, cadmium, and organic solvents (especially trichloroethylene) appears to increase the risk of kidney cancer.

• Soft-tissue sarcomas can be caused by occupational exposure to radiation.

• Liver cancer can be caused by exposure to vinyl chloride in workers involved in its manufacture and in rubber workers.

• Cancer of the lip can be caused by exposure to sunlight.

• Respiratory and urinary tract cancers can be caused by exposure to polycyclic aromatic hydrocarbons (PAHs).

• The National Institute for Occupational Safety and Health (NIOSH) is studying several hazardous workplace substances to determine if they are linked to breast and/or cervical cancers.

Occupations

Farmers appear to be at increased risk for **prostate cancer**, leukemias, and **non-Hodgkin lymphoma**. Farming communities also have higher rates of **multiple myeloma**, soft-tissue sarcomas, and cancers of the skin, lip, stomach, and brain. Since 1993, the **National Cancer Institute**, the National Institute of Environmental Health Sciences, and the Environmental Protection Agency have been investigating relationships between agricultural exposures and cancer as part of the Agricultural Health Study. The NIOSH joined the study in 2000. Exposures to **pesticides**, fertilizers, engine exhausts from farm equipment, chemical solvents, dusts, fuels, animal viruses, and certain other microbes are being examined for potential associations with elevated cancer rates among farm workers and their families.

Various other occupations have been associated with cancers.

• There may be a link between exposure of garment workers to formaldehyde and death from certain types of cancer.

• Workers in aluminum production and iron and steel founding are exposed to carcinogens.

• Dioxins may be a causative factor in a variety of cancers. Dioxins are byproducts of industrial processes utilizing chlorine and hydrocarbons, including incineration and pulp and paper manufacturing.

• Human and veterinary healthcare professionals may handle a variety of carcinogenic chemicals, including chemotherapy and antiviral drugs and hormones. Healthcare workers are also at risk for exposures to body fluids contaminated with hepatitis B and C viruses, which are major causes of liver cancer, and HIV, which causes AIDS and increases the risk of a variety of malignant tumors.

• Both industrial and medical workers may be at exposure risk from radioactive materials or x-ray equipment.

Demographics

Millions of workers in the United States are exposed to substances that have been shown to be carcinogenic in animals, and less than 2% of manufactured or processed chemicals have even been tested for carcinogenicity. An estimated 4%–10% of all cancers in the United States—48,000 cases annually—are caused by occupational exposures. In the United States and other developed countries, workplace regulations have significantly reduced occupational exposures to **carcinogens** in recent decades. However, due to the length of time that may pass between exposure and cancer development, cancer-causing exposures that occurred long ago are only now being recognized. Workplace accidents and safety breaches, as well as exposures to unrecognized hazards, continue to present **cancer** risks. Further, occupational exposures to carcinogens are a major problem in many developing countries, which may have few regulations and even less enforcement.

Causes

Common carcinogens in the workplace include:

• asbestos dust
• benzene
• chromium
• dioxins
• formaldehyde
• nickel compounds
• polychlorinated biphenyls (PCBs)
• secondhand smoke
• some paints and paint solvents
• silica dust
• vinyl chloride
• wood and leather dust

Diagnosis

Symptoms and diagnosis for cancers associated with occupational exposures are generally the same as for the same cancers associated with other causes. However, if occupational exposures are suspected as contributing to symptoms, patients should explain to their healthcare providers their types of jobs and substances they were exposed to in the workplace. They should bring all Material Safety Data Sheets (MSDSs) and other workplace exposure information to appointments. Workers can request further exposure information from their safety officer or human resources manager. Patients may be referred to an occupational medicine specialist or a pulmonary medicine specialist if an occupational lung disease is suspected.

Treatment

Treatments and prognosis will be generally the same as for the same cancers due to other causes and will depend on the type and stage of the cancer and the patient's age.

Prevention

Virtually all occupational exposures are preventable, although workers who learned their trade prior to the establishment of safety measures sometimes find it difficult to change their habits.

QUESTIONS TO ASK YOUR DOCTOR

- Am I likely to have occupational exposures to carcinogens?
- What cancers am I at risk for from my occupation?
- Are my family members at risk for cancer from my occupation?
- How can I protect myself from occupational exposures?
- How can I protect my family from carcinogens that I may bring home from my workplace?

• Workers should ensure that they are not exposed to harmful levels of any substances.

• MSDSs and postings of hazards should warn workers of all possible exposures.

• Workers should be trained in avoiding and preventing occupational exposures.

• Workers should personally ensure that they are not exposed to potentially harmful levels of any substance.

• Exhaust and ventilation systems should be operational.

• Proper procedures should be followed and protective equipment used if necessary.

• If necessary, workers should wear respirators or face masks and protective clothing.

• Cigarette smoke should be avoided.

• Outdoor workers should use sunscreen and wear protective clothing, including long sleeves and pants and wide-brimmed hats.

• Workers at risk for bladder cancer from occupational exposures should drink at least 11 cups (2.6 L) of fluid daily to increase urination and reduce the concentration of carcinogens in the body and the amount of time that carcinogens are in contact with the bladder lining.

Special concerns

Workers' Compensation may pay for medical care and lost income attributed to cancers caused by occupational exposures. Unsafe working conditions should be reported to the Occupational Safety and Health Administration (OSHA). However, it is often very difficult to prove that workplace exposure was a causal factor in the development of a cancer. This can make it harder to obtain work-related compensation and benefits, so financial concerns may be a great burden.

Secondhand exposure of family members to carcinogens brought home from a workplace are of special concern. Fine, carcinogenic dust particles can adhere to workers' clothing, shoes, skin, hair, facial hair, tools, or lunch boxes, as well as the inside and outside of their cars.

Different stresses may affect people with occupation-related cancers, including the possibility that they may have to change jobs or find a new occupation. In addition to the stress of cancer diagnosis and treatment, workers may be disabled and unable to work or may require job retraining. Older workers may be even less employable after surviving cancer. Thus, complementary therapies such as meditation, guided imagery, therapeutic touch, yoga, and t'ai chi may be especially useful.

See also Environmental factors in cancer development.

Resources

BOOKS

Murff, Samuel J. *Safety and Health Handbook for Cytotoxic Drugs*. Lanham, MD: Government Institutes, 2012.

PERIODICALS

Rota, Matteo, et al. "Occupational Exposures to Polycyclic Aromatic Hydrocarbons and Respiratory and Urinary Tract Cancers: An Updated Systematic Review and a Meta-Analysis to 2014." *Archives of Toxicology* 88, no. 8 (August 2014): 1479–90.

OTHER

American Cancer Society. "Occupation and Cancer." http://www.cancer.org/acs/groups/content/@nho/documents/document/occupationandcancerpdf.pdf (accessed August 19, 2014).

WEBSITES

American Cancer Society. "Review Calls for Increased Attention to Cancer Risk from Silica." December 10, 2013. http://pressroom.cancer.org/silica (accessed August 19, 2014).
National Cancer Institute. "Agricultural Health Study." http://www.cancer.gov/cancertopics/factsheet/Risk/ahs (accessed August 19, 2014).
National Institute for Occupational Safety and Health. "Occupational Cancer." Workplace Safety & Health Topics, Centers for Disease Control and Prevention. http://www.cdc.gov/niosh/topics/cancer (accessed August 20, 2014).
National Institute for Occupational Safety and Health. "Women's Safety and Health Issues at Work." Workplace Safety & Health Topics, Centers for Disease Control and Prevention. http://www.cdc.gov/niosh/topics/women/cancer.html (accessed August 20, 2014).
Occupational Safety & Health Administration. "Carcinogens." https://www.osha.gov/SLTC/carcinogens (accessed August 19, 2014).

ORGANIZATIONS

American Cancer Society, 250 Williams Street NW, Atlanta, GA 30303, (800) 227-2345, http://www.cancer.org.
International Agency for Research on Cancer, 150 Cours Albert Thomas, 69372 Lyon CEDEX 08, France, 33 (0)4 72 73 84 85, Fax: 33 (0)4 72 73 85 75, http://www.iarc.fr.
National Cancer Institute, 6116 Executive Boulevard, Suite 300, Bethesda, MD 20892-8322, (800) 4-CANCER (422-6237), http://www.cancer.gov.
National Institute for Occupational Safety and Health, U.S. Centers for Disease Control and Prevention, 1600 Clifton Road, Atlanta, GA 30333, (800) CDC-INFO (232-4636), cdcinfo@cdc.gov, http://www.cdc.gov.
Occupational Safety & Health Administration, U.S. Department of Labor, 200 Constitution Avenue NW, Washington, DC 20210, (800) 321-OSHA (6742), https://www.osha.gov.

Esther Csapo Rastegari, RN, BSN, EdM
REVISED BY MARGARET ALIC, PHD
REVIEWED BY MELINDA GRANGER OBERLEITNER, RN, DNS, APRN, CNS

Octamide *see* **Metoclopramide**
Octreotide *see* **Antidiarrheal agents**

Ofatumumab

Definition

Ofatumumab (Arzerra) is used to treat **chronic lymphocytic leukemia** (CLL), a **cancer** of white blood cells. It is in a class of medications known as **monoclonal antibodies**.

Purpose

Ofatumumab injection was granted accelerated approval in 2009 by the U.S. Food and Drug Administration (FDA) for the treatment of CLL in adults who are have not improved or are no longer responding to **chemotherapy** with **fludarabine** (Fludara) and the monoclonal antibody **alemtuzumab** (Campath). Ofatumumab was approved by the FDA in 2014 for use with **chlorambucil** to treat CLL that has never been treated, in patients for whom fludarabine-based chemotherapy is not appropriate for reasons such as advanced age or coexisting medical conditions. Approval was based on the results of a clinical trial that compared ofatumumab in combination with chlorambucil to chlorambucil alone. The median progression-free survival (PFS)—the length of time that patients survived without their disease worsening—was 22.4 months in the group receiving the combination treatment, compared with 13.1 months in the group receiving chlorambucil alone.

In 2014, ofatumumab failed to demonstrate effectiveness in a phase III clinical trial for treating bulky CLL that does not respond to fludarabine. Ofatumumab was compared to doctors' choices of other therapies. The median PFS with ofatumumab was 5.36 months, compared with 3.61 months for the other therapies. Ofatumumab is being studied for the treatment of other types of cancer and as well as other conditions.

Description

CLL is a disease of immune-system white blood cells, especially B lymphocytes or B cells in the blood and bone marrow. Approximately one-third of adult leukemias are CLL. About 16,000 people are diagnosed with CLL each year in the United States, and about 4,400 die of the disease. CLL usually affects people over age 50, and the majority of patients have at least one other medical condition, such as high blood pressure, diabetes, or cardiovascular disease.

Ofatumumab specifically targets a protein called the CD20 receptor. CD20 is present on the surface of more than 90% of both normal and cancerous B cells but not on other types of cells. When ofatumumab binds to CD20 on B cells that have an overabundance of the protein on their surfaces, the cells become susceptible to attack by the patient's immune system.

Ofatumumab and other monoclonal antibodies are produced by injecting animals, usually mice, with the purified target protein—CD20 in the case of ofatumumab. The animals produce many different antibodies against the target, and the one that binds best to the target and not to other proteins is chosen to be cloned. Monoclonal antibodies are "humanized" by replacing the mouse portions of the antibody molecule with the corresponding portions of human antibodies; thus, the human immune system does not recognize and destroy the drug as "foreign."

U.S. brand names

Ofatumumab is made by GlaxoSmithKline and marketed as Arzerra. It was originally granted accelerated FDA approval in 2009 because it treated CLL at a stage for which there were no other treatments. In 2013, the FDA ordered changes to the prescribing directions to warn of the risk of reactivating latent infections of hepatitis B virus (HBV).

Canadian brand names

Ofatumumab was approved by Health Canada in 2012 under the brand name Arzerra.

International brand names

Ofatumumab was approved by the European Medicines Agency in 2010 under the brand name Arzerra. It

---

---

is also approved for first-line use in Russia. Arzerra is also known as HuMax-CD20.

Recommended dosage

Ofatumumab is a liquid that is added to fluid and is given by infusion into a vein (IV) by a doctor or nurse in a medical office or hospital. For refractory (unresponsive to chemotherapy) CLL, ofatumumab is usually given in 12 doses, with the first eight doses once per week and the last four doses once every four weeks, for a total treatment time of six months. The first dose is 300 milligrams (mg), and subsequent doses are each 2,000 mg. For previously untreated CLL, the recommended dose is 300 mg on Day 1, followed by 1,000 mg on Day 8 (Cycle 1), and then 1,000 mg every 28 days (a 28-day cycle) for at least three cycles until achieving the best response or for a maximum of 12 cycles.

Thirty minutes to two hours before each infusion, patients are given medications, including acetaminophen (Tylenol) by mouth or IV, an antihistamine, and an IV corticosteroid to help reduce the risk of infusion reactions. The first two infusions are given very slowly over about six hours to monitor the patient for reactions. If there are no problems, later infusions are given over about three hours. The treatment may be interrupted if problems develop.

Precautions

Ofatumumab has a "boxed warning" concerning the dangers of reactivated HBV infection and progressive multifocal **leukoencephalopathy** (PML). People can be infected with HBV but have no symptoms. Because ofatumumab suppresses the immune system, a previous HBV infection could be reactivated and become serious or life threatening. Patients are given blood tests for inactive HBV infection before treatment with ofatumumab and, if necessary, HBV can be treated before and during ofatumumab treatment. However, if HBV is reactivated, ofatumumab treatment must be postponed. Reactivation also can occur up to a year or possibly longer after treatment with ofatumumab is ended, so patients are monitored for signs of infection during and for several months after treatment. PML is a rare brain infection for which there is no prevention, treatment, or cure; it usually results in severe disability or death. Some people have developed PML during or after treatment with ofatumumab.

Ofatumumab sometimes causes allergic reactions, especially with the first two treatments. Mild reactions are usually **fever** and chills. Serious reactions are rare but may be dangerous. Symptoms of serious reactions include:

- lightheadedness or dizziness from low blood pressure
- fainting
- headache
- flushing or warmth
- itching
- hives
- shortness of breath
- heart rate changes
- back or abdominal pain
- swelling of the face, tongue, or throat

There are other precautions:

- Ofatumumab can cause tumor lysis syndrome from the rapid killing of large numbers of cancer cells, especially during the first treatment cycle. As the cells die, they release their contents, overwhelming the bloodstream and possibly leading to kidney failure.
- Blood tests will probably be performed throughout treatment to monitor effects on blood counts and bodily organs.
- Ofatumumab can lower white blood cell counts in the weeks after administration and can also have other effects on the immune system, increasing the risk of infection.
- Ofatumumab can lower platelet counts, which may increase the risk of bleeding.
- Patients should not have any immunizations during or after ofatumumab treatment without their doctor's approval, since the drug may make vaccines less effective or lead to serious infection. Patients should try to avoid contact with anyone who has recently received a live virus vaccine, such as oral polio or nasal-spray flu vaccines.
- Rarely, ofatumumab can cause intestinal blockage.
- Doctors should be informed of ofatumumab administration before patients have any type of surgery, including dental surgery.
- It is not known whether ofatumumab affects fertility.

Pediatric

The safety and effectiveness of ofatumumab has not been established in pediatric patients.

Geriatric

In the ofatumumab/chlorambucil combination trial, 68% of patients were 65 or older. They experienced more serious adverse reactions than younger patients, but there were no observable differences in effectiveness. The trial for refractory CLL did not include enough older patients to determine whether they responded differently than younger patients.

Pregnant or breastfeeding

It is not known whether ofatumumab treatment of either a male or female partner causes problems to a fetus at the time of conception or during pregnancy. Ofatumumab should be used during pregnancy only if the potential benefit to the mother outweighs the potential risk to the fetus. It is not known whether ofatumumab is secreted in breast milk, so caution should be exercised in administering it to nursing mothers.

Other conditions and allergies

Trials of ofatumumab were carried out in patients with multiple other medical conditions. Patients should tell their doctors if they:

- are allergic to anything, including medicines, dyes, additives, or foods
- have ever tested positive for HBV
- have any other medical conditions, including kidney, liver, or heart disease; congestive heart failure; breathing problems; diabetes; gout; or infections
- have or have ever had chronic obstructive pulmonary disease

Side effects

Overall, 67% of clinical-trial patients who received ofatumumab experienced one or more symptoms of infusion reaction, and 10% experienced serious reactions. The most common side effects of ofatumumab are:

- mild allergic reactions
- fever
- diarrhea
- nausea
- rash
- fatigue
- shortness of breath
- lowered red blood cell count (anemia)
- lowered white blood cell count with increased risk of infections
- bronchitis, pneumonia, and upper respiratory tract infections

Side effects occurring in at least 5% of patients in the ofatumumab/clorambucil combination trial were:

- infusion reactions
- weakness and fatigue
- headache
- joint pain
- upper abdominal pain
- low white blood cell counts
- respiratory-tract infection
- herpes simplex virus infection

Less common side effects of ofatumumab are:

- allergic reactions with the third or later infusions
- trouble sleeping
- headache
- chills
- swelling in the hands or feet
- cough
- back pain
- changes in blood pressure
- rapid heart rate

- other types of infections

Rare side effects are:

- serious allergic reactions
- lowered platelet count with increased risk of bleeding
- HBV reactivation
- tumor lysis syndrome
- intestinal blockage (obstruction)
- PML
- death due to liver failure, brain infection, or other serious infections

Interactions

Although no serious interactions of ofatumumab with other drugs or foods were known as of 2014, patients should inform their doctors about any prescription or over-the-counter medications, supplements, **vitamins**, and herbs that they are taking. In particular, patients should talk to their doctors before taking any drugs or supplements that could increase the risk of bleeding, including aspirin or aspirin-containing medicines, **warfarin** (Coumadin), or vitamin E.

Resources

BOOKS

Gupta, Ira V., and Roxanne C. Jewell. "Ofatumumab, the First Human Anti-CD20 Monoclonal Antibody for the Treatment of B Cell Hematologic Malignancies." In *Pharmaceutical Science to Improve the Human Condition: Prix Galien 2011*, edited by *Annals of the New York Academy of Sciences* Editorial Office. Malden, MA: Wiley, 2012.

PERIODICALS

Byrd, John C., et al. "Ibrutinib versus Ofatumumab in Previously Treated Chronic Lymphoid Leukemia." *New England Journal of Medicine* 371, no. 3 (July 17, 2014): 213–23.

OTHER

GSK. "Full Prescribing Information." U.S. Food and Drug Administration. http://www.accessdata.fda.gov/drugsatf-da_docs/label/2013/125326s059lbl.pdf (accessed October 20, 2014).

WEBSITES

American Cancer Society. "Ofatumumab." http://www.cancer.org/treatment/treatmentsandsideeffects/guidetocancer-drugs/ofatumumab (accessed September 27, 2014).

National Cancer Institute. "Ofatumumab." http://www.cancer.gov/cancertopics/druginfo/ofatumumab (accessed September 27, 2014).

"Ofatumumab Injection." MedlinePlus. http://www.nlm.nih.gov/medlineplus/druginfo/meds/a610009.html (accessed September 27, 2014).

ORGANIZATIONS

American Cancer Society, 250 Williams Street NW, Atlanta, GA 30303, (800) 227-2345, http://www.cancer.org.

National Cancer Institute, 6116 Executive Boulevard, Suite 300, Bethesda, MD 20892-8322, (800) 4-CANCER (422-6237), http://www.cancer.gov.

U.S. Food and Drug Administration, 10903 New Hampshire Avenue, Silver Spring, MD 20993-0002, (888) INFO-FDA (463-6332), http://www.fda.gov.

Margaret Alic, PhD

Oligodendroglioma

Definition

Oligodendrogliomas are a rare form of **brain tumors**. The brain is made up of many supporting cells that are called glial cells. Any tumor of these glial cells is called a glioma. Oligodendrogliomas are tumors that arise from a type of glial cell called oligodendrocytes. These cells are the specialized cells of the brain that produce the fatty covering of nerve cells (myelin).

Description

Oligodendrogliomas can grow in different parts of the brain, but they are most commonly found in the frontal or temporal lobes of the cerebrum. The frontal lobes are responsible for cognitive thought processes (knowing, thinking, learning, and judging). The temporal lobes are responsible for coordination, speech, hearing, memory, and awareness of time.

There are two types of oligodendroglioma: the well-differentiated tumor, which grows relatively slowly and in a defined shape; and the anaplastic oligodendroglioma,

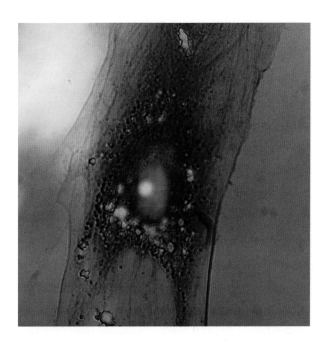

Malignant oligodendroglioma cells from the human brain. *(CECIL FOX/Science Source)*

which grows much more rapidly and does not have a well-defined shape. Anaplastic oligodendrogliomas are much less common than well-differentiated oligodendrogliomas.

More common than either form of pure oligodendroglioma is the mixed glioma, or oligoastrocytoma. These mixed gliomas are a mixture of oligodendroglioma and **astrocytoma**. An astrocytoma is a tumor that arises from the astrocytes, specialized cells in the brain that regulate the chemical environment of the brain and help to form the blood-brain barrier.

Oligodendrogliomas and mixed gliomas account for approximately 4%–5% of all primary brain tumors and 10% of all gliomas. A primary brain tumor is a tumor that begins in the brain, as opposed to a secondary (or metastatic) brain tumor, which originates in another organ and spreads (metastasizes) to the brain.

Demographics

Oligodendrogliomas occur in approximately nine in every one million people. Oligodendrogliomas can occur in people of any age, but most occur in middle-aged adults.

Oligodendrogliomas occur with equal frequency in members of all races and ethnic groups. There does not appear to be any relation of oligodendrogliomas to any geographic region. For unknown reasons, men are affected by oligodendrogliomas in higher numbers than women.

KEY TERMS

Anaplastic oligodendroglioma—A form of oligodendroglioma that does not have a well-defined shape and grows very rapidly and aggressively.

Astrocytoma—A type of brain tumor that arises from the astrocytes, specialized brain cells that regulate the chemical environment of the brain and form the blood-brain barrier. These types of tumors are often mixed with oligodendrogliomas to form oligoastrocytomas.

Frontal lobes—The two lobes of the cerebrum of the brain that are responsible for cognitive thought processes (knowing, thinking, learning, and judging).

Glioma—Any tumor that arises from the supporting cells in the brain called glial cells.

Intracranial hypertension—A higher-than-normal pressure of the fluid in the skull.

Oligoastrocytoma—A type of brain tumor that is a mixture of oligodendroglioma and astrocytoma. This is also called a mixed glioma.

Spinal fluid shunt—A small tube that is surgically implanted to allow excess spinal fluid to drain directly into the abdominal cavity.

Temporal lobes—The two lobes of the cerebrum of the brain that are responsible for coordination, speech, hearing, memory, and awareness of time.

Well-differentiated tumor—A tumor that grows relatively slowly and in a well-defined shape.

Causes and symptoms

The cause, or causes, of oligodendrogliomas are not known; however, most people with these types of tumors have some type of genetic mutation on chromosome 1, chromosome 19, or on both chromosomes 1 and 19. Investigations are ongoing in an attempt to determine if these genetic factors, or other factors, cause oligodendrogliomas. Oligodendrogliomas are not contagious.

The symptoms of oligodendrogliomas are the result of increased pressure in the fluid within the skull (intracranial hypertension). These symptoms include:

• nausea

• vomiting

• irritability

• headache

• vision disturbances

• enlargement of the head

• seizures

Oligodendrogliomas may also be accompanied by a weakness or paralysis on the side of the body opposite to the side of the brain where the tumor is located. When the tumor is located in a frontal lobe, the patient may experience gradual changes in mood and personality. When it is located in a temporal lobe, the patient may experience difficulty with speech, hearing, coordination, and memory.

Diagnosis

The diagnosis of oligodendrogliomas begins in the doctor's office with a basic neurological examination. This examination involves:

• testing eye reflexes, eye movement, and pupil reactions

• testing hearing with a tuning fork or ticking watch

• reflex tests with a rubber hammer

• balance and coordination tests

• pin-prick and cotton ball tests for sense of touch

• sense of smell tests with various odors

• facial muscle tests (e.g., smiling, frowning, etc.)

• tongue movement and gag reflex tests

• head movement tests

• mental status tests (e.g., asking what year it is, who the president is, etc.)

• abstract thinking tests (e.g., asking for the meaning of a common saying, such as "every cloud has a silver lining")

• memory tests (e.g., asking to have a list of objects repeated, asking for details of what a patient ate for dinner last night, etc.)

If the doctor suspects a brain tumor may be present, further diagnostic tests will be ordered. These tests are performed by a neurological specialist. Imaging tests that may be ordered include **computed tomography** (CT) and **magnetic resonance imaging** (MRI). Other tests may include a spinal tap, to examine the cerebrospinal fluid, and an electroencephalogram (EEG), which measures the electrical activity of the brain.

Treatment team

Treatment of any primary brain tumor, including oligodendrogliomas, is different from treating tumors in other parts of the body. Brain surgery requires much more precision than most other surgeries. Also, many medicinal drugs cannot cross the blood-brain barrier. Therefore, the therapies that are used to treat oligodendrogliomas, and the side effects of these therapies, are quite complex.

The most up-to-date treatment opportunities are available from experienced, multi-disciplinary medical professional teams made up of doctors, nurses, and technologists who specialize in **cancer** (oncology), neurology, medical imaging, drug or **radiation therapy**, and anesthesiology.

Clinical staging

Oligodendrogliomas and other primary brain tumors are diagnosed, or staged, in grades of severity from I to IV. Grade I tumors have cells that are not malignant and are nearly normal in appearance. Grade II tumors have cells that appear to be slightly abnormal. Grade III tumors have cells that are malignant and clearly abnormal. Grade IV, the most severe type of brain tumors, contain fast-spreading and abnormal cells. Well-defined oligodendrogliomas are generally stage I or stage II tumors. Anaplastic oligodendrogliomas are generally stage III or stage IV tumors.

Treatment

The standard treatment for all grades of oligodendrogliomas is surgery to remove the tumor completely. This surgery is generally aided by an image guidance system that allows the surgeon to determine the most efficient route to location of the tumor. Approximately half of oligodendroglioma patients gain relief of the increased intracranial pressure after complete removal of their tumors. The other half require a spinal fluid shunt to allow drainage of the excess fluid.

In some instances of oligodendroglioma, the tumor is inoperable or cannot be completely removed. Patients with inoperable oligodendrogliomas are generally treated with radiation therapies. Oligodendrogliomas are among the only brain tumors that can be successfully treated with a type of **chemotherapy** called PCV (**Procarbazine**, CCNU or **lomustine**, and **Vincristine**). Chemotherapy is usually used only in cases of recurrent anaplastic oligodendrogliomas.

Alternative and complementary therapies

There are no effective alternative treatments for oligodendrogliomas.

Prognosis

For patients with well-defined oligodendrogliomas, median survival exceeds 10 years. For patients with anaplastic oligodendrogliomas, median survival ranges from two to five years.

QUESTIONS TO ASK YOUR DOCTOR

- Which type of oligodendroglioma do I have?
- Is my tumor operable?
- What is the likelihood of my type of oligodendroglioma coming back?
- How often should I seek follow-up examinations?

Coping with cancer treatment

Most patients who undergo brain surgery to remove their tumors can resume their normal activities within a few days of the operation.

Clinical trials

There were 48 **clinical trials** underway in 2014 aimed at the treatment of oligodendrogliomas. More information on these trials, including contact information, may be found by conducting a clinical trial search at the website of the **National Cancer Institute**: http://www.cancer.gov/clinicaltrials/search.

Prevention

Because the cause or causes of oligodendrogliomas are not known, there are no known preventions.

Special concerns

Repeat surgery may be necessary for oligodendrogliomas because these tumors sometimes redevelop. Careful monitoring by the medical team will be required. Also, if the tumor is located in the dominant hemisphere of the patient's brain, any treatment, especially surgery, requires special consideration and care not to disrupt the personality or other higher brain functions of the patient.

See also Brain and central nervous system tumors.

Resources

BOOKS

Hayat, M.A. *Tumors of the Central Nervous System, Volume 8: Astrocytoma, Medulloblastoma, Retinoblastoma, Chordoma, Craniopharyngioma, Oligodendroglioma, and Ependymoma.* New York: Springer, 2012.

WEBSITES

Cancer Research UK. "Oligodendroglioma." http://www.cancerresearchuk.org/about-cancer/type/brain-tumour/treatment/types/treatment-for-oligodendroglioma (accessed November 8, 2014).

Dana-Farber Cancer Institute. "Oligodendroglioma." http://www.dana-farber.org/Adult-Care/Treatment-and-Support/Oligodendroglioma.aspx (accessed November 8, 2014).

ORGANIZATIONS

American Brain Tumor Association, 8550 W. Bryn Mawr Ave., Ste. 550, Chicago, IL 60631, (773) 577-8750, (800) 886-2282, Fax: (773) 577-8738, info@abta.org, http://www.abta.org.

National Brain Tumor Society, 55 Chapel St., Ste. 200, Newton, MA 02458, (617) 924-9997, http://www.braintumor.org.

Paul A. Johnson, EdM

Omega-3 fatty acids

Definition

Essential to human health, omega-3 fatty acids are a form of polyunsaturated fats that are not made by the body and must be obtained from a person's food.

Purpose

Eating foods rich in omega-3 fatty acids is part of a healthy diet and helps people maintain their health.

Description

In recent years, a great deal of attention has been placed on the value of eating a low-fat diet. In some cases, people have taken this advice to the extreme by adopting a diet that is far too low in fat or, worse yet, a diet that has no fat at all. But the truth is that not all fat is bad. Although it is true that trans and saturated fats, which are found in high amounts in red meat, butter, whole milk, and some prepackaged foods, have been shown to raise a person's total cholesterol, polyunsaturated fats can actually play a part in keeping cholesterol low. Two especially good fats are the omega-3 fatty acids and the omega-6 fatty acids, which are polyunsaturated.

Two types of omega-3 fatty acids are eicosapentaenoic acid (EPA) and docosahexaenoic acid (DHA), which are found mainly in oily cold-water fish, such as tuna, salmon, trout, herring, sardines, bass, swordfish, and mackerel. With the exception of seaweed, most plants do not contain EPA or DHA. However, alpha-linolenic acid (ALA), which is another kind of omega-3 fatty acid, is found in dark green leafy vegetables, flaxseed oil, fish oil, and canola oil, as well as nuts and beans such as walnuts and soybeans. Enzymes in a person's body can convert ALA to EPA and DHA, which are the two kinds of omega-3 fatty acids easily utilized by the body.

Many experts agree that it is important to maintain a healthy balance between omega-3 fatty acids and omega-6 fatty acids. As Dr. Penny Kris-Etherton and her colleagues reported in their article published in the *American Journal of Nutrition*, an overconsumption of omega-6 fatty acids has resulted in an unhealthy dietary shift in the American diet. The authors point out that what used to be a 1:1 ratio between omega-3 and omega-6 fatty acids is now estimated to be a 10:1 ratio. This poses a problem, researchers say, because some of the beneficial effects gained from omega-3 fatty acids are negated by an overconsumption of omega-6 fatty acids. For example, omega-3 fatty acids have anti-inflammatory properties, whereas omega-6 fatty acids tend to promote inflammation. Cereals, whole grain bread, margarine, and vegetable oils such as corn, peanut, and sunflower oil are examples of omega-6 fatty acids. In addition, people consume a lot of omega-6 fatty acid simply by eating the meat of animals that were fed grain rich in omega-6. Some experts suggest that eating one to four times more omega-6 fatty acids than omega-3 fatty acids is a reasonable ratio. In other words, as dietitians often say, the key to a healthy diet is moderation and balance.

The health benefits of omega-3 fatty acids

There is strong evidence that omega-3 fatty acids protect a person against atherosclerosis and therefore against heart disease and stroke, as well as abnormal heart rhythms that cause sudden cardiac death, and possibly autoimmune disorders, such as lupus and rheumatoid arthritis. Drs. Dean Ornish and Mehmet Oz, renowned heart physicians, said in a 2002 article published in *O Magazine* that the benefits derived from consuming the proper daily dose of omega-3 fatty acids may help to reduce sudden cardiac death by as much as 50%. In an article published by *American Family Physician*, Dr. Maggie Covington, a clinical assistant professor at the University of Maryland, also emphasized the value of omega-3 fatty acids with regard to cardiovascular health and referred to one of the largest **clinical trials** to date, the GISSI-Prevenzione Trial, to illustrate her point. In the study, 11,324 patients with coronary heart disease were divided into four groups: one group received 300 mg of vitamin E, one group received 850 mg of omega-3 fatty acids, one group received the vitamin E and fatty acids, and one group served as the control group. After a little more than three years, "The group given omega-3 fatty acids only had a 45% reduction in sudden death and a 20% reduction in all-cause mortality," as stated by Dr. Covington.

According to the American Heart Association (AHA), the ways in which omega-3 fatty acids may reduce cardiovascular disease are still being studied. However, the AHA indicates that research has shown that omega-3 fatty acids:

- decrease the risk of arrhythmias, which can lead to sudden cardiac death
- decrease triglyceride levels
- decrease the growth rate of atherosclerotic plaque
- lower blood pressure slightly

In fact, numerous studies show that a diet rich in omega-3 fatty acids not only lowers bad cholesterol, known as LDL, but also lowers triglycerides, the fatty material that circulates in the blood. Interestingly, researchers have found that the cholesterol levels of Inuit Eskimos tend to be quite good, despite the fact that they have a high-fat diet. The reason for this, research has found, is that their diet is high in fatty fish, which is loaded with omega-3 fatty acids. The same has often been said about the typical Mediterranean-style diet.

Said to reduce joint inflammation, omega-3 fatty acid supplements have been the focus of many studies attempting to validate its effectiveness in treating rheumatoid arthritis. According to a large body of research in the area, omega-3 fatty acid supplements are clearly effective in reducing the symptoms associated with rheumatoid arthritis, such as joint tenderness and stiffness. In some cases, a reduction in the amount of medication needed by rheumatoid arthritis patients has been noted.

More research needs to be done to substantiate the effectiveness of omega-3 fatty acids in treating eating disorders, attention deficit disorder, and **depression**. Some studies have indicated, for example, that children with behavioral problems and attention deficit disorder have lower than normal amounts of omega-3 fatty acids in their bodies. However, until there is more data in these very important areas of research, a conservative approach should be taken, especially when making changes to a child's diet. Parents should talk to their child's pediatrician to ascertain if adding more omega-3 fatty acids to their child's diet is appropriate. In addition, parents should take special care to avoid feeding their children fish high in mercury. A food list containing items rich in omega-3 fatty acids can be obtained from a licensed dietitian.

A great deal of media attention has been focused on the high mercury levels found in some types of fish. People concerned about fish consumption and mercury levels can review public releases on the subject issued by the U.S. Food and Drug Administration (FDA) and the Environmental Protection Agency. Special precautions exist for children and pregnant or breastfeeding women. They are advised to avoid shark, mackerel, swordfish, and tilefish. However, both the U.S. Food and Drug Administration and the Environmental Protection Agency emphasize the importance of dietary fish. Fish, they caution, should not be eliminated from the diet. Dr. Robert Oh stated in his 2005 article, which was published in *The Journal of the American Board of Family Practice*: "With the potential health benefits of fish, women of childbearing age should be encouraged to eat one to two low-mercury fish meals per week."

Mercury levels and concerns about safety

Other concerns regarding fish safety have also been reported. In 2004, Dr. Ronald A. Hites and his colleagues assessed organic contaminants in salmon in an article published in *Science*. Their conclusion that farmed salmon had higher concentrations of polychlorinated biphenyls than wild salmon prompted public concerns and a response from the American Cancer Society. Farmed fish in Europe was found to have higher levels of mercury than farmed salmon in North and South America; however, the American Cancer Society reminded the public that the "levels of toxins Hites and his colleagues found in the farmed salmon were still below what the U.S. Food and Drug Administration, which regulates food, considers hazardous." The American Cancer Society still continues to promote a healthy, varied diet, which includes fish as a food source.

Recommended dosage

The AHA recommends that people eat two servings of fish, such as tuna or salmon, at least twice a week. A person with coronary heart disease, according to the AHA, should consume 1 gram of omega-3 fatty acids daily through food intake, most preferably through the consumption of fatty fish. The AHA also states that "people with elevated triglycerides may need 2 to 4 grams of EPA and DHA per day provided as a supplement," which is available in liquid or capsule form. Ground or cracked flaxseed can easily be incorporated into a person's diet by sprinkling it over salads, soup, and cereal.

Sources differ, but here are some general examples:

- 3 ounces of pickled herring = 1.2 grams of omega-3 fatty acids
- 3 ounces of salmon = 1.3 grams of omega-3 fatty acids
- 3 ounces of halibut = 1.0 gram of omega-3 fatty acids
- 3 ounces of mackerel = 1.6 grams of omega-3 fatty acids
- 1 1/2 teaspoons of flaxseed = 3 grams of omega-3 fatty acids

Precautions

In early 2004, the U.S. Food and Drug Administration (FDA), along with the Environmental Protection Agency, issued a statement that women who are or may be pregnant, as well as breastfeeding mothers and children, should avoid eating some types of fish thought to contain high levels of mercury. Fish that typically contain high levels of mercury are shark, swordfish, and mackerel, whereas shrimp, canned light tuna, salmon, and catfish are generally thought to have low levels of mercury. Because many people engage in fishing as a hobby, women should be sure before they eat any fish caught by friends and family that the local stream or lake is considered low in mercury.

Conflicting information exists on whether it is safe for patients with macular degeneration to take omega-3 fatty acids in supplement form. Until more data becomes available, it is better for people with macular degeneration to receive their omega-3 fatty acids from the food they eat.

Side effects

Fish oil supplements can cause **diarrhea** and gas. Also, the fish oil capsules tend to have a fishy aftertaste.

Interactions

Although there are no significant drug interactions associated with eating foods containing omega-3 fatty acids, patients who are being treated with blood-thinning medications shouldn't take omega-3 fatty acid supplements without seeking the advice of their physicians. Excessive bleeding could result. For the same reason, some patients who plan to take more than 3 grams of omega-3 fatty acids in supplement form should first seek the approval of their physicians.

Resources

PERIODICALS

Laviano A., Rianda S., Molfino A., and Rossi Fanelli, F. "Omega-3 Fatty Acids in Cancer." *Current Opinion in Clinical Nutrition and Metabolic Care* 16, no. 2 (2013): 156–61. http://www.ncbi.nlm.nih.gov/pubmed/23299701 (accessed November 8, 2014).

Oh, R. "Practical applications of fish oil (omega-3 fatty acids) in primary." *The Journal of the American Board of Family Practice* 18 (2005): 28–36.

WEBSITES

American Cancer Society. "Omega-3 Fatty Acids." http://www.cancer.org/treatment/treatmentsandsideeffects/complementaryandalternativemedicine/dietandnutrition/omega-3-fatty-acids (accessed November 8, 2014).

Lee Ann Paradise

Ommaya reservoir

Definition

The Ommaya reservoir is a plastic, dome-shaped device, with a catheter (thin tubing) attached to the underside used to deliver **chemotherapy** (**anticancer drugs**) to the central nervous system (CNS or brain and spinal cord).

Purpose

Chemotherapy may be administered to patients by various methods, depending on the type of **cancer** being treated. Some cancer types respond well to chemotherapy given by intravenous (IV) injection, and some cancer types may be treated with oral medication. In both cases, the chemotherapy reaches its target site systemically (carried by the blood). Cancers that affect the CNS pose a special challenge. Systemically delivered drugs seldom reach the CNS because of a network of blood vessels that surround the brain. This protective shield is called the blood-brain barrier. It acts as a filtering device for the brain by blocking the passage of foreign substances from the blood to the CNS. To avoid the obstacle created by the blood-brain barrier, alternative delivery treatments must be used. These treatments are collectively called **intrathecal chemotherapy** treatments. These treatments require injecting the chemotherapy directly into the cerebrospinal fluid (CSF). The CSF is the clear fluid surrounding the CNS. An oncologist (a physician specializing in cancer study and treatment) will determine the frequency of the treatment schedule and will decide if it is better for the patient to receive intrathecal chemotherapy injections directly into the spinal column or through an Ommaya reservoir implanted in the brain. The Ommaya reservoir may be used in several ways. Its

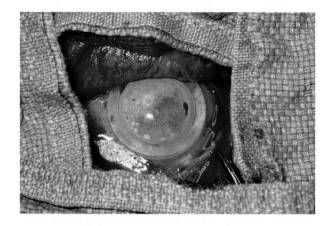

An Ommaya reservoir is used to deliver chemotherapy drugs directly to the central nervous system. *(M. English/ Custom Medical Stock Photo)*

KEY TERMS

Blood-brain barrier—The blood vessel network surrounding the brain that blocks the passage of foreign substances into the brain.

Central nervous system (CNS)—The body system composed of the brain and spinal cord.

Cerebrospinal fluid (CSF)—The fluid surrounding the brain and spinal cord.

Chemotherapy—Anticancer drugs.

Intrathecal chemotherapy—Chemotherapy that must be given directly into the CSF.

primary function is to facilitate the uniform delivery of the intrathecal chemotherapy. By implanting the Ommaya reservoir, multiple rounds of chemotherapy may be given through a single access site, thereby increasing patient comfort and reducing the stress and pain associated with repeated spinal injections. The Ommaya reservoir also serves as a sampling site for removal of CSF. Samples are withdrawn and analyzed for the presence of abnormal cells. Some physicians utilize the reservoir to deliver pain medication, and more recently, trials have been conducted to test the efficacy of using the Ommaya reservoir to deliver **gene therapy** (treating a disease caused by a malfunctioning gene, by introducing a normal gene back into the diseased individual) to cancer patients.

Precautions

High-dose chemotherapy drugs such as **methotrexate** may produce toxic effects if the reservoir or catheter becomes compromised. For infants and children being considered as candidates for an Ommaya reservoir implant, the age of the patient should be considered. Some studies have suggested that infants may be at a higher risk for post-treatment neurologic and endocrinologic problems, cognitive (learning) disabilities, and higher infant mortality when high-dose chemotherapy agents are administered via the Ommaya reservoir. These conditions are significantly reduced in adult patients. Any patient compromised by a pre-existing suppressed immune system should make the physician aware of this condition so the right choice of chemotherapy and specific protocols for administering the drugs are employed.

Description

Placement of the Ommaya reservoir requires a minor surgical procedure with the patient placed under general anesthesia. The procedure is performed in the hospital by a neurosurgeon (a physician specially trained to perform surgery on the brain or spinal cord). The reservoir is placed under the scalp with the catheter positioned into the cavity of the brain where the CSF is formed. Once in place, chemotherapy treatments using the Ommaya reservoir may be conducted as outpatient visits either in the hospital, the home, or a satellite clinic staffed by specially trained healthcare professionals. An Ommaya reservoir tap (CSF sampling and chemotherapy delivery) requires 15–20 minutes with little or no pain to the patient. Basic guidelines for the tap include:

- Remove hair from over the reservoir area.
- Gently pump the reservoir to allow the reservoir to fill with CSF.
- Clean the area with alcohol and iodine solution, maintaining a sterile field.
- The healthcare professional will insert a small needle into the reservoir and slowly withdraw a sample of CSF.
- The chemotherapy will be delivered by slowly injecting the prescribed medication into the reservoir.
- The needle is removed and the site covered with sterile gauze.
- Light pressure is applied, and the reservoir is gently pumped to enhance uniform distribution of the chemotherapy into the CSF.
- The site is covered with a Band-Aid.

Preparation

Placement of the Ommaya reservoir will require a minimal stay in the hospital. The surgeon will provide detailed pre-operative instructions for the patient prior to the hospital visit. Post-operative recovery will monitor vital signs and watch for possible side effects from the anesthesia. Before the patient is discharged, an initial round of chemotherapy administered via the Ommaya reservoir will be performed to assure the device is working properly. No special preparations are required for routine scheduled chemotherapy treatments.

Aftercare

Following an Ommaya tap, the patient may participate in all normal activities. Hair may be washed. There are no special requirements for care of the reservoir site; however, a physician should be notified if symptoms appear such as a spike in **fever**, headaches with or without vomiting, neck stiffness, tenderness, redness, or drainage at the access site of the reservoir.

Risks

The most common risks associated with the use of the Ommaya reservoir primarily deal with complications due to malposition or malfunction of the device. Either condition may result in blockage or leakage of the catheter, leading to improper drug delivery. Lesions may develop along the catheter, infection may develop, and chemotherapy may reach toxic levels. In cancer patients scheduled for surgical intervention who have previously received chemotherapy via an Ommaya reservoir, there is some evidence of increased perioperative morbidity (a diseased condition existing at the time of surgery).

Results

Patients may expect successful delivery of the intrathecal chemotherapy during each treatment session with minimal discomfort. It should be noted, however, that the chemotherapy delivered by the Ommaya reservoir works on cells that are actively growing and dividing. This means both cancer cells and certain normal cell types may be affected and may result in side effects. Depressed blood cell counts may lower resistance to infection and increase susceptibility to bruising and bleeding. There may be an overall decrease in energy levels. Hair loss (**alopecia**) may occur and cells of the digestive tract may be damaged, resulting in bouts of nausea, vomiting, and mouth sores. For female patients, symptoms of menopause may develop, and in males, sperm production may stop.

Abnormal results

Severe complications associated with drug delivery could occur. Due to improper function of the reservoir, toxic levels of chemotherapy could induce behavioral abnormalities, confusion, dementia, irritability, convulsions, sensory impairment, damage to pulmonary and renal function, and patient death.

Resources

PERIODICALS

Szvalb, A.D., Raad II, Weinberg, J.S., Suki, D., Mayer, R., and Viola, G.M. "Ommaya Reservoir-Related Infections: Clinical Manifestations and Treatment Outcomes." *The Journal of Infection* 68, no. 3 (2014): 216–24. http://www.ncbi.nlm.nih.gov/pubmed/24360921 (accessed November 8, 2014).

WEBSITES

Memorial Sloan Kettering Cancer Center. "About Your Ommaya Reservoir Placement Surgery." http://www.mskcc.org/cancer-care/patient-education/resources/about-your-ommaya-reservoir-placement-surgery (accessed November 14, 2014).

National Cancer Institute. "Ommaya Reservoir." http://www.cancer.gov/dictionary?cdrid=46258 (accessed November 14, 2014).

Jane Taylor-Jones, MS, Research Associate

Oncaspar *see* **Pegaspargase**

Oncologic emergencies

Definition

Oncologic or oncological emergencies are serious or life-threatening metabolic, structural, infectious, neurological, cardiovascular, or hematological complications of **cancer** and its treatments. Oncological emergencies necessitate quick action to avoid loss of life or permanent functional compromise.

Description

Oncologic emergencies include a wide variety of conditions. Some develop over a period of months, whereas others develop very quickly and can cause paralysis and death in just a few hours. It is not unusual for cancer to be diagnosed because of an oncologic emergency. Oncologic emergencies may cause severe pain, which is itself an oncologic emergency.

Emergency types

Although oncologic emergencies are sometimes categorized according to their origins or the affected organ(s), most often they are classified as:

- metabolic
- hematologic

Blood urea nitrogen (BUN)—A measurement of the waste product urea in the bloodstream; patients with kidney failure have high BUN levels.

Cardiac tamponade—Compression of the heart by large amounts of fluid or blood.

Electrocardiography (ECG)—Recording of electrical potential during heartbeats.

Electrolytes—Ions such as sodium, potassium, or calcium that are dissolved in bodily fluids such as blood and regulate or affect most metabolic processes.

Extravasation—Escape of chemotherapy drugs during infusion.

Hematologic—Relating to blood.

Hemodialysis—The removal of blood from an artery for purification and its return to a vein.

Hemorrhagic cystitis—Inflammation and bleeding of the urinary bladder.

Hypercalcemia—Excess calcium in the blood.

Hyperkalemia—Excess potassium in the blood.

Hyperphosphatemia—Excess phosphate in the blood.

Hyperuricemia—Excess uric acid in the blood.

Hyperviscosity syndrome—Overly viscous blood that cannot flow easily.

Hypoglycemia—An abnormally low blood glucose level.

Hyponatremia—Blood sodium deficiency.

Intracranial pressure (ICP)—Pressure inside the skull.

Leukocytosis—Increased numbers of circulating white blood cells; an indication of infection.

Necrosis—Tissue death.

Neutropenia—Deficiency of neutrophils.

Neutrophil—The major phagocytic white blood cell of the immune system.

Pancreatitis—Inflammation of the pancreas.

Pericardial effusion—Escape of fluid into the pericardium—the sac that encloses the heart.

Pneumonitis—Lung inflammation.

Superior vena cava (SVC) syndrome—Obstruction or compression of the superior vena cava, the second largest vein in the body that returns blood from the upper part of the body to the atrium of the heart.

Syndrome of inappropriate antidiuretic hormone (SIADH)—Overproduction of antidiuretic hormone by cancer cells or as a side effect of chemotherapy.

Tumor lysis syndrome (TLS)—Excess uric acid, potassium, and phosphate in the blood due to the rapid destruction of large numbers of cancer cells from radiation or chemotherapy.

Uric acid—A nitrogenous waste product in the urine.

• structural or mechanical

• cancer treatment-related or chemotherapy side effects

• neurological

• infections

The most common metabolic oncologic emergencies include:

• TLS, a potentially lethal complication of cancer treatment characterized by excess uric acid, potassium, and phosphate in the blood (hyperuricemia, hyperkalemia, and hyperphosphatemia, respectively), with renal (kidney) failure and hypocalcemia (calcium deficiency) as secondary complications

• hypercalcemia of malignancy

• syndrome of inappropriate antidiuretic hormone (SIADH)

• hyponatremia (low blood sodium)

• hypoglycemia (low blood sugar)

• adrenal failure

• lactic acidosis—the accumulation of lactic acid in body tissues

Hematologic emergencies include febrile **neutropenia**, hyperleukocytosis, and hyperviscosity syndrome, in which the blood thickens and flows sluggishly.

Structural or mechanical emergencies are classified according to the affected organ system:

• Cardiovascular emergencies include superior vena cava (SVC) syndrome (blockage of the vein that returns blood to the heart), malignant pericardial effusion, and cardiac tamponade (the mechanical compression of the heart by fluid or blood).

- Neurologic emergencies include epidural spinal cord compression, increased intracranial pressure (ICP), and status epilepticus (prolonged or recurrent seizures).
- Respiratory emergencies include airway obstruction.
- Urologic emergencies include upper or lower urinary tract obstruction.
- Gastrointestinal emergencies include obstructions of the gastrointestinal tract.

Emergency side effects of **chemotherapy** include extravasation injuries and gastrointestinal emergencies such as severe dehydration. They also include inflammatory conditions—such as inflammation of the lungs (pneumonitis), pancreas (pancreatitis), urinary bladder (hemorrhagic cystitis), or intestines (enterocolitis)—and tissue death (necrosis).

Both cancer and its treatments increase risk of developing acute life-threatening infections by bacteria, viruses, fungi, and parasites. Neutropenic **fever** and septic shock are the most common infectious oncologic emergencies.

Risk factors

Different types of cancer are risk factors for different oncologic emergencies:

- TLS is more common with hematologic malignancies and with bulky, rapidly growing, aggressive, and treatment-sensitive tumors. It is often associated with acute leukemias and high-grade non-Hodgkin lymphomas such as Burkitt lymphoma.
- Hypercalcemia occurs with various cancers. It is most commonly associated with multiple myeloma and cancers of the lung, breast, and kidney. It can occur in children with acute lymphoblastic leukemia, non-Hodgkin lymphoma, neuroblastoma, and various other tumors.
- Hematologic emergencies involving the overproduction of certain types of blood cells are associated with acute leukemia.
- Hyperviscosity syndrome is most common in patients with Waldenström macroglobulinemia, leukemia, or multiple myeloma.
- SVC syndrome is most often the result of lung cancer but can also be caused by other chest tumors or by catheters.
- Most pericardial effusions develop from metastatic lung or breast cancer, but they are also sometimes the side effect of malignant melanoma, leukemia, lymphoma, chemotherapy, or radiation therapy to the chest wall.

- Epidural spinal cord compression is most often associated with breast and lung cancers but also occurs with renal and prostate cancers.
- Airway obstruction is the most common respiratory emergency in children with cancer and is associated with leukemia, lymphoma, Hodgkin lymphoma, rhabdomyosarcoma, and neuroblastoma.

Any type of immunosuppression is a risk factor for infection. Neutropenia from leukemia, chemotherapy, or **radiation therapy** is a major risk factor for bacterial and fungal infections. Corticosteroid treatment, catheters, dysfunction or removal of the spleen, and various other procedures also increase the risk of infection.

Demographics

As both the incidence of cancer and cancer survival rates increase, so does the frequency of oncologic emergencies, although demographic information is limited:

- Tumor lysis syndrome (TLS) is the most common metabolic oncologic emergency in children: 42% of children with intermediate- or high-grade non-Hodgkin lymphomas have laboratory evidence of TLS, although only 6% exhibit symptoms; 70% of children with acute leukemia who receive high-dose chemotherapy for advanced disease have laboratory evidence of TLS, although only 3% have symptoms.
- Hypercalcemia (excess blood calcium) of malignancy affects 20%–30% of all cancer patients and 40%–50% of those with breast cancer or multiple myeloma.
- Febrile (feverish) neutropenia (deficiency of neutrophils, a type of white blood cell) is one of the most common complications related to cancer treatment, especially chemotherapy, and is a contributing factor in 50% of deaths associated with leukemias, lymphomas, and solid tumors.
- Hyperleukocytosis—dangerously high levels of circulating white blood cells—is the most common hematologic (blood cell) overproduction syndrome requiring emergency treatment in pediatric cancer patients. It is present at diagnosis in almost all children with chronic myelogenous leukemia, 13%–22% of those with acute non-lymphocytic leukemia, and 6%–15% of children with acute lymphoid leukemia.
- As many as 10%–15% of cancer patients have some degree of pericardial effusion— leakage of fluid from around the heart. It is a frequent cause of death in patients with otherwise treatable cancers.
- Extravasation injuries—leakage of chemotherapy drugs from a vein into the surrounding tissues—occurs with 0.1%–6.5% of chemotherapy infusions.

- Up to 50% of patients undergoing chemotherapy for colon cancer become severely dehydrated from vomiting, diarrhea, and inflammation of mucous membranes.

Causes and symptoms

Metabolic emergencies

- TLS is caused by the rapid destruction of cancer cells upon the initiation of radiation therapy or chemotherapy. The rapid release into the bloodstream of the contents of large numbers of cancer cells overwhelms the ability of the body to maintain balances of uric acid, potassium, phosphates, and calcium. TLS usually develops within one to five days of treatment.

- Hypercalcemia of malignancy usually results from bone loss (resorption), which disrupts calcium regulation, which results in a variety of symptoms including nausea, vomiting, constipation, progressive decline in mental function, renal failure, and coma.

- SIADH is often the result of the production of antidiuretic hormone by cancer cells. It also can be caused by certain chemotherapy drugs. Symptoms may include anorexia nervosa (loss of appetite), nausea, muscle pain, headaches, and severe neurologic symptoms, including seizures or coma.

- Hyponatremia usually results from water retention combined with normal or excessive administration of fluids. Some chemotherapy drugs interfere with water secretion, causing hyponatremia. Symptoms are primarily neurologic and can be life-threatening.

- Hypoglycemia is most often the result of tumors of the insulin-producing islet cells. Symptoms are neurologic.

Hematologic emergencies

Hematologic emergencies are the result of abnormal blood cell production—most often low production of a particular type of blood cell—or hemorrhage and/or thrombosis (a clot in a blood vessel):

- Underproduction of blood cells is the result of disease infiltration of the bone marrow, bone marrow failure, or treatment, resulting in anemia (red blood cell deficiency), thrombocytopenia (decreased platelets), and neutropenia. Neutropenia is most often a side effect of chemotherapy. Low neutrophil counts leave patients vulnerable to infection.

- Hyperviscosity syndrome is caused by elevated levels of circulating serum immunoglobulins (antibodies) that coat the cells, causing increased blood viscosity, sludging of the blood, and decreased blood flow through the organs. Symptoms include spontaneous bleeding, neurologic defects, and vision changes.

- Symptoms of hyperleukocytosis are usually respiratory and neurologic.

Structural emergencies

Structural emergencies are the result of direct compression, obstruction, or displacement of tissues by cancer:

- The SVC, the second largest vein in the body, returns blood from the upper part of the body to the atrium of the heart. External compression or an internal clot may cause SVC obstruction. SVC compression results in swelling or discoloration of the neck, head, face, or upper extremities. Other symptoms of SVC syndrome may include cough, hoarseness, chest pain, labored breathing, difficulty swallowing, and distension of the superficial veins in the chest wall, progressing to headache, confusion, altered vision, and loss of consciousness.

- Symptoms of pericardial effusions include difficult or labored breathing, especially when lying down; fatigue; heart palpitations; and dizziness. Other symptoms may include a pulse that weakens during inspiration, rapid heart rate, and distended neck veins. Pericardial effusion is often undiagnosed in cancer patients.

- Cardiac tamponade is the inability of the heart ventricle to maintain cardiac output because of external pressure or an intrinsic mass.

- Epidural spinal cord compression is the result of a tumor that compresses the spinal cord, most often in the thoracic spine between the neck and the abdomen. Symptoms include low back pain and pain that worsens when lying down. Late neurologic signs include weakness, incontinence, and sensory defects. Epidural spinal cord compression can result in permanent neurologic impairment if treatment is delayed for even a few hours.

- ICP is associated with cerebral herniation, which can result from an expanding mass in the head or from an obstruction of cerebrospinal fluid circulation. Symptoms include impaired consciousness, abnormal eye movements, abnormal pupil size, nausea, vomiting, and a stiff neck.

- Status epilepticus can result from either mechanical or metabolic perturbation of the central nervous system from a tumor or from treatment.

- Symptoms of gastrointestinal obstruction may include cramping, abdominal pain, an abdominal mass, and currant-jelly stool.

Treatment-related emergencies

Many chemotherapy agents, including anthracyclines and vinca alkaloids, are irritants or blistering agents. Leakage of these agents onto the skin during infusion therapy can result in severe scarring and irreversible damage to joints. Symptoms of extravasation injuries include redness, swelling, and necrosis at the infusion site, usually within hours of chemotherapy.

Dehydration is a serious side effect of cancer treatment that is often overlooked. Up to 30% of cancer patients with delirium are dehydrated.

Severe constipation, characterized by hard stools every three to five days and abdominal pain, is commonly associated with narcotic medications but also sometimes with neurotoxic chemotherapy agents.

Among inflammatory conditions:

- Noninfectious pneumonitis can be a complication of radiation therapy, chemotherapy, stem-cell transplantation, or transfusions. Symptoms range from none to respiratory failure.
- Pancreatitis is a complication of some chemotherapies and systemic steroid treatment. The primary symptom is severe abdominal pain.
- Hemorrhagic cystitis is most often the result of cyclophosphamide and ifosfamide. It also is associated with pelvic irradiation and viral infections. Symptoms can occur anywhere from hours to years after treatment. Painful urination is the major symptom.

Infectious emergencies

Infectious emergencies most often are caused by immunosuppression. The most common causes of bacterial infectious emergencies in cancer patients include:

- *Staphylococcus* spp.
- *Streptococcus* spp.
- *Enterococcus* spp.
- *Pseudomonas aeruginosa*
- *Aeromonas hydrophila*
- *Bacillus* spp.
- *Corynebacterium* spp.
- *Haemophilus influenzae*
- *Neisseria meningitidis*
- *Salmonella* spp.
- *Escherichia coli*
- *Listeria monocytogenes*
- *Legionella* spp.
- *Nocardia* spp.
- *Clostridium difficile*

- *Mycobacterium tuberculosis*
- atypical mycobacteria

Viral infections that can be emergencies in cancer patients include:

- herpes viruses
- influenza
- parainfluenza
- echovirus
- measles virus
- varicella
- respiratory syncytial virus (RSV)
- adenoviruses

Fungal infections in cancer patients often are caused by:

- *Candida* spp.
- *Aspergillus* spp.
- *Fusarium* spp.
- *Cryptococcus neoformans*
- *Coccidioides immitis*
- Mucoraceae

Parasites that result in infectious emergencies include:

- *Giardia lamblia*
- *Cryptosporidium* spp.
- *Toxoplasma gondii*
- *Strongyloides stercoralis*
- *Babesia microti*

Immunosuppression due to cancer or its treatments places cancer patients at very high risk of sepsis, a serious medical condition characterized by an infection that prompts an inflammatory response throughout the entire body, affecting multiple organ systems. Incidence rates of sepsis in cancer patients in North America are estimated at 45%. Mortality rates from sepsis in cancer patients exceed 30%. Although the incidence of sepsis in cancer patients has increased by 2% per year since the early 2000s, a study carried out in three university-related cancer centers reported in 2014 that mortality rates are declining. The cancer patients at highest risk mortality from sepsis are lung cancer patients.

Diagnosis

Examination

Oncologic emergencies are often diagnosed based on symptoms, the type of cancer, and the patient's treatments. Symptoms of bacterial infections include a temperature of at least 101°F (38.3°C).

Tests

A variety of tests are conducted to diagnose oncologic emergencies:

- Tests for TLS include serum electrolyte (potassium, calcium, phosphate, magnesium), blood urea nitrogen (BUN), uric acid, creatinine, and lactic dehydrogenase (LDH) levels and an electrocardiogram (ECG). Elevated levels of uric acid, potassium, phosphate, or LDH before the start of chemotherapy indicate that TLS is already present or impending.
- Laboratory testing for SIADH may reveal hyponatremia, decreased serum osmolarity, and concentrated urine.
- Serum viscosity is measured to diagnose hyperviscosity syndrome.
- SVC syndrome diagnosis may include microscopic examination of the sputum and/or chest fluid obtained via thoracentesis or needle aspiration.
- Hemorrhagic cystitis is suggested by leukocytes and erythrocytes (white and red blood cells, respectively) or clots in the urine.
- Infections are diagnosed by various blood tests and cultures of bodily fluids such as blood, sputum, urine, and/or cerebrospinal fluid (CSF) to identify the organism causing the infection; a complete blood cell count; an absolute neutrophil count (ANC); BUN, serum creatinine, and transaminase measurements; and measurement of procalcitonin. Procalcitonin is a precursor of a hormone known as calcitonin, which regulates calcium levels in the blood. Procalcitonin levels are virtually undetectable in the blood of healthy persons but rise to measurable levels in persons with severe bacterial infections.

Procedures

Diagnostic procedures for oncologic emergencies may include x-rays, **magnetic resonance imaging** (MRI), **computed tomography** (CT) scans, ultrasound, and/or fluoroscopy:

- Although SVC syndrome is a clinical diagnosis, plain radiography, CT scans, and venography (radiography of the vein) help confirm the diagnosis. Bronchoscopy may be used to examine the bronchi.
- Pericardial effusions are diagnosed by echocardiography and fluid samples examined under the microscope.
- Epidural spinal cord compression may be diagnosed by radiography and MRI.

- Chest x-rays are used to diagnose infections with respiratory symptoms.

Treatment

Treatment of oncologic emergencies is initiated as soon as possible.

- TLS treatment includes inpatient monitoring, hyperhydration, urinary alkalinization with sodium bicarbonate, and hemodialysis. Hyperkalemia treatment may include the removal of potassium from IV fluids and administration of sodium polystyrene resin and calcium gluconate. Treatment for hyperphosphatemia may include aluminum hydroxide.
- Hypercalcemia of malignancy is treated with aggressive rehydration and possibly hemodialysis.
- SIADH usually is treated immediately with fluid restriction and slow correction of serum sodium levels as well as treatment of the underlying tumor.
- Hyponatremia is treated with saline administration and management of fluid volume.
- Hypoglycemia is treated with increased feeding and intravenous (IV) dextrose.
- Depressed bone-marrow activity may be treated with transfusion of individual blood components. Severe anemia is treated with blood transfusions.
- Hyperviscosity syndrome is treated with plasmapheresis (removal of blood plasma), followed by targeted chemotherapy.
- Leukocytosis is addressed by anti-leukemic treatments to reduce peripheral leukocytes.
- SVC syndrome treatments include chemotherapy and radiation to reduce the tumor that is causing the obstruction or intravenous stents to open the vein. The head of the patient's bed is elevated.
- Acute symptoms of pericardial effusion are treated with pericardiocentesis (surgical puncture of the pericardium to aspirate the fluid) or a pericardial window procedure. Chemotherapy, radiation, or sclerosis therapy can prevent fluid reaccumulation.
- Most patients with epidural spinal cord compression need radiation treatment or surgery and possibly chemotherapy.
- Gastrointestinal obstruction from external compression is treated with chemotherapy, surgery, radiation therapy, or a combination.
- Extravasation injuries require prompt diagnosis to avoid extensive skin damage. The infusion is halted and the excess drug is aspirated. Depending on the drug, ice or warm packs are applied. Pressure to the site is avoided.
- Dehydration is treated by fluid resuscitation.

- Urinary obstruction may require the removal of clots or placement of a catheter.
- Hemorrhagic cystitis is treated with hyperhydration, continuous bladder irrigation, platelet transfusion, and treatment of impaired blood coagulation.

Drugs

Drug treatments for oncologic emergencies include:

- allopurinol or recombinant urate oxidase to lower uric acid levels and diuretics, insulin, and dextrose for hyperkalemia of TLS
- furosemide, intravenous bisphosphonates, glucocorticoids, calcitonin, plicamycin, gallium nitrate, pamidronate, and zoledronic acid for hypercalcemia of malignancy
- furosemide for SIADH
- demeclocycline for persistent hyponatremia
- corticosteroids and glucagon for hypoglycemia
- broad-spectrum antibiotics, possibly multiple antibiotics or vancomycin and antifungal agents, myeloid growth factors, granulocyte colony-stimulating factor (G-CSF), granulocyte-macrophage colony-stimulating factor (GM-CSF), and androgens for neutropenia
- diuretics, corticosteroids, thrombolytics, and anticoagulants for SVC syndrome
- dexamethasone for neurologic symptoms of epidural spinal cord compression
- antidotes for extravasation injuries
- anti-vomiting agents and antidiarrheals for dehydration
- corticosteroids for noninfectious pneumonitis
- oxybutynin chloride for relief of bladder spasms associated with hemorrhagic cystitis
- antibiotics for bacterial infections
- antiviral agents for viral infections
- anti-fungal agents, especially amphotericin B, for fungal infections

Prognosis

If untreated or if treatment is delayed, most oncologic emergencies lead to severe impairment, irreversible damage, and possibly death. Untreated epidural spinal cord compression can result in permanent paraplegia. Prognoses for treated oncologic emergencies vary tremendously depending on the specific condition, the underlying cancer, and other factors. Hypercalcemia of malignancy has a poor prognosis, with more than 50% of patients dying within 30 days of diagnosis. Patients with SVC syndrome usually have advanced disease and less than 10% survive for more than 30 months following treatment.

QUESTIONS TO ASK YOUR DOCTOR

- What type of oncologic emergency do I have?
- How is it related to my cancer?
- How will my emergency condition be treated?
- How soon can I expect a response to treatment?
- What is my prognosis?

Prevention

Some oncologic emergencies can be foreseen and prevented. Infections may be prevented by prophylactic administration of **antibiotics** and antifungal agents in patients undergoing stem-cell transplants and some types of chemotherapy. Prevention of TLS includes:

- identification of high-risk patients
- allopurinol or urate oxidase to lower uric acid levels
- alkalinization to inhibit the precipitation of uric acid crystals in kidney tubules
- limitation of potassium and phosphorus intake
- hydration to maximize excretion of uric acid, potassium, and phosphate
- ECG monitoring before the start of chemotherapy

See also Infection and sepsis.

Resources

BOOKS

Hazinski, Mary Fran. *Nursing Care of the Critically Ill Child.* 3rd ed. St. Louis, MO: Elsevier/Mosby, 2013.

Kaplan, Marcelle. *Understanding and Managing Oncologic Emergencies: A Resource for Nurses.* 2nd ed. Pittsburgh, PA: Oncology Nursing Society, 2013.

Longo, Dan L., and Tinsley Randolph Harrison. *Harrison's Hematology and Oncology.* 2nd ed. New York: McGraw-Hill Education/Medical, 2013.

Niederhuber, J.E., et al. *Clinical Oncology.* 5th ed. Philadelphia: Elsevier, 2014.

Strange, Gary R. *Pediatric Emergency Medicine: Just the Facts.* 2nd ed. New York: McGraw-Hill Medical, 2012.

Yarbro, Connie Henke, Debra Wujcik, and Barbara Holmes Gobel. *Oncology Nursing Review.* 5th ed. Sudbury, MA: Jones & Bartlett Learning, 2012.

OTHER

"Understanding Side Effects of Drug Therapy." Leukemia & Lymphoma Society. 2013. http://www.lls.org/content/nationalcontent/resourcecenter/freeeducationmaterials/treatments/pdf/understandingdrugtherapy.pdf (accessed August 20, 2014).

WEBSITES

Ikeda, Alan K. "Tumor Lysis Syndrome." Medscape. http://emedicine.medscape.com/article/282171-overview#showall (accessed August 20, 2014).

"SVC Obstruction." MedlinePlus. http://www.nlm.nih.gov/medlineplus/ency/article/001097.htm (accessed August 20, 2014).

ORGANIZATIONS

Leukemia & Lymphoma Society, 1311 Mamaroneck Avenue, Suite 310, White Plains, NY 10605, (914) 949-5213, Fax: (914) 949-6691, (800) 955-4572, infocenter@lls.org, http://www.lls.org.

Margaret Alic, PhD

REVISED BY MARGARET ALIC, PhD

Oncovin *see* **Vincristine**

Ondansetron *see* **Antiemetics**

Ontak *see* **Denileukin diftitox**

Oophorectomy

Definition

Unilateral oophorectomy (also called an ovariectomy) is the surgical removal of an ovary. If one ovary is removed, a woman may continue to menstruate and have children. If both ovaries are removed, a procedure called a bilateral oophorectomy, menstruation stops and a woman loses the ability to have children.

Purpose

Oophorectomy is performed to:

• remove cancerous ovaries

• remove the source of estrogen that stimulates some cancers

• remove a large ovarian cyst

• excise an abscess

• treat endometriosis

In an oophorectomy, one or a portion of one ovary may be removed or both ovaries may be removed. When an oophorectomy is done to treat **ovarian cancer** or other spreading cancers, both ovaries are removed (called a bilateral oophorectomy). Removal of the ovaries and Fallopian tubes is performed in about one-third of hysterectomies (surgical removal of the uterus), often to reduce the risk of ovarian **cancer**.

Oophorectomies are sometimes performed on premenopausal women who have estrogen-sensitive **breast cancer** in an effort to remove the main source of estrogen from their bodies. This procedure has become less common than it was in the 1990s. Today, **chemotherapy** drugs are available that alter the production of estrogen and **tamoxifen** blocks any of the effects any remaining estrogen may have on cancer cells.

Until the 1980s, women over age 40 having hysterectomies routinely had healthy ovaries and Fallopian tubes removed at the same time. This operation is called a bilateral salpingo-oophorectomy. Many physicians reasoned that a woman over 40 was approaching menopause and soon her ovaries would stop secreting estrogen and releasing eggs. Removing the ovaries would

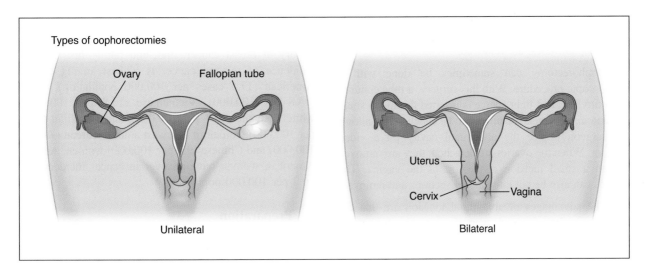

Types of oophorectomies

Ovary — Fallopian tube

Unilateral

Uterus — Cervix — Vagina

Bilateral

In a unilateral oophorectomy, just one ovary is removed; in a bilateral oophorectomy, both ovaries are removed. *(Illustration by Electronic Illustrators Group. © Cengage Learning®.)*

eliminate the risk of ovarian cancer and only accelerate menopause by a few years.

In the 1990s, the thinking about routine oophorectomy began to change. The risk of ovarian cancer in women who have no family history of the disease is less than 1%. Meanwhile, removing the ovaries increases the risk of cardiovascular disease and accelerates osteoporosis unless a woman takes prescribed hormone replacements.

Under certain circumstances, oophorectomy may still be the treatment of choice to prevent breast and ovarian cancer in certain high-risk women. A study done at the University of Pennsylvania and released in 2000 showed that healthy women who carried the BRCA1 or BRCA2 genetic mutations that predisposed them to breast cancer had their risk of breast cancer drop from 80% to 19% when their ovaries were removed before age 40. Women between the ages of 40 and 50 showed less risk reduction, and there was no significant reduction of breast cancer risk in women over age 50. A 2002 study showed that five years after being identified as carrying BRCA1 or BRCA2 genetic mutations, 94% of women who had received a bilateral salpingo-oophorectomy were cancer-free, compared to 79% of women who had not received surgery. However, there are disagreements within the medical community about when and at what age this treatment should be offered.

Description

Oophorectomy is done under general or regional anesthesia. It is often performed through the same type of incision, either vertical or horizontal, as an abdominal hysterectomy. Horizontal incisions leave a less noticeable scar, but vertical incisions give the surgeon a better view of the abdominal cavity. After the incision is made, the abdominal muscles are stretched apart, not cut, so that the surgeon can see the ovaries. Then the ovaries, and often the Fallopian tubes, are removed.

Oophorectomy can sometimes be done with a laparoscopic procedure. With this surgery, a tube containing a tiny lens and light source is inserted through a small incision in the navel. A camera can be attached that allows the surgeon to see the abdominal cavity on a video monitor. When the ovaries are detached, they are removed though a small incision at the top of the vagina. The ovaries can also be cut into smaller sections and removed.

The advantages of abdominal incision are that the ovaries can be removed even if a woman has many adhesions from previous surgery, and the surgeon gets a good view of the abdominal cavity and can check the surrounding tissue for disease. A vertical abdominal incision is mandatory if cancer is suspected. The disadvantages are that bleeding is more likely to be a

complication of this type of operation, the operation is more painful than a laparoscopic operation, and the recovery period is longer. A woman can expect to be in the hospital two to five days and will need three to six weeks to return to normal activities.

Demographics

Overall, ovarian cancer accounts for only 4% of all cancers in women. But the lifetime risk for developing ovarian cancer in women who have mutations in BRCA1 is significantly increased over the general population and may cause an ovarian cancer risk of 30% by age 60. For women at increased risk, oophorectomy may be considered after the age of 35 if childbearing is complete.

Other factors that increase a woman's risk of developing ovarian cancer include age (most ovarian cancers occur after menopause), the number of menstrual periods a woman has had (affected by age of onset, pregnancy, breast-feeding, and oral contraceptive use), history of breast cancer, diet, and family history. The incidence of ovarian cancer is highest among Native American (17.5 cases per 100,000 population), white (15.8 per 100,000), Vietnamese (13.8 per 100,000), white Hispanic (12.1 per 100,000), and Hawaiian (11.8 per 100,000) women; it is lowest among Korean (7.0 per 100,000) and Chinese (9.3 per 100,000) women. African American women have an ovarian cancer incidence of 10.2 per 100,000 population.

Preparation

Before surgery, the doctor will order blood and urine tests, and any additional tests such as ultrasound or **x-rays** to help the surgeon visualize the woman's condition. The woman may also meet with the anesthesiologist to evaluate any special conditions that might affect the administration of anesthesia. A colon preparation may be done, if extensive surgery is anticipated.

On the evening before the operation, the woman should eat a light dinner, then take nothing by mouth, including water or other liquids, after midnight.

Aftercare

After surgery a woman will feel discomfort. The degree of discomfort varies and is generally greatest with abdominal incisions, because the abdominal muscles must be stretched out of the way so that the surgeon can reach the ovaries. In order to minimize the risk of postoperative infection, **antibiotics** will be given.

When both ovaries are removed, women who do not have cancer are started on hormone replacement therapy to ease the symptoms of menopause that occur because estrogen produced by the ovaries is no longer present. If even part of one ovary remains, it will produce enough estrogen that a woman will continue to menstruate, unless her uterus was removed in a hysterectomy. To help offset the higher risks of heart and bone disease after loss of the ovaries, women should get plenty of exercise, maintain a low-fat diet, and ensure intake of calcium is adequate.

Return to normal activities takes anywhere from two to six weeks, depending on the type of surgery. When women have cancer, chemotherapy or radiation are often given in addition to surgery. Some women have emotional trauma following an oophorectomy, and can benefit from counseling and support groups.

Risks

Oophorectomy is a relatively safe operation, although, like all major surgery, it does carry some risks. These include an unanticipated reaction to anesthesia, internal bleeding, blood clots, accidental damage to other organs, and post-surgery infection.

Complications after an oophorectomy include changes in sex drive, hot flashes, and other symptoms of menopause if both ovaries are removed. Women who have both ovaries removed and who do not take estrogen replacement therapy run an increased risk for cardiovascular disease and osteoporosis. Women with a history of psychological and emotional problems before an oophorectomy are more likely to experience psychological difficulties after the operation.

Complications may arise if the surgeon finds that cancer has spread to other places in the abdomen. If the cancer cannot be removed by surgery, it must be treated with chemotherapy and radiation.

QUESTIONS TO ASK YOUR DOCTOR

- Why is an oophorectomy being recommended?
- How will the procedure be performed?
- Will I have a remaining ovary (or portion of ovary)?
- What alternatives to oophorectomy are available to me?

Results

If the surgery is successful, the ovaries will be removed without complication, and the underlying problem resolved. In the case of cancer, all the cancer will be removed. A woman will become infertile following a bilateral oophorectomy.

Morbidity and mortality rates

Studies have shown that the complication rate following oophorectomy is essentially the same as that following hysterectomy. The rate of complications associated with hysterectomy differs by the procedure performed. Abdominal hysterectomy is associated with a higher rate of complications (9.3%), while the overall complication rate for vaginal hysterectomy is 5.3%, and 3.6% for laparoscopic vaginal hysterectomy. The risk of death is about one in every 1,000 women having a hysterectomy. The rates of some of the more commonly reported complications are:

- excessive bleeding (hemorrhaging): 1.8%–3.4%
- fever or infection: 0.8%–4.0%
- accidental injury to another organ or structure: 1.5%–1.8%

Because of the cessation of hormone production that occurs with a bilateral oophorectomy, women who lose both ovaries also prematurely lose the protection these hormones provide against heart disease and osteoporosis. Women who have undergone bilateral oophorectomy are seven times more likely to develop coronary heart disease and much more likely to develop bone problems at an early age than are premenopausal women whose ovaries are intact.

Alternatives

Depending on the specific condition that warrants an oophorectomy, it may be possible to modify the surgery so at least a portion of one ovary remains, allowing the woman to avoid early menopause. In the case of prophylactic oophorectomy, drugs such as tamoxifen may be administered to block the effects that estrogen may have on cancer cells.

Health care team roles

Oophorectomies are usually performed in a hospital operating room by a gynecologist, a medical doctor who has completed specialized training in the areas of women's general health, pregnancy, labor and childbirth, prenatal testing, and genetics.

Resources

PERIODICALS

Laughlin-Tommaso, Shannon K., et al. "Incidence, Time Trends, Laterality, Indications, and Pathological Findings of Unilateral Oophorectomy before Menopause." *Menopause* (September 24, 2013): e-pub ahead of print. http://dx.doi.org/10.1097/GME.0b013e3182a3ff45 (accessed October 3, 2014).

WEBSITES

FORCE. "Oophorectomy." MayoClinic.com. http://www.facingourrisk.org/info_research/risk-management/oophorectomy/index.php (accessed October 3, 2014).

Mayo Clinic staff. "Oophorectomy (Ovary Removal Surgery)." MayoClinic.com. http://www.mayoclinic.com/health/oophorectomy/MY00554 (accessed October 3, 2014).

ORGANIZATIONS

American Cancer Society, 250 Williams St. NW, Atlanta, GA 30303, (800) 227-2345, http://www.cancer.org.

American Congress of Obstetricians and Gynecologists, 409 12th St. SW, Washington, DC 20024-2188, (202) 638-5577, (800) 673-8444, resources@acog.org, http://www.acog.org.

FORCE: Facing Our Risk of Cancer Empowered, 16057 Tampa Palms Blvd. W, PMB #373, Tampa, FL 33647, (866) 288-RISK (7475), info@facingourrisk.org, http://www.facingourrisk.org.

National Cancer Institute, 6116 Executive Blvd., Ste. 300, Bethesda, MD 20892-8322, (800) 4-CANCER (422-6237), http://cancer.gov.

Tish Davidson, AM
Stephanie Dionne Sherk

Opioids

Definition

Opioids are narcotics prescribed for managing moderate to severe pain, especially pain from **cancer** or its treatments. Natural opioids are derived from the

Asian opium poppy *Palaver somniferous*; however, today most opioids are at least partially synthesized. Opioids function in the body much like endorphins, the body's own natural painkillers.

Purpose

About 70% of cancer patients experience pain at some point, and opioids are the most effective drugs available for relieving pain. Between 30% and 40% of patients undergoing cancer treatment report pain, and 70%–90% of those with advanced cancer have pain. However, fewer than 50% of cancer patients receive adequate treatment for their pain. Furthermore, studies have shown that pain in cancer survivors often goes unreported, unrecognized, or is not adequately treated.

The World Health Organization (WHO) has developed an "analgesic ladder" for cancer pain relief:

• Step 1 for patients with mild-to-moderate pain is a non-opioid analgesic, such as acetaminophen or a nonsteroidal, anti-inflammatory drug (NSAID), and an adjuvant drug if indicated.

• Step 2—for patients with moderate-to-severe pain or who failed to achieve adequate pain relief in step 1—is an opioid typically used for moderate pain, a non-opioid analgesic or NSAID, and an adjuvant drug as indicated.

• Step 3—for patients with severe pain or who failed to achieve adequate pain relief in step 2—is an opioid typically used for severe pain and possibly a non-opioid analgesic and/or adjuvant drug.

Rapid-onset opioids are used to treat breakthrough pain in patients who are taking opioids on a regular schedule. Sometimes called rescue medicines, they act quickly for a short period of time. They are taken as needed immediately upon experiencing breakthrough pain or as a preventive if the breakthrough is predictable.

Description

Opioids depress the central nervous system by binding with receptors to block the transmission of nerve impulses and pain perception. Natural opioids (opiates) are derived directly from the sap of unripe seedpods of the opium poppy, but most prescription opioids are synthesized or semi-synthesized. Opioids are widely prescribed for cancer patients in the developed world. However, in much of the world, most patients are not presented for treatment until their cancers are advanced, and pain relief is the only treatment possible. According to the WHO, in most developing countries cancer pain relief is limited by national drug laws that severely restrict access to opioids. The WHO estimates that more than 80% of the global population have little or no access to opioid analgesics to treat pain from cancer and other end-of-life conditions.

Common opioids

Codeine and morphine are the most frequently prescribed natural or semi-synthetic opioids. Since codeine concentrations in the opium poppy are low, most codeine is manufactured by chemical alteration of morphine sap. Morphine sulfate is a white powder that dissolves in water. It is administered as a tablet or by injection into a muscle or vein (intravenously). Intravenous (IV) injection is effective almost immediately. Oxycodone (OxyContin) and fentanyl are common synthetic opioids. Oxycodone is available in tablets of various strengths, including controlled-release formulas for continuous pain relief. Oxycodone is also a street drug with high potential for abuse. Fentanyl is used for breakthrough pain in cancer patients who are taking regular doses of another narcotic. It is available as a lozenge absorbed through the mouth or as a tablet, film, or patch. The most commonly prescribed formulations of codeine, morphine, oxycodone, and hydrocodone also contain acetaminophen or an NSAID (aspirin or ibuprofen) and often caffeine. Fast-acting oral morphine is also used for breakthrough pain. Hydromorphone (Dilaudid),

synthesized from morphine and available in tablets or as an injectable solution, is commonly prescribed for terminally ill patients. Zohydro is the first long-acting formulation of hydrocodone for severe, continuous pain from advanced cancer. Because of its high strength, it has been controversial since it first entered the U.S. market in March 2014. Propoxyphene, which is similar to **meperidine** (Demerol), was removed from the U.S. market in 2010 because of its potential to cause life-threatening heart disturbances.

Common opioids prescribed for moderate cancer pain include:

• codeine

• hydrocodone

• dihydrocodeine

• oxycodone

• tramadol

Common opioids prescribed for severe cancer pain include:

• fentanyl

• hydromorphone

• levorphanol

• methadone

• morphine

• oxycodone

• oxymorphone

Recommended dosage

Opioids and their various formulations are prescribed in different strengths, and there is no correct opioid dosage for treating cancer pain. The goal is to control the pain, whatever it takes. Every patient is medicated differently depending, in part, on the type of cancer, the type of pain and its severity, and other medications used. Different pain medications are more effective for some people than for others. In a 2014 study comparing oral and sublingual (dissolved under the tongue) fentanyl for breakthrough pain in cancer patients taking regularly scheduled opioids, optimal doses varied from 133 micrograms (ug) to 800 ug.

Opioids may be administered orally (in pill or liquid form), by injection, through an IV line, as an anal suppository, as a skin patch, or through an implanted patient-controlled delivery system. Extended-release opioids are taken on a regular schedule, usually every 8–12 hours or via a skin patch. It is most important that opioids be taken as prescribed to prevent pain from starting or becoming worse, since it is harder to control pain that has already started, and it is much easier to control pain when it is mild.

Cancer patients who take their pain medications as prescribed rarely become addicted to them, nor do their bodies become immune to pain medication, so there is no reason to avoid or delay taking stronger doses. Dosages of even strong opioids can be safely raised to ease pain. Decreasing pain relief can be caused by increasing pain, advancing cancer, or tolerance to the medication. Tolerance is a common problem for cancer patients, although many patients never develop tolerance to opioids. Tolerance may require increasing the dose or frequency, changing medications, or adding a medication. If pain relief does not last long enough, an extended-release form of morphine or oxycodone or a slow-release fentanyl skin patch may be prescribed.

Precautions

Opioids cause some people to feel drowsy, dizzy, or lightheaded. It may be unsafe to drive, operate machinery, or perform activities that require alertness, especially when first taking an opioid, before the body has had an opportunity to adjust. Narcotics can cause lethargy and interfere with the ability to function normally. Studies have found that while opioids are helpful for pain relief if taken for less than three months, long-term use does not improve daily functioning in patients with chronic pain.

Although many cancer patients find it necessary to increase their opioid doses, this should only be done under the supervision of their physician. Opioids are broken down by the liver, and people with liver damage may not detoxify them readily, which can lead to accidental overdose. It is also very important that pain medications be prescribed by only one doctor. Patients with multiple doctors should make sure that all their doctors are aware of all medications they are taking, including tranquilizers, sleeping pills, barbiturates, seizure medications, muscle relaxants, antidepressants, antihistamines, cold medicines, other prescription and over-the-counter pain medications, certain anesthetics including some dental anesthetics, or any other medications that cause drowsiness or depress the central nervous system, including alcohol. Even small doses of opioids in combination with alcohol or tranquilizers can cause overdoses that may lead to unconsciousness, coma, or death. Other symptoms of overdose include:

- weakness
- difficulty breathing
- anxiety
- dizziness
- severe drowsiness
- confusion

Opioids should not be halted abruptly. They must be tapered off gradually to allow the body to adjust. Abruptly halting opioids can cause flu-like symptoms, including sweating and **diarrhea**. These symptoms usually go away in a few days to a few weeks.

Two 2012 studies indicated that opioids for relieving pain in postoperative and chronic cancer patients may stimulate the growth and spread of tumors. Opioids can also interfere with or exacerbate certain medical conditions including:

- alcohol abuse
- drug dependency, especially dependency on narcotics
- brain disease or head injury
- colitis
- emotional problems
- emphysema, asthma, or other chronic lung disease
- enlarged prostate
- gallstones or gallbladder disease
- heart disease
- kidney disease
- liver disease
- problems with urination
- seizures
- underactive thyroid

Side effects

The most common side effects of opioids are drowsiness and constipation. Drowsiness is usually temporary and sometimes occurs in patients who have been unable to sleep because of pain and need to catch up. Most people are constipated when taking opioids, because the drugs slow movement of stool through the intestinal tract, causing it to harden. Dietary fiber in whole grains, **laxatives**, stool softeners, or other treatments can often prevent or control constipation. **Nausea and vomiting** usually disappear after the first few days on an opioid.

Less common side effects that may require a different type of medication, a different dose, or different timing of administration include:

- dizziness or fainting
- itching
- urine retention
- slow or shallow breathing
- mental effects such as nightmares, confusion, or hallucinations
- abnormally fast or slow heartbeat
- blurred or double vision

QUESTIONS TO ASK YOUR DOCTOR

- How should I take this pain medication?
- Can I take more if my pain does not go away?
- How long does the medication take to work?
- For how long is a dose effective?
- What if I miss a dose?
- Can I drink alcohol or drive a car on this medication?
- Will this medication interact with my other drugs?
- What side effects might I experience?

- cold, clammy skin
- depression or other mood changes
- dry mouth
- hives
- loss of appetite
- pinpoint pupils
- redness or flushing of the face
- restlessness
- rigid muscles
- ringing or buzzing in the ears
- seizures
- severe drowsiness
- skin reaction at the site of injection
- stomach cramps or pain
- sweating
- trouble sleeping (insomnia)
- yellowing of the skin or whites of the eyes

Interactions

Opioids should not be taken in combination with any prescription or over-the-counter drug or herbal remedy without consulting one's physician. It is particularly important that the prescribing physician be aware of **radiation therapy** or the use of any of the following drugs that can interact with opioids:

- central nervous system depressants
- carbamazepine, an antiepileptic
- monoamine oxidase (MAO) inhibitors (a class of antidepressants), such as furazolidone, isocarboxazid, pargyline, phenelzine, procarbazine, or tranylcypromine

- tricyclic antidepressants, such as amitriptyline, amoxapine, clomipramine, desipramine, doxepin, imipramine, nortriptyline, protriptyline, or trimipramine
- naltrexone, an opioid antagonist
- rifampin, a tuberculosis drug
- zidovudine, an antiviral drug
- some chemotherapy drugs

Resources

BOOKS

Bennett, Sally, Geoffrey Mitchell, and Jenny Strong. "Cancer Pain." In *Pain: A Textbook for Health Professionals*, edited by Hubert Van Griensven, Jenny Strong, and Anita M. Unruh. 2nd ed. New York: Churchill Livingstone Elsevier, 2014.

Davies, Andrew. *Cancer-Related Breakthrough Pain*. Oxford, UK: Oxford University, 2012.

Fallon, Marie. "Cancer Pain." In *ABC of Pain*, edited by Lesley Colvin and Marie Fallon. Hoboken, NJ: Wiley-Blackwell/BMJ, 2012.

Gaguski, Michele E., and Susan D. Bruce. *Cancer Pain Management Scenarios*. Pittsburgh, PA: Oncology Nursing Society, 2013.

Hanna, Magdi, and Zbigniew Zylicz. *Cancer Pain*. London, UK: Springer, 2013.

Hester, Joan, Nigel Sykes, and Sue Peat. *Interventional Pain Control in Cancer Pain Management*. New York: Oxford University, 2012.

Sharma, Manohar. *Practical Management of Complex Cancer Pain*. Oxford, UK: Oxford University, 2014.

PERIODICALS

Gibbins, Jane, et al. "What Do Patients with Advanced Incurable Cancer Want from the Management of Their Pain? A Qualitative Study." *Palliative Medicine* 28, no. 1 (January 2014): 71–78.

Husain, S. Asra, Marty Skemp Brown, and Martha A. Maurer. "Do National Drug Control Laws Ensure the Availability of Opioids for Medical and Scientific Purposes?" *Bulletin of the World Health Organization* 92, no. 2 (February 2014): 108–16.

Loftus, Peter. "Doctors Split on Benefits of Longer-Lasting New Painkiller." *Wall Street Journal* (May 27, 2014): D1.

Meier, Barry. "F.D.A. Urging a Tighter Rein on Painkillers." *New York Times* (October 25, 2013): A1.

Novotna, Stanislava, et al. "Fentanyl Citrate (Fentanyl Ethypharm) for Breakthrough Pain in Opioid-Treated Patients with Cancer." *Clinical Therapeutics* 36, no. 3 (March 2014): 357–67.

"Palliative Care: A Peaceful, Humane Global Campaign Is Needed." *Lancet* 383, no. 9916 (February 8, 2014): 487.

OTHER

"Guide to Controlling Cancer Pain." American Cancer Society. June 10, 2014. http://www.cancer.org/acs/groups/cid/documents/webcontent/002906-pdf.pdf (accessed October 12, 2014).

WEBSITES

Department of Pain Medicine & Palliative Care. "Pain." StopPain.org. http://www.stoppain.org/palliative%5Fcare/content/symptom/pain.asp (accessed October 12, 2014).

"Medicines to Treat Cancer Pain." National Cancer Institute. May 16, 2014. http://www.cancer.gov/cancertopics/coping/paincontrol/page6 (accessed October 12, 2014).

"Opioid Pain Medicines." American Cancer Society. June 10, 2014. http://www.cancer.org/treatment/treatmentsandsideeffects/physicalsideeffects/pain/paindiary/pain-control-opioid-pain-medicines (accessed October 12, 2014).

"Pain." Cancer Support Community. http://www.cancersupportcommunity.org/MainMenu/About-Cancer/Treatment/Treatment-Side-Effects/Pain.html (accessed October 12, 2014).

"Pain Control: Support for People with Cancer." National Cancer Institute. July 16, 2012. http://www.cancer.gov/cancertopics/coping/paincontrol (accessed October 12, 2014).

"WHO's Cancer Pain Ladder for Adults." World Health Organization. http://www.who.int/cancer/palliative/painladder/en (accessed October 12, 2014).

ORGANIZATIONS

American Cancer Society, 250 Williams Street NW, Atlanta, GA 30303, (800) 227-2345, http://www.cancer.org.

National Cancer Institute, 6116 Executive Boulevard, Suite 300, Bethesda, MD 20892-8322, (800) 4-CANCER (422-6237), http://www.cancer.gov.

World Health Organization, Avenue Appia 20, 1211 Geneva, Switzerland 27, 41 22 791 21 11, Fax: 41 22 791 31 11, info@who.int, http://www.who.int/en.

Paul A. Johnson, EdM
Margaret Alic, PhD

Opium tincture *see* **Antidiarrheal agents**

Oprelvekin

Definition

Oprelvekin, also known as Neumega, is a hematopoietic stimulant used as supportive care after myelosuppressive **chemotherapy** to combat thrombopenia.

Purpose

Oprelvekin is a prescription medication used following the administration of myelosuppressive chemotherapy drugs such as **azathioprine** and **mercaptopurine**. Myelosuppressive chemotherapy acts on bone marrow and causes a decrease in the amount of white blood cells (leukopenia) and platelets (thrombopenia). Oprelvekin acts as a growth factor stimulating stem cells to

---

KEY TERMS

Growth factor—A body-produced substance that regulates cell division and cell survival. It can also be produced in a laboratory for use in biological therapy.

Hematopoietic—Related to the formation of blood cells.

Thrombopenia—Decreased number of platelets.

Papilledema—Swelling around the optic disk.

---

proliferate. The result is an increase in the amount of platelets (or thrombocytes).

Description

Oprelvekin is a recombinant human interleukin. Further, it is a synthetic version of the naturally occurring interleukin-11, which is produced by the cells of the bone marrow. It is a growth factor that stimulates the formation of platelets, which are necessary in the process of blood clot formation. Oprelvekin is therefore important in increasing platelet formation after treatment with **cancer** medications that cause **thrombocytopenia**.

The U.S. Food and Drug Administration approved oprelvekin for prevention of severe thrombocytopenia, which is observed after chemotherapy. Oprelvekin is in **clinical trials** for treatment support and therapy for acute myelocytic leukemia.

Recommended dosage

This drug is available by injection. The dose is different from person to person and is dependent on the patient's body weight. Generally, 50 mcg/kg is given once daily in either the abdomen, thigh, or hip. This medication should be taken at the same time every day for best results. If a dosage of oprelvekin is missed, the patient should skip the missed dose and take the next dose at the scheduled time.

Precautions

Although oprelvekin is effective at increasing the number of platelets in patients following chemotherapy, patients should understand that there are a number of precautions that should be taken when their physician is prescribing oprelvekin.

If the patient has any existing medical problems, he or she should tell the doctor prior to beginning treatment with oprelvekin. Congestive heart failure may be worsened when taking oprelvekin as it causes increased water retention. Oprelvekin can also cause atrial arrhythmias that result in heart rhythm problems. It should also be used with caution in patients with preexisting papilledema or with tumors that involve the central nervous system.

Oprelvekin has not been studied in pregnant women, women who are nursing, or children. However, animal testing has shown that oprelvekin can have negative effects on the fetus and can cause joint and tendon problems in children. It is eliminated primarily by the kidneys and should be used carefully in patients with renal impairment.

Side effects

Although oprelvekin is a synthetic version of a naturally occurring growth factor, there are side effects associated with taking it. The side effects should be weighed against the needed effects of this medication. Some side effects do not require medical attention and others do.

The following are side effects that do not require medical attention and could gradually go away as treatment progresses:

• red eyes
• weakness
• numb extremities such as the hands and feet
• skin reactions such as rash and discoloration

If patients encounter any of the following side effects, they should contact their physicians immediately:

• rapid heartbeat
• irregular heartbeat
• short breath
• white spots in the mouth or on the tongue
• swelling feet and legs
• bloody eye
• blurred vision
• heart rhythm problems

If the patient notices any other side effects not listed, a physician should be contacted immediately.

Interactions

There are no known interactions with oprelvekin.

Resources

BOOKS

Chu, Edward, and Vincent T. DeVita Jr. *Physicians' Cancer Chemotherapy Drug Manual 2014*. Burlington, MA: Jones & Bartlett Learning, 2014.

WEBSITES

American Cancer Society. "Oprelvekin." http://www.cancer.org/treatment/treatmentsandsideeffects/guidetocancer-drugs/oprelvekin (accessed November 10, 2014).
The Scott Hamilton CARES Initiative. "Oprelvekin." Chemo care.com. http://chemocare.com/chemotherapy/drug-info/Oprelvekin.aspx (accessed November 10, 2014).

Sally C. McFarlane-Parrott

Oral cancers

Definition

A **cancer** that occurs in the mouth or the oral cavity and the oropharynx is referred to as an oral cancer.

Description

The oral cavity, known more commonly as the mouth, includes a broad array of parts including the lips; the lining of the lips and cheeks (buccal mucosa); the teeth and gums; and the tongue, floor of the mouth, and hard palate. The oropharynx is a group of structures behind the oral cavity: it includes the back of the tongue, the soft palate, and the tonsils. The oral cavity also contains salivary glands; secretions from these glands are called saliva and aid in the digestion of food. There are three major pairs of salivary glands: the parotid glands, which lie behind the jaw close to the ears; the submandibular glands, which lie beneath the floor of the mouth and produce about two-thirds of the total

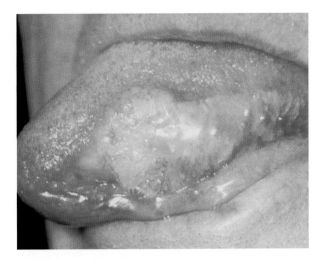

Close-up of large cancerous tumor on the tongue. *(Biophoto Associates/Science Source)*

KEY TERMS

Biopsy—Removal of a portion of tissue or cells for microscopic examination. Incisional biopsy is removal of a small tissue sample. Excisional biopsy is removal of entire tumor or lesion. Fine-needle biopsy is the removal of a tissue sample or fluid with a needle.

Brachytherapy—A form of radiation therapy in which small pellets of radioactive material are placed inside or near the area to be treated. It is also known as internal radiation therapy or sealed-source radiotherapy.

Buccal—Pertaining to the mouth or cheeks. It is derived from the Latin word for cheek.

Erythroplakia—A flat red patch or lesion in the mouth.

Leukoplakia—A flat, whitish-colored area of the oral mucosa that is not caused by thrush or any other specific disease.

Lymph node—Bean-shaped mass of lymphatic tissue surrounded by connective tissue. Lymph nodes contain lymphocytes, which are cells that help to maintain the immune system.

Mandible—The medical term for the lower jaw or jawbone.

Maxilla—The medical term for the upper jaw, which is formed by the fusion of two bones at the center of the roof of the mouth.

Mohs surgery—A form of microscopically controlled surgery that allows for the precise removal of cancerous tissue. It is commonly used to treat various types of skin cancer, particularly in areas of the body where maximum tissue preservation is essential. Mohs surgery is also known as micrographic surgery.

Oropharynx—A set of structures behind the oral cavity that lies between the upper portion of the pharynx and the lower portion of the throat. The oropharynx contains the tonsils, the base of the tongue, and the soft palate.

Otolaryngologist—A physician who diagnoses and treats disorders of the head and neck; sometimes called an ear, nose, and throat specialist or ENT.

Palliative care—Care intended to relieve pain and other symptoms of cancer rather than cure the disease.

Prosthesis—An artificial device used to replace a missing body part.

Squamous cell—A flat, scale-like cell found in epithelial tissue. Squamous cells are polygon-shaped when viewed from above.

Squamous cell carcinoma—A malignancy that arises from outer skin cells.

Targeted therapy—A type of drug treatment for cancer that blocks tumors by interfering with specific molecules that the cancer cells need for growth. Also called biologic therapy, targeted therapy is less harmful to normal cells than traditional chemotherapy.

---

volume of saliva; and the sublingual glands, which lie beneath the tongue.

Under normal circumstances, the oral cavity and oropharynx comprise several types of tissues and cells; tumors can develop from any of these cells. These tumors may be benign (they do not spread to the adjoining tissues), or the tumor may invade other tissues of the body. Any potential growth of a benign tumor into a cancerous (malignant) tumor is referred to as a precancerous condition. Leukoplakia or erythroplakia, which are abnormal areas in the oral cavity, may develop as the first stage in many of the oral cancers. Leukoplakia refers to white areas that are usually benign, but approximately 5% of leukoplakias develop into cancer. Erythroplakia refers to red bumpy areas in the mouth that

bleed when scraped; they have a greater potential to develop into cancer if not treated.

Benign tumors are those that are not invasive and thus incapable of spreading. Examples of benign tumors of the oral cavity include keratoacanthoma, leiomyoma, osteochondroma, neurofibroma, papilloma, schwannoma, and odontogenic tumors. These tumors are generally harmless and can be surgically removed. Recurrence of these tumors after surgical removal is very rare.

More than 90% of malignant tumors of the oral cavity and oropharynx are squamous cell carcinomas. Squamous cells form the lining of the oral cavity and oropharynx; morphologically, they appear flat and scale-like. When the cancer appears only in the lining of the oral cavity, it is referred to as **carcinoma** in situ and marks the initial stages of the squamous cell cancer. Appearance of cancer cells on deeper layers of the oral cavity or oropharynx refers to invasive squamous cell cancer, which is a more serious condition. Verrucous carcinomas are a wart-like type of squamous cell carcinoma that seldom metastasize but can spread to the adjoining tissues. Thus a surgeon might suggest removal of a wide area of surrounding tissues in addition to removal of the cancerous tissue. The chance of developing a second cancer in the oral region (oral cavity or pharynx) at a later time in life is about 10%–40%, thus necessitating thorough follow-up examinations. In addition, refraining from smoking and drinking will help to prevent recurrence. Among other types of malignant tumors of the oral cavity are salivary gland cancers and **Hodgkin lymphoma**. The former affects the salivary glands, which are present throughout the mucosal lining of the oral cavity and oropharynx. The latter is the cancer that develops in the lymphoid tissue of the tonsils and base of the tongue.

Demographics

The American Cancer Society estimates that about 37,000 new cases of oral cavity and pharyngeal cancers were diagnosed in the United States in the year 2014, with 7,300 deaths. The estimated number of cases worldwide was about 450,000. Men have twice the risk of oral cancer as women, and men over age 50 are at greatest risk. There does not seem to be much disparity in the prevalence of oral cancer among different racial or ethnic groups in the United States. The demographics of oral cancer are changing, however—nonsmokers below the age of 50 represent the fastest-growing group among people recently diagnosed with oral cancer. It is thought that the spread of **human papillomavirus** (HPV) among younger people is a major factor in this demographic shift.

Certain geographic differences affect the incidence of oral cavity cancers. Hungary and France report higher incidences of the disease than the United States. However, the disease is less common in Japan and Mexico, suggesting that environmental factors may play a key role in the incidence of the disease. Local customs may also affect the rate of oral cancer; for example, the custom in Southeast Asia of chewing betel leaf or gutka, a combination of betel leaf and tobacco, is believed to increase the risk of oral cancer.

About 15% of patients diagnosed with either oral or **oropharyngeal cancer** are known to develop cancer of the adjoining organs (or tissues) including the larynx, esophagus, or lung. The chance of developing a second cancer in the oral region (oral cavity or pharynx) for survivors in later life is about 10%–40%. Thus, a person once diagnosed with cancer of the oral cavity must continue to have follow-up examinations, even if cured completely. In addition, avoiding the use of alcohol and tobacco is believed to lower the risk of recurrence.

Causes and symptoms

Smoking and alcohol consumption are major risk factors for oral and oropharyngeal cancers. These two factors account for approximately 75% of all oral cavity cancers reported in the United States. Smokeless tobacco (chewing tobacco) is yet another important risk factor. Each dip or chew of tobacco contains five times as much nicotine as one cigarette, in addition to 28 potential other **carcinogens**. Infection with human papillomavirus (HPV)—particularly HPV16—is a recently recognized risk factor for oral cancer. Oral HPV infection is more common in men than in women. The risk of oral HPV infection is linked to such sexual behaviors as open-mouth kissing and oral-genital contact (oral sex). The risk of HPV16 infection also increases with the number of a person's sexual partners.

For **lip cancer**, exposure to sunlight appears to be one of the risk factors. Geographical location and sex are also risk factors. While oral cancer is ranked as the sixth-leading cancer among men in the United States, it is the fourth-leading cancer in African American men. About 7% of oral cancers are thought to result from a genetic predisposition; two inherited syndromes linked to an increased risk of oral cancer are **Fanconi anemia** and dyskeratosis congenita. A family history of oral cancer is an additional risk factor.

Other factors that increase the risk of oral cancer include disorders of the immune system, including HIV infection. Certain medications taken following organ transplantation also weaken the immune system and increase risk.

Common symptoms of oral cancer include:

- mouth sores that do not heal
- persistent pain in the mouth
- thickening in the mouth
- white or red patches on the tongue, gums, tonsils, or lining of the mouth
- sore throat or a feeling that something is stuck in the back of the throat
- difficulty in chewing or swallowing
- difficulty in moving the jaw or tongue
- numbness in the gums, tongue, or any other area of the mouth
- swelling of the jaw

- ear pain
- loosening of the teeth
- hoarseness or changes in the voice
- unexplained or unintended weight loss
- presence of a lumpy mass in the neck

Patients with any of the above symptoms that persist for more than a few weeks should seek medical attention.

Diagnosis

Routine screening or examination of the oral cavity by a physician or a dentist is the key to early detection of oral and oropharyngeal cancers; there is, however, no **screening test** for oral HPV infection that has been approved by the Food and Drug Administration (FDA) as of 2014. Thorough self-examination may also help detect abnormal growth in the oral cavity or neck in the early stages. If any of the signs listed above suggest the presence of oral cancer, the physician or dentist may recommend additional tests or procedures to confirm the diagnosis and refer the patient to a specialist, usually an oral surgeon or an otolaryngologist.

Head and neck examination

In addition to thorough physical examinations, physicians focus special attention on the neck and head area. Highly sophisticated fiberoptic scopes inserted through the mouth or nose are used to view the oropharynx. Since patients with oral cancers are at greater risk for additional cancers, physicians carefully examine other parts of the head and neck, including nose, larynx, and lymph nodes. The terms for these procedures are pharyngoscopy, **laryngoscopy**, or nasopharyngoscopy, depending on the specific part that is examined.

Panendoscopy and biopsy

After considering a patient's risk factors, the surgeon may suggest an extensive examination of the oral cavity, oropharynx, larynx, esophagus, trachea, and the bronchi. This overall examination, called panendoscopy, is performed under general anesthesia to avoid discomfort to the patient and to allow a thorough inspection of the neck and head regions. A **biopsy** of the suspected tissue is completed to determine the severity of the cancer. The specimen analyzed in the biopsy might be a scraping from the suspected area, which is then smeared onto a slide, stained, and examined under the microscope. This technique is easy, inexpensive, and offers information about the abnormal lesions. Incisional biopsy is another alternative, which involves the removal of a small piece of tissue from the tumor area. This relatively simple procedure is performed either in the doctor's office or in

the operating room, depending upon the area of the tumor to be removed. The biopsy tissue samples are subjected to various procedures before the cells can be viewed under the microscope. Fine-needle aspiration biopsy (FNAB) is the aspiration of fluid from a mass, lump, or cyst in the neck. This would also include excisional biopsy. Depending upon the type of cells recognized in the aspiration, the pathologist is able to determine whether the cancer is related to the neck or oral region or whether it has metastasized from a distant organ. FNAB may also determine whether a neck mass is benign. Finally, a tissue sample from a biopsy can be tested for the presence of HPV.

Computed tomography and PET scan

A **computed tomography** or CT scan is a sophisticated x-ray that scans parts of the body in cross-section. This procedure is carried out by administering a dye that aids in locating abnormalities. CT scans help physicians judge to what extent the cancer has spread to lymph nodes, the lower mandible, and the neck. A **positron emission tomography** or PET scan involves the injection of a radioactive sugar into the patient's blood. Since cancerous cells use sugar at a higher rate than normal tissue, they emit higher levels of radioactivity. Levels of radioactivity are detected by the PET scanner. Some machines are designed to perform both a CT scan and a PET scan simultaneously.

Magnetic resonance imaging (MRI)

This type of imaging is used for evaluating soft tissue cancers of the tonsil and the base of the tongue. MRIs use radio waves and strong magnets to image structures within the body.

Panorex

Also called a dental panoramic radiograph, a Panorex is a rotating x-ray of the upper and lower jawbones that determines changes that occur from the result of cancers in the oral cavity.

In addition to the imaging tests already discussed, chest **x-rays** help to check for lung cancers in oral cancer patients who smoke. A barium swallow is a commonly performed series of x-rays to assess cancers of the digestive tract in patients with oral cancer. A radionuclide bone scan may be suggested if the physician suspects that the cancer may have spread to the bones.

Other tests may include blood tests to provide a complete blood analysis, including determination of **anemia**, liver disease, kidney disease, and red and white blood cell counts.

Treatment team

The cancer care team typically involves a specialist surgeon, usually either an otolaryngologist or oral surgeon; a dentist; a medical oncologist; oncology nurses; and a radiation therapist. Because treatment of oral cancers often involves adjustments to the patient's diet, a dietitian is commonly consulted. If cancer treatment involves facial disfigurement, a plastic surgeon may perform follow-up surgery.

Clinical staging

The TNM system of the **American Joint Committee on Cancer** is used in staging the cancer, in which the size (T), spread to regional lymph nodes (N), and **metastasis** to other organs (M) are classified.

T classification

- Tx: Information not known and thus tumor cannot be assessed.
- T0: No evidence of primary tumor.
- Tis: Carcinoma in situ, which means the cancer has affected the epithelial cells lining the oral cavity or the oropharynx but the tumor is not deep.
- T1: Tumor is 2 cm (1 cm equals 0.39 inches) or smaller.
- T2: Tumor is larger than 2 cm but smaller than 4 cm.
- T3: Tumor is larger than 4 cm.
- T4: The tumor is any size and has invaded adjacent structures, such as the larynx, bone, connective tissues, or muscles.

N classification

- Nx: Information not known, cannot be assessed.
- N0: No metastasis in the regional lymph node.
- N1: Metastasis in one lymph node on the same side of the primary tumor and smaller than 3 cm.
- N2: Divided into 3 subgroups. N2a is metastasis in one lymph node larger than 3 cm and smaller than 6 cm. N2b is metastasis in multiple lymph nodes on the same side of the tumor, none larger than 6 cm. N2c denotes one or more lymph nodes, which may or may not be on the side of the primary tumor, none larger than 6 cm.
- N3: Metastasis in lymph node larger than 6 cm.

M classification

- Mx: Distant metastasis cannot be assessed, information not known.
- M0: No distant metastasis.
- M1: Distant metastasis present.

Stage grouping

- Stage 0: Carcinoma in situ. The cancer has not invaded deeper layers of tissue, spread to nearby lymph nodes, or spread to distant sites.
- Stage I: The tumor is 2 cm across or smaller, and has not spread to nearby structures, lymph nodes, or distant sites.
- Stage II: The tumor is larger than 2 cm across but smaller than 4 cm. It has not spread to nearby structures, lymph nodes, or distant sites.
- Stage III: The tumor is larger than 4 cm across but has not spread to nearby lymph nodes or distant sites; or it has spread to one lymph node on the same side of the head or neck but not to distant sites.
- Stage IVA: The tumor is growing into nearby structures and can be any size. It has either not spread to nearby lymph nodes or has spread to one lymph node on the same side of the head or neck but not to distant sites; or the tumor is any size and may or may not grow into nearby structures but has spread either to two or more lymph nodes, to one lymph node on the same side of the neck that is between 3 cm and 6 cm across, or to a lymph node on the opposite side of the neck that is no more than 6 cm across.
- Stage IVB: The tumor is growing into deeper areas or tissues; it may or may not have spread to lymph nodes but has not spread to distant sites; or the tumor is any size and may or may not have grown into other structures but has spread to one or more lymph nodes larger than 6 cm across. It has not spread to distant sites.
- Stage IVC: The tumor is any size, and it may or may not have spread to nearby lymph nodes, but it has spread to distant sites, most commonly the lungs.

Treatment

After the cancer is diagnosed and staged, the medical team will discuss treatment options. Cancers of the oral cavity are generally treated with surgery first, followed by **radiation therapy** or **chemotherapy**. Cancers of the oropharynx are usually treated either with trans-oral robotic surgery (TORS) or with a combination of radiation therapy and chemotherapy. Treatment decisions are reached on the basis of the stage of the disease, the physical health of the patient, and the possible impact of the treatment on the patient's speech, swallowing, chewing, or general appearance.

Surgery

Primary tumor resection involves removal of the entire tumor with some normal adjacent tissue surrounding the tumor to ensure that all of the residual cancerous mass is removed. Partial mandible resection is carried out in cases where involvement of the jawbone is suspected, even though the x-ray does not reveal evidence. Full mandible resection is performed when the x-rays indicate destruction of the jawbone. Cancers of the oropharynx may be treated by resection using trans-oral robotic surgery or TORS. In the past, these cancers were difficult to treat with open-throat surgery due to high incidence of postoperative complications. TORS, however, allows the surgeon to remove cancerous tissue from the oropharynx through the mouth, thus avoiding open-throat procedures.

Maxillectomy is the removal of the hard palate. A special denture called a prosthesis can alter the defect in the hard palate that results from the surgery. **Mohs surgery** involves removal of thin sections of lip tumors. Immediate examination of the sections for potential cancer cells allows the surgeon to determine whether the cancer has been completely removed.

Laryngectomy is the surgical removal of the larynx (voice box). It is performed when removal of tumors of the tongue or oropharynx increases the risk of food entering the trachea and infecting the lungs. By removing the larynx, the trachea is attached to the skin of the neck, thus eliminating the risk of infecting the lung and potential **pneumonia**.

Neck dissection is a surgical procedure involving the removal of lymph nodes in the neck known to contain cancer cells. The side effects of this surgery include numbness of the ear, difficulty in raising the arm above the head, and discomfort to the lower lip—all of which may result from nerve damage during surgery.

Tracheostomy is an incision made in the trachea to facilitate breathing for oral cancer patients who may develop considerable swelling when a tumor in the oral cavity is surgically removed. This procedure prevents obstruction in the throat and allows easy breathing.

In addition to these surgical procedures, dental extractions and removal of large tumors in oral cancer patients may require later **reconstructive surgery**.

Radiation therapy

Radiation therapy is the use of high-energy rays to kill or reduce the growth of cancer cells. Small tumors are sometimes treated with radiation only, or radiation therapy may be combined with surgery to destroy deposits of cancer cells. Radiation is also suggested for relief of cancer symptoms, including bleeding and difficulty swallowing. Radiation may be administered either externally or internally. External radiation (also called external beam radiation therapy) delivers radiation to oral or oropharyngeal cancers from outside the body. Brachytherapy, or internal radiation, involves the surgical implant of metal rods that deliver radioactive materials in or near the cancer.

Chemotherapy

Chemotherapy involves the administration of **anti-cancer drugs** parenterally or orally. Chemotherapy may be suggested in combination with radiation therapy for some large tumors of the head and neck to avoid surgery in those regions. Some studies indicate that chemotherapy is ideal for shrinking the size of the tumor before surgery or initiation of radiation therapy. This form of chemotherapy is termed neoadjuvant chemotherapy. The drugs most often used in chemotherapy for oral cancers include 5-fluorouracil, **bleomycin**, **cisplatin**, **carboplatin**, paclitaxel, **methotrexate**, and **docetaxel**.

Targeted therapy

A newer form of pharmacotherapy is targeted therapy (sometimes called biologic therapy), which uses drugs that block the growth of cancer cells by targeting specific molecules needed by cancer cells for growth and reproduction. The targeted drug used most often to treat oral cancer is **cetuximab**, which may be combined with radiation therapy for earlier-stage cancers or with cisplatin for advanced-stage oral cancers. Cetuximab works by targeting the epidermal growth factor receptor (EGFR), a protein on the surface of certain cells that helps those cells grow and divide. Cancers of the oral cavity usually have greater than normal amounts of EGFR, which increases the effectiveness of cetuximab. Other drugs that target EGFR are currently under investigation as treatments for oral cancer.

Palliative care

Patients for whom all treatments for oral cancer have failed often benefit from palliative care, or care intended to control pain and relieve other symptoms, rather than cure the disease. At the end of life, patients and their families may consider **hospice care**, available at home as well as in a separate hospice facility.

Treatment choices by stage and prognosis

Depending on the stage of cancer spread, different treatment options are recommended for oral cancer.

Stage 0: Surgical stripping or thin resection is suggested at this stage, before the cancer has become invasive. If there is repeated recurrence, radiation therapy is an option. More than 95% of the patients at this stage survive for years without requiring further surgery on their oral cavity.

QUESTIONS TO ASK YOUR DOCTOR

- What is a cancer of the oral cavity or the oropharynx?
- How far has the cancer spread beyond its primary site?
- What is the stage of the cancer?
- What are the available treatment options?
- What are the chances of survival?
- What are the side effects of treatment?
- What are the potential risks of specific treatments?
- How long will it take to recover from treatment?
- What are the chances of recurrence?
- What is the benefit of one treatment over the other in terms of recurrence?
- How should I prepare for treatment?
- Should I get a second opinion?

Stages I and II: Surgery or radiation therapy is the treatment of choice, depending on the location of the tumor in the oral cavity and oropharynx.

Stages III and IV: Therapy that combines either surgery and radiation, radiation and chemotherapy, or all three types of treatment may be required for these advanced stages of cancer. About 20%–50% of patients who undergo a combination of surgery and radiation for stages III and IV oral cavity and oropharyngeal cancers will survive for five years after treatment.

Alternative and complementary therapies

While there are no alternative or complementary therapies that claim to cure oral cancers, patients may find such complementary treatments as guided imagery, prayer or meditation, journaling, relaxation techniques, massage therapy, or music therapy helpful in coping with the emotional stress of a cancer diagnosis and the side effects of cancer treatments.

Coping with cancer treatment

Cancer of any type is a psychologically stressful journey from the time of diagnosis through treatment and recovery. Coping with the side effects of treatment both physically and emotionally is a challenge to the patient, the family, and the medical team. Oral cancers are further complicated by the fact that surgery most often leads to

disfigurement, which may be devastating in a society that attaches great importance to physical appearance. Reconstructive surgeries or facial prostheses may be psychologically helpful, and the cancer care team may advise on this issue. Laryngectomy or removal of the voice box leaves the person without speech, and breathing through a stoma (artificial opening in the neck). A stoma cover helps in hiding the mucus that the stoma secretes and also serves as a filter in the absence of the nose's natural filter. In addition to laryngectomy, surgery on the jaw, plate, or tongue can also disrupt speech. The cancer care team can usually help the patient make contact with a certified speech therapist and a local support group.

Side effects of chemotherapy may include **fatigue** and hair loss (**alopecia**) and may affect a patient's quality of life. Some patients wear a wig for cosmetic purposes to hide the hair loss. Studies have concluded that abstaining from smoking and drinking helps patients gradually regain their health after chemotherapy.

Clinical trials

A clinical trial is the evaluation on a selected patient population of a potential treatment for a disease. As of mid-2014, there were 1,622 open studies in the United States for patients with oral or oropharyngeal cancer. These studies included new imaging techniques; **investigational drugs**; applications of transoral robotic surgery to a wider range of **head and neck cancers**; further research into the relationship between HPV and oral cancers; and studies of various therapies to treat the side effects of chemotherapy or radiation therapy for oral cancer.

Prevention

Since oral cavity and oropharyngeal cancer patients are at risk of recurrence or of developing secondary cancers in the head and neck area, close follow-up is mandatory. A thorough examination every month in the first year, at least every three months in the following year, and yearly thereafter is the recommended schedule to facilitate early detection of the cancer's recurrence. Various chemopreventive drugs are being tested to prevent the occurrence of secondary tumors in the neck and head region.

Tobacco (smoking, chewing, spitting) and alcohol consumption are major risk factors for oral and oropharyngeal cancers. Public knowledge regarding the risk factors for oral cancers and the signs of early detection is limited. Only 25% of U.S. adults can detect early signs of an abnormal oral cavity; and only 13% understand the implications of regular alcohol consumption in developing oral cancer. **Cancer prevention** and control programs are growing rapidly with screening services for high-risk populations, health promotion, education, and intervention strategies. National Spit Tobacco Education Program (NSTEP), an initiative of Oral Health America, educates the public about dangers of spit tobacco and its link to oral cancer.

Since exposure to sun may cause lip cancers, regular use of lip balm is important to protect the lips. Smoking a pipe also increases the risk of this type of cancer.

Special concerns

Surgical treatment for oral cancer may affect normal speech and swallowing. A speech pathologist will educate patients and suggest remedies to alleviate speech and swallowing problems. In addition, a dietitian may help patients select more palatable foods in the event of chewing and swallowing problems. Physicians may recommend saliva supplements if patients experience extreme dryness.

Advances in reconstructive surgery of the mouth and lower face have significantly improved patients' appearance and quality of life after treatment for oral cancer. Some of these reconstructive procedures can now be performed by transoral robotic surgery.

The side effects of cancer treatment often include fatigue. Taking ample time to recover will help improve energy in the long-term. **Smoking cessation**, elimination of alcohol, and maintenance of a balanced diet that includes fruits, vegetables, and whole grains are key to the return to a normal life for patients suffering from oral cancers.

See also Cancer biology; Cancer genetics; Cigarettes.

Resources

BOOKS

Cummings, Louise, ed. *The Cambridge Handbook of Communication Disorders*. Cambridge, UK: Cambridge University Press, 2014.

Harrison, Louis B., et al, eds. *Head and Neck Cancer: A Multidisciplinary Approach*. 4th ed. Philadelphia, PA: Wolters Kluwer Health/Lippincott Williams and Wilkins, 2013.

Hinni, Michael L., and David G. Lott, eds. *Contemporary Transoral Surgery for Primary Head and Neck Cancer*. San Diego, CA: Plural Publishing, 2015.

Kesting, Marco. *Oral Cancer Surgery: A Visual Guide*. New York: Thieme, 2014.

Ward, Elizabeth C., and Corina J. van As-Brooks, eds. *Head and Neck Cancer: Treatment, Rehabilitation, and Outcomes*, 2nd ed. San Diego, CA: Plural Publishing, 2015.

PERIODICALS

Baumeister, P., et al. "Surgically Treated Oropharyngeal Cancer: Risk Factors and Tumor Characteristics." *Journal of Cancer Research and Clinical Oncology* 140 (June 2014): 1011–1019.

Brickman, D., and N.D. Gross. "Robotic Approaches to the Pharynx: Tonsil Cancer." *Otolaryngologic Clinics of North America* 47 (June 2014): 359–372.

Fried, J.L. "Confronting Human Papilloma Virus/Oropharyngeal Cancer: A Model for Interprofessional Collaboration." *Journal of Evidence-based Dental Practice* 14, suppl. (June 2014): 136–146.e1.

Hayes, D.N., et al. "An Exploratory Subgroup Analysis of Race and Gender in Squamous Cancer of the Head and Neck: Inferior Outcomes for African American Males in the LORHAN Database." *Oral Oncology* 50 (June 2014): 605–610.

Mirghani, H., et al. "Human Papilloma Virus Testing in Oropharyngeal Squamous Cell Carcinoma: What the Clinician Should Know." *Oral Oncology* 50 (January 2014): 1–9.

Sasahira, T., T. Kirita, and H. Kuniyasu. "Update of Molecular Pathobiology in Oral Cancer: A Review." *International Journal of Clinical Oncology* 19 (June 2014): 431–436.

Seiwert, T.Y., et al. "A Randomized, Phase 2 Study of Afatinib versus Cetuximab in Metastatic or Recurrent Squamous Cell Carcinoma of the Head and Neck." *Annals of Oncology* 25, no. 9 (2014): 1813–20.

Selber, J.C., et al. "Transoral Robotic Reconstructive Surgery." *Seminars in Plastic Surgery* 28 (February 2014): 35–38.

Vainshtein, J.M., et al. "Refining Risk Stratification for Locoregional Failure after Chemoradiotherapy in Human Papillomavirus-associated Oropharyngeal Cancer." *Oral Oncology* 50 (May 2014): 513–519.

OTHER

American Cancer Society (ACS). "Oral Cavity and Oropharyngeal Cancer." http://www.cancer.org/acs/groups/cid/documents/webcontent/003128-pdf.pdf (accessed May 15, 2014).

National Cancer Institute (NCI). "What You Need to Know about Oral Cancer." http://www.cancer.gov/cancertopics/wyntk/oral/WYNTK_oral.pdf (accessed June 21, 2014).

WEBSITES

American Dental Association (ADA). "Oral Cancer." http://www.ada.org/en/member-center/oral-health-topics/oral-cancer (accessed June 21, 2014).

National Cancer Institute (NCI). "Oral Cancer." http://www.cancer.gov/cancertopics/types/oral (accessed May 15, 2014).

Oral Cancer Foundation (OCF). "Oral Cancer Facts." http://www.oralcancerfoundation.org/facts/ (accessed June 21, 2014).

Scully, Crispian. "Cancers of the Oral Mucosa." Medscape Reference. http://emedicine.medscape.com/article/1075729-overview (accessed May 15, 2014).

WebMD. "Oral Cancer." http://www.webmd.com/oral-health/guide/oral-cancer (accessed June 21, 2014).

ORGANIZATIONS

American Academy of Facial Plastic and Reconstructive Surgery (AAFPRS), 310 South Henry Street, Alexandria, VA 22314, (703) 299-9291, Fax: (703) 299-8898, info@aafprs.org, http://www.aafprs.org/.

American Academy of Otolaryngology—Head and Neck Surgery, 1650 Diagonal Road, Alexandria, VA 22314-2857, (703) 836-4444, http://entnet.org/content/contact_us, http://entnet.org/.

American Cancer Society (ACS), 250 Williams Street NW, Atlanta, GA 30303, (800) 227-2345, http://www.cancer.org/aboutus/howwehelpyou/app/contact-us.aspx, http://www.cancer.org/index.

American Dental Association (ADA), 211 East Chicago Ave., Chicago, IL 60611-2678, (312) 440-2500, http://www.ada.org/en.

National Cancer Institute (NCI), BG 9609 MSC 9760, 9609 Medical Center Drive, Bethesda, MD 20892-9760, (800) 4-CANCER (422-6237), http://www.cancer.gov/global/contact/email-us, http://www.cancer.gov/.

Oral Cancer Foundation, 3419 Via Lido #205, Newport Beach, CA 92663, (949) 723-4400, http://www.oralcancerfoundation.org/contact/index.html, http://www.oralcancerfoundation.org/.

Support for People with Oral and Head and Neck Cancer (SPOHNC), P.O. Box 53, Locust Valley, NY 11560-0053, (800) 377-0928, Fax: (516) 671-8794, info@spohnc.org, http://www.spohnc.org/.

Kausalya Santhanam, PhD
Rebecca J. Frey, PhD

Ora-Testryl *see* **Fluoxymesterone**

Orbital exenteration *see* **Exenteration**

Orchiectomy

Definition

Orchiectomy is the surgical removal of one or both testicles, or testes, in the human male. It is also called an orchidectomy, particularly in British publications. The removal of both testicles is known as a bilateral orchiectomy, or castration, because the person is no longer able to reproduce.

Purpose

An orchiectomy is done to treat **cancer** or to lower the level of **testosterone**, the primary male sex hormone, in the body. Surgical removal of a testicle is the usual treatment if a tumor is found within the gland itself, but an orchiectomy may also be performed to treat **prostate cancer** or cancer of the male breast, as testosterone causes these cancers to grow and metastasize (spread to other parts of the body). An orchiectomy is sometimes done to prevent cancer when an undescended testicle is found in a patient who is beyond the age of puberty.

Description

There are three basic types of orchiectomy: simple, subcapsular, and inguinal (or radical). The first two types are usually done under local or epidural anesthesia and take about 30 minutes to perform. An inguinal orchiectomy is sometimes done under general anesthesia and takes between 30–60 minutes to complete.

Simple orchiectomy

A simple orchiectomy is performed as part of gender reassignment surgery or as palliative treatment for advanced cancer of the prostate. The patient lies flat on an operating table with the penis taped against the abdomen. After the anesthetic has been given, the surgeon makes an incision in the midpoint of the scrotum and cuts through the underlying tissue. The surgeon removes the testicles and parts of the spermatic cord through the incision. The incision is closed with two layers of sutures and covered with a surgical dressing. If the patient desires, a prosthetic testicle can be inserted before the incision is closed to give the appearance of a normal scrotum from the outside.

Subcapsular orchiectomy

A subcapsular orchiectomy is also performed for treatment of prostate cancer. The operation is similar to a simple orchiectomy, with the exception that the glandular tissue is removed from the lining of each testicle rather than the entire gland being removed. This type of orchiectomy is done primarily to keep the appearance of a normal scrotum.

Inguinal orchiectomy

An inguinal orchiectomy, which is sometimes called a radical orchiectomy, is done when **testicular cancer** is suspected. It may be either unilateral, involving only one testicle, or bilateral. This procedure is called an inguinal orchiectomy because the surgeon makes the incision, which is about 3 in. (7.6 cm) long, in the patient's groin area rather than directly into the scrotum. It is called a radical orchiectomy because the surgeon removes the entire spermatic cord as well as the testicle itself. The reason for this complete removal is that testicular cancers frequently spread from the spermatic cord into the lymph nodes near the kidneys. A long nonabsorbable suture is

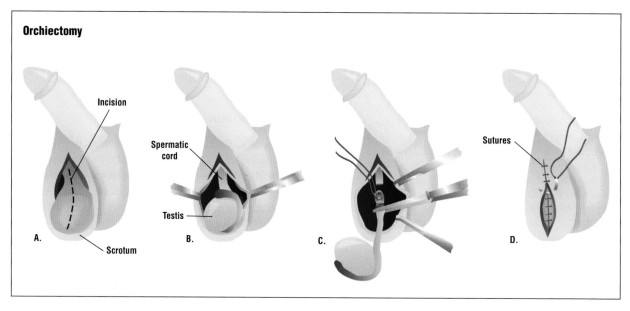

Orchiectomy

A. Incision — Scrotum

B. Spermatic cord — Testis

C.

D. Sutures

In an orchiectomy, the scrotum is cut open (A). The testicle covering is cut to expose the testis and spermatic cord (B). The cord is tied and cut, removing the testis (C), and the wound is repaired (D). *(Illustration by GGS Information Services. © Cengage Learning®.)*

left in the stump of the spermatic cord in case later surgery is necessary.

After the cord and testicle have been removed, the surgeon washes the area with saline solution and closes the various layers of tissues and skin with various types of sutures. The wound is then covered with sterile gauze and bandaged.

Diagnosis

The doctor may suspect that a patient has prostate cancer from feeling a mass in the prostate in the course of a rectal examination, from the results of a transrectal ultrasound (TRUS), or from elevated levels of prostate-specific antigen (PSA) in the patient's blood. PSA is a tumor marker, or chemical, in the blood that can be used to detect cancer and monitor the results of therapy. A definite diagnosis of prostate cancer, however, requires a tissue **biopsy**. The tissue sample can usually be obtained with the needle technique. Testicular cancer is suspected when the doctor feels a mass in the patient's scrotum, which may or may not be painful. In order to perform a biopsy for definitive diagnosis, however, the doctor must remove the affected testicle by radical orchiectomy.

Preparation

All patients preparing for an orchiectomy will have standard blood and urine tests before the procedure. They are asked to discontinue aspirin-based medications for a week before surgery and all **nonsteroidal anti-inflammatory drugs** (NSAIDs) two days before the procedure. Patients should not eat or drink anything for the eight hours before the scheduled time of surgery.

Most surgeons ask patients to shower or bathe on the morning of surgery using a special antibacterial soap. They should take extra time to lather, scrub, and rinse their genitals and groin area.

Patients who are anxious or nervous before the procedure are usually given a sedative to help them relax.

Patients who are having an orchiectomy as treatment for testicular cancer should consider banking sperm if they plan to have children following surgery. Although it is possible to father a child if only one testicle is removed, some surgeons recommend banking sperm as a precaution in case the other testicle should develop a tumor at a later date.

Aftercare

Patients who are having an orchiectomy in an ambulatory surgery center or other outpatient facility must have a friend or family member to drive them home after the procedure. Most patients can go to work the following day, although some may need an additional day of rest at home. Even though it is normal for patients to feel nauseated after the anesthetic wears off, they should start eating regularly when they get home. Some pain and swelling is also normal; the doctor will usually prescribe a pain-killing medication to be taken for a few days.

KEY TERMS

Androgen—Any substance that promotes the development of masculine characteristics in a person. Testosterone is one type of androgen; others are produced in the adrenal glands located above the kidneys.

Bilateral—On both sides. A bilateral orchiectomy is the removal of both testicles.

Capsule—A general medical term for a structure that encloses another structure or body part. The capsule of the testicle is the membrane that surrounds the glandular tissue.

Castration—Removal or destruction by radiation of both testicles (in a male) or both ovaries (in a female), making the individual incapable of reproducing.

Cryptorchidism—A developmental disorder in which one or both testes fail to descend from the abdomen into the scrotum before birth.

Emasculation—Another term for castration of a male.

Epidural—A type of regional anesthetic delivered by injection into the area around the patient's lower spine. An epidural numbs the body below the waist but allows the patient to remain conscious throughout the procedure.

Gender identity disorder (GID)—A condition in which a person strongly identifies with the other sex and feels uncomfortable with his or her biological sex. It occurs more often in males than in females.

Gender reassignment surgery—The surgical alteration and reconstruction of a person's sex organs to resemble those of the other sex as closely as possible; it is sometimes called sex reassignment surgery.

Inguinal—Referring to the groin area.

Metastasis—A process in which a malignant tumor transfers cells to a part of the body not directly connected to its primary site. A cancer that has spread from its original site to other parts of the body is said to be metastatic.

Oophorectomy—Removal of one or both ovaries in a woman.

Orchiectomy—Surgical removal of one or both testicles in a male. It is also called an orchidectomy.

Scrotum—The pouch of skin on the outside of the male body that holds the testes.

Spermatic cord—A tube-like structure that extends from the testicle to the groin area. It contains blood vessels, nerves, and a duct to carry spermatic fluid.

Subcapsular—Inside the outer tissue covering of the testicle. A subcapsular orchiectomy is a procedure in which the surgeon removes the inner glandular tissue of the testicle while leaving the outer capsule intact.

Testis (plural, testes)—The medical term for a testicle.

Testosterone—The major male sex hormone, produced in the testes.

Tumor marker—A circulating biochemical compound that indicates the presence of cancer. Tumor markers can be used in diagnosis and in monitoring the effectiveness of treatment.

Urology—The branch of medicine that deals with disorders of the urinary tract in both males and females, and with the genital organs in males.

Other recommendations for aftercare include:

• Drink extra fluids for the next several days, except for caffeinated and alcoholic beverages.

• Avoid sexual activity, heavy lifting, and vigorous exercise until the follow-up appointment with the doctor.

• Take a shower rather than a tub bath for a week following surgery to minimize the risk of absorbable stitches dissolving prematurely.

• Apply an ice pack to the groin area for the first 24–48 hours.

• Wear a jock strap or snug briefs to support the scrotum for two weeks after surgery.

Some patients may require psychological counseling following an orchiectomy as part of their long-term aftercare. Many men have very strong feelings about any procedure involving their genitals, and may feel depressed or anxious about their bodies or their relationships after genital surgery. In addition to individual psychotherapy, support groups are often helpful. There are active networks of prostate cancer support groups in Canada and the United States as well as support groups for men's issues in general.

Long-term aftercare for patients with testicular cancer includes frequent checkups in addition to radiation treatment or **chemotherapy**. Patients with prostate cancer may be given various hormonal therapies or radiation treatment.

Risks

Some of the risks for an orchiectomy done under general anesthesia are the same as for other procedures. They include deep venous thrombosis, heart or breathing problems, bleeding, infection, or reaction to the anesthesia. If the patient is having epidural anesthesia, the risks include bleeding into the spinal canal, nerve damage, or a spinal headache.

Specific risks associated with an orchiectomy include:

• loss of sexual desire (can be treated with hormone injections or gel preparations)

• impotence

• hot flashes similar to those in menopausal women, controllable by medication

• weight gain of 10–15 lb. (4.5–6.8 kg)

• mood swings or depression

• enlargement and tenderness in the breasts

• fatigue

• loss of sensation in the groin or the genitals

• osteoporosis (men taking hormone treatments for prostate cancer are at greater risk)

An additional risk specific to cancer patients is recurrence of the cancer.

Results

Normal results depend on the location and stage of the patient's cancer at the time of surgery. Most prostate cancer patients, however, report rapid relief from cancer symptoms after an orchiectomy. Patients with testicular cancer have a 95% survival rate five years after surgery if the cancer had not spread beyond the testicle. Metastatic testicular cancer, however, has a poorer prognosis.

Alternatives

There is no effective alternative to radical orchiectomy in the treatment of testicular cancer; radiation and chemotherapy are considered follow-up treatments rather than alternatives.

QUESTIONS TO ASK YOUR DOCTOR

• How effective is an orchiectomy in preventing a recurrence of my cancer?

• What side effects of this procedure am I most likely to experience?

• How many orchiectomies have you performed?

• Can you recommend a local men's network or support group?

There are, however, several alternatives to orchiectomy in the treatment of prostate cancer, including:

• watchful waiting

• hormonal therapy, usually either medications that oppose the action of male sex hormones (antiandrogens, usually flutamide or nilutamide) or medications that prevent the production of testosterone (goserelin or leuprolide acetate)

• radiation treatment

• chemotherapy

Health care team roles

Orchiectomy performed as part of cancer therapy may be done in a hospital under general anesthesia, but is most often done as an outpatient procedure in a urology clinic or similar facility. Most surgeons who perform orchiectomies to treat cancer are board-certified urologists or general surgeons.

Resources

PERIODICALS

Fedyanin, Mikhail, et al. "Effect of the Timing of Orchiectomy on Survival in Patients with Metastatic Germ Cell Tumors of Testis." *Urologic Oncology: Seminars and Original Investigations* (April 29, 2013): e-pub ahead of print. http://dx.doi.org/10.1016/j.urolonc.2012.12.001 (accessed October 3, 2014).

Louda, M., et al. "Psychosocial Implications and the Duality of Life Outcomes for Patients with Prostate Carcinoma after Bilateral Orchiectomy." *Neuro Endocrinology Letters* 33, no. 8 (2012): 761–64.

WEBSITES

National Cancer Institute. "Testicular Cancer Treatment (PDQ®)." http://www.cancer.gov/cancertopics/pdq/treatment/testicular/HealthProfessional (accessed October 3, 2014).

Papanikolaou, Frank. "Orchiectomy, Radical." Medscape Reference. http://emedicine.medscape.com/article/449033-overview (accessed October 3, 2014).

UPMC CancerCenter. "Orchiectomy." http://www.upmccancercenter.com/cancer/prostate/hormoneorchtherapy.cfm (accessed October 3, 2014).

ORGANIZATIONS

American Board of Urology, 600 Peter Jefferson Pkwy., Ste. 150, Charlottesville, VA 22911, (434) 979-0059, Fax: (434) 979-0266, http://www.abu.org.

American Cancer Society, 250 Williams St. NW, Atlanta, GA 30303, (800) 227-2345, http://www.cancer.org.

American Prostate Society, 10 E. Lee St., Ste. 1504, Baltimore, MD 21202, (410) 837-3735, Fax: (410) 837-8510, info@americanprostatesociety.com, http://americanprostatesociety.com.

National Cancer Institute, 6116 Executive Blvd., Ste. 300, Bethesda, MD 20892-8322, (800) 4-CANCER (422-6237), http://cancer.gov.

Rebecca Frey, PhD

Oropharyngeal cancer

Definition

Oropharyngeal **cancer** is an uncontrolled growth of cells that begins in the oropharynx, the area at the back of the mouth.

Description

The oropharynx is the passageway at the back of the mouth. It connects the mouth to the esophagus (tube through which food passes) and to the pharynx (the channel for the flow of air into and out of the lungs). It takes its name from the way it ties the oral cavity (hence the oro) to the rest of the pharynx, one part of which extends toward the back of the nose (nasopharynx). The base of the tongue, the soft palate (the soft roof of the mouth, above the base of the tongue), and the tonsils are part of the oropharynx.

If the oropharynx is blocked or injured in any way, the condition presents a threat to life because it interferes with both eating and breathing. Thus, an obstruction caused by oropharyngeal cancer is in itself a problem. Oropharyngeal cancer also contributes to problems with chewing and talking because of the importance of the oropharynx in these activities. If the oropharyngeal cancer spreads to the bone, muscle, and soft tissue in the neck, there is a severe effect on the ability of the neck

---

KEY TERMS

Biopsy—Tissue sample taken from the body for examination.

Bronchi—Branches of the trachea that distribute air to the air sacs (alveoli) of the lungs.

Computed tomography (CT)—X-rays are aimed at slices of the body (by rotating equipment) and results are assembled with a computer to give a three-dimensional picture of a structure.

Endoscope—Instrument designed to allow direct visual inspection of body cavities, a sort of microscope in a long access tube.

Fiberoptics—Cool, refracted (bounced) light passes (bounces) along extremely small diameter glass tubes; used to illuminate body cavities, such as the oropharynx, with high intensity and almost heatless light.

Larynx—Commonly known as the voice box, the place between the pharynx and the trachea where the vocal cords are located.

Magnetic resonance imaging (MRI)—Magnetic fields and radio frequency waves are used to take pictures of the inside of the body.

Salivary glands—Structures in the mouth that make and release (secrete) saliva that helps with digestion.

Tonsils—Lymph nodes in the throat that are partly encapsulated (enclosed). They are components of the lymphatic system, which functions in immunity and removes the excess fluid around cells and returns it to cells.

Trachea—Tube ringed with cartilage that connects the larynx with the bronchi.

---

to support the head. In individuals with oropharyngeal cancer that has spread, surgical options might be limited.

Oropharyngeal cancer usually begins in the squamous cells of the epithelial tissue. The squamous cells are flat, and often layered. The epithelial tissue forms coverings for the surfaces of the body. Skin, for example, has an outer layer of epithelial tissue. Throughout the oropharynx there are some very small salivary glands and one or more of them sometimes becomes the site of tumor growth.

Many times cancer that begins in the oropharynx spreads to the base of the tongue. Oropharyngeal cancer can spread to the muscle and bone in the neck, and also to the soft tissue that fills the space around the muscle and bone.

Demographics

In the United States, about 4,000 cases of oropharyngeal cancer are diagnosed each year. Most of the cancer is found in people who are more than 50 years old. A history of tobacco or alcohol use, especially heavy use, is typically linked to the diagnosis. Men are three to five times more likely to be diagnosed than women.

Some benign tumors arise in the oropharynx. Although they are benign, many studies suggest the growths indicate the person is at greater risk for a malignant tumor growth in the future.

Causes and symptoms

The cause of oropharyngeal cancer is not known, but the risk factors for oropharyngeal cancer are understood. Three important lifestyle choices increase the chance a person will be diagnosed with cancer of the oropharynx. They are tobacco use, alcohol consumption, and certain sexual practices.

Anything that passes into the lungs or stomach through the nose and mouth must move through the oropharynx. (Air moves through the nasopharynx to reach the oropharynx.) Long periods of exposure to substances such as tobacco byproducts and alcohol somehow trigger cells to begin uncontrolled growth, or cancer. About 90% of all cancer of the oropharynx starts in a squamous cell.

Since tobacco and alcohol come into direct contact with the squamous cells of the oropharynx as they move through the cavity, they might change the genetic material (DNA) of cells. If a cell cannot repair damage to DNA, a cancerous growth can begin.

A serious interaction occurs between tobacco and alcohol. Individuals who smoke and drink alcoholic beverages are at much greater risk for oropharyngeal cancer. They have as much as 30 to 40 times the normal risk. The estimate is difficult to make because not all individuals diagnosed are accurate in the statements they make to physicians about their use of these substances. Patients often say they used less tobacco or less alcohol than they actually did.

Viral infection increases the risk of oropharyngeal cancer. So does reduced immunity, which is a condition that may be caused by viral infection. Individuals with human papillomaviruses, which are sexually transmitted, are known to be at greater risk, particularly those infected by HPV-16. The virus increases a person's risk of cancer because it inactivates the TP53 gene, which regulates the cycle of cell division by keeping cells from dividing in an uncontrolled fashion. The specific sexual practices associated with an increased risk of oropharyngeal cancer include a high lifetime number of sexual partners, oral-genital sex, and oral-anal sex.

Marijuana seems to be linked with oropharyngeal cancer too. Vitamin A deficiency, or specifically, the absence of the carotene (from fruits and vegetables) that the body uses to make vitamin A, might also be a contributing factor.

Symptoms of oropharyngeal cancer include:

- difficulty swallowing
- difficulty chewing
- change in voice
- loss of weight
- lump in the throat
- lump in the neck

Diagnosis

Cells grow old and flake off regularly from epithelial tissues. The first step in diagnosing oropharyngeal cancer often makes use of the natural process. It is given the name exfoliative **cytology**. A physician scrapes cells from the part of the oropharynx where a cancer is suspected and smears them on a slide. The cells are then treated with chemicals so they can be studied with a microscope. If they do not appear normal, a **biopsy**, or a tissue sample from a deeper layer of cells, is taken for examination.

Different sorts of biopsies are used. An incision, or cut, is made to obtain tissue. Or, a needle with a small diameter is inserted into the neck to obtain cells, especially if there is a lump in the neck.

Computed tomography (CT) and **magnetic resonance imaging** (MRI) scans are also used. They help determine whether the cancer has spread from the walls of the oropharynx. MRI offers a good way to examine the tonsils and the back of the tongue, which are soft tissues. CT is used as a way of studying the jaw, which is bone.

Many extremely specialized means of determining the condition of the oropharynx have been developed. One of them relies on the same sort of light wave technology that now powers much of the communications world, fiberoptics. A fiber (a bundle of glass fibers, actually) with a very small diameter is inserted in the oropharynx and the area is probed with light that is reflected on mirrors for interpretation. Lighting up the oropharynx with the high intensity, very low heat illumination of fiberoptics, a physician can get a good look at the cavity.

Another special way of getting a good look at the oropharynx involves studying it from within by inserting an endoscope into the oropharynx and weaving it through adjacent connecting structures. The structures include the trachea, the bronchi, the larynx, and the esophagus. The patient is given an anesthetic, local or general, for this procedure. When several organs are examined at the same time, the procedure is called a panendoscopy. The tool used is generally named for the organ for which it is most closely designed. For example, there is a laryngoscope.

Because oropharyngeal cancer often spreads, bones near the oropharynx must be examined carefully. Some special types of equipment are used. A rotating x-ray called Panorex provides for close inspection of the jaw.

Oropharyngeal cancer also spreads to the esophagus, so physicians usually examine the esophagus when they diagnose oropharyngeal cancer. To do so, they ask the patient to drink a liquid containing barium, a chemical that can be seen on x-rays. Then, they can x-ray the esophagus and look for bulges or lumps that indicate cancer there.

Treatment team

Generally, physicians with special training in the organs of the throat take responsibility for the care of a patient with oropharyngeal cancer. They are called otolaryngologists or occasionally otorhinolaryngologists.

In abbreviation, otolaryngologists are usually labeled ENT (for ear, nose, and throat) specialists. An ENT specializing in cancer will probably lead the team. Some ENTs have a specialty in surgery. Some have a specialty in oncology. Some have a specialty in both.

Nurses, as well as a nutritionist, speech therapist, and social worker will also be part of the team. Depending on the extent of the cancer when diagnosed, some surgery and treatments result in extensive changes in the throat, neck, and jaw. The social worker, speech therapist, and nutritionist are important in helping the patient cope with the changes caused by surgery and radiation treatment. If there is great alteration to the neck because of surgery, rehabilitation will also be part of the recovery process and a rehabilitation therapist will be added to the team.

The treatment team may also include a psychiatrist, as patients with oropharyngeal cancer have extremely high rates of **depression** compared with other cancer patients. A study carried out at Memorial Sloan Kettering Cancer Center in New York reported in 2004 that as many as 57% of patients with oropharyngeal cancer suffer an episode of major depression, compared to 50%

of **pancreatic cancer** patients, 46% of **breast cancer** patients, and 44% of lung cancer patients.

Clinical staging

Stage 0 indicates some cells with the potential to grow erratically have been discovered. But the cells have not multiplied beyond the surface layer of the epithelial tissue of the oropharynx. Stage I describes a cancer less than approximately 2.5 cm (about one inch in diameter) that has not spread. Stage II describes a bigger cancer, up to about 5 cm (about two inches), that has not spread.

Stage III oropharyngeal cancer is either larger than two inches or has spread to one lymph node. The lymph node is enlarged but not much larger than an inch.

In Stage IV, one or more of several things happens. There is either a spread of cancer to a site near the original site. Or, there is more than one lymph node with cancer. Or, the cancer has spread to other parts of the body, such as the larynx, the trachea, the bronchi, the esophagus, or even more distant points, such as the lungs.

Besides categories, or stages, that indicate how far the disease has progressed, there are many categories that are used to describe the kind, or grade, of tumor. The grades take into account such factors as the density of a tumor. Eventually, physicians hope information about tumor grade will make it possible to match treatment and condition very precisely.

Treatment

For stage I and stage II, surgical removal or **radiation therapy** of the affected area is sometimes all that is required to halt the cell growth. Decisions about which method to use depend on many factors. The tolerance a patient has for radiation or **chemotherapy** and the size of the tumor are crucial to the decision process.

Surgical removal can interfere with speech, eating, and breathing. So, if nonsurgical treatment is an option, it is a good one to try. The larger the tumor, the more urgent its removal. Smaller tumors can be treated with radiation or chemotherapy to shrink them before surgery. Some smaller tumors can be removed completely with a carbon dioxide laser. In some cases, surgery might be avoided. For stage III cancer with lymph node involvement, the lymph nodes with the cancer are also removed.

Chemotherapy might be used at any stage, but it is particularly important for stage IV cancer. In some cases, chemotherapy is used before surgery, just as radiation is, to try to eliminate the cancer without cutting, or at least to make it smaller before it is cut out (excised). After surgery, radiation therapy and chemotherapy are both used to treat patients with stage IV oropharyngeal cancer, sometimes in combination. Treatments vary in Stage IV patients depending on the extent of the spread.

Some tumors are so large they cannot be completely removed by surgery. Often, the most promising treatment option for a person with such a tumor is a clinical trial. One technique that has had some success with recurrent or advanced oropharyngeal tumors is **radiofrequency ablation**. In radiofrequency ablation, the tumor is heated by the application of 90–150 watts of energy to an internal temperature of 60°–110°C (140°–230°F) for a period of 5 to 15 minutes.

Coping with cancer treatment

The patient should be an active member of the treatment team, listening to information and making decisions about which course of treatment to take. Premier cancer centers encourage such a role.

Prior to surgery, discuss the need for a way to communicate if speech is impaired after surgery. A pad and pencil might be all that are needed for a short interval. If there will be a long period of difficulty, the patient should be ready with other means, including special phone service.

A change in appearance after the removal of part of the oropharynx, whether part of the tongue or soft palate or some other portion, can lead to concerns about **body image**. Social interaction might suffer. A support group can help. Discussions with a social worker also can be beneficial.

If any part of the oropharynx is removed, speech therapy might be necessary to relearn how to make certain sounds. If the surgery requires the removal of some or all of the tongue, a person's speech will be greatly impaired.

Appetite might be affected before, during, and after treatment. Before treatment, the presence of a tumor can interfere with chewing and swallowing food, and food might not seem as appealing as it once did. During treatment, particularly radiation treatment, the treated oropharynx will be sore and eating and breathing will be difficult, or impossible.

In some cases, a patient requires a feeding tube (inserted at the opening of the esophagus, through the mouth), a stomach tube (inserted directly in the stomach, if there is no access to the opening of the esophagus), or a breathing tube (inserted directly in the trachea) for some interval of time. The tubes bypass the normal entryways to the stomach and lungs. Liquid food is put directly into the esophagus or stomach. Air is taken directly into the trachea during breathing. The incision or cut in the trachea is called a tracheotomy and the opening in the neck around

the trachea is a **tracheostomy**. Air that enters the trachea directly is not warmed or moistened, and the dry, cold air in the lungs can lead to respiratory complications. Attachments are now available that are positioned at the opening in the neck and filter and add moisture to the air entering the tracheal tube. Learning how to care for the tracheotomy and tracheostomy, how to keep the openings clean, and what to do if the tube pops out relieves anxiety and improves ease of breathing.

After treatment, a loss of sensation in the part of the oropharynx affected, or a loss of part of the tongue or the jaw, can reduce appetite. A nutritionist can help with supplements for people who experience significant **weight loss** and who do not have an appetite (**anorexia**).

Patients who are dependent on tobacco or alcohol products and want to reduce or eliminate their intake will have to deal with the psychological effects of substance withdrawal in addition to the side-effects from treatment. A support group for tobacco or alcohol dependence might be considered and joined before treatment begins.

Clinical trials

There are a number of **clinical trials** in progress. For example, the better researchers understand the nature of cancer cells, the better they are able to design drugs that attack only cancer cells. Or, in some cases, drugs that make it easier to kill cancer cells have also been designed.

Prevention

Avoiding smoking, drinking alcohol, and having oral sex with a large number of partners are important in the prevention of oropharyngeal cancer. Including lots of fruits and vegetables in the diet is also an important step to preventing cancer. (Even though the importance of fruits and vegetables is not proven to prevent oropharyngeal cancer, overall fruits and vegetables are demonstrated cancer fighters.) Carotene, which the body uses to make vitamin A, seems to be important in the diet of people who are less likely to be diagnosed with oropharyngeal cancer. Any precaution that is taken to avoid contracting sexually transmitted diseases, such as the use of condoms, also offers protection from oropharyngeal cancer.

Special concerns

Growths sometimes develop in the oropharynx that are not cancerous. The benign tumors can be removed by surgery. They usually do not recur. The surgeon should be able to give a patient an accurate appraisal identifying the noncancerous growth, and whether it is likely to indicate future problems.

22314, (703) 299-9291, Fax: (703) 299-8898, info@aafprs.org, http://www.aafprs.org.

American Society of Plastic Surgeons, 444 E. Algonquin Rd., Arlington Heights, IL 60005, (847) 228-9900, (800) 514-5058, memserv@plasticsurgery.org, http://www.plastic-surgery.org.

Support for People with Oral and Head and Neck Cancer (SPOHNC), PO Box 53, Locust Valley, NY 11560-0053, (800) 377-0928, Fax: (516) 671-8794, info@spohnc.org, http://www.spohnc.org.

Diane M. Calabrese
Rebecca J. Frey, PhD

Oropharyngeal cancer frequently recurs in patients who have been treated for the condition. Thus, after treatment, patients must be examined monthly for one year. They also must be committed to telling their physician if they notice any changes. By the second year, examinations can be at two-month intervals; and then, three-month intervals by the third year and six-month intervals beyond that.

Mouthwash has been suspected as a cancer-causing agent for oropharyngeal cancer. Studies are not conclusive. One line of reasoning suggests alcohol-based mouthwashes add to the effects of alcohol consumed by heavy drinkers. Alcohol-based mouthwashes can be avoided.

See also Cigarettes; Oral cancer; Nasopharyngeal cancer; Smoking cessation.

Resources

BOOKS

Beers, Mark H., MD, and Robert Berkow, MD, editors. "Disorders of the Oral Region: Neoplasms." *The Merck Manual of Diagnosis and Therapy*. Whitehouse Station, NJ: Merck Research Laboratories, 2007.

PERIODICALS

Baumeister, P., et al. "Surgically Treated Oropharyngeal Cancer: Risk Factors and Tumor Characteristics." *Journal of Cancer Research and Clinical Oncology* 140, no. 6 (2014): 1011–9. http://www.ncbi.nlm.nih.gov/pubmed/24615330 (accessed November 10, 2014).

WEBSITES

American Society of Clinical Oncology. "Oral and Oropharyngeal Cancer." Cancer.net. http://www.cancer.net/cancer-types/oral-and-oropharyngeal-cancer (accessed November 10, 2014).

ORGANIZATIONS

American Academy of Facial Plastic and Reconstructive Surgery (AAFPRS), 310 S. Henry St., Alexandria, VA

Osteosarcoma

Definition

Osteosarcoma, also called osteogenic **sarcoma**, is a type of **cancer** that develops from bone. Osteosarcoma is destructive in its original area and is likely to spread to other parts of the body.

Description

Osteosarcoma is a malignant (cancerous) tumor that arises from bone itself, and is thus called a primary bone cancer. Primary bone cancers are relatively rare overall in humans; interestingly, osteosarcomas are ten times more common in dogs than in humans. Approximately 800 new cases of osteosarcoma occur in the United States each year; about half of these are diagnosed in children and adolescents. Osteosarcomas account for about 3% of **childhood cancers**.

Osteosarcoma occurs most frequently during childhood or adolescence. Most cases of this disease develop between the ages of 10 and 30; the average age at diagnosis is 15. The incidence of osteosarcoma rises again among people in their 60s; about 10% of osteosarcomas are diagnosed in this age group.

Osteosarcoma may occur in any bone, but develops most commonly in long bones, particularly near the knee or upper arm. About 60% of osteosarcomas develop at the knee, 15% at the hip, 10% at the shoulder, 8% at the pelvis, and 7% at the jaw. There are two major types of osteosarcomas: medullary or central osteosarcomas, and peripheral or surface osteosarcomas. Most osteosarcomas are conventional central osteosarcomas. In these, the cancer starts growing within a bone and forms an expanding ball-like mass. The tumor eventually breaks through the surface of the bone and begins to invade such

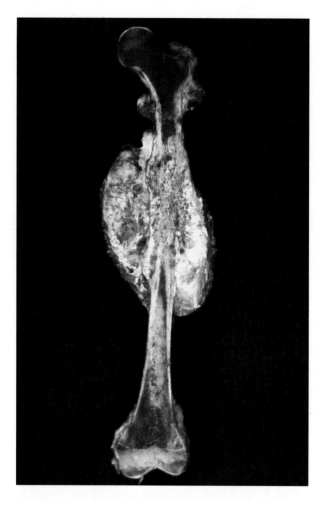

This excised specimen of a femur thigh bone shows the decaying and dryness caused by cancer. *(ST BARTHOLOMEW HOSPITAL /Science Source)*

adjoining structures as muscles. If untreated, the disease usually appears elsewhere in the same limb and metastasizes to such distant parts of the body as the lungs.

Causes and symptoms

Cancers of childhood are different from cancers found primarily in adults in that they typically are caused by DNA mutations that arise early in life or even before birth, and do not have close associations with lifestyle choices or environmental factors, such as occupational exposure to hazardous chemicals. Although the causes of osteosarcoma are not yet fully understood, several risk factors have been identified:

• Age: The risk of osteosarcoma is highest between the ages of 10 and 30, most often during the period of growth of the long bones. This finding suggests that the cancer may develop when the body loses its ability to control the multiplication of certain bone cells.

• Sex: In the United States and Canada, 5.5 boys develop osteosarcoma for every 4 girls.

• Being taller than average for one's age. This finding also suggests a link between osteosarcomas and rapid bone growth.

• Race/ethnicity: African Americans have the highest rate of osteosarcoma, followed by Hispanics/Latinos and Caucasians.

• Genetic factors: These include children with hereditary retinoblastoma (a form of eye cancer), caused by mutations in the *RB1* gene; children with Li-Fraumeni syndrome, caused by a mutation in the *TP53* tumor suppressor gene; and children with Rothmund-Thomson syndrome, caused by a mutation in the *REQL4* gene.

• A history of Paget's disease of bone or hereditary multiple osteochondromas, a bone disease in which many small benign tumors called osteochondromas develop in the bone and cartilage. Osteochondromas sometimes develop into osteosarcomas.

• History of radiation therapy for another cancer.

The most common early symptoms of osteosarcoma are often vague. There may be pain or swelling at the site of the tumor, but these symptoms initially may not seem serious in a young, active person. Thus the patient or medical personnel may attribute the symptoms to growing pains or an injury from sports, for example, and the diagnosis may be delayed. During an office physical examination, the doctor may feel the affected area is warm to the touch, and the affected joint will usually have a decreased range of motion. Eventually, it is possible to feel a firm lump on the bone, and this lump will be uncomfortable to the touch.

In some cases, the child may complain of pain in the affected area that is worse at night. Children whose osteosarcomas are in the long bones of the legs may start to walk with a limp. A relatively rare subtype of osteosarcoma called telangiectatic osteosarcoma may cause unexpected fractures of the weakened bone. In rare cases, children with an osteosarcoma in the pelvis may complain of back pain or have difficulty with bowel or bladder control.

Diagnosis

The complete diagnosis of osteosarcoma is a complicated process, requiring a variety of tests and the help of many different medical specialists. There were no screening tests for osteosarcomas as of 2014; these cancers are usually found when the patient experiences symptoms. Physicians must determine the stage of the cancer (the extent to which it has spread) and the grade of the cancer (the degree of cancerous qualities shown by its

KEY TERMS

Alkaline phosphatase (Alk phos)—A body protein, measurable in the blood, that often appears in high amounts in patients with osteosarcoma. However, many other conditions also elevate the level of alkaline phosphatase.

Chemotherapy—A type of treatment for cancer that attempts to kill tumor cells with doses of powerful, often toxic, chemicals.

Grade—As a noun: a classification of the cancerous qualities of an individual tumor. A higher grade indicates a more serious disease than does a lower grade. As a verb: to classify the cancerous qualities of an individual tumor.

Li-Fraumeni syndrome—A hereditary cancer predisposition syndrome that increases a person's risk of breast cancer, brain cancer, and osteosarcoma.

Malignant—Cancerous.

Medullary osteosarcoma—An osteosarcoma located within the bone. It is also called a central osteosarcoma.

Metastasize—To spread to another part of the body.

Monoclonal antibody—A protein produced in large quantities in a laboratory, designed to attack a specific target in the body.

Osteoblasts—Cells that build up bone by forming the bone matrix.

Osteochondromas—Small benign tumors that develop in the bone and cartilage in people with a hereditary form of this disorder. Osteochondromas are a risk factor for later osteosarcoma.

Osteogenic—Creating bone.

Osteogenic sarcoma—Another name for osteosarcoma.

Paget's disease—A noncancerous disease marked by excessive growth of abnormal bone material.

Peripheral osteosarcoma—An osteosarcoma that develops on the surface of the bone.

Retinoblastoma—A cancerous tumor of the eye.

Rothmund-Thomson syndrome—A rare disorder characterized by short stature, early hair loss, skin rashes, and noncancerous abnormalities of the bones. It is a risk factor for osteosarcoma.

Sarcoma—Any cancer that develops in bone, fat, muscle, cartilage, or soft tissue.

Stage—As a noun: the extent to which an individual cancer has spread. A higher stage indicates a more serious disease than does a lower stage. As a verb: to determine the extent to which an individual cancer has spread.

Tumor—An abnormal growth of cells in the body. Tumors may be benign (non-cancerous) or malignant.

cells in a **biopsy** specimen). About 20% of osteosarcomas have metastasized at the time of diagnosis. A higher grade or stage indicates a more serious disease than does a lower grade or stage. Osteosarcomas are usually staged as localized, metastatic, or recurrent. Localized osteosarcomas are divided into two groups: resectable (removable with surgery) and unresectable.

Initial diagnosis begins with x-ray images of the affected area. These images will show a destructive growth within the bone that is often described as having a "moth-eaten appearance." The patient then requires such further imaging tests as **computed tomography** (CT, CAT), **positron emission tomography** (PET), or magnetic resonance imaging (MRI) scans of the tumor; a chest x-ray series or chest CT; and a nuclear medicine scan of the entire skeleton (bone scan). Blood tests to measure alkaline phosphatase (alk phos) provide additional information. These tests all help determine the stage of the cancer.

Finally, physicians require a biopsy sample of the diseased bone, obtained with a needle or by a surgical procedure, to ensure that the disease is truly cancer and to identify its grade. There are numerous tests, mostly involving examinations under the microscope, to perform on this biopsy specimen.

Treatment

Before the 1980s, limb **amputation** was the standard treatment for osteosarcoma. By that time, the tumor had usually spread elsewhere in the body—most often to the lungs—and the patient eventually died of the disease.

Newer medical developments make it possible to avoid amputation and still treat many patients with osteosarcoma successfully. Patients almost always receive **chemotherapy** with more than one drug (multidrug therapy) before surgery to shrink the original cancer and reduce the likelihood of spread to other areas. This preoperative administration of chemotherapy is known as neoadjuvant therapy. Drugs used in chemotherapy for osteosarcoma include **ifosfamide**, **epirubicin**, **cisplatin** or **carboplatin**, **methotrexate**, **doxorubicin**, **gemcitabine**, or **topotecan**.

Techniques known as limb-sparing surgery often allow removal of the tumor while saving the rest of the extremity. Afterward, patients usually continue to receive chemotherapy, and may require bone grafts or prosthetic devices to replace parts of bones or joints that have been removed. It takes about a year of intensive **physical therapy** for a child to walk again on a leg that has undergone limb-sparing surgery. In addition, most children and adolescents will require some type of psychotherapy or counseling to cope with the effects of treatment on their physical appearance and functioning.

Radiation therapy may be used in patients whose tumors cannot be completely removed via surgery.

Future treatments under investigation include **monoclonal antibodies** that destroy specific cancer cells, techniques to slow cancer growth by controlling certain cellular genes, and bone-seeking substances that directly target areas of active bone growth. There were 77 open **clinical trials** of osteosarcoma therapies in the United States as of mid-2014; most were trials of **investigational drugs**.

Alternative and complementary therapies

Complementary and alternative medicine techniques may improve a patient's sense of well-being and help him or her cope with the side effects of treatment, but will not cure this destructive type of cancer.

Prognosis

Prognosis for an individual patient reflects the complexity of many factors, including the extent to which the cancer has already spread at the time of diagnosis, the aggressiveness of the cells within the cancer, and the response to chemotherapy. Early detection is extremely important. The best chance of cure occurs when a tumor shows no sign of **metastasis** at the time of original surgery, is well-confined within a single bone, is completely removed, and has a good response to chemotherapy.

The five-year survival rate for osteosarcoma in a long bone of a limb is about 60%–80% in patients who undergo chemotherapy and surgery, and have no metastases. Girls generally have a better prognosis than boys, and children with osteosarcomas on the arm or leg have a better prognosis than those with an osteosarcoma on the hip. Survival rates for patients with metastases to the lungs or other bones are 15%–30% even when the affected tissues are successfully removed. A problem unsolved as of 2014 is the poor prognosis for metastatic relapse or recurrence of osteosarcoma. All patients must be followed closely by a physician to watch for cancer recurrence.

Prevention

Prevention of osteosarcoma is difficult because the disease is not related to such adult lifestyle choices as smoking or sun exposure, and the only known environmental factor linked to this form of cancer is radiation therapy for a previous cancer. Further research may improve prevention strategies. Early detection of the disease remains vital. Anyone with persistent pain in a bone or limb should report this to a physician. People with special risk factors including Paget's disease, exposure to significant amounts of radiation, or a family history of certain types of cancer must be especially vigilant.

Resources

BOOKS

Choy, Edwin, and Dana Farber, eds. *Osteosarcoma: Symptoms, Diagnosis and Treatment Options*. Hauppauge, NY: Nova Science Publishers, 2014.

Kleinerman, Eugenie S. *Current Advances in Osteosarcoma*. New York: Springer, 2014.

PERIODICALS

Ando, K., et al. "Current Therapeutic Strategies and Novel Approaches in Osteosarcoma." *Cancers (Basel)* 5 (May 24, 2013): 591–616.

Botter, S.M., D. Neri, and B. Fuchs. "Recent Advances in Osteosarcoma." *Current Opinion in Pharmacology* 16C (June 2014): 15–23.

Loh, A.H., et al. "Management of Local Recurrence of Pediatric Osteosarcoma Following Limb-sparing Surgery." *Annals of Surgical Oncology* 21 (June 2014): 1948–1955.

Luetke, A., et al. "Osteosarcoma Treatment—Where Do We Stand? A State of the Art Review." *Cancer Treatment Reviews* 40 (May 2014): 523–532.

Yamamoto, N., and H. Tsuchiya. "Chemotherapy for Osteosarcoma—Where Does It Come From? What Is It? Where Is It Going?" *Expert Opinion on Pharmacotherapy* 14 (November 2013): 2183–2193.

OTHER

American Cancer Society (ACS). "Osteosarcoma." http://www.cancer.org/acs/groups/cid/documents/webcontent/003129-pdf.pdf (accessed July 7, 2014).

WEBSITES

Cancer.Net. "Osteosarcoma–Childhood." http://www.cancer.net/cancer-types/osteosarcoma-childhood (accessed July 9, 2014).

Cripe, Timothy M. "Pediatric Osteosarcoma." Medscape Reference. http://emedicine.medscape.com/article/988516-overview (accessed July 8, 2024).

Nemours Foundation. "Childhood Cancer: Osteosarcoma." http://kidshealth.org/parent/medical/cancer/cancer_osteosarcoma.html (accessed July 8, 2014).

University of Chicago Corner Children's Hospital. "Osteosarcoma." http://www.uchicagokidshospital.org/specialties/cancer/sarcoma/osteosarcoma/ (accessed July 8, 2014).

ORGANIZATIONS

American Cancer Society (ACS), 250 Williams Street NW, Atlanta, GA 30303, (800) 227-2345, http://www.cancer.org/aboutus/howwehelpyou/app/contact-us.aspx, http://www.cancer.org/index.

American Society of Clinical Oncology (ASCO), 2318 Mill Road, Suite 800, Alexandria, VA 22314, (571) 483-1300, (888) 651-3038, contactus@cancer.net, http://www.asco.org/.

Children's Oncology Group (COG), 222 E. Huntington Drive, Suite 100, Monrovia, CA 91016, (626) 447-0064, Fax: (626) 445-4334, HelpDesk@childrensoncologygroup.org, http://www.childrensoncologygroup.org/.

National Cancer Institute (NCI), BG 9609 MSC 9760, 9609 Medical Center Drive, Bethesda, MD 20892-9760, (800) 4-CANCER (422-6237), http://www.cancer.gov/global/contact/email-us, http://www.cancer.gov/.

Kenneth J. Berniker, MD
REVISED BY ABIGAIL V. BERNIKER, BA
REVISED BY REBECCA J. FREY, PhD

Ovarian cancer

Definition

Ovarian **cancer** is cancer of the ovaries, the egg-releasing and hormone-producing organs of the female reproductive tract. In ovarian cancer, malignant (cancerous) cells divide and multiply in an uncontrolled, abnormal fashion to form a tumor.

Description

The ovaries are small almond-shaped organs located in the pelvic region, one on either side of the uterus. During a woman's childbearing years, the ovaries

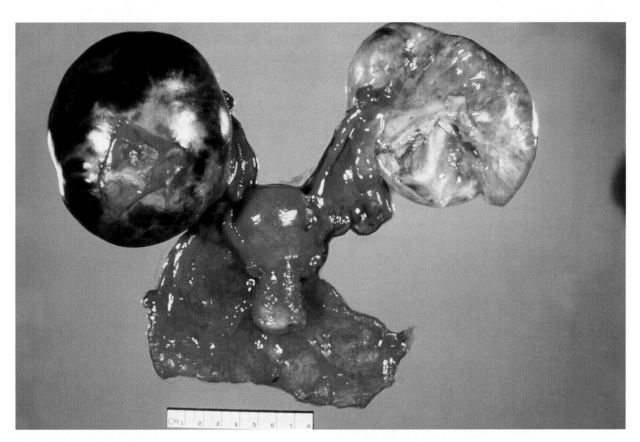

Excised female reproductive organs, showing a cancerous ovary (left, black). *(ST BARTHOLOMEW HOSPITAL/Science Source)*

generally alternate to produce and release one egg each month as part of the normal menstrual cycle. The released egg is shunted into the adjacent Fallopian tube and moves downward to the uterus where, if fertilized, it will implant and develop into a fetus, and if unfertilized will be shed along with menstrual blood. The ovaries also secrete the female hormones estrogen and progesterone, which help regulate the menstrual cycle and pregnancy, as well as support the development of the secondary female sexual characteristics (i.e., breasts, body shape, vocal pitch, and body hair). During pregnancy and when women take certain medications, mainly oral contraceptives, the ovaries do not produce eggs.

Types of ovarian tumors

The ovaries contain three main types of cells: epithelial cells, stromal cells, and germ cells. About 90% of all ovarian cancers develop from epithelial cells covering the surface of the ovaries. About 15% of tumors that develop from epithelial cells are considered low malignant potential (LMP) tumors. These tumors occur more often in younger women, are more likely to be diagnosed early, and thus have a better prognosis.

Stromal cells are located inside the ovary and produce the hormones estrogen and progesterone. About 1% of ovarian cancers begin in the stromal cells.

Germ cells also are located within the ovary. **Germ cell tumors** develop in the cells that would become eggs (ova). They account for about 2% of ovarian tumors. Many germ cell tumors are benign (noncancerous). These tumors often occur in teenaged girls and young women. The prognosis is good if they are found early, but as with other ovarian cancers, early detection is difficult.

Risk factors

Age is one of the greatest risk factors in developing ovarian cancer, with risk increasing after menopause. Another risk factor is a family or personal history of cancers of the female reproductive tract or breast that is caused by an inherited mutation in the genes *BRCA1* or *BRCA2*. Not all women with *BRCA1* or *BRCA2* mutations will develop ovarian cancer. By age 70, a woman who has the *BRCA1* mutation carries about a 40%–60% risk of developing ovarian cancer. Women with the mutation in *BRCA2* have a 15% risk of developing ovarian cancer. However, these gene mutations play a role in only about 5% of all ovarian cancer cases.

Another inherited syndrome that increases a woman's risk of ovarian cancer is hereditary nonpolyposis colorectal cancer or HNPCC. It is also called Lynch syndrome. While the greatest risk of HNPCC is colorectal cancer, women with the syndrome have a 12% lifetime risk of developing ovarian or uterine cancer. Up to 1% of all ovarian epithelial cancers are caused by Lynch syndrome.

Less common genetic disorders that increase a woman's risk of ovarian cancer include:

- Cowden's disease. Women with this disease have thyroid problems and an increased risk of breast cancer as well as ovarian cancer. Cowden's disease is caused by mutations in the *PTEN* gene.
- Peutz-Jeghers syndrome. Also called hereditary intestinal polyposis syndrome, it is a genetic disorder caused by a mutation in the *STK11* gene and characterized by brown freckles around the mouth and benign polyps known as hamartomas in the digestive tract. People with this syndrome are at greatly increased risk of colon cancer as well as ovarian cancer, and at a relatively young age.
- *MUTYH*-associated polyposis. Women with this syndrome develop small polyps in the colon and small intestine. They are at increased risk of colon cancer as well as ovarian cancer. The syndrome is caused by a mutation in the *MUTYH* gene.

Early menarche (first menstruation; before age 12) and late menopause also seem to put women at a higher risk of ovarian cancer. Other risk factors include: eating a diet high in saturated fats; treatment with androgens (male hormones); treatment with the fertility drug clomiphene citrate for longer than a year; never having been pregnant (nulliparity); or having the first child after age 30. Conversely, having been pregnant, breastfeeding, and using oral contraceptives decrease the risk of developing ovarian cancer. It has been suggested that taking aspirin or acetaminophen lowers the risk of ovarian cancer, but this association had not been proven as of 2014.

Other risk factors for ovarian cancer include:

- Family history: having a first-degree relative (mother or sister) with ovarian cancer.
- Obesity.
- Use of hormone replacement therapy (HRT) for treating symptoms of menopause.

Demographics

Ovarian cancer can develop at any age, but is most likely to occur in women who are 50 or older. Most women are diagnosed after menopause. More than half the cases are among women who are over age 63. Industrialized countries have the highest incidence of ovarian cancer. Caucasian women, especially those of Ashkenazi Jewish descent, are at somewhat higher risk; African American and Asian women are at a slightly lower risk.

Adjuvant therapy—Treatment involving radiation, chemotherapy (drug treatment), hormone therapy, biotherapeutics, or a combination of any of these given after the primary treatment in order to rid the body of residual microscopic cancer.

Ascites—Accumulation of fluid within the peritoneal cavity.

Biomarker—A biochemical substance that can be detected in blood samples and indicates the presence of a cancerous tumor.

Debulking—The surgical removal of part of a cancerous tumor that cannot be completely excised, in order to improve the effectiveness of radiation therapy or chemotherapy.

Estrogen—Any of several steroid hormones, produced mainly in the ovaries, that stimulate the development of the endometrium and the development of female secondary sexual characteristics.

Hysterectomy—Surgical removal of the uterus.

Lymphatic system—A connected network of nodes, or glands that carry lymph throughout the body. Lymph is a fluid that contains the infection-fighting white blood cells that form part of the body's immune system. Because the network goes throughout the body, cancer cells that enter the lymphatic

system can travel to and be deposited at any point into the tissues and organs and form new tumors there.

Menarche—The medical term for a girl's first menstrual period.

Omentum—The layer of peritoneal tissue that covers the abdominal organs. Its name comes from the Latin word for apron.

Oophorectomy—Surgical removal of the ovaries.

Pap (Papanicolaou) smear—Pap test; removal of cervical cells to screen for cancer. The test was invented by and named for a Greek physician, George Papanicolaou, who was an early pioneer in cancer detection.

Placebo—A pill or liquid given during the study of a drug or dietary supplement that contains no medication or active ingredient. Usually study participants do not know if they are receiving a pill containing the drug or an identical-appearing placebo.

Targeted therapy—In cancer treatment, a type of drug therapy that blocks tumors by interfering with specific molecules that the cancer cells need for growth. Also called biologic therapy, targeted therapy is less harmful to normal cells than traditional chemotherapy.

In 2014, ovarian cancer was the ninth most common cancer among women in the United States. It accounted for about 2.8% of all new cancers in American women. However, because of poor early detection, ovarian cancer is the fifth most common cause of cancer death among women. About 1 in 71 American women will develop ovarian cancer during her lifetime, and 1 in 95 will die from it. The rate of new cases of ovarian cancer in the United States has been declining at the rate of about 1% per year since 2006, and the death rate has been declining about 1.6% each year since 2001. Rates are thought to be similar worldwide. The American Cancer Society estimated that about 21,980 new cases of ovarian cancer would be diagnosed in the United States in 2014, with 14,270 deaths.

Causes and symptoms

Cells in ovarian tissue normally divide and grow according to controls and instructions by proteins produced by various genes. If certain genes develop

changes (mutations), instructions for cellular growth and division may go awry. Abnormal, uncontrolled cell growth may occur, causing cancer. Most of these genetic changes are not inherited. Instead, they are sporadic, unexplained changes. Most ovarian cancers occur later in life after years of exposure to various environmental factors (e.g., the body's own hormones, asbestos exposure, or smoking) that may cause sporadic genetic alterations.

Ovarian cancer is often called a silent killer because it produces few symptoms in its early stages. Only 20% of ovarian cancers are diagnosed early. Most women are unaware they have the disease until it has progressed to advanced stages. Most early symptoms are vague and either abdominal or gastrointestinal in nature. These symptoms may not be properly diagnosed or may be recognized as ovarian in nature only after a significant length of time has passed and the cancer has advanced.

The following symptoms are warning signs of ovarian cancer, but these symptoms can also be due to many other causes. Symptoms that persist for two to three weeks or symptoms that are unusual for the particular woman should be evaluated by a doctor.

- digestive symptoms such as gas, indigestion, constipation, or a feeling of fullness after a light meal
- bloating, distention, or cramping
- abdominal or low-back discomfort
- pelvic pressure or frequent urination
- unexplained changes in bowel habits
- nausea or vomiting
- pain or swelling in the abdomen
- loss of appetite (anorexia)
- fatigue
- unexplained weight gain or loss
- pain during intercourse
- vaginal bleeding in postmenopausal women

Diagnosis

In the best-case scenario, a woman is diagnosed with ovarian cancer while it is still contained in just one ovary. Early detection can bring the five-year survival to about 94%. Advanced ovarian cancer is at stage III or stage IV, and it has already spread (metastasized) to other organs. A physical examination and pelvic exam generally do not reveal early-stage ovarian cancer.

Tests

If ovarian cancer is suspected, several of the following tests and examinations will be necessary to make a definitive diagnosis.

- a complete medical history to assess all the risk factors
- a thorough bimanual pelvic examination
- CA-125 assay
- one or more various imaging procedures
- a lower GI series or barium enema
- diagnostic laparoscopy for definitive diagnosis

BIMANUAL PELVIC EXAMINATION. The exam should include feeling the following organs for any abnormalities in shape or size: the ovaries, Fallopian tubes, uterus, vagina, bladder, and rectum. Because the ovaries are located deep within the pelvic area, it is unlikely that a manual exam will detect any abnormality while the cancer is still localized. However, a full examination provides the practitioner with a more complete picture. An enlarged ovary does not confirm cancer, as the ovary may be large because of a cyst or endometriosis. While women should have an annual **Pap test** to detect **cervical cancer**, this test is ineffective in detecting ovarian cancer.

CA-125 ASSAY. This is a blood test to determine the level of CA-125, a biomarker or tumor marker. A tumor marker is a measurable protein-based substance given off by the tumor. A series of CA-125 tests may be done to see if the amount of the marker in the blood is stable, increasing, or decreasing. A rising CA-125 level often indicates cancer, while a stable or declining value is more characteristic of a cyst. The CA-125 level should never be used alone to diagnose ovarian cancer. It can be normal in 50% of women with early-stage ovarian cancer. It is elevated in about 80% of women with late-stage ovarian cancer, but in 20% of cases is not elevated. In addition, CA-125 is a general biomarker and can be elevated because of a non-ovarian cancer, or from such nonmalignant gynecologic conditions as endometriosis or ectopic pregnancy. During menstruation the CA-125 level may be elevated, so the test is best done when the woman is not menstruating.

Other biomarkers that may be measured include human chorionic gonadotropin (HCG), alpha-fetoprotein (AFP), or lactate dehydrogenase (LDH), if the patient is suspected of having a germ cell ovarian tumor. High levels of estrogen and **testosterone** may point to a stromal tumor.

IMAGING. Several different imaging techniques are used in evaluating ovarian cancer. Ultrasound uses high-frequency sound waves that create a visual pattern of echoes of the structures at which they are aimed. It often can distinguish between a fluid-filled structure (such as a cyst) and a solid structure (such as a tumor). Ultrasound is painless and harmless; it is the same technique used to check a developing fetus in the womb. Ultrasound may be done externally through the abdomen and lower pelvic area, or with a transvaginal probe (**transvaginal ultrasound**).

Other painless imaging techniques are **computed tomography** (CT) and **magnetic resonance imaging** (MRI). Color Doppler analysis provides additional contrast and accuracy in distinguishing masses. A **positron emission tomography** (PET) scan may also be used to look for metastatic ovarian cancer. PET scans involve the use of radioactive glucose to look for cancer cells, as cancers take up sugar more rapidly than normal tissues. These imaging techniques allow better visualization of the internal organs and can detect abnormalities without having to perform surgery.

LOWER GI SERIES. A lower GI series, or **barium enema**, uses a series of **x-rays** to highlight the colon and rectum. To provide contrast, the patient drinks a chalky liquid containing barium. This test might be done to see whether cancer has spread to these areas.

DIAGNOSTIC LAPAROSCOPY. This technique uses a thin hollow lighted instrument inserted through a small incision in the abdomen to visualize the organs inside of the abdominal cavity. If the ovary is believed to be malignant, the entire ovary may be removed (**oophorectomy**) and its tissue sent for evaluation to the pathologist, even though only a small piece of the tissue is needed for evaluation. If cancer is present, great care must be taken not to cause the rupture of the malignant tumor, as this could spread cancer cells to adjacent organs. If the cancer is completely contained in the ovary, its removal also functions as the treatment. If the cancer has spread or is suspected to have spread, then a saline solution may be instilled into the cavity and then drawn out again. This technique is called peritoneal lavage. The aspirated fluid will be evaluated for the presence of cancer cells. If peritoneal fluid is present—a condition called ascites—a sample of this fluid will also be drawn and examined for malignant cells. If cancer cells are present in the peritoneum, then treatment will be directed at the abdominal cavity as well.

Treatment team

A family practice physician or a gynecologist may perform a women's initial pelvic exam. Once diagnosed, a specialist in cancers of the female reproductive system, known as a gynecologic oncologist, will likely lead the treatment team. Other members of the team may include a radiation oncologist, an oncology nurse, and/or a medical oncologist to administer **chemotherapy**. Women with ovarian cancer may also wish to consult with a social worker and a registered dietitian.

Clinical staging

Staging is the term used to determine whether the cancer is localized or has spread, and, if so, how far and to where. Staging helps define the cancer and will determine the course of suggested treatment. Staging involves examining any tissue samples (biopsies) that have been taken from the ovary, nearby lymph nodes, and any structures where **metastasis** is suspected. Samples may be taken from the diaphragm, lungs, stomach, intestines, and omentum (the tissue covering internal organs), and any fluid as described above.

The **National Cancer Institute** staging system uses the Tumor/Node/Metastasis (TNM) system for staging ovarian cancer. Other staging systems, such as the International Federation of Gynecology and Obstetrics (FIGO) staging system, may also be used. The TNM staging system is summarized as follows:

- Stage I: Cancer is confined to one or both ovaries.
- Stage II: Cancer is found in one or both ovaries and/or has spread to the uterus, Fallopian tubes, and/or other body parts within the pelvic cavity. It has not spread to lymph nodes, the lining of the abdomen, or distant sites.
- Stage III: Cancer is found in one or both ovaries and has spread to lymph nodes or other body parts within the abdominal cavity, such as the surfaces of the liver or intestines.
- Stage IV: Cancer is found in one or both ovaries and has spread to such other distant organs as the lungs or the interior of the liver.

Individual stages are further subdivided; the FIGO subdivision of the stages was revised in January 2014. Accurate staging is important in determining a treatment plan.

Treatment

Treatment is based on the stage of cancer at diagnosis and the woman's age.

Surgery

Surgery is done to remove as much of the tumor as possible (called tissue debulking), usually followed by chemotherapy and/or radiation (adjuvant therapy) to target cancer cells that have remained in the body without jeopardizing the woman's health. Maintaining health can be hard to achieve, however, once the cancer has spread. Removal of the ovary is called oophorectomy, and removal of both ovaries is called bilateral oophorectomy. Unless it is very clear that the cancer has not spread, the Fallopian tubes are removed as well (salpingo-oophorectomy). Removal of the uterus is called hysterectomy.

If the woman is young and wishes to have children, all attempts will be made to spare the uterus. It is crucial that a woman discuss with her surgeon her childbearing plans before surgery. Ovarian cancer spreads easily and often swiftly throughout the reproductive tract, so it may be necessary to remove all reproductive organs as well as part of the lining of the peritoneum to provide the woman with the best possible chance of long-term survival. Fertility-sparing surgery can be successful if the ovarian cancer is diagnosed very early.

Side effects of the surgery will depend on the extent of the surgery, but may include pain and temporary difficulty with bladder and bowel function, as well as reaction to the loss of hormones produced by the organs removed. A hormone replacement patch may be applied to the woman's skin in the recovery room to help with the transition. An emotional side effect involves the feeling of loss stemming from the removal of reproductive organs.

Additional surgical procedures may be performed to help relieve conditions caused by the cancer, such as **ascites** (fluid in the abdomen) or urethral obstruction. Such procedures include:

- paracentesis
- catheterization
- thoracentesis
- pleurodesis
- video-assisted thoracoscopy
- ureteral or intestinal stenting
- nephrostomy
- gastrostomy tube insertion
- removal of intestinal obstruction

Chemotherapy

Chemotherapy is used to target cells that have traveled to other organs, and throughout the body via the lymphatic system or the bloodstream (metastasized). Chemotherapy drugs are designed to kill cancer cells, but they can also cause harm to healthy cells. Chemotherapy may be administered through a vein in the arm (intravenous, IV), may be taken in tablet form (orally), and/or may be given through a thin tube called a catheter directly into the abdominal cavity (intraperitoneal, IP). IV and oral chemotherapy drugs travel throughout the body; intraperitoneal chemotherapy is localized in the abdominal cavity.

Side effects of chemotherapy vary greatly depending on the drugs used. Currently, chemotherapy drugs are often used in combinations to treat advanced ovarian cancer, and usually the combination includes a platinum-based drug (such as **cisplatin**) with a taxol agent, such as paclitaxel. Some of the combinations used or being studied include: carboplatin/paclitaxel, cisplatin/paclitaxel, cisplatin/topotecan, and cisplatin/carboplatin. Such **antineoplastic agents** as **topotecan** (Hycamtin) or **gemcitabine** (Gemzar) that interfere with the ability of the tumor cells to reproduce may also be given. Other drugs that have been used to treat ovarian cancer include **melphalan**, **ifosfamide**, **pemetrexed**, and **vinorelbine**.

The goal of chemotherapy is to maximize effectiveness with a minimum of side effects. One serious side effect is an adverse reaction to the drug(s) used. Severe reactions may result in anaphylaxis, which can be fatal if not treated immediately. Other side effects include **nausea and vomiting**, **diarrhea**, decreased appetite and resulting **weight loss**, **fatigue**, headaches, loss of hair, and numbness and tingling (paresthesia) in the hands or feet. Managing these side effects is an important part of cancer treatment.

After the full course of chemotherapy has been given, the surgeon may perform a "second look" surgery to examine the abdominal cavity again to evaluate the success of treatment.

Radiation

Radiation is not used as a primary treatment in most patients with ovarian cancer. For patients with incurable ovarian cancer, radiation may be used to shrink tumor masses to provide pain relief and improve quality of life (palliative care).

Following treatment, regular follow-up appointments will be scheduled to monitor for any long-term side effects, relapse, or metastases.

Targeted therapy

Targeted therapy is a newer form of pharmacotherapy that treats cancers with drugs that target the changes in genes or proteins that cause cancer cells to grow and spread. As of 2014, targeted therapy is most often used to treat advanced or metastatic ovarian cancer. The drug most often used to treat ovarian cancer is **bevacizumab**, a drug that works by blocking the growth of new blood vessels that nourish the tumor. It can be given together with chemotherapy. Although bevacizumab has been approved by the Food and Drug Administration (FDA) to treat other cancers, it had not been approved specifically for the treatment of ovarian cancer as of 2014. Other targeted therapy drugs are presently being researched; for example, pazopanib is a newer drug in this class that shows promise in treating ovarian cancer.

Hormone therapy

Hormone therapy is used more often to treat stromal tumors than other types of ovarian cancer. The patient may be given luteinizing hormone-releasing hormone (LHRH) agonists. These drugs work by opposing the production of estrogen in the ovaries and are given to premenopausal women. They include leuprolide and goserelin. **Tamoxifen** is another drug with anti-estrogen activity that may be used to keep any estrogens circulating in the woman's bloodstream from stimulating the growth of new cancer cells. The third group of drugs used in hormone therapy for ovarian cancer is known as **aromatase inhibitors**. They block an enzyme called aromatase from turning other hormones in the woman's body into estrogen. The aromatase inhibitors include letrozole, exemestane, and anastrozole.

Clinical trials

Clinical trials are human research studies. Their goal is to evaluate the effectiveness of new ways to treat cancer. There are many different designs, and they target different aspects of care. For example, some may investigate the response of different chemotherapy drugs, while another study may compare different types of treatment/chemotherapy combinations.

Research studies are often designed to compare the effectiveness of a new treatment method against the standard method or the effectiveness of a drug against a placebo (an inert substance that would be expected to have no effect on the outcome). Since the research is experimental in nature, there are no guarantees about the outcome. New drugs being used may have harmful, unknown side effects. Some people participate to help further knowledge about their disease. For others, the study may provide a possible treatment that is not yet available otherwise. Although there is no cost to participate, participants have to meet certain criteria before being admitted into the study. It is important to fully understand one's role in the study, and weigh the potential risks versus benefits when deciding whether or not to participate.

There were 348 open clinical trials for ovarian cancer in the United States as of mid-2014: some are studies of imaging modalities to detect occult (hidden) ovarian cancer; others are trials of new chemotherapy drugs and targeted therapy drugs; one is a trial of a potential screening method for ovarian cancer that uses a special tampon to collect cell samples to be tested for DNA; and several are psychological and demographic studies of long-term survivors of ovarian cancer.

Alternative and complementary therapies

The term *alternative therapy* refers to therapy used instead of conventional treatment. By definition, these treatments have not been scientifically proven or investigated as thoroughly and by the same standards as conventional treatments. The terms *complementary* or *integrative therapy* denote practices used in conjunction with rather than instead of conventional treatment. Patients should inform their doctors of any alternative or complementary therapies being used or considered as some alternative and complementary therapies adversely affect the effectiveness of conventional treatments. Some common complementary and alternative medicine therapies include:

• prayer and faith healing

• meditation

• such mind/body techniques as support groups, visualization, guided imagery, and hypnosis

• Therapeutic Touch, Reiki, and other energy therapies

• acupuncture and traditional Chinese medicine

• yoga, massage, and t'ai chi

• vitamin, mineral, and/or herbal supplements

• special diets: vegetarian, vegan, or macrobiotic

Coping with cancer treatment

While the cancer may be in only part of the body, it is very much a full mind/body experience. Strategies for coping with the treatment need to address the entire range of the experience. Each woman will have different needs. She might want to create a personal support team of friends. They can provide support by:

• Finding helpful information in the library or on the Internet about clinical trials, new therapies or treatments, different treatment centers, etc.

• Providing transportation to and from appointments. A diagnosis of cancer can be overwhelming. In such a stressful and distracted state it is often hard to remember what a doctor has said, or even to remember the questions to be asked. Having a second set of ears during this stressful time can be helpful.

• Helping with household duties so that the woman can rest after treatments and have more energy to devote to her family.

• Assisting with childcare. Children are very much affected by a parent's cancer diagnosis, whether or not they have been fully informed of what is taking place. Friends and relatives who can help care for children assist in providing a sense of normality and security.

• Being available to participate in activities and conversations not centering on the cancer. While in the midst of cancer treatments, it is important to talk about noncancer issues as well and to maintain social relationships and activities.

A woman may wish to join a support group of women with ovarian cancer. This group can provide the environment to talk about the diagnosis, the treatments, the side effects, and the impact the diagnosis has on her life with others who can empathize. If there is no support group nearby, she may be able to join one on the Internet. Support groups also may exist for caregivers and loved ones.

Prognosis

Prognosis for ovarian cancer depends largely on the stage at which it is first diagnosed. Stage I ovarian cancer has the best survival rate, although ovarian cancer is rarely diagnosed at this stage. As of 2014, the five-year survival rates for the four stages of ovarian cancer were: stage I, 92.3%; stage II, 66%; stage III, 37%; stage IV, 18%.

QUESTIONS TO ASK YOUR DOCTOR

- What tests will be used to look for and diagnose my cancer?
- How should I prepare for the tests?
- What will take place during the test? Will it be painful? What can I do to decrease the pain?
- When will I learn the results?
- Once the results are in, what do these results mean?
- What type and stage is my cancer?
- What are my treatment options?
- Who will be involved in my care?
- Are there clinical trials that might benefit me?
- What changes in my ability to work or perform my daily functions should I expect during treatment?
- How long will my treatment last?
- What side effects should I expect from treatment?
- Are there any conventional or alternative therapies that can diminish the side effects of treatments?
- During treatment will I need a caregiver or will I be able to care for myself?
- How soon after treatment will I be able to resume my regular activities?
- What is the plan for my follow-up care?

Prevention

Since the cause of ovarian cancer is not known as of 2014, it is not possible to fully prevent the disease. There are, however, ways to reduce one's risks of developing the disease.

Decrease ovulation

Pregnancy temporarily stops ovulation, and multiple pregnancies appear to further reduce the risk of ovarian cancer. The research is not clear as to whether the pregnancy must result in a term delivery to have full benefit. Women who breastfeed their children also appear to have a lower risk of developing the disease. Since oral contraceptives also suppress ovulation, women who take birth control pills have a lower incidence of ovarian cancer. It appears that the longer a woman takes

oral contraceptives, the lower her risk of ovarian cancer. However, since oral contraceptives alter a woman's hormonal status, her risk for other hormonally related cancers may change. The woman should discuss the risks and benefits of oral contraceptives with her healthcare provider.

Genetic testing

Genetic testing is available that can help determine whether a woman carries certain genes that increase her risk of breast and ovarian cancer. If the woman tests positive for a *BRCA1* or *BRCA2* mutation, then she may wish to consider having her ovaries removed as a preventive measure (prophylactic oophorectomy).

Surgery

Such procedures as tubal ligation (in which the Fallopian tubes are blocked or tied) and hysterectomy (in which the uterus is removed) appear to reduce the risk of ovarian cancer. However, any removal of the reproductive organs has surgical as well as hormonal side effects.

Screening

There were no definitive tests or screening procedures approved by the FDA as of 2014 to detect ovarian cancer in its early stages. Women at high risk should consult their physicians about possible regular screenings, which may include a transvaginal ultrasound and a blood test for the CA-125 protein. The American Cancer Society recommends annual pelvic examinations for all women after age 40, in order to increase the chances of early detection of both cervical and ovarian cancer.

Early detection remains the focal point in increasing survival rates for ovarian cancer because the more ovarian cancer has spread, the poorer the chance for survival past one or two years. As women and healthcare practitioners become more alert to vague early warning signs and seek out more accurate family histories, earlier awareness may begin to lead to earlier detection and improved survival rates.

Resources

BOOKS

Akin, Oguz, ed. *Atlas of Gynecologic Oncology Imaging*. New York: Springer, 2014.

Farghaly, Samir A., ed. *Advances in Diagnosis and Management of Ovarian Cancer*. New York: Springer, 2013.

Hesse-Biber, Sharlene. *Waiting for Cancer to Come: Women's Experiences with Genetic Testing and Medical Decision Making for Breast and Ovarian Cancer*. Ann Arbor: University of Michigan Press, 2014.

Malek, Anastasia, and Oleg Tchernitsa, eds. *Ovarian Cancer: Methods and Protocols*. New York: Humana Press and Springer, 2013.

Odunse, Kunle, and Tanja Pejovic, eds. *Gynecologic Cancers: A Multidisciplinary Approach to Diagnosis and Management*. New York: Demos Medical Publishing, 2013.

PERIODICALS

Aravantinos, G., and D. Pectasides. "Bevacizumab in Combination with Chemotherapy for the Treatment of Advanced Ovarian Cancer: A Systematic Review." *Journal of Ovarian Research* 7 (May 19, 2014): 57.

Davidson, B., C. G. Trope, and R. Reich. "The Role of the Tumor Stroma in Ovarian Cancer." *Frontiers in Oncology* 4 (May 13, 2014): 104.

Davidson, B. A., and A. A. Secord. "Profile of Pazopanib and Its Potential in the Treatment of Epithelial Ovarian Cancer." *International Journal of Women's Health* 6 (March 13, 2014): 289–300.

Decruze, S. B. "Paracentesis in Ovarian Cancer: A Study of the Physiology during Free Drainage of Ascites." *Journal of Palliative Medicine* 13, no. 3 (2010): 251–54. http://dx. doi.org/10.1089/jpm.2009.0158 (accessed September 2, 2014).

Friebel, T. M., S. M. Domchek, and T. R. Rebbeck. "Modifiers of Cancer Risk in BRCA1 and BRCA2 Mutation Carriers: Systematic Review and Meta-analysis." *Journal of the National Cancer Institute* 106 (June 2014): dju091.

Grisham, R. N., D. M. Hyman, and G. Iyer. "Targeted Therapies for Treatment of Recurrent Ovarian Cancer." *Clinical Advances in Hematology and Oncology* 12 (March 2014): 158–162.

Hodeib, M., R. Eskander, and R. F. Bristow. "New Paradigms in the Surgical and Adjuvant Treatment of Ovarian Cancer." *Minerva Ginecologica* 66 (April 2014): 179–192.

Jayson, G. C., et al. "Ovarian Cancer." *Lancet* 384, no. 9951 (2014): 1376–81.

Miccò, M., et al. "Role of Imaging in the Pretreatment Evaluation of Common Gynecological Cancers." *Women's Health (London, England)* 10 (May 2014): 299–321.

Poveda, A., et al. "Emerging Treatment Strategies in Recurrent Platinum-sensitive Ovarian Cancer: Focus on Trabectedin." *Cancer Treatment Reviews* 40 (April 2014): 366–375.

Syrios, J., S. Banerjee, and S. B. Kaye. "Advanced Epithelial Ovarian Cancer: From Standard Chemotherapy to Promising Molecular Pathway Targets—Where Are We Now?" *Anticancer Research* 34 (May 2014): 2069–2077.

Yokoyama, A., and H. Mizunuma. "Recurrent Epithelial Ovarian Cancer and Hormone Therapy." *World Journal of Clinical Cases* 1 (September 16, 2013): 187–190.

OTHER

American Cancer Society (ACS). "Ovarian Cancer." http://www.cancer.org/acs/groups/cid/documents/webcontent/003130-pdf.pdf (accessed September 2, 2014).

Society of Gynecologic Oncology (SGO). "Revised FIGO Ovarian Cancer Staging." https://www.sgo.org/wp-content/uploads/2012/09/FIGO-Ovarian-Cancer-Staging_1.10.14.pdf (accessed September 2, 2014).

WEBSITES

Foundation for Women's Cancer. "Working with Your Treatment Team." http://www.foundationforwomenscancer.org/types-of-gynecologic-cancers/ovarian/working-with-your-treatment-team (accessed September 2, 2014).

National Cancer Institute (NCI). "Ovarian Cancer." http://www.cancer.gov/cancertopics/types/ovarian/ (accessed September 2, 2014).

Ovarian Cancer National Alliance. "About Ovarian Cancer." http://www.ovariancancer.org/about/ (accessed September 2, 2014).

Society of Gynecologic Oncology (SGO). "Ovarian Cancer." https://www.sgo.org/ovarian-cancer/ (accessed September 2, 2014).

ORGANIZATIONS

American Cancer Society (ACS), 250 Williams Street NW, Atlanta, GA 30303, (800) 227-2345, http://www.cancer.org/aboutus/howwehelpyou/app/contact-us.aspx, http://www.cancer.org/index.

American Congress of Obstetricians and Gynecologists (ACOG), PO Box 70620, Washington, DC 20024-9998, (202) 638-5577, (800) 673-8444, resources@acog.org, http://www.acog.org/.

American Society of Clinical Oncology (ASCO), 2318 Mill Road, Suite 800, Alexandria, VA 22314, (571) 483-1300, (888) 651-3038, contactus@cancer.net, http://www.asco.org/.

Foundation for Women's Cancer, 230 W. Monroe, Suite 2528, Chicago, IL 60606-4902, (312) 578-1439, (800) 444-4441, Fax: (312) 578-9769, info@foundationforwomenscancer.org, http://www.foundationforwomenscancer.org/.

National Cancer Institute (NCI), BG 9609 MSC 9760, 9609 Medical Center Drive, Bethesda, MD 20892-9760, (800) 4-CANCER (422-6237), http://www.cancer.gov/global/contact/email-us, http://www.cancer.gov/.

Office of Cancer Complementary and Alternative Medicine (OCCAM), 9609 Medical Center Dr., Room 5-W-136, Rockville, MD 20850, (240) 276-6595, Fax: (240) 276-7888, ncioccam1-r@mail.nih.gov, http://cam.cancer.gov/.

Ovarian Cancer National Alliance, 1101 14th Street NW, Suite 850, Washington, DC 20005, (202) 331-1332, (866) 399-6262, Fax: (202) 331-2292, http://www.ovariancancer.org/.

Society of Gynecologic Oncology (SGO), 230 W. Monroe St., Suite 710, Chicago, IL 60606-4703, (312) 235-4060, Fax: (312) 235-4059, sgo@sgo.org, https://www.sgo.org/.

Esther Csapo Rastegari, RN, BSN, EdM
REVISED BY TISH DAVIDSON, AM
REVISED BY REBECCA J. FREY, PhD

Ovarian epithelial cancer

Definition

Ovarian epithelial **cancer** is a type of cancer that develops in the cells that line the surface of the ovaries.

Description

Part of the female reproductive system, the ovaries are a pair of almond-shaped organs that are located on either side of the uterus, just above the pelvic bone. The ovaries produce estrogen and progesterone, which are female hormones. At birth, each ovary contains thousands of eggs. During a woman's fertile years, one ripened egg (or sometimes more) is released each month into a Fallopian tube. As the egg takes its journey toward the uterus, a sperm can fertilize it. When a baby is conceived, it stays in the uterus until birth. During the birth process, powerful muscles in the uterus help to push the baby out through the cervix and vagina.

When an ovarian cell becomes cancerous, it tends to multiply quickly, forming a growth (or tumor). The resulting tumor may interfere with the way the ovary normally functions, but not in every case. Sometimes the cancer cells break off from the tumor and spread contiguously, which means they spread to nearby organs, such as to other areas of the pelvis.

Demographics

Although **ovarian cancer** rates differ significantly from country to country, Europe has been recognized as having one of the highest incidence rates of ovarian cancer in the world. Having carefully studied the ovarian cancer trends of 28 European countries, Freddie Bray and his colleagues reported in a 2004 article published by the *International Journal of Cancer* that European countries with the highest ovarian cancer rates in the past included the Nordic countries, Austria, Germany, and the United Kingdom, but current trends in these and other northern European countries showed a decline in ovarian cancer rates, especially with regard to mortality. However, the opposite was found to be true with regard to some of the southern and eastern European countries. In the Czech Republic and Hungry, there has been a drop in the mortality rates associated with ovarian cancer, but not a drop in the number of cases diagnosed. Bray and his colleagues reported that "recent trends in ovarian cancer have led to a leveling of rates across various areas of the [European] continent, although a 2.5-fold variation was still observed in the late 1990s between the highest mortality rate of 9.3/100,000 in Denmark and the lowest one of 3.6 in Portugal."

The American Cancer Society estimated that 21,980 cases of ovarian cancer were diagnosed in the United States in 2014, resulting in approximately 14,270 deaths. Rarely seen in women under the age of 30, the risk of developing ovarian cancer increases with age. Nearly 90% of all the cases of ovarian cancer are ovarian epithelial cancer. Ranked fifth as the most frequent cause of cancer death in women, ovarian epithelial cancer most commonly occurs in women over the age of 65.

Causes and symptoms

The presence of mutations in the *BRCA1* and *BRCA2* genes increase a woman's risk of developing breast or ovarian cancer, including ovarian epithelial cancer. When these gene mutations are not present in a woman who has ovarian epithelial cancer, it is difficult to identify the cause. Several factors may increase a woman's risk of developing ovarian epithelial cancer, such as having a close relative with the disease or a personal history of **breast cancer**.

There seems to be a connection between the development of ovarian epithelial cancer and the number of times a woman ovulates in her lifetime. Statistics show that a woman who ovulates less seems to have less risk. For example, a woman who has had a child may have a decreased risk of developing ovarian epithelial cancer, because she has had a nine-month break in ovulation. On the other hand, a woman who has used birth control pills may lessen her risk for the same reason, because she, too, has had a break in ovulation.

Ovarian epithelial cancer often produces no symptoms in its early stages; therefore, by the time it is discovered, the disease is often widespread. In addition, women often ignore the symptoms, because they do not identify them with anything serious. Some of the symptoms include:

• gas and indigestion

• bloating

• swelling of the abdomen

• constipation, nausea, and vomiting

- fullness or pressure in the pelvis
- abnormal bleeding from the vagina
- lower abdominal pain (such as cramps)

Diagnosis

A variety of tests and examinations are used to diagnose ovarian epithelial cancer.

Pelvic exam

Many women are familiar with this exam and schedule one on a yearly basis along with a pap smear. The exam is usually performed by a gynecologist, but is also sometimes performed by a physician specializing in family or internal medicine. Many women think a **Pap test** will detect ovarian cancer, but, in truth, it is the pelvic examination that helps a physician diagnose ovarian epithelial cancer, whereas the Pap test is useful in detecting **cervical cancer**.

To perform a pelvic examination, the physician inserts one or two lubricated, gloved fingers of one hand into a woman's vagina while pressing down on her abdomen with the other hand. By touch, the physician examines the uterus and ovaries, checking for any abnormalities in shape, size, or position. This examination only takes a few minutes and is not painful, although some women may feel some pressure or minor discomfort. The patient should tell the physician immediately if any pain is experienced. As part of the examination, the physician will also insert a lubricated, gloved finger into the rectum to feel for lumps.

Ultrasound

Often referred to as a sonogram, ultrasound is a completely painless procedure performed by a radiologist in which high-energy sound waves are bounced off internal organs.

Magnetic resonance imaging (MRI)

Although an expensive test, an MRI is often covered by many insurance plans. Using a magnetic field and imaging waves, an MRI scans a specific portion of the body from any angle. Painless and noninvasive, MRI testing does not require the use of contrast dye. However, the MRI is an unnerving machine for anyone claustrophobic, because the machine surrounds almost the entire body. Claustrophobic patients should ask their physician to refer them to the nearest Open Air MRI facility. The open design of an Open Air MRI provides access from all four sides and allows patients to feel more comfortable during their exam.

Blood test

A test that measures the level of CA-125 in the blood is often recommended if ovarian epithelial cancer is suspected. An increased level of CA-125 may be a sign that cancer is present in the body.

Barium enema

In this procedure—sometimes referred to as a lower GI—a liquid that contains barium is put into the rectum, which coats the gastrointestinal tract so that x-rays can be taken. It is usually performed by an x-ray technician or radiologist and is considered by many people to be as unpleasant as a normal enema.

Intravenous pyelogram (IVP)

The purpose of this test, which normally takes about 30 minutes to an hour, is to see if any abnormalities exist in the kidneys and bladder. An IVP is essentially a series of x-rays. A contrast dye, which is injected into the patient's vein, enhances the x-ray images that are taken to see if there are any blockages.

The night before the exam, the patient will be asked to fast (not eat any food) and to take a mild laxative, such as a teaspoon of castor oil. Patients who suspect they might be pregnant should inform their physicians prior to having an IVP. Although it is often not necessary for patients to remove their clothing, they will often be asked to remove any jewelry that might interfere with the images.

An IVP itself is painless, although some patients experience nausea and/or a metallic taste in their mouth as the dye is being inserted. Both the nausea and metallic taste tend to go away as the patient's body gets used to the dye. Some patients develop hives, which is an allergic reaction to the dye. The radiologist, who performs the test, will have medication on hand to treat the hives. When the test is completed, the radiologist will examine the x-rays and write up a report for the referring physician who will deliver the results to the patient.

Computed tomography (CT) scan

A CT scan, also referred to as a CAT scan, is a procedure that takes a series of detailed pictures of the inside of the body and is considered one of the best tools available for studying abdominal tissue, especially with regard to the presence of a tumor.

Like an IVP, a contrast dye is injected into a vein to help the organs and surrounding tissue show up more clearly. In some cases, the contrast dye is swallowed by the patient rather than injected. A computer linked to an x-ray machine generates the pictures. The test is painless and generally takes about 30 minutes to an hour, depending on how many images are needed. Unlike the IVP, however, the x-ray technician or radiologist will not remain in the room while the x-rays are being taken. The patient will be able to hear and speak to the person performing the test, which is either an x-ray technician or radiologist. Because of the radiation used to perform a CT scan, patients that suspect they are pregnant should tell their physicians prior to having the test. If the images show a tumor, many different specialists, such as a radiologist, oncologist, surgeon, and the referring physician, will often work together to arrive at a suitable course of treatment.

Biopsy

A physician may recommend that a **biopsy** be performed, which is a surgical procedure to remove tissue or cells from the surface of the ovary to see if they are cancerous.

Treatment team

The treatment team is comprised of physicians from a variety of medical specialties. For example, a patient diagnosed with ovarian epithelial cancer may have a treatment team that includes the patient's primary care physician and her gynecologist, as well as a radiologist, oncologist, surgeon, and **pain management** specialist. At-home caretakers are also part of the treatment team, providing important physical and emotional support to the patient. Physicians and patients that value a holistic approach to fighting cancer may add a variety of other advisors to the treatment team, such as psychologists, pastors, and alternative medicine specialists.

Clinical staging

After ovarian epithelial cancer has been diagnosed, it is classified as being in one of four stages based on whether the cancer cells have or have not spread within the ovaries or to other parts of the body. To determine the stage of the disease, the patient is placed under general anesthesia and a surgical procedure called a laparotomy is performed. By making an incision through the abdomen, the surgeon can inspect the ovaries and adjacent organs for cancer. A biopsy is often done at that time and the cells are viewed under a microscope by the surgeon who often specializes in oncology. If there are clear indications that cancerous tissue is present, the surgeon will usually remove it and any effected organs during the laparotomy. A tissue sample is also sent to a lab where a pathologist can further classify the sample

and confirm the diagnosis. It can take several days to receive the pathologist's report.

The **National Cancer Institute** explains the four main stages of ovarian epithelial cancer as follows:

- Stage I: The cancer is present in one or both ovaries, but the cancer has not spread.
- Stage II: The cancer is present in one or both ovaries and has spread to the pelvis.
- Stage III: The cancer is present in one or both ovaries and has spread to other parts of the abdomen.
- Stage IV: The cancer is not only in one or both ovaries, but it has spread beyond the abdomen to other parts of the body.

All four stages have subcategories A, B, and C, which further indicate the characteristics and severity of the cancer within each stage. For example, according to the National Cancer Institute, in Stage IIIB, "The cancer has spread to the peritoneum but is 2 centimeters or smaller in diameter, whereas in Stage IIIC, the cancer has spread to the peritoneum and is larger than 2 centimeters and/or has spread to lymph nodes in the abdomen."

Treatment

Depending on the patient and the stage of the cancer, there are a variety of treatment options for patients with ovarian epithelial cancer. The three conventional treatment options are surgery, **radiation therapy**, and **chemotherapy**. As the National Cancer Institute states, "Most patients have surgery to remove as much of the tumor as possible." Although ovarian epithelial cancer usually does not strike young women, it does pose a special concern for young women hoping to have a family. In the event that the disease is caught early enough, it might be possible to perform a unilateral salpingo-oophorectomy, which is the removal of only the involved ovary and Fallopian tube, thereby giving the woman a chance to have children someday. However, in many cases, it is necessary to remove both ovaries, as well as the uterus, Fallopian tubes, and nearby lymph glands. Sometimes it is even necessary to remove the omentum, which is a fold of the peritoneum.

Depending on the stage of cancer, radiation therapy may be recommended. There are generally two types of radiation therapy: external radiation therapy, which comes from a machine outside of the body, and internal radiation therapy, such as implant radiation or brachytherapy. Chemotherapy is a commonly known cancer treatment that utilizes strong drugs to stop the growth of cancer cells. Chemotherapy is either given intravenously or orally; it often involves combination drug therapy. The administration and combination of chemotherapy drugs utilized is largely dependant on the extent of the cancer and the patient's medical profile.

Prognosis

The survival rate depends on a variety of factors, such as the patient's age and general health as well as the type and stage of tumor. When ovarian epithelial cancer is found early, the five-year survival rate is approximately 60%–80%. However, because ovarian epithelial cancer is often found late in its development, the overall survival rate is 30%–40%. In addition, ovarian epithelial cancer can recur after it has been treated.

Coping with cancer treatment

Patients having difficulty coping with the pain associated with cancer and chemotherapy might find it helpful to be referred to a physician who specializes in pain management or a pain clinic. Physicians specializing in the treatment of pain come from a variety of medical backgrounds, such as anesthesiology, obstetrics and gynecology, neurology, and surgery. Because of the complicated nature of cancer and cancer-related pain, ideally a pain management team should be formed that works with the patient's primary care physician, oncologist, and radiologist to provide comprehensive care to the patient.

Much has been written about coping with the physical side effects of cancer treatment; however, patients with ovarian epithelial cancer also face emotional challenges associated with their treatment. For example, women who are still in their reproductive years and need to have both ovaries removed must deal with an abrupt end to their reproductive choices. Women of all ages will have to deal with a variety of psychological issues, such as **body image** versus self-image. Some woman may need to be reminded, especially by family members and friends, that they are more than a collection of body parts. The spirit of their womanhood remains even if their ovaries do not.

It is important for cancer patients to understand that they are not alone. Support groups exist to help patients cope not only with the physical aspects of having cancer, but with the psychological ones as well. Patients should be encouraged to talk about their feelings. The positive support (both emotional and otherwise) provided by caregivers can help to improve a patient's quality of life. In addition, support groups on the Internet have made it possible for women, even those in rural or remote areas, to reach out to one another in ways that allow anonymity.

QUESTIONS TO ASK YOUR DOCTOR

- What clinical trials do you recommend?
- Will I be able to have children?
- When will I be able to return to work?
- Are there any local cancer support groups?
- How will the treatment affect my sex life?
- Are there any medications that could alter the test or treatment results?
- What prescription and over-the-counter medications should be avoided during treatment?

Clinical trials

Patients should ask their doctor if there are any **clinical trials** being conducted in their area that they should consider joining. Clinical trials are conducted to improve current methods of treatment or to develop new treatments. Patients with cancer who participate in clinical trials may improve their chances of survival.

Prevention

Women with a strong family history of ovarian epithelial cancer should be sure to have regular pelvic examinations, because an early diagnosis increases the chance of survival. However, there really is no way to prevent ovarian epithelial cancer, other than to have both ovaries removed before cancer has had a chance to grow, which is an extremely controversial prevention method. Nonetheless, some women with a high risk of developing ovarian epithelial cancer who have had the chance to have a family have elected to have a prophylactic **oophorectomy**, which is the medical name for the procedure that refers to the removal of healthy ovaries. Women considering this procedure need to know that it isn't necessarily a guarantee against ovarian cancer.

Resources

BOOKS

Almadrones-Cassidy, Lois, ed. *Gynecologic Cancers*. Pittsburgh, PA: Oncology Nursing Society, 2010.

WEBSITES

National Cancer Institute. "General Information about Ovarian Epithelial Cancer." http://www.cancer.gov/cancertopics/pdq/treatment/ovarianepithelial/HealthProfessional/page1 (accessed November 10, 2014).

National Ovarian Cancer Coalition. "Types & Stages of Ovarian Cancer." http://www.ovarian.org/types_and_stages.php (accessed November 10, 2014).

ORGANIZATIONS

American Cancer Society, 250 Williams St. NW, Atlanta, GA 30303, (800) 227-2345, http://www.cancer.org.

National Cancer Institute, 9609 Medical Center Dr., BG 9609 MSC 9760, Bethesda, MD 20892-9760, (800) 4-CANCER (422-6237), http://www.cancer.gov.

Lee Ann Paradise

Oxycodone *see* **Opioids**